COMPREHENSIVE OPHTHALMOLOGY

COMPREHENSIVE

OPHTHALMOLOGY

5th Edition

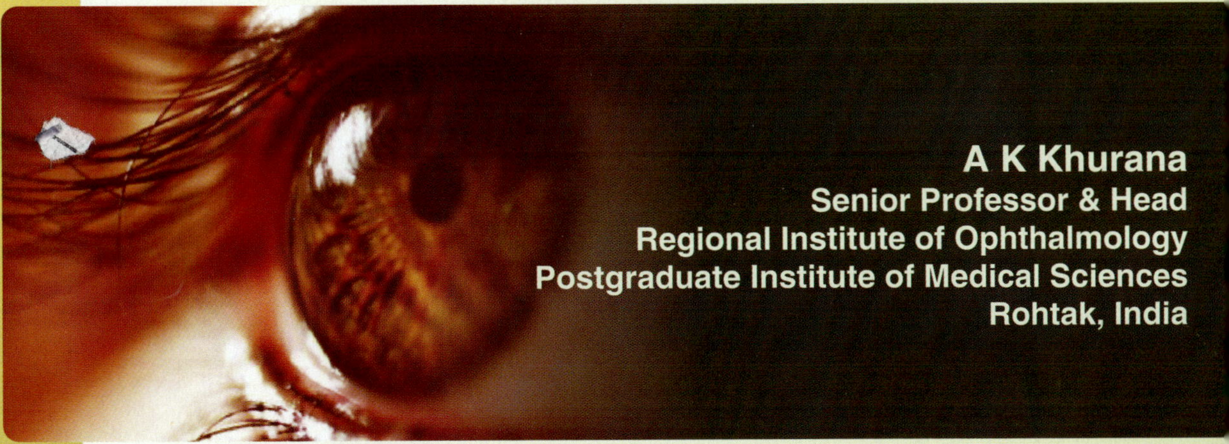

A K Khurana
Senior Professor & Head
Regional Institute of Ophthalmology
Postgraduate Institute of Medical Sciences
Rohtak, India

Aruj K Khurana
DNB (Ophthal)
(Sankra Nethralaya, Chennai, India)

Bhawna Khurana
MS
(GNEC, MAMC, New Delhi, India)

Anshan
6 Newlands Road
Tunbridge Wells
Kent, UK

Co-published in the UK in 2014

ANSHAN LTD
6 Newlands Road
Tunbridge Wells
Kent, UK

Tel:+44(0) 1892 557767
e-mail: info@anshan.co.uk
Web Site: www.anshan.co.uk

ISBN: 978-184-8290-723

British Library Cataloguing in Publication Data

A Catalogue record for this book is available from the British Library

Printed in India at Rakesh Press

Dedicated

To my parents and teachers for their blessings

To my students for their encouragement

To my children for their patience

To my wife for her understanding

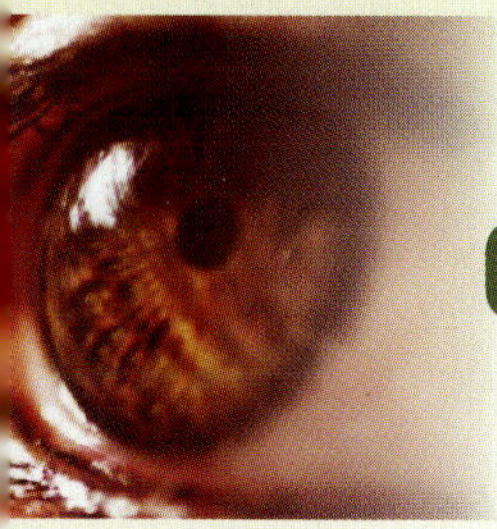

Contents

Section-I

Anatomy, Physiology and Diseases of the Eye

1 CHAPTER

Anatomy and Development of the Eye

ANATOMY OF THE EYE

This chapter gives only a brief account of the anatomy of eyeball and its related structures. The detailed anatomy of different structures is described in the relevant chapters.

THE EYEBALL

Each eyeball (Fig. 1.1) is a cystic structure kept distended by the pressure inside it. Although, generally referred to as a globe, the eyeball is not a sphere but an oblate spheroid. The central point on the maximal convexities of the anterior and posterior curvatures of the eyeball is called the *anterior* and *posterior pole,* respectively. The *equator* of the eyeball lies at the mid plane between the two poles (Fig. 1.2).

Dimensions of an adult eyeball

- Anteroposterior diameter 24 mm
- Horizontal diameter 23.5 mm
- Vertical diameter 23 mm
- Circumference 75 mm
- Volume 6.5 ml
- Weight 7 gm

Coats of the eyeball

The eyeball comprises three coats: outer (fibrous coat), middle (vascular coat) and inner (nervous coat).

1. *Fibrous coat*. It is a dense strong wall which protects the intraocular contents. Anterior 1/6th of this fibrous coat is transparent and is called *cornea*. Posterior 5/6th opaque part is called *sclera*. Cornea is set into the sclera like a watch glass. Junction of the cornea and sclera is called *limbus*. Conjunctiva is firmly attached at the limbus.

2. *Vascular coat (uveal tissue)*. It supplies nutrition to the various structures of the eyeball. It consists of three parts, from anterior to posterior, which are : iris, ciliary body and choroid.

3. *Nervous coat (retina)*. It is concerned with visual functions.

Segments and chambers of the eyeball

The eyeball can be divided into two segments: anterior and posterior.

1. *Anterior segment*. It includes crystalline lens (which is suspended from the ciliary body by zonules), and structures anterior to it, viz., iris, cornea and two aqueous humour-filled spaces : anterior and posterior chambers.

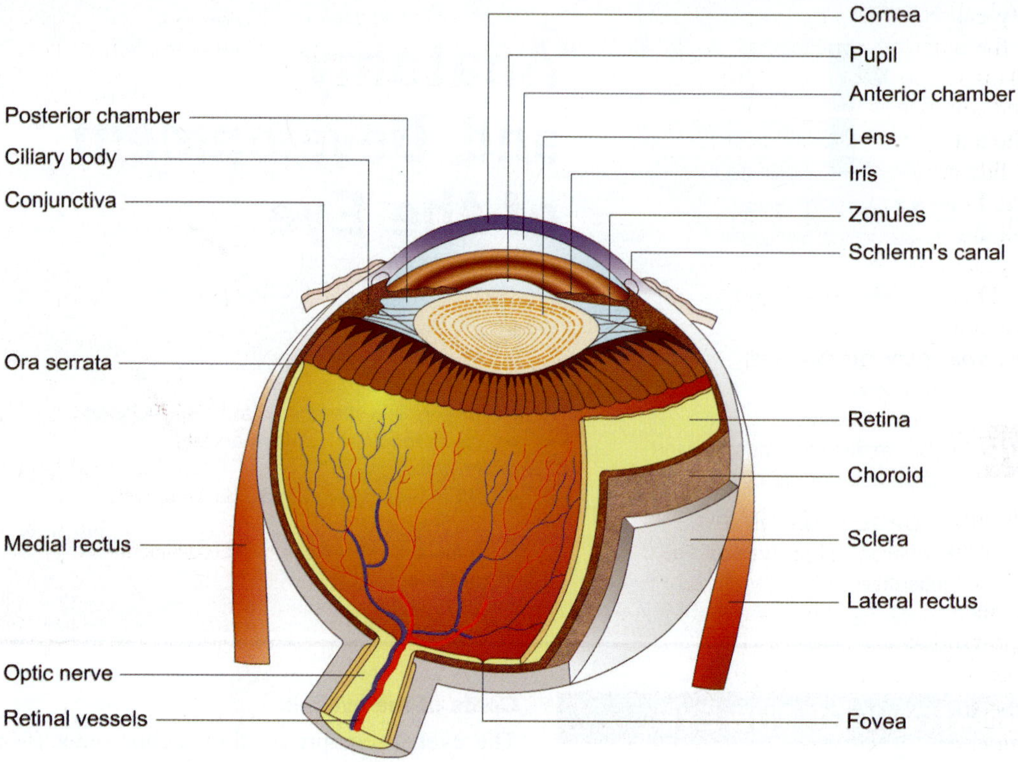

Fig. 1.1. Gross anatomy of the eyeball.

- *Anterior chamber*. It is bounded anteriorly by the back of cornea, and posteriorly by the iris and part of ciliary body. The anterior chamber is about 2.5 mm deep in the centre in normal adults. It is slightly shallower in hypermetropes and deeper in myopes, but is almost equal in the two eyes of the same individual. It contains about 0.25 ml of the aqueous humour.

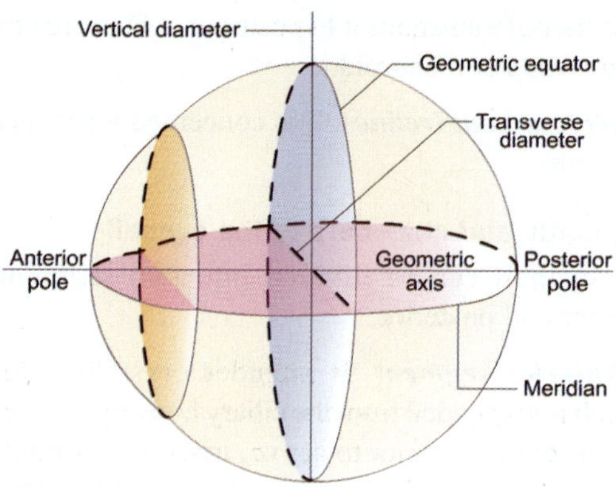

Fig. 1.2. Poles and equators of the eyeball.

- *Posterior chamber*. It is a triangular space containing 0.06 ml of aqueous humour. It is bounded anteriorly by the posterior surface of iris and part of ciliary body, posteriorly by the crystalline lens and its zonules, and laterally by the ciliary body.

2. *Posterior segment*. It includes the structures posterior to lens, viz., vitreous humour (a gel like material which fills the space behind the lens), retina, choroid and optic disc.

VISUAL PATHWAY

Each eyeball acts as a camera; it perceives the images and relays the sensations to the brain (occipital cortex) via visual pathway which comprises optic nerves, optic chiasma, optic tracts, geniculate bodies and optic radiations (Fig. 1.3).

ORBIT, EXTRAOCULAR MUSCLES, AND APPENDAGES OF THE EYE

Each eyeball is suspended by extraocular muscles and fascial sheaths in a quadrilateral pyramid-shaped bony cavity called *orbit* (Fig. 1.4). Each eyeball is located in the anterior orbit, nearer to the roof and lateral wall than to the floor and medial wall. Each eye is protected anteriorly by two shutters called the *eyelids.* The anterior part of the sclera and posterior surface of lids are lined by a thin membrane called *conjunctiva.* For smooth functioning, the cornea and conjunctiva are to be kept moist by tears which are produced by lacrimal gland and drained by the lacrimal passages. These structures (eyelids, eyebrows, conjunctiva and lacrimal apparatus) are collectively called '*the appendages of the eye*'.

DEVELOPMENT OF THE EYE

The development of eyeball can be considered to commence around day 22 when the embryo has eight pairs of somites and is around 2 mm in length. The eyeball and its related structures are derived from the following primordia:

- *Optic vesicle,* an outgrowth from prosencephalon (a neuroectodermal structure),
- *Lens placode,* a specialised area of surface ectoderm, and the surrounding surface ectoderm,
- *Mesenchyme* surrounding the optic vesicle, and
- *Visceral mesoderm* of maxillary processes.

Before going into the development of individual structure, it will be helpful to understand the formation of optic vesicle, lens placode, optic cup and changes in the surrounding mesenchyme, which play a major role in the development of the eye and its related structures.

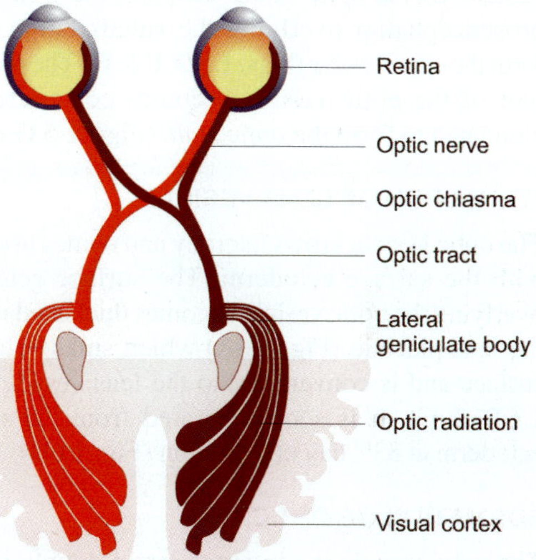

Fig. 1.3. Gross anatomy of the visual pathway.

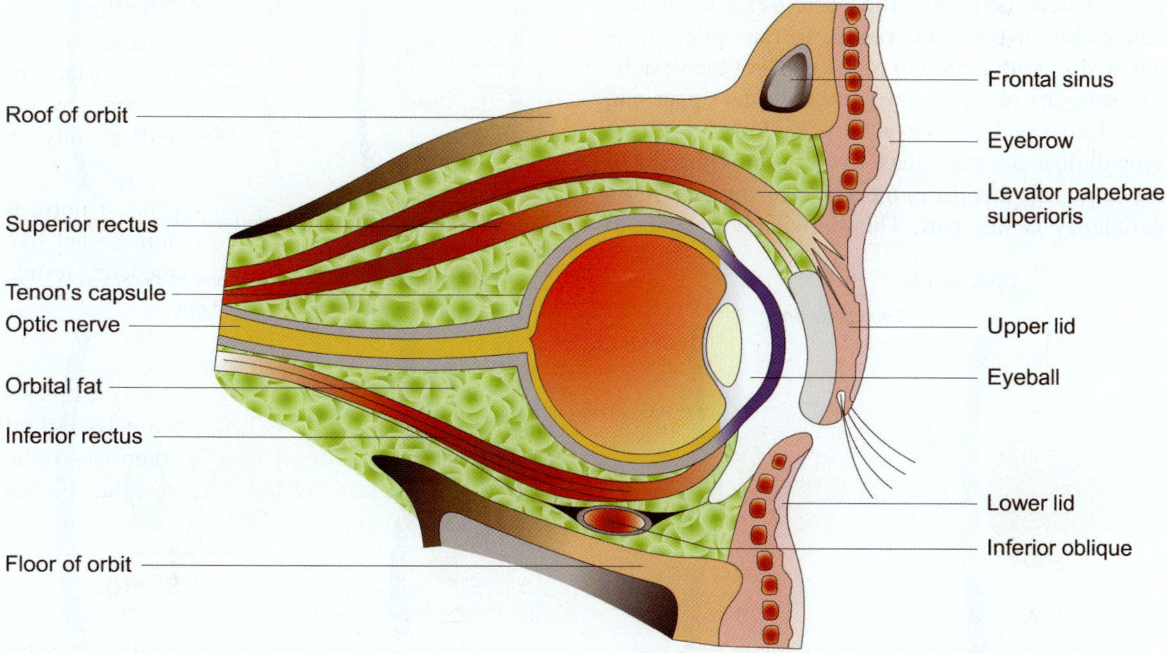

Fig. 1.4. Section of the orbital cavity to demonstrate eyeball and its accessory structures.

FORMATION OF OPTIC VESICLE AND OPTIC STALK

The area of neural plate (Fig. 1.5 A) which forms the prosencephalon develops a linear thickened area on either side (Fig. 1.5B), which soon becomes depressed to form the optic sulcus (Fig. 1.5 C). Meanwhile the neural plate gets converted into prosencephalic vesicle. As the optic sulcus deepens, the walls of the prosencephalon overlying the sulcus bulge out to form the *optic vesicle* (Figs. 1.5 D, E & F). The proximal part of the optic vesicle becomes constricted and elongated to form the *optic stalk* (Figs. 1.5 G & H).

FORMATION OF LENS VESICLE

The optic vesicle grows laterally and comes in contact with the surface ectoderm. The surface ectoderm, overlying the optic vesicle becomes thickened to form the lens placode (Fig. 1.6A) which sinks below the surface and is converted into the lens vesicle (Figs. 1.6 B & C). It is soon separated from the surface ectoderm at 33rd day of gestation (Fig. 1.6D).

FORMATION OF OPTIC CUP

The optic vesicle is converted into a double-layered *optic cup*. It appears from Fig. 1.6 that this has happened because the developing lens has invaginated itself into the optic vesicle. In fact conversion of the optic vesicle to the optic cup is due to differential growth of the walls of the vesicle. The margins of optic cup grow over the upper and lateral sides of the lens to enclose it. However, such a growth does not take place over the inferior part of the lens, and therefore, the walls of the cup show deficiency in this part. This deficiency extends to

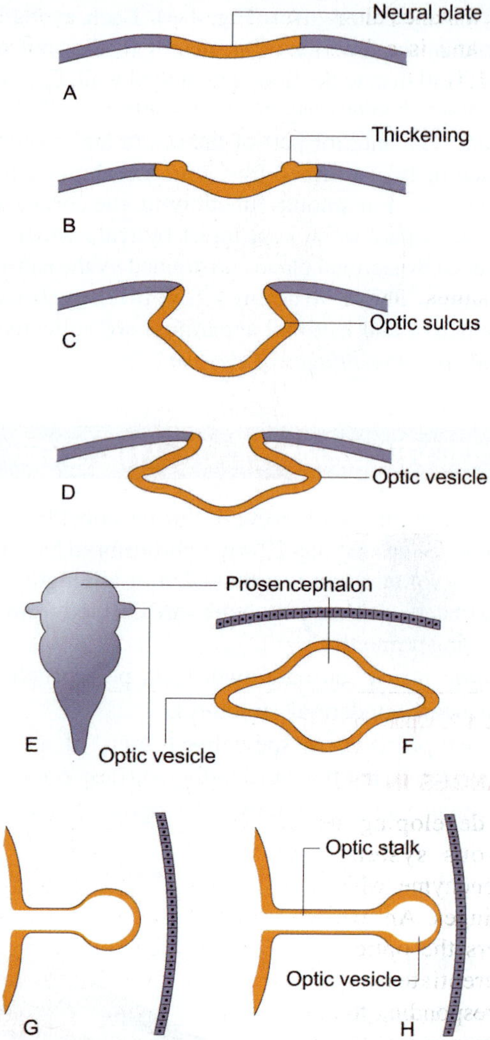

Fig. 1.5. Formation of the optic vesicle and optic stalk.

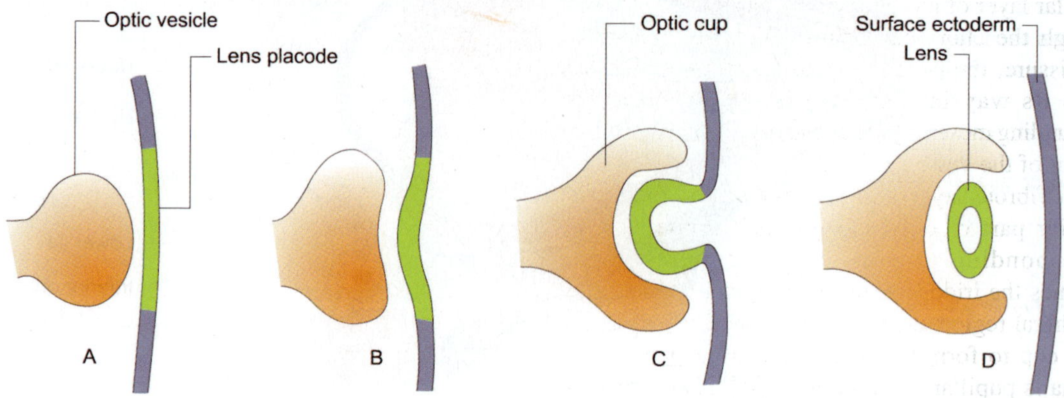

Fig. 1.6. Formation of lens vesicle and optic cup.

some distance along the inferior surface of the optic stalk and is called the *choroidal or fetal fissure* (Fig. 1.7).

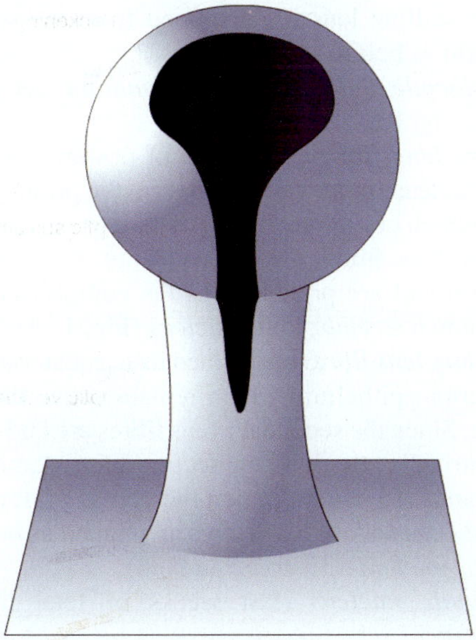

Fig. 1.7. Optic cup and stalk seen from below to show the choroidal fissure.

CHANGES IN THE ASSOCIATED MESENCHYME

The developing neural tube (from which central nervous system develops) is surrounded by mesenchyme, which subsequently condenses to form meninges. An extension of this mesenchyme also covers the optic vesicle. Later, this mesenchyme differentiates to form a superficial fibrous layer (corresponding to dura) and a deeper vascular layer (corresponding to pia-arachnoid) (Fig. 1.8).

With the formation of optic cup, part of the inner vascular layer of mesenchyme is carried into the cup through the choroidal fissure. With the closure of this fissure, the portion of mesenchyme which has made its way into the eye is cut off from the surrounding mesenchyme and gives rise to the hyaloid system of the vessels (Fig. 1.9).

The fibrous layer of mesenchyme surrounding the anterior part of optic cup forms the cornea. The corresponding vascular layer of mesenchyme becomes the iridopupillary membrane, which in the peripheral region attaches to the anterior part of the optic cup to form the iris. The central part of this lamina is pupillary membrane which also forms the tunica vasculosa lentis (Fig. 1.9).

In the posterior part of optic cup the surrounding fibrous mesenchyme forms sclera and extraocular muscles, while the vascular layer forms the choroid and ciliary body.

DEVELOPMENT OF VARIOUS OCULAR STRUCTURES

Retina

Retina is developed from the two walls of the optic cup, namely: (a) nervous retina from the inner wall, and (b) pigment epithelium from the outer wall (Fig. 1.10).

(a) *Nervous retina.* The inner wall of the optic cup is a single-layered epithelium. It divides into several layers of cells which differentiate into the following three layers (as also occurs in neural tube):

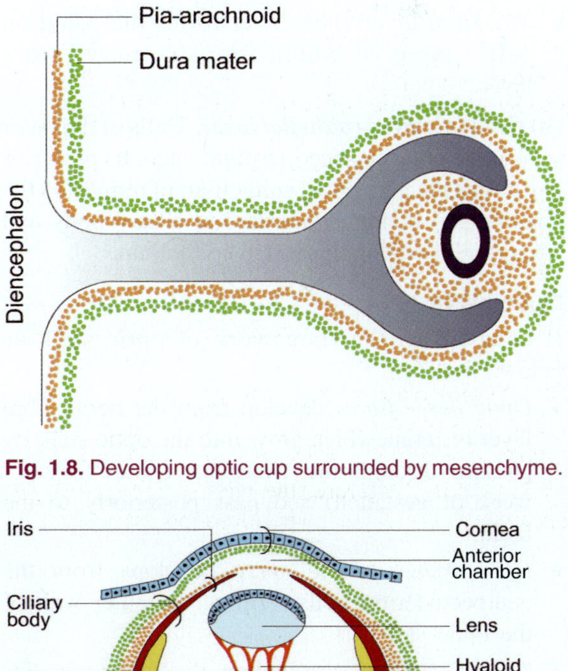

Fig. 1.8. Developing optic cup surrounded by mesenchyme.

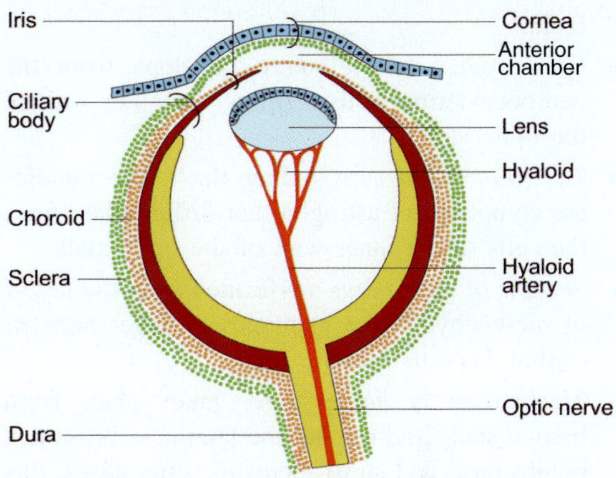

Fig. 1.9. Derivation of various structures of the eyeball.

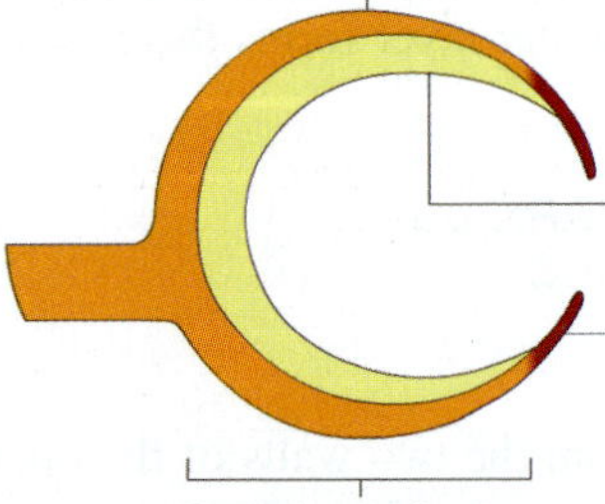

Fig. 1.10. Development of the retina.

- *Matrix cell layer.* Cells of this layer form the rods and cones.
- *Mantle layer.* Cells of this layer form the bipolar cells, ganglion cells, other neurons of retina and the supporting tissue.
- *Marginal layer.* This layer forms the ganglion cells, axons of which form the nerve fibre layer.

(b) ***Outer pigment epithelial layer.*** Cells of the outer wall of the optic cup become pigmented. Its posterior part forms the pigmented epithelium of retina and the anterior part continues forward in ciliary body and iris as their anterior pigmented epithelium.

Optic nerve

It develops in the framework of optic stalk as below:

- *Optic nerve fibres* develop from the nerve fibre layer of retina which grow into the optic stalk by passing through the choroidal fissure (by 6th week of gestation) and pass posteriorly to the brain.
- *Glial system of the nerve* develops from the neuroectodermal cells forming the outer wall of the optic stalk.
- *The glial septa* surrounding the nerve bundles are composed of astroglia that differentiate from the cells of the inner wall of the optic stalk.
- *Sheaths of optic nerve* are formed from the layers of mesenchyme like meninges of other parts of central nervous system.
- *Myelination of nerve fibres* takes place from brain distally and reaches the lamina cribrosa just before birth and stops there. In some cases, this extends up to around the optic disc and presents as congenital opaque nerve fibres. These develop after birth.

Crystalline lens

The crystalline lens is developed from the surface ectoderm as below :

Lens placode and lens vesicle formation (see pages 5, 6 and Fig. 1.6).

Primary lens fibres. The cells of posterior wall of lens vesicle elongate rapidly to form the primary lens fibres which obliterate the cavity of lens vesicle. The primary lens fibres are formed upto 3rd month of gestation and are preserved as the compact core of lens, known as *embryonic nucleus* (Fig. 1.11).

Secondary lens fibres are formed from equatorial cells of anterior epithelium which remain active through out life. Since the secondary lens fibres are laid down concentrically, the lens on section has a laminated appearance. Depending upon the period of development, the secondary lens fibres are named as below :

- *Fetal nucleus* (3rd to 8th month),
- *Infantile nucleus* (last weeks of fetal life to puberty),
- *Adult nucleus* (after puberty), and
- *Cortex* (superficial lens fibres of adult lens)

Lens capsule is a true basement membrane produced by the lens epithelium on its external aspect.

Cornea (Fig. 1.9)

1. ***Epithelium*** is formed from the surface ectoderm.

2. ***Other layers viz.*** endothelium, Descemet's membrane, stroma and Bowman's layer are derived from the fibrous layer of mesenchyme lying anterior to the optic cup (Fig. 1.9).

Sclera

Sclera is developed from the fibrous layer of mesenchyme surrounding the optic cup (corresponding to dura of CNS) (Fig. 1.9).

Choroid

It is derived from the inner vascular layer of mesenchyme that surrounds the optic cup (Fig. 1.9).

Ciliary body

- The two layers of *epithelium* of ciliary body develop from the anterior part of the two layers of optic cup (neuroectodermal).
- *Stroma of ciliary body,* ciliary muscle and blood vessels are developed from the vascular layer of mesenchyme surrounding the optic cup (Fig. 1.9).

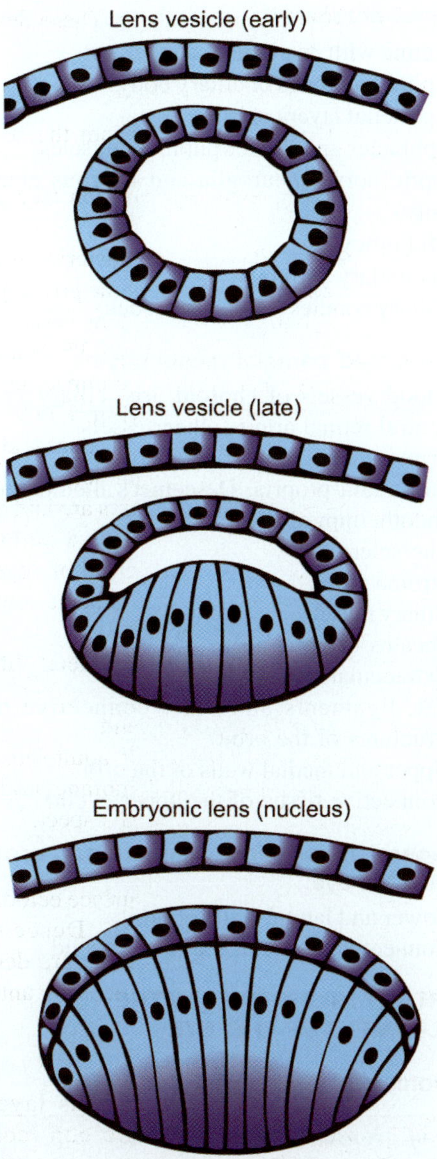

Fig. 1.11. Development of the crystalline lens.

Iris

- Both layers of *epithelium* are derived from the marginal region of optic cup (neuroectodermal) (Fig. 1.9).
- *Sphincter and dilator pupillae* muscles are derived from the anterior epithelium (neuroectodermal).
- *Stroma and blood vessels* of the iris develop from the vascular mesenchyme present anterior to the optic cup.

Vitreous

1. *Primary or primitive vitreous* is mesenchymal in origin and is a vascular structure having the hyaloid system of vessels.
2. *Secondary or definitive or vitreous proper* is secreted by neuroectoderm of optic cup. This is an avascular structure. When this vitreous fills the cavity, primitive vitreous with hyaloid vessels is pushed anteriorly and ultimately disappears.
3. *Tertiary vitreous* is developed from neuroectoderm in the ciliary region and is represented by the ciliary zonules.

Eyelids

Eyelids are formed by reduplication of surface ectoderm above and below the cornea (Fig. 1.12). The folds enlarge and their margins meet and fuse with each other. The lids cut off a space called the *conjunctival sac*. The folds thus formed contain some mesoderm which would form the muscles of the lid and the tarsal plate. The lids separate after the seventh month of intra-uterine life.

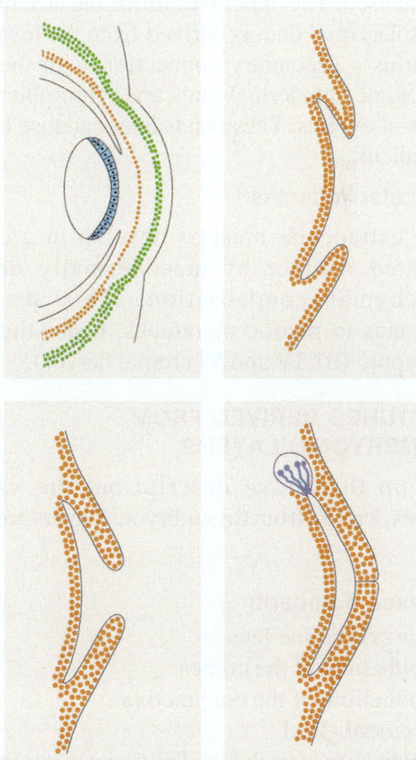

Fig. 1.12. Development of the eyelids, conjunctiva and lacrimal gland.

- *Tarsal glands* are formed by ingrowth of a regular row of solid columns of ectodermal cells from the lid margins.
- *Cilia* develop as epithelial buds from lid margins.

Conjunctiva

Conjunctiva develops from the ectoderm lining the lids and covering the globe (Fig. 1.12).

- *Conjunctival glands* develop as growth of the basal cells of upper conjunctival fornix. Fewer glands develop from the lower fornix.

The lacrimal apparatus

Lacrimal gland is formed from about 8 cuneiform epithelial buds which grow by the end of 2nd month of fetal life from the superolateral side of the conjunctival sac (Fig. 1.12).

Lacrimal sac, nasolacrimal duct and canaliculi. These structures develop from the ectoderm of nasolacrimal furrow. It extends from the medial angle of eye to the region of developing mouth. The ectoderm gets buried to form a solid cord. The cord is later canalised. The upper part forms the lacrimal sac. The nasolacrimal duct is derived from the lower part as it forms a secondary connection with the nasal cavity. Some ectodermal buds arise from the medial margins of eyelids. These buds later canalise to form the canaliculi.

Extraocular muscles

All the extraocular muscles develop in a closely associated manner by mesodermally derived mesenchymal condensation. This probably corresponds to preotic myotomes, hence the triple nerve supply (III, IV and VI cranial nerves).

STRUCTURES DERIVED FROM THE EMBRYONIC LAYERS

Based on the above description, the various structures derived from the embryonic layers are given below :

1. Surface ectoderm

- The crystalline lens
- Epithelium of the cornea
- Epithelium of the conjunctiva
- Lacrimal gland
- Epithelium of eyelids and its derivatives viz., cilia, tarsal glands and conjunctival glands.
- Epithelium lining the lacrimal apparatus.

2. Neural ectoderm

- Retina with its pigment epithelium
- Epithelial layers of ciliary body
- Epithelial layers of iris
- Sphincter and dilator pupillae muscles
- Optic nerve (neuroglia and nervous elements only)
- Melanocytes
- Secondary vitreous
- Ciliary zonules (tertiary vitreous)

3. Associated paraxial mesenchyme

- Blood vessels of choroid, iris, ciliary vessels, central retinal artery, other vessels.
- Primary vitreous
- Substantia propria, Descemet's membrane and endothelium of cornea
- The sclera
- Stroma of iris
- Ciliary muscle
- Sheaths of optic nerve
- Extraocular muscles
- Fat, ligaments and other connective tissue structures of the orbit
- Upper and medial walls of the orbit
- Connective tissue of the upper eyelid

4. Visceral mesoderm of maxillary process below the eye

- Lower and lateral walls of orbit
- Connective tissue of the lower eyelid

IMPORTANT MILESTONES IN THE DEVELOPMENT OF THE EYE

Embryonic and fetal period

Stage of growth	*Development*
2.6 mm (3 weeks)	Optic pits appear on either side of cephalic end of forebrain.
3.5 mm (4 weeks)	Primary optic vesicle invaginates.
5.5 to 6 mm	Development of embryonic fissure
10 mm (6 weeks)	Retinal layers differentiate, lens vesicle formed.
20 mm (9 weeks)	Sclera, cornea and extraocular muscles differentiate.

25 mm (10 weeks)	Lumen of optic nerve obliterated.
50 mm (3 months)	Optic tracts completed, pars ciliaris retina grows forwards, pars iridica retina grows forward and lid folds develop.
60 mm (4 months)	Hyaloid vessels atrophy, iris sphincter, dilator and ciliary muscles develop.
230-265 mm (8th month)	Fetal nucleus of lens is complete, all layers of retina nearly developed and macula starts differentiation.
265-300mm (9th month)	Except macula, retina is fully developed, infantile nucleus of lens begins to appear, pupillary membrane and hyaloid vessels disappear. Medulation of optic nerve reaches lamina cribrosa.

Eye at birth

- *Anteroposterior diameter* of the eyeball is about 16.5 mm (70% of adult size which is attained by 7-8 years).
- *Corneal diameter* is about 10 mm. Adult size (11.7 mm) is attained by 2 years of age.
- *Anterior chamber* is shallow and angle is narrow.
- *Pupil* is small and does not dilate fully.
- *Lens* is spherical at birth. Infantile nucleus is present.
- *Retina.* Apart from macular area the retina is fully differentiated. Macula differentiates 4-6 months after birth.
- *Myelination* of optic nerve fibres has reached the lamina cribrosa.
- *Newborn* is usually hypermetropic by +2 to +3 D.
- *Orbit* is more divergent (50°) as compared to adult (45°).
- *Lacrimal gland* is still underdeveloped and tears are not secreted.

Postnatal period

- *Fixation* starts developing in first month and is completed in 6 months.
- *Macula* is fully developed by 4-6 months.
- *Fusional reflexes,* stereopsis and accommodation is well developed by 4-6 months.
- *Cornea* attains normal adult diameter by 2 years of age.
- *Lens* grows throughout life.

CHAPTER 2

Physiology of Eye and Vision

INTRODUCTION

Sense of vision is a complex function of the two eyes and their central connections. The physiological activities involved in the normal functioning of the eyes are :

- Maintenance of clear ocular media,
- Maintenance of normal intraocular pressure,
- The image forming mechanism,
- Physiology of vision,
- Physiology of binocular vision,
- Physiology of pupil, and
- Physiology of ocular motility.

MAINTENANCE OF CLEAR OCULAR MEDIA

The main prerequisite for visual function is the maintenance of clear refractive media of the eye. The major factor responsible for transparency of the ocular media is their avascularity. The structures forming refractive media of the eye from anterior to posterior are :

- Tear film,
- Cornea,
- Aqueous humour,
- Crystalline lens, and
- Vitreous humour

PHYSIOLOGY OF TEARS

Tear film plays a vital role in maintaining the transparency of cornea. The physiological aspects of the tears and tear film are described in the chapter on diseases of the lacrimal apparatus (see page 388).

PHYSIOLOGY OF CORNEA

The cornea forms the main refractive medium of the eye. Physiological aspects in relation to cornea include:

- Transparency of cornea,
- Nutrition and metabolism of cornea,
- Permeability of cornea, and
- Corneal wound healing.

(For details see page 90).

PHYSIOLOGY OF CRYSTALLINE LENS

The crystalline lens is a transparent structure playing main role in the focussing mechanism for vision. Its physiological aspects include :

- Lens transparency
- Metabolic activities of the lens and
- Accommodation.

(For details see page 40 and 178).

PHYSIOLOGY OF AQUEOUS HUMOUR AND MAINTENANCE OF INTRAOCULAR PRESSURE

The aqueous humour is a clear watery fluid filling the anterior chamber (0.25 ml) and the posterior chamber (0.06 ml) of the eyeball. In addition to its role in maintaining a proper intraocular pressure it also plays an important metabolic role by providing substrates and removing metabolities from the avascular cornea and the crystalline lens. For details see pages 219-222.

PHYSIOLOGY OF VISION

Physiology of vision is a complex phenomenon which is still poorly understood. The main mechanisms involved in physiology of vision are :

- *Initiation of vision* (Phototransduction), a function of photoreceptors (rods and cones),
- *Processing and transmission of visual sensation,* a function of image processing cells of retina and visual pathway, and
- *Visual perception,* a function of visual cortex and related areas of cerebral cortex.

PHOTOTRANSDUCTION

The rods and cones serve as sensory nerve endings for visual sensation. Light falling upon the retina causes photochemical changes which in turn trigger a cascade of biochemical reactions that result in generation of electrical changes. Photochemical changes occuring in the rods and cones are essentially similar but the changes in rod pigment (rhodopsin or visual purple) have been studied in more detail. This whole phenomenon of conversion of light energy into nerve impulse is known as phototransduction.

Photochemical changes

The photochemical changes include :

Rhodopsin bleaching. Rhodopsin refers to the visual pigment present in the rods – the receptors for night (scotopic) vision. Its maximum absorption spectrum is around 500 nm. Rhodopsin consists of a colourless protein called *opsin* coupled with a carotenoid called *retinine* (Vitamin A aldehyde or 11-*cis-retinal).* Light falling on the rods converts 11-cis-retinal component of rhodopsin into *all-trans-retinal* through various stages (Fig. 2.1). The all-trans-retinal so formed is soon separated from the opsin. This process of separation is called *photodecomposition* and the rhodopsin is said to be bleached by the action of light.

Rhodopsin regeneration. The 11-cis-retinal is regenerated from the all-trans-retinal separated from the opsin (as described above) and vitamin-A (retinal) supplied from the blood. The 11-cis-retinal then reunites with opsin in the rod outer segment to form the rhodopsin. This whole process is called *rhodopsin regeneration* (Fig. 2.1). Thus, the bleaching of the rhodopsin occurs under the influence of light, whereas the regeneration process is independent of light, proceeding equally well in light and darkness.

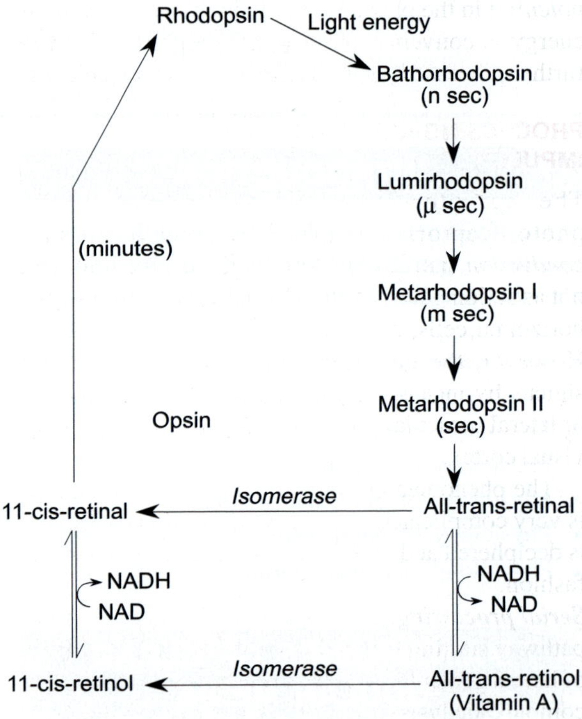

Fig. 2.1. Light induced changes in rhodopsin.

Visual cycle. In the retina of living animals, under constant light stimulation, a steady state must exist under which the rate at which the photochemicals are bleached is equal to the rate at which they are regenerated. This equilibrium between the photodecomposition and regeneration of visual pigments is referred to as *visual cycle* (Fig. 2.2).

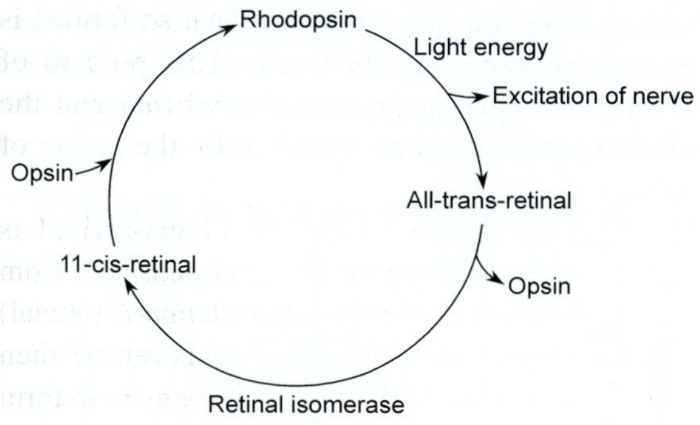

Fig. 2.2. Visual cycle.

Electrical changes

The activated rhodopsin, following exposure to light, triggers a cascade of complex biochemical reactions which ultimately result in the generation of *receptor potential* in the photoreceptors. In this way, the light energy is converted into electrical energy which is further processed and transmitted via visual pathway.

PROCESSING AND TRANSMISSION OF VISUAL IMPULSE

The receptor potential generated in the photoreceptors is transmitted by *electrotonic conduction* (i.e., direct flow of electric current, and not as action potential) to other cells of the retina viz. horizontal cells, amacrine cells, and ganglion cells. However, the ganglion cells transmit the visual signals by means of action potential to the neurons of lateral geniculate body and the later to the primary visual cortex.

The phenomenon of processing of visual impulse is very complicated. It is now clear that visual image is deciphered and analyzed in both serial and parallel fashion.

Serial processing. The successive cells in the visual pathway starting from the photoreceptors to the cells of lateral geniculate body are involved in increasingly complex analysis of image. This is called sequential or serial processing of visual information.

Parallel processing. Two kinds of cells can be distinguished in the visual pathway starting from the ganglion cells of retina including neurons of the lateral geniculate body, striate cortex, and extrastriate cortex. These are large cells (magno or M cells) and small cells (parvo or P cells). There are striking differences between the sensitivity of M and P cells to stimulus features (Table 2.1).

Table 2.1. Differences in the sensitivity of M and P cells to stimulus features

Stimulus feature	*Sensitivity*	
	M cell	*P cell*
Colour contrast	No	Yes
Luminance contrast	Higher	Lower
Spatial frequency	Lower	Higher
Temporal frequency	Higher	Lower

The visual pathway is now being considered to be made of two lanes: one made of the large cells is called *magnocellular pathway* and the other of small cells is called *parvocellular pathway*. These can be compared to two-lanes of a road. The M pathway and P pathway are involved in the *parallel processing* of the image i.e., analysis of different features of the image.

VISUAL PERCEPTION

It is a complex integration of light sense, form sense, sense of contrast and colour sense. The receptive field organization of the retina and cortex are used to encode this information about a visual image.

1. The light sense

It is awareness of the light. The minimum brightness required to evoke a sensation of light is called the *light minimum*. It should be measured when the eye is dark adapted for at least 20-30 minutes.

The human eye in its ordinary use throughout the day is capable of functioning normally over an exceedingly wide range of illumination by a highly complex phenomenon termed as the *visual adaptation*. The process of visual adaptation primarily involves :

- Dark adaptation (adjustment in dim illumination), and
- Light adaptation (adjustment to bright illumination).

Dark adaptation

It is the ability of the eye to adapt itself to decreasing illumination. When one goes from bright sunshine into a dimly-lit room, one cannot perceive the objects in the room until some time has elapsed. During this period, eye is adapting to low illumination. The time taken to see in dim illumination is called *'dark adaptation time'*.

The rods are much more sensitive to low illumination than the cones. Therefore, rods are used more in dim light (*scotopic vision*) and cones in bright light (*photopic vision*).

Dark adaptation curve (Fig. 2.3) plotted with illumination of test object in vertical axis and duration of dark adaptation along the horizontal axis shows that visual threshold falls progressively in the darkened room for about half an hour until a relative constant value is reached. Further, the dark adaptation curve consists of two parts: the initial small curve represents the adaptation of cones and the remainder of the curve represents the adaptation of rods.

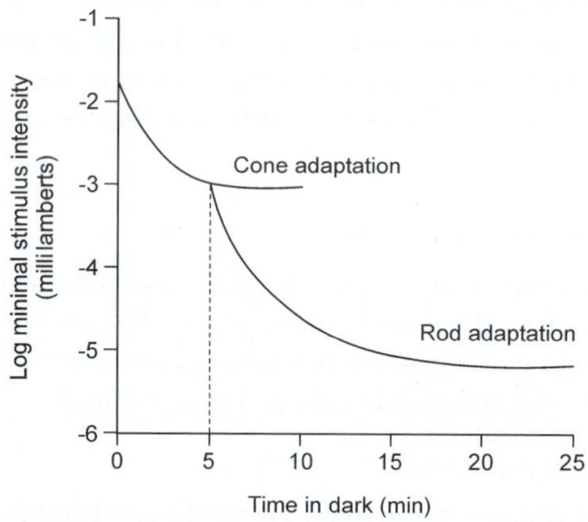

Fig. 2.3. Dark adaptation curve plotted with illumination of test object in vertical axis and duration of dark adaptation along the horizontal axis.

When fully dark adapted, the retina is about one lakh times more sensitive to light than when bleached.

Delayed dark adaptation occurs in diseases of rods e.g., retinitis pigmentosa and vitamin A deficiency.

Light adaptation

When one passes suddenly from a dim to a brightly lighted environment, the light seems intensely and even uncomfortably bright until the eyes adapt to the increased illumination and the visual threshold rises. The process by means of which retina adapts itself to bright light is called *light adaptation*. Unlike dark adaptation, the process of light adaptation is very quick and occurs over a period of 5 minutes. Strictly speaking, light adaptation is merely the disappearance of dark adaptation.

2. The form sense

It is the ability to discriminate between the shapes of the objects. Cones play a major role in this faculty. Therefore, form sense is most acute at the fovea, where there are maximum number of cones and decreases very rapidly towards the periphery (Fig. 2.4). Visual acuity recorded by Snellen's test chart is a measure of the form sense.

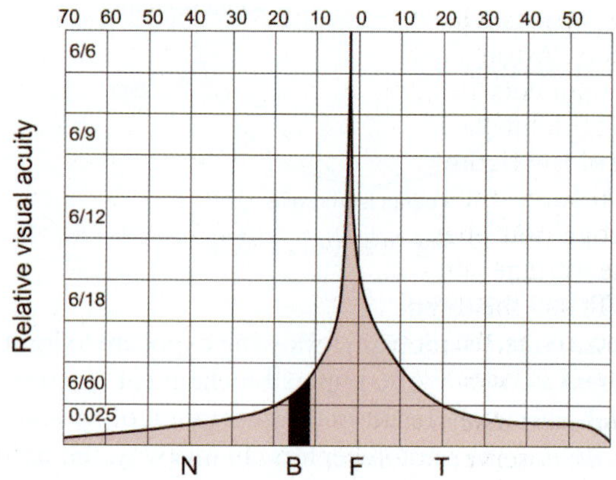

Fig. 2.4. Visual acuity (form sense) in relation to the regions of the retina: N, nasal retina; B, blind spot; F, foveal region; and T, temporal retina.

Components of visual acuity. In clinical practice, measurement of the threshold of discrimination of two spatially separated targets (a function of the fovea centralis) is termed *visual acuity*. However, in theory, visual acuity is a highly complex function that consists of the following components :

Minimum visible. It is the ability to determine whether an object is present or not.

Resolution (ordinary visual acuity). Discrimination of two spatially separated targets is termed resolution. The minimum separation between the two points, which can be discriminated as two, is known as *minimum resolvable*. Measurement of the threshold of discrimination is essentially an assessment of the function of the fovea centralis and is termed *ordinary visual acuity*. Histologically, the diameter of a cone in the foveal region is 0.004 mm and this, therefore, represents the smallest distance between two cones. It is reported that in order to produce an image of minimum size of 0.004 mm (resolving power of the eye) the object must subtend a visual angle of 1 minute at the nodal point of the eye. It is called the *minimum angle of resolution (MAR)*.

The clinical tests determining visual acuity measure the form sense or reading ability of the eye. Thus, broadly, resolution refers to the ability to identify the spatial characteristics of a test figure. The test targets in these tests may either consist of letters (Snellen's chart) or broken circle (Landolt's ring). More complex targets include gratings and checker board patterns.

Recognition. It is that faculty by virtue of which an individual not only discriminates the spatial characteristics of the test pattern but also identifies the patterns with which he has had some experience. Recognition is thus a task involving cognitive components in addition to spatial resolution. For recognition, the individual should be familiar with the set of test figures employed in addition to being able to resolve them. The most common example of recognition phenomenon is identification of faces. The average adult can recognize thousands of faces.

Thus, the form sense is not purely a retinal function, as, the perception of its composite form (e.g., letters) is largely psychological.

Minimum discriminable refers to spatial distinction by an observer when the threshold is much lower than the ordinary acuity. The best example of minimum discriminable is *vernier acuity*, which refers to the ability to determine whether or not two parallel and straight lines are aligned in the frontal plane.

3. Sense of contrast

It is the ability of the eye to perceive slight changes in the luminance between regions which are not separated by definite borders. Loss of contrast sensitivity results in mild fogginess of the vision.

Contrast sensitivity is affected by various factors like age, refractive errors, glaucoma, amblyopia, diabetes, optic nerve diseases and lenticular changes. Further, contrast sensitivity may be impaired even in the presence of normal visual acuity.

Measurement of contrast sensitivity: In clinical practice the contrast sensitivity can be measured by using any of the following charts with letters or stripes represented in various shades of gray:

- Arden gratings,
- Cambridge low-contrast gratings,
- Pelli-Robson contrast sensitivity chart which consists of low contrast letters with same size (Fig. 2.5),
- The Visitach chart, and
- Functional acuity contrast test (FACT).

4. Colour sense

It is the ability of the eye to discriminate between different colours excited by light of different wavelengths. Colour vision is a function of the cones and thus better appreciated in photopic vision. In dim light (scotopic vision), all colours are seen grey and this phenomenon is called *Purkinje shift.*

Theories of colour vision

The process of colour analysis begins in the retina and is not entirely a function of brain. Many theories have been put forward to explain the colour perception, but two have been particularly influential:

1. *Trichromatic theory.* The trichromacy of colour vision was originally suggested by Young and subsequently modified by Helmholtz. Hence it is called *Young-Helmholtz theory*. It postulates the existence of three kinds of cones, each containing a different photopigment which is maximally sensitive to one of the three primary colours viz. red, green and blue. The sensation of any given colour is determined by the relative frequency of the impulse from each of the three cone systems. In other words, a given colour consists of admixture of the three primary colours in different proportion. The correctness of the Young-Helmholtz's trichromacy theory of colour vision has now been demonstrated by the identification and chemical characterization of each of the three pigments by recombinant DNA technique, each having different absorption spectrum as below (Fig. 2.6):

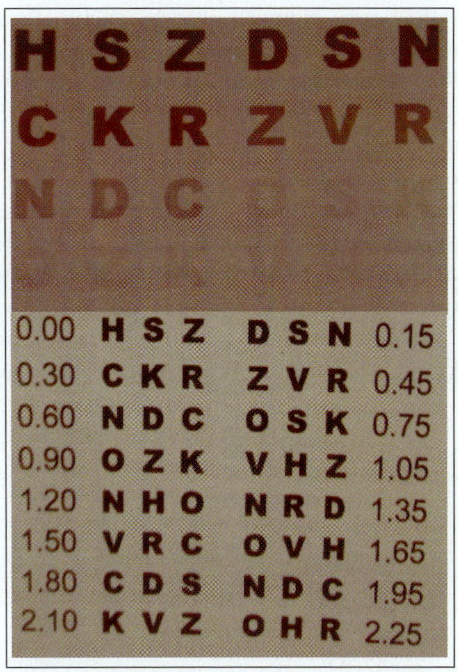

Fig. 2.5. Pelli-Robson contrast sensitivity chart: A. Photograph; B. Log contrast sensitivity score of each patient.

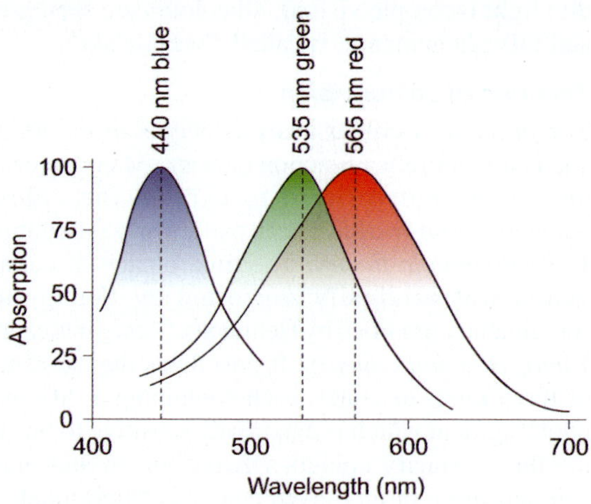

Fig. 2.6. Absorption spectrum of three cone pigments.

- *Red sensitive cone pigment,* also known as *erythrolabe* or long wave length sensitive (LWS) cone pigment, absorbs maximally in a yellow portion with a peak at 565 nm. But its spectrum extends far enough into the long wavelength to sense red.
- *Green sensitive cone pigment*, also known as *chlorolabe* or medium wavelength sensitive (MWS) cone pigment, absorbs maximally in the green portion with a peak at 535 nm.
- *Blue sensitive cone pigment*, also known as *cyanolabe* or short wavelength sensitive (SWS) cone pigment, absorbs maximally in the blue-violet portion of the spectrum with a peak at 440 nm.

Thus, the Young-Helmholtz theory concludes that blue, green and red are primary colours, but the cones with their maximal sensitivity in the yellow portion of the spectrum are at a lower threshold than green.

It has been studied that the gene for human rhodopsin is located on chromosome 3, and the gene for the blue-sensitive cone is located on chromosome. The genes for the red and green sensitive cones are arranged in tandem array on the q arm of the X chromosomes.

2. *Opponent colour theory of Hering.* The opponent colour theory of Hering points out that some colours appear to be 'mutually exclusive'. There is no such colour as 'reddish-green', and such phenomenon can be difficult to explain on the basis of trichromatic theory alone. In fact, it seems that both theories are useful in that:

- The colour vision is trichromatic at the level of photoreceptors, and
- Colour opponency occurs at ganglion cell onward.

According to opponent colour theory, there are two main types of colour opponent ganglion cells:

- *Red-green opponent colour cells* use signals from red and green cones to detect red/green contrast within their receptive field.
- *Blue-yellow opponent colour cells* obtain a yellow signal from the summed output of red and green cones, which is contrasted with the output from blue cones within the receptive field.

Colour vision tests

(See page 326)

PHYSIOLOGY OF OCULAR MOTILITY AND BINOCULAR VISION

PHYSIOLOGY OF OCULAR MOTILITY

See page 333.

PHYSIOLOGY OF BINOCULAR SINGLE VISION

See page 338.

3 CHAPTER

Optics and Refraction

OPTICS

LIGHT

Light is the visible portion of the electromagnetic radiation spectrum. It lies between ultraviolet and infrared portions, from 400 nm at the violet end of the spectrum to 700 nm at the red end. The white light consists of seven colours denoted by VIBGYOR (violet, indigo, blue, green, yellow, orange and red).

Light ray is the term used to describe the radius of the concentric wave forms. A group of parallel rays of light is called a *beam of light.*

Important facts to remember about light rays are :

- The media of the eye are uniformally permeable to the visible rays between 600 nm and 390 nm.
- Cornea absorbs rays shorter than 295 nm. Therefore, rays between 600 nm and 295 nm only can reach the lens.
- Lens absorbs rays shorter than 350 nm. Therefore, rays between 600 and 350 nm can reach the retina in phakic eye; and those between 600 nm and 295 nm in aphakic eyes.

GEOMETRICAL OPTICS

The behaviour of light rays is determined by ray-optics. A ray of light is the straight line path followed by light in going from one point to another. The ray-optics, therefore, uses the geometry of straight lines to account for the macroscopic phenomena like rectilinear propagation, reflection and refraction. That is why the ray-optics is also called geometrical optics.

The knowledge of geometrical optics is essential to understand the optics of eye, errors of refraction and their correction. Therefore, some of its important aspects are described in the following text.

Reflection of light

Reflection of light is a phenomenon of change in the path of light rays without any change in the medium (Fig. 3.1). The light rays falling on a reflecting surface are called *incident rays* and those reflected by it are *reflected rays.* A line drawn at right angle to the surface is called the *normal.*

Laws of reflection are (Fig. 3.1):

1. The incident ray, the reflected ray and the normal at the point of incident, all lie in the same plane.
2. The angle of incidence (i) is equal to the angle of reflection (r).

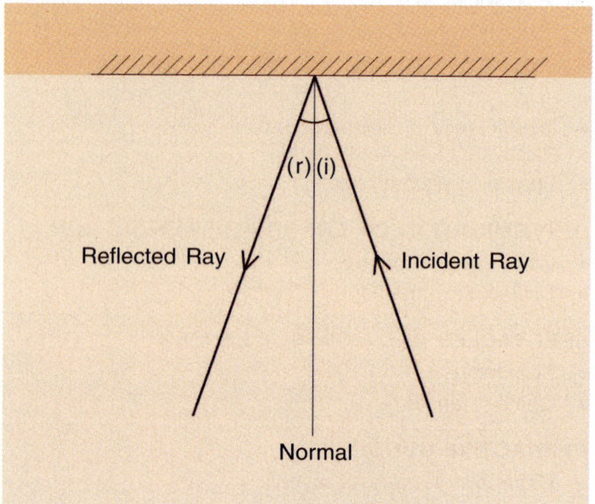

Fig. 3.1. Laws of reflection.

Mirrors

A smooth and well-polished surface which reflects regularly most of the light falling on it is called a mirror.

Types of mirrors

Mirrors can be plane or spherical.

1. *Plane mirror.* The features of an image formed by a plane mirror (Fig. 3.2) are: (i) it is of the same size as the object; (ii) it lies at the same distance behind the mirror as the object is in front; (iii) it is laterally inverted; and (iv) virtual in nature.

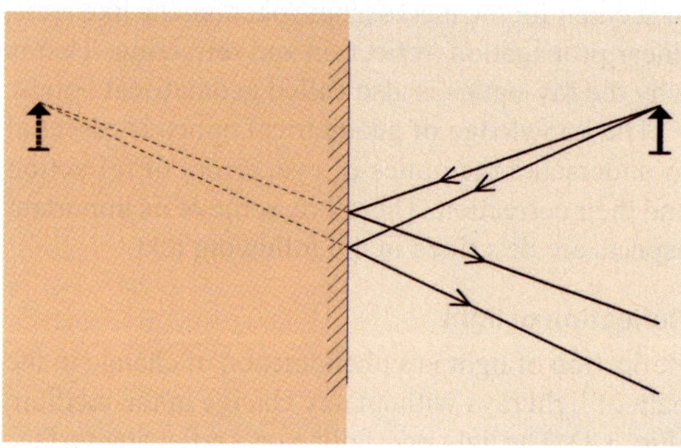

Fig. 3.2. Image formation with a plane mirror.

2. *Spherical mirror.* A spherical mirror (Fig. 3.3) is a part of a hollow sphere whose one side is silvered and the other side is polished. The two types of spherical mirrors are : *concave mirror* (whose reflecting surface is towards the centre of the sphere) and *convex mirror* (whose reflecting surface is away from the centre of the sphere).

Cardinal data of a spherical mirror (Fig. 3.3)

- *Centre of curvature* (C) and *radius of curvature* (R) of a spherical mirror are the centre and radius, respectively, of the sphere of which the mirror forms a part.
- *Normal* to the spherical mirror at any point is the line joining that point to the centre of curvature (C) of the mirror.
- *Pole* of the mirror (P) is the centre of the reflecting surface.
- *Principal axis of the mirror* is the straight line joining the pole and centre of curvature of spherical mirror and extended on both sides.

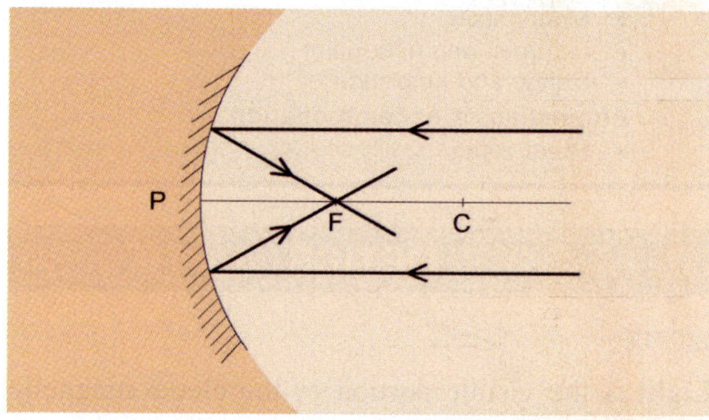

Fig. 3.3. Cardinal points of a concave mirror.

- *Principal focus* (F) of a spherical mirror is a point on the principal axis of the mirror at which, ray incident on the mirror in a direction parallel to the principal axis actually meet (in concave mirror) or appear to diverge (as in convex mirror) after reflection from the mirror.
- *Focal length* (f) of the mirror is the distance of principal focus from the pole of the spherical mirror.

Images formed by a concave mirror

As a summary, Table 3.1 gives the position, size and nature of images formed by a concave mirror for different positions of the object. Figures 3.4 a, b, c, d, e and f illustrate various situations.

Table 3.1. Images formed by a concave mirror for different positions of object

No.	Position of the object	Position of the image	Nature and size of the image	Ray diagram
1.	At infinity	At the principal focus (F)	Real, very small and inverted	Fig. 3.4 (a)
2.	Beyond the centre of curvature (C)	Between F & C	Real, diminished in size, and inverted	Fig. 3.4 (b)
3.	At C	At C	Real, same size as object and inverted	Fig. 3.4 (c)
4.	Between F & C	Beyond C	Real, enlarged and inverted	Fig. 3.4 (d)
5.	At F	At infinity	Real, very large and inverted	Fig. 3.4 (e)
6.	Between pole of the mirror (P) and focus (F)	Behind the mirror	Virtual, enlarged and erect	Fig. 3.4 (f)

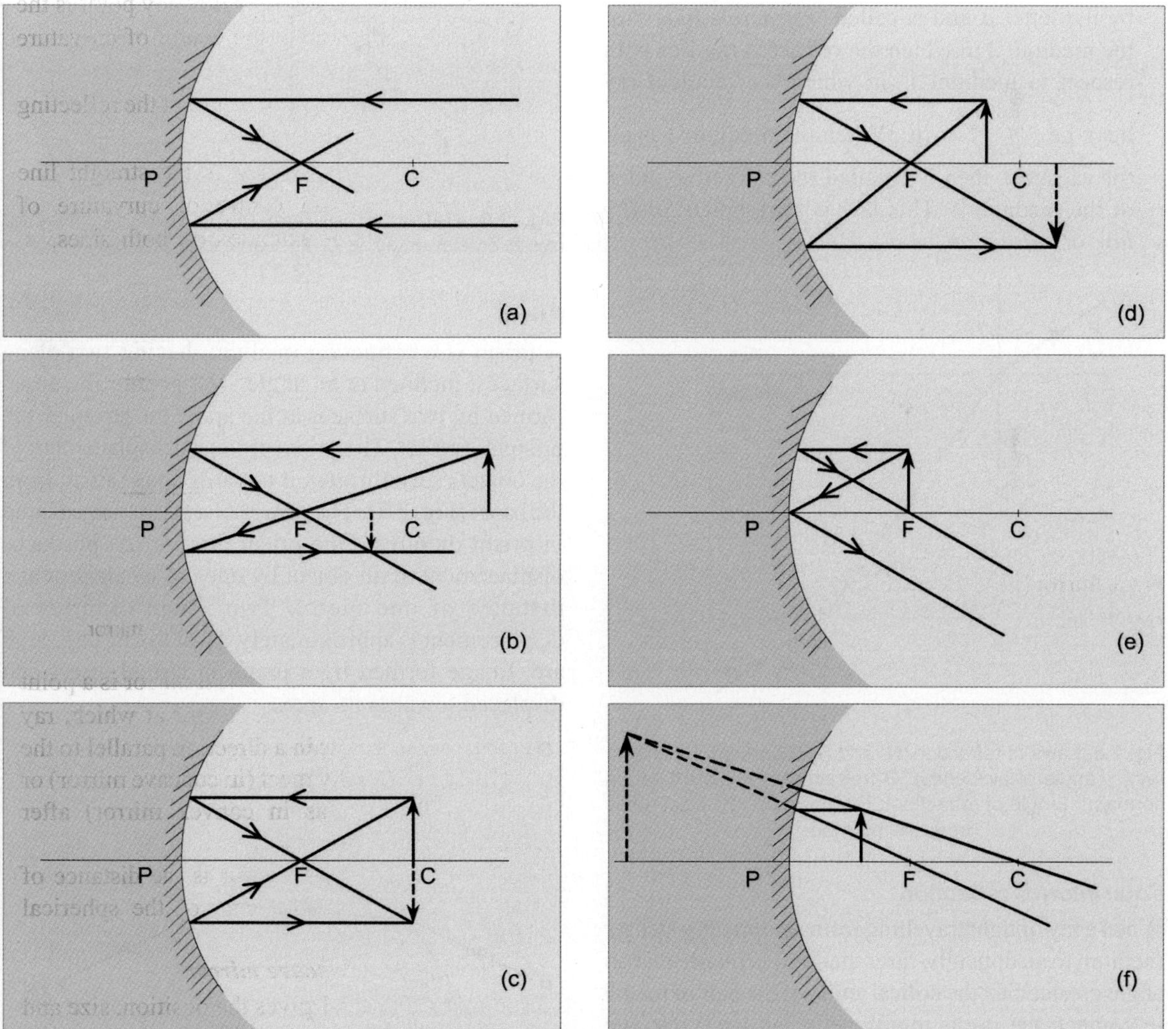

Fig. 3.4. Images formed by a concave mirror for different positions of the object : (a) at infinity; (b) between infinity and C; (c) at C; (d) between C and F; (e) at F; (f) between F and P.

Refraction of light

Refraction of light is the phenomenon of change in the path of light, when it goes from one medium to another. The basic cause of refraction is change in the velocity of light in going from one medium to the other.

Laws of refraction are (Fig. 3.5):

1. The incident (i) and refracted (r) rays are on opposite sides of the normal (N) and all the three are in the same plane.
2. The ratio of sine of angle of incidence (i) to the sine of angle of refraction (r) is constant for the part of media in contact. This constant is denoted by the letter μ and is called '*refractive index*' of the medium 2 in which the refracted ray lies with respect to medium 1 (in which the incident ray lies), i.e., $\frac{\sin i}{\sin r} = {}^1\mu_2$. When the medium 1 is air (or vaccum), then n is called the refractive index of the medium 2. This law is also called *Snell's law of refraction.*

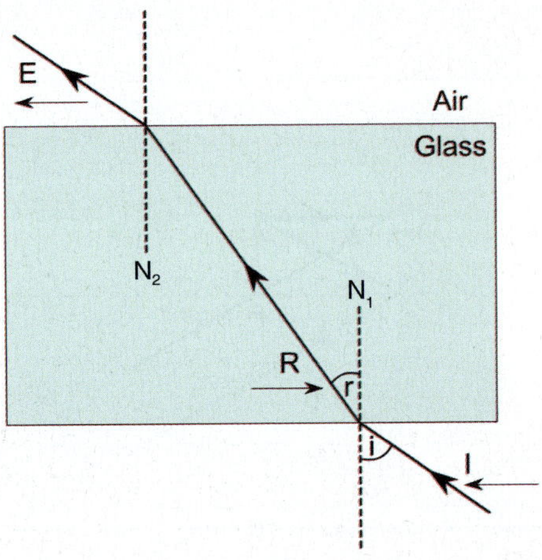

Fig. 3.5. Laws of refraction. N_1 and N_2 (normals); I (incident ray); i (angle of incidence); R (refracted ray, bent towards normal); r (angle of refraction); E (emergent ray, bent away from the normal).

Total internal reflection

When a ray of light travelling from an optically-denser medium to an optically-rarer medium is incident at an angle greater than the critical angle of the pair of media in contact, the ray is totally reflected back into the denser medium (Fig. 3.6). This phenomenon is called *total internal reflection.*

Critical angle refers to the angle of incidence in the denser medium, corresponding to which angle of refraction in the rare medium is 90°. It is represented by C and its value depends on the nature of media in contact.

The principle of total internal reflection is utilized in many optical equipments; such as fibroptic lights, applanation tonometer, and gonioscope.

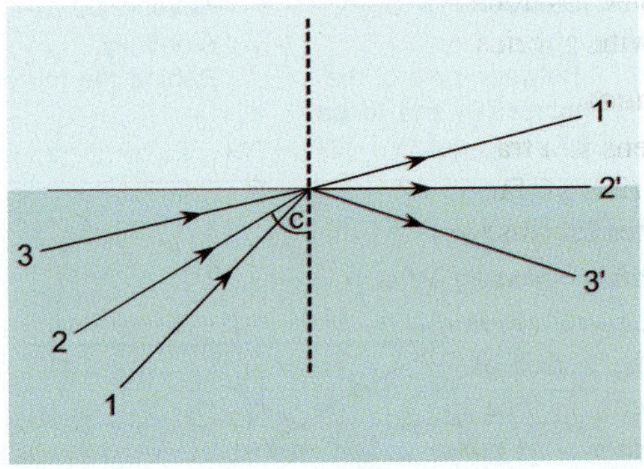

Fig. 3.6. Refraction of light (1-1'); path of refracted ray at critical angle, c (2-2'); and total internal reflection (3-3').

Prism

A prism is a refracting medium, having two plane surfaces, inclined at an angle. The greater the angle formed by two surfaces at the apex, the stronger the prismatic effect. The prism produces displacement of the objects seen through it towards apex (away from the base) (Fig. 3.7). The power of a prism is measured in prism dioptres. One prism dioptre (Δ) produces displacement of an object by one cm when kept at a distance of one metre. Two prism dioptres of displacement is approximately equal to one degree of arc. Image formed by a prism is virtual, erect and displaced towards its apex.

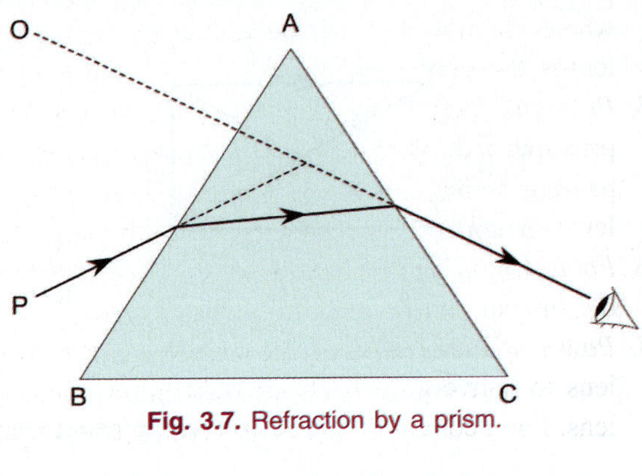

Fig. 3.7. Refraction by a prism.

Uses. In ophthalmology, prisms are used for :

1. Objective measurement of angle of deviation (Prism bar cover test, Krimsky test).
2. Measurement of fusional reserve and diagnosis of microtropia.
3. Prisms are also used in many ophthalmic equipments such as gonioscope, keratometer, applanation tonometer.
4. Therapeutically, prisms are prescribed in patients with phorias and diplopia.

Lenses

A lens is a transparent refracting medium, bounded by *two* surfaces which form a part of a sphere (spherical lens) or a cylinder (cylindrical or toric lens).

Cardinal data of a lens (Fig. 3.8)

1. *Centre of curvature* (C) of the spherical lens is the centre of the sphere of which the refracting lens surface is a part.
2. *Radius of curvature* of the spherical lens is the radius of the sphere of which the refracting surface is a part.

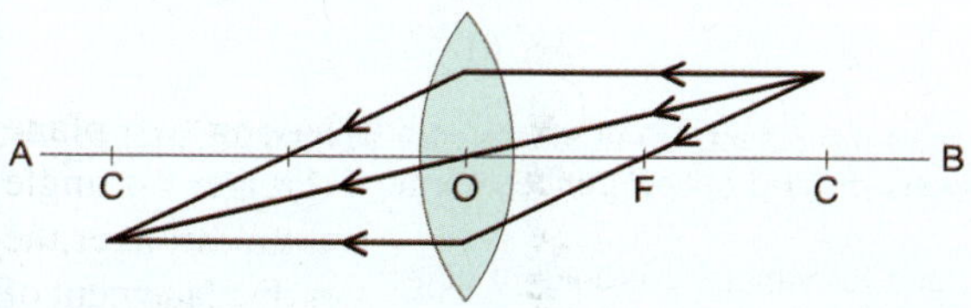

Fig. 3.8. Cardinal points of a convex lens: optical centre (O); principal focus (F); centre of curvature (C); and principal axis (AB).

3. *Principal axis* (AB) of the lens is the line joining the centres of curvatures of its surfaces.
4. *Optical centre* (O) of the lens corresponds to the nodal point of a thick lens. It is a point on the principal axis in the lens, the rays passing from where do not undergo deviation. In meniscus lenses the optical centre lies outside the lens.
5. *Principal focus* (F) of a lens is that point on the principal axis where parallel rays of light, after passing through the lens, converge (in convex lens) or appear to diverge (in concave lens).
6. *Focal length* (*f*) of a lens is the distance between the optical centre and the principal focus.
7. *Power of a lens* (P) is defined as the ability of the lens to converge a beam of light falling on the lens. For a converging (convex) lens the power is taken as positive and for a diverging (concave) lens power is taken as negative. It is measured as reciprocal of the focal length in metres i.e. P = 1/f. The unit of power is dioptre (D). One dioptre is the power of a lens of focal length one metre.

Types of lenses

Lenses are of two types: the spherical and cylindrical (toric or astigmatic).

1. ***Spherical lenses.*** Spherical lenses are bounded by two spherical surfaces and are mainly of two types : convex and concave.

(i) ***Convex lens*** or plus lens is a converging lens. It may be of biconvex, plano-convex or concavo-convex (meniscus) type (Fig. 3.9).

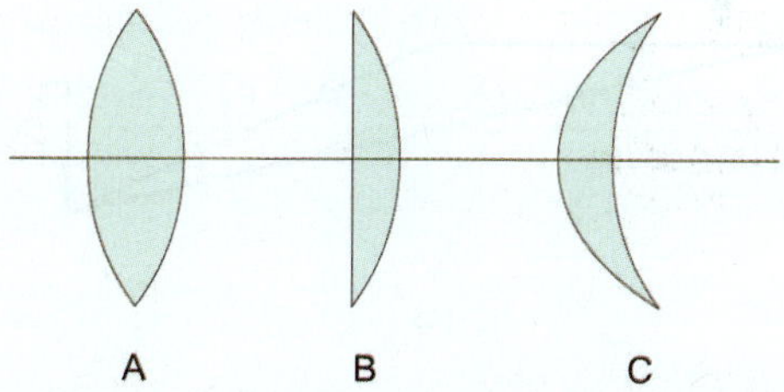

Fig. 3.9. Basic forms of a convex lens: (A) biconvex; (B) plano-convex; (C) concavo-convex.

Identification of a convex lens. (i) The convex lens is thick in the centre and thin at the periphery (ii) An object held close to the lens, appears magnified. (iii) When a convex lens is moved, the object seen through it moves in the opposite direction to the lens.

Uses of convex lens. It is used (i) for correction of hypermetropia, aphakia and presbyopia; (ii) in oblique illumination (loupe and lens) examination, in indirect ophthalmoscopy, as a magnifying lens and in many other equipments.

Image formation by a convex lens. Table 3.2 and Fig. 3.10 provide details about the position, size and the nature of the image formed by a convex lens.

(ii) ***Concave lens*** or minus lens is a diverging lens. It is of three types: biconcave, plano-concave and convexo-concave (meniscus) (Fig. 3.11).

Identification of concave lens. (i) It is thin at the centre and thick at the periphery. (ii) An object seen through it appears minified. (iii) When the lens is moved, the object seen through it moves in the same direction as the lens.

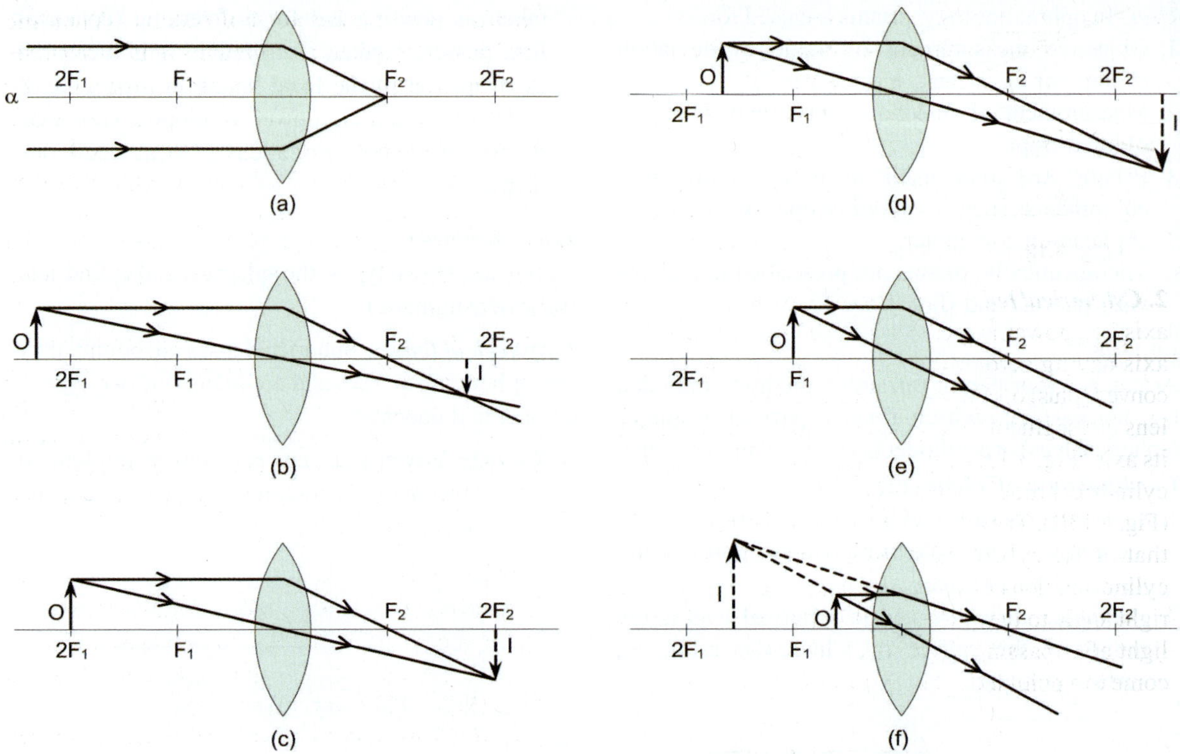

Fig. 3.10. Images formed by a convex lens for different positions of the object, (a) at infinity ; (b) beyond $2F_1$; (c) at $2F_1$; (d) between F_1 and $2F_1$; (e) at F_1; (f) between F_1 and optical centre of lens.

Table 3.2. Images formed by a convex lens for various positions of object

No.	*Position of the object*	*Position of the image*	*Nature and size of the image*	*Ray diagram*
1.	At infinity	At focus (F_2)	Real, very small and inverted	Fig. 3.10 (a)
2.	Beyond $2F_1$	Between F_2 and $2F_2$	Real, diminished and inverted	Fig. 3.10 (b)
3.	At $2F_1$	At $2F_2$	Real, same size and inverted	Fig. 3.10 (c)
4.	Between F_1 and $2F_1$	Beyond $2F_2$	Real, enlarged and inverted	Fig. 3.10 (d)
5.	At focus F_1	At infinity	Real, very large and inverted	Fig. 3.10 (e)
6.	Between F_1 and the optical centre of the lens	On the same side of lens	Virtual, enlarged and erect	Fig. 3.10 (f)

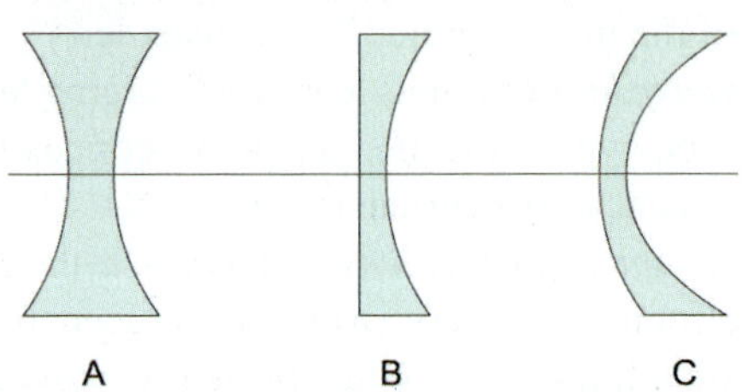

Fig. 3.11. Basic forms of a concave lens: biconcave (A); plano-concave (B); and convexo-concave (C).

Uses of concave lens. It is used (i) for correction of myopia; (ii) as Hruby lens for fundus examination with slit-lamp.

Image formation by a concave lens. A concave lens always produces a virtual, erect image of an object (Fig. 3.12).

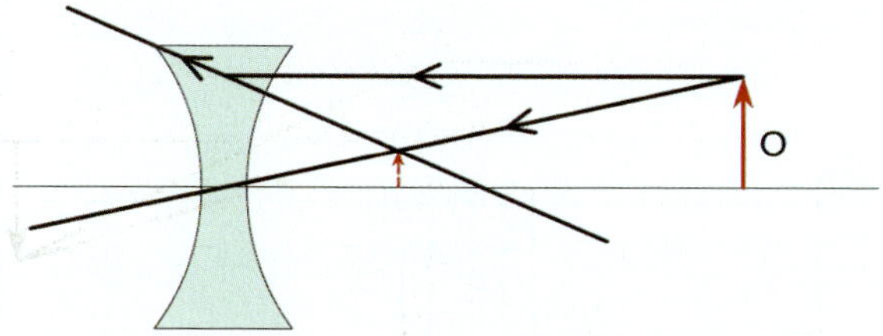

Fig. 3.12. Image formation by a concave lens.

2. *Cylindrical lens.* A cylindrical lens acts only in one axis i.e., power is incorporated in one axis, the other axis having zero power. A cylindrical lens may be convex (plus) or concave (minus). A convex cylindrical lens is a segment of a cylinder of glass cut parallel to its axis (Fig. 3.13A). Whereas a lens cast in a convex cylindrical mould is called concave cylindrical lens (Fig. 3.13B). The axis of a cylindrical lens is parallel to that of the cylinder of which it is a segment. The cylindrical lens has a power only in the direction at right angle to the axis. Therefore, the parallel rays of light after passing through a cylindrical lens do not come to a point focus but form a focal line (Fig. 3.14).

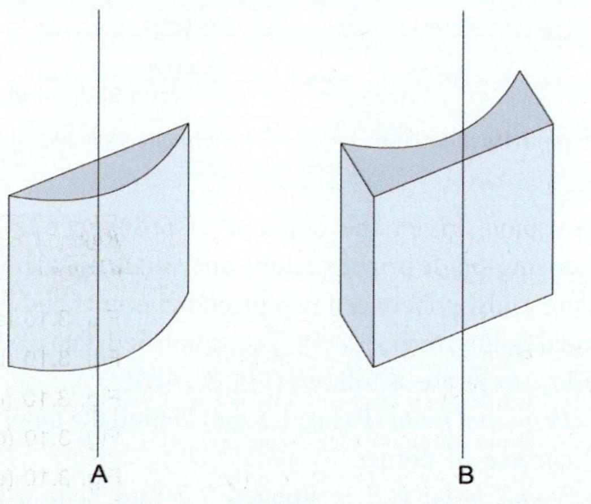

Fig. 3.13. Cylindrical lenses: convex (A) and concave (B).

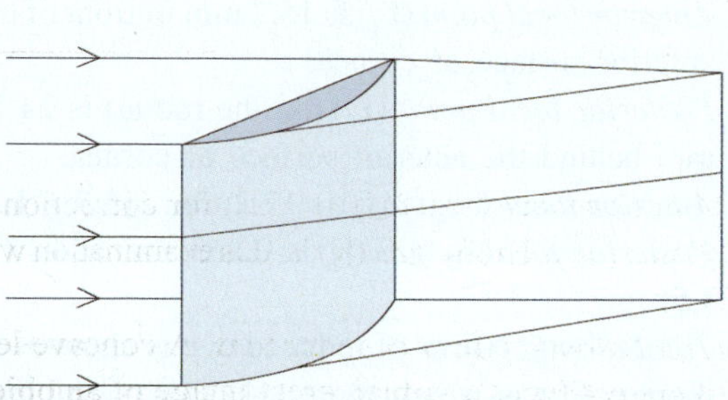

Fig. 3.14. Refraction through a convex cylindrical lens.

Identification of a cylindrical lens. (i) When the cylindrical lens is rotated around its optical axis, the object seen through it becomes distorted. (ii) The cylindrical lens acts in only one axis, so when it is moved up and down or sideways, the objects will move with the lens (in concave cylinder) or opposite to the lens (in convex cylinder) only in one direction.

Uses of cylindrical lenses. (i) Prescribed to correct astigmatism (ii) As a cross cylinder used to check the refraction subjectively.

Images formed by cylindrical lenses. Cylindrical or astigmatic lens may be simple (curved in one meridian only, either convex or concave), compound (curved unequally in both the meridians, either convex or concave). The compound cylindrical lens is also called *sphericylinder.* In mixed cylinder one meridian is convex and the other is concave.

Sturm's conoid

The configuration of rays refracted through a toric surface is called the Sturm's conoid. The shape of bundle of the light rays at different levels in Sturm's conoid (Fig. 3.15) is as follows:

- *At point A*, the vertical rays (V) are converging more than the horizontal rays (H); so the section here is a horizontal oval or an oblate ellipse.
- *At point B*, (first focus) the vertical rays have come to a focus while the horizontal rays are still converging and so they form a horizontal line.
- *At point C*, the vertical rays are diverging and their divergence is less than the convergence of the horizontal rays; so a horizontal oval is formed here.

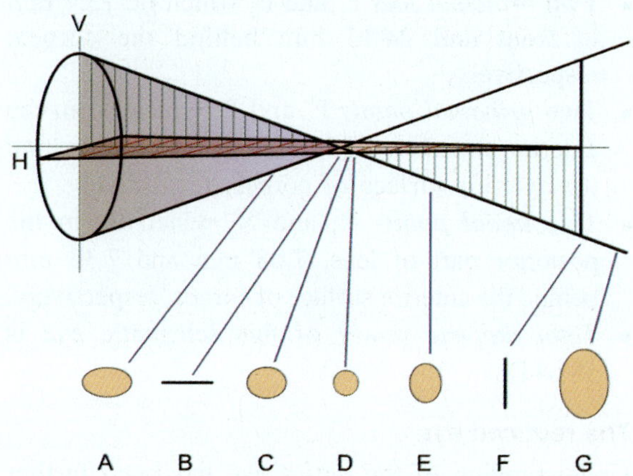

Fig. 3.15. Sturm's conoid.

- *At point D*, the divergence of vertical rays is exactly equal to the convergence of the horizontal rays from the axis. So here the section is a circle, which is called the *circle of least diffusion.*
- *At point E*, the divergence of vertical rays is more than the convergence of horizontal rays; so the section here is a vertical oval.
- *At point F*, (second focus), the horizontal rays have come to a focus while the vertical rays are divergent and so a vertical line is formed here.
- *Beyond F*, (as at point G) both horizontal and vertical rays are diverging and so the section will always be a vertical oval or prolate ellipse.
- The distance between the two foci (B and F) is called the *focal interval of Sturm.*

OPTICS OF THE EYE

As an optical instrument, the eye is well compared to a camera with retina acting as a unique kind of 'film'. Focusing system of the eye is composed of several refracting structures which (with their refractive indices given in parentheses) include cornea (1.37), aqueous humour (1.33), crystalline lens (1.42), and vitreous humour (1.33). These constitute a homocentric system of lenses, which when combined in action form a very strong refracting system of a short focal length.

Schematic eye: Cardinal points

The complex optics of eye, forming a homocentric lens system, has been simplified by Gullstrand by resolving it into six cardinal points (schematic eye) as follows (Fig. 3.16A):

- Two *principal foci* F_1 and F_2 which lie 15.7 mm in front and 24.13 mm behind the cornea, respectively.
- Two *principal points* P_1 and P_2 which lie in the anterior chamber, 1.35 mm and 1.60 mm behind the anterior surface of cornea, respectively.
- Two *nodal points* N_1 and N_2 which lie in the posterior part of lens, 7.08 mm and 7.33 mm behind the anterior surface of cornea, respectively.
- *Total dioptric power* of this schematic eye is 58.64 D.

The reduced eye

Understanding of the optics eye has been further simplified by Listing and Donder. From schematic eye, they have given the concept of reduced eye by choosing single principal point and single nodal point lying midway between two principal points and two nodal points, respectively. The simplified data of this reduced eye are as follows (Fig. 3.16B):

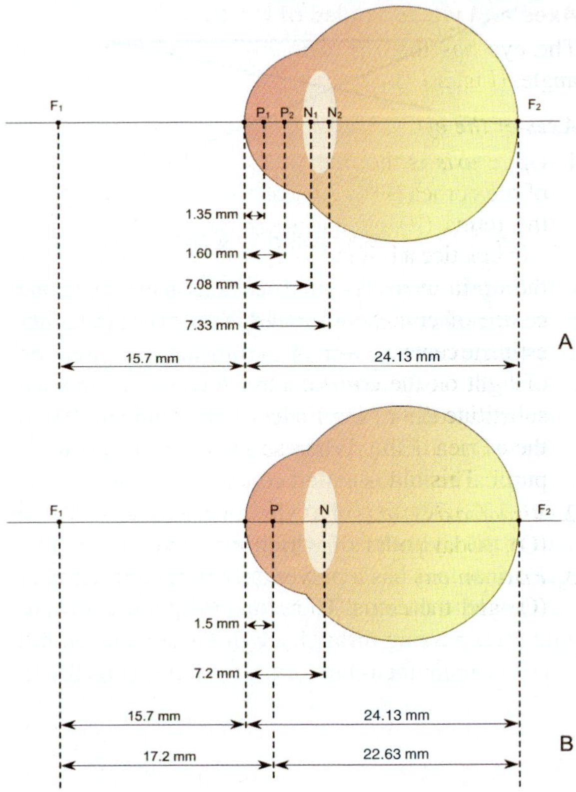

Fig. 3.16. Cardinal points of schematic eye (A); and reduced eye (B).

- *Principal point* (P) lies 1.5 mm behind the anterior surface of cornea.
- *Nodal point* (N) is situated 7.2 mm behind the anterior surface of cornea.
- *Anterior focal point* (F_1) is 15.7 mm in front of the anterior surface of cornea.
- *Posterior focal point* (F_2) (on the retina) is 24.13 mm behind the anterior surface of cornea.
- *Anterior focal length* (f_1) is 17.2 mm (15.7 + 1.5)
- *Posterior focal length* (f_2) is 22.63 mm (24.13 – 1.5).
- *Total dioptic power* of reduced eye is about + 60 dioptre. Out of which about + 43 D is contributed by the cornea and + 17 D by the crystalline lens.

Axes and visual angles of the eye

The eye has three principal axes and three visual angles (Fig. 3.17).

Axes of the eye

1. *Optic axis* is the line passing through the centre of the cornea (P), centre of the lens (N) and meets the retina (R) on the nasal side of the fovea.

   In practice it is impossible to determine accurately the optic axis, since we cannot know the exact centre of cornea. However, it is much easier to estimate center of the pupil, for example by an image of light on the cornea. Therefore, in practice we substitute the optic axis by a line perpendicular to the cornea at the point coinciding to the center of pupil. This line is called *pupillary line*.
2. *Visual axis* is the line joining the fixation point (O), nodal point (N), and the fovea (F).
3. *Fixation axis* is the line joining the fixation point (O) and the centre of rotation (C).

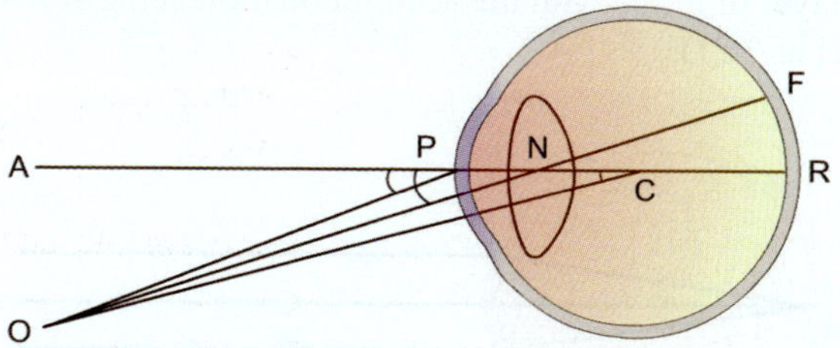

Fig. 3.17. Axis of the eye: optic axis (AR); visual axis (OF); fixation axis (OC) and visual angles : angle alpha (ONA, between optical axis and visual axis at nodal point N); angle kappa (OPA, between optical axis and pupillary line – OP); angle gamma (OCA, between optical axis and fixation axis).

Visual angles (Fig. 3.17)

1. *Angle alpha.* It is the angle (ONA) formed between the optic axis (AR) and visual axis (OF) at the nodal point (N).
2. *Angle gamma.* It is the angle (OCA) between the optic axis (AR) and fixation axis (OC) at the centre of rotation of the eyeball (C).
3. *Angle kappa.* It is the angle (OPA) formed between the visual axis (OF) and pupillary line (AP). The point P on the centre of cornea is considered equivalent to the centre of pupil.

Practically only the angle kappa can be measured and is of clinical significance. A positive angle kappa results in pseudo-exotropia and a negative angle kappa in pseudo-esotropia.

Optical aberrations of the normal eye

The eye, in common with many optical systems in practical use, is by no means optically perfect; the lapses from perfection are called *aberrations*. Fortunately, the eyes possess those defects to so small a degree that, for functional purposes, their presence is immaterial.

Natural mechanisms to decrease abberations in the human eye include:

- Cutting off of the peripheral rays by iris,
- High refractive index of the core of nucleus of the lens than that of the peripheral cortex.
- Low sensitivity of the peripheral retina, and
- Stiles Crawford effect i.e. more sensitivity of the retina to perpendicular rays than the oblique rays.

It has been said that despite imperfections the overall performance of the eye is little short of astonishing. Physiological optical defects in a normal eye include the following :

1. *Diffraction of light.* Diffraction refers to the bending of light rays caused by the edge of an aperture or the rim of a lens. The actual pattern of a diffracted image point produced by a lens with a circular aperture or pupil is a series of concentric bright and dark rings with a bright spot in the centre. Such a pattern is termed as the *Airy disc*. (Fig. 3.18)

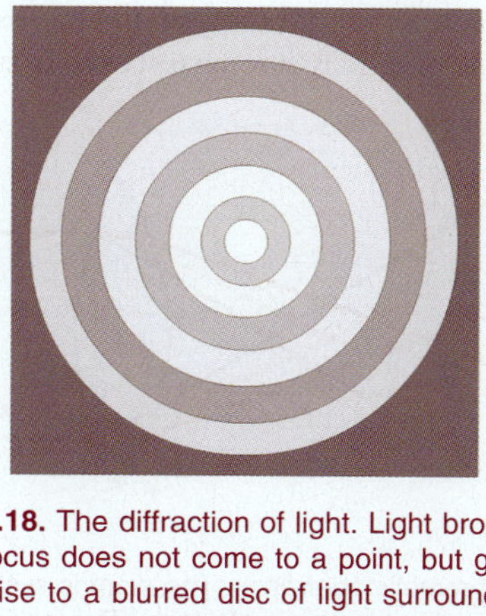

Fig. 3.18. The diffraction of light. Light brought to a focus does not come to a point, but gives rise to a blurred disc of light surrounded by several dark and light bands (the 'Airy disc').

2. *Spherical aberrations.* Spherical aberrations occur owing to the fact that spherical lens refracts peripheral rays more strongly than paraxial rays which in the case of a convex lens brings the more peripheral rays to focus closer to the lens (Fig. 3.19).

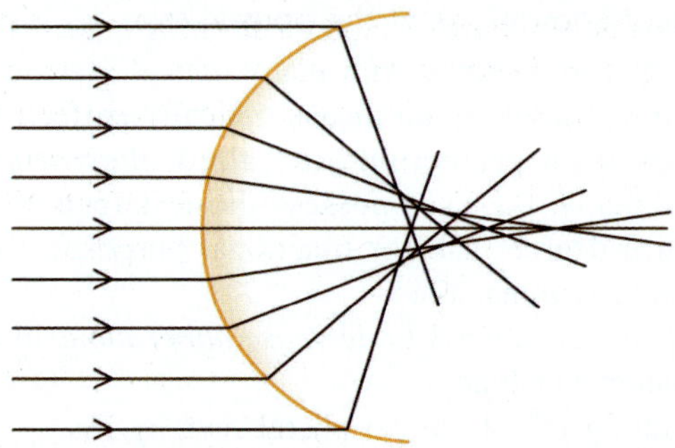

Fig. 3.19. Spherical aberration. Because there is greater refraction at periphery of spherical lens than near centre, incoming rays of light do not truly come to a point focus.

The human eye, having a power of about +60 D, was long thought to suffer from various amounts of spherical aberrations. However, results from aberroscopy have revealed the fact that the dominant aberration of human eye is not spherical aberration but rather a coma-like aberration.

3. ***Chromatic aberrations.*** Chromatic aberrations result owing to the fact that the index of refraction of any transparent medium varies with the wavelength of incident light. In human eye, which optically acts as a convex lens, blue light is focussed slightly in front of the red (Fig. 3.20). In other words, the emmetropic eye is in fact slightly hypermetropic for red rays and myopic for blue and green rays. This in fact forms the basis of bichrome test used in subjective refraction.

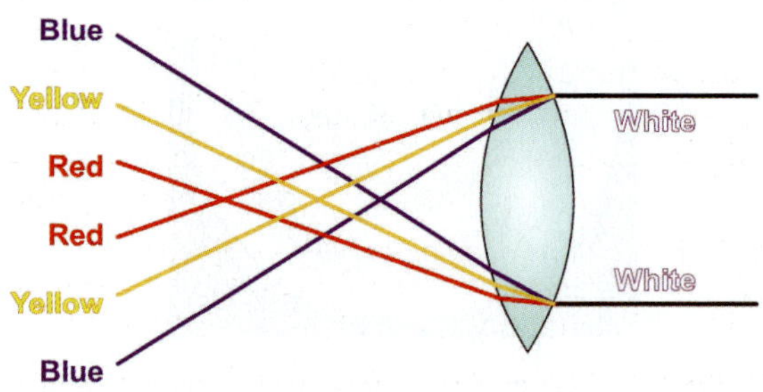

Fig. 3.20. Chromatic aberration. The dioptric system of the eye is represented by a simple lens. The yellow light is focussed on the retina, and the eye is myopic for blue, and hypermetropic for red.

4. ***Decentring.*** The cornea and lens surfaces alter the direction of incident light rays causing them to focus on the retina. Actually these surfaces are not centred on a common axis. The crystalline lens is usually slightly decentred and tipped with respect to the axis of the cornea and the visual axis of the eye. It has been reported that the centre of curvature of cornea is situated about 0.25 mm below the axis of the lens. However, the effects of deviation are usually so small that they are functionally neglected.

5. ***Oblique aberration.*** Objects in the peripheral field are seen by virtue of obliquely incident narrow pencil of rays which are limited by the pupil. Because of this, the refracted pencil shows oblique astigmatism.

6. ***Coma.*** Different areas of the lens will form foci in planes other than the chief focus. This produces in the image plane a 'coma effect' from a point source of light.

ERRORS OF REFRACTION

Emmetropia (optically normal eye) can be defined as a state of refraction, where in the parallel rays of light coming from infinity are focused at the sensitive layer of retina with the accommodation being at rest (Fig. 3.21).

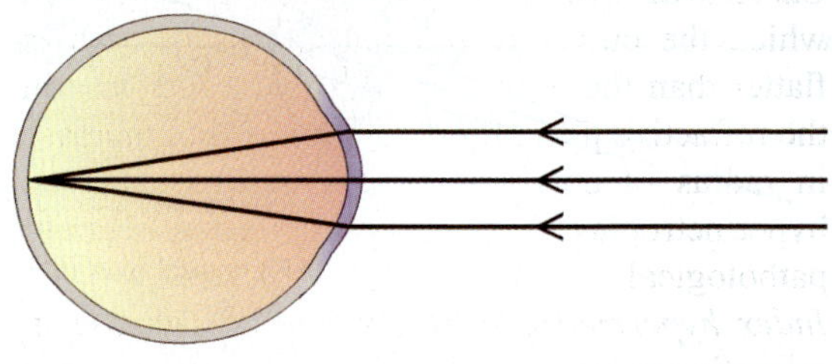

Fig. 3.21. Refraction in an emmetropic eye.

Ametropia (a condition of refractive error), is defined as a state of refraction, when the parallel rays of light coming from infinity (with accommodation at rest), are focused either in front or behind the sensitive layer of retina, in one or both the meridians. The ametropia includes *myopia, hypermetropia* and *astigmatism.* The related conditions aphakia and pseudophakia are also discussed here.

HYPERMETROPIA

Hypermetropia (hyperopia) or long-sightedness is the refractive state of the eye wherein parallel rays of light coming from infinity are focused behind the retina with accommodation being at rest (Fig. 3.22). Thus, the posterior focal point is behind the retina, which, therefore, receives a blurred image.

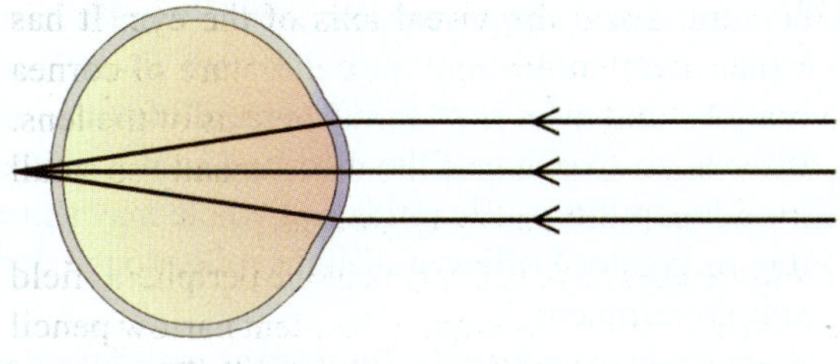

Fig. 3.22. Refraction in a hypermetropic eye.

Etiology

Hypermetropia may be axial, curvatural, index, positional and due to absence of crystalline lens.

1. *Axial hypermetropia* is by far the commonest form. In this condition the total refractive power of eye is normal but there is an axial shortening of eyeball. About 1mm shortening of the antero-posterior diameter of the eye results in 3 dioptres of hypermetropia. Axial hypermetropia may be developmental or pathological. High hypermetropia occurs in microopthalmos and nanophthalmos due to markedly short axial length (usually less than 20 mm).
2. *Curvatural hypermetropia* is the condition in which the curvature of cornea, lens or both is flatter than the normal resulting in a decrease in the refractive power of eye. About 1 mm increase in radius of curvature results in 6 dioptres of hypermetropia. It may be developmental or rarely pathological.
3. *Index hypermetropia* occurs due to decrease in refractive index of the lens in old age. It may also occur in diabetics under treatment.
4. *Positional hypermetropia* results from posteriorly placed crystalline lens.
5. *Absence of crystalline lens* either congenitally or acquired (following surgical removal or posterior dislocation) leads to aphakia — a condition of high hypermetropia.

Clinical types

There are three clinical types of hypermetropia:

1. *Simple or developmental hypermetropia* is the commonest form. It results from normal biological variations in the development of eyeball. It includes:

- Developmental, axial hypermetropia, and
- Developmental curvatural hypermetropia.

2. *Pathological hypermetropia* results due to either congenital or acquired conditions of the eyeball which are outside the normal biological variations of the development. It includes:

- *Index hypermetropia* due to acquired cortical sclerosis,
- *Positional hypermetropia* due to posterior subluxation of lens,
- *Aphakia* i.e., congenital or acquired, absence of lens,
- *Consecutive hypermetropia* due to surgically over-corrected myopia.
- *Pathological axial hypermetropia* due to forward displacement of the retina as seen in retinal detachment, central serous retinopathy and orbital tumours.
- *Pathological curvatural hypermetropia* may occur due to post traumatic or post inflammatory corneal flattening.
- *Pseudophakic hypermetropia* occurs due to implantation of an underpowered intraocular lens.

3. *Functional hypermetropia* results from paralysis of accommodation as seen in patients with third nerve paralysis and internal ophthalmoplegia.

Components of hypermetropia (effect of accommodation)

Nomenclature for various components of the hypermetropia vis-a-vis accommodation is as follows:

Total hypermetropia is the total amount of refractive error, which is estimated after complete cycloplegia with atropine. It consists of latent and manifest hypermetropia.

1. *Latent hypermetropia* implies the amount of hypermetropia (about 1D) which is normally corrected by the inherent tone of ciliary muscle. The degree of latent hypermetropia is high in children and gradually decreases with age. The latent hypermetropia is disclosed when refraction is carried after abolishing the tone with atropine.

2. *Manifest hypermetropia* is the remaining portion of total hypermetropia, which is not corrected by the ciliary tone. It consists of two components, the facultative and the absolute hypermetropia.

i. *Facultative hypermetropia* constitutes that part which can be corrected by the patient's accommodative effort.

ii. *Absolute hypermetropia* is the residual part of manifest hypermetropia which cannot be corrected by the patient's accommodative efforts.

Thus, briefly:

Total hypermetropia = latent + manifest (facultative + absolute).

Age and Hypermetropia

At birth, the eyeball is relatively short, having +2 to +3 hypermetropia. This is gradually reduced until by the age of 5-7 years, the eye is emmetropic and remains so till the age of about 50 years. After this, there is tendency to develop hypermetropia again, which gradually increases until at the extreme of life the eye has the same +2 to +3 with which it started. This senile hypermetropia is due to changes in the crystalline lens.

Clinical picture

Symptoms

In patients with hypermetropia, the symptoms vary depending upon the age of patient and the degree of refractive error. These can be grouped as under:

1. *Asymptomatic.* A small amount of refractive error in young patients is usually corrected by mild accommodative effort without producing any symptom.
2. *Asthenopic symptoms.* At times the hypermetropia is fully corrected by use of accommodation. Thus vision is normal, but due to sustained accommodative efforts patient develops asthenopic symptoms. These include: tiredness of eyes, frontal or fronto-temporal headache, watering and mild photophobia. These asthenopic symptoms are especially associated with near work and increase towards evening.
3. *Defective vision with asthenopic symptoms.* When the amount of hypermetropia is such that it is not fully corrected by the voluntary accommodative efforts, then the patients complain of defective vision which is more for near than distance and is associated with asthenopic symptoms due to sustained accommodative efforts.
4. *Defective vision only.* When the amount of hypermetropia is very high, the patients usually do not accommodate (especially adults) and there occurs marked defective vision for near and distance.

Signs

1. *Size of eyeball* may appear small as a whole.
2. *Cornea* may be slightly smaller than the normal.
3. *Anterior chamber* is comparatively shallow.
4. *Retinoscopy* and *autorefractometry* reveals hypermetropia.
5. *Fundus examination* reveals a small optic disc which may look more vascular with ill-defined margins and even may simulate papillitis (though there is no swelling of the disc, and so it is called pseudopapillitis). The retina as a whole may shine due to greater brilliance of light reflections (shot silk appearance).
6. *A-scan ultrasonography* (biometry) may reveal a short antero-posterior length of the eyeball in axial hypermetropia.

Grading of hypermetropia

American Optometric Association (AOA) has defined three grades of hypermetropia as below:

- *Low hypermetropia*, when the error is $\leq +2$D.
- *Moderate hypermetropia*, when the error is between +2 to + 5D.
- *High hypermetropia*, when the error is $\geq +5$D.

Complications

If hypermetropia is not corrected for a long time the following complications may occur:

1. *Recurrent styes, blepharitis or chalazia* may occur, probably due to infection introduced by repeated rubbing of the eyes, which is often done to get relief from fatigue and tiredness.
2. *Accommodative convergent squint* may develop in children (usually by the age of 2-3 years) due to excessive use of accommodation.
3. *Amblyopia* may develop in some cases. It may be anisometropic (in unilateral hypermetropia), strabismic (in children developing accommodative squint) or ametropic (seen in children with uncorrected bilateral high hypermetropia).
4. *Predisposition to develop primary narrow angle glaucoma.* The eye in hypermetropes is small with a comparatively shallow anterior chamber. Due to regular increase in the size of the lens with increasing age, these eyes become prone to an attack of narrow angle glaucoma. This point should be kept in mind while instilling mydriatics in elderly hypermetropes.

Treatment

A. *Optical treatment.* Basic principle of treatment is to prescribe convex (plus) lenses, so that the light rays are brought to focus on the retina (Fig. 3.23).

Fundamental rules for prescribing glasses in hypermetropia include:

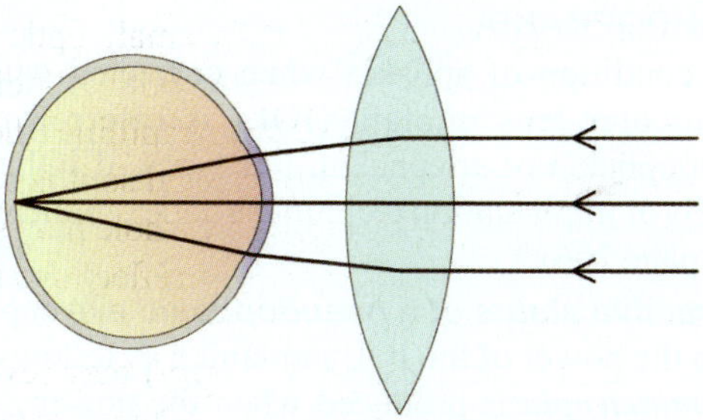

Fig. 3.23. Refraction in a hypermetropic eye corrected with convex lens

1. Total amount of hypermetropia should always be discovered by performing refraction under complete cycloplegia.
2. The spherical correction given should be comfortably acceptable to the patient. However, the astigmatism should be fully corrected.
3. Gradually increase the spherical correction at 6 months interval till the patient accepts manifest hypermetropia.
4. In the presence of accommodative convergent squint, full cycloplegic correction should be given at the first sitting.
5. If there is associated amblyopia, full correction with occlusion therapy should be started.

Modes of prescription of convex lenses

1. *Spectacles* are most comfortable, safe and easy method of correcting hypermetropia.
2. *Contact lenses* are indicated in unilateral hypermetropia (anisometropia). For cosmetic reasons, contact lenses should be prescribed once the prescription has stabilised, otherwise, they may have to be changed many a times.

B. *Surgical treatment* (See page 49).

APHAKIA

Aphakia literally means 'absence of crystalline lens' from the eye. However, from the optical point of view, it may be considered a condition in which the lens is absent from the pupillary area. Aphakia produces a high degree of hypermetropia.

Causes

1. *Congenital* absence of lens. It is a rare condition.
2. *Surgical aphakia* occurring after removal of lens is the commonest presentation.
3. *Aphakia due to absorption of lens matter* is noticed rarely after trauma in children.
4. *Traumatic extrusion* of lens from the eye also constitutes a rare cause of aphakia.
5. *Posterior dislocation* of lens in vitreous causes optical aphakia.

Optics of aphakic eye

Following optical changes occur after removal of crystalline lens:

1. Eye becomes highly hypermetropic.
2. Total power of eye is reduced to about +44 D from +60 D.
3. The anterior focal point becomes 23.2 mm in front of the cornea. (Normal: 15.7 mm)
4. The posterior focal point is about 31 mm behind the cornea i.e., about 7 mm behind the eyeball. (The antero-posterior length of eyeball is about 24 mm)
5. There occurs total loss of accommodation.

Clinical features

Symptoms.

1. *Defective vision.* Main symptom in aphakia is marked defective vision for both far and near due to high hypermetropia and absence of accommodation.
2. *Erythropsia and cyanopsia* i.e., seeing red and blue images. This occurs due to excessive entry of ultraviolet and infrared rays in the absence of crystalline lens.

Signs of aphakia include:

1. *Limbal scar* may be seen in surgical aphakia.
2. *Anterior chamber* is deeper than normal.
3. *Iridodonesis* i.e., tremulousness of iris can be demonstrated.
4. *Pupil* is jet black in colour.
5. *Purkinje's image test* shows only two images (normally four images are seen- see page 506 and Fig. 21.10).
6. *Fundus examination* shows hypermetropic small disc.
7. *Retinoscopy* and *autorefractometry* reveals high hypermetropia.

Treatment

Optical principle is to correct the error by convex lenses of appropriate power so that image is formed on the retina (Fig. 3.23).

Modalities for correcting aphakia include: (1) spectacles, (2) contact lens, (3) intraocular lens, and (4) refractive corneal surgery.

1. *Spectacles* prescription has been the most commonly employed method of correcting aphakia in the past, especially in developing countries. Presently, use of aphakic spectacles has decreased markedly. Roughly, about +10 D with cylindrical lenses for surgically induced astigmatism are required to correct aphakia in previously emmetropic patients. However, exact number of glasses will differ in individual case and should be estimated by refraction. An addition of +3 to +4 D is required for near vision to compensate the loss of accommodation.

Disadvantages of spectacles. (i) Image is magnified by 30 percent, so not useful in unilateral aphakia (produce diplopia). (ii) Problem of spherical and chromatic aberrations of thick lenses. (iii) Field of vision is limited. (iv) Prismatic effect of thick glasses. (v) 'Roving ring Scotoma' (Jack in the box phenomenon). (vi) Cosmetic blemish especially in young aphakes.

2. *Contact lenses*. Advantages of contact lenses over spectacles include: (i) Less magnification of image. (ii) Elimination of aberrations and prismatic effect of thick glasses. (iii) Wider and better field of vision. (iv) Cosmetically more acceptable. (v) Better suited for uniocular aphakia.

Disadvantages of contact lenses are: (i) more cost; (ii) cumbersome to wear, especially in old age and in childhood; and (iii) corneal complications may be associated.

3. *Intraocular lens implantation* is the best available method of correcting aphakia. Therefore, it is the commonest modality being employed now-a-days.

- *Primary intraocular lens implantation* is done during cataract surgery.
- *Secondary intraocular lens implantation* is done in already aphakic patients.

(For detail see page 206).

4. *Refractive corneal surgery.* It includes:

- *Keratophakia and Epikeratophakia* have been tried without much success. In *keratophakia* a lenticule prepared from the donor cornea is placed between the lamellae of patient's cornea and in *epikeratophakia*, the lenticule prepared from the donor cornea is stitched over the surface of cornea after removing the epithelium.
- *Hyperopic Lasik* may be tried in cases where secondary IOL cannot be implanted (see page 49)

PSEUDOPHAKIA

The condition of aphakia when corrected with an intraocular lens implant (IOL) is referred to as pseudophakia or artephakia. For types of IOLs and details of implantation techniques and complications (see page 206).

Refractive status of a pseudophakic eye depends upon the power of the IOL implanted as follows:

1. *Emmetropia* is produced when the power of the IOL implanted is exact. It is the most ideal situation. Such patients need plus glasses for near vision only.

2. *Consecutive myopia* occurs when the IOL implanted overcorrects the refraction of eye. Such patients require glasses to correct the myopia for distance vision and may or may not need glasses for near vision depending upon the degree of myopia.

3. *Consecutive hypermetropia* develops when the under-power IOL is implanted. Such patients require plus glasses for distance vision and additional +2 to +3 D for near vision.

Note: Varying degree of surgically-induced astigmatism is also present in pseudophakia

Signs of pseudophakia (with posterior chamber IOL).

1. *Surgical scar* may be seen near the limbus.
2. *Anterior chamber* is slightly deeper than normal.
3. *Mild iridodonesis* (tremulousness) of iris may be demonstrated.
4. *Purkinje image test* shows four images.
5. *Pupil* is blackish in colour but when light is thrown in pupillary area shining reflexes are observed. When examined under magnification after dilating the pupil, the presence of IOL is confirmed (see Fig. 8.26).
6. *Visual status and refraction* will vary depending upon the power of IOL implanted as described above.

MYOPIA

Myopia or short-sightedness is a type of refractive error in which parallel rays of light coming from infinity are focused in front of the retina when accommodation is at rest (Fig. 3.24).

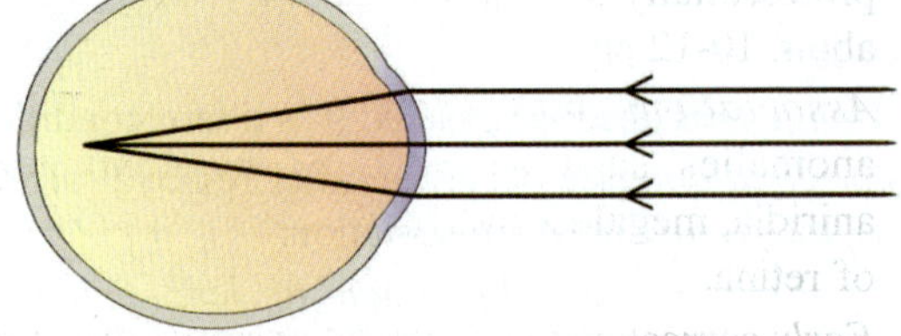

Fig. 3.24. Refraction in a myopic eye.

Etiological classification

1. *Axial myopia* results from increase in antero-posterior length of the eyeball. It is the commonest form.
2. *Curvatural myopia* occurs due to increased curvature of the cornea, lens or both.
3. *Positional myopia* is produced by anterior placement of crystalline lens in the eye.
4. *Index myopia* results from increase in the refractive index of crystalline lens associated with nuclear sclerosis.
5. *Myopia due to excessive accommodation* occurs in patients with spasm of accommodation.

Grading of myopia

American Optometric Association (AOA) has defined three grades of myopia:

- *Low myopia*, when the error is ≤ –3D.
- *Moderate myopia*, when the error is between –3D to –6D.
- *High myopia*, when the error is ≥ –6D.

Clinical varieties of myopia

1. Congenital myopia
2. Simple or developmental myopia
3. Pathological or degenerative myopia
4. Acquired myopia which may be: (i) post-traumatic; (ii) post-keratitic; (iii) drug-induced, (iv) pseudomyopia; (v) space myopia; (vii) night myopia; and (viii) consecutive myopia.

1. Congenital myopia

- *Present since birth*, the congenital myopia, is usually diagnosed by the age of 2-3 years.
- *Anisometropia* is usually present, hence most of the time the error is unilateral. Rarely, it may be bilateral.
- *High degree of error*, about 8 to 10D, is usually present, which mostly remains constant.
- *Convergent squint* may develop in order to preferentially see clear at its far point (which is about 10-12 cms).
- *Associations* may include other congenital anomalies such as cataract, microphthalmos, aniridia, megalocornea, and congenital separation of retina.
- *Early correction* of congenital myopia is desirable.

2. Simple myopia

Simple or developmental myopia is the commonest variety. It is considered as a physiological error not associated with any disease of the eye. Overall reported prevalence is 20-40% of population. Since the sharpest rise occurs at school going age i.e., between 8 year to 12 years so, it is also called *school myopia*.

Etiology. It results from normal biological variation in the development of eye which may or may not be genetically determined. Some factors associated with simple myopia are as follows:

- *Axial type of simple myopia* may signify just a physiological variation in the length of the eyeball or it may be associated with precocious neurological growth during childhood.
- *Curvatural type* of simple myopia is considered to be due to underdevelopment of the eyeball.
- *Role of diet* in early childhood has also been reported without any conclusive results.
- *Role of genetics.* Genetics plays some role in the biological variation of the development of eye, as prevalence of myopia is more in children with both parents myopic (20%) than the children with one parent myopic (10%) and children with no parent myopic (5%).
- *Theory of excessive near work in* childhood was also put forward, but did not gain much importance. In fact, there is no truth in the folklore that myopia is aggravated by close work, watching television and by not using glasses.

Clinical picture

Symptoms

- *Poor vision for distance* (short-sightedness) is the main symptom of myopia.
- *Asthenopic symptoms* may occur in patients with small degree of myopia.
- *Half shutting* of the eyes may be complained by parents of the child. The child does so to achieve the greater clarity of stenopaeic vision.

Signs

- *Prominent eyeballs.* The myopic eyes typically are large and somewhat prominent.
- *Anterior chamber* is slightly deeper than normal.

- *Pupils* are somewhat large and a bit sluggishly reacting.
- *Fundus* is normal; rarely temporal myopic crescent may be seen.
- *Magnitude of refractive error.* Simple myopia usually occurs between 5 and 10 years of age and it keeps on increasing till about 18-20 years of age at a rate of about –0.5 ± 0.30 every year. In simple myopia, usually the error is low to moderate i.e. does not exceed – 6 D.

Diagnosis is confirmed by performing refraction (page 579).

3. Pathological myopia

Pathological/degenerative/progressive myopia, as the name indicates, is a rapidly progressive error which starts in childhood at 5-10 years of age and results in high myopia (≥ –6 D) during early adult life which is usually associated with degenerative changes in the eye. It is much less common (about 2% of population)

Etiology. It is unequivocal that the pathological myopia results from a rapid axial growth of the eyeball which is outside the normal biological variations of development. To explain this spurt in axial growth various theories have been put forward. So far no satisfactory hypothesis has emerged to explain the etiology of pathological myopia. However, it is definitely linked with (i) heredity and (ii) general growth process.

1. *Role of heredity.* It is now confirmed that genetic factors play a major role in the etiology, as the progressive myopia is: (i) familial; (ii) more common in certain races like Chinese, Japanese, Arabs and Jews, and (iii) uncommon among Negroes, Nubians and Sudanese. It is presumed that heredity-linked growth of retina is the determinant in the development of myopia. The sclera due to its distensibility follows the retinal growth but the choroid undergoes degeneration due to stretching, which in turn causes degeneration of retina.

2. *Role of general growth process,* though minor, cannot be denied on the progress of myopia. Lengthening of the posterior segment of the globe commences only during the period of active growth and probably ends with the termination of the active growth. Therefore, the factors (such as nutritional deficiency, debilitating diseases, endocrinal disturbances and indifferent general health) which affect the general growth process will also influence the progress of myopia.

The etiological hypothesis for pathological myopia is summarised in Fig. 3.25:

Genetic factors (play major role) ↓   General growth process (plays minor role) ↙

More growth of retina

↓

Stretching of sclera

→ Increased axial length
→ Degeneration of choroid
→ Degeneration of retina
→ Degeneration of vitreous

} Features of pathological myopia

Fig. 3.25. Etiological hypothesis for pathological myopia.

Clinical picture

Symptoms

1. *Defective vision.* There is considerable failure in visual function as the error is usually high. Further, due to progressive degenerative changes, an uncorrectable loss of vision may occur.
2. *Muscae volitantes* i.e., floating black opacities in front of the eyes are also complained by many patients. These occur due to degenerated liquified vitreous.
3. *Night blindness* may be complained by very high myopes having marked degenerative changes.

Signs

1. *Prominent eye balls.* The eyes are often prominent, appearing elongated and even simulating an exophthalmos, especially in unilateral cases. The elongation of the eyeball mainly affects the posterior pole and surrounding area; the part of the eye anterior to the equator may be normal (Fig. 3.26).
2. *Cornea* is large.
3. *Anterior chamber* is deep.
4. *Pupils* are slightly large and react sluggishly to light.
5. *Fundus examination* reveals following characteristic signs :

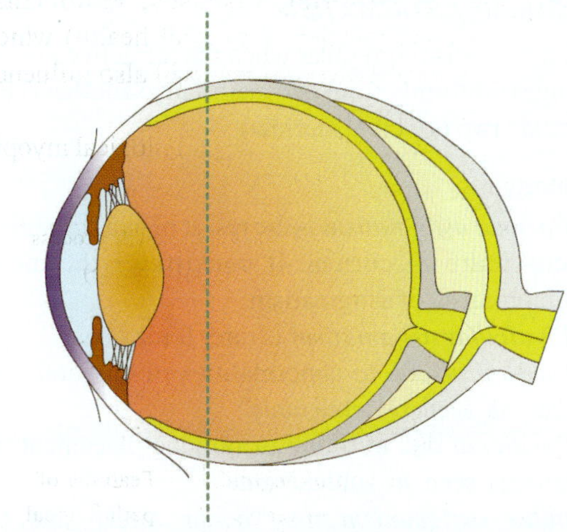

Fig. 3.26. Elongation of the eyeball posterior to equator in pathological myopia.

(a) *Optic disc* appears large and pale and at its temporal edge a characteristic myopic crescent is present (Fig. 3.27). Sometimes peripapillary crescent encircling the disc may be present, where the choroid and retina is distracted away from the disc margin. A super-traction crescent (where the retina is pulled over the disc margin) may be present on the nasal side.

(b) *Degenerative changes in retina and choroid* are common in progressive myopia (Fig. 3.28).

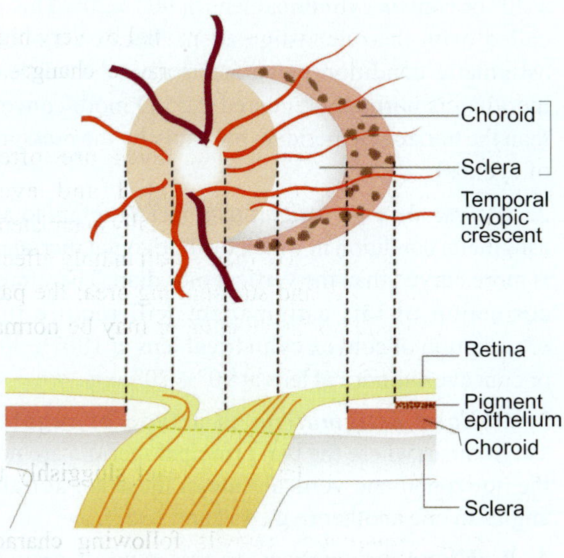

Fig. 3.27. Myopic crescent.

These are characterised by white atrophic patches at the macula with a little heaping up of pigment around them. *Foster-Fuchs'* spot (dark red circular patch due to sub-retinal neovascularization and choroidal haemorrhage) may be present at the macula. *Cystoid degeneration* may be seen at the periphery. In an advanced case there occurs total retinal atrophy, particularly in the central area.

(c) *Posterior staphyloma* due to ectasia of sclera at posterior pole may be apparent as an excavation with the vessels bending backward over its margins.

(d) *Degenerative changes in vitreous* include: liquefaction, vitreous opacities, and posterior vitreous detachment (PVD) appearing as Weiss' reflex.

6. *Visual fields* may show contraction and in some cases ring scotoma may be seen.
7. *ERG* may reveal subnormal electroretinogram due to chorioretinal atrophy.

Complications

(i) Retinal detachment; (ii) complicated cataract; (iii) vitreous haemorrhage; (iv) choroidal haemorrhage (v) Strabismus fixus convergence.

Treatment of myopia

1. *Optical treatment of myopia* constitutes prescription of appropriate concave lenses, so that clear image is formed on the retina (Fig. 3.29). The *basic rule of correcting myopia* is converse of that in hypermetropia, i.e., the minimum acceptance providing maximum vision should be

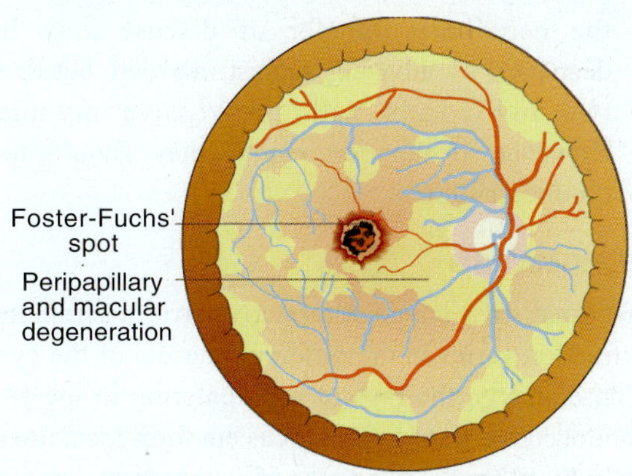

Fig. 3.28. Fundus changes in pathological myopia.

prescribed. In very high myopia undercorrection is always better to avoid the problem of near vision and that of minification of images.

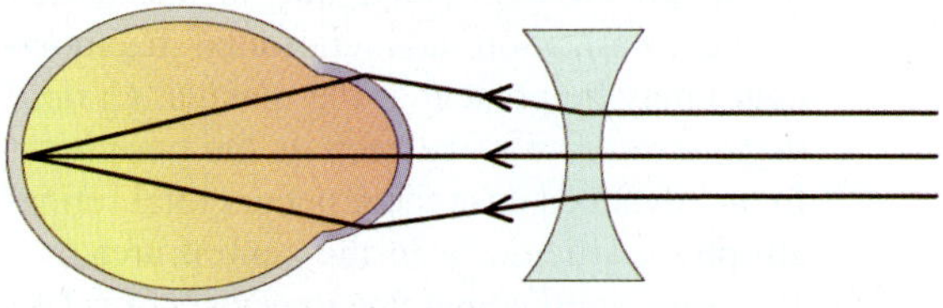

Fig. 3.29. Refraction in a myopic eye corrected with concave lens.

Modes of prescribing concave lenses are spectacles and contact lenses. Their advantages and disadvantages over each other are the same as described for hypermetropia. Contact lenses are particularly justified in cases of high myopia as they avoid peripheral distortion and minification produced by strong concave spectacle lens.

2. *Surgical treatment of myopia* is becoming very popular now-a-days. (For details see page 47).
3. *General measures* empirically believed to effect the progress of myopia (unproven usefulness) include balanced diet rich in vitamins and proteins and early management of associated debilitating disease.
4. *Low vision aids* (LVA) are indicated in patients of progressive myopia with advanced degenerative changes, where useful vision cannot be obtained with spectacles and contact lenses.
5. *Prophylaxis (genetic counselling)*. As the pathological myopia has a strong genetic basis, the hereditary transfer of disease may be decreased by advising against marriage between two individuals with progressive myopia. However, if they do marry, they should not produce children.

ASTIGMATISM

Astigmatism is a type of refractive error wherein the refraction varies in the different meridia of the eye. Consequently, the rays of light entering in the eye cannot converge to a point focus but form focal lines. Broadly, there are two types of astigmatism: regular and irregular.

REGULAR ASTIGMATISM

The astigmatism is regular when the refractive power changes uniformly from one meridian to another (i.e., there are two principal meridia).

Etiology

1. ***Corneal astigmatism*** is the result of abnormalities of curvature of cornea. It constitutes the most common cause of astigmatism.
2. ***Lenticular astigmatism*** is rare. It may be:
   - i. *Curvatural* due to abnormalities of curvature of lens as seen in lenticonus.
   - ii. *Positional* due to tilting or oblique placement of lens as seen in subluxation.
   - iii. *Index astigmatism* may occur rarely due to variable refractive index of lens in different meridia.
3. ***Retinal astigmatism*** due to oblique placement of macula may also be seen occasionally.

Types of regular astigmatism

Depending upon the axis and the angle between the two principal meridia, regular astigmatism can be classified into the following types :

1. ***With-the-rule astigmatism (WTR).*** In this type the two principal meridia are placed at right angles to one another but the vertical meridian is more curved than the horizontal. Thus, correction of this astigmatism will require the concave cylinder at 180° ± 20° or convex cylindrical lens at 90° ± 20°. This is called 'with-the-rule' astigmatism, because similar astigmatic condition exists normally (the vertical meridian is normally rendered 0.25 D more convex than the horizontal meridian probably by the pressure of eyelids).

2. ***Against-the-rule astigmatism (ATR)*** refers to an astigmatic condition in which the horizontal meridian is more curved than the vertical meridian. Therefore, correction of this astigmatism will require the prescription of convex cylindrical lens at 180° ± 20° or concave cylindrical lens at 90° ± 20° axis.

3. ***Oblique astigmatism*** is a type of regular astigmatism where the two principal meridia are not the horizontal and vertical though these are at right angles to one another (e.g., 45° and 135°).

4. ***Bioblique astigmatism.*** In this type of regular astigmatism the two principal meridia are not at right

angle to each other e.g., one may be at 30° and other at 100°.

Optics of regular astigmatism

As already mentioned, in regular astigmatism the parallel rays of light are not focused on a point but form two focal lines. The configuration of rays refracted through the astigmatic surface (toric surface) is called *Sturm's conoid* and the distance between the two focal lines is known as *focal interval* of Sturm. The shape of bundle of rays at different levels (after refraction through astigmatic surface) has been described earlier (see page 25, Fig. 3.15).

Refractive types of regular astigmatism

Depending upon the position of the two focal lines in relation to retina, the regular astigmatism is further classified into three types:

1. *Simple astigmatism,* wherein the rays are focused on the retina in one meridian and either in front (*simple myopic astigmatism* – Fig. 3.30A) or behind (*simple hypermetropic astigmatism* – Fig. 3.30B) the retina in the other meridian.

2. *Compound astigmatism.* In this type the rays of light in both the meridia are focused either in front or behind the retina and the condition is labelled as *compound myopic* or *compound hypermetropic astigmatism*, respectively (Figs. 3.30C and D).

3. *Mixed astigmatism* refers to a condition wherein the light rays in one meridian are focused in front and in other meridian behind the retina (Fig. 3.30E). Thus in one meridian eye is myopic and in another hypermetropic. Such patients have comparatively less symptoms as 'circle of least *diffusion*' is formed on the retina (see Fig. 3.15).

Symptoms

1. *Asthenopia* (tiredness of eyes relieved by closing the eyes) characterised by difficulty in focussing, transient blurred vision, dull ache in eyes frontal headache and sometimes nausea and even drowsiness is especially marked in low astigmatism ≤ 1D.
2. *Blurred vision and defective vision* is reported when the astigmatism is ≥ 1D.
3. *Elongation of objects* proportionate to the degree and type of astigmatism may be noticed in high astigmatism.

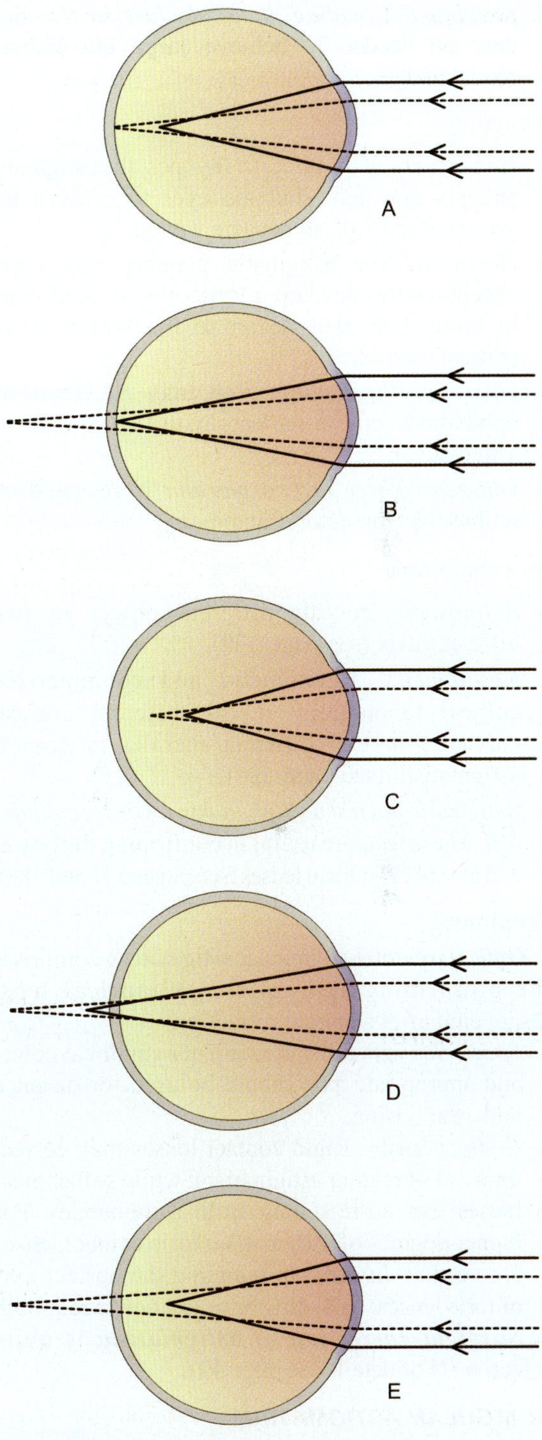

Fig. 3.30. Types of astigmatism : simple myopic (A); simple hypermetropic (B); compound myopic (C); compound hypermetropic (D); and mixed (E).

4. *Keeping the reading material close to the eyes* may be needed to achieve large but blurred retinal image.

Signs

1. *Half closure of the lid.* Like myopes, the astigmatic patients may half shut the eyes to achieve the greater clarity of stenopaeic vision.
2. *Head tilt.* The astigmatic patients may (very exceptionally) develop a torticollis in an attempt to bring their axes nearer to the horizontal or vertical meridians.
3. *Oval or tilted optic disc* may be seen on ophthalmoscopy in patients with high degree of astigmatism.
4. *Different power in two meridia* is revealed on retinoscopy or autorefractometry.

Investigations

1. *Retinoscopy* reveals different power in two different axis (see page 579).
2. *Keratometry.* Keratometry and computerized corneal topotograpy reveal different corneal curvature in two different meridia in corneal astigmatism (see page 586).
3. *Astigmatic fan test* and (4) *Jackson's cross cylinder test.* These tests are useful in confirming the power and axis of cylindrical lenses (see pages 587 and 588).

Treatment

1. *Optical treatment* of regular astigmatism comprises the prescribing appropriate cylindrical lens, discovered after accurate refraction.

i. *Spectacles* with full correction of cylindrical power and appropriate axis should be used for distance and near vision.
ii. *Contact lenses.* Rigid contact lenses may correct upto 2-3 of regular astigmatism, while soft contact lenses can correct only little astigmatism. For higher degrees of astigmatism toric contact lenses are needed. In order to maintain the correct axis of toric lenses, ballasting or truncation is required.

2. *Surgical correction of astigmatism* is quite effective. (For details see page 49).

IRREGULAR ASTIGMATISM

It is characterized by an irregular change of refractive power in different meridia. There are multiple meridia which admit no geometrical analysis.

Etiological types

1. *Curvatural irregular astigmatism* is found in patients with extensive corneal scars or keratoconus.
2. *Index irregular astigmatism* due to variable refractive index in different parts of the crystalline lens may occur rarely in patients with cataract.

Clinical picture

Symptoms of irregular astigmatism include:

- Defective vision,
- Distortion of objects and
- Polyopia (seeing multiple images).

Signs depicted on investigations are as below:

1. *Retinoscopy* reveals irregular pupillary reflex
2. *Slitlamp examination* may reveal corneal irregularity or *Keratoconus.*
3. *Placido's disc test* reveals distorted circles (see page 501).
4. *Photokeratoscopy and computerized corneal topography* give photographic record of irregular corneal curvature.

Treatment

1. *Optical treatment* of irregular astigmatism consists of contact lens which replaces the anterior surface of the cornea for refraction.
2. *Phototherapeutic keratectomy* (PTK) performed with excimer laser may be helpful in patients with superficial corneal scar responsible for irregular astigmatism.
3. *Surgical treatment* is indicated in extensive corneal scarring (when vision does not improve with contact lenses) and consists of penetrating keratoplasty.

ANISOMETROPIA

The optical state with equal refraction in the two eyes is termed *isometropia.* When the total refraction of the two eyes is unequal the condition is called *anisometropia.* Small degree of anisometropia is of no concern. A difference of 1 D in two eyes causes a 2 percent difference in the size of the two retinal images. A difference up to 5 percent in retinal images of two eyes is well tolerated. In other words, an anisometropia up to 2.5 is well tolerated and that between 2.5 and 4 D can be tolerated depending upon the individual sensitivity. However, if it is more than 4 D, it is not tolerated and is a matter of concern.

Etiology

1. *Congenital and developmental anisometropia* occurs due to differential growth of the two eyeballs.
2. *Acquired anisometropia* may occur due to asymmetric age change uniocular aphakia after removal of cataractous lens or due to implantation of IOL of wrong power.

Clinical types

1. *Simple anisometropia.* In this, one eye is normal (emmetropic) and the other either myopic (simple myopic anisometropia) or hypermetropic (simple hypermetropic anisometropia).
2. *Compound anisometropia.* wherein both eyes are either hypermetropic (compound hypermetropic anisometropia) or myopic (compound myopic anisometropia), but one eye is having higher refractive error than the other.
3. *Mixed anisometropia.* In this, one eye is myopic and the other is hypermetropic. This is also called *antimetropia.*
4. *Simple astigmatic anisometropia.* When one eye is normal and the other has either simple myopic or hypermetropic astigmatism.
5. *Compound astigmatic anisometropia.* When both eyes are astigmatic but of unequal degree.

Status of binocular vision in anisometropia

Three possibilities are there:

1. *Binocular single vision* is present in small degree of anisometropia (less than 3).
2. *Uniocular vision.* When refractive error in one eye is of high degree, that eye is suppressed and develops anisometropic amblyopia. Thus, the patient has only uniocular vision.
3. *Alternate vision* occurs when one eye is hypermetropic and the other myopic. The hypermetropic eye is used for distant vision and myopic for near.

Diagnosis

It is made after retinoscopic examination and/or autorefractometry in patients with defective vision.

Treatment

1. *Spectacles.* The corrective spectacles can be tolerated up to a maximum difference of 4 D. After that there occurs diplopia.
2. *Contact lenses* are advised for higher degrees of anisometropia.
3. *Aniseikonic glasses* are also available, but their clinical results are often disappointing.
4. *Other modalities of treatment* include:

- *Intraocular lens implantation* for uniocular aphakia.
- *Refractive corneal surgery* for unilateral high myopia, astigmatism and hypermetropia.
- *Phakic Refractive Lenses* (PRL) and *Refractive Lens Exchange* (RLE) are quite useful in very high degree anisometropia.

Note: Efforts should be made to fully correct the anisometropia in children to prevent anisometropic amblyopia. In adults with amblyopia under correction of more ametropic eye may be required to avoid ocular discomfort.

ANISEIKONIA

Aniseikonia is defined as a condition wherein the images projected to the visual cortex from the two retinae are abnormally unequal in size and/or shape. Up to 5 per cent aniseikonia is well tolerated.

Etiological types

1. *Optical aniseikonia* may occur due to either inherent or acquired anisometropia of high degree.
2. *Retinal aniseikonia* may develop due to: displacement of retinal elements towards the nodal point in one eye due to stretching or oedema of the retina.
3. *Cortical aniseikonia* implies asymmetrical simultaneous perception inspite of equal size of images formed on the two retinae.

Clinical types

Clinically, aniseikonia may be of different types (Fig. 3.31):

1. ***Symmetrical aniseikonia***
   i. *Spherical,* image may be magnified or minified equally in both meridia (Fig. 3.31A)
   ii. *Cylindrical,* image is magnified or minified symmetrically in one meridian (Fig. 3.31 B).

2. ***Asymetrical aniseikonia***
   i. *Prismatic* In this image difference increases progressively in one direction (Fig. 3.31C).
   ii. *Pincushion.* In this image distortion increases progressively in both directions, as seen with high plus correction in aphakia (Fig. 3.31D).
   iii. *Barrel distortion.* In this image distortion decreases progressively in both directions, as seen with high minus correction (Fig. 3.31E).
   iv. *Oblique distortion.* In this, the size of image is same, but there occurs an oblique distortion of shape (Fig. 3.31F).

Symptoms

1. *Asthenopia*, i.e., eyeache, browache and tiredness of eyes.
2. *Diplopia* due to difficult binocular vision when the difference in images of two eyes is more than 5 percent.
3. *Difficulty in depth perception* is often noticed.

Treatment

1. *Optical aniseikonia* may be corrected by aniseikonic glasses, contact lenses or intraocular lenses or other refractive surgery depending upon the situation.
2. *Retinal aniseikonia* may be corrected by treating the cause.
3. *Cortical aniseikonia* is very difficult to treat.

ACCOMMODATION AND ITS ANOMALIES

ACCOMMODATION

Definition. As we know that in an emmetropic eye, parallel rays of light coming from infinity are brought to focus on the retina, with accommodation being at rest. However, our eyes have been provided with a unique mechanism by which we can even focus the diverging rays coming from a near object on the retina in a bid to see clearly (Fig. 3.32). This mechanism is

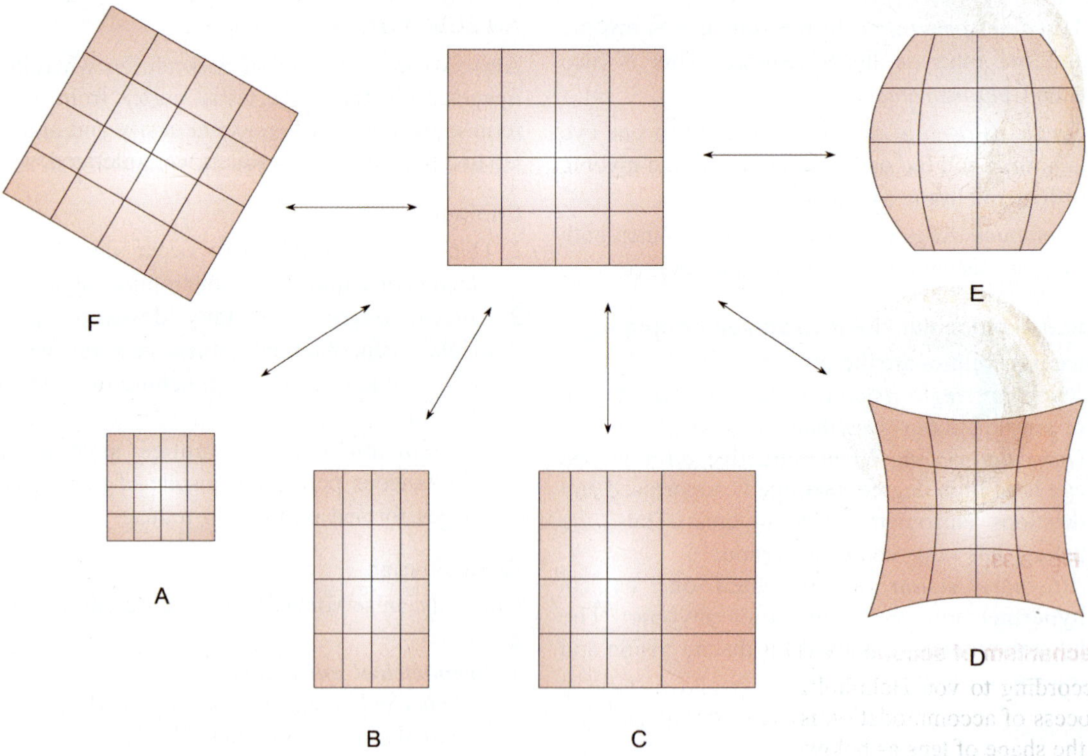

Fig. 3.31. Types of aniseikonia : A, spherical; B, cylindrical; C, prismatic; D, pin-cushion; E, barrel distortion; and F, oblique distortion.

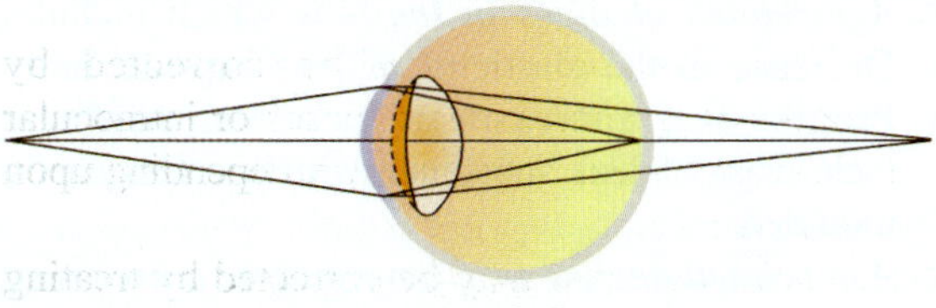

Fig. 3.32. Effect of accommodation on divergent rays entering the eye.

called *accommodation.* In this increase in the power of crystalline lens occurs due to increase in curvature of its surfaces (Fig. 3.33).

At rest the radius of curvature of anterior surface of the lens is 10 mm and that of posterior surface is 6 mm (Fig. 3.33A). During accommodation, curvature of the posterior surface remains almost the same but that of anterior surface changes. In strong accommodation radius of curvature of anterior surface also becomes 6 mm (Fig. 3.33B).

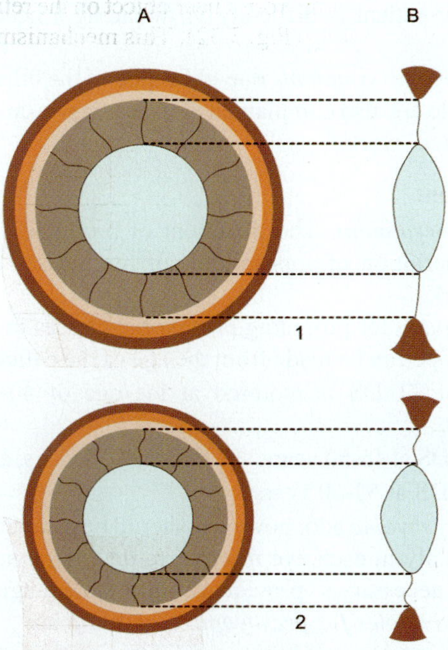

Fig. 3.33. Changes in the crystalline lens during accommodation.

Mechanism of accommodation

According to von Helmholtz's capsular theory the process of accommodation is achieved by a change in the shape of lens as below:

- *When the eye is at rest* (unaccomodated), the ciliary ring is large and keeps the zonules tense. Because of zonular tension the lens is kept compressed (flat) by the capsule (Fig. 3.33A).
- *Contraction of the ciliary muscle* causes the ciliary ring to shorten and thus releases zonular tension on the lens capsule. This allows the elastic capsule to act unrestrained to deform the lens substance. The lens then alters its shape to become more convex or conoidal (to be more precise) (Fig. 3.33B). The lens assumes conoidal shape due to configuration of the anterior lens capsule which is thinner at the center and thicker at the periphery.

Far point and near point

The nearest point at which small objects can be seen clearly is called *near point* or *punctum proximum* and the distant (farthest) point is called *far point* or *punctum remotum.*

Far point and near point of the eye. These vary with the static refraction of the eye as shown below (Fig. 3.34):

- In an *emmetropic* eye far point is infinity (Fig. 3.34A) and near point varies with age.
- In *hypermetropic* eye far point is virtual and lies behind the eye (Fig. 3.34B).

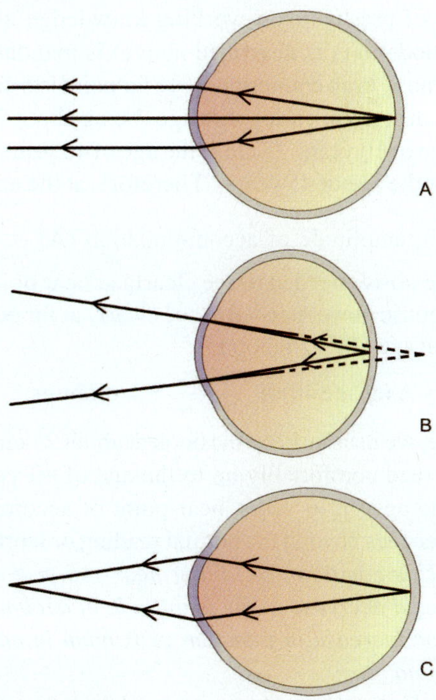

Fig. 3.34. Far point in emmetropic eye (A); hypermetropic eye (B); and myopic eye (C).

- In *myopic* eye, it is real and lies in front of the eye (Fig. 3.34C).

Range and amplitude of accommodation

Range of accommodation. The distance between the near point and the far point is called the *range of accommodation.*

Amplitude of accommodation. The difference between the dioptric power needed to focus at near point (P) and far point (R) is called *amplitude of accommodation* (A). Thus A = P – R.

ANOMALIES OF ACCOMMODATION

Anomalies of accommodation are not uncommon. These include: (1) Presbyopia, (2) Insufficiency of accommodation, (3) Paralysis of accommodation, and (4) Spasm of accommodation.

PRESBYOPIA

Pathophysiology and causes

Presbyopia (eye sight of old age) is not an error of refraction but a condition of physiological insufficiency of accommodation leading to a progressive fall in near vision.

Pathophysiology. To understand the pathophysiology of presbyopia a working knowledge about accommodation (as described above) is mandatory. As we know, in an emmetropic eye far point is infinity (∞) and near point varies with age (being about 7 cm at the age of 10 years, 25 cm at the age of 40 years and 33 cm at the age of 45 years). Therefore, at the age of 10 years, amplitude of accommodation (A) = $\frac{100}{7}$ (dioptric power needed to see clearly at near point) - 1/∞ (dioptric power needed to see clearly at far point) i.e., A (at age 10) = 14 dioptres;

similarly A (at age 40) = $\frac{100}{25} - \frac{1}{\infty}$ = 4 dioptres.

Since, we usually keep the book at about 25 cm, so we can read comfortably up to the age of 40 years. After the age of 40 years, near point of accommodation recedes beyond the normal reading or working range. *This condition of failing near vision due to age-related decrease in the amplitude of accommodation or increase in punctum proximum is called presbyopia.*

Causes. Decrease in the accommodative power of crystalline lens with increasing age, leading to presbyopia, occurs due to:

1. *Age-related changes in the lens* which include:
   - Decrease in the elasticity of lens capsule, and
   - Progressive, increase in size and hardness (sclerosis) of lens substance which is less easily moulded.
2. *Age related decline in ciliary muscle power* may also contribute in causation of presbyopia.

Causes of premature presbyopia are:

1. Uncorrected hypermetropia.
2. Premature sclerosis of the crystalline lens.
3. General debility causing pre-senile weakness of ciliary muscle.
4. Chronic simple glaucoma.

Symptoms

1. *Difficulty in near vision.* Patients usually complaint of difficulty in reading small prints (to start with in the evening and in dim light and later even in good light). Another important complaint of the patient is difficulty in threading a needle etc.
2. *Asthenopic symptoms* due to fatigue of the ciliary muscle are also complained after reading or doing any near work.

Treatment

Optical treatment. The treatment of presbyopia is the prescription of appropriate convex glasses for near work.

Rough guide for providing presbyopic glasses in an emmetrope can be made from the age of the patient.

- About +1 DS is required at the age of 40-45 years,
- +1.5 DS at 45-50 years, + 2 DS at 50-55 years, and
- +2.5 DS at 55-60 years.

Exact presbyopic add, however, should be estimated individually in each eye in order to determine how much is necessary to provide a comfortable range.

Basic principles for presbyopic correction are:

1. Always find out refractive error for distance and first correct it.
2. Find out the presbyopic correction needed in each eye separately and add it to the distant correction.
3. Near point should be fixed by taking due consideration for profession of the patient.
4. The weakest convex lens with which an individual can see clearly at the near point should be

prescribed, since overcorrection will also result in asthenopic symptoms.

Presbyopic spectacles may be unifocal, bifocal or varifocal (see page 44).

Surgical treatment of presbyopia also being considered (see page 49).

INSUFFICIENCY OF ACCOMMODATION

The term insufficiency of accommodation is used when the accommodative power is significantly less than the normal physiological limits for the patient's age. Therefore, it should not be confused with presbyopia in which the physiological insufficiency of accommodation is normal for the patient's age.

Causes

1. Premature sclerosis of lens.
2. Weakness of ciliary muscle due to systemic causes of muscle fatigue such as debilitating illness, anaemia, toxaemia, malnutrition, diabetes mellitus, pregnancy, stress and so on.
3. Weakness of ciliary muscle associated with primary open-angle glaucoma.

Clinical features

All the symptoms of presbyopia are present, but those of asthenopia are more prominent than the blurring of vision.

Treatment

1. The treatment is essentially that of the systemic cause.
2. *Near vision spectacles* in the form of weakest convex lens which allows adequate vision should be given till the power of accommodation improves.
3. *Accommodation exercises* help in recovery, if the underlying debility has passed.

PARALYSIS OF ACCOMMODATION

Paralysis of accommodation also known as *cycloplegia* refers to complete absence of accommodation.

Causes

1. *Drug induced cycloplegia* results due to the effect of atropine, homatropine or other parasympatholytic drugs.
2. *Internal ophthalmoplegia* (paralysis of ciliary muscle and sphincter pupillae) may result from neuritis associated with diphtheria, syphilis, diabetes, alcoholism, cerebral or meningeal diseases.
3. *Paralysis of accommodation as a component of complete third nerve paralysis* may occur due to intracranial or orbital causes. The lesions may be traumatic, inflammatory or neoplastic in nature.

Clinical features

1. *Blurring of near vision* is the main complaint in previously emmetropic or hypermetropic patients. Blurring of near vision may not be marked in myopic patients.
2. *Photophobia* (glare) due to accompanying dilatation of pupil (mydriasis) is usually associated with blurring of near vision.
3. Examination reveals abnormal receding of near point and markedly decreased range of accommodation.

Treatment

1. *Self-recovery* occurs in drug-induced paralysis and in diphtheric cases (once the systemic disease is treated).
2. *Dark-glasses* are effective in reducing the glare.
3. *Convex lenses* for near vision may be prescribed if the paralysis is permanent.

SPASM OF ACCOMMODATION

Spasm of accommodation refers to exertion of abnormally excessive accommodation.

Causes

1. *Drug induced spasm* of accommodation is known to occur after use of strong miotics such as echothiophate and DFP.
2. *Spontaneous spasm* of accommodation is occasionally found in children who attempt to compensate for a refractive anomaly that impairs their vision. It usually occurs when the eyes are used for excessive near work in unfavourable circumstances such as bad illumination, bad reading position, lowered vitality, state of neurosis, mental stress or anxiety.

Clinical features

1. Defective vision due to induced myopia.
2. Asthenopic symptoms are more marked than the visual symptoms.

Diagnosis

It is made with refraction under atropine.

Treatment

1. Relaxation of ciliary muscle by atropine for few weeks and prohibition of near work allow prompt recovery from spasm of accommodation.
2. Correction of associated causative factors prevent recurrence.
3. Assurance and if necessary psychotherapy.

DETERMINATION AND CORRECTION OF REFRACTIVE ERRORS

For details see page 579 .

SPECTACLES AND CONTACT LENSES

SPECTACLES

The lenses fitted in a frame constitute the spectacles. It is a common, cheap and easy method of prescribing corrective lenses in patients with refractive errors and presbyopia. Some important aspects of the spectacles are as follows:

Lens materials

1. *Crown glass* of refractive index 1.5223 is very commonly used for spectacles. It is ground to the appropriate curvature and then polished to await the final cutting that will enable it to fit the desired spectacle frame.
2. *Resin lenses* made of allyldiglycol carbonate is an alternative to crown glass. The resin lenses are light, unbreakable and scratch resistant.
3. *Plastic lenses* are readily prepared by moulding. They are unbreakable and light weight but have the disadvantages of being readily scratched and warped.
4. *Triplex lenses* are also light, they will shatter but not splinter.

Lens shapes

1. *Meniscus lenses* are used for making spectacles in small or moderate degree of refractive errors. The standard curved lenses are ground with a concave posterior surface (–1.25 D in the periscopic type or –6.0 D in the deep meniscus type) and the spherical correction is then added to the anterior surface.
2. *Lenticular form lenses* are used for high plus and high minus lenses. In this type the central portion is corrective and the peripheral surfaces are parallel to one another.
3. *Aspheric lenses* are also used to make high plus aphakic lenses by modifying the lens curvature peripherally to reduce aberrations and provide better peripheral vision.

Single versus multiple power lenses

1. *Single vision lens* refers to a lens having the same corrective power over the entire surface. These are used to correct myopia, hypermetropia, astigmatism or presbyopia.
2. *Bifocal lenses* have different powers to upper (for distant vision) and lower (for near vision) segments. Different styles of bifocal lenses shown in Fig. 3.35 are:
   - Two piece bifocals,
   - Cemented supplementary wafer,
   - Inserted wafer,
   - Fused bifocals, and
   - Solid bifocals.

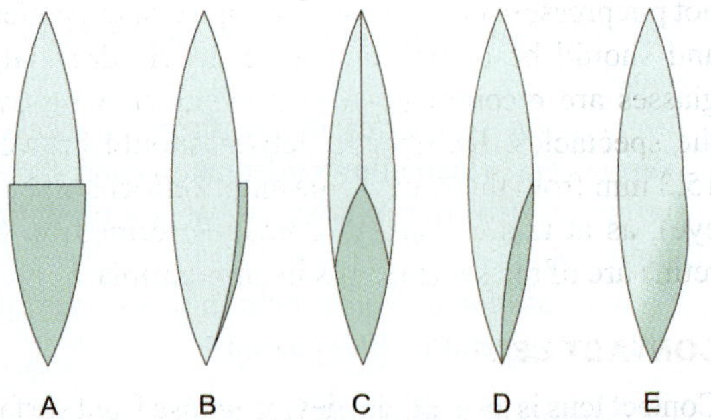

Fig. 3.35. Bifocal lenses. (A) two-piece; (B) cemented supplementary wafer; (C) inserted wafer; (D) fused; (E) solid.

3. *Trifocal lenses* have three portions, upper (for distant vision), middle (for intermediate range vision) and lower (for near vision).
4. *Multifocal* (varifocal) or progressive lenses having many portions of different powers are also available.

Tinted lenses

Tinted glasses reduce the amount of light they transmit and provide comfort, safety and cosmetic effect. They are particularly prescribed in patients with albinism, high myopia and glare prone patients. Good tinted glasses should be dark enough to absorb 60-80 percent of the incident light in the visible part of the spectrum and almost all of the ultraviolet and infrared rays.

Photochromatic lenses alter their colour according to the amount of ultraviolet exposure. These lenses do not function efficiently indoors and in automobiles.

Centring and decentring

- *For proper centring*, the visual axis of the patient and the optical centre of the spectacle lens should correspond, otherwise prismatic effect will be introduced. The distance between the visual axes is measured as interpupillary distance (IPD).
- *Decentring* of the lens is indicated where prismatic effect is required. One prism dioptre effect is produced by 1 cm decentring of a 1 D lens.
- *Reading glasses* should be decentred by about 2.5 mm medially and about 6.5 mm downward as the eyes are directed down and in during reading.

Frames

The spectacle frame selected should be comfortable i.e. neither tight nor loose, light in weight and should not put pressure on the nose or temples of the patient, and should be of optimum size. In children large glasses are recommended to prevent viewing over the spectacles. Ideally, the lenses should be worn 15.3 mm from the cornea (the anterior focal plane of eye), as at this distance the images formed on the retina are of the same size as in emmetropia.

CONTACT LENSES

Contact lens is an artificial device whose front surface substitutes the anterior surface of the cornea. Therefore, in addition to correction of refractive error, the irregularities of the front surface of cornea can also be corrected by the contact lenses.

Parts, curves, and nomenclature for contact lens

To understand the contact lens specifications following standard nomenclature has been recommended (Fig. 3.36).

1. *Diameters of the lens* are as follows :

i. *Overall diameter* (OD) of the lens is the linear measurement of the greatest distance across the physical boundaries of the lens. It is expressed in millimetres. (It should not be confused as being twice the radius of curvature).

ii. *Optic zone diameter* (OZ) is the dimension of the central optic zone of lens which is meant to focus rays on the retina.

2. Curves of the lens are as follows :

i. *Base curve* (BC) or central posterior curve (CPC) is a curve on the back surface of the lens to fit the front surface of cornea.

ii. *Peripheral curves.* These are concentric to base curve and include intermediate posterior curve (IPC) and peripheral posterior curve (PPC). These are meant to serve as reservoir of tears and to form a ski for lens movements.

iii. *Central anterior curve* (CAC) or front curve (FC) is the curve on the anterior surface of the optical zone of the lens. Its curvature determines the power of contact lens.

iv. *Peripheral anterior curve* (PAC) is a slope on the periphery of anterior surface which goes up to the edge.

v. *Intermediate anterior curve* (IAC) is fabricated only in the high power minus and plus lenses. It lies between the CAC and PAC.

3. *Edge of the lens.* It is the polished and blended union of the peripheral posterior and anterior curves of the lens.

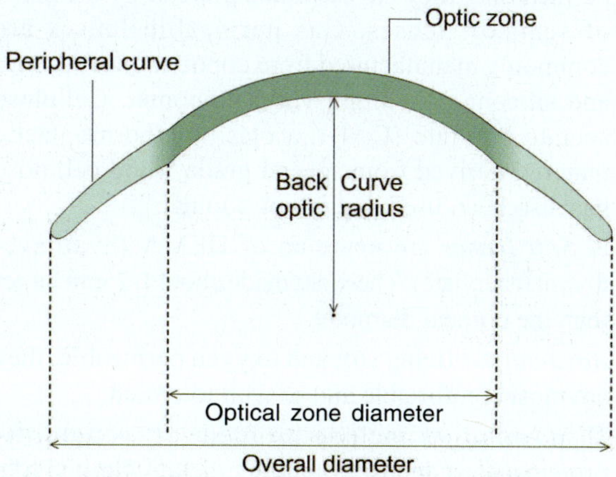

Fig. 3.36. A contact lens.

4. ***Power of the lens.*** It is measured in terms of posterior vertex power in dioptres.

5. ***Thickness of the lens.*** It is usually measured in the centre of the lens and varies depending upon the posterior vertex power of the lens.

6. ***Tint.*** It is the colour of the lens.

Types of contact lenses

Depending upon the nature of the material used in their manufacturing, the contact lenses can be divided into following three types:

1. Hard lenses,
2. Rigid gas permeable lenses, and
3. Soft lenses.

1. ***Hard lenses*** are manufactured from PMMA (polymethylmethacrylate). The PMMA has a high optical quality, stability and is light in weight, non-toxic, durable and cheap. The hard corneal lenses have a diameter of 8.5-10 mm. Presently these are not used commonly.

Disadvantages of PMMA hard contact lenses. (i) PMMA is practically impermeable to O_2 thus restricting the tolerance. (ii) Being hard, it can cause corneal abrasions. (iii) Being hydrophobic in nature, resists wetting but a stable tear film can be formed over it.

Note : PMMA contact lenses are sparingly used in clinical practice because of poor patient acceptance.

2. ***Rigid gas permeable (RGP) lenses*** are made up of materials which are permeable to oxygen. Basically these are also hard, but somehow due to their O_2 permeability they have become popular by the name of semisoft lenses. Gas permeable lenses are commonly manufactured from copolymer of PMMA and silicone containing vinyl monomer. Cellulose acetate butyrate (CAB), a class of thermoplastic material derived from special grade wood cellulose has also been used, but is not popular.

3. ***Soft lenses*** are made up of HEMA (hydroxyethylmethacrylate). These are made about 1-2 mm larger than the corneal diameter.

Advantages: Being soft and oxygen permeable, they are most comfortable and so well tolerated.

Disadvantages include problem of wettability, proteinaceous deposits, getting cracked, limited life, inferior optical quality, more chances of corneal infections and inability to correct astigmatism of more than 2 dioptres.

Note: In clinical practice soft lenses are most frequently prescribed.

Indications of contact lens use

1. ***Optical indications.*** Optically contact lenses can be used by every patient having refractive error, if so required, for cosmetic purposes. However, the absolute indications include anisometropia, unilateral aphakia, high myopia, keratoconus and irregular astigmatism.

Advantages of contact lenses over spectacles: (i) Irregular corneal astigmatism which is not possible to correct with glasses can be corrected with contact lenses. (ii) Contact lenses provide normal field of vision. (iii) Aberrations associated with spectacles (such as peripheral aberrations and prismatic distortions) are eliminated. (iv) Binocular vision can be retained in high anisometropia (e.g., unilateral aphakia) owing to less magnification of the retinal image. (v) Rain and fog do not condense upon contact lenses as they do on spectacles. (vi) Cosmetically more acceptable especially by females and all patients with thick glasses in high refractive errors.

2. ***Therapeutic indications*** are as follows :

i. *Corneal diseases* e.g., non-healing corneal ulcers, bullous keratopathy, filamentary keratitis and recurrent corneal erosion syndrome.
ii. *Diseases of iris* such as aniridia, coloboma and albinism to avoid glare.
iii. In *glaucoma* as vehicle for drug delivery.
iv. In *amblyopia*, opaque contact lenses are used for occlusion.
v. *Bandage soft contact lenses* are used following keratoplasty and in microcorneal perforation.

3. ***Preventive indications*** include (i) prevention of symblepharon and restoration of fornices in chemical burns; (ii) exposure keratitis; and (iii) trichiasis.

4. ***Diagnostic indications*** include use during (i) gonioscopy; (ii) electroretinography; (iii) examination of fundus in the presence of irregular corneal astigmatism; (iv) fundus photography; (v) Goldmann's 3 mirror examination.

5. ***Operative indications.*** Contact lenses are used during (i) goniotomy operation for congenital

glaucoma; (ii) vitrectomy; and (iii) endocular photocoagulation.

6. *Cosmetic indications* include (i) unsightly corneal scars (colour contact lenses); (ii) ptosis (haptic contact lens); and (iii) cosmetic scleral lenses in phthisis bulbi.

7. *Occupational indications* include use by (i) sportsmen; (ii) pilots; and (iii) actors.

Contraindications for contact lens use

(i) Mental incompetence, and poor motivation; (ii) chronic dacryocystitis; (iii) chronic blepharitis and recurrent styes; (iv) chronic conjunctivitis; (v) dry-eye syndromes; (vi) corneal dystrophies and degenerations; and (vii) recurrent diseases like episcleritis, scleritis and iridocyclitis.

Principles of fitting and care of lenses

It is beyond the scope of this chapter. Interested readers are advised to consult some textbook on contact lenses.

REFRACTIVE SURGERY

Surgery to correct refractive errors has become very popular. It should be performed after the error has stabilized; preferably after 20 years of age. Various surgical techniques in vogue are described below:

REFRACTIVE SURGERY OF MYOPIA

I. Cornea based procedures

1. *Radial keratotomy (RK)* refers to making deep (90 percent of corneal thickness) radial incisions in the peripheral part of cornea leaving the central 4 mm optical zone (Fig 3.37). These incisions on healing; flatten the central cornea thereby reducing its refractive power. This procedure gives good correction in low to moderate myopia (2 to 6 D).

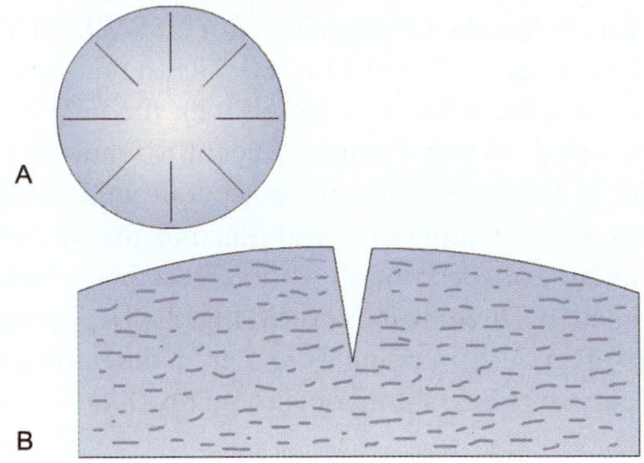

Fig. 3.37. Radial keratotomy. (A) configuration of radial incisions; (B) depth of incision.

However, because of its disadvantages and advent of safe techniques (LASIK and PRK) RK is not recommended presently.

Disadvantages of RK: (i) Cornea is weakened, so chances of globe rupture following trauma are more after RK than after PRK. This point is particularly important for patients who are at high risk of blunt trauma, e.g., sports persons, athletes and military personnel. (ii) Rarely, uneven healing may lead to irregular astigmatism. (iii) Patients may feel glare at night.

2. *Photorefractive keratectomy (PRK).* In this technique, to correct myopia a central optical zone of anterior corneal stroma is photoablated using *excimer laser* (193-nm UV flash) to cause flattening of the central cornea (Fig. 3.38). Like RK, the PRK also gives very good correction for –2 to –6 D of myopia.

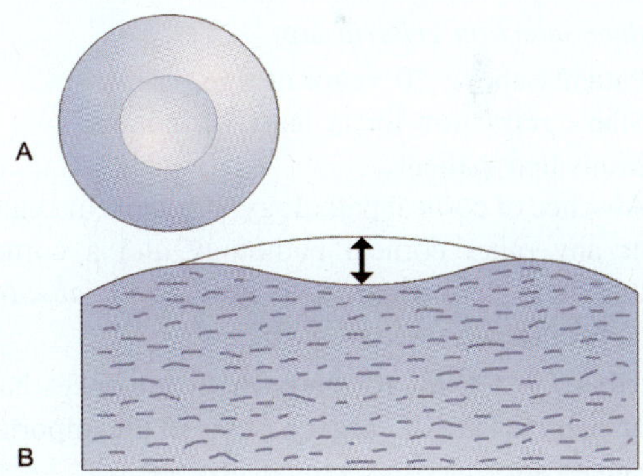

Fig. 3.38. Photorefractive keratectomy (PRK) for myopia as seen (A) from front; (B) in cross section.

Disadvantages. (i) Postoperative recovery is slow. Healing of the epithelial defect may delay return of good vision and patient may experience pain or discomfort for several weeks. (ii) There may occur some residual corneal haze in the centre affecting vision. (iii) PRK is more expensive than RK. *Note:* Because of its disadvantages PRK is not preferred presently.

3. *Laser in-situ keratomileusis (LASIK).* In this technique first a flap of 130-160 micron thickness of anterior corneal tissue is raised with the help of an automated microkeratome. Recently femtosecond laser is being used for more accurate and smooth flaps. After creating a corneal flap midstromal tissue is ablated directly with an excimer laser beam, ultimately flattening the cornea (Fig. 3.39). Currently this procedure is being considered the refractive surgery of choice for myopia of up to – 8 D.

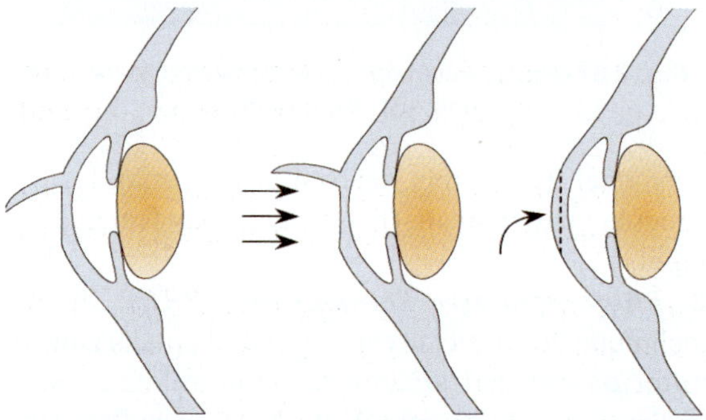

Fig. 3.39. Procedure of laser *in-situ* keratomileusis (LASIK).

Patient selection criteria are:

- Patients above 20 years of age,
- Stable refraction for at least 12 months.
- Motivated patient.
- Absence of corneal pathology. Presence of ectasia or any other corneal pathology and a corneal thickness less than 450 µm is an *absolute contraindication* for LASIK.

Advances in LASIK. Recently many advances have been made in LASIK surgery. Some of the important advances are:

- *Customized (C) LASIK.* C-LASIK is based on the wave front technology. This technique, in addition to spherical and cylindrical correction, also corrects the aberrations present in the eye and gives vision beyond 6/6 i.e., 6/5 or 6/4
- *Epi-(E) LASIK.* In this technique instead of corneal stromal flap only the epithelial sheet is separated mechanically with the use of a customized device (Epiedge Epikeratome). Being an advanced surface ablation procedure, it is devoid of complications related to corneal stromal flap.

Advantages of LASIK. (i) Minimal or no postoperative pain. (ii) Recovery of vision is very early as compared to PRK. (iii) No risk of perforation during surgery and later rupture of globe due to trauma unlike RK. (iv) No residual haze unlike PRK where subepithelial scarring may occur. (v) LASIK is effective in correcting myopia of – 8 D.

Disadvantages. 1. LASIK is much more expensive. 2. It requires greater surgical skill than RK and PRK. 3. There is potential risk of flap related complications which include (i) intraoperative flap amputation, (ii) wrinkling of the flap on repositioning, (iii) postoperative flap dislocation/subluxation, (iv) epithelization of flap-bed interface, and (v) irregular astigmatism.

4. *Intercorneal ring (ICR) implantation* into the peripheral cornea at approximately 2/3 stromal depth is being considered. It results in a vaulting effect that flattens the central cornea, decreasing myopia. The ICR procedure has the advantage of being reversible.

5. *Orthokeratology* is a non-surgical reversible method of molding the cornea with overnight wear of unique rigid gas permeable contact lenses. It is being considered for correction of myopia upto –5D. It can be used even in patients below 18 year of age.

II. Lens based procedures

1. *Refractive lens exchange.* Extraction of clear crystalline lens (Fucala's operation) has been advocated long back for myopia of –16 to –18 D, especially in unilateral cases. Recently, clear lens extraction with intraocular lens (IOL) implantation of appropriate power, i.e. refractive lens exchange (RLE) is being recommended as the refractive surgery for myopia of more than 12 D.

2. *Phakic refractive lens* (PRL) or implantable contact lens (ICL) is also being considered for correction of myopia of >8D. In this technique, a special type of intraocular lens (IOL) is implanted in the anterior chamber or posterior chamber anterior to the natural crystalline lens.

REFRACTIVE SURGERY FOR HYPEROPIA

In general, refractive surgery for hyperopia is not as effective or reliable as for myopia. However, following procedures are used:

I. Cornea based procedures

1. *Thermal laser keratoplasty* (TLK) has been used for low degree of hyperopia. In this technique, 8 laser spots are applied in a ring at the periphery to produce central steepening with mid-infrared energy from Thallium-Holmium-Chromium (THC): YAG laser. Regression effect and induced astigmatism are the main problems.

2. *Hyperopic PRK* using excimer laser has also been tried. Regression effect and prolonged epithelial healing are the main problems encountered.

3. *Hyperopic LASIK* is effective in correcting hypermetropia upto +4D.

4. *Conductive keratoplasty (CK)* is nonablative and nonincisional procedure in which cornea is steepened by collagen shrinkage through the radiofrequency energy applied through a fine tip inserted into the peripheral corneal stroma in a ring pattern. This technique is effective for correcting hyperopia of upto 3D.

II. Lens based procedures

1. *Phakic refractive lens (PRL)* or *Implantable Contact Lens (ICL)* is being considered a surgical option for hyperopia of more than + 4D.

2. *Refractive lens exchange (RLE)* is a good option for high hyperopia especially in presbyopic age.

REFRACTIVE SURGERY FOR ASTIGMATISM

Refractive surgical techniques employed for myopia can be adapted to correct astigmatism alone or simultaneously with myopia as follows:

1. *Astigmatic keratotomy (AK)* refers to making transverse cuts in the mid periphery of the steep corneal meridian (Fig. 3.40). AK can be performed alone (for astigmatism only) or along with RK (for associated myopia).

2. *Photo-astigmatic refractive keratotomy (PARK)* is performed using excimer laser.

3. *LASIK* procedure can also be adapted to correct astigmatism upto 5D.

MANAGEMENT OF POST-KERATOPLASTY ASTIGMATISM

1. *Selective removal of sutures* in steep meridians may improve a varying degree of astigmatism and should be tried first of all.

Note: Other procedures mentioned below should be performed only after all the sutures are out and refraction is stable.

2. *Arcuate relaxing incisions* in the donor cornea along the steep meridian may correct astigmatism up to 4-6 D.

3. *Relaxing incisions combined with compression* sutures may correct astigmatism up to 10 D.

4. *Corneal wedge resection* with suture closure of the wound may be performed in the flat meridian to correct astigmatism greater than 10 D.

5. *LASIK procedure* can also be adopted to correct post-keratoplasty astigmatism.

REFRACTIVE SURGERY FOR PRESBYOPIA

Refractive surgery for presbyopia, still under trial, includes :

I. Cornea based procedures

- *Monovision LASIK,* i.e., one eye is corrected for distance and other is made slightly near sighted.
- *Monovision conductive keratoplasty (CK)* is being considered increasingly to correct

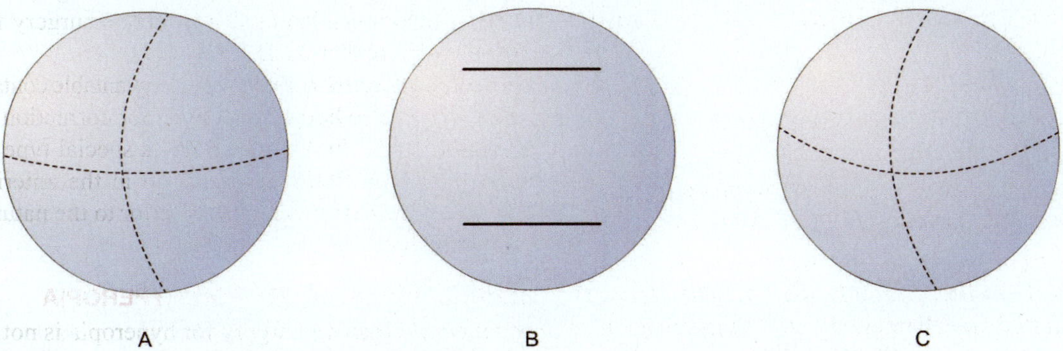

Fig. 3.40. Astigmatic keratotomy. (A) showing flat and deep meridians of cornea; (B) paired transverse incisions to flattern the steep meridian; (C) showing correction of astigmatism after astigmatic keratotomy.

presbyopia in one eye (non-dominant). Principle is same as for correction of hypermetropia (see page 48).

- *Presbyopic bifocal LASIK or LASIK-PARM* i.e., LASIK by *Presbyopia Avalos Rozakis Method* is a technique undertrial in which the shape of the cornea is altered to have two concentric vision zones that help the presbyopic patient to focus on near and distant objects.

II. Lens based procedures

- *Bifocal or multifocal or accommodating IOL* implantation after lens extraction especially in patients with cataract or high refractive errors (refractive lens exchange) correct far as well as near vision.
- *Monovision with intraocular lenses,* i.e., correction of one eye for distant vision and other for near vision with IOL implantation after bilateral cataract extraction also serves as a solution for far and near correction. Similarly, monovision with clear lens extraction and intraocular lens implantation (refractive lens exchange i.e. RLE) is also being considered increasingly in presbyopic patients with associated higher refractive errors.

III. Sclera based procedures

Following scleral expansion procedures are being tried, but results are controversial.

- *Anterior ciliary sclerotomy (ACS), with tissue barriers* is currently under trial. With initial encouraging results, multi-site clinical studies are planned for US and Europe to evaluate this technique.
- *Scleral spacing procedures* and *scleral ablation* with erbium: YAG laser are other sclera-based procedures still under trial.

4 CHAPTER

Diseases of the Conjunctiva

APPLIED ANATOMY
- Parts
- Structure
- Glands

INFLAMMATIONS OF CONJUNCTIVA
- Infective conjunctivitis
  - Bacterial
  - Chlamydial
  - Viral
  - Granulomatous
- Allergic conjunctivitis
- Cicatricial conjunctivitis
- Toxic conjunctivitis

DEGENERATIVE CONDITIONS
- Pinguecula
- Pterygium
- Concretions

SYMPTOMATIC CONDITIONS OF CONJUNCTIVA
- Hyperaemia
- Chemosis
- Ecchymosis
- Xerosis
- Discoloration

CYSTS AND TUMOURS
- Cysts of conjunctiva
- Tumours of conjunctiva

APPLIED ANATOMY

Conjunctiva is a translucent mucous membrane which lines the posterior surface of the eyelids and anterior aspect of the eyeball. The name conjunctiva (conjoin: to join) has been given to this mucous membrane owing to the fact that it joins the eyeball to the lids. It stretches from the lid margin to the limbus, and encloses a complex space called *conjunctival sac* which is open in front at the palpebral fissure.

Parts of conjunctiva

Conjunctiva can be divided into three parts (Fig. 4.1):

1. *Palpebral conjunctiva.* It lines the lids and can be subdivided into marginal, tarsal and orbital conjunctiva.

i. *Marginal conjunctiva* extends from the lid margin to about 2 mm on the back of lid up to a shallow groove, the *sulcus subtarsalis.* It is actually a transitional zone between skin and the conjunctiva proper.

ii. *Tarsal conjunctiva* is thin, transparent and highly vascular. It is firmly adherent to the whole tarsal plate in the upper lid. In the lower lid, it is adherent only to half width of the tarsus. The tarsal glands are seen through it as yellow streaks.

iii. *Orbital part* of palpebral conjunctiva lies loose between the tarsal plate and fornix.

2. *Bulbar conjunctiva.* It is thin, transparent and lies loose over the underlying structures and thus can be moved easily. It is separated from the anterior sclera by episcleral tissue and Tenon's capsule. A 3-mm ridge of bulbar conjunctiva around the cornea is called *limbal conjunctiva.* In the area of limbus, the conjunctiva, Tenon's capsule and the episcleral tissue are fused into a dense tissue which is strongly adherent to the underlying corneoscleral junction. At the limbus, the epithelium of conjunctiva becomes continuous with that of cornea.

3. *Conjunctival fornix.* It is a continuous circular cul-de-sac which is broken only on the medial side by caruncle and the plica semilunaris. Conjunctival fornix joins the bulbar conjunctiva with the palpebral

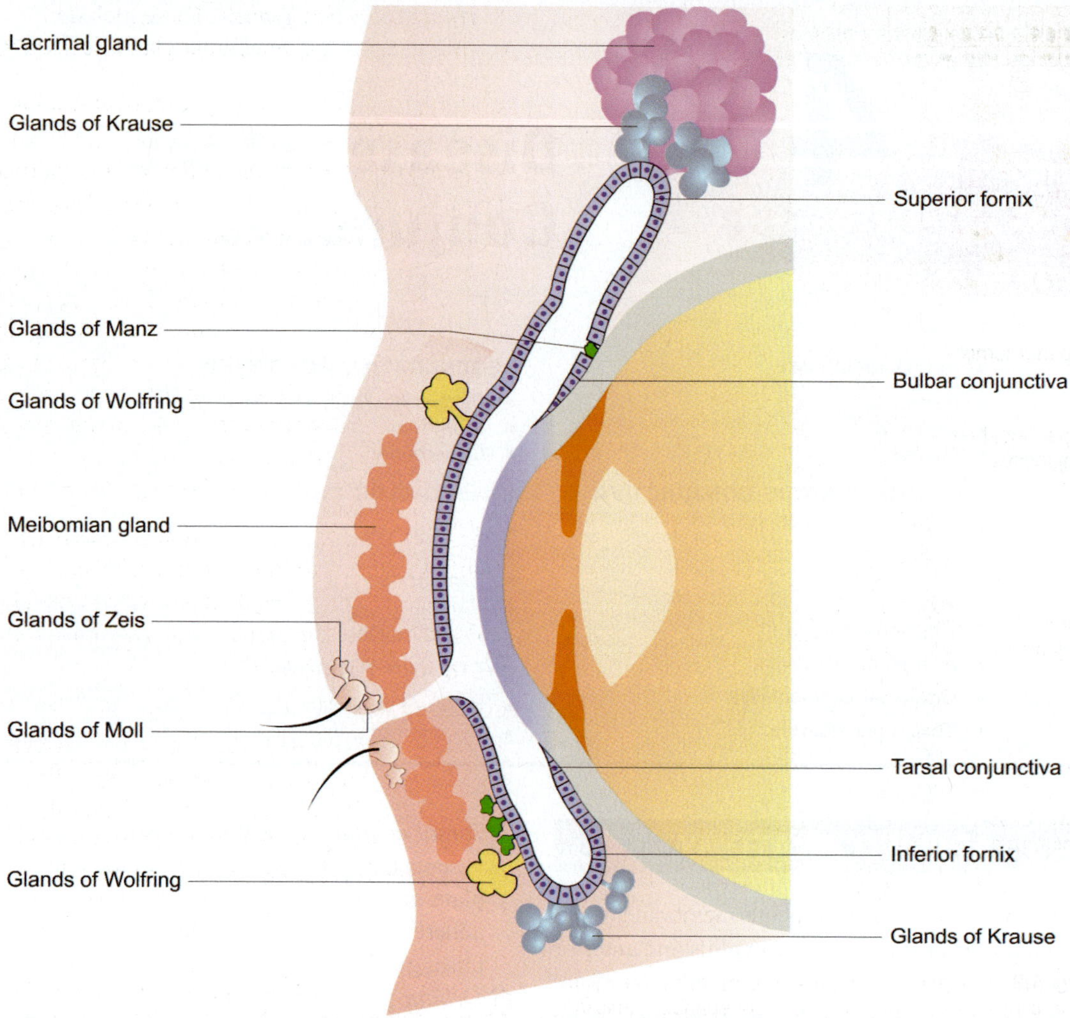

Fig. 4.1. Parts of conjunctiva and conjunctival glands.

conjunctiva. It can be subdivided into superior, inferior, medial and lateral fornices.

Structure of conjunctiva

Histologically, conjunctiva consists of three layers namely, epithelium, adenoid layer, and fibrous layer (Fig. 4.2).

1. *Epithelium.* This is a 2-5 layered, non-keratinized epithilium. It also contains goblet cells which constitute about 10% of epithelium. The layer of epithelial cells in conjunctiva varies from region to region and in its different parts as follows:

- *Marginal conjunctiva* has 5-layered stratified squamous type of epithelium.
- *Tarsal conjunctiva* has 2-layered epithelium: superficial layer of cylindrical cells and a deep layer of flat cells.
- *Fornix and bulbar conjunctiva* have 3-layered epithelium: a superficial layer of cylindrical cells, middle layer of polyhedral cells and a deep layer of cuboidal cells.
- *Limbal conjunctiva* has again many layered (5 to 6) stratified squamous epithelium.

2. *Adenoid layer.* It is also called *lymphoid layer* and consists of fine connective tissue reticulum in the meshes of which lie lymphocytes. This layer is most developed in the fornices. It is not present since

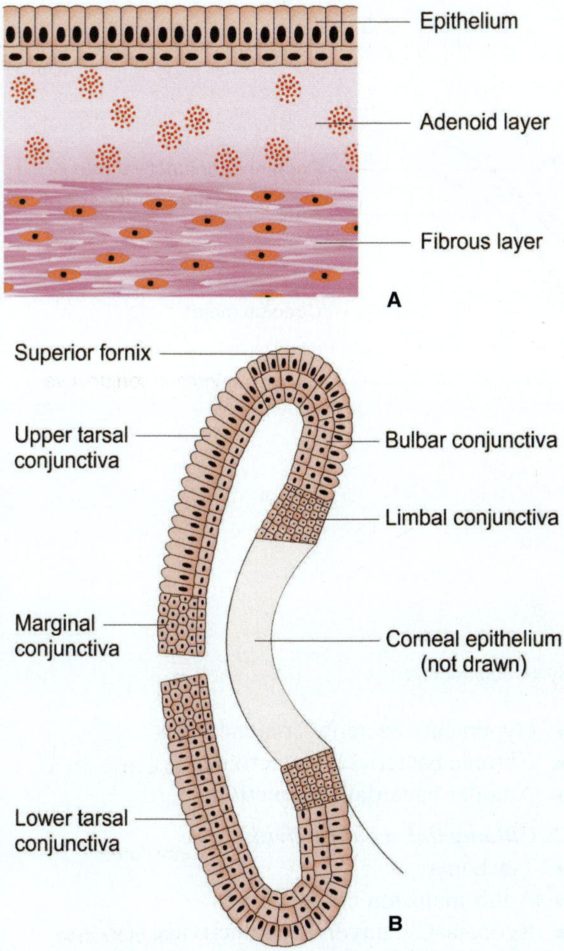

Fig. 4.2. Microscopic structure of conjunctiva showing three layers (A), and arrangement of epithelial cells in different regions of conjunctiva (B).

birth but develops after 3-4 months of life. For this reason, conjunctival inflammation in an infant does not produce follicular reaction.

3. *Fibrous layer.* It consists of a meshwork of collagenous and elastic fibres. It is thicker than the adenoid layer, except in the region of tarsal conjunctiva, where it is very thin. This layer contains vessels and nerves of conjunctiva. It blends with the underlying Tenon's capsule in the region of bulbar conjunctiva.

Glands of conjunctiva

The conjunctiva contains *two types* of glands (Fig. 4.1):

1. *Mucin secretory glands.* These include:
- *Goblet cells* (the unicellular glands located within the epithelium),
- *Crypts of Henle* (present in the tarsal conjunctiva), and
- *Glands of Manz* (found in limbal conjunctiva).

These glands secrete mucus which is essential for wetting the cornea and conjunctiva.

2. *Accessory lacrimal glands.* These are:
- *Glands of Krause* (present in subconjunctival connective tissue of fornices, about 42 in the upper fornix and 8 in the lower fornix) and
- *Glands of Wolfring*, present along the upper border of superior tarsus and along the lower border of inferior tarsus.

Plica semilunaris

It is a pinkish crescentric fold of conjunctiva, present in the medial canthus. Its lateral free border is concave. It is a vestigeal structure in human beings and represents the nictitating membrane (or third eyelid) of lower animals.

Caruncle

The caruncle is a small, ovoid, pinkish mass, situated in the inner canthus, just medial to the plica semilunaris. In reality, it is a piece of modified skin and so is covered with stratified squamous epithelium and contains sweat glands, sebaceous glands and hair follicles.

Blood supply of conjunctiva

Arteries supplying the conjunctiva are derived from three sources (Fig. 4.3): (1) peripheral arterial arcade of the eyelid; (2) marginal arcade of the eyelid; and (3) anterior ciliary arteries.

- *Palpebral conjunctiva and fornices* are supplied by branches from the peripheral and marginal arterial arcades of the eyelids.
- *Bulbar conjunctiva* is supplied by two sets of vessels: the *posterior conjunctival arteries* which are branches from the arterial arcades of the eyelids; and the *anterior conjunctival* arteries which are the branches of anterior ciliary arteries. Terminal branches of the posterior conjunctival arteries anastomose with the anterior conjunctival *arteries* to form the pericorneal plexus.

Veins from the conjunctiva drain into the venous plexus of eyelids and some around the cornea into the anterior ciliary veins.

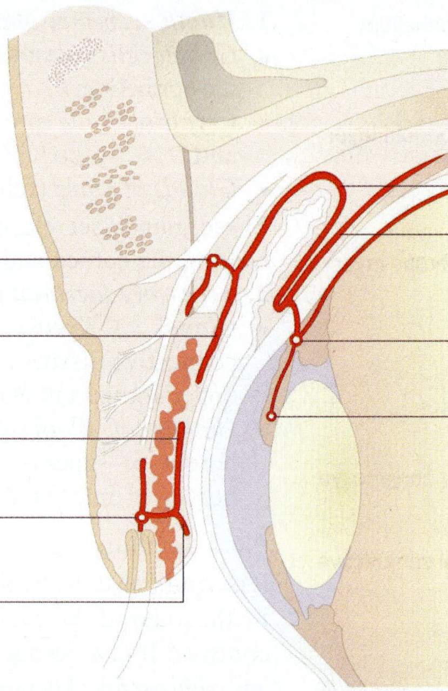

Fig. 4.3. Blood supply of conjunctiva.

Lymphatics of the conjunctiva are arranged in two layers: a superficial and a deep. Lymphatics from the lateral side drain into *preauricular lymph nodes* and those from the medial side into the *submandibular lymph nodes.*

Nerve supply of conjunctiva

A circumcorneal zone of conjunctiva is supplied by the branches from long ciliary nerves which supply the cornea. Rest of the conjunctiva is supplied by the branches from lacrimal, infratrochlear, supratrochlear, supraorbital and frontal nerves.

INFLAMMATIONS OF CONJUNCTIVA

Inflammation of the conjunctiva (conjunctivitis) is classically defined as conjunctival hyperaemia associated with a discharge which may be watery, mucoid, mucopurulent or purulent.

TYPES OF CONJUNCTIVITIS

Common types of conjunctivitis include:

A. Infective conjunctivitis

1. ***Bacterial conjunctivitis***
- Acute bacterial conjunctivitis
- Hyperacute bacterial conjunctivitis
- Chronic bacterial conjunctivitis
- Angular bacterial conjunctivitis

2. ***Chlamydial conjunctivitis***
- Trachoma
- Adult inclusion conjunctivitis
- Neonatal Chlamydial conjunctivitis

3. ***Viral conjunctivitis***
- Adenovirus conjunctivitis
  - Epidemic keratoconjunctivitis
  - Pharyngoconjunctival fever
- Enterovirus conjunctivitis
- Molluscum contagiosum conjunctivitis
- Herpes simplex conjunctivitis

4. ***Opthalmia neonatorum*** (A separate entity)
5. ***Granulomatous conjunctivitis***
- Parinaud oculoglandular syndrome

B. Allergic Conjunctivitis

1. ***Simplex allergic conjunctivitis***
- Hay fever conjunctivitis (rhino conjunctivitis)
- Seasonal allergic conjunctivitis (SAC)
- Perennial allergic conjunctivitis (PAC)

2. ***Vernal keratoconjunctivitis*** (VKC)
3. ***Atopic keratoconjunctivitis***
4. ***Giant papillary conjunctivitis*** (GPC)

5. ***Phlyctenular conjunctivitis*** (PKC)
6. ***Contact dermoconjunctivitis*** (drop conjunctivitis)

C. Cicatricial conjunctivitis

- Ocular mucous membrane pemphigoid (OMMP),
- Stevens Johnson syndrome (SJS),
- Toxic epidermal necrolysis (TeN), and
- Secondary cicatricial conjunctivitis.

D. Toxic conjunctivitis

A. Infective Conjunctivitis

Infective conjunctivitis, i.e., inflammation of the conjunctiva caused by microorganisms is the commonest variety. This is in spite of the fact that the conjunctiva has been provided with *natural protective mechanisms* in the form of :

- Low temperature due to exposure to air,
- Physical protection by lids,
- Flushing action of tears,
- Antibacterial activity of lysozymes and
- Humoral protection by the tear immunoglobulins.

BACTERIAL CONJUNCTIVITIS

There has occurred a relative decrease in the incidence of bacterial conjunctivitis in general and those caused by *Gonococcus* and *Corynebacterium Diphtheriae* in particular. However, in developing countries it still continues to be the commonest type of conjunctivitis. It can occur as sporadic and epidemics cases. Outbreaks of bacterial conjunctivitis epidemics are quite frequent during monsoon season.

Etiology

A. *Predisposing factors* for bacterial conjunctivitis, especially epidemic forms, are flies, poor hygienic conditions, hot dry climate, poor sanitation and dirty habits. These factors help the infection to establish, as the disease is highly contagious.

B. *Causative organisms.* It may be caused by a wide range of organisms in the following approximate order of frequency :

- *Staphylococcus aureus* is the most common cause of bacterial conjunctivitis and blepharo-conjunctivitis.
- *Staphylococcus epidermidis* is an innocuous flora of lid and conjunctiva. It can also produce blepharoconjunctivitis.
- *Streptococcus pneumoniae* (pneumococcus) produces acute conjunctivitis usually associated with petechial subconjunctival haemorrhages. The disease has a self-limiting course of 9-10 days.
- *Streptococcus pyogenes* (haemolyticus) is virulent and usually produces pseudomembranous conjunctivitis.
- *Haemophilus influenzae* (aegyptius, Koch- Weeks bacillus). It classically causes epidemics of mucopurulent conjunctivitis, known as 'red-eye' especially in semitropical countries.
- *Moraxella lacunate* (Moraxella Axenfeld Bacillus) is most common cause of angular conjunctivitis and angular blepharoconjunctivitis.
- *Pseudomonas pyocyanea* is a virulent organism. It readily invades the cornea.
- *Neisseria gonorrhoeae* typically produces acute purulent conjunctivitis in adults and ophthalmia neonatorum in new born. It is capable of invading intact corneal epithelium.
- *Neisseria meningitidis* (meningococcus) may produce mucopurulent conjunctivitis.
- *Corynebacterium diphtheriae* causes acute membranous conjunctivitis. Such infections are rare now-a-days.

C. *Mode of infection.* Conjunctiva may get infected from three sources, viz, exogenous, local surrounding structures and endogenous, by following modes :

1. *Exogenous infections* may spread: (i) directly through close contact, as air-borne infections or as water-borne infections; (ii) through vector transmission (e.g., flies); or (iii) through material transfer such as infected fingers of doctors, nurses, common towels, handkerchiefs, and infected tonometers.
2. *Local spread* may occur from neighbouring structures such as infected lacrimal sac, lids, and nasopharynx. In addition to these, a change in the character of relatively innocuous organisms present in the conjunctival sac itself may cause infections.
3. *Endogenous infections* may occur very rarely through blood e.g., gonococcal and meningococcal infections.

Pathology

Pathological changes of bacterial conjunctivitis consist of :

1. *Vascular response.* It is characterised by congestion and increased permeability of the

conjunctival vessels associated with proliferation of capillaries.

2. *Cellular response.* It is in the form of exudation of polymorphonuclear cells and other inflammatory cells into the substantia propria of conjunctiva as well as in the conjunctival sac.
3. *Conjunctival tissue repsonse.* Conjunctiva becomes oedematous. The superficial epithelial cells degenerate, become loose and even desquamate. There occurs proliferation of basal layers of conjunctival epithelium and increase in the number of mucin secreting goblet cells.
4. *Conjunctival discharge.* It consists of tears, mucus, inflammatory cells, desquamated epithelial cells, fibrin and bacteria. If the inflammation is very severe, diapedesis of red blood cells may occur and discharge may become blood stained.

Severity of pathological changes varies depending upon the severity of inflammation and the causative organism. The changes are thus more marked in purulent conjunctivitis than mucopurulent conjunctivitis.

CLINICAL TYPES OF BACTERIAL CONJUNCTIVITIS

Depending upon the causative bacteria and the severity of infection, bacterial conjunctivitis may present in following clinical forms:

- Acute bacterial conjunctivitis
- Hyperacute bacterial conjunctivitis
- Chronic bacterial conjunctivitis
- Angular bacterial conjunctivitis

ACUTE BACTERIAL CONJUNCTIVITIS

Acute bacterial conjunctivitis is characterised by marked conjunctival hyperaemia and mucopurulent discharge from the eye. So clinically it is called acute mucopurulent conjunctivitis. It is the most common type of bacterial conjunctivitis.

Common causative bacteria are: *Staphylococcus aureus*, *Koch-Weeks Bacillus*, *Pneumococcus* and *Streptococcus*. Mucopurulent conjunctivitis generally accompanies exanthemata such as measles and scarlet fever.

Clinical picture

Symptoms

- *Discomfort and foreign body sensation* due to engorgement of vessels.
- *Mild photophobia,* i.e., difficulty to tolerate light.
- *Mucopurulent discharge* from the eyes.
- *Sticking together of lid margins* with discharge during sleep.
- *Slight blurring of vision* due to mucous flakes in front of cornea.
- Sometimes patient may complain of *coloured halos* due to prismatic effect of mucus present on cornea.

Signs (Fig. 4.4)

- *Flakes of mucopus* seen in the fornices, canthi and lid margins is a critical sign.
- *Conjunctival congestion,* which is more marked in palpebral conjunctiva, fornices and peripheral part of bulbar conjunctiva, giving the appearance of 'fiery red eye'. The congestion is typically less marked in circumcorneal zone.

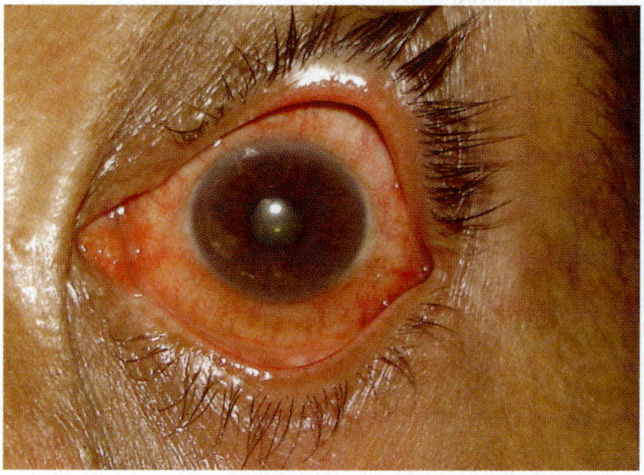

Fig. 4.4. Signs of acute mucopurulent conjunctivitis.

- *Chemosis* i.e., swelling of conjunctiva.
- *Papillae* of fine type may be seen.
- *Petechial* haemorrhages are seen when the causative organism is *pneumococcus.*
- *Cilia* are usually matted together with yellow crusts.
- *Eyelids* maybe slightly oedematous.

Clinical course. Mucopurulent conjunctivitis reaches its height in three to four days. If untreated, in mild cases the infection may be overcome and the condition is cured in 10-15 days; or it may pass to less intense form, the 'chronic catarrhal conjunctivitis'.

Complications. Occasionally the disease may be complicated by superficial punctate epitheliopathy, marginal corneal ulceration, superficial keratitis, blepharitis, or dacryocystitis.

Table 4.1. Differentiating features of common types of conjunctivitis

	Bacterial	*Viral*	*Allergic*	*Chlamydial (TRIC)*
[A] CLINICAL SIGNS				
1. Congestion	Marked	Moderate	Mild to moderate	Moderate
2. Chemosis	++	±	++	±
3. Subconjunctival haemorrhages	±	±	–	–
4. Discharge	Purulent or mucopurulent	Watery	Ropy/ watery	Mucopurulent
5. Papillae	±	–	++	±
6. Follicles	–	+	–	++
7. Pseudomembrane	±	±	–	–
8. Pannus	–	–	– (Except vernal)	+
9. Pre-auricular lymph nodes	+	++	–	±
[B] CYTOLOGICAL FEATURES				
1. Neutrophils	+	+ (Early)	–	+
2. Eosinophils	–	–	+	–
3. Lymphocytes	–	+	–	+
4. Plasma cells	–	–	–	+
5. Multinuclear cells	–	+	–	–
6. Inclusion bodies :				
Cytoplasmic	–	+ (Pox)	–	+
Nuclear	–	+ (Herpes)	–	–
7. Micro-organisms	+	–	–	–

Differential diagnosis

1. *From other causes of acute red eye* (see page 154).
2. *From other types of conjunctivitis.* It is made out from the typical clinical picture of disease and is confirmed by conjunctival cytology and bacteriological examination of secretions and scrapings (Table 4.1).

Treatment

1. *Topical antibiotics* to control the infection constitute the main treatment of acute bacterial conjunctivitis. Ideally, the antibiotic should be selected after culture and sensitivity tests but in practice, it is difficult. However, in routine, most of the patients respond well to broad spectrum antibiotics. Therefore, treatment may be started with chloramphenicol (1%), or gentamycin (0.3%), or tobramycin 0.3% or framycetin 0.3% eye drops 3-4 hourly in day and ointment used at night will not only provide antibiotic cover but also help to reduce the early morning stickiness. If the patient does not respond to these antibiotics, then the quinolone antibiotic drops such as ciprofloxacin (0.3%), ofloxacin (0.3%), gatifloxacin (0.3%) or moxifloxacin (0.5%) may be used.
2. *Irrigation of conjunctival sac* with sterile warm saline once or twice a day will help by removing the deleterious material. Frequent eyewash (as advocated earlier) is, however, contraindicated as it will wash away the lysozyme and other protective proteins present in the tears.
3. *Dark goggles* should be used to prevent photophobia.
4. *No bandage* should be applied in patients with mucopurulent conjunctivitis. Exposure to air keeps the temperature of conjunctival cul-de-sac low which inhibits the bacterial growth; while after bandaging, conjunctival sac is converted into an incubator, and thus infection flares to a severe degree within 24 hours. Further, bandaging of eye will also prevent the escape of discharge.
5. *No steroids* should be applied, otherwise infection will flare up and bacterial corneal ulcer may develop.

6. *Anti-inflammatory and analgesic drugs* (e.g. ibuprofen and paracetamol) may be given orally for 2-3 days to provide symptomatic relief from mild pain especially in sensitive patients.

HYPERACUTE BACTERIAL CONJUNCTIVITIS

Hyperacute bacterial conjunctivitis also known as acute purulent conjunctivities or *acute blenorrhea* is characterised by a violent inflammatory response. It occurs in two forms:

1. Adult purulent conjunctivitis and
2. Ophthalmia neonatorum in newborn (see page 69).

HYPERACUTE CONJUNCTIVITIS OF ADULTS (GONOCOCCAL CONJUNCTIVITIS)

Etiology

The disease affects adults, predominantly males. Gonococcal infection directly spreads from genitals to eye. Presently incidence of gonococcal conjunctivitis has markedly decreased.

Clinical picture

Onset is hyperacute (12 to 24 hrs.)

Symptoms include:

- *Pain* which is moderate to severe
- *Purulent discharge*, is usually copious
- *Swelling of eyelids*, usually marked

Signs are as follows: (Fig. 4.5)

- *Eyelids* are tense and swollen
- *Tenderness* is marked
- *Discharge* is thick purulent, copius trickling down the cheeks.

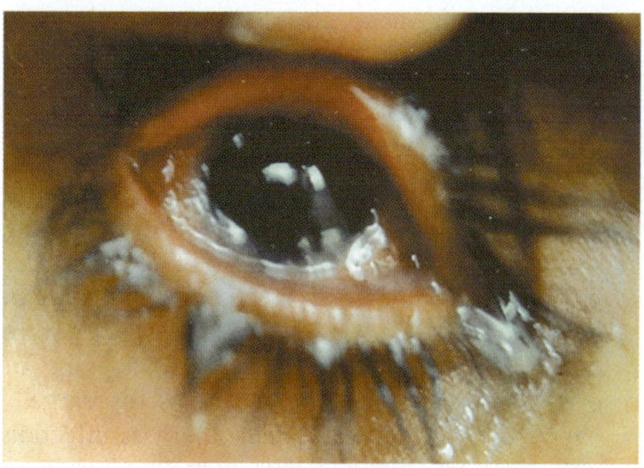

Fig. 4.5. Hyperacute conjunctivitis.

- *Conjunctiva* shows marked chemosis, congestion and papillae, giving bright red velvety appearence, Frequently a pseudomembrane may be seen on the conjunctival surface (Fig. 4.6)
- *Preauricular lymph nodes* are usually enlarged and tender.

Associations. Gonococcal conjunctivitis is usually associated with urethritis and arthritis.

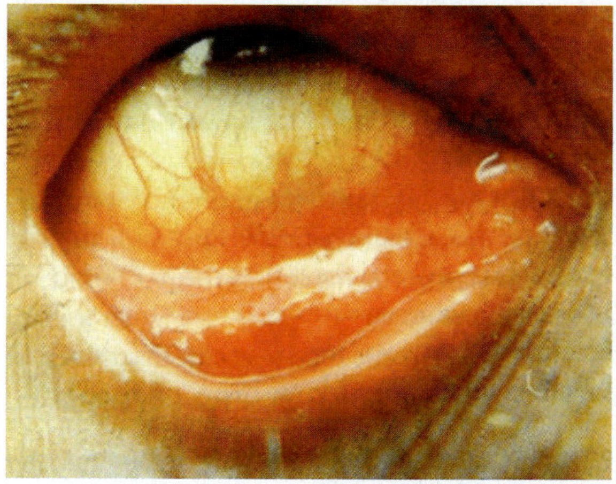

Fig. 4.6. Pseudomembranous conjunctivitis.

Complications

1. *Corneal involvement* is quite frequent as the *gonococcus* can invade the normal cornea through an intact epithelium. It may occur in the form of diffuse haze and oedema, central necrosis, corneal ulceration or even perforation.
2. *Iridocyclitis* may also occur, but is not as common as corneal involvement.
3. *Systemic complications,* though rare, include gonorrhoea arthritis, endocarditis and septicaemia.

Treatment

1. *Systemic therapy* is far more critical than the topical therapy for the infections caused by *N. gonorrhoeae*. Because of the resistant strains penicillin and tetracyline are no longer adequate as first-line treatment. Any of the following regimes can be adopted:
   - Norfloxacin 1.2 gm orally qid for 5 days
   - Cefoxitim 1.0 gm or cefotaxime 500 mg. IV qid or ceftriaxone 1.0 gm IM qid, all for 5 days; or
   - Spectinomycin 2.0 gm IM for 3 days.

   All of the above regimes should then be followed by a one week course of either doxycycline 100 mg bid or erythromycin 250-500 mg orally qid.

2. *Topical antibiotic therapy* presently recommended includes ofloxacin, ciprofloxacin or tobramycin eye drops or bacitracin or erythromycin eye ointment every 2 hours for the first 2-3 days and then 5 times daily for 7 days. Because of the resistant strains, intensive therapy with penicillin drops is not reliable.
3. *Irrigation* of the eyes frequently with sterile saline is very therapeutic in washing away infected debris.
4. *Other general measures* are similar to acute mucopurulent conjunctivitis.
5. *Topical atropine* 1 per cent eye drops should be instilled once or twice a day if cornea is involved.

Note: Sexual partner should also be treated with systemic antibiotics. Further, both the patient and the sexual partner should be referred for evaluation of other sexually transmitted diseases.

CHRONIC BACTERIAL CONJUNCTIVITIS

Chronic bacterial conjuctivitis also known as '*Chronic catarrhal conjunctivitis*' or '*simple chronic conjunctivitis*' is characterised by mild catarrhal inflammation of the conjunctiva.

Etiology

A. *Predisposing factors*

1. *Chronic exposure* to dust, smoke, and chemical irritants.
2. *Local cause of irritation* such as trichiasis, concretions, foreign body and seborrhoeic scales.
3. *Eye strain* due to refractive errors, phorias or convergence insufficiency.
4. *Abuse of alcohol,* insomnia and metabolic disorders.

B. *Causative organisms*

- *Staphylococcus aureus* is the commonest cause of chronic bacterial conjunctivitis.
- *Gram negative rods* such as *Proteus mirabilis, Klebsiella pneumoniae, Escherichia coli* and *Moraxella lacunata* are other rare causes.

C. *Source and mode of infection*. Chronic conjunctivitis may occur:

1. *As continuation of acute mucopurulent conjunctivitis* when untreated or partially treated.
2. *As chronic infection* from associated chronic dacryocystitis, chronic rhinitis or chronic upper respiratory catarrh.
3. *As a mild exogenous infection* which results from direct contact, air-borne or material transfer of infection.

Clinical picture

Symptoms of simple chronic conjunctivitis include:

- *Burning and grittiness* in the eyes, especially in the evening.
- *Mild chronic redness* in the eyes.
- *Feeling of heat and dryness* on the lid margins.
- Difficulty in keeping the eyes open.
- *Mild mucoid discharge* especially in the canthi.
- Off and on lacrimation.
- Feeling of sleepiness and tiredness in the eyes.

Signs. Grossly the eyes look normal but careful examination may reveal following signs:

- *Congestion* of posterior conjunctival vessels.
- Mild papillary hypertrophy of the palpebral conjunctiva.
- Surface of the conjunctiva looks sticky.
- Lid margins may be congested.

Treatment

1. *Eliminate predisposing factors* when associated.
2. *Topical antibiotics* such as chloramphenicol, tobramycin or gentamycin should be instilled 3-4 times a day for about 2 weeks to eliminate the mild chronic infection.
3. *Astringent eye drops* such as zinc-boric acid drops provide symptomatic relief.

ANGULAR BACTERIAL CONJUNCTIVITIS

It is a type of chronic conjunctivitis characterised by mild grade inflammation confined to the conjunctiva and lid margins near the angles (hence the name) associated with maceration of the surrounding skin.

Etiology

1. *Predisposing factors* are same as for 'simple chronic conjunctivitis'.
2. *Causative organisms. Moraxella Axenfeld* is the commonest causative organism. MA bacilli are placed end to end, so the disease is also called 'diplobacillary conjunctivitis'. Rarely, staphylococci may also cause angular conjunctivitis.
3. *Source of infection* is usually nasal cavity.

4. *Mode of infection.* Infection is transmitted from nasal cavity to the eyes by contaminated fingers or handkerchief.

Pathology

The causative organism, i.e., MA bacillus produces a proteolytic enzyme which acts by macerating the epithelium. This proteolytic enzyme collects at the angles by the action of tears and thus macerates the epithelium of the conjunctiva, lid margin and the skin the surrounding angles of eye. The maceration is followed by vascular and cellular responses in the form of mild grade chronic inflammation. Skin may show eczematous changes.

Clinical picture

Symptoms

- Irritation, smarting sensation and feeling of discomfort in the eyes.
- History of collection of dirty-white foamy discharge at the angles.
- Redness in the angles of eyes.

Signs (Fig. 4.7) include:

- *Hyperaemia of bulbar conjunctiva* near the canthi.
- *Hyperaemia* of *lid margins* near the angles.
- *Excoriation of the skin* around the angles.
- *Foamy mucopurulent discharge* at the angles is usually present.

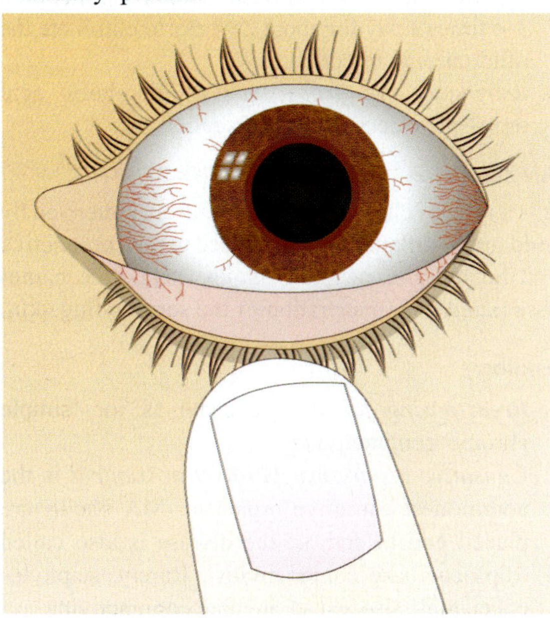

Fig. 4.7. Signs of angular conjunctivitis.

Complications include: blepharitis and shallow marginal catarrhal corneal ulceration.

Treatment

A. ***Prophylaxis*** includes treatment of associated nasal infection and good personal hygiene.

B. ***Curative treatment*** consists of :

1. *Oxytetracycline* (1%) eye ointment, 2-3 times a day for 9-14 days will eradicate the infection.
2. *Zinc lotion* instilled in day time and zinc oxide ointment at bed time inhibits the proteolytic ferment and thus helps in reducing the maceration.

CHLAMYDIAL CONJUNCTIVITIS

Chlamydia lie midway between bacteria and viruses, sharing some of the properties of both. Like viruses, they are obligate intracellular and filterable, whereas like bacteria they contain both DNA and RNA, divide by binary fission and are sensitive to antibiotics.

The *Chlamydia* combinedly form the PLT group (*Psittacosis*, *Lymphogranuloma venereum* and *Trachomatis* group).

Life cycle of the chlamydia. The infective particle invades the cytoplasm of epithelial cells, where it swells up and forms the *'initial body'*. The initial bodies rapidly divide into *'elementary bodies'* embedded in glycogen matrix which are liberated when the cells burst. Then the 'elementary bodies' infect other cells where the whole cycle is repeated.

Ocular infections produced by chlamydia in human beings are summarised in Table 4.2.

TRACHOMA

Trachoma (previously known as *Egyptian ophthalmia*) is a chronic keratoconjunctivitis, primarily affecting the superficial epithelium of conjunctiva and cornea simultaneously. It is characterised by a mixed follicular and papillary response of conjunctival tissue. It is still one of the leading causes of preventable blindness in the world. The word 'trachoma' comes from the Greek word for 'rough' which describes the surface appearance of the conjunctiva in chronic trachoma.

Etiology

A. *Causative organism.* Trachoma is caused by a Bedsonian organism, the Chlamydia trachomatis

Table 4.2. Summary of ocular infections caused by chlamydia

Genus	Chlamydia			
Species	C. trachomatis (TRIC agent) (Humans)		C. lymphogranulomatis (Humans)	C. psittacosis (Animals)
Serotype	A, B, Ba, C	D to K	L1, L2, L3	
Ocular disease	Hyperendemic trachoma	Paratrachoma (– neonatal and adult inclusion conjunctivitis)	Lymphogranuloma venereum conjunctivitis	
Transmission	Eye to eye	Genitals to eye	Genitals to eye	

belonging to the Psittacosis-lymphogranuloma-trachoma (PLT) group. The organism is epitheliotropic and produces intracytoplasmic inclusion bodies called H.P. bodies (*Halberstaedter* Prowazeke bodies). Presently, 11 serotypes of Chlamydia, (A, B, Ba, C, D, E, F, G, H, J and K) have been identified using microimmunofluorescence techniques. Sero types A, B, Ba and C are associated with hyper-endemic (blinding) trachoma, while serotypes D-K are associated with paratrachoma (oculogenital chlamydial disease).

B. *Predisposing factors.* These include age, sex, race, climate, socioeconomic status and environmental factors.

1. *Age.* The infection is usually contracted during infancy and early childhood. Otherwise, there is no age bar.
2. *Sex.* As far as sex is concerned, there is general agreement that preponderance exists in the females both in number and in severity of disease.
3. *Race.* No race is immune to trachoma, but the disease is very common in Jews and comparatively less common among Negroes.
4. *Climate.* Trachoma is more common in areas with dry and dusty weather.
5. *Socioeconomic status.* The disease is more common in poor classes owing to unhygienic living conditions, overcrowding, unsanitary conditions, abundant fly population, paucity of water, lack of materials like separate towels and handkerchiefs, and lack of education and understanding about spread of contagious diseases.
6. *Environmental factors* like exposure to dust, smoke, irritants, sunlight etc. increase the risk of contracting disease. Therefore, outdoor workers are more affected in comparison to office workers.

C. *Source of infection.* In trachoma endemic zones the main source of infection is the conjunctival discharge of the affected person. Therefore, super-imposed bacterial infections help in trans-mission of the disease by increasing the conjunctival secretions.

D. *Modes of infection.* Infection may spread from eye to eye by any of the following modes:

1. *Direct spread* of infection may occur through contact by air-borne or water-borne modes.
2. *Vector transmission* of trachoma is common through flies.
3. *Material transfer* plays an important role in the spread of trachoma. Material transfer can occur through contaminated fingers of doctors, nurses and contaminated tonometers. Other sources of material transfer of infection are use of common towel, handkerchief, bedding and *surma*-rods.

Prevalence

Trachoma is a worldwide disease but it is highly prevalent in North Africa, Middle East and certain regions of South-East Asia. It is believed to affect some 500 million people in the world. There are about 150 million cases with active trachoma and about 30 million having trichiasis, needing lid surgery. Trachoma is responsible for 15-20 percent of the world's blindness, being second only to cataract.

Clinical profile of trachoma

Incubation period of trachoma varies from 5-21 days. Onset of disease is usually insidious (subacute), however, rarely it may present in acute form.

Clinical course of trachoma is determined by the presence or absence of secondary infection. In the absence of such an infection, a pure trachoma is so mild and symptomless that the disease is usually neglected. But, mostly the picture is complicated by secondary infection and may start with typical symptoms of acute conjunctivitis. In the early stages it is clinically indistinguishable from the bacterial conjunctivitis and the term *'trachoma-dubium'* (doubtful trachoma) is sometimes used for this stage.

Natural history. In an endemic area natural history of trachoma is characterized by the development of acute disease in the first decade of life which continues with slow progression, until the disease becomes inactive in the second decade of life. The sequelae occur at least after 20 years of the disease. Thus, the peak incidence of blinding sequelae is seen in the fourth and fifth decade of life.

Symptoms

- *In the absence of secondary infection*, symptoms are minimal and include mild foreign body sensation in the eyes, occasional lacrimation, slight stickiness of the lids and scanty mucoid discharge.
- *In the presence of secondary infection*, typical symptoms of acute mucopurulent conjunctivitis develop.

Signs

A. ***Conjunctival signs***

1. *Congestion* of upper tarsal and forniceal conjunctiva.
2. *Conjunctival follicles.* Follicles (Figs. 4.8 and 4.9) look like boiled sagograins and are commonly seen on upper tarsal conjunctiva and fornix; but may also be present in the lower fornix, plica semilunaris and caruncle. Sometimes, (follicles may be seen on the bulbar conjunctiva (pathognomic of trachoma).

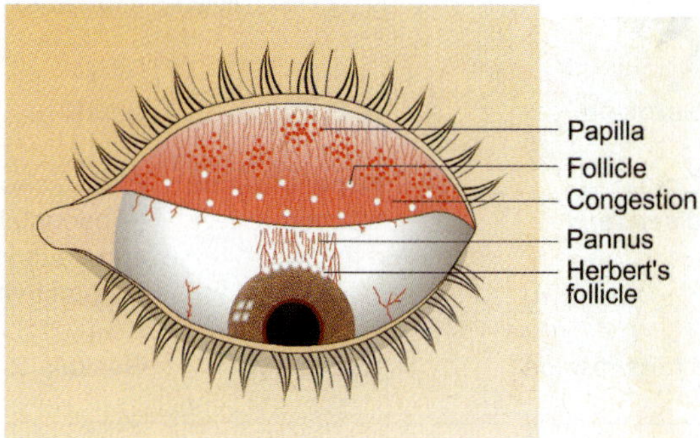

Fig. 4.8. Signs of active trachoma (diagrammatic).

Structure of follicle. Follicles are formed due to scattered aggregation of lymphocytes and other cells in the adenoid layer. Central part of each follicle is made up of mononuclear histiocytes, few lymphocytes and large multinucleated cells called *Leber cells.* The cortical part is made up of a zone of lymphocytes showing active proliferation. Blood vessels are present in the most peripheral part. In later stages signs of necrosis are also seen. Presence of Leber cells and signs of necrosis differentiate trachoma follicles from follicles of other forms of follicular conjunctivitis.

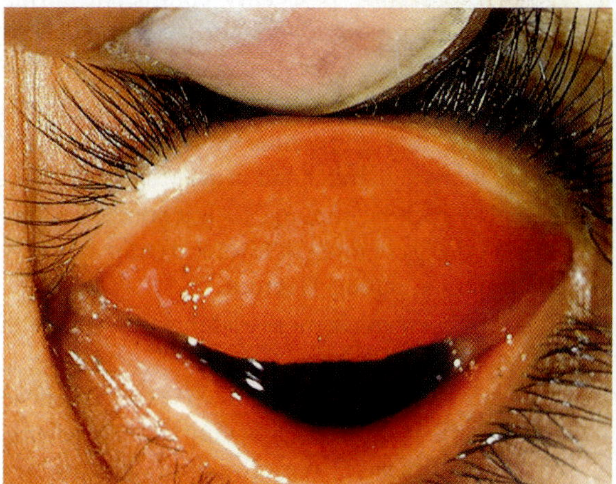

Fig. 4.9. Trachomatous inflammation follicular (TF)

3. *Papillary hyperplasia.* Papillae are reddish, flat topped raised areas which give red and velvety appearance to the tarsal conjunctiva (Fig. 4.10). Each papilla consists of central core of numerous dilated blood vessels surrounded by lymphocytes and covered by hypertrophic epithelium.

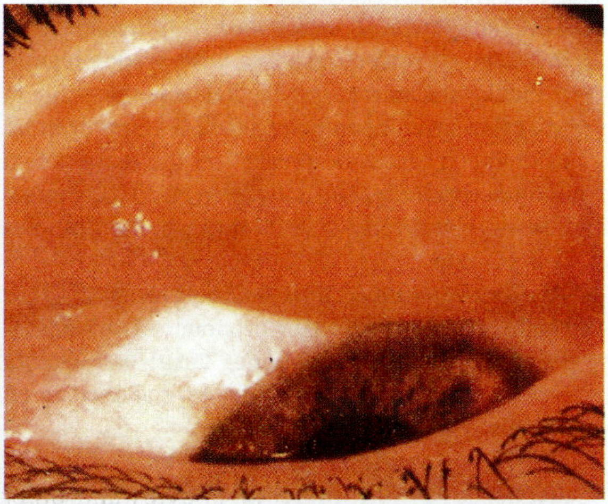

Fig. 4.10. Trachomatous inflammation intense (TI)

4. *Conjunctival scarring* (Fig. 4.11), which may be irregular, star-shaped or linear. Linear scar present in the sulcus subtarsalis is called *Arlt's line.*

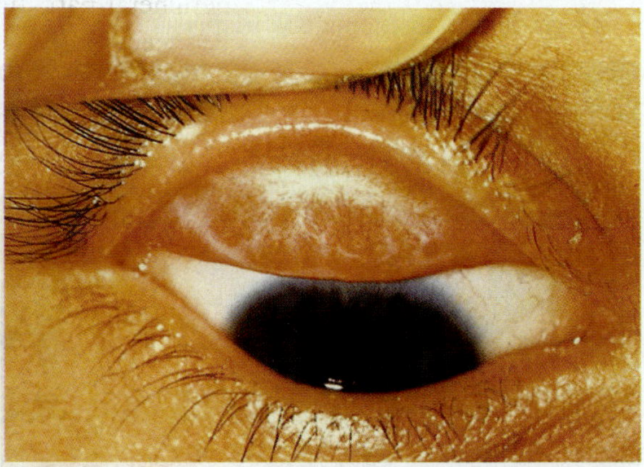

Fig. 4.11. Trachomatous scarring (TS)

5. *Concretions* are hard looking whitish deposits varying from pin point to 2mm in size (Fig. 4.12). These are not calcareous deposits, but are formed due to accumulation of dead epithelial cells and inspissated mucus in the depressions called *glands of Henle*. Hence the name is misnomer.

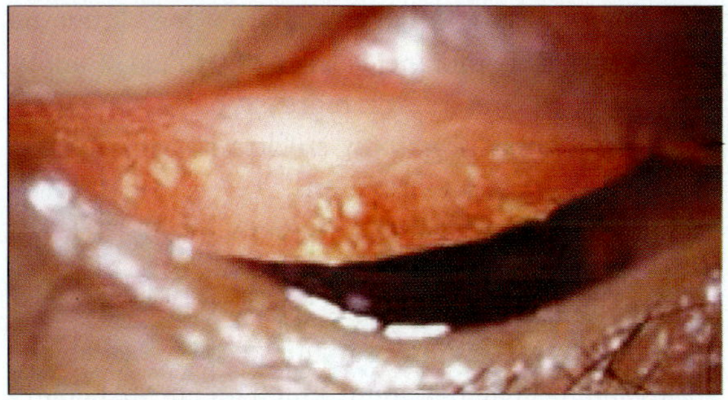

Fig. 4.12. Concretions in upper palpebral conjunctiva

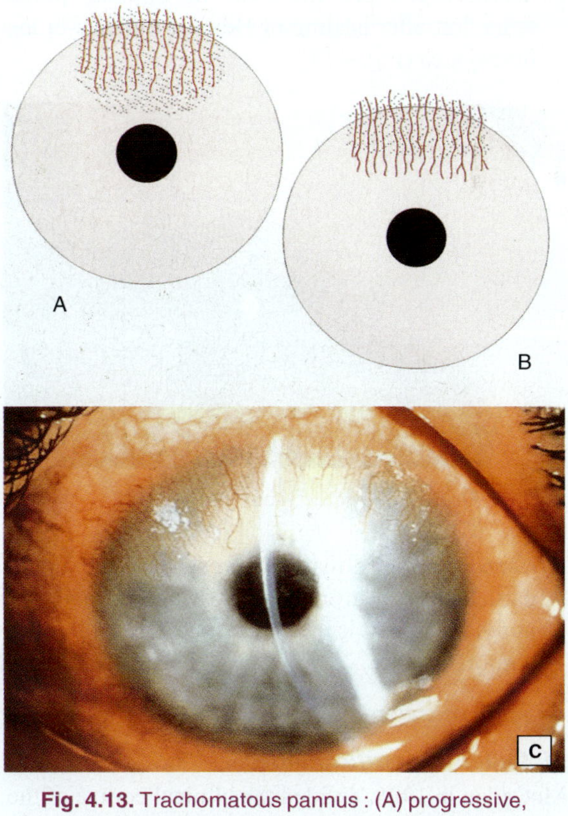

Fig. 4.13. Trachomatous pannus : (A) progressive, (B) regressive (diagrammatic) and (C) clinical photograph

B. *Corneal signs*

1. *Superficial keratitis* may be present in the upper part.
2. *Herbert follicles* refer to typical follicles present in the limbal area. These are histologically similar to conjunctival follicles.
3. *Pannus* i.e., infiltration of the cornea associated with vascularization is seen in upper part (Fig. 4.13). The vessels are superficial and lie between

epithelium and Bowman's membrane. Later on Bowman's membrane is also destroyed. Pannus may be progressive or regressive.

- In *progressive pannus,* infiltration of cornea is ahead of vascularization.
- In *regressive pannus* (pannus siccus) vessels extend a short distance beyond the area of infiltration.

4. *Corneal ulcer* may sometime develop at the advancing edge of pannus. Such ulcers are usually shallow which may become chronic and indolent.
5. *Herbert pits* are the oval or circular pitted scars, left after healing of Herbert follicles in the limbal area (Fig. 4.14).

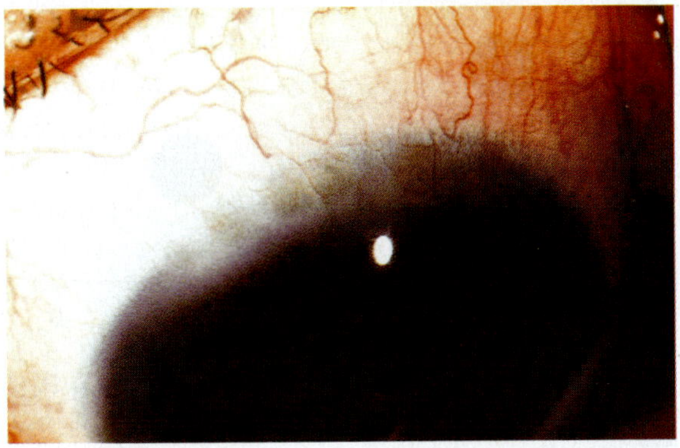

Fig. 4.14. Trachomatous Herbert's pits.

6. *Corneal opacity* may be present in the upper part. It may even extend down and involve the pupillary area. It is the end result of trachomatous corneal lesions.

Grading of trachoma

McCallan's classification

McCallan in 1908, divided the clinical course of the trachoma into four stages:

- *Stage* I (Incipient trachoma or stage of infiltration). It is characterized by hyperaemia of palpebral conjunctiva and immature follicles.
- *Stage* II (Established trachoma or stage of florid infiltration). It is characterized by appearance of mature follicles, papillae and progressive corneal pannus.
- *Stage* III (Cicatrising trachoma or stage of scarring). It includes obvious scarring of palpebral conjunctiva.
- *Stage* IV (Healed trachoma or stage of sequelae). The disease is quiet and cured but sequelae due to cicatrisation, give rise to symptoms.

WHO classification

The latest classification suggested by WHO in 1987 is as follows (FISTO):

1. *TF: Trachomatous inflammation-follicular.* It is the stage of active trachoma with predominantly follicular inflammation. To diagnose this stage at least five or more follicles (each 0.5 mm or more in diameter) must be present on the upper tarsal conjunctiva (Fig. 4.9). Further, the deep tarsal vessels should be visible through the follicles and papillae.
2. *TI: Trachomatous inflammation intense.* This stage is diagnosed when pronounced inflammatory thickening of the upper tarsal conjunctiva obscures more than half of the normal deep tarsal vessels (Fig. 4.10).
3. *TS: Trachomatous scarring.* This stage is diagnosed by the presence of scarring in the tarsal conjunctiva. These scars are easily visible as white, bands or sheets (fibrosis) in the tarsal conjunctiva (Fig. 4.11).
4. *TT: Trachomatous trichiasis.* TT is labelled when at least one eyelash rubs the eyeball. Evidence of recent removal of inturned eyelashes should also be graded as trachomatous trichiasis (Fig. 4.15).

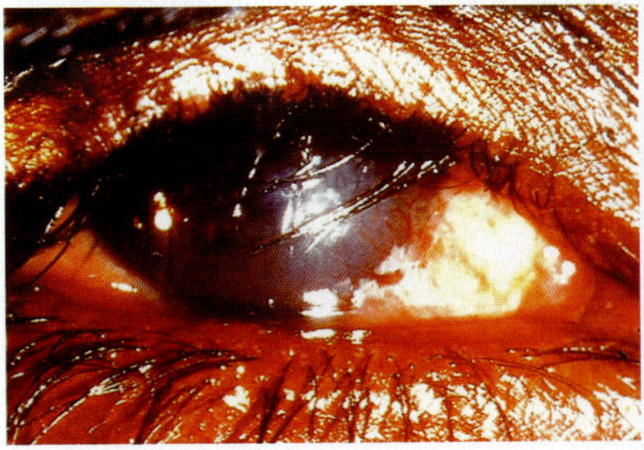

Fig. 4.15. Trachomatous trichiasis (TT).

5. *CO: Corneal opacity.* This stage is labelled when easily visible corneal opacity is present over the pupil. This sign refers to corneal scarring that is so dense that at least part of pupil margin is blurred when seen through the opacity. The

definition is intended to detect corneal opacities that cause significant visual impairment (less than 6/18).

Sequelae of trachoma

1. *Sequelae in the lids* may be trichiasis (Fig. 4.15), entropion, tylosis (thickening of lid margin), ptosis, madarosis and ankyloblepharon.
2. *Conjunctival sequelae* include concretions, pseudocyst, xerosis and symblepharon.
3. *Corneal sequelae* may be corneal opacity, ectasia, corneal xerosis and total corneal pannus (blinding sequelae).
4. *Other sequelae* may be chronic dacryocystitis, and chronic dacryoadenitis.

Complications

The only complication of trachoma is corneal ulcer which may occur due to rubbing by concretions, or trichiasis with superimposed bacterial infection.

Diagnosis

A. *Clinical diagnosis* of trachoma is made from its typical signs. Clinical grading of each case should be done as per WHO classification into TF, TI, TS, TT or CO.

B. *Laboratory diagnosis*. Advanced laboratory tests are employed for research purposes only. Laboratory diagnosis of trachoma includes :

1. *Conjunctival cytology.* Giemsa stained smears showing a predominantly polymorphonuclear reaction with presence of plasma cells and Leber cells is suggestive of trachoma.
2. *Detection of inclusion bodies* in conjunctival smear may be possible by Giemsa stain, iodine stain or immunofluorescent staining, specially in cases with active trachoma.
3. *Enzyme-linked immunosorbent assay* (ELISA) for chlamydial antigens.
4. *Polymerase chain reaction* (PCR) is also useful.
5. *Isolation of Chlamydia* is possible by yolk-sac inoculation method and tissue culture technique. Standard single-passage McCoy cell culture requires at least 3 days.
6. *Serotyping of TRIC agents* is done by detecting specific antibodies using microimmuno-fluorescence (micro-IF) method. *Direct monoclonal fluorescent antibody microscopy* of conjunctival smear is rapid and inexpensive.

Differential diagnosis

1. *Trachoma with follicular hypertrophy* must be differentiated from acute adenoviral follicular conjunctivitis (epidemic keratoconjunctivitis) as follows :

- *Distribution of follicles* in trachoma is mainly on upper palpebral conjunctiva and upper fornix, while in EKC lower palpebral conjunctiva and lower fornix is predominantly involved.
- *Associated signs* such as papillae and pannus are characteristic of trachoma.
- *Laboratory diagnosis* of trachoma helps in differentiation of clinically indistinguishable cases.

2. *Trachoma with predominant papillary hypertrophy* needs to be differentiated from palpebral form of spring catarrh as follows:

- *Papillae* are large in size and usually there is typical cobble-stone arrangement in spring catarrh.
- *pH of tears* is usually alkaline in spring catarrh, while in trachoma it is acidic,
- *Discharge* is ropy in spring catarrh.
- *Follicles and pannus* may also be present in trachoma.
- *Conjunctival cytology* and other laboratory tests for trachoma usually help in diagnosis in clinically indistinguishable cases.

Management

Management of trachoma should involve curative as well as control measures.

A. *Treatment of active trachoma*

Antibiotics for treatment of active trachoma may be given locally or systemically, but topical treatment is preferred because:

- It is cheaper,
- There is no risk of systemic side-effects, and
- Local antibiotics are also effective against bacterial conjunctivitis which may be associated with trachoma.

Therapeutic regimes recommended are:

1. *Topical therapy regimes* are best for individual cases and consist of:

- Tetracycline (1%) or erythromycin (1%) eye ointment 4 times a day for 6 weeks or

- Sulfacetamide (20%) eye drops three times a day along with 1 percent tetracycline eye ointment at bed time for 6 weeks.

  The *continuous treatment* for active trachoma should be followed by an *intermittent treatment* especially in endemic or hyperendemic area.

2. *Systemic therapy regimes* include:
- Tetracycline or erythromycin 250 mg orally, four times a day for 3-4 weeks or
- Doxycycline 100 mg orally twice daily for 3-4 weeks or
- Azithromycin 1 gm stat or 250 mg od × 4 days. It is presently considered the first drug of choice.

3. *Combined topical and systemic therapy regime.* It is preferred when the ocular infection is severe (TI) or when there is associated genital infection. It includes: (i) Tetracycline (1%) or erythromycin eye ointment 4 times a day for 6 weeks; and (ii) Tetracycline or erythromycin 250 mg orally 4 times a day for 2 weeks.

B. *Treatment of trachoma sequelae*

1. *Concretions* should be removed with a hypodermic needle.
2. *Trichiasis* may be treated by epilation, electrolysis or cryolysis (see page 370).
3. *Entropion* should be corrected surgically (see page 371).
4. *Xerosis* should be treated by artificial tears.

C. *Prophylaxis for trachoma infection*

Since, immunity is very poor and short lived, so reinfections and recurrences are likely to occur. Following prophylactic measures may be helpful against infection of trachoma.

1. *Hygienic measures.* These help a great deal in decreasing the transmission of disease, as trachoma is closely associated with personal hygiene and environmental sanitation. Therefore, health education on trachoma should be given to public. The use of common towel, handkerchief, surma rods etc. should be discouraged. A good environmental sanitation will reduce the flies. A good water supply would improve washing habits.
2. *Early treatment of conjunctivitis.* Every case of conjunctivitis should be treated as early as possible to reduce transmission of disease.
3. *Blanket antibiotic therapy (intermittent treatment).* WHO has recommended this regime to be carried out in endemic areas to minimise the intensity and severity of disease. The regime is to apply 1 percent tetracycline eye ointment twice daily for 5 days in a month for 6 months.

D. *Prevention of trachoma blindness*

(See page 478).

ADULT INCLUSION CONJUNCTIVITIS

It is a type of acute follicular conjunctivitis associated with mucopurulent discharge. It usually affects the sexually active young adults.

Etiology

Inclusion conjunctivitis is caused by serotypes D to K of *Chlamydia trachomatis*. The primary source of infection is urethritis in males and cervicitis in females. The transmission of infection may occur to eyes either through contaminated fingers or more commonly through contaminated water of swimming pools (hence the name *swimming pool conjunctivitis).*

Clinical features

Incubation period of the disease is 4-12 days.

Symptoms are similar to acute mucopurulent conjunctivitis and include:

- Ocular discomfort, foreign body sensation,
- Mild photophobia, and
- Mucopurulent discharge from the eyes.

Signs of inclusion conjunctivitis are:

- Conjunctival hyperaemia, more marked in fornices.
- Acute follicular hypertrophy predominantly of lower palpebral conjunctiva .
- Superficial keratitis in upper half of cornea. Sometimes, superior micropannus may also occur.
- Pre-auricular lymphadenopathy is a usual finding.

Clinical course. The disease runs a benign course and often evolves into the chronic follicular conjunctivitis.

Differential diagnosis must be made from other causes of acute follicular conjunctivitis.

Treatment

1. *Topical therapy.* It consists of tetracycline (1%) eye ointment 4 times a day for 6 weeks.
2. *Systemic therapy* is very important, since the condition is often associated with an asympto-

matic venereal infection. Commonly employed antibiotics are:

- Tetracycline 250 mg four times a day for 3-4 weeks, or
- Erythromycin 250 mg four times a day for 3-4 weeks (only when the tetracycline is contraindicated e.g., in pregnant and lactating females), or
- Doxycycline 100 mg twice a day for 1-2 weeks or 200 mg weekly for 3 weeks is an effective alternative to tetracycline, or
- Azithromycin 1 gm as a single dose is also effective.

Prophylaxis

Improvement in personal hygiene and regular chlorination of swimming pool water will definitely decrease the spread of disease. Patient's sexual partner should be examined and treated.

VIRAL CONJUNCTIVITIS

Most of the viral infections tend to affect the epithelium, both of the conjunctiva and cornea; so, the typical viral lesion is a 'keratoconjunctivitis'. In some viral infections, conjunctival involvement is more prominent (e.g., pharyngo-conjunctival fever), while in others cornea is more involved (e.g., herpes simplex).

Viral infections of conjunctiva include:

- Adenovirus conjunctivitis
- Herpes simplex keratoconjunctivitis
- Herpes zoster conjunctivitis
- Molluscum contagiosum conjunctivitis
- Pox virus conjunctivitis
- Myxovirus conjunctivitis
- Paramyxovirus conjunctivitis
- ARBOR virus conjunctivitis

Clinical presentations. Acute viral conjunctivitis may present in two clinical forms:

1. Acute follicular conjunctivitis
2. Acute haemorrhagic conjunctivitis

ACUTE FOLLICULAR CONJUNCTIVITIS

It is an acute catarrhal conjunctivitis associated with marked follicular hyperplasia especially of the lower fornix and lower palpebral conjunctiva.

General clinical features

Symptoms are similar to acute catarrhal conjunctivitis and include: redness, watering, mild mucoid discharge, mild photophobia and feeling of discomfort and foreign body sensation.

Signs are conjunctival hyperaemia, associated with multiple follicles, more prominent in lower lid than the upper lid (Fig. 4.16).

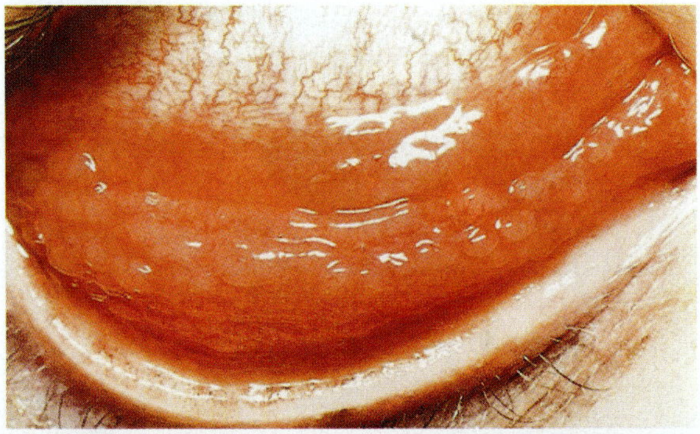

Fig. 4.16. Signs of acute follicular conjunctivitis.

Etiological types

Etiologically, acute follicular conjunctivitis is of the following types:

- Adult inclusion conjunctivitis (see page 66).
- Epidemic keratoconjunctivitis
- Pharyngoconjunctival fever
- Newcastle conjunctivitis
- Acute herpetic conjunctivitis.

Epidemic Keratoconjunctivitis (EKC)

It is a type of acute follicular conjunctivitis mostly associated with superficial punctate keratitis and usually occurs in epidemics, hence the name EKC.

Etiology. EKC is mostly caused by adenoviruses type 8 and 19. The condition is markedly contagious and spreads through contact with contaminated fingers, solutions and tonometers.

Clinical picture. *Incubation period* after infection is about 8 days and virus is shed from the inflamed eye for 2-3 weeks.

Clinical stages. The condition mainly affects young adults. Clinical picture can be arbitrarily divided into three stages for the purpose of description only.

- The first phase is of *acute serous conjunctivitis* which is characterised by non-specific conjunctival hyperaemia, mild chemosis and lacrimation.

- Soon it is followed by second phase of *typical acute follicular conjunctivitis*, characterised by formation of follicles which are more marked in lower lid (Fig. 4.16).
- In severe cases, third phase of *'acute pseudomembranous conjunctivitis'* is recognised due to formation of a pseudomembrane on the conjunctival surface (Fig. 4.17).

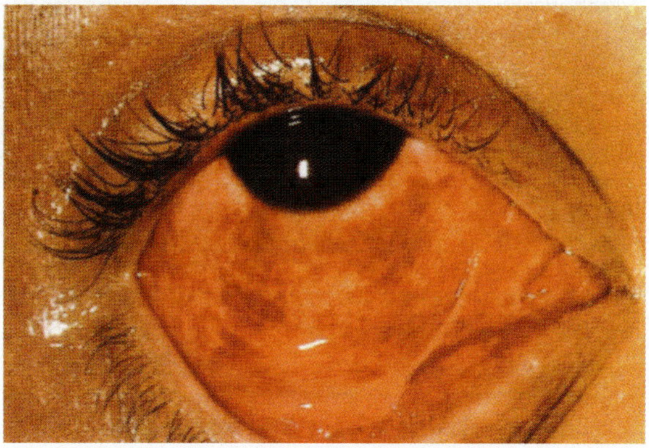

Fig. 4.17. Pseudomembrane in acute epidemic keratoconjunctivitis (EKC)

- *Corneal involvement* in the form of '*superficial punctate keratitis*', which is a distinctive feature of EKC, becomes apparent after 1 week of the onset of disease.
- *Preauricular lymphadenopathy* is associated in almost all cases.

Treatment. It is usually supportive. Antiviral drugs are ineffective. Recently, promising results are reported with adenine arabinoside (Ara-A). Corticosteroids should not be used during active stage.

Pharyngoconjunctival fever (PCF)

Etiology. It is an adenoviral infection commonly associated with subtypes 3 and 7.

Clinical picture. Pharyngoconjunctival fever is characterised by an acute follicular conjunctivitis, associated with pharyngitis, fever and preauricular lymphadenopathy. The disease primarily affects children and appears in epidemic form. Corneal involvement in the form of superficial punctate keratitis is seen only in 30 percent of cases.

Treatment is usually supportive.

Newcastle conjunctivitis

Etiology. It is a rare type of acute follicular conjunctivitis caused by Newcastle virus. The infection is derived from contact with diseased owls; and thus the condition mainly affects poultry workers.

Clinically the condition is similar to pharyngoconjunctival fever.

Acute herpetic conjunctivitis

Acute herpetic follicular conjunctivitis is always an accompaniment of the 'primary herpetic infection', which mainly occurs in small children and in adolescents.

Etiology. The disease is commonly caused by herpes simplex virus type 1 and spreads by kissing or other close personal contacts. HSV type 2 associated with genital infections, may also involve the eyes in adults as well as children, though rarely.

Clinical picture. Acute herpetic follicular conjunctivitis is usually a unilateral affection with an incubation period of 3-10 days. It may occur in two clinical forms the typical and atypical.

- In *typical form,* the follicular conjunctivitis is usually associated with other lesions of primary infection such as vesicular lesions of face and lids.
- In *atypical form,* the follicular conjunctivitis occurs without lesions of the face, eyelid and the condition then resembles epidemic keratoconjunctivitis. The condition may evolve through phases of non-specific hyperaemia, follicular hyperplasia and pseudomembrane formation.
- *Corneal involvement,* though rare, is not uncommon in primary herpes. It may be in the form of fine or coarse epithelial keratitis or typical dendritic keratitis.
- *Preauricular lymphadenopathy* occurs almost always.

Treatment. Primary herpetic infection is usually self-limiting. The topical antiviral drugs control the infection effectively and prevent recurrences.

ACUTE HAEMORRHAGIC CONJUNCTIVITIS

It is an acute inflammation of conjunctiva characterised by multiple conjunctival haemorrhages, conjunctival hyperaemia and mild follicular hyperplasia.

Etiology. The disease is caused by picornaviruses (enterovirus type 70) which are RNA viruses of small (pico) size. The disease is very contagious and is transmitted by direct hand-to-eye contact.

Clinical picture. The disease has occurred in an epidemic form in the far East, Africa and England and hence the name 'epidemic haemorrhagic conjunctivitis (EHC)' has been suggested. An epidemic of the disease was first recognized in Ghana in 1969 at the time when Apollo XI spacecraft was launched, hence the name 'Apollo conjunctivitis'.

- *Incubation period* of EHC is very short (1-2 days).
- *Symptoms* include pain, redness, watering, mild photophobia, transient blurring of vision and lid swelling.
- *Signs* of EHC are conjunctival congestion, chemosis, multiple haemorrhages in bulbar conjunctiva, mild follicular hyperplasia, lid oedema and pre-auricular lymphadenopathy. (Fig. 4.18)

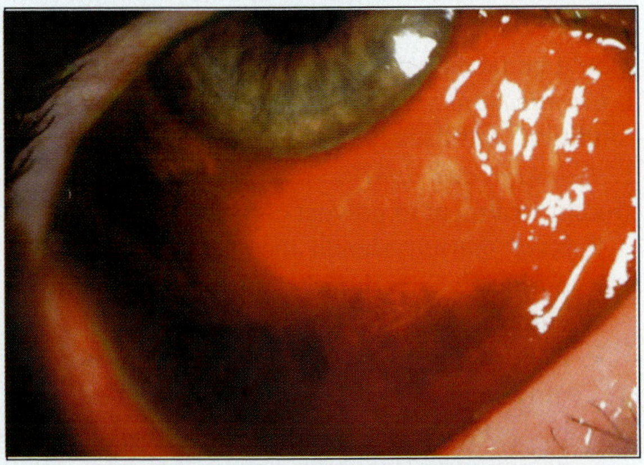

Fig. 4.18. Acute haemorrhagic conjunctivitis

- *Corneal involvement* may occur in the form of fine epithelial keratitis.

Treatment. EHC is very infectious and poses major potential problems of cross-infection. Therefore, prophylactic measures are very important. No specific effective curative treatment is known. However, broad spectrum antibiotic eye drops may be used to prevent secondary bacterial infections. Usually the disease has a self-limiting course of 5-7 days.

OPHTHALMIA NEONATORUM

Ophthalmia neonatorum is the name given to bilateral inflammation of the conjunctiva occurring in an infant, less than 30 days old. It is a preventable disease usually occurring as a result of carelessness at the time of birth. As a matter of fact *any discharge or even watering from the eyes in the first week of life should arouse suspicion of ophthalmia neonatorum,* as tears are not formed till then.

Etiology

Source and mode of infection

Infection may occur in three ways: before birth, during birth or after birth.

1. *Before birth* infection is very rare through infected liquor amnii in mothers with ruptured membrances.
2. *During birth.* It is the most common mode of infection from the infected birth canal especially when the child is born with face presentation or with forceps.
3. *After birth.* Infection may occur during first bath of newborn or from soiled clothes or fingers with infected lochia.

Causative agents

1. *Chemical conjunctivitis* It is caused by silver nitrate or antibiotics used for prophylaxis.
2. *Gonococcal infection* was considered a serious disease in the past, as it used to be responsible for 50 per cent of blindness in children. But, recently the decline in the incidence of gonorrhoea as well as effective methods of prophylaxis and treatment have almost eliminated it in developed countries. However, in many developing countries it still continues to be a problem.
3. *Other bacterial infections,* responsible for ophthalmia neonatorum are *Staphylococcus aureus*, *Streptococcus haemolyticus*, and *Streptococcus pneumoniae*.
4. *Neonatal inclusion conjunctivitis* caused by serotypes D to K of *Chlamydia trachomatis* is the commonest cause of ophthalmia neonatorum in developed countries.
5. *Herpes simplex ophthalmia neonatorum* is a rare condition caused by herpes simplex-II virus.

Clinical features

Incubation period

It varies depending on the type of the causative agent as shown below:

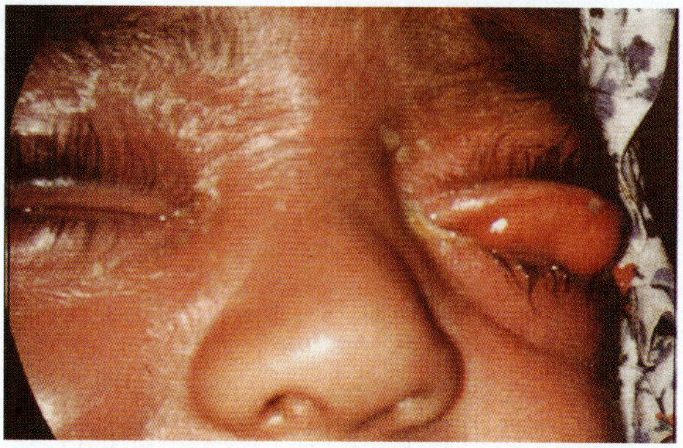

Fig. 4.19. Ophthalmia neonatorum.

	Causative agent	*Incubation period*
1.	Chemical	4-6 hours
2.	Gonococcal	2-4 days
3.	Other bacterial	4-5 days
4.	Neonatal inclusion conjunctivitis	5-14 days
5.	Herpes simplex	5-7 days

Symptoms and signs (Fig. 4.19)

1. *Pain* and *tenderness* in the eyeball.
2. *Conjunctival discharge*. It is purulent in gonococcal ophthalmia neonatorum and mucoid or mucopurulent in other bacterial cases and neonatal inclusion conjunctivitis.
3. *Lids* are usually swollen.
4. *Conjunctiva* may show hyperaemia and chemosis. There might be mild papillary response in neonatal inclusion conjunctivitis and herpes simplex ophthalmia neonatorum.
5. *Corneal involvement*, though rare, may occur in the form of superficial punctate keratitis especially in herpes simplex ophthalmia neonatorum.

Complications

Untreated cases, especially of gonococcal ophthalmia neonatorum, may develop corneal ulceration, which may perforate rapidly resulting in corneal opacification or staphyloma formation.

Treatment

Prophylactic treatment is always better than curative.

A. *Prophylaxis* needs antenatal, natal and postnatal care.

1. *Antenatal measures* include thorough care of mother and treatment of genital infections when suspected.
2. *Natal measures* are of utmost importance, as mostly infection occurs during childbirth.
   - Deliveries should be conducted under hygienic conditions taking all aseptic measures.
   - The newborn baby's closed lids should be thoroughly cleansed and dried.
3. *Postnatal measures* include :
   - Use of either 1 percent tetracycline ointment or 0.5 percent erythromycin ointment or 1 percent silver nitrate solution (Crede's method) into the eyes of the babies immediately after birth.
   - Single injection of ceftriaxone 50 mg/kg IM or IV (not to exceed 125 mg) should be given to infants born to mothers with untreated gonococcal infection.

B. *Curative treatment.* As a rule, conjunctival cytology samples and culture sensitivity swabs should be taken before starting the treatment.

1. *Chemical ophthalmia neonatorum* is a self-limiting condition, and does not require any treatment.

2. *Gonococcal ophthalmia neonatorum* needs prompt treatment to prevent complications.

i. *Topical therapy* should include :
   - *Saline lavage* hourly till the discharge is eliminated.
   - *Bacitracin eye ointment* 4 times/day. Because of resistant strains topical penicillin therapy is not reliable. However in cases with proved penicillin susceptibility, penicillin drops 5000 to 10000 units per ml should be instilled every minute for half an hour, every five minutes for next half an hour and then half hourly till the infection is controlled.
   - If cornea is involved then atropine sulphate ointment should be applied.

ii. *Systemic therapy*. Neonates with gonococcal ophthalmia should be treated for 7 days with one of the following regimes:
   - Ceftriaxone 75-100 mg/kg/day IV or IM, QID or
   - Cefotaxime 100-150 mg/kg/day IV or IM, 12 hourly or
   - Ciprofloxacin 10-20 mg/kg/day or Norfloxacin 10 mg/kg/day or

- If the gonococcal isolate is proved to be susceptible to penicillin, crystalline benzyl penicillin G 50,000 units to full term, normal weight babies and 20,000 units to premature or low weight babies should be given intramuscularly twice daily for 3 days.

3. *Other bacterial ophthalmia neonatorum* should be treated by broad spectrum antibiotic drops and ointments for 2 weeks.

4. *Neonatal inclusion conjunctivitis* responds well to topical tetracycline 1 per cent or erythromycin 0.5 per cent eye ointment QID for 3 weeks. However, systemic erythromycin (125 mg orally, QID for 3 weeks should also be given since the presence of chlamydia agents in the conjunctiva implies colonization of upper respiratory tract as well. Both parents should also be treated with systemic erythromycin.

5. *Herpes simplex conjunctivitis* is usually a self-limiting disease. However, topical antiviral drugs control the infection more effectively and may prevent the recurrence.

GRANULOMATOUS CONJUNCTIVITIS

Granulomatous conjunctivitis is the term used to describe certain specific chronic inflammations of the conjunctiva, characterised by proliferative lesions which usually tend to remain localized to one eye and are mostly associated with regional lymphadenitis.

Common granulomatous conjunctival inflammations are:

- Tuberculosis of conjunctiva
- Sarcoidosis of conjunctiva
- Syphilitic conjunctivitis
- Leprotic conjunctivitis
- Conjunctivitis in tularaemia
- Ophthalmia nodosa

Parinaud's oculoglandular syndrome

It is the name given to a group of conditions characterised by:

1. Unilateral granulomatous conjunctivitis (nodular elevations surrounded by follicles),
2. Preauricular lymphadenopathy, and
3. Fever.

Its common ***causes*** are tularaemia, cat-scratch disease, tuberculosis, syphilis and lymphogranuloma venereum.

This term (Parinaud's oculoglandular syndrome) is largely obsolete, since the infecting agents can now be usually determined.

Ophthalmia nodosa (Caterpillar hair conjunctivitis)

It is a granulomatous inflammation of the conjunctiva characterized by formation of a nodule on the bulbar conjunctiva in response to irritation caused by the retained *hair of caterpillar*. The disease is, therefore, common in summers. The condition may be often mistaken for a tubercular nodule.

Histopathological examination reveals hair surrounded by giant cells and lymphocytes.

Treatment consists of excision biopsy of the nodule.

B. Allergic Conjunctivitis

It is the inflammation of conjunctiva due to allergic or hypersensitivity reactions which may be immediate (humoral) or delayed (cellular). The conjunctiva is ten times more sensitive than the skin to allergens.

Types

1. Simple allergic conjunctivitis
   - Hay fever conjunctivitis
   - Seasonal allergic conjunctivitis (SAC)
   - Perennial allergic conjunctivitis (PAC)
2. Vernal keratoconjunctivitis (VKC)
3. Atopic keratoconjunctivitis (AKC)
4. Giant papillary conjunctivitis (GPC)
5. Phlyctenular keratoconjunctivitis (PKC)
6. Contact dermoconjunctivitis (CDC)

SIMPLE ALLERGIC CONJUNCTIVITIS

It is a mild, non-specific allergic conjunctivitis characterized by itching, hyperaemia and mild papillary response. Basically, it is an acute or subacute urticarial reaction.

Etiology

It is seen in following forms:

1. *Hay fever conjunctivitis*. It is commonly associated with hay fever (allergic rhinitis). The common allergens are pollens, grass and animal dandruff.
2. *Seasonal allergic conjunctivitis* (SAC). SAC is a response to seasonal allergens such as grass pollens. It is of very common occurrence.

3. *Perennial allergic conjunctivitis (PAC)* is a response to perennial allergens such as house dust and mite. It is not so common.

Pathology

Pathological features of simple allergic conjunctivitis comprise vascular, cellular and conjunctival responses.

1. *Vascular response* is characterised by sudden and extreme vasodilation and increased permeability of vessels leading to exudation.
2. *Cellular response* is in the form of conjunctival infiltration and exudation in the discharge of eosinophils, plasma cells and mast cells producing histamine and histamine-like substances.
3. *Conjunctival response* is in the form of boggy swelling of conjunctiva followed by increased connective tissue formation and mild papillary hyperplasia.

Clinical picture

Symptoms include intense itching and burning sensation in the eyes associated with watery discharge and mild photophobia.

Signs. (a) *Hyperaemia and chemosis* which give a swollen juicy appearance to the conjunctiva. (b) Conjunctiva may also show mild papillary reaction. (c) Oedema of lids.

Diagnosis

Diagnosis is made from : (1) typical symptoms and signs; (2) normal conjunctival flora; and (3) presence of abundant eosinophils in the discharge.

Treatment

1. *Elimination of allergens* if possible.
2. *Local palliative measures* which provide immediate relief include:
   i. *Vasoconstrictors* like adrenaline, ephedrine, and naphazoline.
   ii. *Sodium cromoglycate* drops are very effective in preventing recurrent atopic cases.
   iii. *Steroid eye drops* should be avoided. However, these may be prescribed for short duration in severe and non-responsive patients.
3. *Systemic antihistaminic drugs* are useful in acute cases with marked itching.
4. *Desensitization* has been tried without much rewarding results. However, a trial may be given in recurrent cases.

VERNAL KERATOCONJUNCTIVITIS (VKC) OR SPRING CATARRH

It is a recurrent, bilateral, interstitial, self-limiting, allergic inflammation of the conjunctiva having a periodic seasonal incidence.

Etiology

It is considered a hypersensitivity reaction to some exogenous allergen, such as grass pollens. VKC is thought to be an atopic allergic disorder in many cases, in which IgE-mediated mechanisms play an important role. Such patients may give personal or family history of other atopic diseases such as hay fever, asthma or eczema and their peripheral blood shows eosinophilia and increased serum IgE levels.

Predisposing factors

1. *Age and sex.* 4-20 years; more common in boys than girls.
2. *Season.* More common in summer; hence the name spring catarrh seems to be a misnomer. Recently it is being labelled as '*Warm weather conjunctivitis*'.
3. *Climate.* More prevalent in tropics, less in temperate zones and almost non-existent in cold climate.

Pathology

1. *Conjunctival epithelium* undergoes hyperplasia and sends downward projections into the subepithelial tissue.
2. *Adenoid layer* shows marked cellular infiltration by eosinophils, plasma cells, lymphocytes and histiocytes.
3. *Fibrous layer* shows proliferation which later on undergoes hyaline changes.
4. *Conjunctival vessels* also show proliferation, increased permeability and vasodilation.

All these pathological changes lead to formation of multiple papillae in the upper tarsal conjunctiva.

Clinical picture

Symptoms. Spring catarrh is characterised by marked burning and itching sensation which is usually intolerable and accentuated when patient comes in a warm humid atmosphere. Itching is more marked with palpebral form of disease.

Other associated symptoms include: mild photophobia, lacrimation, stringy (ropy) discharge and heaviness of lids.

Signs of vernal keratoconjunctivitis can be described in following three clinical forms:

1. *Palpebral form.* Usually upper tarsal conjunctiva of both eyes is involved. The typical lesion is characterized by the presence of hard, flat topped, papillae arranged in a '*cobble-stone*' or '*pavement stone*', fashion (Fig. 4.20). In severe cases, papillae may hypertrophy to produce cauliflower like excrescences of 'giant papillae'. Conjunctival changes are associated with white ropy discharge.
2. *Bulbar form.* It is characterised by: (i) dusky red triangular congestion of bulbar conjunctiva in palpebral area; (ii) gelatinous thickened accumulation of tissue around the limbus; and (iii) presence of discrete whitish raised dots along the limbus (Tranta's spots) (Fig. 4.21).
3. *Mixed form.* It shows combined features of both palpebral and bulbar forms (Fig. 4.22).

Vernal keratopathy. Corneal involvement in VKC may be primary or secondary due to extension of limbal lesions. Vernal keratopathy includes following 5 types of lesions:

1. *Punctate epithelial keratitis* involving upper cornea is usually associated with palpebral form of disease. The lesions always stain with rose bengal and invariably with fluorescein dye.
2. *Ulcerative vernal keratitis* (*shield ulceration*) presents as a shallow transverse ulcer in upper part of cornea. The ulceration results due to epithelial macroerosions. It is a serious problem which may be complicated by bacterial keratitis.
3. *Vernal corneal plaques* result due to coating of bare areas of epithelial macroerosions with a layer of altered exudates (Fig. 4.23).
4. *Subepithelial scarring* occurs in the form of a ring scar.
5. *Pseudogerontoxon* is characterised by a classical 'cupid's bow' outline.

Clinical course of disease is often self-limiting and usually burns out spontaneously after 5-10 years.

Differential diagnosis. Palpebral form of VKC needs to be differentiated from trachoma with pre-dominant papillary hypertrophy (see page 65).

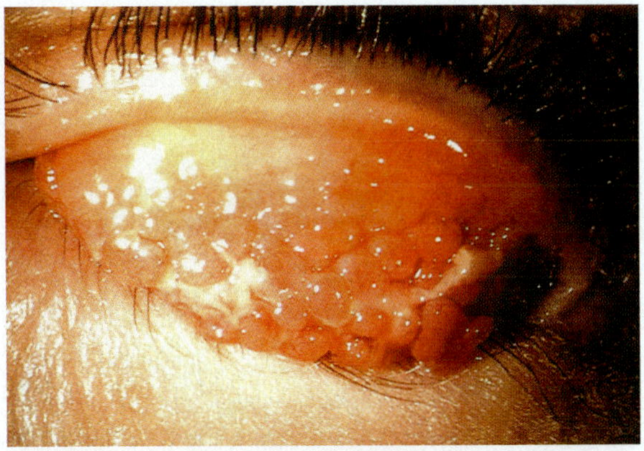

Fig. 4.20. Palpebral form of vernal keratoconjunctivitis.

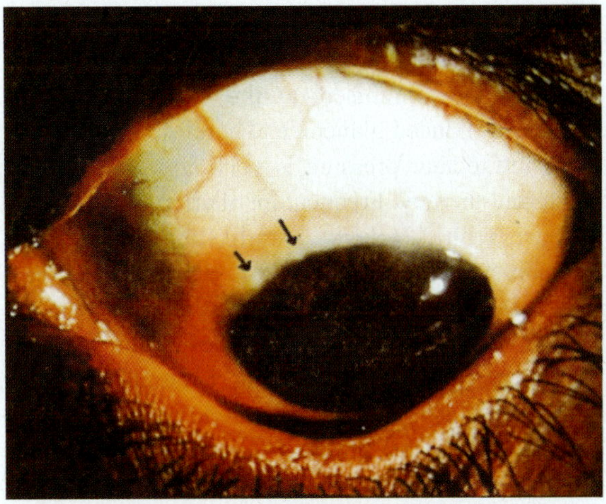

Fig. 4.21. Bulbar form of vernal keratoconjunctivitis.

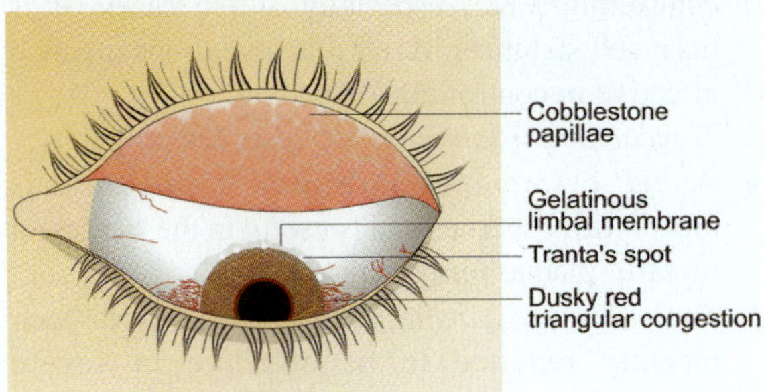

Fig. 4.22. Artist's diagram of mixed form of vernal keratoconjunctivitis.

Treatment

A. *Local therapy*

1. *Topical steroids.* These are effective in all forms of spring catarrh. However, their use

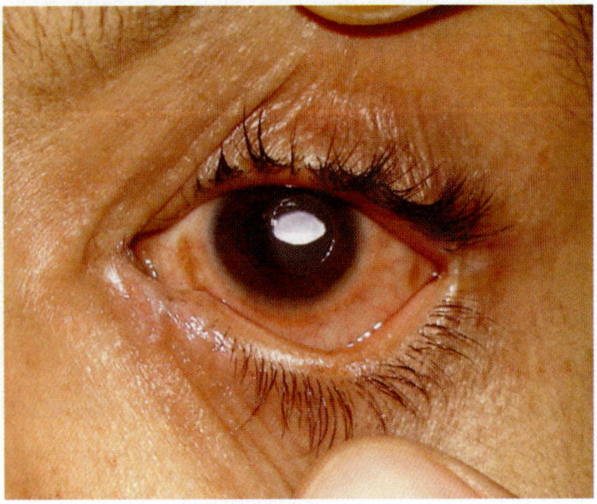

Fig. 4.23. Vernal corneal plaque.

should be minimised, as they frequently cause steroid induced glaucoma. Therefore, monitoring of intraocular pressure is very important during steroid therapy. Frequent instillation (4 hourly) to start with (2 days) should be followed by maintenance therapy for 3-4 times a day for 2 weeks.

Commonly used steroid solutions are of fluorometholone medrysone, betamethasone or dexamethasone. Medrysone and fluorometholone are safest of all these.

2. *Mast cell stabilizers* such as sodium cromoglycate (2%) drops 4-5 times a day are quite effective in controlling VKC, especially atopic cases. It is mast cell stabilizer. Azelastine eye drops are also effective in controlling VKC.
3. *Topical antihistaminics* are also effective.
4. *Acetyl cysteine* (0.5%) used topically has mucolytic properties and is useful in the treatment of early plaque formation.
5. *Topical cyclosporine* (1%) drops have been recently reported to be effective in severe unresponsive cases.

B. *Systemic therapy*

1. *Oral antihistaminics* may provide some relief from itching in severe cases.
2. *Oral steroids* for a short duration have been recommended for advanced, very severe, non-responsive cases.

C. *Treatment of large papillae.* Very large (giant) papillae can be tackled either by :

- *Supratarsal injection* of long acting steroid, or
- Cryo application
- Surgical excision is recommended for extra-ordinarily large papillae.

D. *General measures* include :

- Dark goggles to prevent photophobia.
- Cold compresses and ice packs have soothing effects.
- Change of place from hot to cold area is recommended for recalcitrant cases.

E. *Desensitization* has also been tried without much rewarding results.

F. *Treatment of vernal keratopathy*

- *Punctate epithelial keratitis* requires no extra treatment except that instillation of steroids should be increased.
- *A large vernal plaque* requires surgical excision by superficial keratectomy.
- *Severe shield ulcer* resistant to medical therapy may need surgical treatment in the form of debridment, superficial keratectomy, excimer laser therapeutic kerateotomy as well as amniotic membrane transplantation to enhance re-epithelialization.

Atopic keratoconjunctivitis (AKC)

It can be thought of as an adult equivalent of vernal keratoconjunctivitis and is often associated with atopic dermatitis. Most of the patients are young atopic adults, with male predominance.

Symptoms include:

- Itching, soreness, dry sensation.
- Mucoid discharge.
- Photophobia or blurred vision.

Signs

- *Lid margins* are chronically inflamed with rounded posterior borders.
- *Tarsal conjunctiva* has a milky appearance. There are very fine papillae, hyperaemia and scarring with shrinkage.
- *Cornea* may show punctate epithelial keratitis, often more severe in lower half. There may also occur corneal vascularization, thinning and plaques.

Clinical course. Like the dermatitis with which it is associated, AKC has a protracted course with exacerbations and remissions. Like vernal kerato-conjunctivitis it tends to become inactive when patient reaches the fifth decade.

Associations may be keratoconus and atopic cataract.

Treatment is often frustrating.

- Treat facial eczema and lid margin disease.
- Sodium cromoglycate drops, steroids and tear supplements may be helpful for conjunctival lesions.

GIANT PAPILLARY CONJUNCTIVITIS (GPC)

It is the inflammation of conjunctiva with formation of very large sized papillae.

Etiology. It is a localised allergic response to a physically rough or deposited surface (contact lens, prosthesis, left out nylon sutures). Probably it is a sensitivity reaction to components of the plastic leached out by the action of tears.

Symptoms. Itching, stringy discharge and reduced wearing time of contact lens or prosthetic shell.

Signs. Papillary hypertrophy (1 mm in diameter) of the upper tarsal conjunctiva, similar to that seen in palpebral form of VKC with hyperaemia are the main signs (Fig. 4.24).

Treatment

1. *The offending cause should be removed.* After discontinuation of contact lens or artificial eye or removal of nylon sutures, the papillae resolve over a period of one month.

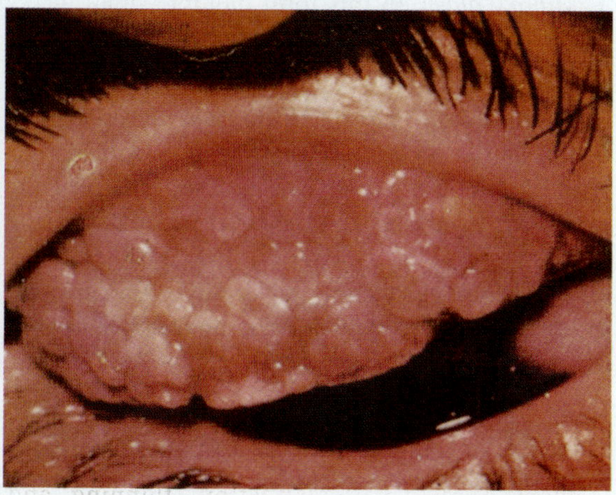

Fig. 4.24. Giant papillary conjunctivities (GPC).

2. *Disodium cromoglycate* is known to relieve the symptoms and enhance the rate of resolution.
3. *Steroids* are not of much use in this condition.

PHLYCTENULAR KERATOCONJUNCTIVITIS

Phlyctenular keratoconjunctivitis is a characteristic nodular affection occurring as an allergic response of the conjunctival and corneal epithelium to some endogenous allergens to which they have become sensitized. Phlyctenular conjunctivitis is of worldwide distribution. However, its incidence is higher in developing countries.

Etiology

It is believed to be a delayed hypersensitivity (Type IV-cell mediated) response to endogenous microbial proteins.

I. *Causative allergens*

1. *Tuberculous proteins* were considered, previously, as the most common cause.
2. *Staphylococcus proteins* are now thought to account for most of the cases.
3. *Other allergens* may be proteins of Moraxella Axenfeld bacillius and certain parasites (worm infestation).

II. *Predisposing factors*

1. *Age.* Peak age group is 3-15 years.
2. *Sex.* Incidence is higher in girls than boys.
3. *Undernourishment.* Disease is more common in undernourished children.
4. *Living conditions.* Overcrowded and unhygienic.
5. *Season.* It occurs in all climates but incidence is high in spring and summer seasons.

Pathology

1. *Stage of nodule formation.* In this stage there occurs exudation and infiltration of leucocytes into the deeper layers of conjunctiva leading to a nodule formation. The central cells are polymorphonuclear and peripheral cells are lymphocytes. The neighbouring blood vessels dilate and their endothelium proliferates.
2. *Stage of ulceration.* Later on necrosis occurs at the apex of the nodule and an ulcer is formed. Leucocytic infiltration increases with plasma cells and mast cells.

3. *Stage of granulation.* Eventually floor of the ulcer becomes covered by granulation tissue.
4. *Stage of healing.* Healing occurs usually with minimal scarring.

Clinical picture

Symptoms in simple phlyctenular conjunctivitis are few, like mild discomfort in the eye, irritation and reflex watering. However, usually there is associated mucopurulent conjunctivitis due to secondary bacterial infection.

Signs. The phlyctenular conjunctivitis can present in three forms: simple, necrotizing and miliary.

1. *Simple phylctenular conjunctivitis.* It is the most commonly seen variety. It is characterised by the presence of a typical pinkish white nodule surrounded by hyperaemia on the bulbar conjunctiva, usually near the limbus. Most of the times there is solitary nodule but at times there may be two nodules (Fig. 4.25). In a few days the nodule ulcerates at apex which later on gets epithelised. Rest of the conjunctiva is normal.

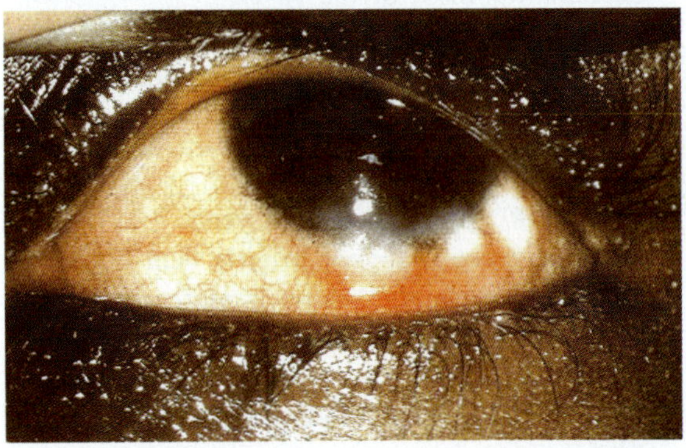

Fig. 4.25. Phylctenular conjunctivitis.

2. *Necrotizing phlyctenular conjunctivitis* is characterised by the presence of a very large phlycten with necrosis and ulceration leading to a severe pustular conjunctivitis.
3. *Miliary phlyctenular conjunctivitis* is characterised by the presence of multiple phlyctens which may be arranged haphazardly or in the form of a ring around the limbus and may even form a ring ulcer.

Phlyctenular keratitis. Corneal involvement may occur secondarily from extension of conjunctival phlycten; or rarely as a primary disease. It may present in two forms: the 'ulcerative phlyctenular keratitis' or 'diffuse infiltrative keratitis'.

A. *Ulcerative phlyctenular keratitis* may occur in the following three forms:

1. *Sacrofulous ulcer* is a shallow marginal ulcer formed due to breakdown of small limbal phlycten. It differs from the catarrhal ulcer in that there is no clear space between the ulcer and the limbus and its long axis is frequently perpendicular to limbus. Such an ulcer usually clears up without leaving any opacity.
2. *Fascicular ulcer* has a prominent parallel leash of blood vessels (Fig. 4.26). This ulcer usually remains superficial but leaves behind a band-shaped superficial opacity after healing.

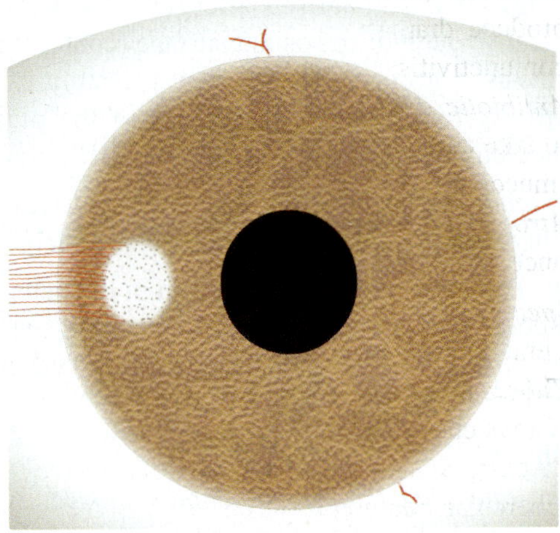

Fig. 4.26. Fascicular corneal ulcer.

3. *Miliary ulcer.* In this form multiple small ulcers are scattered over a portion of or whole of the cornea.

B. *Diffuse infiltrative phlyctenular keratitis* may appear in the form of central infiltration of cornea with characteristic rich vascularization from the periphery, all around the limbus. It may be superficial or deep.

Clinical course is usually self-limiting and phlycten disappears in 8-10 days leaving no trace. However, recurrences are very common.

Differential diagnosis

Phlyctenular conjunctivitis needs to be differentiated from the *episcleritis, scleritis,* and conjunctival *foreign body granuloma.*

Presence of one or more whitish raised nodules on the bulbar conjunctiva near the limbus, with hyperaemia usually of the surrounding conjunctiva, in a child living in bad hygienic conditions (most of the times) are the diagnostic features of the phlyctenular conjunctivitis.

Management

It includes treatment of phlyctenular conjunctivitis by local therapy, investigations and specific therapy aimed at eliminating the causative allergen and general measures to improve the health of the child.

1. *Local therapy*.

i. *Topical steroids,* in the form of eye drops or ointment (dexamethasone or betamethasone) produce dramatic effect in phlyctenular kerato-conjunctivitis.

ii. *Antibiotic drops* and ointment should be added to take care of the associated secondary infection (mucopurulent conjunctivitis).

iii. *Atropine (1%)* eye ointment should be applied once daily when cornea is involved.

2. *Specific therapy*. Attempts must be made to search and eradicate the following causative conditions:

i. *Tuberculous* infection should be excluded by X-rays chest, Mantoux test, TLC, DLC and ESR. In case, a tubercular focus is discovered, anti-tubercular treatment should be started to combat the infection.

ii. *Septic focus,* in the form of tonsillitis, adenoiditis, or caries teeth, when present should be adequately treated by systemic antibiotics and necessary surgical measures.

iii. *Parasitic infestation* should be ruled out by repeated stool examination and when discovered should be adequately treated for complete eradication.

3. *General measures* aimed to improve the health of child are equally important. Attempts should be made to provide high protein diet supplemented with vitamins A, C and D.

CONTACT DERMOCONJUNCTIVITIS

It is an allergic disorder, involving conjunctiva and skin of lids along with surrounding area of face.

Etiology

It is in fact a delayed hypersensitivity (type IV) response to prolonged contact with chemicals and drugs. A few common topical ophthalmic medications known to produce contact dermoconjunctivitis are atropine, penicillin, neomycin, soframycin and gentamycin.

Clinical picture

1. *Cutaneous involvement* is in the form of weeping eczematous reaction, involving all areas with which medication comes in contact.
2. *Conjunctival response* is in the form of hyperaemia with a generalised papillary response affecting the lower fornix and lower palpebral conjunctiva more than the upper.

Diagnosis is made from:

- Typical clinical picture.
- Conjunctival cytology shows a lymphocytic response with masses of eosinophils.
- Skin test to the causative allergen is positive in most of the cases.

Treatment consists of:

1. Discontinuation of the causative medication,
2. Topical steroid eye drops to relieve symptoms, and
3. Application of steroid ointment on the involved skin.

C. Cicatricial Conjunctivitis

OCULAR MUCOUS MEMBRANE PEMPHIGOID (OMMP)

Etiology

- OMMP is thought to be a *type II hypersensitivity* reaction involving basement membrane of epithelial cells of conjunctiva, other mucosal surfaces and even skin.
- *Age*. Usually occurs after 60 years of age, but may occur in adolescence.
- *Sex*. Slightly more common in female than male.

Pathology

It is chronic inflammatory subepithelial blistering disease with subsequent cicatrization of the involved mucosa.

Clinical features

I. ***Ocular features***

Symptoms include insidious onset of bilateral redness, foreign body sensation, watering and photophobia

Signs progress as below:

- *Inflammatory signs* include hyperaemia, chronic papillae and subconjunctival vesicles which later ulcerate.
- *Cicatrization signs* include loss of plica semilunaris and fornices, formation of symblepharon (usually inferior and ankyloblepharon) ending in severe dry eye syndrome.
- *Corneal involvement* occurs as superficial punctate keratitis, secondary microbial keratitis, corneal neovascularization and even perforation.
- *Lid sequelae* include trichiasis and entropion formation.

II. ***Systemic features***

- Mucosa of oral cavity, anus, vagina and urethra may be involved
- Desquamative gingivitis is common association
- Cutaneous vesicles, bullae and scar formation may occur
- Involvement of trachea and esophagus is potentially life threatening

Differential diagnosis need to be made from Stevens Johnson syndrome and other cicatrizing disorders.

Treatments

I. ***Topical treatment*** comprise:

- Tear substitutes, to be used frequently
- Antibiotics for secondary infection
- Steroids may help in reducing inflammation (caution for corneal melting)

II. ***Systemic immunosuppression*** is typically required to suppress the acute phase of disease.

- *Mild disease*—use dapsone
- *Moderate disease*—use methotrexate or azathiopirone
- *Severe disease*—use intravenous methylprednisolone with or without cyclophosphamide

III. ***Surgical Intervention*** required in late stage (depending upon the condition) may be:

- Punctal occlusion
- Silicon hydrogel contact lens use
- Correction of trichiasis and entropion
- Ocular surface reconstruction for advanced scarring
- Corneal transplantation, and
- Kerotoprothesis in extensive corneal and ocular surface scarring

STEVENS-JOHNSON SYNDROME AND TOXIC EPIDERMAL NECROSIS

Stevens-Johnson syndrome (SJS) and toxic epidermal necrosis (TEN) are acute mucocutaneous blistering diseases usually associated with severe ocular complications.

Etiology

These conditions are thought to result from a type-III hypersensitivity response to certain drugs (such as sulfonamides, anticonvulsants and allopurinol) and infectious agents (such as mycoplasma, pneumoniae, herpes simplex virus and adenovirus)

Clinical features

Symptoms include acute onset of fever, skin rash, red eyes, malaise, arthralgia and respiratory tract symptoms.

Systemic signs

- Classic 'target' skin lesions are maculopapules with a red crator and white surrounding area or bullae
- Hemorrhagic inflammation of mucous membranes, e.g., hemorrhagic lip crusting
- Ulcerative stomatitis
- Sloughing of epidermal surface (seen in TEN) is called Nikolsky sign

Ocular signs

Acute disease is characterized by papillary or mucopurulant or pseudomembranous conjunctivitis, episcleritis, and iritis.

Late disease is characterized by:

- Conjunctival scarring and symblepharon formation
- Trichiasis and lid deformities
- Dry eye resulting from loss of Goblet cells and destruction of lacrimal gland ductules
- Corneal neovascularization, ulceration, perforation and scarring

Treatment

Systemic treatment in acute phase include:

- Removal (e.g. causative drugs) or treatment (e.g. of causative infection) of the inciting factor
- Intravenous immunoglobulin

- Role of systemic steroids is controversial
- Maintenance of hydration
- Debridement and replacement of sloughing skin

Ocular treatment during acute phase includes:

- Topical tear drops and prevention of exposure
- Topical antibiotics and steroid eye drops
- Daily pseudomembrane peel and symblepharon lysis with glass rod or moistened cotton swab

Late stage interventions are similar to OMMP (see page 78).

SECONDARY CICATRICIAL CONJUNCTIVITIS

Cicatricial conjunctivitis may occur secondary to:

- *Injuries* (such as thermal, radiational or chemical burns) and
- *Infective conjunctivitis* (such as trachoma and viral pseudomembranous conjunctivitis).

D. Toxic Conjunctivitis

1. *Toxic conjunctivitis secondary to molluscum contagiosum.* It is a type of chronic follicular conjunctivitis that occurs as a response to toxic cellular debris desquamated into the conjunctival sac from the molluscum contagiosum nodules present on the lid margin (the primary lesion).

2. *Chemical toxic conjunctivitis*. It is an irritative follicular conjunctival response which occurs after prolonged administration of topical medication. The common topical preparations associated with chronic follicular conjunctivitis are: idoxuridine (IDU), eserine, pilocarpine, DFP adrenaline, neomycin and preservatives including contact lens solutions.

DEGENERATIVE CONDITIONS

PINGUECULA

Pinguecula is an extremely common degenerative condition of the conjunctiva. It is characterized by formation of a yellowish-white patch on the bulbar conjunctiva near the limbus. This condition is termed pinguecula, because of its resemblance to fat, which means pinguis.

Etiology of pinguecula is not known exactly. It has been considered as *an age-change,* occurring more commonly in persons exposed to strong sunlight, dust and wind. It is also considered a precursor of pterygium.

Pathology. There is an elastotic degeneration of collagen fibres of the substantia propria of conjunctiva, coupled with deposition of amorphous hyaline material in the substance of conjunctiva.

Clinical features. Pinguecula is a bilateral, usually stationary condition, presenting as yellowish-white triangular patch near the limbus (Fig. 4.27) . Apex of the triangle is away from the cornea. It affects the nasal side first and then the temporal side. When conjunctiva is congested, it stands out as an avascular prominence.

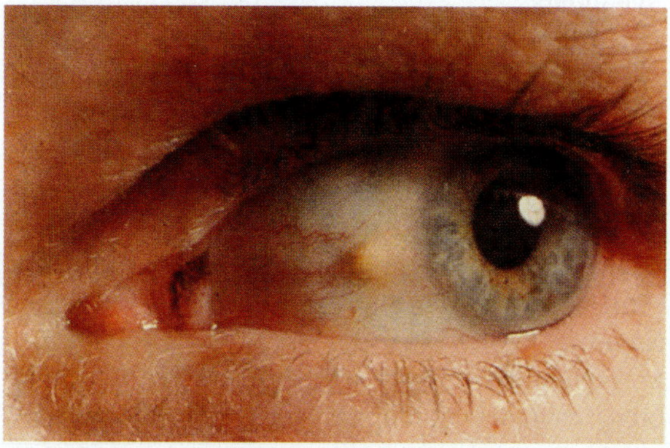

Fig. 4.27. Pinguecula.

Complications of pinguecula include its inflammation, intraepithelial abscess formation and rarely calcification and conversion into pterygium.

Treatment. In routine no treatment is required for pinguecula. However, if so desired, it may be excised. When inflamed it is treated with topical steroid.

PTERYGIUM

Pterygium (L. Pterygion = a wing) is a wing-shaped fold of conjunctiva encroaching upon the cornea from either side within the interpalpebral fissure.

Etiology. Etiology of pterygium is not definitely known. But the disease is more common in people living in hot climates. Therefore, the most accepted view is that it is a response to prolonged effect of environmental factors such as exposure to sun (ultraviolet rays), dry heat, high wind and abundance of dust.

Pathology. Pathologically pterygium is a degenerative and hyperplastic condition of conjunctiva. The subconjunctival tissue undergoes elastotic degeneration and proliferates as vascularised granulation tissue under the epithelium, which ultimately encroaches the cornea. The corneal epithelium, Bowman's layer and superficial stroma are destroyed.

Clinical features

Demography

- *Age:* Usually seen in old age
- *Sex:* More common in males doing outdoor work than females.
- *Laterality:* It may be unilateral or bilateral. Usually present on the nasal side but may also occur on the temporal side.

Symptoms

- *Cosmetic intolerance* may be the only issue in otherwise asymptomatic condition in early stages.
- *Foreign body sensation* may be experienced
- *Defective vision* occurs when it encroaches the pupillary area or due to corneal astigmatism induced by fibrosis in the regressive stage.
- *Diplopia* may occur occasionally due to limitation of ocular movements.

Signs

Pterygium presents as a triangular fold of conjunctiva encroaching on the cornea in the area of palpebral aperture usually on the nasal side (Fig. 4.28) but may also occur on the temporal side. Very rarely, both nasal and temporal sides are involved (*primary double pterygium*).

Parts of a fully developed pterygium are as follows: (Fig. 4.28):

- *Head:* Apical part present on the cornea,
- *Neck:* Constricted part present in the limbal area, and
- *Body:* Scleral part, extending between limbus and the canthus.
- *Cap:* Semilunar whitish infiltrate present just in front of the head.

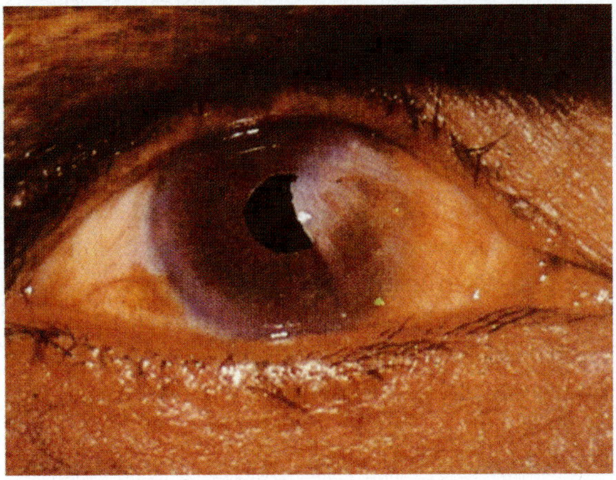

Fig. 4.28. Pterygium

Types. Depending upon the progression it may be progressive or regressive pterygium.

- *Progressive pterygium* is thick, fleshy and vascular with a few infiltrates in the cornea, in front of the head of the pterygium (called cap of pterygium).
- *Regressive pterygium* is thin, atrophic, attenuated with very little vascularity. There is no cap, but deposition of iron (Stocker's line) may be seen sometimes, just anterior to the head of pterygium. Ultimately it becomes membranous but never disappears.

Complications

- *Cystic degeneration and infection* are infrequent.
- *Neoplastic change* to epithelioma, fibrosarcoma or malignant melanoma, may occur rarely.

Differential diagnosis

Pterygium must be differentiated from pseudopterygium.

Pseudopterygium is a fold of bulbar conjunctiva attached to the cornea. It is formed due to adhesions of chemosed bulbar conjunctiva to the marginal corneal ulcer. It usually occurs following chemical burns of the eye.

Differences between pterygium and pseudopterygium are given in Table 4.3.

Table 4.3. Differences between pterygium and pseudopterygium

	Pterygium	*Pseudopterygium*
1. Etiology	Degenerative process	Inflammatory process
2. Age	Usually occurs in elder persons	Can occur at any age
3. Site	Always situated in the palpebral aperture	Can occur at any site
4. Stages	Either progressive, regressive or stationary	Always stationary
5. Probe test	Probe cannot be passed underneath	A probe can be passed under the neck

Treatment

Surgical excision is the only satisfactory treatment, which may be indicated for: (1) cosmetic reasons, (2) continued progression threatening to encroach onto the pupillary area (once the pterygium has encroached pupillary area, wait till it crosses on the other side), (3) diplopia due to interference in ocular movements.

Recurrence of the pterygium after surgical excision is the main problem (30-50%). However, it can be reduced by any of the following measures:

- *Surgical excision with free conjunctival limbal autograft* (CLAU) taken from the same eye or other eye is presently the preferred technique.
- *Surgical excision with amniotic membrane graft* and mitomycin-C (MMC) (0.02%) application may be required in recurrent pterygium or when dealing with a very large pterygium.
- *Surgical excision, with lamellar keratectomy and lamellar keratoplasty* may be required in deeply infiltrating recurrent recalcitrant pterygia.
- *Old methods to prevent recurrence* (not preferred now) included transplantation of pterygium in the lower fornix (McRaynold's operation) and postoperative use of beta irradiation.

Surgical technique of pterygium excision

1. After topical anaesthesia, eye is cleansed, draped and exposed using universal eye speculum.
2. Head of the pterygium is lifted and dissected off the cornea very meticulously (Fig. 4.29A).
3. The main mass of pterygium is then separated from the sclera underneath and the conjunctiva superficially.
4. Pterygium tissue is then excised taking care not to damage the underlying medial rectus muscle (Fig. 4.29B).
5. *Haemostasis* is achieved and the episcleral tissue exposed is cauterised thoroughly.
6. *Conjunctival limbal autograft (CLAU)* transplantation to cover the defect after pterygium excision (Fig. 4.29C). It is the latest and most effective technique in the management of pterygium.

CONCRETIONS

Etiology. Concretions are formed due to accumulation of inspissated mucus and dead epithelial cell debris into the conjunctival depressions called *loops of Henle*. They are commonly seen in elderly people in a degenerative condition and also in patients with scarring stage of trachoma. The name concretion is a misnomer, as they are not calcareous deposits.

Clinical features. Concretions are seen on palpebral conjunctiva, more commonly on upper than the lower. They may also be seen in lower fornix. These are yellowish white, hard looking, raised areas, varying

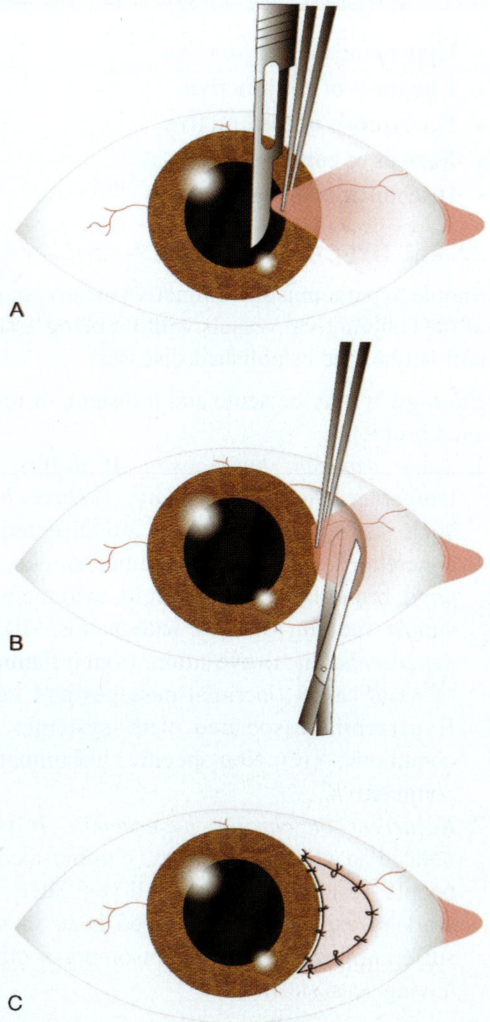

Fig. 4.29. Surgical technique of pterygium excision : A, dissection of head from the cornea; B, excision of pterygium tissue under the conjunctiva; C, conjunctival limbal autograft after excising the pterygium.

in size from pin point to pin head (Fig. 4.12). Being hard, they may produce foreign body sensations and lacrimation by rubbing the corneal surface. Occasionally they may even cause corneal abrasions.

Treatment. It consists of their removal with the help of a hypodermic needle under topical anaesthesia.

SYMPTOMATIC CONDITIONS OF CONJUNCTIVA

- **Hyperaemia of conjunctiva**
- **Chemosis of conjunctiva**
- **Ecchymosis of conjunctiva**
- **Xerosis of conjunctiva**
- **Discoloration of conjunctiva**

SIMPLE HYPERAEMIA OF CONJUNCTIVA

Simple hyperaemia of conjunctiva means congestion of the conjunctival vessels without being associated with any of the established diseases.

Etiology. It may be acute and transient, or recurrent and chronic.

1. *Acute transient hyperaemia.* It results due to temporary irritation caused by: (i) *Direct irritants* such as a foreign body, misdirected cilia, concretions, dust, chemical fumes, smoke, stormy wind, bright light, extreme cold, extreme heat and simple rubbing of eyes with hands; (ii) *Reflex hyperaemia* due to eye strain, from inflammations of nasal cavity, lacrimal passages and lids; (iii) Hyperaemia associated with systemic febrile conditions; (iv) Non-specific inflammation of conjunctiva.
2. *Recurrent or chronic hyperaemia.* It is often noticed in chronic smokers, chronic alcoholics, people residing in dusty, ill-ventilated rooms, workers exposed to prolonged heat, in patients suffering from rosacea and insomnia or otherwise having less sleep.

Clinical features. Patients with simple hyperaemia usually complain of a feeling of discomfort, heaviness, grittiness, tiredness and tightness in the eyes. There may be associated mild lacrimation and minimal mucoid discharge. On cursory examination, the conjunctiva often looks normal. However, eversion of the lids may reveal mild to moderate congestion being more marked in fornices.

Treatment. It consists of *removal of the cause* of hyperaemia. In acute transient hyperaemia the removal of irritants (e.g., misdirected cilia) gives prompt relief. *Symptomatic relief* may be achieved by use of topical decongestants (e.g., 1:10000 adrenaline drops) or naphazoline drops.

CHEMOSIS OF CONJUNCTIVA

Chemosis or oedema of the conjunctiva is of frequent occurrence owing to laxity of the tissue.

Causes. The common causes of chemosis can be grouped as under:

1. *Local inflammatory conditions.* These include conjunctivitis, corneal ulcers, fulminating iridocyclitis, endophthalmitis, panophthalmitis, styes, acute meibomitis, orbital cellulitis, acute dacryoadenitis, acute dacryocystitis, tenonitis and so on.
2. *Local obstruction to flow of blood and/or lymph.* It may occur in patients with orbital tumours, cysts, endocrine exophthalmos, orbital pseudotumours, cavernous sinus thrombosis, carotico-cavernous fistula, blockage of orbital lymphatics following orbital surgery, acute congestive glaucoma etc.
3. *Systemic causes.* These include severe anaemia and hypoproteinaemia, congestive heart failure, nephrotic syndrome, urticaria, and angioneurotic oedema.

Clinical features and management of chemosis depends largely upon the causative factor.

ECCHYMOSIS OF CONJUNCTIVA

Ecchymosis or subconjunctival haemorrhage is of very common occurrence. It may vary in extent from small petechial haemorrhage to an extensive one spreading under the whole of the bulbar conjunctiva and thus making the white sclera of the eye invisible. The condition though draws the attention of the patients immediately as an emergency but is most of the time trivial.

Etiology. Subconjunctival haemorrhage may be associated with following conditions:

1. *Trauma.* It is the most common cause of subconjunctival haemorrhage. It may be in the

form of (i) local trauma to the conjunctiva including that due to surgery and subconjunctival injections, (ii) retrobulbar haemorrhage which almost immediately spreads below the bulbar conjunctiva. Mostly, it results from a retrobulbar injection and from trauma involving various walls of the orbit.

2. *Inflammations of the conjunctiva.* Petechial subconjunctival haemorrhages are usually associated with acute haemorrhagic conjunctivitis caused by picornaviruses, pneumococcal conjunctivitis and leptospirosis, icterohaemorrhagica conjunctivitis.
3. *Sudden venous congestion of head.* The subconjunctival haemorrhages may occur owing to rupture of conjunctival capillaries due to sudden rise in pressure. Common conditions are whooping cough, epileptic fits, strangulation or compression of jugular veins and violent compression of thorax and abdomen as seen in crush injuries.
4. *Spontaneous rupture of fragile capillaries* may occur in vascular diseases such as arteriosclerosis, hypertension and diabetes mellitus.
5. *Local vascular anomalies* like telengiectasia, varicosities, aneurysm or angiomatous tumour.
6. *Blood dyscrasias* like anaemias, leukaemias and dysproteinaemias.
7. *Bleeding disorders* like purpura, haemophilia and scurvy.
8. *Acute febrile systemic infections* such as malaria, typhoid, diphtheria, meningococcal septicaemia, measles and scarlet fever.
9. *Vicarious bleeding* associated with menstruation is an extremely rare cause of subconjunctival haemorrhage.

Clinical features. Subconjunctival haemorrhage per se is symptomless. However, there may be symptoms of associated causative disease. On examination subconjunctival haemorrhage looks as a flat sheet of homogeneous bright red colour with well defined limits (Fig. 4.30). In traumatic subconjunctival haemorrhage, posterior limit is visible when it is due to local trauma to eyeball, and not visible when it is due to head injury or injury to the orbit. Most of the time it is absorbed completely within 7 to 21 days. During absorption colour changes are noted from bright red to orange and then yellow. In severe cases, some pigmentation may be left behind after absorption.

Treatment. (i) Treat the cause when discovered. (ii) Placebo therapy with astringent eye drops. (iii) Psychotherapy and assurance to the patient is most important part of treatment. (iv) Cold compresses to check the bleeding in the initial stage and hot compresses may help in absorption of blood in late stages.

XEROSIS OF CONJUNCTIVA

Xerosis of the conjunctiva is a symptomatic condition in which conjunctiva becomes dry and lustreless. Normal conjunctiva is kept moist by its own secretions, mucin from goblet cells and aqueous solution from accessory lacrimal glands. Therefore, even if the main lacrimal gland is removed, xerosis does not occur. Depending upon the etiology, conjunctival xerosis can be divided into two groups, parenchymatous and epithelial xerosis.

1. *Parenchymatous xerosis.* It occurs following cicatricial disorganization of the conjunctiva due to local causes which can be in the form of (i) widespread destructive interstitial conjunctivitis as seen in trachoma, diptheric membranous conjunctivitis, Steven-Johnsons syndrome, pemphigus or pemphigoid conjunctivitis, thermal, chemical or radiational burns of conjunctiva, (ii) exposure of conjunctiva to air as seen in marked degree of proptosis, facial palsy, ectropion, lack of blinking (as in coma), and lagophthalmos due to symblepharon.

2. *Epithelial xerosis.* It occurs due to hypovitaminosis -A. Epithelial xerosis may be seen in association with night blindness or as a part and

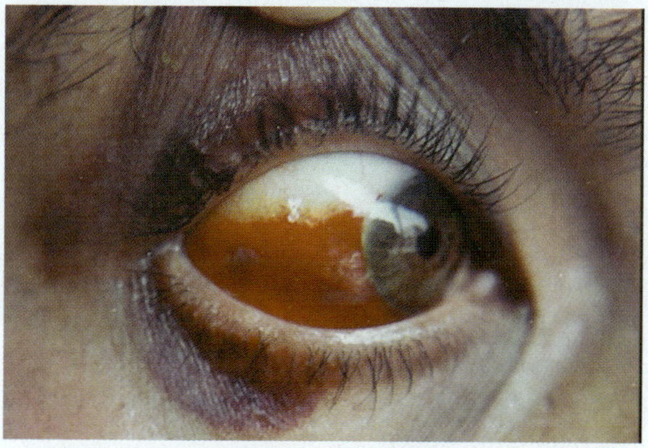

Fig. 4.30. Subconjunctival haemorrhage.

parcel of the xerophthalmia (the term which is applied to all ocular manifestations of vitamin A deficiency which range from night blindness to keratomalacia (see pages 463-466).

Epithelial xerosis typically occurs in children and is characterized by varying degree of conjunctival thickening, wrinkling and pigmentation.

Treatment. Treatment of conjunctival xerosis consists of (i) treatment of the cause, and (ii) symptomatic local treatment with artificial tear preparations (0.7% methyl cellulose or 0.3% hypromellose or polyvinyl alcohol), which should be instilled frequently.

DISCOLORATION OF CONJUNCTIVA

Normal conjunctiva is a thin transparent structure. In the bulbar region, underlying sclera and a fine network of episcleral and conjunctival vessels can be easily visualized. In the palpebral region and fornices, it looks pinkish because of underlying fibrovascular tissue.

Causes. Conjunctiva may show discoloration in various local and systemic diseases given below:

1. *Red discoloration.* A bright red homogeneous discoloration suggests subconjunctival haemorrhage (Fig. 4.30).
2. *Yellow discoloration.* It may occur due to: (i) bile pigments in jaundice, (ii) blood pigments in malaria and yellow fever, (iii) conjunctival fat in elder and Negro patients.
3. *Greyish discoloration.* It may occur due to application of Kajal (surma or soot) and mascara in females.
4. *Brownish grey discoloration.* It is typically seen in argyrosis, following prolonged application of silver nitrate for treatment of chronic conjunctival inflammations. The discoloration is most marked in lower fornix.
5. *Blue discoloration.* It is usually due to ink tattoo from pens or effects of manganese dust. Blue discoloration may also be due to pseudopigmentation as occurs in patients with blue sclera and scleromalacia perforans.
6. *Brown pigmentation.* Its common causes can be grouped as under:

(a) *Non-melanocytic pigmentation*

i. *Endogenous pigmentation.* It is seen in patients with Addison's disease and ochronosis.

ii. *Exogenous pigmentation.* It may follow long-term use of adrenaline for glaucoma. Argyrosis may also present as dark brown pigmentation.

(b) *Melanocytic pigmentation*

i. *Conjunctival epithelial melanosis.* It develops in early childhood, and then remains stationary. It is found in 90 percent of the blacks. The pigmented spot freely moves with the movement of conjunctiva. It has got no malignant potential and hence no treatment is required.

ii. *Subepithelial melanosis.* It may occur as an isolated anomaly of conjunctiva (congenital melanosis oculi, Fig. 4.31) or in association with the ipsilateral hyperpigmentation of the face (oculodermal melanosis or Naevus of Ota).

iii. *Pigmented tumours.* These can be benign naevi, precancerous melanosis or malignant melanoma.

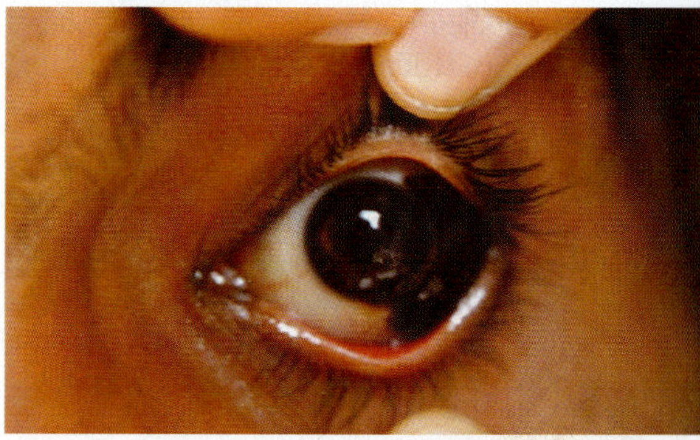

Fig. 4.31. Conjunctival melanosis.

CYSTS AND TUMOURS

CYSTS OF CONJUNCTIVA

The common cystic lesions of the conjunctiva are:

1. *Congenital cystic lesions.* These are of rare occurrence and include congenital corneoscleral cyst and cystic form of epibulbar dermoid.
2. *Lymphatic cysts of conjunctiva.* These are common and usually occur due to dilatation of

lymph spaces in the bulbar conjunctiva. Lymphangiectasis is characterized by a row of small cysts. Rarely, lymphangioma may occur as a single multilocular cyst.

3. *Retention cysts.* These occur occasionally due to blockage of ducts of accessory lacrimal glands of Krause in chronic inflammatory conditions, viz., trachoma and pemphigus. Retention cysts are more common in upper fornix.
4. *Epithelial implantation cyst* (traumatic cyst). It may develop following implantation of conjunctival epithelium in the deeper layers, due to surgical or non-surgical injuries of conjunctiva.
5. *Epithelial cysts due to downgrowth of epithelium* are rarely seen in chronic inflammatory or degenerative conditions, e.g. cystic change in pterygium.
6. *Aqueous cyst.* It may be due to healing by cystoid cicatrix formation, following surgical or non-surgical perforating limbal wounds.
7. *Pigmented epithelial cyst.* It may be formed sometimes following prolonged topical use of cocaine or epinephrine.
8. *Parasitic cysts* such as subconjunctival cysticercus (Fig. 4.32), hydatid cyst and filarial cyst are not infrequent in developing countries.

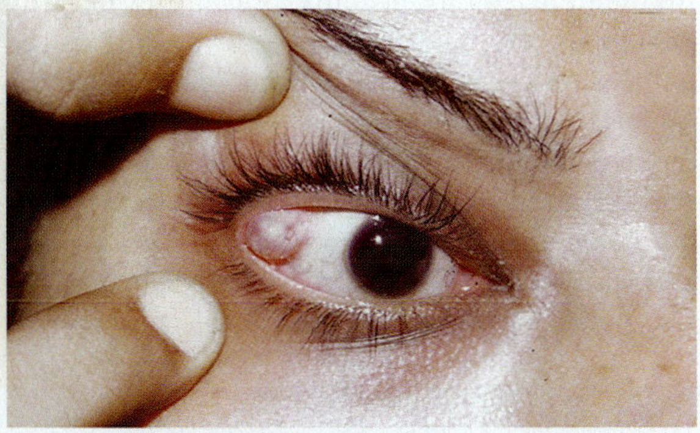

Fig. 4.32. Cysticercosis of conjunctiva.

Treatment

Conjunctival cysts need a careful surgical excision. The excised cyst should always be subjected to histopathological examination.

TUMOURS OF CONJUNCTIVA

Classification

Non-pigmented tumours

I. *Congenital:* dermoid and lipodermoid (choristomas).
II. *Benign:* simple granuloma, papilloma, adenoma, fibroma and angiomas.
III. *Premalignant:* intraepithelial epithelioma (Bowen's disease).
IV. *Malignant:* epithelioma or squamous cell carcinoma, basal cell carcinoma.

Pigmented tumours

I. *Benign:* naevi or congenital moles.
II. *Precancerous melanosis:* superficial spreading melanoma and lentigo maligna (Hutchinson's freckle).
III. *Malignant:* primary melanoma (malignant melanoma).

A. Non-pigmented Tumours

I. *Congenital tumours*

1. *Dermoids.* These are common congenital tumours which usually occur at the limbus. They appear as solid white masses, firmly fixed to the cornea (Fig. 4.33). Dermoid consists of collagenous connective tissue, sebaceous glands and hair, lined by epidermoid epithelium. *Treatment* is simple excision.

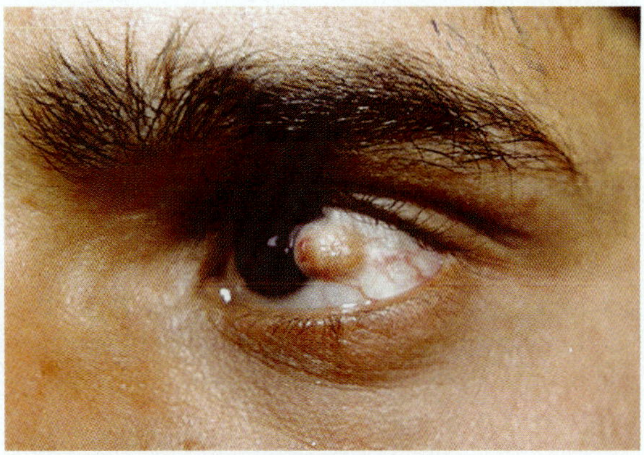

Fig. 4.33. Limbal dermoid.

2. *Lipodermoid* (Fig. 4.34). It is a congenital tumour, usually found at the limbus or outer canthus. It appears as soft, yellowish white, movable sub-conjunctival mass. It consists of fatty tissue and the surrounding dermis-like connective tissue, hence the name lipodermoid.

Sometimes the epibulbar dermoids or lipodermoids may be associated with accessory auricles and other congenital defects (*Goldenhar's syndrome*).

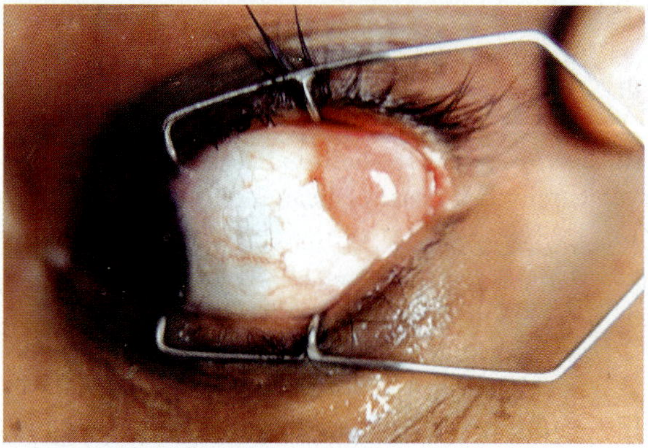

Fig. 4.34. Lipodermoid.

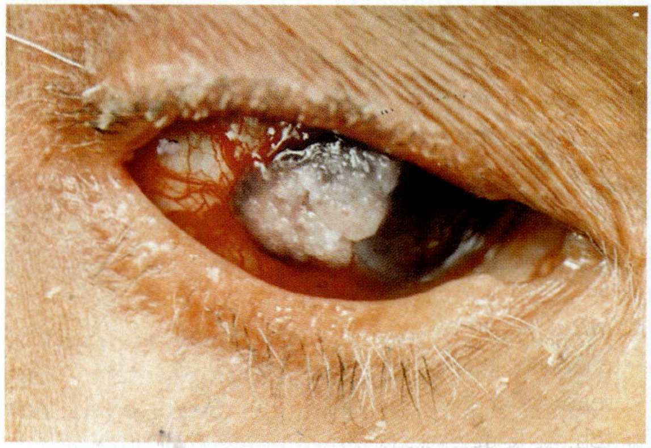

Fig. 4.35. Squamous cell carcinoma at the limbus.

II. *Benign tumours*

1. *Simple granuloma.* It consists of an extensive polypoid, cauliflower-like growth of granulation tissue. Simple granulomas are common following squint surgery, as foreign body granuloma and following inadequately scraped chalazion.

Treatment consists of complete surgical removal.

2. *Papilloma.* It is a benign polypoid tumour usually occurring at inner canthus, fornices or limbus. It may resemble the cocks comb type of conjunctival tubercular lesion. It has a tendency to undergo malignant change and hence needs complete excision.

3. *Fibroma.* It is a rare soft or hard polypoid growth usually occurring in lower fornix.

III. *Pre-malignant tumours*

Bowen's intraepithelial epithelioma (carcinoma *in-situ*). It is a rare, precancerous condition, usually occurring at the limbus as a flat, reddish grey, vascularised plaque. Histologically, it is confined within the epithelium. It should be treated by complete local excision.

IV. *Malignant tumours*

1. *Squamous cell carcinoma* (epithelioma) (Fig. 4.35). It usually occurs at the transitional zones i.e. at limbus and the lid margin. The tumour invades the stroma deeply and may be fixed to underlying tissues. Histologically, it is similar to squamous cell carcinomas occurring elsewhere (see page 384). *Treatment.* Early cases may be treated by complete local excision combined with extensive diathermy cautery of the area. However, in advanced and recurrent cases radical excision including enucleation or even exenteration may be needed along with postoperative radiotherapy.

2. *Basal cell carcinoma.* It may invade the conjunctiva from the lids or may arise pari-passu from the plica semilunaris or caruncle. Though it responds very favourably to radiotherapy, the complete surgical excision, if possible, should be preferred to avoid complications of radiotherapy.

B. Pigmented tumours

1. *Naevi or congenital moles.* These are common pigmented lesions, usually presenting as grey gelatinous, brown or black, flat or slightly raised nodules on the bulbar conjunctiva, mostly near the limbus (Fig. 4.36). They usually appear during early childhood and may increase in size at puberty or during pregnancy. Histologically, they resemble their cutaneous brethren. Malignant change is very rare and when occurs is indicated by sudden increase in size or increase in pigmentation or appearance of signs

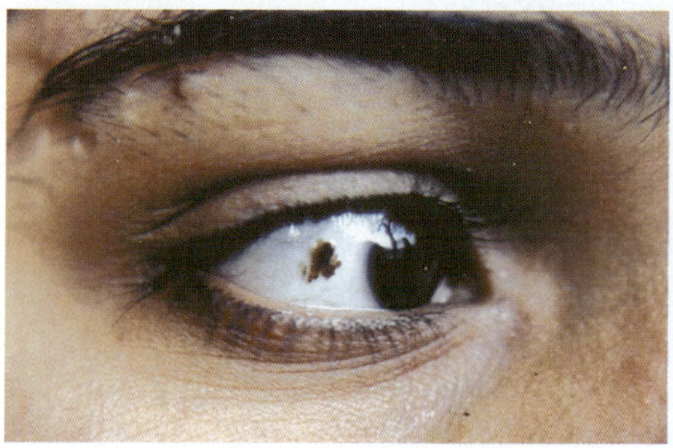

Fig. 4.36. Conjunctival naevus.

of inflammation. Therefore, excision is usually indicated for cosmetic reasons and rarely for medical reasons. Whatever may be the indication, excision should be complete.

2. *Precancerous melanosis.* Precancerous melanosis (intraepithelial melanoma) of conjunctiva occurs in adults as 'superficial spreading melanoma'. It never arises from a congenital naevus.

Clinically a small pigmented tumour develops at any site on the bulbar or palpebral conjunctiva, which spreads as a diffuse, flat, asymptomatic pigmented patch. As long as it maintains its superficial spread, it does not metastasize. However, ultimately in about 20 percent cases it involves the subepithelial tissues and proceeds to frank malignant change.

Treatment. In early stages local excision with postoperative radiotherapy may be sufficient. But in case of recurrence, it should be treated as malignant melanoma.

3. *Malignant melanoma (primary melanoma).* Malignant melanoma of the conjunctiva mostly arises *de-novo*, usually near the limbus, or rarely it may occur due to malignant change in pre-existing naevus. The condition usually occurs in elderly patients.

Clinically it may present as pigmented or non-pigmented mass near limbus or on any other part of the conjunctiva. It spreads over the surface of the globe and rarely penetrates it. Distant metastasis occurs elsewhere in the body, commonly in liver.

Histologically, the neoplasm may be alveolar, round-celled or spindle-celled.

Treatment. Once suspected, enucleation or exenteration is the treatment of choice, depending upon the extent of growth.

5 CHAPTER

Diseases of the Cornea

ANATOMY AND PHYSIOLOGY

APPLIED ANATOMY

Cornea is a transparent, avascular, watch-glass like structure. It forms anterior one-sixth of the outer fibrous coat of the eyeball.

Dimensions

- *Anterior surface* of cornea is elliptical with an average horizontal diameter of 11.7 mm and vertical diameter of 11 mm.
- *Posterior surface* of cornea is circular with an average diameter of 11.5 mm.
- *Thickness of* cornea in the centre varies from 0.5 to 0.6 mm while at the periphery it varies from 1 to 1.2 mm.
- *Radius of curvature.* The central 5 mm area of the cornea forms the powerful refracting surface of the eye. The anterior and posterior radii of curvature of this central part of cornea are 7.8 mm and 6.5 mm, respectively.
- *Refractive index* of the cornea is 1.376.
- *Refractive power* of the cornea is about 45 dioptres, which is roughly three-fourth of the total refractive power of the eye (60 dioptres).

Histology

Histologically, the cornea consists of five distinct layers. From anterior to posterior these are: epithelium, Bowman's membrane, substantia propria (corneal stroma), Descemet's membrane and endothelium (Fig. 5.1).

1. *Epithelium.* It is of stratified squamous type and becomes continuous with epithelium of bulbar conjunctiva at the limbus. It consists of 5-6 layers of cells. The deepest (basal) layer is made up of columnar cells, next 2-3 layers of wing or umbrella cells and the most superficial two layers are made of flattened cells. Tight junctions between superficial epithelial cells prevent penetration of tear fluid into the stroma.

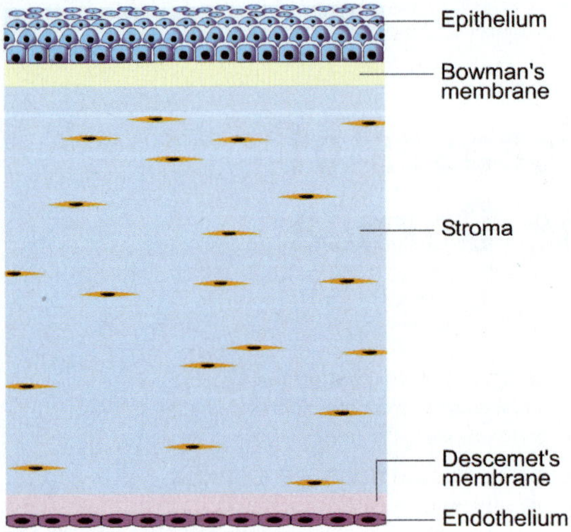

Fig. 5.1. Microscopic structure of the cornea.

Limbal epithelium. The basal epithelial cells of the limbal area constitute the limbal stem cells which amplify, proliferate, and differentiate into corneal epithelium. Damage to this area results in the invasion of conjunctival epithelium on to the cornea.

2. *Bowman's membrane.* This layer consists of acellular mass of condensed collagen fibrils. It is about 12 μm in thickness and binds the corneal stroma anteriorly with basement membrane of the epithelium. It is not a true elastic membrane but simply a condensed superficial part of the stroma. It shows considerable resistance to infection. But *once destroyed, it is unable to regenerate and, therefore, heals by scarring.*

3. *Stroma (substantia propria).* This layer is about 0.5 mm in thickness and constitutes most of the cornea (90% of total thickness). It consists of collagen fibrils (type-I and type-V fibrillae interwined with filaments of type-VI collagen) embedded in hydrated matrix of proteoglycans (chondroitin sulphate and keratan sulphate). The lamellae are arranged in many layers. In each layer they are not only parallel to each other but also to the corneal plane and become continuous with scleral lamellae at the limbus. The alternating layers of lamellae are at right angle to each other. Among the lamellae are present keratocytes (modified fibroblasts), wandering macrophages, histiocytes and a few leucocytes.

4. *Descemet's membrane (posterior elastic lamina).* The Descemet's membrane is a strong homogenous basement membrane of the corneal endothelium which bounds the stroma posteriorly. It is very resistant to chemical agents, trauma and pathological processes. Therefore, '*Descemetocele'* can maintain the integrity of eyeball for long. Descemet's membrane consists of collagen and glycoproteins. Unlike Bowman's membrane *it can regenerate*. Normally it remains in a state of tension and when torn, it curls inwards on itself. In the periphery it appears to end at the anterior limit of trabecular meshwork as Schwalbe's line (ring).

5. *Endothelium.* It consists of a single layer of flat polygonal (mainly hexagonal) epithelial cells (misnamed as endothelium) which on slit lamp biomicroscopy appear as a mosaic. The cell density of endothelium is around 3000 cells/mm^2 in young adults, which decreases with the advancing age. The human endothelium cells do not proliferate *in-vivo* and the cell loss with age is compensated by enlargement (polymegathism) and migration of neighbouring cells. There is a considerable functional reserve for the endothelium. Therefore, corneal decompensation occurs only after more than 75 percent of the cells are lost. The endothelial cells contain 'active-pump' mechanism.

Blood supply

Cornea is an avascular structure. Small loops derived from the anterior ciliary vessels invade its periphery for about 1 mm. Actually these loops are not in the cornea but in the subconjunctival tissue which overlaps the cornea.

Nerve supply

Cornea is supplied by anterior ciliary nerves which are branches of ophthalmic division of the 5th cranial nerve. After going about 2 mm in cornea the nerves lose their myelin sheath and divide dichotomously and form three plexuses — the stromal, subepithelial and intraepithelial.

APPLIED PHYSIOLOGY

The two primary physiological functions of the cornea are (i) to act as a major refracting medium; and (ii) to protect the intraocular contents. Cornea performs these functions by maintaining its transparency and replacement of its tissues.

Corneal transparency

The transparency is the result of :

- Peculiar arrangement of corneal lamellae (lattice theory of Maurice),
- Avascularity,
- Relative state of dehydration (78% water content), which is maintained by barrier effects of epithelium and endothelium and the active Na^+ K^+ ATPase pump of the endothelium, and
- Swelling pressure (SP) of the stroma which counters the imbibition effect of intraocular pressure (IOP).

For these processes, cornea needs some energy.

Source of nutrients

1. *Solutes* (glucose and others) enter the cornea by either simple diffusion or active transport through aqueous humour and by diffusion from the perilimbal capillaries.
2. *Oxygen* is derived directly from air through the tear film. This is an active process undertaken by the epithelium.

Metabolism of cornea

The most actively metabolising layers of the cornea are epithelium and endothelium, the former being 10 times thicker than the latter requires a proportionately larger supply of metabolic substrates. Like other tissues, the epithelium can metabolize glucose both aerobically and anaerobically into carbon dioxide and water and lactic acid, respectively. Thus, under anaerobic conditions lactic acid accumulates in the cornea.

CONGENITAL ANOMALIES

Megalocornea

Definition. Horizontal diameter of cornea at birth is about 10 mm and the adult size of about 11.7 mm is attained by the age of 2 years. Megalocornea is labelled when the horizontal diameter of cornea is of adult size at birth or 13 mm or greater after the age of 2 years.

Salient features. The cornea is usually clear with normal thickness and vision. The condition is not progressive.

Systemic associations include Marfan's, Apert, Ehlers Danlos and Down syndromes.

Differential diagnosis

1. *Buphthalmos.* In this condition IOP is raised and the eyeball is enlarged as a whole. The enlarged cornea is usually associated with central or peripheral clouding and Descemet's tears (Haab's striae).
2. *Keratoglobus.* In this condition, there is thinning and excessive protrusion of cornea, which seems enlarged; but its diameter is usually normal.

Microcornea

In microcornea, the horizontal diameter is less than 10 mm since birth. The condition may occur as an isolated anomaly (rarely) or in association with *nanophthalmos* (normal small eyeball) or *microphthalmos* (abnormal small eyeball).

Cornea plana

This is a rare anomaly in which bilaterally cornea is comparatively flat since birth. It may be associated with microcornea. Cornea plana usually results in marked astigmatic refractive error.

Congenital cloudy cornea

The acronym 'STUMPED' helps to remember the common conditions to be included in differential diagnosis of neonatal cloudy cornea. The conditions are as follows:

- Sclerocornea
- Tears in Descemet's membrane
- Ulcer
- Metabolic conditions
- Posterior corneal defect
- Endothelial dystrophy
- Dermoid

INFLAMMATIONS OF THE CORNEA

Inflammation of the cornea (keratitis) is characterised by corneal oedema, cellular infiltration and ciliary congestion.

Classification

It is difficult to classify and assign a group to each and every case of keratitis; as overlapping or concurrent findings tend to obscure the picture. However, the following simplified topographical and etiological classifications provide a workable knowledge.

Topographical (morphological) classification

(A) ***Ulcerative keratitis (corneal ulcer)***

Corneal ulcer can be further classified variously:

1. *Depending on location*
   - Central corneal ulcer
   - Peripheral corneal ulcer
2. *Depending on purulence*
   - Purulent corneal ulcer or suppurative corneal ulcer (most bacterial and fungal corneal ulcers are suppurative).
   - Non-purulent corneal ulcers (most of viral, chlamydial and allergic corneal ulcers are non-suppurative).
3. *Depending upon association of hypopyon*
   - Simple corneal ulcer (without hypopyon)
   - Hypopyon corneal ulcer
4. *Depending upon depth of ulcer*
   - Superficial corneal ulcer
   - Deep corneal ulcer
   - Corneal ulcer with impending perforation
   - Perforated corneal ulcer
5. *Depending upon slough formation*
   - Non-sloughing corneal ulcer
   - Sloughing corneal ulcer

(B) ***Non-ulcerative keratitis***

1. *Superficial keratitis*
   - Diffuse superficial keratitis
   - Superficial punctate keratitis (SPK)
2. *Deep keratitis*
   - (a) Non-suppurative
     - Interstitial keratitis
     - Disciform keratitis
     - Keratitis profunda
     - Sclerosing keratitis
   - (b) Suppurative deep keratitis
     - Central corneal abscess
     - Posterior corneal abscess

Etiological classification

1. *Infective keratitis*
   - Bacterial
   - Viral
   - Fungal
   - Chlamydial
   - Protozoal
   - Spirochaetal
2. *Allergic keratitis*
   - Phlyctenular keratitis
   - Vernal keratitis
   - Atopic keratitis
3. *Trophic keratitis*
   - Exposure keratitis
   - Neurotrophic keratopathy
   - Keratomalacia
   - Atheromatous ulcer
4. *Keratitis associated with diseases of skin and mucous membrane.*
5. *Keratitis associated with systemic collagen vascular disorders.*
6. *Traumatic keratitis*, which may be due to mechanical trauma, chemical trauma, thermal burns, radiations.
7. *Idiopathic keratitis* e.g.,
   - Mooren's corneal ulcer
   - Superior limbic keratoconjunctivitis
   - Superficial punctate keratitis of Thygeson

ULCERATIVE KERATITIS

Corneal ulcer may be defined as discontinuation in normal epithelial surface of cornea associated with necrosis of the surrounding corneal tissue. Pathologically, it is characterised by oedema and cellular infiltration. Common types of corneal ulcers are described below.

INFECTIVE KERATITIS

BACTERIAL CORNEAL ULCER

Being the most anterior part of eyeball, the cornea is exposed to atmosphere and hence prone to get infected easily. At the same time cornea is protected from day-to-day minor infections by the normal defence mechanisms present in tears in the form of lysozyme, betalysin and other protective proteins. Therefore, infective corneal ulcer may develop when:

- either the local ocular defence mechanism is jeopardised, or
- there is some local ocular predisposing disease, or host's immunity is compromised, or
- the causative organism is very virulent.

Etiology

There are two main factors in the production of purulent corneal ulcer:

- Damage to corneal epithelium; and
- Infection of the eroded area.

However, following three pathogens can invade the intact corneal epithelium and produce ulceration: *Neisseria gonorrhoeae, Corynebacterium diphtheriae* and *Neisseria meningitidis.*

1. ***Corneal epithelial damage***. It is a prerequisite for most of the infecting organisms to produce corneal ulceration. It may occur in following conditions:

i. *Corneal abrasion* due to small foreign body, misdirected cilia, concretions and trivial trauma in contact lens wearers or otherwise.
ii. *Epithelial drying* as in xerosis and exposure keratitis.
iii. *Necrosis of epithelium* as in keratomalacia.
iv. *Desquamation of epithelial cells* as a result of corneal oedema as in bullous keratopathy.
v. *Epithelial damage due to trophic changes* as in neuroparalytic keratitis.

2. ***Source of infection*** include:

i. *Exogenous infection.* Most of the times corneal infection arises from exogenous source like conjunctival sac, lacrimal sac (dacryocystitis), infected foreign bodies, infected vegetative material and water-borne or air-borne infections.
ii. *From the ocular tissue.* Owing to direct anatomical continuity, diseases of the conjunctiva readily spread to corneal epithelium, those of sclera to stroma, and of the uveal tract to the endothelium of cornea.
iii. *Endogenous infection.* Owing to avascular nature of the cornea, endogenous infections are of rare occurrence.

3. ***Causative organisms.*** Common bacteria associated with corneal ulceration are: *Staphylococcus aureus, Pseudomonas pyocyanea, Streptococcus pneumoniae, E. coli, Proteus, Klebsiella, N. gonorrhoea, N. meningitidis* and *C. diphtheriae.*

Pathogenesis and pathology of corneal ulcer

i. Once the damaged corneal epithelium is invaded by the offending agents the sequence of pathological changes which occur during development of corneal ulcer can be described under four stages:
   - Stage of progressive infiltration
   - Stage of active ulceration
   - Stage of regression
   - Stage of cicatrization
ii. The terminal course of corneal ulcer depends upon the virulence of infecting agent, host defence mechanism and the treatment received.
iii. Depending upon the prevalent circumstances the course of corneal ulcer may take one of the three forms:
   - Ulcer may become localised and heal;
   - Penetrate deep leading to corneal perforation;
   - Spread fast in the whole cornea as sloughing corneal ulcer.

The salient pathological features of these are as under:

[A] *Pathology of localised corneal ulcer*

1. ***Stage of progressive infiltration*** (Fig. 5.2A). It is characterised by the infiltration of polymor-

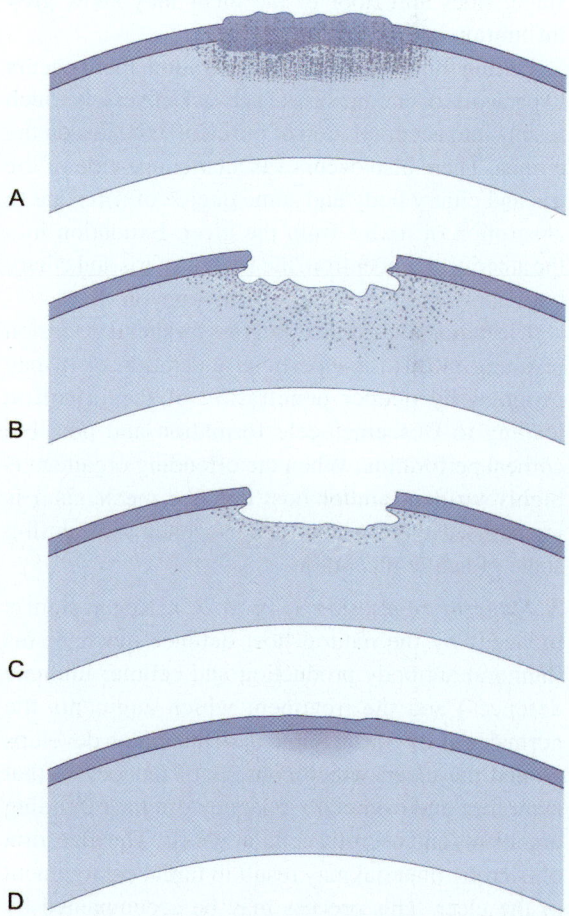

Fig. 5.2. Pathology of corneal ulcer : A, stage of progressive infiltration; B, stage of active ulceration; C, stage of regression; D, stage of cicatrization.

phonuclear and/or lymphocytes into the epithelium from the peripheral circulation supplemented by similar cells from the underlying stroma if this tissue is also affected. Subsequently, necrosis of the involved tissue may occur, depending upon the virulence of offending agent and the strength of host defence mechanism.

2. *Stage of active ulceration* (Fig. 5.2B). Active ulceration results from necrosis and sloughing of the epithelium, Bowman's membrane and the involved stroma. The walls of the active ulcer project owing to swelling of the lamellae by the imbibition of fluid and the packing of masses of leucocytes between them. This zone of infiltration may extend to a considerable distance both around and beneath the ulcer. At this stage, sides and floor of the ulcer may show grey infiltration and sloughing.

During this stage of active ulceration, there occurs hyperaemia of circumcorneal network of vessels which results into accumulation of purulent exudates on the cornea. There also occurs vascular congestion of the iris and ciliary body and some degree of iritis due to absorption of toxins from the ulcer. Exudation into the anterior chamber from the vessels of iris and ciliary body may lead to formation of hypopyon.

Ulceration may further progress by lateral extension resulting in diffuse superficial ulceration or it may progress by deeper penetration of the infection leading to Descemetocele formation and possible corneal perforation. When the offending organism is highly virulent and/or host defence mechanism is jeopardised there occurs deeper penetration during stage of active ulceration.

3. *Stage of regression* (Fig. 5.2C). Regression is induced by the natural host defence mechanisms (humoral antibody production and cellular immune defences) and the treatment which augments the normal host response. A line of demarcation develops around the ulcer, which consists of leucocytes that neutralize and eventually phagocytose the offending organisms and necrotic cellular debris. The digestion of necrotic material may result in initial enlargement of the ulcer. This process may be accompanied by superficial vascularization that increases the humoral and cellular immune response. The ulcer now begins to heal and epithelium starts growing over the edges.

A

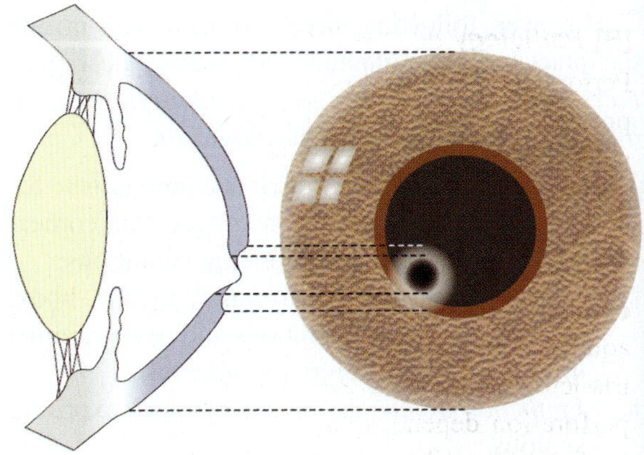

B

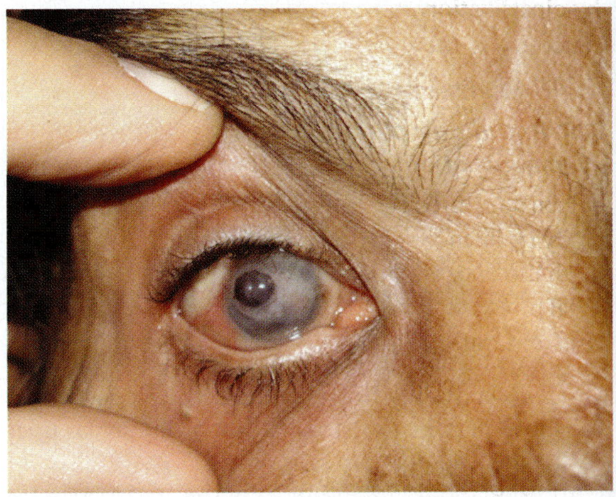

Fig. 5.3. Descemetocele : A, Diagrammatic depiction; B.Clinical photographs.

4. *Stage of cicatrization* (Fig. 5.2D). In this stage healing continues by progressive epithelization which forms a permanent covering. Beneath the epithelium, fibrous tissue is laid down partly by the corneal fibroblasts and partly by the endothelial cells of the new vessels. The stroma thus thickens and fills in under the epithelium, pushing the epithelial surface anteriorly.

The degree of scarring from healing varies. If the ulcer is very superficial and involves epithelium only, it heals without leaving any opacity behind. When ulcer involves Bowman's membrane and few superficial stromal lamellae, the resultant scar is called a 'nebula'. Macula and leucoma result after healing of ulcers involving up to one-third and more than that of corneal stroma, respectively.

[B] *Pathology of perforated corneal ulcer*

Perforation of corneal ulcer occurs when the ulcerative process deepens and reaches up to Descemet's membrane. This membrane is tough and bulges out as Descemetocele (Fig. 5.3). At this stage, any exertion on the part of patient, such as coughing, sneezing, straining for stool etc., will perforate the corneal ulcer. Immediately after perforation, the aqueous escapes, intraocular pressure falls and the iris-lens diaphragm moves forward. The effects of perforation depend upon the position and size of perforation. When the perforation is small and opposite to iris tissue, it is usually plugged and healing by cicatrization proceeds rapidly (Fig. 5.4). Adherent leucoma is the commonest end result after such a catastrophe.

[C] *Pathology of sloughing corneal ulcer and formation of anterior staphyloma*

When the infecting agent is highly virulent and/or body resistance is very low, the whole cornea sloughs with the exception of a narrow rim at the margin and total prolapse of iris occurs. The iris becomes inflamed and exudates block the pupil and cover the iris surface; thus a *false cornea* is formed. Ultimately these exudates organize and form a thin fibrous layer over which the conjunctival or corneal epithelium rapidly grows and thus a *pseudocornea* is formed. Since the pseudocornea is thin and cannot withstand the intraocular pressure, so it usually bulges forward along with the plastered iris tissue. This ectatic cicatrix is called *anterior staphyloma* which, depending upon its extent, may be either partial or total. The bands of scar tissue on the staphyloma vary in breadth and thickness, producing a lobulated surface often blackened with iris tissue which resembles a bunch of black grapes (hence the name staphyloma).

Clinical picture

In bacterial infections the outcome depends upon the virulence of organism, its toxins and enzymes, and the response of host tissue.

Broadly bacterial corneal ulcers may manifest as:

i. Purulent corneal ulcer without hypopyon; or
ii. Hypopyon corneal ulcer.

A

B

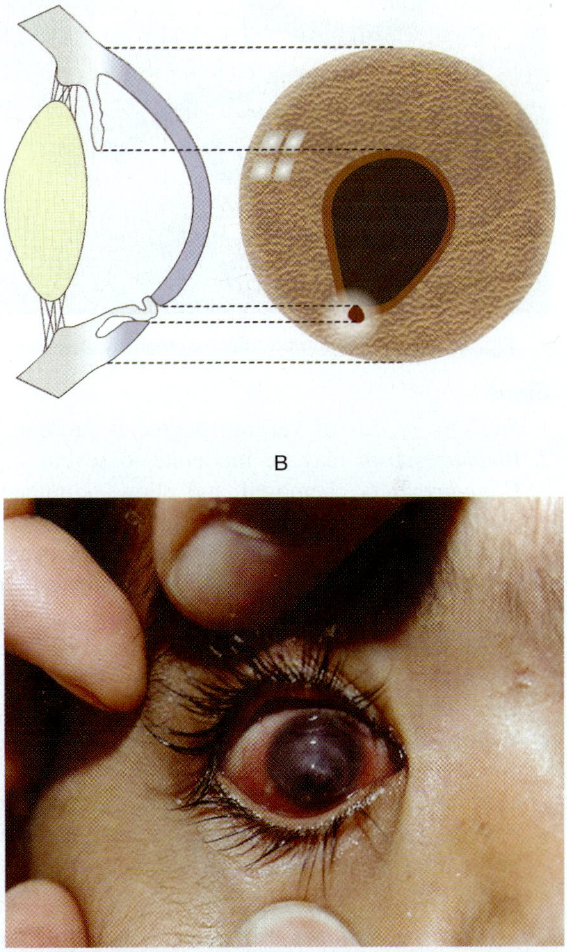

Fig. 5.4. Perforated corneal ulcer with prolapse of iris: A, diagrammatic depiction; B, clinical photograph.

In general, following symptoms and signs may be present :

Symptoms

1. *Pain* and foreign body sensation occurs due to mechanical effects of lids and chemical effects of toxins on the exposed nerve endings.
2. *Watering* from the eye occurs due to reflex hyperlacrimation.
3. *Photophobia,* i.e., intolerance to light results from stimulation of nerve endings.
4. *Blurred vision* results from corneal haze.
5. *Redness of eyes* occurs due to congestion of circumcorneal vessels.

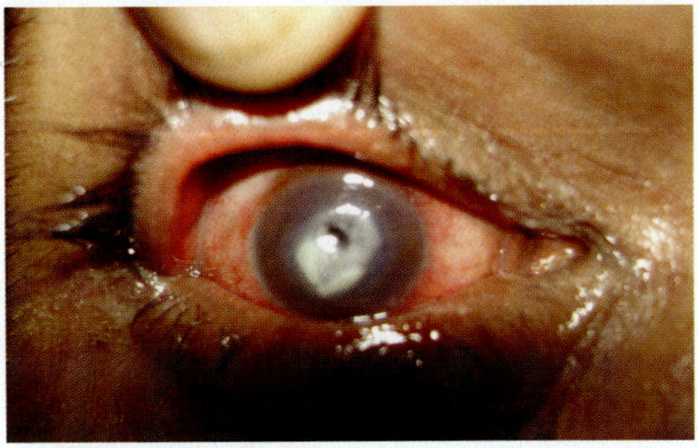

Fig. 5.5. Bacterial corneal ulcer without hypopyon.

Signs

1. *Swelling of lids* of varying degree is present.
2. *Blepharospasm* may be moderate to severe.
3. *Conjunctiva* is chemosed and shows conjunctival hyperaemia and ciliary congestion.
4. *Corneal ulcer* usually starts as an epithelial defect associated with greyish-white circumscribed infiltrate (seen in early stage). Soon the epithelial defect and infiltrate enlarges and stromal oedema develops. A well established bacterial ulcer is characterized by (Fig. 5.5):

- Yellowish-white area of ulcer which may be oval or irregular in shape.
- Margins of the ulcer are swollen and over hanging.
- Floor of the ulcer is covered by necrotic material.
- Stromal oedema is present surrounding the ulcer area.

Characteristic features produced by some of the causative bacteria are as follows:

- *Staphylococcal aureus and streptococcus pneumoniae* usually produce an oval, yellowish white densely opaque ulcer which is surrounded by relatively clear cornea.
- *Pseudomonas species* usually produce an irregular sharp ulcer with thick greenish mucopurulent exudate, diffuse liquefactive necrosis and semiopaque (ground glass) surrounding cornea. Such ulcers are usually associated with hypopyon, spread very rapidly and may even perforate within 48 to 72 hours.
- *Enterobacteriae* (*E. coli*, *Proteus sp.*, and *Klebsiella sp.*) usually produce a shallow ulcer with greyish white pleomorphic suppuration and diffuse stromal opalescence. The endotoxins produced by these Gram –ve bacilli may produce ring-shaped corneal infilterate.

5. *Anterior chamber* may or may not show pus (hypopyon). In bacterial corneal ulcers the hypopyon remains sterile so long as the Descemet's membrane is intact.
6. *Iris* may be slightly muddy in colour.
7. *Pupil* may be small due to associated toxin–induced iritis.
8. *Intraocular pressure* may sometimes be raised (inflammatory glaucoma).

Hypopyon corneal ulcer

Etiopathogenesis

Causative organisms. It is customary to reserve the term 'hypopyon corneal ulcer' for the characteristic ulcer caused by *Pneumococcus* and the term 'corneal ulcer with hypopyon' for the ulcers associated with hypopyon due to other organisms such as *Staphylococci*, *Streptococci*, *Gonococci*, *Moraxella* and *Pseudomonas pyocyanea*. The characteristic hypopyon corneal ulcer caused by *Pneumococcus* is called *ulcus serpens.*

Source of infection for pneumococcal infection is usually the chronic dacryocystitis.

Factors predisposing to development of hypopyon. Two main factors which predispose to development of hypopyon in a patient with corneal ulcer are the virulence of the infecting organism and the resistance of the tissues. Hence, hypopyon ulcers are much more common in old debilitated or alcoholic subjects.

Mechanism of development of hypopyon. Corneal ulcer is often associated with some iritis owing to diffusion of bacterial toxins. When the iritis is severe the outpouring of leucocytes from the vessels is so great that these cells gravitate to the bottom of the anterior chamber to form a hypopyon. Thus, it is important to note that the hypopyon is sterile since the outpouring of polymorphonuclear cells is due to the toxins and not due to actual invasion by bacteria. Once the ulcerative process is controlled, the hypopyon is absorbed.

Clinical features

Symptoms are same as described above for bacterial corneal ulcer. However, it is important to note that during initial stage of ulcus serpens there is remarkably little pain. As a result the treatment is often unduly delayed.

Signs. In general the signs are same as described above for the bacterial ulcer.

Characteristic features of ulcus serpens:

- Ulcus serpens is a greyish white or yellowish disc shaped ulcer occuring near the centre of cornea (Fig. 5.6).
- The ulcer has a tendency to creep over the cornea in a serpiginous fashion. One edge of the ulcer, along which the ulcer spreads, shows more infiltration. The other side of the ulcer may be undergoing simultaneous cicatrization and the edges may be covered with fresh epithelium.
- Violent iridocyclitis is commonly associated with a definite hypopyon.

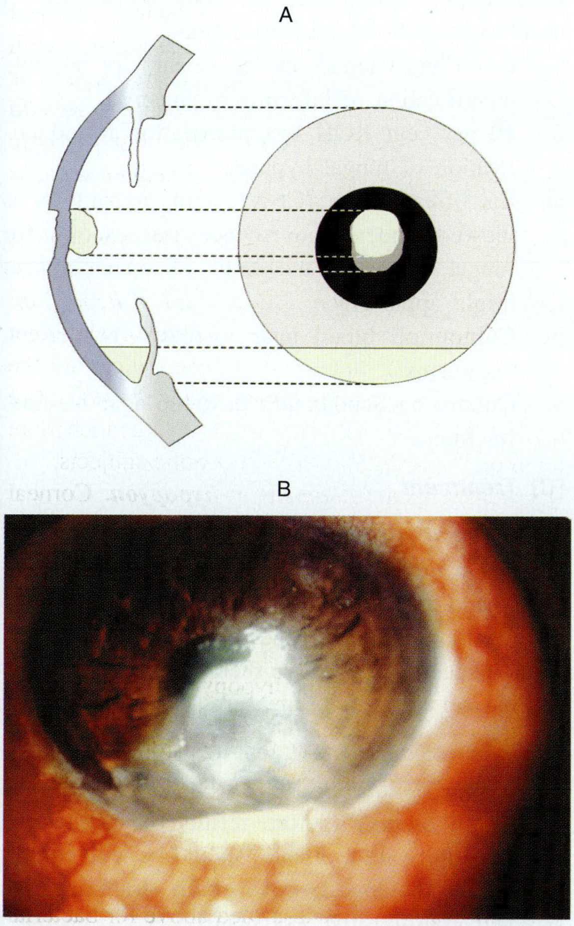

Fig. 5.6. Hypopyon corneal ulcer : A, Diagrammatic depiction; B, Clinical photograph.

- Hypopyon increases in size very rapidly and often results in secondary glaucoma.
- Ulcer spreads rapidly and has a great tendency for early perforation.

Management

Management of hypopyon corneal ulcer is same as for other bacterial corneal ulcer.

Special points which need to be considered are :

- *Secondary glaucoma* should be anticipated and treated with 0.5% timolol maleate, B.I.D. eye drops and oral acetazolamide.
- *Source of infection,* i.e., chronic dacryocystitis if detected, should be treated by dacryocystectomy.

Complications of corneal ulcer

1. *Toxic iridocyclitis.* It is usually associated with cases of purulent corneal ulcer due to absorption of toxins in the anterior chamber.

2. *Secondary glaucoma.* It occurs due to fibrinous exudates blocking the angle of anterior chamber (inflammatory glaucoma).

3. *Descemetocele.* Some ulcers caused by virulent organisms extend rapidly up to Descemet's membrane, which gives a great resistance, but due to the effect of intraocular pressure it herniates as a transparent vesicle called the descemetocele or keratocele (Fig. 5.3). This is a sign of impending perforation and is usually associated with severe pain.

4. *Perforation of corneal ulcer.* Sudden strain due to cough, sneeze or spasm of orbicularis muscle may convert impending perforation into actual perforation (Fig. 5.4). Following perforation, immediately pain is decreased and the patient feels some hot fluid (aqueous) coming out of eyes.

Sequelae of corneal perforation include :

i. *Prolapse of iris.* It occurs immediately following perforation in a bid to plug it.

ii. *Subluxation or anterior dislocation of lens* may occur due to sudden stretching and rupture of zonules.

iii. *Anterior capsular cataract.* It is formed when the lens comes in contact with the ulcer following a perforation in the pupillary area.

iv. *Corneal fistula.* It is formed when the perforation in the pupillary area is not plugged by iris and is lined by epithelium which gives way repeatedly. There occurs continuous leak of aqueous through the fistula.

v. *Purulent uveitis, endophthalmitis* or even *panophthalmitis* may develop due to spread of intraocular infection.

vi. *Intraocular haemorrhage* in the form of either vitreous haemorrhage or expulsive choroidal haemorrhage may occur in some patients due to sudden lowering of intraocular pressure.

5. *Corneal scarring.* It is the usual end result of healed corneal ulcer. Corneal scarring leads to permanent visual impairment ranging from slight blurring to total blindness. Depending upon the clinical course of ulcer, corneal scar noted may be nebula, macula, leucoma, ectatic cicatrix or kerectasia, adherent leucoma or anterior staphyloma (for details see page 128).

Management of a case of corneal ulcer

Since corneal ulcer is sight threatening, it needs urgent treatment by identification and eradication of causative bacteria. Preferably such patients should be hospitalized. The management includes:

- Clinical evaluation
- Laboratory investigations
- Treatment

[A] *Clinical evaluation*

Each case with corneal ulcer should be subjected to:

1. *Thorough history taking* to elicit mode of onset, duration of disease and severity of symptoms.

2. *General physical examination,* especially for built, nourishment, anaemia and any immuno-compromising disease.

3. *Ocular examination* should include:

i. *Diffuse light examination* for gross lesions of lids, conjunctiva and cornea including testing for sensations.

ii. *Regurgitation test* and *syringing* to rule out lacrimal sac infection.

iii. *Biomicroscopic examination* after staining of corneal ulcer with 2 per cent freshly prepared aqueous solution of fluorescein dye or sterilised fluorescein impregnated filter paper strip. Ulcer area stains as brilliant green, which looks opaque green when seen with blue filter. Note site, size, shape, depth, margin, floor and vascularization of corneal ulcer. On biomicroscopy also note presence of keratic precipitates at the back of cornea, depth and contents of anterior chamber, colour and pattern of iris and condition of crystalline lens.

[B] *Laboratory investigations*

1. *Routine laboratory investigations* such as haemoglobin, TLC, DLC, ESR, blood sugar, complete urine and stool examination should be carried out in each case.

2. *Microbiological investigations*. These studies are essential to identify causative organism, confirm the diagnosis and guide the treatment to be instituted. Material for such investigations is obtained by scraping the base and margins of the corneal ulcer (under local anaesthesia, using 2 percent xylocaine or preferably paracain) with the help of a modified Kimura spatula or by simply using the bent tip of a 20 gauge hypodermic needle. The material obtained is used for the following investigations:

i. Gram and Giemsa stained smears for possible identification of infecting organisms.

ii. 10 per cent KOH wet preparation for identification of fungal hyphae.

iii. Calcofluor white (CFW) stain preparation is viewed under fluorescence microscope for fungal filaments, the walls of which appear bright apple green.

iv. Culture on blood agar medium for aerobic organisms.

v. Culture on Sabouraud's dextrose agar medium for fungi.

[C] *Treatment*

I. *Treatment of uncomplicated corneal ulcer*

Treatment of corneal ulcer can be discussed under three headings:

- Specific treatment for the cause.
- Non-specific supportive therapy.
- Physical and general measures.

1. *The specific treatment*

(a) *Topical antibiotics.*

- *Initial therapy* (before results of culture and sensitivity are available) should be with combination therapy to cover both gram-negative and gram-positive organisms.

  To begin with any of the following two drugs may be instilled:

– Fortified Cefazoline, 5% i.e. 50 mg/ml freshly prepared by adding sterile water to 500 mg powder to make 10 ml solution, and fortified tobramycin, 1.3%, i.e 13.6 mg/ml (prepared by adding 2 ml of tobramycin injection (40 mg/ml in 5 ml bottle of commercially available 0.3% tobramycin drops.

or

– Freshly prepared fortified vancomycin 5%, i.e. 50 mg/ml, (prepared by adding sterile water to 500 mg vancomycin powder to form 10 ml solution) and one of commercially available fluoroquinolones eye drops (.3% ciprofloxacin, or 0.3% ofloxacin or 0.3% gatifloxacin or 0.5% moxifloxacin)

Frequency of instillation. The chosen two drugs should be instilled alternately as below:

– 1 hourly round the clock for first 48 hours.
– 2 hourly during day and 4 hourly at night till healing is ensured
– 4-6 hourly till healing occurs
– Once the favourable response is obtained, the fortified drops can be substituted by the commercially available eye-drops.

- *Subsequent therapy.* There is no need to change initial antibiotics, if the response is good. However, if the response is poor, immediately change the antibiotics as per culture and sensitivity report.

(b) *Systemic antibiotics* are usually not required. However, a cephalosporine and an aminoglycoside or oral ciprofloxacin (750 mg twice daily) may be given in fulminating cases with perforation or when sclera is also involved.

2. *Non-specific treatment*

(a) *Cycloplegic drugs.* Preferably 1 percent atropine eye ointment or drops should be used to reduce pain from ciliary spasm and to prevent the formation of posterior synechiae from secondary iridocyclitis. Atropine also increases the blood supply to anterior uvea by relieving pressure on the anterior ciliary arteries and so brings more antibodies in the aqueous humour. It also reduces exudation by decreasing hyperaemia and vascular permeability. Other cycloplegic which can be used is 2 per cent homatropine eye drops.

(b) *Systemic analgesics* and *anti-inflammatory drugs* such as paracetamol and ibuprofen relieve the pain and decrease oedema.

(c) *Vitamins* (A, B-complex and C) help in early healing of ulcer.

3. *Physical and general measures*

(a) *Hot fomentation.* Local application of heat (preferably dry) gives comfort, reduces pain and causes vasodilatation.

(b) *Dark goggles* may be used to prevent photophobia.

(c) *Rest, good diet* and *fresh air* may have a soothing effect.

II. *Treatment of non-healing corneal ulcer*

If the ulcer progresses despite the above therapy the following additional measures should be taken:

1. *Removal of any known cause of non-healing ulcer.* A thorough search for any already missed cause not allowing healing should be made and when found, such factors should be eliminated. *Common causes of non-healing ulcers are as under:*
   i. *Local causes.* Associated raised intraocular pressure, concretions, misdirected cilia, impacted foreign body, dacryocystitis, inadequate therapy, wrong diagnosis, lagophthalmos and excessive vascularization of ulcer.
   ii. *Systemic causes:* Diabetes mellitus, severe anaemia, malnutrition, chronic debilitating diseases and patients on systemic steroids.
2. *Mechanical debridement of ulcer* to remove necrosed material by scraping floor of the ulcer with a spatula under local anaesthesia may hasten the healing.
3. *Cauterisation of the ulcer* may also be considered in non-responding cases. Cauterisation may be performed with pure carbolic acid or 10-20 per cent trichloracetic acid.
4. *Bandage soft contact lens* may also help in healing.
5. *Peritomy,* i.e., severing of perilimbal conjunctival vessels may be performed when excessive corneal vascularization is hindering healing.

III. *Treatment of impending perforation*

When ulcer progresses and perforation seems imminent, the following additional measures may help to prevent perforation and its complications:

1. *No strain.* The patient should be advised to avoid sneezing, coughing and straining during stool etc. He should be advised strict bed rest.
2. *Pressure bandage* should be applied to give some external support.
3. *Lowering of intraocular pressure* by simultaneous use of acetazolamide 250 mg QID orally, intravenous mannitol (20%) drip stat, oral glycerol twice a day, 0.5% timolol eyedrops twice a day, and even paracentesis with slow evacuation of aqueous from the anterior chamber may be performed if required.
4. *Tissue adhesive glue* such as cyanoacrylate is helpful in preventing perforation.
5. *Bandage soft contact lens* may also be used.
6. *Conjunctival flap.* The cornea may be covered completely or partly by a conjunctival flap to give support to the weak tissue.
7. *Amniotic membrane transplantation* may also be considered as an option.
8. *Penetrating therapeutic keratoplasty* (tectonic graft) may be undertaken in suitable cases, when available.

IV. *Treatment of perforated corneal ulcer*

Best is to prevent perforation. However, if perforation has occurred, immediate measures should be taken to restore the integrity of perforated cornea. Depending upon the size of perforation and availability, measures like use of tissue adhesive glues, covering with conjunctival flap, use of bandage soft contact lens or therapeutic keratoplasty should be undertaken. Best option is an urgent therapeutic keratoplasty.

Marginal catarrhal ulcer

These superficial ulcers situated near the limbus are frequently seen especially in old people.

Etiology

Marginal catarrhal ulcer is thought to be caused by a hypersensitivity reaction to Staphylococcal toxins. It occurs in association with chronic Staphylococcal blepharoconjunctivitis. Moraxella and Haemophilus are also known to cause such ulcers.

Clinical features

1. Patient usually presents with mild ocular irritation, pain, photophobia and watering.
2. The ulcer is shallow, slightly infiltrated and often multiple, usually associated with Staphylococcal conjunctivitis (Fig. 5.7).

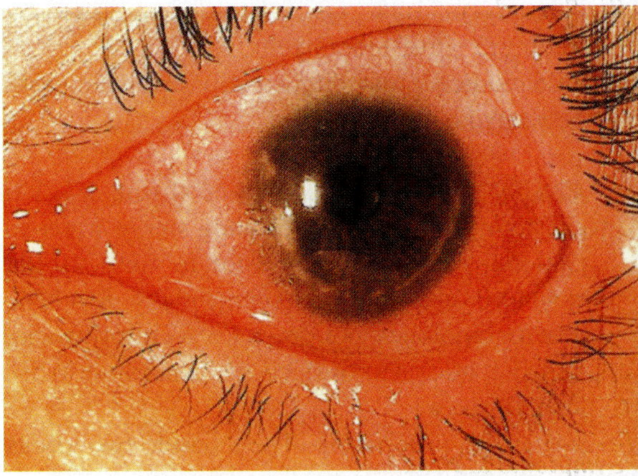

Fig. 5.7. Marginal corneal ulcer in a patient with acute conjunctivitis.

3. Soon vascularization occurs followed by resolution. Recurrences are very common.

Treatment

1. A short course of topical corticosteroid drops along with adequate antibiotic therapy often heals the condition.
2. Adequate treatment of associated blepharitis and chronic conjunctivitis is important to prevent recurrences.

MYCOTIC CORNEAL ULCER

The incidence of suppurative corneal ulcers caused by fungi has increased in the recent years due to injudicious use of antibiotics and steroids.

Etiology

1. *Causative fungi*. The fungi which may cause corneal infections are :

i. *Filamentous fungi* e.g., *Aspergillus*, *Fusarium*, *Alternaria*, *Cephalosporium*, *Curvularia* and *Penicillium*.
ii. *Yeasts* e.g., *Candida* and *Cryptococcus*.

Note: The fungi commonly responsible for mycotic corneal ulcers are *Aspergillus* (most common), *Candida* and *Fusarium*.

2. *Modes of infection*

i. *Injury by vegetative material* such as crop leaf, branch of a tree, straw, hay or decaying vegetable matter. Common sufferers are field workers especially during harvesting season.

ii. *Injury by animal tail* is another mode of infection.

iii. *Secondary fungal ulcers* are common in patients who are immunosuppressed systemically or locally such as patients suffering from dry eye, herpetic keratitis, bullous keratopathy or postoperative cases of keratoplasty.

3. *Role of antibiotics and steroids*. Antibiotics disturb the symbiosis between bacteria and fungi; and the steroids make the fungi facultative pathogens which are otherwise symbiotic saprophytes. Therefore, excessive use of these drugs predisposes the patients to fungal infections.

Clinical features

Symptoms are similar to the central bacterial corneal ulcer (see page 95), but in general they are less marked than the equal-sized bacterial ulcer and the overall course is slow and torpid.

Signs. A typical fungal corneal ulcer has following salient features (Fig. 5.8):

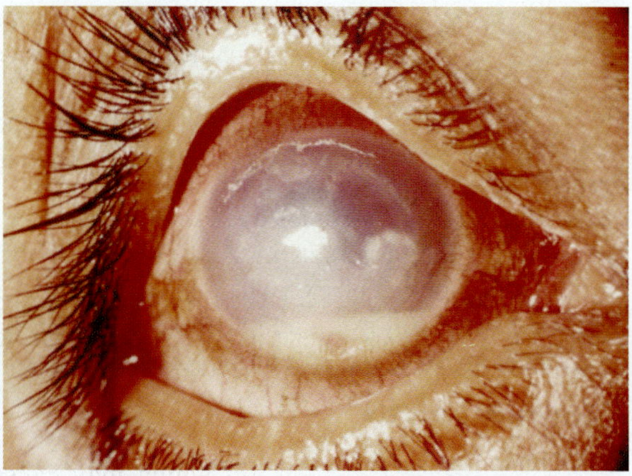

Fig. 5.8. Fungal corneal ulcer.

- Corneal ulcer is *dry-looking*, greyish white, with elevated rolled out margins.
- Delicate *feathery finger-like extensions* are present into the surrounding stroma under the intact epithelium.
- A *sterile immune ring* (yellow line of demarcation) may be present where fungal antigen and host antibodies meet.
- Multiple, small *satellite lesions* may be present around the ulcer.
- Usually a *big hypopyon* is present even if the ulcer is very small. Unlike bacterial ulcer, the hypopyon may not be sterile as the fungi can penetrate into the anterior chamber without perforation.
- *Perforation* in mycotic ulcer is rare but can occur.
- *Corneal vascularization* is conspicuously absent.

Diagnosis

1. *Typical clinical manifestations* associated with history of injury by vegetative material are diagnostic of a mycotic corneal ulcer.
2. *Chronic ulcer worsening* inspite of most efficient treatment should arouse suspicion of mycotic involvement.
3. *Laboratory investigations* required for confirmation, include examination of wet KOH, Calcofluor white, Gram's and Giemsa- stained films for fungal hyphae and culture on Sabouraud's agar medium.

Treatment

I. *Specific treatment* includes antifungal drugs:

1. *Topical antifungal eye drops* should be used for a long period (6 to 8 weeks). These include:

- *Natamycin* (5%), Amphotericin B (10-1.25 mg/ml), and either Fluconalzole (0.2%), or miconazole (10mg/ml) or voriconazole (10%) eye drops to be instilled initially one hourly around the clock, then taper slowly over 6 to 8 weeks. These are effective against *Aspergillus* and *Fusarium*.
- *Nystatin* (3.5%) eye ointment, five times a day is effective against *Candida*.

(For details see page 450).

2. *Systemic antifungal drugs* may be required for severe cases of fungal keratitis. Tablet fluconazole or ketoconazole may be given for 2-3 weeks.

II. *Non specific treatment.* *Non-specific treatment* and general measures are similar to that of bacterial corneal ulcer (see page 99).

III. *Therapeutic penetrating keratoplasty* may be required for nonresponsive cases.

VIRAL CORNEAL ULCERS

Incidence of viral corneal ulcers has become much greater especially because of the role of antibiotics in eliminating the pathogenic bacterial flora. Most of the viruses tend to affect the epithelium of both the conjunctiva and cornea, hence the typical viral lesions constitute the viral keratoconjunctivitis.

Common viral infections include herpes simplex keratitis, herpes zoster ophthalmicus and adenovirus keratitis.

HERPES SIMPLEX KERATITIS

Ocular infections with herpes simplex virus (HSV) are extremely common and constitute herpetic keratoconjunctivitis and iritis.

Etiology

Herpes simplex virus (HSV). It is a DNA virus. Its only natural host is man. Basically HSV is epitheliotropic but may become neurotropic. According to different clinical and immunological properties, HSV is of two types: HSV type I typically causes infection above the waist and HSV type II below the waist (herpes genitalis). HSV-II has also been reported to cause ocular lesions.

Mode of Infection

- *HSV-1 infection.* It is acquired by kissing or coming in close contact with a patient suffering from herpes labialis.
- *HSV-II infection.* It is transmitted to eyes of neonates through infected genitalia of the mother.

Ocular lesions of herpes simplex

Ocular involvement by HSV occurs in two forms, primary and recurrent; with following lesions:

A. *Primary herpes*

1. Skin lesions
2. Conjunctiva-acute follicular conjunctivitis
3. Cornea
   i. Fine epithelial punctate keratitis
   ii. Coarse epithelial punctate keratitis
   iii. Dendritic ulcer

B. *Recurrent herpes*

1. *Active epithelial keratitis*
   i. Punctate epthelial keratitis
   ii. Dendritic ulcer
   iii. Geographical ulcer
2. *Stromal keratitis*
   i. Disciform keratitis
   ii. Diffuse stromal necrotic keratitis
3. *Trophic keratitis (meta-herpetic)*
4. *Herpetic iridocyclitis*

A. Primary ocular herpes

Primary infection (first attack) involves a nonimmune person. It typically occurs in children of 6 months till 5 years of age and in teenagers.

Clinical features

1. *Skin lesions.* Vesicular lesions may occur involving skin of lids, periorbital region and the lid margin (vesicular blepharitis).
2. *Acute follicular conjunctivitis* with regional lymphadenitis is the usual and sometimes the only manifestation of the primary infection.
3. *Keratitis.* Cornea is involved in about 50 percent of the cases. The keratitis can occur as a coarse punctate or diffuse branching epithelial keratitis that does not usually involve the stroma.

Note: Primary infection is usually self-limiting but virus travels up to the trigeminal ganglion and establishes the latent infection.

B. Recurrent ocular herpes

The virus which lies dormant in the trigeminal ganglion, periodically reactivates and causes recurrent infection.

Predisposing stress stimuli which trigger an attack of herpetic keratitis include fever such as malaria, flu, exposure to ultraviolet rays, general ill health, emotional or physical exhaustion, mild trauma, menstrual stress following administration of topical or systemic steroids and immunosuppressive agents.

1. *Epithelial keratitis*

Symptoms

Symptoms of epithelial HSV keratitis include redness, pain, photophobia, tearing and decreased vision.

Signs

Three distinct patterns of epithelial keratitis seen are: punctate epithelial keratitis, dendritic ulcer and geographical ulcer.

i. *Punctate epithelial keratitis* (Fig. 5.9A). The initial epithelial lesions of recurrent herpes resemble those seen in primary herpes and may be either in the form of fine or coarse superficial punctate lesions.

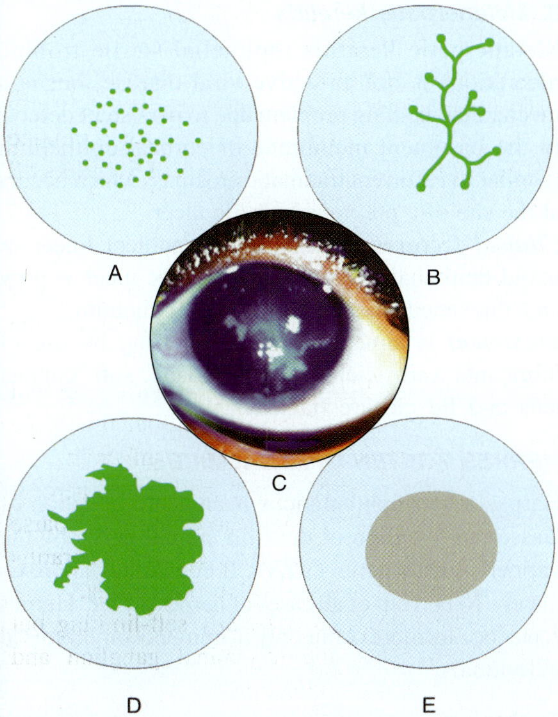

Fig. 5.9. Lesions of recurrent herpes simplex keratitis: A, Punctate epithelial keratitis; B and C, Dendritic ulcer; Diagramatics depiction and Clinical photograph; D, Geographical ulcer; and E, Disciform keratitis.

ii. *Dendritic ulcer* (Figs. 5.9B and C). Dendritic ulcer is a typical lesion of recurrent epithelial keratitis. The ulcer is of an irregular, zigzag linear branching shape. The branches are generally knobbed at the ends. Floor of the ulcer stains with fluorescein and the virus-laden cells at the margin take up rose bengal. There is an associated marked diminution of corneal sensations.

iii. *Geographical ulcer* (Fig. 5.9D). Sometimes, the branches of dendritic ulcer enlarge and coalesce to form a large epithelial ulcer with a 'geographical' or 'amoeboid' configuration, hence the name. The use of steroids in dendritic ulcer hastens the formation of geographical ulcer.

I. *Specific treatment*

1. *Antiviral drugs* are the first choice presently. Always start with one drug first and see the response. Usually after 4 days the lesion starts healing which is completed by 10 days. After healing, taper the drug and withdraw in 5 days. If after 7 days of initial therapy, there is no response, it means the virus is resistant to this drug. So change the drug and/or do mechanical debridement. Commonly used antiviral drugs with their dose regime is given below (for details see page 448).

i. *Acycloguanosine* (Aciclovir) 3 percent ointment: 5 times a day until ulcer heals and then 3 times a day for 5 days. It is least toxic and most commonly used antiviral drug. It penetrates intact corneal epithelium and stroma, achieving therapeutic levels in aqueous humour, and can therefore be used to treat herpetic keratitis.

ii. *Ganciclovir* (0.15% gel), 5 times a day until ulcer heals and then 3 times a day for 5 days. It is more toxic than aciclovir.

iii. *Triflurothymidine* 1 percent drops: Two hourly until ulcer heals and then 4 times a day for 5 days.

iv. *Adenine arabinoside* (Vidarabine) 3 percent ointment: 5 times a day until ulcer heals and then 3 times a day for 5 days.

2. *Mechanical debridement* of the involved area along with a rim of surrounding healthy epithelium with the help of sterile cotton applicator under magnification helps by removing the virus-laden cells.

Before the advent of antiviral drugs, it used to be the treatment of choice. Now it is reserved for resistant cases, cases with non-compliance and those allergic to antiviral drugs.

3. *Systemic antiviral drugs* for a period of 10 to 21 days are increasingly being considered for recurrent and even acute cases in following doses:

- Acyclovir 400 mg p.o. tid to bid, or
- Famcyclovir 250 mg p.o. bid, or
- Valacyclovir 500 mg p.o. bid.

II. *Non-specific supportive therapy* and physical and general measures are same as for bacterial corneal ulcer (see page 99).

2. *Stromal keratitis*

i. *Disciform keratitis*

Pathogenesis. It is due to delayed hypersensitivity reaction to the HSV antigen. Primarily, there occurs endothelitis. Endothelial damage results in disci form corneal stromal oedema due to imbibition of aqueous humour.

Signs. Disciform keratitis is characterized by (Fig. 5.9E):

- Focal disc-shaped patch of stromal oedema without necrosis, usually with an intact epithelium,
- Folds in Descemet's membrane,
- Keratic precipitates,
- Ring of stromal infilterate (Wessley immune ring) may be present surrounding the stromal oedema. It signifies the junction between viral antigen and host antibody.
- Corneal sensations are diminished.
- Intraocular pressure (IOP) may be raised despite only mild anterior uveitis. In severe cases, anterior uveitis may be marked.

Important note. During active stage diminished corneal sensations and keratic precipitates are the differentiating points from other causes of stromal oedema.

Treatment consists of diluted steroid eye drops instilled 4-5 times a day with an antiviral cover (aciclovir 3%) twice a day. Steroids should be tapered over a period of several weeks. When disciform keratitis is present with an infected epithelial ulcer, antiviral drugs should be started 5-7 days before the steroids.

ii. *Necrotizing intestitial keratitis (IK).* It is a type of interstitial keratitis caused by active viral invasion and tissue destruction.

Symptoms. Pain, photophobia and redness are common symptoms.

Signs

- *Corneal lesions* include necrotic, blotchy, cheesy white infiltrates that may lie under the epithelial ulcer or may present independently under the intact epithelium.
- *Mild iritis* and keratic precipitates are usually associated (herpetic keratouveitis).
- *Stromal vascularization* may occur.

Treatment is similar to disciform keratitis but frequently the results are unsatisfactory.

- *Systemic antiviral drugs* for 10 to 21 days are being considered in recurrent cases and in those with associated herpetic uveitis.
- *Keratoplasty* should be deferred until the eye has been quiet with little or no steroidal treatment for several months; because viral interstitial keratitis is the form of herpes which is most likely to recur in a new graft.

3. *Metaherpetic keratitis*

Metaherpetic keratitis (epithelial sterile trophic ulceration) is not an active viral disease, but is a mechanical healing problem due to persistent defects in the basement membrane of corneal epithelium (similar to recurrent traumatic erosions) which occurs at the site of a previous herpetic ulcer.

Clinical features presents as an indolent linear or ovoid epithelial defect. Margin of the ulcer is grey and thickened due to heaped up epithelium.

Treatment is aimed to promote healing by use of lubricants (artificial tears), bandage soft contact lens and lid closure (tarsorrhaphy).

HERPES ZOSTER OPHTHALMICUS

Herpes zoster ophthalmicus is an acute infection of Gasserian ganglion of the fifth cranial nerve by the varicella-zoster virus (VZV). It constitutes approximately 10 percent of all cases of herpes zoster. Herpes zoster occurs more commonly in immunocompromised individuals.

Etiology

Varicella -zoster virus. It is a DNA virus and produces acidophilic intranuclear inclusion bodies. It is neurotropic in nature.

Pathogenesis. The infection is contracted in childhood, which manifests as chickenpox and the child develops immunity. The virus then remains dormant in the sensory ganglion of trigeminal nerve. It is thought that, usually in elderly people (can occur at any age) with depressed cellular immunity, the virus reactivates, replicates and travels down along one or more of the branches of the ophthalmic division of the fifth nerve to produce cutaneous and ocular lesions.

Clinical features

- In herpes zoster ophthalmicus, frontal nerve is more frequently affected than the lacrimal and nasociliary nerves.
- About 50 percent cases of herpes zoster ophthalmicus get ocular complications.
- *Hutchinson's rule*, which implies that ocular involvement is frequent if the side or tip of nose presents vesicles (cutaneous involvement of nasociliary nerve), is useful but not infallible.

- Lesions of herpes zoster are strictly limited to one side of the midline of head.

Clinical phases of H. zoster ophthalmicus are:

I. *Acute*, which may totally resolve within few weeks.

II. *Chronic,* which may persist for years.

III. *Relapsing,* where the acute or chronic lesions reappear sometimes years later.

I. *Acute phase lesions.*

A. *General features*. The onset of illness is sudden with fever, malaise and severe neuralgic pain along the course of the affected nerve. The distribution of pain is so characteristic of zoster that it usually arouses suspicion of the nature of the disease before appearance of vesicles.

B. *Cutaneous lesions*. Cutaneous lesions (Fig. 5.10) in the area of distribution of the involved nerve appear usually after 3-4 days of the onset of disease. To begin with, the skin of lids and other affected areas become red and oedematous (mimicking erysipelas), followed by vesicle formation. In due course of time vesicles are converted into pustules, which subsequently burst to become crusting ulcers. When crusts are shed, permanent pitted scars are left. The active eruptive phase lasts for about 3 weeks. Main symptom is severe neuralgic pain which usually diminishes with the subsidence of eruptive phase.

C. *Ocular lesions*. Ocular complications usually appear at the subsidence of skin eruptions and may present as a combination of two or more of the following lesions:

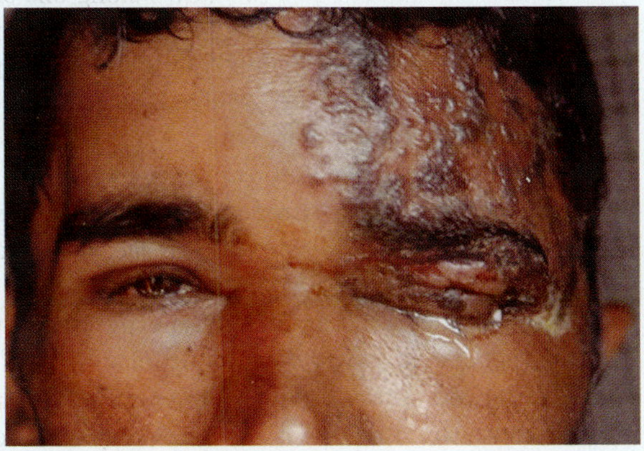

Fig. 5.10. Cutaneous lesions of herpes zoster ophthalmicus.

1. *Conjunctivitis* is one of the most common complication of herpes zoster. It may occur as mucopurulent conjunctivitis with petechial haemorrhages or acute follicular conjunctivitis with regional lymphadenopathy. Sometimes, severe necrotizing membranous inflammation may be seen.

2. *Zoster keratitis* occurs in 40 percent of all patients and sometimes may precede the neuralgia or skin lesions. It may occur in several forms (Fig. 5.11):

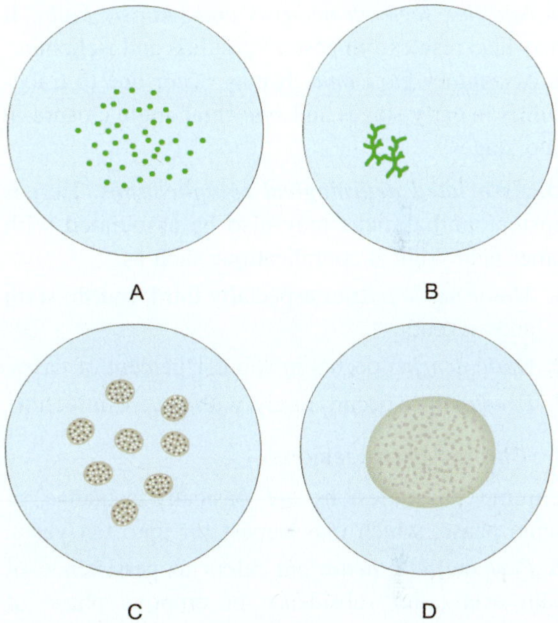

Fig. 5.11. Types of zoster keratitis : A, Punctate epithelial keratitis; B, Microdendritic epithelial ulcer; C, Nummular keratitis; D, Disciform keratitis.

- *Epithelial keratitis.* To begin with there occurs fine or coarse *punctate epithelial keratitis.* It is followed by *microdendritic epithelial ulcers* which unlike dendritic ulcers of herpes simplex are usually peripheral and stellate rather than exactly dendritic in shape. In contrast to Herpes simplex dendrites, they have tapered ends which lack bulbs.
- *Anterior stromal infiltrates nummular keratitis* is seen in about one-third number of total cases. It typically occurs as multiple tiny granular deposits surrounded by a halo of stromal haze. After healing 'nummular scars' are left behind.
- *Disciform keratitis* occurs in about 50 percent of cases and is always preceded by nummular keratitis.

3. *Episcleritis and scleritis* occur in about one-half of the cases. These usually appear at the onset of the rash but are frequently concealed by the overlying conjunctivitis.

4. *Iridocyclitis* is of a frequent occurrence and may or may not be associated with keratitis. There may be associated hypopyon and hyphaema (acute haemorrhagic uveitis).

5. *Acute retinal necrosis* may occurs in some cases.

6. *Anterior segment necrosis and phthisis bulbi.* It may also result from zoster vasculitis and ischemia.

7. *Secondary glaucoma.* It may occur due to trabeculitis in early stages and synechial angle closure in late stages.

D. *Associated neurological complications.* Herpes zoster ophthalmicus may also be associated with other neurological complications such as:

1. *Motor nerve palsies* especially third, fourth, sixth and seventh.
2. *Optic neuritis* occurs in about 1 percent of cases.
3. *Encephalitis* occurs rarely with severe infection.

II. *Chronic phase lesions*

Chronic phase lesions are basically sequelae of acute phase, which may persist for upto ten years.

1. *Post herpetic neuralgia* refers to persistence of pain even after subsidence of eruptive phase of zostar which occurs in about 10% cases. Pain is mild to moderate in intensity, worsens at night and is aggravated by touch and heat. But sometimes it may persist for years with little diminution of intensity. There occurs some anaesthesia of the affected skin which when associated with continued post-herpetic neuralgia is called anaesthesia dolorosa.

2. *Lid lesions* which occur as sequalae of scarring include ptosis, trichiasis, entropion and notching.

3. *Conjunctival lesions* include chronic mucous secreting conjunctivitis.

4. *Corneal lesions* are as below:

- *Neuroparalytic ulceration* may occur as a sequelae of acute infection and Gasserian ganglion destruction.
- *Exposure keratitis* may supervene in some cases due to associated facial palsy.
- *Mucous plaque keratitis* develops in 5% of cases between 3rd and 5th months and is characterised by sudden development of elevated mucous plaque which stain brilliantly with rose bengal.

5. *Scleritis* and *Uveitis* may persist in chronic form.

III. *Relapsing phase lesions*

Relapsing phase lesions, which may recur even after ten years of acute phase include nummular keratitis, mucous plaque keratitis, episcleritis, scleritis and secondary glaucoma.

Treatment

Therapeutic approach to herpes zoster ophthalmicus should be vigorous and aimed at preventing severe devastating ocular complications and promoting rapid healing of the skin lesions without the formation of massive crusts which result in scarring of the nerves and postherpetic neuralgia. The following regime may be followed:

I. *Systemic therapy for herpes zoster*

1. *Oral antiviral drugs.* These significantly decrease pain, curtail vesiculation, stop viral progression and reduce the incidence as well as severity of keratitis and iritis. In order to be effective, the treatment should be started immediately after the onset of rash. It has no effect on post herpetic neuralgia.
   - *Acyclovir* in a dose of 800 mg 5 times a day for 10 days, or
   - *Valaciclovir* in a dose of 500 mg TDS
2. *Analgesics.* Pain during the first 2 weeks of an attack is very severe and should be treated by analgesics such as combination of mephenamic acid and paracetamol or pentazocin or even pethidine (when very severe).
3. *Systemic steroids.* They appear to inhibit development of post-herpetic neuralgia when given in high doses. However, the risk of high doses of steroids in elders should always be taken into consideration. Steroids are commonly recommended in cases developing neurological complications such as third nerve palsy and optic neuritis.
4. *Cimetidine* in a dose of 300 mg QID for 2-3 weeks starting within 48-72 hours of onset has also

been shown to reduce pain and pruritis in acute zoster - presumably by histamine blockade.

5. *Amitriptyline* should be used to relieve the accompanying depression in acute phase.

II. *Local therapy for skin lesions*

1. *Antibiotic-corticosteroid skin ointment or lotions.* These should be used three times a day till skin lesions heal.
2. *No calamine lotion.* Cool zinc calamine application, as advocated earlier, is better avoided, as it promotes crust formation.

III. *Local therapy for ocular lesions*

1. *For zoster keratitis, iridocyctitis and scleritis*
   i. Topical steroid eye drops 4 times a day.
   ii. Cycloplegics such as cyclopentolate eyedrops BD or atropine eye ointment OD.
   iii. Topical acyclovir 3 percent eye ointment should be instilled 5 times a day for about 2 weeks.
2. *To prevent secondary infections* topical antibiotics are used.
3. *For secondary glaucoma*
   i. 0.5 percent timolol or 0.5% betaxolol drops, BD.
   ii. Acetazolamide 250 mg, QID.
4. *For mucous plaques*, add topical mucolytics e.g. acetyl cysteine 5 to 10%, three times a day.
5. *For persistent epithelial defects* use:
   i. Lubricating artificial tear drops, and
   ii. Bandage soft contact lens.
6. *For neuroparalytic corneal ulcer* caused by herpes zoster, lateral tarsorrhaphy should be performed. Amniotic membrane transplantation (AMT) or conjunctival flap should be considered for non-healing cases.
7. *Keratoplasty.* It may be required for visual rehabilitation of zoster-patients with dense scarring. However, these are poor risk patients.

PROTOZOAL KERATITIS

ACANTHAMOEBA KERATITIS

Acanthamoeba keratitis has recently gained importance because of its increasing incidence, difficulty in diagnosis and unsatisfactory treatment.

Etiology

Acanthamoeba castellani, the causative organism is a free lying amoeba found in soil, fresh water, well water, sea water, sewage and air. It exists in trophozoite and encysted forms.

Mode of infection. Corneal infection with acanthamoeba results from direct corneal contact with any material or water contaminated with the organism. Following situations of contamination have been described:

1. *Contact lens wearers* using home-made saline (from contaminated tap water and saline tablets) is the commonest situation recognised for acanthamoeba infection in western countries.
2. *Non-contact lens related situations* include mild trauma associated with contaminated vegetable matter, salt water diving, wind blown contaminant and hot tub use. Trauma with organic matter and exposure to muddy water are the major (90% cases) predisposing factors in developing countries.
3. *Opportunistic infection.* Acanthamoeba keratitis can also occur as opportunistic infection in patients with herpetic keratitis, bacterial keratitis, bullous keratopathy and neuroparalytic keratitis.

Clinical features

Symptoms. These vary from asymptomatic to foreign body sensation, mild pain to severe pain (out of proportion to the degree of inflammation), watering, photophobia, blepharospasm and blurred vision.

Signs. Acanthamoeba keratitis evolves over several months as a gradual worsening keratitis with periods of temporary remission. Presentation is markedly variable, making diagnosis difficult. Characteristic features are described below:

1. *Initial lesions* include:

- Limbitis, reported in 94% cases,
- Radial keratoneuritis reported in 30% cases, and
- Epitheliopathy of any of the following forms:
  - punctate epitheliopathy
  - epithelial ridges
  - pseudo or true dendrites, or
  - irregular epitheliopathy

2. *Advanced case* of acanthamoeba keratitis are characterized by:

- Patchy stromal infiltrates,
- Satellite infiltrates,
- Central or paracentral ring infiltrates with overlying epithelial defects (Fig. 5.12A)

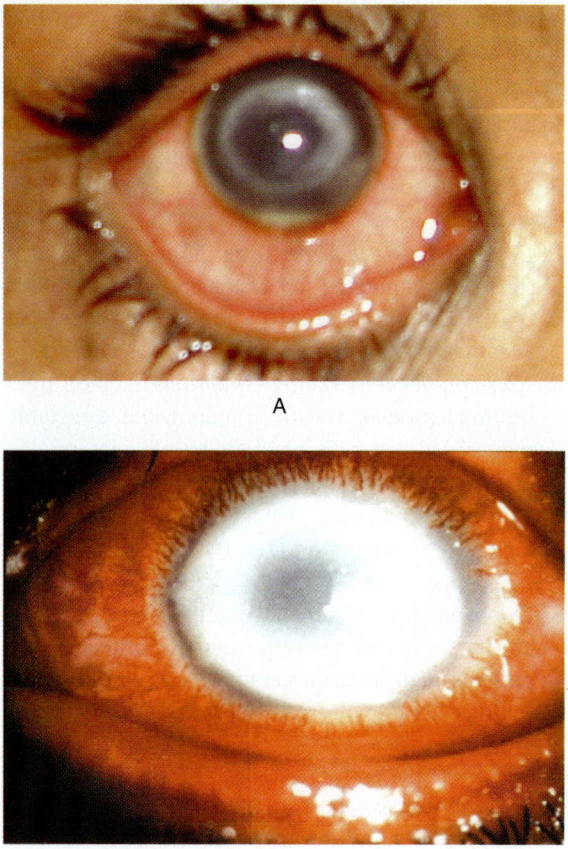

Fig. 5.12. Ring infiltrate (A) and ring abscess (B) in a patient with advanced acanthamoeba keratitis.

- Hypopyon may also be seen in advanced cases

3. *Severe cases* may develop:
- Ring abscess (Fig. 5.12B) associated with
- Hypopyon, and Stromal necrosis

Diagnosis

1. *Clinical diagnosis.* It is difficult and usually made by exclusion with strong clinical suspicion out of the non-responsive patients being treated for herpetic, bacterial or fungal keratitis.

2. *Laboratory diagnosis.* Corneal scrapings may be helpful in some cases as under:

i. *Confocal microscopy*, when available allows direct visualization of the cysts, which is diagnostic.
ii. *Potassium hydroxide(KOH) mount* is reliable in experienced hands for recognition of acanthamoeba cysts.
iii. *Calcofluor white stain* is a fluorescent brightener which stains the cysts of acanthamoeba bright apple green under fluorescence microscope.
iv. *Lactophenol cotton blue stained* film is also useful for demonstration of acanthamoeba cysts in the corneal scrapings.
v. *Culture on non-nutrient agar* (*E. coli* enriched) may show trophozoites within 48 hours, which gradually turn into cysts.

Treatment

It is usually unsatisfactory.

1. ***Non-specific treatment*** is on the general lines for corneal ulcer (see page 99).
2. ***Specific treatment***

i. *Topical Antiamoebic agents*: include
- *Diamidines*: Propamidine isethionate (0.1%), and hexamidine (0.1%)
- *Biguanides*: Polyhexamethylene biguanide (PHMB), 0.02% and chlorhexidine, 0.02%,
- *Aminoglycosides*: Neomycin, and Paromycin
- *Imidazoles*: Clotrimazole and miconazole

Multiple drug therapy is needed for a long time (3-4 months) for early epithelial lesions and 6-12 months for stromal lesions. Any of the following combination may be choosen: Propamidine or hexamidine + PHMB or chlorhexidine + Neomycin or Paromycin + clotrimazole or miconazole or itraconazole.
Frequency of instillation: hourly for a week, then taper slowly 3-4 months for epithelial lesions and 6-12 months for stromal lesions

ii. *Oral ketoconazole* 200 mg BID, or itraconazole 100 mg BD may be added in advanced cases.

3. Long term prophylactic therapy with PHMB, twice a day for a year is recommended.
4. *Penetrating keratoplasty* is frequently required in non-responsive cases. Surgery should be performed after a full course of maximum medical therapy and a quiescent phase of atleast six months.

ALLERGIC KERATITIS

1. Phlyctenular keratitis (page 76)
2. Vernal keratitis (page 73)
3. Atopic keratitis (page 74)

TROPHIC CORNEAL ULCERS

Trophic corneal ulcers develop due to disturbance in metabolic activity of epithelial cells. This group includes: Neurotrophic keratopathy and Exposure keratopathy.

NEUROTROPHIC KERATOPATHY

Neurotrophic keratopathy occurs due to decreased corneal sensations owing to damage of sensory nerve supply of the cornea.

Causes

I. *Congenital*
  1. Familial dysautonomia (Riley-Day syndrome)
  2. Congenital insensitivity to pain.
  3. Anhidrotic ectodermal dysplasia.

II. *Acquired*
  1. Following alcohol-block or electrocoagulation of Gasserian ganglion or section of the sensory root of trigeminal nerve for trigeminal neuralgia.
  2. A neoplasm pressing on Gasserian ganglion.
  3. Gasserian ganglion destruction due to acute infection in herpes zoster ophthalmicus.
  4. Acute infection of Gasserian ganglion by herpes simplex virus.
  5. Syphilitic (luetic) neuropathy.
  6. Involvement of corneal nerves in leprosy.
  7. Injury to Gasserian ganglion.

Pathogenesis

Exact pathogenesis is not clear; presumably, the disturbances in the corneal sensations occur due to damage to sensory nerves. As a consequence metabolic activity of corneal epithelium is disturbed, leading to accumulation of metabolites; which in turn cause oedema and exfoliation of epithelial cells followed by ulceration. Corneal changes can occur in the presence of a normal blink reflex and normal lacrimal secretions.

Clinical features

Symptoms

- Red eye, swollen eyelids and defective vision are common complaints.
- No pain, and no tearing are characteristic features.

Signs

1. *Ciliary congestion* is marked,
2. *Corneal* signs,

- Sensations are decreased,
- Sheen is lost (dull sheen),
- Punctate epithelial erosions involving the interpalpabral area are initial lesions, which soon converts into,
- Frank epithelial defects due to exfoliation of corneal epithelium, later followed by
- Corneal ulcer formation, which is typically horizontally oval, located in the lower one-half of the cornea and have grey heaped-up epithelial borders.

Note: Relapses are very common, even the healed scars quickly breakdown again.

Treatment

- *Conventional treatment* with antibiotics, cycloplegics, lubricating drops and patching should be started immediately.
- *Special treatment* recommended is topical nerve growth factor drops and autologous serum drops.
- *Amniotic membrane transplantation* is recommended when patients present with large non healing ulcers.
- *Lateral tarsorrhaphy* is usually required to promote healing and prevent relapses. It should be kept at least for one year alongwith and prolonged use of artificial tears is also recommended.

EXPOSURE KERATOPATHY

Normally cornea is covered by eyelids during sleep and is constantly kept moist by blinking movements during awaking. When eyes are covered insufficiently by the lids and there is loss of protective mechanism of blinking, the condition of exposure keratopathy (keratitis lagophthalmos) develops.

Causes

Following factors which produce lagophthalmos may lead to exposure keratopathy:

1. *Extreme proptosis* due to any cause will allow inadequate closure of lids.
2. *Bell's palsy* or any other cause of facial palsy.
3. *Ectropion* of severe degree.
4. *Symblepharon* causing lagophthalmos.
5. *Deep coma* associated with inadequate closure of lids.
6. *Physiological lagophthalmos.* Occasionally, lagophthalmos during sleep may occur in healthy individuals.

Pathogenesis

Due to exposure the corneal epithelium dries up followed by dessication. After the epithelium is cast off, invasion by infective organisms may occur.

Clinical features

Symptoms & signs of the causative disease are evident

Symptoms of exposure keratopathy include ocular irritation, burning, foreign body sensation and redness. Symptoms are usually worse in the morning.

Signs of exposure keratopathy are:

- *Drying of cornea* occurs to begin with due to inadequate blinking or closure of the lids .
- *Punctate epithelial defects* develop in the lower third of cornea or as a horizontal band in the region of palpebral fissure.
- *Corneal ulceration* may develop soon due to necrosis followed by bacterial superinfection. If neglected, corneal ulcer may even perforate soon.

Treatment

1. *Prophylaxis.* Once lagophthalmos is diagnosed following measures should be taken to prevent exposure keratitis.

- *Artificial tears* should be instilled frequently.
- *Instillation of ointment* and closure of lids by a tape or bandage during sleep.
- *Soft bandage contact lens* with frequent instillation of artificial tears is required in cases of moderate exposure.
- *Treatment of the cause of exposure:* e.g. proptosis, ectropion, symblepharon should be taken up.

2. *Treatment of the corneal ulcer* once developed is on the general lines (see page 98).

- *Tarsorrhaphy* is invariably required when it is not possible to treat the cause or when recovery of the cause (e.g., facial palsy) is not anticipated.

PERIPHERAL ULCERATIVE KERATOPATHIES

Peripheral ulcerative keratopathies (PUKs), characterized by peripheral corneal thinning, infiltrates and ulceration, includes various conditions with different etiologies. Some of the PUKs are as follows:

- Peripheral ulcerative keratitis associated with connective tissue disorders,
- Mooren's ulcer,
- Rosacea keratitis,
- Marginal keratitis (catarrhal ulcer) of Staphylococcal hypersensitivity (see page 100),
- Terrien marginal degeneration (see page 119),
- Pellucid marginal degeneration (see page 119),
- Phlyctenular keratitis (see page 76), and
- Dellen

PERIPHERAL ULCERATIVE KERATITIS ASSOCIATED WITH CONNECTIVE TISSUE DISEASES (MARGINAL KERATOLYSIS)

Causes

Peripheral corneal ulceration and/or melting of corneal tissue is not of infrequent occurrence in patients suffering from connective tissue diseases such as:

- Rheumatoid arthritis,
- Systemic lupus erythematosus (SLE),
- Polyarteritis nodosa, and
- Wegener's granulomatosis.

Clinical features

- Unilateral/bilateral peripheral acute corneal ulceration with rapid progression, usually in one sector, associated with inflammation at the limbus.
- Peripheral corneal guttering or thinning may involve entire corneal periphery (contact lens cornea)
- Peripheral corneal melting may result in descemetocele formation or even perforation.
- Corneal ulceration may be the first manifestation of the systemic disease and there may be associated systemic features of any of the causative disease.

Treatment

Such corneal ulcers are usually indolent and difficult to treat

1. *Topical medication* include, antibiotics, cycloplegics and frequent instillation of lubricating drops. Topical steroids may be used with great caution, but not in the presence of significant thinning.
2. *Systemic medication* includes immunosuppresants (corticosteroids, or methotrexate, cyclophosphamide), doxycycline and oral vitamin C (to promote a healing stromal environment).
3. *Surgical measures* needed include:
   - Excision of adjacent inflamed conjunctiva,
   - Bandage contact lens or conjunctival flap for impending perforation,

- Application of cynoacrylate tissue adhesive or peripheral tectonic keratoplasty for actual perforation.

MOOREN'S ULCER

The Mooren's ulcer (chronic serpiginous or rodent ulcer) is a severe inflammatory peripheral ulcerative keratitis.

Etiology

Exact etiology is not known. Most probably it is an *autoimmune disease* (antibodies against corneal epithelium have been demonstrated in serum).

Clinical picture

Two clinical varieties of Mooren's ulcer have been recognised.

1. *Benign or limited form* which is usually unilateral, affects the elderly Caucasians and is characterised by a relative slow progress.
2. *Virulent type* also called the *progressive form* is bilateral, more often occurs in young African patients. The ulcer is rapidly progressive with a high incidence of scleral involvement.

Symptoms. These include severe pain, photophobia, lacrimation and defective vision.

Signs. Features of Mooren's ulcer are shown in Fig. 5.13.

- It is a superficial ulcer which starts at the corneal margin as patches of grey infiltrates which coalesce to form a shallow furrow over the whole cornea.
- Peripheral ulcer is associated with undermining of the epithelium and superficial stromal lamellae at the advancing border which forms a characteristic whitish overhanging edge. Base of the ulcer soon becomes vascularized. The spread may be self-limiting or progressive.
- At the end-stage, the cornea is thinned and conjunctivised.
- The ulcer rarely perforates and the sclera remains uninvolved.

Treatment

Since exact etiology is still unknown, its treatment is highly unsatisfactory. Following measures may be tried:

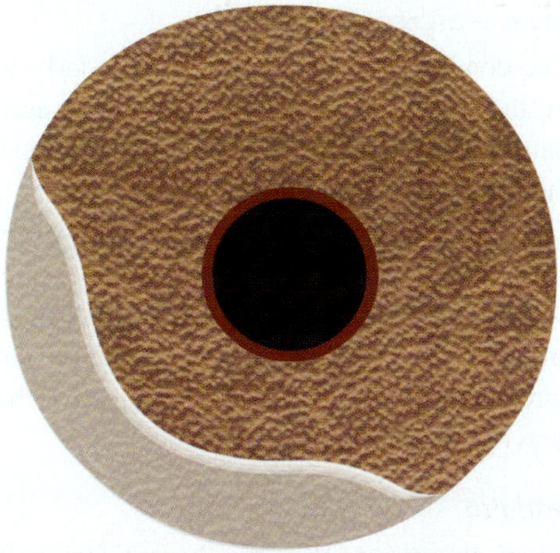

A

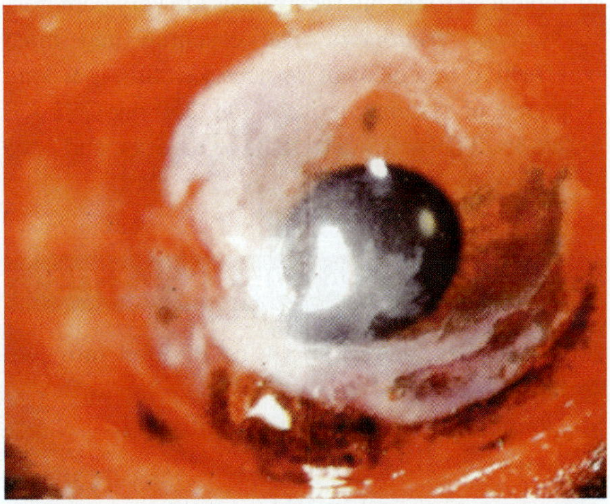

B

Fig. 5.13. Mooren's ulcer : A, diagrammatic depiction; B, clinical photograph.

1. *Topical corticosteroids* instilled every 2-3 hours are tried as initial therapy with limited success.
2. *Immunosuppressive therapy* with systemic steroids may be of help. Immunosuppression with *cyclosporin* or other cytotoxic agents may be quite useful in virulent type of disease.
3. *Soft contact lenses* have also been used with some relief in pain.
4. *Lamellar or full thickness corneal grafts* often melt or vascularize.

ROSACEA KERATITIS

Corneal ulceration is seen in about 10 percent cases of acne rosacea, which is primarily a disease of the sebaceous glands of the skin.

Clinical features

1. The condition typically occurs in elderly women in the form of *facial eruptions* presenting as butterfly configuration, predominantly involving the malar and nasal area of face.
2. *Ocular lesions* include chronic blepharo-conjunctivitis and keratitis. Rosacea keratitis occurs as yellowish white marginal infiltrates, and small ulcers that progressively advance across the cornea and almost always become heavily vascularised.

Treatment

1. *Local treatment.* Rosacea keratitis responds to topical steroids, but recurrences are very common.
2. *Systemic treatment.* The essential and most effective treatment of rosacea keratitis is a long course of systemic tetracycline (250 mg QID × 3 weeks, TDS × 3 weeks, BID × 3 weeks, and once a day for 3 months).

NON-ULCERATIVE KERATITIS

Non-ulcerative keratitis can be divided into two groups:

- Non-ulcerative superficial keratitis and
- Non-ulcerative deep keratitis.

NON-ULCERATIVE SUPERFICIAL KERATITIS

This group includes a number of conditions of varied etiology. Here the inflammatory reaction is confined to epithelium, Bowman's membrane and superficial stromal lamellae. Non-ulcerative superficial keratitis may present in two forms:

- Diffuse superficial keratitis and
- Superficial punctate keratitis

DIFFUSE SUPERFICIAL KERATITIS

Diffuse inflammation of superficial layers of cornea occurs in two forms, acute and chronic.

1. *Acute diffuse superficial keratitis*

Etiology. Mostly of infective origin, may be associated with Staphylococcal or gonococcal infections.

Clinical features. It is characterised by faint diffuse epithelial oedema associated with grey farinaceous appearance being interspersed with relatively clear area. Epithelial erosions may be formed at places. If uncontrolled, it usually converts into ulcerative keratitis.

Treatment. It consists of frequent instillation of antibiotic eyedrops such as tobramycin or gentamycin 2-4 hourly.

2. *Chronic diffuse superficial keratitis*

It may be seen in rosacea, phlyctenulosis and is typically associated with pannus formation.

SUPERFICIAL PUNCTATE KERATITIS (SPK)

Superficial punctate keratitis is characterised by occurrence of multiple, spotty lesions in the superficial layers of cornea. It may result from a number of conditions, identification of which (causative condition) might not be possible most of the times.

Causes

Some important causes of superficial punctate keratitis are listed here.

1. *Viral infections* are the chief cause. Of these more common are: herpes zoster, adenovirus infections, epidemic keratoconjunctivitis, pharyngo-conjunctival fever and herpes simplex.
2. *Chlamydial infections* include trachoma and inclusion conjunctivitis.
3. *Toxic lesions* e.g., due to Staphylococcal toxin in association with blepharoconjunctivitis.
4. *Trophic lesions* e.g., exposure keratitis and neuroparalytic keratitis.
5. *Allergic lesions* e.g., vernal keratoconjunctivitis.
6. *Irritative lesions* e.g., effect of some drugs such as idoxuridine.
7. *Disorders of skin and mucous membrane,* such as acne rosacea and pemphigoid.
8. *Dry eye syndrome,* i.e., keratoconjunctivitis sicca.
9. *Specific type of idiopathic SPK* e.g., Thygeson's superficial punctate keratitis and Theodore's superior limbic keratoconjunctivitis.
10. *Photo-ophthalmitis.*

Morphological types (Fig. 5.14)

1. Punctate epithelial erosions (multiple superficial erosions).
2. Punctate epithelial keratitis.

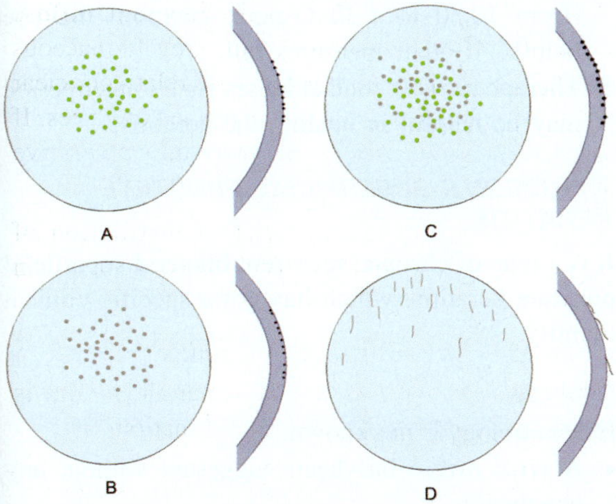

Fig. 5.14. Morphological types of superficial punctate keratitis.

3. Punctate subepithelial keratitis.
4. Punctate combined epithelial and subepithelial keratitis.
5. Filamentary keratitis.

Clinical features

Superficial punctate keratitis may present as different morphological types as enumerated above. Punctate epithelial lesions usually stain with fluorescein, rose bengal and other vital dyes. The condition mostly presents with acute pain, photophobia and lacrimation; and is usually associated with conjunctivitis.

Treatment

Treatment of most of these conditions is symptomatic.

1. *Topical steroids* have a marked suppressive effect.
2. *Artificial tears* have soothing effect.
3. *Specific treatment* of cause should be instituted whenever possible e.g., antiviral drugs in cases of herpes simplex.

PHOTO-OPHTHALMIA

Photo-ophthalmia refers to occurrence of multiple epithelial erosions due to the effect of ultraviolet rays especially from 311 to 290 μ.

Causes

1. Exposure to bright light of a short circuit.
2. Naked arc light exposure as in industrial welding and cinema operators.
3. *Snow blindness* due to reflected ultraviolet rays from snow surface.

Pathogenesis

After an interval of 4-5 hours (latent period) of exposure to ultraviolet rays, there occurs desquamation of corneal epithelium leading to formation of multiple epithelial erosions.

Clinical features

- Typically, patient presents with severe burning pain, lacrimation, photophobia, blepharospasm, swelling of palpebral conjunctiva and retrotarsal folds.
- There is history of exposure to ultraviolet rays 4-5 hours earlier.
- On fluorescein staining multiple spots are demonstrated on both corneas.

Prophylaxis

Crooker's glass which cuts off all infrared and ultraviolet rays should be used by those who are prone to exposure e.g., welding workers, cinema operators etc.

Treatment

1. Cold compresses.
2. Patching with antibiotic ointment for 24 hours, heals most of the cases.
3. Oral analgesics may be given if pain is intolerable.
4. Single dose of tranquilliser may be given to apprehensive patients.

SUPERIOR LIMBIC KERATOCONJUNCTIVITIS

Superior limbic keratoconjunctivitis of Theodore is the name given to inflammation of superior limbic, bulbar and tarsal conjunctiva associated with punctate keratitis of the superior part of cornea.

Etiology

Exact etiology is not known. It occurs with greater frequency in patients with hyperthyroidism and is more common in females.

Clinical features

Clinical course is chronic with remissions and exacerbations.

Symptoms include :

- Bilateral ocular irritation.

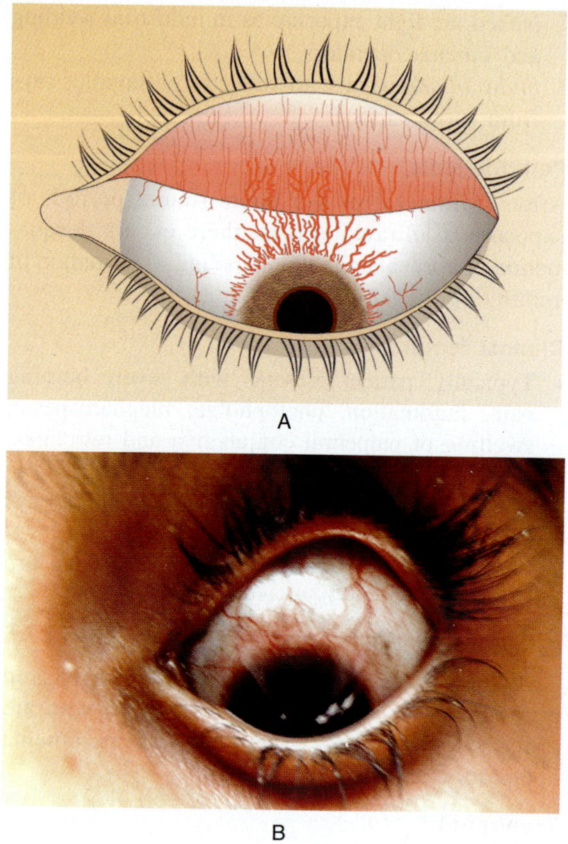

Fig. 5.15. Superior limbic keratoconjunctivitis : A, diagramatic depiction; B, clinical photograph.

- Mild photophobia, and
- Redness in superior bulbar conjunctiva.

Signs (Fig. 5.15) include
- *Congestion* of superior limbic, bulbar and tarsal conjunctiva.
- *Punctate keratitis* which stains with fluorescein and rose bengal stain is seen in superior part of cornea.
- *Corneal filaments* are also frequently seen in the involved area.

Treatment

1. Topical artificial tears.
2. Low doses of topical corticosteroids may reduce the symptoms temporarily.
3. Faint diathermy of superior bulbar conjunctiva in a checker board pattern gives acceptable results.
4. Recession or resection of a 3-4 mm wide perilimbal strip of conjunctiva from the superior limbus (from 10.30 to 1.30 O'clock position) may be helpful, if other measures fail.
5. Therapeutic soft contact lenses for a longer period may be helpful in healing the keratitis.

THYGESON'S SUPERFICIAL PUNCTATE KERATITIS

It is a type of chronic, recurrent bilateral superficial punctate keratitis, which has got a specific clinical identity.

Etiology

Exact etiology is not known.
- A *viral origin* has been suggested without any conclusion.
- An *allergic* or dyskeratotic nature also has been suggested owing to its response to steroids.

Clinical features

- *Age and sex.* It may involve all ages with no sex predilection.
- *Laterality.* Usually bilateral.
- *Course.* It is a chronic disease characterised by remissions and exacerbations.

Symptoms

It may be asymptomatic, but is usually associated with foreign body sensation, photophobia and lacrimation.

Signs

1. *Conjunctiva* is uninflamed (no conjunctivitis).
2. *Corneal lesions.* There are coarse punctate epithelial lesions (snow flake) circular, oval or stellate in shape, slightly elevated and situated in the central part (pupillary area) of cornea. Each lesion is a cluster of heterogeneous granular grey dots.

Treatment

1. The disease is self-limiting with remissions and may permanently disappear in a period of 5-6 years.
2. During exacerbations the lesions and associated symptoms usually respond quickly to topical steroids (so, should be tapered rapidly).
3. Therapeutic soft contact lenses may be required in steroid-resistant cases.

FILAMENTARY KERATITIS

It is a type of superficial punctate keratitis, associated with formation of corneal epithelial filaments.

Pathogenesis

Corneal filaments which essentially consist of a tag of elongated epithelium are formed due to aberrant epithelial healing. Therefore, any condition that leads to focal epithelial erosions may produce filamentary keratopathy.

Causes

The common conditions associated with filamentary keratopathy are:

1. Keratoconjunctivitis sicca (KCS).
2. Superior limbic keratoconjunctivitis.
3. Epitheliopathy due to radiation keratitis.
4. Following epithelial erosions as in herpes simplex keratitis, Thygeson's superficial punctate keratitis, recurrent corneal erosion syndrome and trachoma.
5. Prolonged patching of the eye particularly following ocular surgery like cataract.
6. Systemic disorders like diabetes mellitus, ectodermal dysplasia and psoriasis.
7. Idiopathic.

Clinical features

Symptoms. Patients usually experience moderate pain, ocular irritation, lacrimation and foreign body sensation.

Signs. Corneal examination reveals.

- *Filaments* i.e., fine tags of elongated epithelium which are firmly attached at the base, intertwined with mucus and degenerated cells. The filament is freely movable over the cornea.
- *Superficial punctate keratitis* of varying degree is usually associated with corneal filaments.

Treatment

1. *Management of filaments* include their mechanical debridement and patching for 24 hours followed by lubricating drops.
2. *Therapeutic soft contact lenses* may be useful in recurrent cases.
3. *Treatment of the underlying cause* to prevent recurrence.

DEEP KERATITIS

An inflammation of corneal stroma with or without involvement of posterior corneal layers constitutes deep keratitis, which may be non-suppurative or suppurative.

- *Non-suppurative deep keratitis* includes, interstitial keratitis, disciform keratitis, keratitis profunda and sclerosing keratitis.
- *Suppurative deep keratitis* includes central corneal abscess and posterior corneal abscess, which are usually metastatic in nature.

INTERSTITIAL KERATITIS

Interstitial keratitis denotes an inflammation of the corneal stroma without primary involvement of the epithelium or endothelium.

Causes. Its common causes are:

- Congenital syphilis
- Tuberculosis
- Cogan's syndrome
- Acquired syphilis
- Trypanosomiasis
- Malaria
- Leprosy
- Sarcoidosis

Syphilitic (luetic) interstitial keratitis

Syphilitic interstitial keratitis is associated more frequently (90 percent) with congenital syphilis than the acquired syphilis. The disease is generally bilateral in inherited syphilis and unilateral in acquired syphilis. In congenital syphilis, manifestations develop between 5-15 years of age.

Pathogenesis

It is now generally accepted that the disease is a manifestation of local antigen-antibody reaction. It is presumed that *Treponema pallidum* invades the cornea and sensitizes it during the period of its general diffusion throughout the body in the foetal stage. Later a small-scale fresh invasion by *Treponema* or toxins excite the inflammation in the sensitized cornea. The inflammation is usually triggered by an injury or an operation on the eye.

Clinical features

Interstitial keratitis characteristically forms one of the late manifestations of congenital syphilis. Many times it may be a part of *Hutchinson's triad*, which includes interstitial keratitis, *Hutchinson's teeth* and vestibular deafness.

The clinical picture of interstitial keratitis can be divided into three stages: initial progressive stage, florid stage and stage of regression.

1. *Initial progressive stage.* The disease begins with oedema of the endothelium and deeper stroma, secondary to anterior uveitis, as evidenced by the presence of keratic precipitates (KPs). There is associated pain, lacrimation, photophobia, blepharospasm and circumcorneal injection followed by a diffuse corneal haze giving it a *ground glass appearance*. This stage lasts for about 2 weeks.

2. *Florid stage.* In this stage eye remains acutely inflamed. Deep vascularization of cornea, consisting of radial bundle of brush-like vessels develops. Since these vessels are covered by hazy cornea, they look dull reddish pink which is called *'Salmon patch appearance'*. There is often a moderate degree of superficial vascularization. These vessels arising from the terminal arches of conjunctival vessels, run a short distance over the cornea. These vessels and conjunctiva heap at the limbus in the form of *epulit.* This stage lasts for about 2 months.

3. *Stage of regression.* The acute inflammation resolves with the progressive appearance of vascular invasion. Clearing of cornea is slow and begins from periphery and advances centrally. Resolution of the lesion leaves behind some opacities and *ghost vessels*. This stage may last for about 1 to 2 years.

Diagnosis

The diagnosis is usually evident from the clinical profile. A positive VDRL or *Treponema pallidum* immobilization test confirms the diagnosis.

Treatment

The treatment should include topical treatment for keratitis and systemic treatment for syphilis.

1. *Local treatment.* *Topical corticosteroid drops* e.g., dexamethasone 0.1% drops every 2-3 hours. As the condition is allergic in origin, corneal clearing occurs with steroids if started well in time and a useful vision is obtained.

- *Atropine eye ointment* 1 percent 2-3 times a day.
- *Dark goggles* to be used for photophobia.
- *Keratoplasty* is required in cases where dense corneal opacities are left.

2. *Systemic treatment*

- *Penicillin* in high doses should be started to prevent development of further syphilitic lesions. However, an early treatment of congenital syphilis usually does not prevent the onset of keratitis at a later stage.
- *Systemic steroids* may be added in refractory cases of keratitis.

Tuberculous interstitial keratitis

The features of tubercular interstitial keratitis are similar to syphilitic interstitial keratitus except that it is more frequently unilateral and sectorial (usually involving a lower sector of cornea).

Treatment consists of systemic antitubercular drugs, topical steroids and cycloplegics.

Cogan's syndrome

This syndrome comprises the interstitial keratitis of unkown etiology, acute tinnitus, vertigo, and deafness. It typically occurs in middle-aged adults and is often bilateral.

Treatment consists of topical and systemic *corticosteroids*. An early treatment usually prevents permanent deafness and blindness.

CORNEAL DEGENERATIONS

Corneal degenerations refers to the conditions in which the normal cells undergo some degenerative changes under the influence of age or some pathological condition.

CLASSIFICATION

A. *Depending upon location*

I. *Axial corneal degenerations*
   1. Fatty degeneration
   2. Hyaline degeneration
   3. Amyloidosis
   4. Calcific degeneration (Band keratopathy)
   5. Salzmann's nodular degeneration.

II. *Peripheral degenerations*
   1. Arcus senilis
   2. Vogt's white limbal girdle
   3. Hassal-Henle bodies
   4. Terrien's marginal degeneration

5. Mooren's ulcer
6. Pellucid marginal degeneration
7. Furrow degeneration (senile marginal degeneration).

B. *Depending upon etiology*

I. *Age related degenerations.* Arcus senilis, Vogt's white limbal girdle, Hassal-Henle bodies, Mosaic degeneration.

II. *Pathological degenerations:* Fatty degeneration, amyloidosis, calcific degeneration, Salzmann's nodular degeneration, Furrow degeneration, spheroidal degeneration, Pellucid marginal degeneration, Terrien's marginal degeneration, Mooren's ulcer.

I. AGE-RELATED CORNEAL DEGENERATIONS

Arcus senilis

Arcus senilis refers to an annular lipid infiltration of corneal periphery. This is an age-related change occurring bilaterally in 60 percent of persons between 40 and 60 years of age and in nearly all individuals over the age of 80. Sometimes, similar changes may occur in young persons (*arcus juvenilis*) which may or may not be associated with hyperlipidemia.

Clinical features

- The arcus starts in the superior and inferior quadrants and then progresses circumferentially to form a ring which is about 1 mm wide. Peripheral border of this ring opacity is sharp while central border is diffuse.
- This ring of opacity is separated from the limbus by a clear zone (*the lucid interval of Vogt*) (Fig. 5.16).

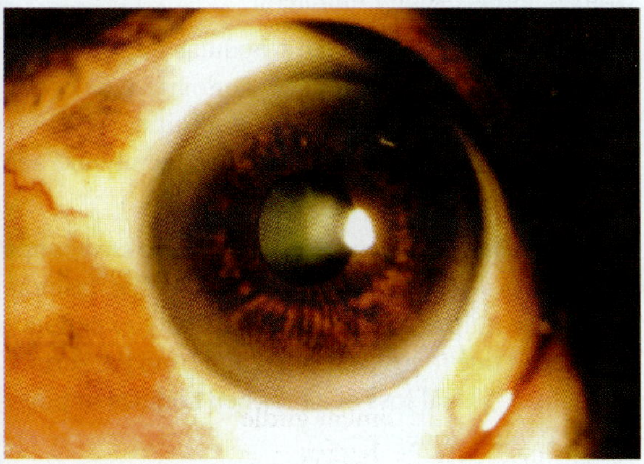

Fig. 5.16. Arcus senilis.

- Sometimes there may be double ring of arcus.

Vogt's white limbal girdle

It is also an age-related change seen frequently in elderly people. It appears as bilateral chalky white opacities in the interpalpebral area both nasally and temporally. There may or may not be a clear area between opacity and the limbus. The opacity is at the level of Bowman's membrane.

Hassal-Henle bodies

Hassal-Henle bodies are drop-like excrescences of hyaline material projecting into the anterior chamber around the corneal periphery. These arise from Descemet's membrane. These form the commonest senile change seen in the cornea. In pathological conditions they become larger and invade the central area and the condition is called *cornea guttata.*

II. PATHOLOGICAL CORNEAL DEGENERATIONS

Fatty degeneration (Lipoid keratopathy)

Fatty degeneration of cornea is characterised by whitish or yellowish deposits. The fat deposits mostly consist of cholesterol and fatty acids. Initially fat deposits are intracellular but some become extracellular with necrosis of stromal cells. Lipid keratopathy can be primary or secondary.

1. *Primary lipid keratopathy* is a rare condition which occurs in a cornea free of vascularization. Serum lipid levels are normal in such patients.
2. *Secondary lipid keratopathy* occurs in vascularised cornea secondary to diseases such as corneal infections, interstitial keratitis, ocular trauma, glaucoma, and chronic iridocyclitis.

Treatment is usually unsatisfactory. In some cases slow resorption of lipid infiltrate can be induced by argon laser photocoagulation of the new blood vessels.

Hyaline degeneration

Hyaline degeneration of cornea is characterised by deposition of hyaline spherules in the superficial stroma and can be primary or secondary.

1. *Primary hyaline degeneration* is bilateral and noted in association with granular dystrophy.

2. *Secondary hyaline degeneration* is unilateral and associated with various types of corneal diseases including old keratitis, long-standing glaucoma, trachomatous pannus. It may be complicated by recurrent corneal erosions.

Treatment of the condition when it causes visual disturbance is keratoplasty.

Amyloid degeneration

Amyloid degeneration of cornea is characterised by deposition of amyloid material underneath its epithelium. It is very rare condition and occurs in primary (in a healthy cornea) and secondary forms (in a diseased cornea).

Calcific degeneration (Band shape keratopathy)

Band shape keratopathy (BSK) is essentially a degenerative change associated with deposition of calcium salts in Bowman's membrane, most superficial part of stroma and in deeper layers of epithelium.

Etiology

- *Ocular diseases* complicated by band keratopathy include chronic uveitis in adults, children with Still's disease, phthisis bulbi, chronic glaucoma, chronic keratitis and ocular trauma.
- *Age related* BSK is common and affects otherwise healthy cornea.
- *Primary BSK is familial.*
- *Metabolic conditions* rarely associated with BSK include hypercalcaemia, hyperphosphataemia, hyperuricemia and chronic renal failure.

Clinical features. It typically presents as a band-shaped opacity in the interpalpebral zone with a clear interval between the ends of the band and the limbus (Fig. 5.17). The condition begins at the periphery and gradually progresses towards the centre. The opacity is beneath the epithelium which usually remains intact. Surface of this opaque band is stippled due to holes in the calcium plaques in the area of nerve canals of Bowman's membrane. In later stages, transparent clefts due to cracks or tears in the calcium plaques may also be seen.

Treatment. It consists of :

1. *Chelation*, i.e., chemical removal of deposited calcium salts is an effective treatment. First of all corneal epithelium is scraped under local anaesthesia. Then 0.01 molar solution of EDTA (chelating agent) is applied to the denuded cornea with the help of a cotton swab for about 10 minutes. This removes most of the deposited calcium. Pad and bandage is then applied for 2-3 days to allow the epithelium to regenerate.
2. *Phototherapeutic keratectomy* (PTK) with excimer laser is very effective in clearing the cornea.
3. *Keratoplasty* may be performed when the band keratopathy is obscuring useful vision.
4. Treatment of underlying causative disease.

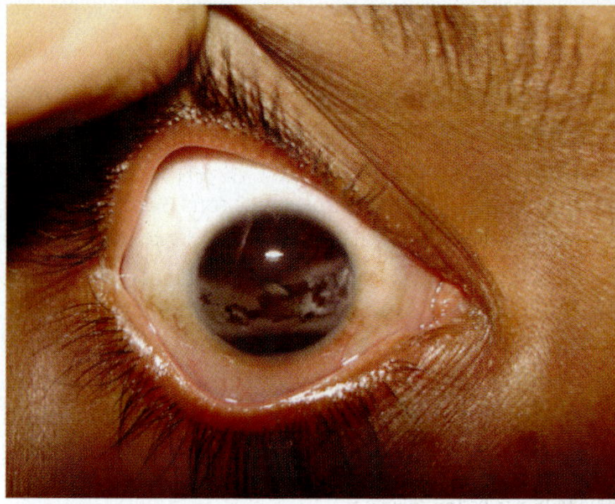

Fig. 5.17. Band-shaped keratopathy in a patient with chronic uveitis.

Salzmann's nodular degeneration

Etiology. This condition occurs in eyes with recurrent attacks of phlyctenular keratitis, rosacea keratitis and trachoma. The condition occurs more commonly in women and is usually unilateral.

Pathogenesis. In Salzmann's nodular degeneration, raised hyaline plaques are deposited between epithelium and Bowman's membrane. There is associated destruction of Bowman's membrane and the adjacent stroma.

Clinical features. Clinically, one to ten bluish white elevations (nodules), arranged in a circular fashion, are seen within the cornea. Patient may experience discomfort due to loss of epithelium from the surface of nodules. Visual loss occurs when nodules impinge on the central zone.

Treatment is essential by keratoplasty.

Furrow degeneration (Senile marginal degeneration)

In this condition thinning occurs at the periphery of cornea leading to formation of a furrow. In the presence of arcus senilis, the furrow occupies the area of lucid interval of Vogt. Thinning occurs due to fibrillar degeneration of the stroma.

Patient develops defective vision due to induced astigmatism.

Treatment is usually not necessary.

Spheroid degeneration

(Climatic droplet keratopathy/Labrador keratopathy/ Bietti's nodular dystrophy)/corneal elastosis.

Etiology. It typically occurs in men who work outdoors, especially in hostile climates. Its occurrence has been related to exposure to ultraviolet rays and/ or ageing and/or corneal disease.

Clinical features. In this condition amber-coloured spheroidal granules (small droplets) accumulate at the level of Bowman's membrane and anterior stroma in the interpalpebral zone. In marked degeneration, the vision is affected.

Treatment in advanced cases is by corneal transplantation.

Pellucid marginal degeneration

It is characterised by corneal thinning involving the periphery of lower cornea. It induces marked astigmatism which is corrected by scleral type contact lenses.

Terrien's marginal degeneration

Terrien's marginal degeneration is non-ulcerative thinning of the marginal cornea.

Clinical features are as follows :

1. Predominantly affects males usually after 40 years of age.
2. Mostly involves superior peripheral cornea.
3. Initial lesion is asymptomatic corneal opacification separated from limbus by a clear zone.
4. The lesion progresses very slowly over many years with thinning and superficial vascularization. Dense yellowish white deposits may be seen at the sharp leading edge. Patient experiences irritation and defective vision (due to astigmatism).

Complications such as perforation (due to mild trauma) and pseudopterygia may develop.

Treatment is non-specific. In severe thinning, a patch of corneal graft may be required.

CORNEAL DYSTROPHIES

Corneal dystrophies are inherited disorders in which the cells have some inborn defects due to which pathological changes may occur with passage of time leading to development of corneal haze in otherwise normal eyes that are free from inflammation or vascularization. There is no associated systemic disease. Dystrophies occur bilaterally, manifesting occasionally at birth, but more usually during first or second decade and sometimes even later in life.

Note: Recent studies have revealed that all the above definitions are not true for every type of corneal dystrophy. However, the International Committee for Classification of Corneal Dystrophies (2008) has decided to continue with the above given customary definition of corneal dystrophies.

CLASSIFICATION

The International Committee for Classification of Corneal Dystrophies(IC3D) in 2008 has proposed a new classification of corneal dystrophies, which in addition to the anatomic basis (site primarily involved) also incorporates the current clinical, pathological and genetic basis. Therefore, dystrophies with a common genetic basis, i.e., TGFb1 dystrophies have been grouped together (irrespective of the primary location of the lesion). The new IC3D classification of corneal dystrophies is as below:

I. *Epithelial and Subepithelial Dystrophies*

1. Epithelial basement membrane dystrophy (EBMD)
2. Epithelial recurrent erosion dystrophy (ERED)
3. Subepithelial mucinous corneal dystrophy (SMCD)
4. Mutation in keratin genes: Meesmann corneal dystrophy (MECD)
5. Lisch epithelial corneal dystrophy (LECD)
6. Gelatinous drop-like corneal dystrophy (GDLD)

II. *Bowman Layer Dystrophies*

1. Reis–Bucklers corneal dystrophy (RBCD)—Granular corneal dystrophy type 3
2. Thiel–Behnke corneal dystrophy (TBCD)
3. Grayson –Wilbrandt corneal dystrophy (GWCD)

III. *Stromal Dystrophies*

1. TGFBI corneal dystrophies

A. *Lattice corneal dystrophy*

i. Classic lattice corneal dystrophy (LCD1)

ii. Lattice corneal dystrophy, gelsolin type (LCD2)

B. *Granular corneal dystrophy*

i. Granular corneal dystrophy, type 1 (classic) (GCD1)

ii. Granular corneal dystrophy, type 2 (granular-lattice) (GCD2)

iii. Granular corneal dystrophy, type 3 (RBCD)

2. Macular corneal dystrophy (MCD)
3. Schnyder corneal dystrophy (SCD)
4. Congenital stromal corneal dystrophy (CSCD)
5. Fleck corneal dystrophy (FCD)
6. Posterior amorphous corneal dystrophy (PACD)
7. Central cloudy dystrophy of Francois (CCDF)
8. Pre-Descemet corneal dystrophy (PDCD)

IV. *Descemet Membrane and Endothelial Dystrophies*

1. Fuchs endothelial corneal dystrophy (FECD)
2. Posterior polymorphous corneal dystrophy (PPCD)
3. Congenital hereditary endothelial dystrophy 1 (CHED1)
4. Congenital hereditary endothelial dystrophy 2 (CHED2)
5. X-linked endothelial corneal dystrophy (XECD)

1. EPITHELIAL AND SUBEPITHELIAL DYSTROPHIES

1. Epithelial basement membrane dystrophy

Epithelial basement membrane dystrophy (EBMD) is also known as map-dot-fingerprint dystrophy or Cogan microcystic epithelial dystrophy or anterior basement membrane dystrophy.

Inheritance. Most cases have no inheritance documented.

Genetic locus and gene are 5q31 and TGFBI, respectively.

Onset,course and symptoms. Presents in adult life, rarely seen in children. Asymptomatic or recurrent erosions with pain, lacrimation and blurred vision are observed. Except for the bleb pattern, on-axis lesions may also cause blurred vision due to irregular astigmatism. Location and degree of pathology can fluctuate with time.

Signs. Typical lesions include:

- *Maps.* Irregular islands of thickened, gray, hazy epithelium with scalloped, circumscribed borders, particularly affecting the central or paracentral cornea. Isolated or combined with other signs.
- *Dots* (Cogan). Irregular round, oval or comma-shaped, non-staining, putty-gray opacities. Clustered like an archipelago in the central cornea. Typically combined with other signs, especially with maps.
- *Fingerprint lines.* Parallel, curvilinear lines, usually paracentral, best seen in retro illumination. They may be isolated or combined with other signs, especially maps.
- *Bleb pattern* (Bron). A subepithelial pattern like pebbled glass, best seen by retro-illumination. Isolated or combined with other signs

Note: Poor adhesion of basal epithelial cells to abnormal basal laminar material is thought predisposition to recurrent erosions.

2. Epithelial recurrent erosion dystrophy

Onset and course. Epithelial recurrent erosion dystrophy (ERED), also known as corneal erosions or recurring hereditary dystrophy, usually occurs in first decade of life.

Inheritance is autosomal dominant.

Genetic locus and gene involved are unknown.

Onset and course. Recurrent corneal erosions appear typically at 4–6 years of age but occasionally as early as 8 months of age. Attacks generally decline in frequency in intensity and cease by the age of 50 years.

Signs include:

- *Corneal erosions* are seen during the attack recurrent corneal erosions appear typically at 4–6 years of age but occasionally as early as 8 months of age. Attacks generally decline in frequency and intensity and cease by the age of 50 years.
- *Subepithelial haze or blebs* may be seen between the attacks
- *Central subepithelial corneal opacities,* may appear as early as 7 years of age. These vary from subepithelial fibrosis to protruding keloid-like nodules.

Symptoms are precipitated by minimal trauma or occur spontaneously and are in the form of attacks of redness, photophobia, epiphora and ocular pain.

Treatment. About 25% of the patients may eventually need corneal grafts at the mean age of 45 years.

3. Subepithelial mucinous corneal dystrophy

Inheritance is autosomal dominant.

Genetic locus and gene is unknown

Onset and course. Onset is in the first decade of life and progressive loss of vision occurs in adolescence.

Signs include bilateral subepithelial opacities and haze, most dense centrally, involving the entire cornea.

Symptoms include painful episodes of recurrent corneal erosions, which decrease during adolescence

4. Mutations in keratin genes: Meesmann corneal dystrophy

Onset and course. Meesmann corneal dystrophy (MECD) also known as juvenile hereditary epithelial dystrophy occurs in early childhood and the condition is slowly progressive. Its variant is Stocker-Holt dystrophy.

Inheritance is autosomal dominant.

Genetic loci are 12q13 (KRT3) and 17q12 (KRT12) for Stocker–Holt variant .

Genes involved are Keratin K3 (KRT3) and Keratin K12 (KRT12) for Stocker–Holt variant.

Signs. Characteristic lesions include:

- *Multiple, tiny epithelial vesicles* which extend to the limbus and are most numerous in the interpalpebral area with clear surrounding epithelium.
- *Whorled and wedge-shaped epithelial patterns* have also been reported.
- *Corneal thinning* and reduction in corneal sensation may be noted.
- *In Stocker–Holt variant,* the entire cornea demonstrates fine, grayish punctuate epithelial opacities that stain with fluorescein and fine linear opacities that may appear in a whorl pattern.

Symptoms. Patients are typically asymptomatic or may have mild visual reduction, although some patients complain of glare and light sensitivity. Recurrent painful punctiform epithelial erosions may occur. Rarely, blurred vision results from corneal irregularity and scarring.

5. Lisch epithelial corneal dystrophy

Onset and course. Lisch epithelial corneal dystrophy (LECD) also known as band-shaped and whorled microcystic dystrophy of the corneal epithelium occurs in childhood and there occurs slow progression of opacities with possible deterioration in vision.

Inheritance is X-chromosomal dominant.

Signs are as below.

- *Direct illumination* shows localized gray opacities in different patterns: whorl-like, radial, band shaped, flame/ feathery shaped, and club shaped.
- *Indirect illumination* demonstrates multiple, densely crowded clear cysts with clear surrounding epithelium.

Symptoms. The condition is asymptomatic, blurring of vision occurs if the pupillary zone is involved.

6. Gelatinous drop-like corneal dystrophy (GDLD)

Onset and course. Gelatinous drop-like corneal dystrophy (GDLD) also known as subepithelial amyloidosis or primary familial amyloidosis (Grayson) occurs in the first decade of life and the condition is progressive.

Genetic locus is 1p32 and ***gene*** involved is tumor-associated calcium signal transducer 2 (TACSTD2)

Inheritance is autosomal recessive.

Signs include:

- *Subepithelial lesions which* appear initially may be similar to band-shaped keratopathy or there may be groups of small multiple nodules, that is, mulberry configuration.
- *Superficial vascularization* is frequently seen.
- *Stromal opacification* or larger nodular lesions, that is, kumquat-like lesions may appear in later life.

Symptoms include significant decrease in vision, photophobia, irritation, redness, and tearing.

II. BOWMAN LAYER DYSTROPHIES

1. Reis–Bucklers corneal dystrophy

Onset and course. Reis–Bucklers corneal dystrophy (RBCD) also known as corneal dystrophy of Bowman layer, type I (CDB I) or geographic corneal dystrophy (Weidle), occurs in childhood and causes slowly progressive deterioration of vision.

Genetic locus is 5q31 and the ***gene*** involved is TGFBI.

Inheritance is autosomal dominant.

Signs include confluent irregular and coarse geographic-like opacities with varying densities which develop at the level of Bowman layer and superficial stroma, initially separated from one another. Opacities may extend to the limbus and deeper stroma with time.

Symptoms. Vision is impaired from childhood. Recurrent corneal erosions cause ocular discomfort and pain in the first decade but may become less severe from the end of the second decade.

2. Thiel–Behnke corneal dystrophy

Onset and course. Thiel–Behnke corneal dystrophy (TBCD) also known as corneal dystrophy of Bowman layer, type II (CDB2) or honeycomb-shaped corneal dystrophy occurs in childhood and causes slowly progressive deterioration of vision.

Genetic locus is 5q31 and the ***gene*** involved is TGFBI.

Inheritance is autosomal dominant.

Onset and course. Occurs in childhood and there occurs slowly progressive deterioration of vision from increasing corneal opacification.

Signs include symmetrical subepithelial reticular *(honeycomb)* opacities with peripheral cornea typically uninvolved, which can progress to deep stromal layers and corneal periphery.

Symptoms. Recurrent corneal erosions cause ocular discomfort and pain in the first and second decade. Gradual visual impairment develops later.

3. Grayson–Wilbrandt corneal dystrophy (GWCD)

Onset and course. Occurs during first to second decade of life and the condition is progressive.

Inheritance is autosomal dominant.

Signs. Bowman layer demonstrates variable patterns of opacification from diffuse mottling to diffuse gray-white opacities, which extend anteriorly into the epithelium. The cornea between the deposits is clear. Refractile bodies are described in corneal stroma.

Symptoms. Decreased to normal visual acuity. Recurrent corneal erosions may cause ocular discomfort and pain.

III. STROMAL CORNEAL DYSTROPHIES

1. TGFBI corneal dystrophies.

These include:

A. *Lattice corneal dystrophy*, which is of two types:
- i. Classic lattice corneal dystrophy (LCD1)
- ii. Lattice corneal dystrophy, gelsolin type (LCD2)

B. *Granular corneal dystrophy*, which is of three types:
- i. Granular corneal dystrophy, type 1 (classic) (GCD1)
- ii. Granular corneal dystrophy, type 2 (granular-lattice) (GCD2)
- iii. Granular corneal dystrophy, type 3 (RBCD)

A. Lattice corneal dystrophy

i. Classical lattice corneal dystrophy:

Classic lattice corneal dystrophy (LCD1) is also known as Biber-Haab-Dimmer dystrophy.

Genetic locus is 5q31 and the ***gene*** involved is TGFBI.

Inheritance is autosomal dominant.

Onset, symptoms and course. It appears at the age of 2 years and the condition is progressive. Recurrent erosions are frequent and ocular discomfort and pain occurs sometimes starting as early as in the first decade of life. Progressive clouding of central cornea is apparent by the age of 20 years. Soon, visual acuity is impaired. Usually penetrating keratoplasty is required by the age of 30-40 years.

Signs. The disease is characterised by branching spider-like amyloid deposits forming an irregular lattice work in the corneal stroma, sparing the periphery. The number of lattice lines may differ between the 2 eyes and the dystrophy may be difficult to diagnose in some younger patients.

ii. Lattice corneal dystrophy, Gelsolin Type (LCD2)

Lattice corneal dystrophy, Gelsolin type is also known as Familial amyloidosis of Finnish (FAF) or Meretoja syndrome.

Genetic locus is 9q34 and the ***gene*** involved is Gelsolin GSN.

Inheritance is autosomal dominant.

Onset and course. Onset occurs in third to fourth decade of life, the condition is slowly progressive and the majority of patients are in good health even in the seventh decade.

Signs include:
- *Lattice lines* appear in the corneal stroma (spreading centripetally from the limbus) which are more peripheral and less numerous than those of lattice dystrophy, type I. The central cornea is relatively spared.
- *Corneal sensitivity* is reduced or absent.

Symptoms include:
- *Dry eye symptoms* are frequent, and corneal erosions may occur late in life.
- *Visual acuity* is usually normal until the sixth decade because the dystrophy progresses from the peripheral to central cornea.

B. Granular dystrophy

i. Granular corneal dystrophy, Type 1(Classic) (GCD1)

Onset and course Granular corneal dystrophy, Type 1(Classic) (GCD1), also known Corneal dystrophy Groenouw type I occurs in childhood, may be seen as early as 2 years of age. As the condition progresses, the opacities become more confiuent in the superficial cornea.

Genetic locus is 5q31 and the ***gene*** involved is TGFBI.

Inheritance is autosomal dominant.

Signs. The condition is characterised by milky-granular hyaline deposits in anterior stroma. Intervening stroma is clear. Opacities do not extend to the limbus.In children, there may be a vortex pattern of brownish granules superficial to Bowman layer. In later life, granules may extend into the deeper stroma down to Descemet membrane.

Symptoms include:

- *Glare and photophobia* are early symptoms.
- *Recurrent erosions* occur frequently causing ocular discomfort, pain and watering.
- *Visual acuity* decreases as opacification progresses with age.

ii. Granular corneal dystrophy, Type 2 (Granular-Lattice) (GCD2)

Onset and course Granular corneal dystrophy, Type 2 (Granular-Lattice) (GCD2) also known as combined granular–lattice corneal dystrophy or Avellino corneal dystrophy, occurs in first decade, may be as early as 3 years of age and the condition is generally progressive.

Genetic locus is 5q31and ***gene*** involved is TGFBI.

Inheritance is autosomal dominant.

Signs include*:*

- *Subtle superficial stromal tiny whitish dots* are initial lesions.
- *Rings or stellate-shaped snowflake stromal opacities* appearing between the superficial stroma and the mid stroma are next lesions.
- *Lattice lines* in deeper cornea may be seen in some patients. Typically, these lines are located deeper than the snowflake stromal opacity.
- *Superficial, translucent flattened breadcrumb opacities* are seen in the final stages, which may coalesce in the anterior stroma.

Symptoms.

- *Vision* decreases with age as the central visual axis becomes affected.
- *Pain and ocular discomfort* may accompany mild corneal erosions.

2. Macular corneal dystrophy

Onset and course. Macular corneal dystrophy (MCD), also known as Groenouw corneal dystrophy type II or Fehr spotted dystrophy, occurs in childhood and is slowly progressive.

Genetic locus is 16q22 and ***gene*** involved is carbohydrate sulfotransferase 6 gene—CHST6.

Inheritance is autosomal recessive.

Signs include:

- *Diffuse stromal haze* extending to the limbus is the initial lesion .
- *Macules,* i.e. superficial, central, elevated, irregular whitish opacities develop later and give the condition its name.
- Posterior peripheral white lesions are also seen.
- Corneal sensitivity is reduced.

Symptoms

- *Recurrent corneal erosions* cause photophobia and pain.
- *Visual impairment,* usually severe, occurs between 10 and 30 years of age.

3. Schnyder corneal dystrophy

Schnyder corneal dystrophy (SCD) is also known as hereditary crystalline stromal dystrophy of Schnyder. Affected patients and non-affected members of the pedigrees may have hyperlipoproteinemia.

Genetic locus is 1p36 and the ***gene*** involved is UbiA prenyltransferase domain containing 1—UBIAD1.

Inheritance is autosomal dominant.

Onset and course. The dystrophy appears in early infancy or at birth or sometimes in the first decade of life. It is slowly progressive and usually asymptomatic.

Signs include:

- *Round ring-shaped central corneal stromal opacities* due to deposition of fine needle-like cholesterol crystals, which may be white to yellow or polychromatic in colour are characteristic lesions.
- *Corneal sensations* decrease with age.

Symptoms include:

- *Visual acuity* progressively decreases with age. Although scotopic vision may be remarkably good, photopic vision may be disproportionately decreased.
- *Glare* which increase with age.

4. Congenital stromal corneal dystrophy

Onset and course. Congenital stromal corneal dystrophy (CSCD), also known as congenital hereditary stromal dystrophy occurs congenitally and

is a non-progressive or slowly progressive condition.
Genetic locus is 12q21.33 and the ***gene*** involved is decorin—DCN.
Inheritance is autosomal dominant.
Signs and symptoms. The characteristic lesions are diffuse, bilateral, corneal clouding with flake-like, whitish stromal opacities throughout the stroma, causing moderate to severe visual loss.

5. Fleck corneal dystrophy

Onset and course. Fleck corneal dystrophy (FCD) also known as Francois-Neetens speckled corneal dystrophy occurs congenitally and is a non-progressive condition.
Gene locus is 2q35and the ***gene*** involved is phosphatidylinositol-3-phosphate/phosphatidylinositol 5-Kinase type III—PIP5K3.
Inheritance is autosomal dominant.
Signs and symptoms. The condition is asymptomatic characterized by small, translucent, discoid opacities or discrete, flat, gray-white, dandruff-like (sometimes ring-shaped) opacities scattered sparsely throughout any level of the otherwise clear stroma.

6. Posterior amorphous corneal dystrophy

Onset and course. Posterior amorphous corneal dystrophy (PACD), also known as Posterior amorphous stromal dystrophy, often occurs in the first decade of life. It has been noted as early as 16 weeks, suggesting a congenital nature. The condition is non or slowly progressive.
Inheritance is autosomal dominant.
Signs and symptoms. It presents as diffuse gray-white, sheet-like opacities that can involve any layer of the stroma but are most prominent posteriorly. The condition is largely asymptomatic except for mild decrease in visual acuity (usually better than 6/12).

7. Central cloudy dystrophy of Francois

Onset and course. Central cloudy dystrophy of Francois (CCDF) occurs in first decade and is non-progressive,
Inheritance is unknown.
Signs and symptoms. The condition is mostly asymptomatic and is characterized by cloudy central polygonal or rounded stromal opacities that fade anteriorly and peripherally and are surrounded by clear tissue.

8. Pre-descemet corneal dystrophy

Onset and course. Onset usually occurs after 30 years of age but has been found in children as young as 3 years. The condition is usually non-progressive, some conditions may show progression.
Inheritance is unknown
Signs and symptoms. The condition is usually asymptomatic and is characterized by focal, fine, gray opacities in the deep stroma immediately anterior to Descemet membrane with a variety of shapes.

IV. DESCEMET MEMBRANE AND ENDOTHELIAL DYSTROPHIES

1. Fuchs endothelial corneal dystrophy

Onset and course. Fuchs endothelial corneal dystrophy (FECD), also known as endoepithelial corneal dystrophy, is frequently seen as a slowly progressive bilateral condition affecting females more than males (F:M::4:1), usually between fifth and seventh decade of life. Primary open angle glaucoma is its common association.

Inheritance. It may be autosomal dominant or sporadic(more common) in nature.

Genetic locus is 13p. No gene has been associated.

Clinical features can be divided into following four stages:

1. *Stage of cornea guttata.* It is characterised by the presence of Hassal-Henle type of excrescenses in the central part of cornea. A gradual increase of central guttae with peripheral spread and confluence gives rise to the so called '*beaten-metal*' appearance. This stage is asymptomatic.
2. *Oedematous stage or stage of endothelial decompensation* is characterised by the occurrence of early stromal oedema and epithelial dystrophy. Patients complaint of blurring vision.
3. *Stage of bullous keratopathy.* This stage follows long-standing stromal oedema and is characterised by marked epithelial oedema with formation of bullae, when rupture cause pain, discomfort and irritation with associated decreased visual acuity.
4. *Stage of scarring.* In this stage epithelial bullae are replaced by scar tissue and cornea becomes opaque and vascularized. The condition may sometimes be complicated by occurrence of secondary infection or glaucoma.

Specular microscopy reveals decreased endothelial cell count, increased average cell diameter, decreased hexagons and increased variation in cell size.

Treatment is as follows:

1. *Hypertonic saline:* (5 percent sodium chloride) may be of some use in early oedematous stage.
2. *Warm air* blown on the eyes (e.g. hair dryer) helps in reducing edema.
3. *Intraocular pressure lowering drugs* e.g. 0.5% timolol or others should be used to treat associated ocular hypertension.
4. *Bandage soft contact lenses* provide some relief from disturbing symptoms in bullous keratopathy stage.
5. *Penetrating keratoplasty* is the treatment of choice when the visual acuity is reduced markedly.

2. Posterior polymorphous corneal dystrophy (PPCD)

Onset and course: Posterior polymorphous corneal dystrophy (PPCD) also known as Schlichting dystrophy occurs in early childhood and is very slowly progressive.

Inheritance is autosomal dominant.

Genetic Loci are PPCD 1—20p11.2–q11.2; PPCD 2—1p34.3–p32.3; PPCD 3—10p11.2.

Genes involved are: PPCD 1—unknown; PPCD 2—collagen type VIII alpha 2, COL8A2 and PPCD 3—two-handed zinc-finger homeodomain transcription factor 8—ZEB1.

Signs and symptoms. The condition is often asymptomatic. The signs include:

- *Deep corneal lesions* of various shapes including nodular, vesicular (isolated, in clusters, or confluent) and blister-like lesions.
- *Railroad tracks* appearance lesions (multiple and isolated)
- *Varying gray tissue* at the level of Descemet membrane.

3. Congenital hereditary endothelial dystrophy 1

Onset and course. Congenital hereditary endothelial dystrophy 1 (CHED1) occurs in first or second year of life, occasionally congenital. Progression of corneal clouding occurs over 1–10 years.

Genetic Locus is 20p 11.2–q11.2 (pericentromeric region) and ***gene*** is unknown.

Inheritance is autosomal dominant.

Signs and symptoms include

- *Endothelial changes* in form of moon crater–like appearance and peau d'orange texture may be seen (Such patients are asymptomatic).
- *Corneal clouding* ranging from a diffuse haze to a ground-glass, milky appearance with occasional focal gray spots causing blurred vision associated with photophobia and watering. Vision is characteristically worse in the morning.
- *Thickening* of the cornea, can be 2–3 times of normal thickness.
- *Subepithelial band keratopathy* may be seen ocassionally.
- IOP may be elevated rarely.

4. Congenital hereditary endothelial dystrophy 2

Onset and course. Congenital hereditary endothelial dystrophy 2 (CHED2) also called as Maumenee corneal dystrophy occurs congenitally and is a relatively stationary condition.

Genetic locus is 20p13 (telomeric portion) and the ***gene*** involved is solute carrier family 4, sodium borate transporter, member 11—SLC4A11.

Inheritance is autosomal recessive.

Signs and symptoms are similar to CHED1 except :

- The condition is more common and severe than CHED 1.
- Nystagmus is often associated.

5. X-linked endothelial corneal dystrophy

Onset and course. X-linked endothelial corneal dystrophy (XECD) occurs congenitally and is a progressive condition in males and non-progressive in females.

Genetic locus is Xq25 and the ***gene*** involved is unknown.

Inheritance is X-chromosomal dominant.

Signs and symptoms

Male patients have blurring of vision associated with:

- *Corneal clouding* since birth ranging from a diffuse haze to a ground-glass, milky appearance.
- *Moon crater–like* endothelial changes.
- *Subepithelial band keratopathy* combined with moon crater–like endothelial changes.
- *Nystagmus* may be associated.

Female patients are asymptomatic having only *moon crater–like* endothelial changes.

ECTATIC CONDITIONS OF CORNEA

KERATOCONUS

Keratoconus (conical cornea) (Fig. 5.18) is a non-inflammatory bilateral (85%) ectatic condition of cornea in its axial part. It usually starts at puberty and progresses slowly.

Etiopathogenesis. It is still not clear. Various theories proposed so far label it as developmental condition, degenerative condition, hereditary dystrophy and endocrine anomaly. Essential pathological changes are thinning and ectasia which occur as a result of defective synthesis of mucopolysaccharide and collagen tissue.

Clinical features. *Symptoms.* Patient presents with a defective vision due to progressive myopia and irregular astigmatism, which does not improve fully despite full correction with glasses.

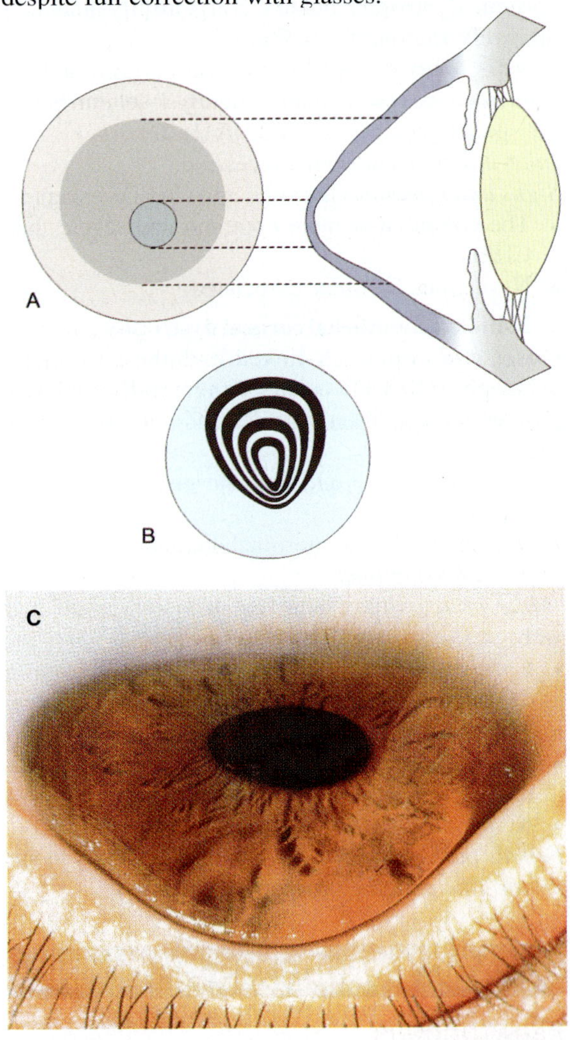

Fig. 5.18. Keratoconus showing: A, configuration of cone-shaped cornea; B, irregular circles on Placido disc examination; C, clinical photograph (note Munson's sign).

Signs. Following signs may be elicited:

1. *Window reflex* is distorted.
2. *Placido disc examination* shows irregularity of the circles (Fig. 5.18B).
3. *Keratometry* depicts extreme malalignment of *mires.*
4. *Photokeratoscopy* reveals distortion of circles.
5. *Slit lamp examination* (Fig. 5.18C) may show thinning and ectasia of central cornea, opacity at the apex and Fleischer's ring at the base of cone, folds in Descemet's and Bowman's membranes. Very fine, vertical, deep stromal striae (Vogt lines) which disappear with external pressure on the globe are peculiar feature.
6. *On retinoscopy* a yawning reflex (scissor reflex) and high oblique or irregular astigmatism is obtained.
7. *On distant direct ophthalmoscopy* an annular dark shadow (due to total internal reflection of light) is seen which separates the central and peripheral areas of cornea (oil droplet reflex).
8. *Munson's sign*, i.e. localised bulging of lower lid when patient looks down is positive in late stages.

Morphological classification. Depending upon the size and shape of the cone, the keratoconus is of three types:

- *Nipple cone* has a small size (<5mm) and steep curvature.
- *Oval cone* is larger (5-6 mm) and ellipsoid in shape.
- *Globus cone* is very large (>6 mm) and globe like.

Complications. Keratoconus may be complicated by development of *acute hydrops* due to rupture of Descemet's membrane. The condition is characterised by sudden development of corneal oedema associated with marked defective vision, pain, photophobia and lacrimation.

Associations. Keratoconus may be associated with :

- *Ocular conditions* e.g. ectopia lentis, congenital cataract, aniridia, retinitis pigmentosa, and vernal keratoconjunctivitis (VKC).
- *Systemic conditions* e.g., Marfan's syndrome, atopy, Down's syndrome, Ehlers-Danlos syndrome, osteogenesis imperfecta and mitral valve prolapse.

Treatment modalities include:

- *Spectacle correction* may improve vision in very early cases. However, later in the course of disease the falling vision may not be corrected by glasses due to irregular astigmatism.
- *Contact lenses* (rigid gas permeable) usually improve the vision in early cases.
- *Intacs,* the intracorneal ring segments, are reported to be useful in early cases.
- *Corneal collagen cross linking* with riboflavin (C3R) may slow the progression of disease.
- *Keratoplasty* may be required in later stages. Deep anterior lamellar keratoplasty (DALK) or Penetrating keratoplasty (PK) may be perform

KERATOGLOBUS

It is a familial and hereditary bilateral congenital disorder characterised by thinning and hemispherical protrusion of the entire cornea. It is non-progressive and inherited as an autosomal recessive trait. It must be differentiated from congenital buphthalmos, where increased corneal size is associated with raised intraocular pressure, angle anomaly and/or cupping of optic disc.

KERATOCONUS POSTERIOR

In this extremely rare condition there is slight cone-like bulging of the posterior surface of the cornea. It is non-progressive.

ABNORMALITIES OF CORNEAL TRANSPARENCY

Normal cornea is a transparent structure. Any condition which upsets its anatomy or physiology causes loss of its transparency to some degree.

Common causes of loss of corneal transparency are:

- Corneal oedema
- Drying of cornea
- Depositions on cornea
- Inflammations of cornea
- Corneal degenerations
- Dystrophies of cornea
- Vascularization of cornea
- Scarring of cornea (corneal opacities)

Most of the conditions responsible for decreased transparency of cornea have been described earlier. However, some important *symptomatic conditions of the cornea* such as corneal oedema, corneal opacity and vascularization of cornea are described here.

CORNEAL OEDEMA

The water content of normal cornea is 78 percent. It is kept constant by a balance of factors which draw water in the cornea (e.g., intraocular pressure and swelling pressure of the stromal matrix = 60 mm of Hg) and the factors which draw water out of cornea (viz. the active pumping action of corneal endothelium, and the mechanical barrier action of epithelium and endothelium).

Disturbance of any of the above factors leads to corneal oedema, wherein its hydration becomes above 78 percent, central thickness increases and transparency reduces.

Causes of corneal oedema

1. Raised intraocular pressure
2. Endothelial damage
   - Due to injuries, such as birth trauma (forceps delivery), surgical trauma during intraocular operation, contusion injuries and penetrating injuries.
   - Endothelial damage associated with corneal dystrophies such as, Fuchs dystrophy, congenital hereditary endothelial dystrophy and posterior polymorphous dystrophy.
   - Endothelial damage secondary to inflammations such as uveitis, endophthalmitis and corneal graft infection.
3. Epithelial damage due to :
   - mechanical injuries
   - chemical burns
   - radiational injuries

Clinical features

Initially there occurs stromal haze with reduced vision. In long-standing cases with chronic endothelial failure (e.g., in Fuch's dystrophy) there occurs permanent oedema with epithelial vesicles and bullae formation (*bullous keratopathy*). This is associated with marked loss of vision, pain, discomfort and photophobia, due to periodic rupture of bullae.

Treatment

1. *Treat the cause* wherever possible, e.g., raised IOP and ocular inflammations.

2. *Dehydration of cornea* may be tried by use of:
- Hypertonic agents e.g., 5 percent sodium chloride drops or ointments or anhydrous glycerine may provide sufficient dehydrating effect.
- Hot forced air from hair dryer may be useful.

3. *Therapeutic soft contact lenses* may be used to get relief from discomfort of bullous keratopathy.
4. *Penetrating keratoplasty* is required for long-standing cases of corneal oedema, non-responsive to conservative therapy.

CORNEAL OPACITY

The word '*corneal opacification*' literally means loss of normal transparency of cornea, which can occur in many conditions. Therefore, the term '*corneal opacity*' is used particularly for the loss of transparency of cornea due to scarring.

Causes

1. Congenital opacities may occur as developmental anomalies or following birth trauma.
2. Healed corneal wounds.
3. Healed corneal ulcers.

Clinical features

Corneal opacity may produce loss of vision (when dense opacity covers the pupillary area) or blurred vision (due to astigmatic effect).

Types of corneal opacity

Depending on the density, corneal opacity is graded as nebula, macula and leucoma.

1. *Nebular corneal opacity.* It is a faint opacity which results due to superficial scars involving Bowman's layer and superficial stroma (Figs. 5.19A and 5.20A). A thin, diffuse nebula covering the pupillary area interferes more with vision than the localised leucoma away from pupillary area. Further, the nebula produces more discomfort to patient due to blurred image owing to irregular astigmatism than the leucoma which completely cuts off the light rays.
2. *Macular corneal opacity.* It is a semi-dense opacity produced when scarring involves about half the corneal stroma (Figs. 5.19B and 5.20B).
3. *Leucomatous corneal opacity* (leucoma simplex). It is a dense white opacity which results due to scarring of more than half of the stroma (Figs. 5.19C and 5.20C).
4. *Adherent leucoma:* It results when healing occurs after perforation of cornea with incarceration of iris (Figs. 5.19D and 5.20D).
5. *Corneal facet.* Sometimes the corneal surface is depressed at the site of healing (due to less fibrous tissue); such a scar is called facet.
6. *Kerectasia.* In this condition corneal curvature is increased at the site of opacity (bulge due to weak scar).
7. *Anterior staphyloma.* An ectasia of psuedocornea (the scar formed from organised exudates and fibrous tissue covered with epithelium) which results after total sloughing of cornea, with iris plastered behind it is called *anterior staphyloma* (Figs. 5.21 A and B).

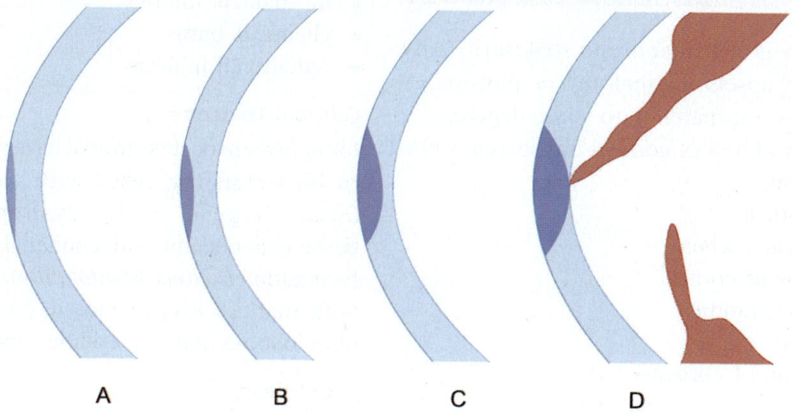

Fig. 5.19. Diagramatic depiction of corneal opacity: A, nebular; B, macular; C, leucomatous; D, adherent leucoma.

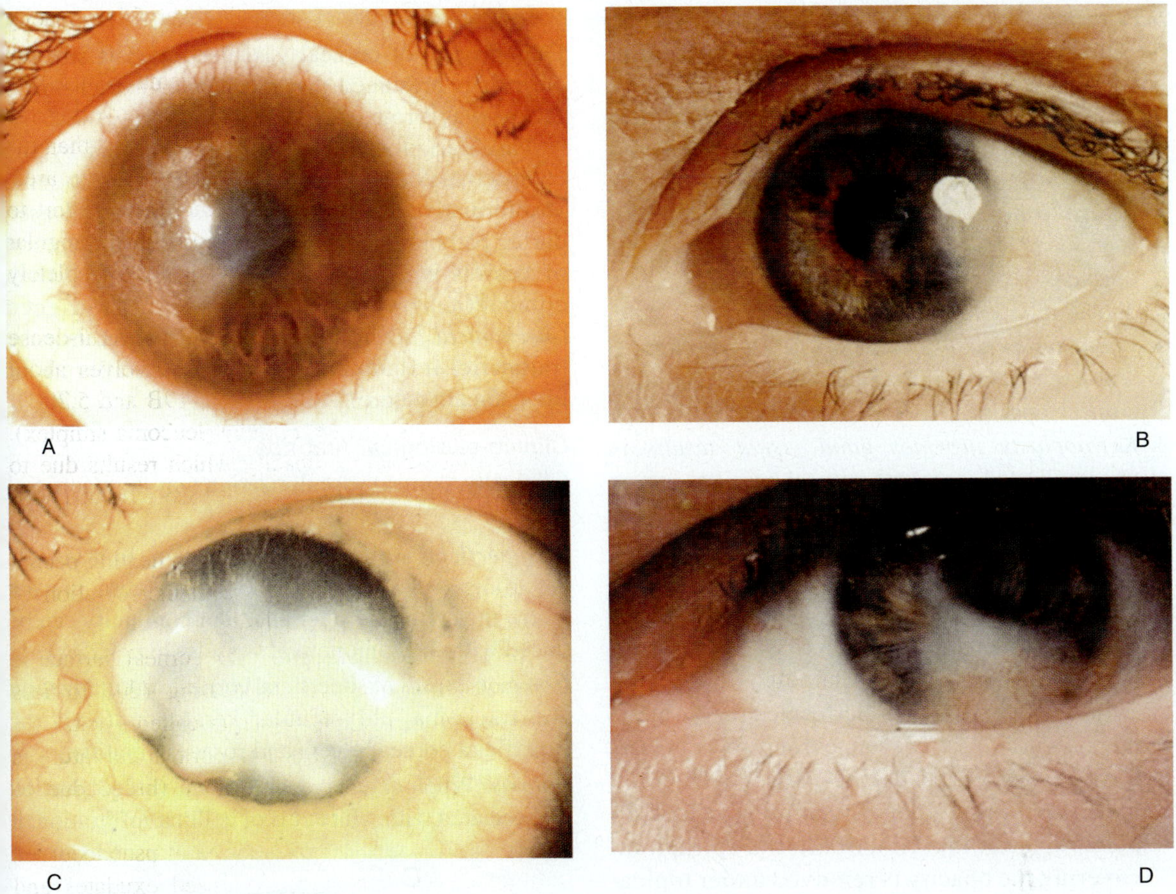

Fig. 5.20. Clinical photographs of corneal opacity: A, nebular; B, bacular; C, leucomatous; D, adherent leucoma.

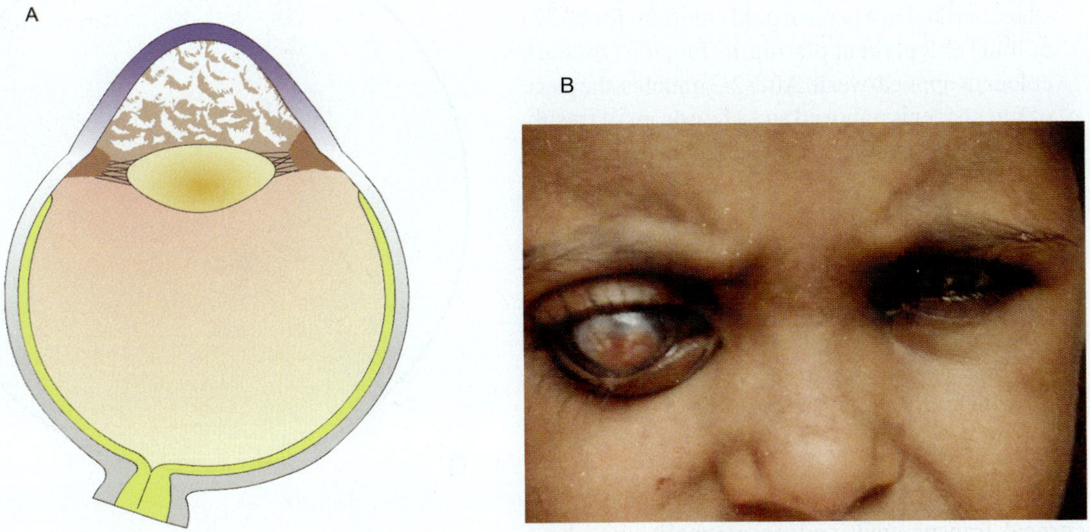

Fig. 5.21. Anterior staphyloma : A, diagrammatic cross-section; B, clinical photograph.

Secondary changes in corneal opacity which may be seen in long-standing cases include: hyaline degeneration, calcareous degeneration, pigmentation and atheromatous ulceration.

Treatment

1. *Optical iridectomy.* It may be performed in cases with central macular or leucomatous corneal opacities, provided vision improves with pupillary dilatation.
2. *Phototherapeutic keratectomy* (PTK) performed with excimer laser is useful in superficial (nebular) corneal opacities.
3. *Keratoplasty provides good visual results* in uncomplicated cases with corneal opacities, where optical iridectomy is not of much use.
4. *Cosmetic coloured contact lens* gives very good cosmetic appearance in an eye with ugly scar having no potential for vision. Presently, this is considered the best option, even over and above the tatooing for cosmetic purpose.
5. *Tattooing of scar.* It was performed for cosmetic purposes in the past. It is suitable only for firm scars in a quiet eye without useful vision. For tattooing Indian black ink, gold or platinum may be used. To perform tattooing, first of all, the epithelium covering the opacity is removed under topical anaesthesia (2 percent or 4 percent xylocaine). Then a piece of blotting paper of same size and shape, soaked in 4 percent gold chloride (for brown colour) or 2 percent platinum chloride (for dark colour) is applied over it. After 2-3 minutes, the piece of filter paper is removed and a few drops of freshly prepared 2% hydrazine hydrate solution are poured over it. Lastly, eye is irrigated with normal saline and patched after instilling antibiotic and atropine eye ointment. Epithelium grows over the pigmented area.

CORNEAL VASCULARIZATION

Normal cornea is avascular except for small capillary loops which are present in the periphery for about 1 mm. In pathological states, it can be invaded by vessels as a defence mechanism against the disease or injury. However, vascularization interferes with corneal transparency and occasionally may be a source of irritation.

Pathogenesis

Pathogenesis of corneal vascularization is still not clear. It is presumed that mechanical and chemical factors play a role.

Vascularization is normally prevented by the compactness of corneal tissue. Probably due to some vasoformative stimulus (*chemical factor*) released during pathological states, there occurs proliferation of vessels which invade from the limbus; when compactness of corneal tissue is loosened (*mechanical factor*) due to oedema (which may be traumatic, inflammatory, nutritional, allergic or idiopathic in nature).

Clinico-etiological features

Clinically, corneal vascularization may be superficial or deep.

1. *Superficial corneal vascularization*. In it vessels are arranged usually in an arborising pattern, present below the epithelial layer and their continuity can be traced with the conjunctival vessels (Fig. 5.22A).

Common causes of superficial corneal vascularization are: trachoma, phlyctenular keratoconjunctivitis, superficial corneal ulcers and rosacea keratitis.

Pannus. When extensive superficial vascularization is associated with white cuff of cellular infiltration, it

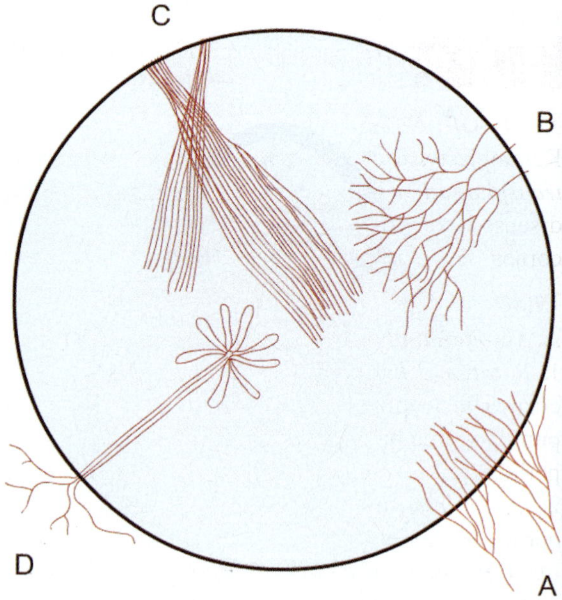

Fig. 5.22. Corneal vascularization : A, superficial B, terminal loop type C, brush type D, umbel type

is termed as *pannus*. In progressive pannus, corneal infiltration is ahead of vessels while in *regressive pannus* it lags behind.

2. *Deep vascularization*. In this vessels are generally derived from anterior ciliary arteries and lie in the corneal stroma. These vessels are usually straight, not anastomosing and their continuity cannot be traced beyond the limbus. Deep vessels may be arranged as terminal loops (Fig. 5.22B), brush (Fig. 5.22C), parasol, umbel (Fig. 5.22D), network or interstitial arcade.

Common causes of deep vascularization are: interstitial keratitis, disciform keratitis, deep corneal ulcer, chemical burns and sclerosing keratitis and grafts.

Treatment

Treatment of corneal vascularization is usually unsatisfactory. Vascularization may be *prevented* by timely and adequate treatment of the causative conditions. *Corticosteroids* may have vasoconstrictive and suppressive effect on permeability of capillaries. Application of *irradiation* is more useful in superficial than the deep vascularization. *Surgical treatment* in the form of peritomy may be employed for superficial vascularization.

CORNEAL SURGERY

KERATOPLASTY

Keratoplasty, also called *corneal grafting* or *corneal transplantation*, is an operation in which the patient's diseased cornea is replaced by the healthy clear cornea.

Types

A. *Autokeratoplasty*, which can be:

1. *Rotational keratoplasty*, in which patient's own cornea is trephined and rotated to transfer the pupillary area having a small corneal opacity to the periphery.
2. *Contralateral keratoplasty*. It is indicated when cornea of one eye of the patient is opaque and the other eye is blind due to posterior segment disease (e.g., optic atrophy and retinal detachment etc.) with clear cornea. In contralateral autokeratoplasty cornea of the two eyes are exchanged with each other.

B. *Allografting or Allo-keratoplasty*. In it, patient's diseased cornea is replaced by the donor's healthy cornea. It can be of following types:

1. *Penetrating Keratoplasty* (PK) (full-thickness grafting)
2. *Lamellar Keratoplasty* (partial-thickness grafting) which may be:
   - *Deep anterior lamellar keratoplasty* (DLK). It is performed when endothelium and Descemet's membrane are normal e.g. keratoconus.
   - *Descemet's stripping endothelial keratoplasty* (DSEK). It is performed when only endothelium is defective e.g. after the surgical trauma during phacoemulsification.
3. *Small patch graft* (for small defects), which may be full thickness or partial thickness.

Indications

1. *Optical*, i.e., to improve vision. Important indications are: corneal opacity, bullous keratopathy, corneal dystrophies, advanced keratoconus.
2. *Therapeutic*, i.e., to replace inflamed cornea not responding to conventional therapy.
3. *Tectonic graft*, i.e., to restore integrity of eyeball e.g. after corneal perforation and in marked corneal thinning.
4. *Cosmetic*, i.e., to improve the appearance of the eye.

Donor tissue

The donor eye should be removed as early as possible (within 6 hours of death). It should be stored under sterile conditions.

Evaluation of donor cornea. Biomicroscopic examination of the whole globe, before processing the tissue for media storage, is very important. The donor corneal tissue is graded into excellent, very good, good, fair, and poor depending upon the condition of corneal epithelium, stroma, Descemet's membrane and endothelium (Table 5.1).

Methods of corneal preservation

1. *Short-term storage* (up to 48 hours). The whole globe is preserved at 4°C in a moist chamber.
2. *Intermediate storage* (up to 2 weeks) of donor cornea can be done in McCarey-Kaufman (MK) medium and various chondroitin sulfate enriched media such as optisol medium.
3. *Long-term storage* up to 35 days is done by organ culture method or by cryopreservation at –70°C.

Table 5.1. Grading of donor cornea on slit-lamp biomicroscopic examination

			Grade of donor corneal tissue		
Parameter	*Grade I (Excellent)*	*Grade II (Very good)*	*Grade III (Good)*	*Grade IV (Fair)*	*Grade V (Poor)*
Epithelial defects and haze	None	Slight epithelial haze or defects	Obvious moderate epithelial defects		
Corneal stromal clarity	Crystal clear	Clear	Slight cloudiness	Moderate cloudiness	Marked cloudiness
Arcus senilis	None	Slight	Moderate (<2.5mm)	Heavy (>2.5mm-4mm)	Very heavy (>4 mm)
Descemet's membrane	No folds	Few shallow folds	Numerous shallow folds	Numerous deep folds	Marked deep folds
Endothelium	No defect	No defect	Few vacuolated cells	Moderate guttate	Marked guttate

Surgical technique of penetrating keratoplasty

1. *Excision of donor corneal button* (Fig. 5.23A). The donor corneal button should be cut 0.25 mm larger than the recipient, taking care not to damage the endothelium.
2. *Excision of recipient corneal button.* With the help of a corneal trephine (7.5 mm to 8 mm in size) a partial thickness incision is made in the host cornea (Fig. 5.23B). Then, anterior chamber is entered with the help of a razor blade knife and excision is completed using corneo-scleral scissors (Fig. 5.23C).
3. *Suturing of corneal graft into the host bed* (Fig. 5.23D) is done with either continuous (Fig. 5.23E) or interrupted (Fig. 5.23F) 10-0 nylon sutures.

Complications

1. *Early complications.* These include flat anterior chamber, iris prolapse, infection, secondary glaucoma, epithelial defects and primary graft failure.
2. *Late complications.* These include graft rejection, recurrence of disease and astigmatism.

Graft rejection. It refers to the immunological response of the host to the donor corneal tissue. It can occur as early as 2 weeks and upto several years after grafting. Graft rejection is classically believed to be a delayed type of hypersensitivity response.

Risk factors include younger age of recipient, previous graft failure, corneal vascularization, larger graft size, donor epithelium and massive blood transfusion.

Clinical presentations include:

- *Epithelial rejection* characterized by an elevated epithelial rejection line which stains with fluorescein.
- *Subepithelial infiltrates* known as Kayes dots.
- *Stromal rejection* is characterized by sudden onset of full thickness stromal haze in a previously clear graft.
- *Endothelial rejection* may present as:
  - Khodadaust line demarcating healthy and damaged endothelium
  - Diffuse endothelial rejection with lot of Keratic precipitates.

REFRACTIVE CORNEAL SURGERY

Refractive corneal surgery includes:

- Radial Keratotomy (RK),
- Astigmatic Keratotomy (AK),
- Photorefractive Keratotomy (PRK),
- Laser assisted *in-situ* Keratomileusis (LASIK) and its varieties,

- Thermal laser Keratoplasty (TLK),
- Conductive Keratoplasty (CK),
- Orthokeratoplasty, and
- Intracorneal ring (ICR) implants

(For details see page 47 to 50).

PHOTOTHERAPEUTIC KERATECTOMY

Phototherapeutic Keratectomy (PTK) refers to the ablation of superficial corneal lesion with the help of excimer laser (198 nm).

Indications include:

- Superficial corneal scars
- Corneal degenerations, e.g. band shaped Keratopathy, Salzman nodular degeneration and oil droplet keratopathy.
- Epithelial dystrophies (e.g. Reis-Buckler dystrophy)
- Recurrent corneal erosions

Procedure. The modern excimer laser machines have two modes for PTK:

- *Spot mode*, where a small spot (<1 mm) can be ablated, and
- *Shapping mode,* which allows uniform removal of corneal tissue from a large zone.

Contraindications include:

- Excessive thin corneas,
- Moderate to severe dry eye, and
- Deep corneal lesions

Complications. Faint corneal haze is a usual end result of the PTK. Other complications include:

- Secondary infections,
- Induced hypermetropia, and
- Secondary Keractesia

KERATOPROSTHESIS

Keratoprosthesis refers to an artificial corneal device used in patients unsuitable for keratoplasty.

Types. Keratoprosthesis basically consists of a central optical cylindrical part made of polymethyl-methaacrylate (PMMA). Based on the surrounding fixation device, the keratoprosthesis of various designs have been devised:

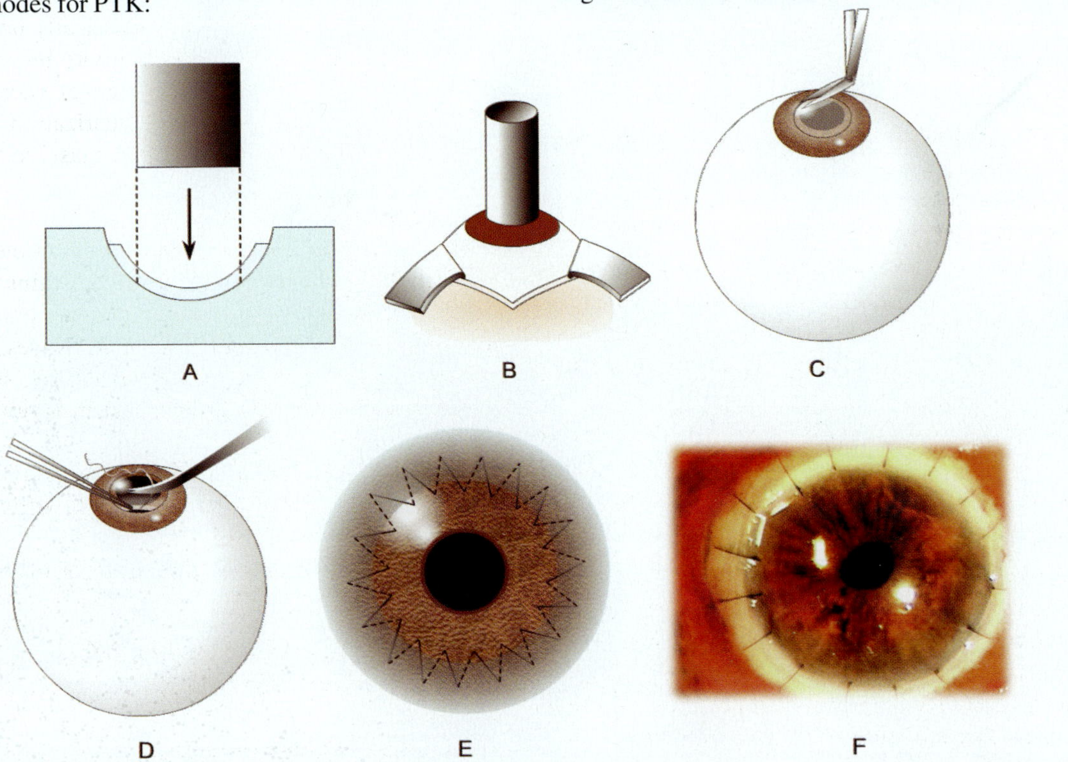

Fig. 5.23. Technique of keratoplasty : A, excision of donor corneal button; B & C, excision of recipient corneal button; D, suturing of donor button into recipient's bed; E, showing pattern of continuous sutures in keratoplasty; F, Clinical photograph of a patient with interrupted sutures in keratoplasty.

- *Osteo-odonto-Kertaoprosthesis* is fixed with the help of patients own tooth root and alveolar bone.
- *Chondro- Keratoprosthesis,* is fixed with patients own cartilage.
- *Onycho- Keratoprosthesis,* is fixed with patient's nails.
- *Singh and Worst Collar-stud keratoprosthesis* is fixed with stainless steel sutures.

Indications. Prerequisites for keratoprosthesis include bilateral blindness due to corneal diseases (not suitable for keratoplasty) with accurate perception of light, normal electrophysiological tests and absence of gross posterior segment disorders on ultrasonography. e.g.,:

- Stevens-Johnson syndrome,
- Chemical burns,
- Ocular cicatricial pemphigoid,
- Severe trachoma
- Multiple previous failed corneal grafts

Complications include:

- Extrusion of prosthesis,
- Intractable glaucoma,
- Retroprosthetic membrane formation,
- Uveitis, and
- Retinal detachment.

6

CHAPTER

Diseases of the Sclera

APPLIED ANATOMY

INFLAMMATIONS OF THE SCLERA

- Episcleritis
- Scleritis
  - Anterior
  - Posterior
- Blue Sclera

STAPHYLOMAS

- Anterior
- Intercalary
- Ciliary
- Equatorial
- Posterior

APPLIED ANATOMY

Sclera forms the posterior five-sixth opaque part of the external fibrous tunic of the eyeball. Its whole outer surface is covered by Tenon's capsule. In the anterior part it is also covered by bulbar conjunctiva. Its inner surface lies in contact with choroid with a potential suprachoroidal space in between. In its anterior most part near the limbus there is a furrow which encloses the canal of Schlemm.

Thickness of sclera varies considerably in different individuals and with the age of the person. It is generally thinner in children than the adults and in females than the males. Sclera is thickest posteriorly (1mm) and gradually becomes thin when traced anteriorly. It is thinnest at the insertion of extraocular muscles (0.3 mm). Lamina cribrosa is a sieve-like sclera from which fibres of optic nerve pass.

Apertures. Sclera is pierced by three sets of apertures (Fig. 6.1).

1. *Posterior apertures* are situated around the optic nerve and transmit long and short ciliary nerves and vessels.
2. *Middle apertures* (four in number) are situated slightly posterior to the equator; through these pass the four vortex veins (vena verticosae).
3. *Anterior apertures* are situated 3 to 4 mm away from the limbus. Anterior ciliary vessels and branches from long ciliary nerves pass through these apertures.

Microscopic structure. Histologically, sclera consists of following three layers:

1. *Episcleral tissue.* It is a thin, dense vascularised layer of connective tissue which covers the sclera proper. Fine fibroblasts, macrophages and lymphocytes are also present in this layer.
2. *Sclera proper.* It is an avascular structure which consists of dense bundles of collagen fibres. The bands of collagen tissue cross each other in all directions.

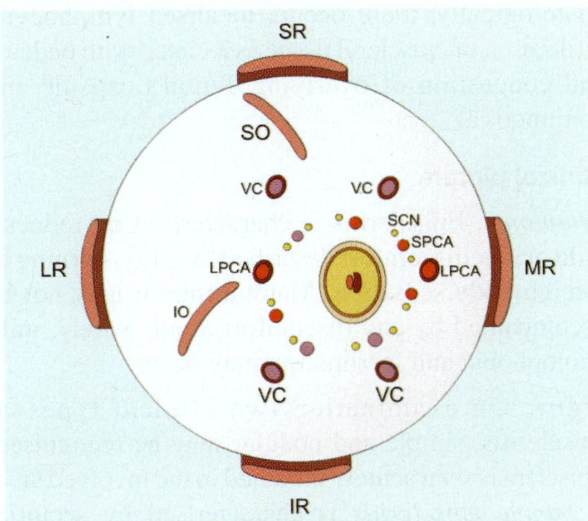

Fig. 6.1. Apertures in the sclera. (posterior view) for: SCN, short ciliary nerve; SPCA, short posterior ciliary artery; LPCA, long posterior ciliary artery; VC, vena verticosa

3. *Lamina fusca.* It is the innermost part of sclera which blends with suprachoroidal and supraciliary laminae of the uveal tract. It is brownish in colour owing to the presence of pigmented cells.

Nerve supply. Sclera is supplied by branches from the long ciliary nerves which pierce it 2-4 mm from the limbus to form a plexus.

INFLAMMATIONS OF THE SCLERA

EPISCLERITIS

Episcleritis is benign recurrent inflammation of the episclera, involving the overlying Tenon's capsule but not the underlying sclera. It typically affects young adults, being twice as common in women than men.

Etiology

1. ***Idiopathic.*** Exact etiology is not known in many cases.
2. ***Systemic diseases*** associated with episcleritis, include gout, rosacea, psoriasis and connective tissue diseases.
3. ***Hypersensitivity reaction*** to endogenous tubercular or streptococcal toxins is also reported.
4. ***Infectious episcleritis*** may be caused by herpes zoster virus, syphillis, Lyme disease and tuberculosis.

Pathology

Histologically, there occurs localised lymphocytic infiltration of episcleral tissue associated with oedema and congestion of overlying Tenon's capsule and conjunctiva.

Clinical picture

Symptoms. Episcleritis is characterised by redness, mild ocular discomfort described as gritty, burning or foreign body sensation. Many a time it may not be accompanied by any discomfort at all. Rarely, mild photophobia and lacrimation may occur.

Signs. On examination two clinical types of episcleritis, simple and nodular may be recognised. Episclera is seen acutely inflamed in the involved area.

- *Simple episcleritis* is characterised by sectorial (occasionally diffuse) inflammation of episclera. The engorged episcleral vessels are large and run in radial direction beneath the conjunctiva (Fig. 6.2A).
- *Nodular episcleritis* is characterised by a pink or purple flat nodule surrounded by injection, usually situated 2-3 mm away from the limbus (Fig. 6.2B). The nodule is firm, tender, can be moved separately from the sclera and the overlying conjunctiva also moves freely.

Clinical course. Episcleritis runs a limited course of 10 days to 3 weeks and resolves spontaneously. However, recurrences are common and tend to occur in bouts. Rarely, a fleeting type of disease *(episcleritis periodica)* may occur.

Differential diagnosis

- *Simple episcleritis* may be confused rarely with conjunctivitis.

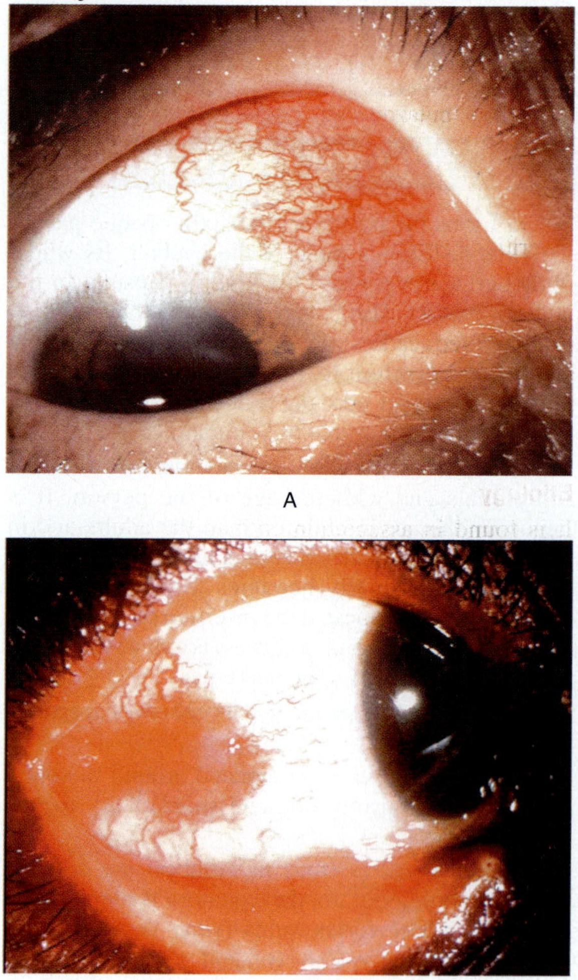

A

B

Fig. 6.2. Episcleritis: A, diffuse; B, nodular.

- *Nodular episcleritis* may be confused with inflamed pinguecula, swelling and congestion due to foreign body lodged in bulbar conjunctiva and very rarely with scleritis.

Treatment

1. *Topical artificial tears* e.g. 0.5% carboxy methyl cellulose have soothing effect.
2. *Topical NSAIDs* e.g. ketorolac 0.3% may be useful.
3. *Topical mild corticosteroid eyedrops* e.g., fluorometholone or loteprednol instilled 2-3 hourly, render the eye more comfortable and resolve the episcleritis within a few days.
4. *Cold compresses* applied to the closed lids may offer symptomatic relief from ocular discomfort.
5. *Systemic non-steroidal anti-inflammatory drugs (NSAIDs)* such as flurbiprofen (300 mg OD), indomethacin (25 mg three times a day), or oxyphenbutazone may be required in recurrent cases.

SCLERITIS

Scleritis refers to a chronic inflammation of the sclera proper. It is a comparatively serious disease which may cause visual impairment and even loss of the eye if treated inadequately. Fortunately, its incidence is much less than that of episcleritis. It usually occurs in elderly patients (40-70 years) involving females more than the males.

Etiology

It is found in association with multiple conditions which are as follows:

1. *Autoimmune collagen disorders,* especially rheumatoid arthritis, is the most common association. Overall about 5% cases of scleritis are associated with some connective tissue disease. About 0.5 percent of patients (1 in 200) suffering from seropositive rheumatoid arthritis develop scleritis. Other associated collagen disorders are Wegener's granulomatosis, polyarteritis nodosa (PAN), systemic lupus erythematosus (SLE) and ankylosing spondylitis.
2. *Metabolic disorders* like gout and thyrotoxicosis have also been reported to be associated with scleritis.
3. *Some infections,* particularly herpes zoster ophthalmicus, chronic staphylococcal and streptococcal infection have also been known to cause scleritis.
4. *Granulomatous diseases* like tuberculosis, syphilis, sarcoidosis, leprosy can also cause scleritis.
5. *Miscellaneous conditions* like irradiation, chemical burns, Vogt-Koyanagi-Harada syndrome, Behcet's disease and rosacea are also implicated in the etiology.
6. *Surgically induced scleritis* (SIS) is a rare complication of ocular surgery. It occurs within 6 months postoperatively. Exact mechanism not known, may be precipitation of underlying systemic cause.
7. *Idiopathic.* In many cases of scleritis, cause is unknown.

Pathology

Histopathological changes are that of a chronic granulomatous disorder characterised by fibrinoid necrosis, destruction of collagen together with infiltration by polymorphonuclear cells, lymphocytes, plasma cells and macrophages. The granuloma is surrounded by multinucleated epitheloid giant cells and old and new vessels, some of which may show evidence of vasculitis.

Classification

Scleritis can be classified as follows:

I. *Anterior scleritis* (98%)
   1. Non-necrotizing scleritis (85%)
      (a) Diffuse
      (b) Nodular
   2. Necrotizing scleritis (13%)
      (a) with inflammation
      (b) without inflammation (scleromalacia perforans)

II. *Posterior scleritis* (2%)

Clinical features

Symptoms of scleritis are:

- *Pain:* Patients complain of moderate to severe pain which is deep and boring in character and often wakes the patient early in the morning. Ocular pain radiates to the jaw and temple.
- *Redness* may be localized or diffuse.
- *Photophobia* and *lacrimation* may be mild to moderate.
- *Diminution of vision* may occur occasionally.

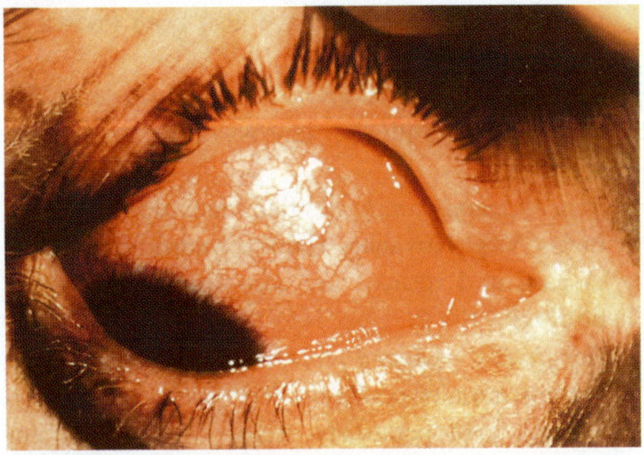

Fig. 6.3. Non-necrotizing anterior diffuse scleritis.

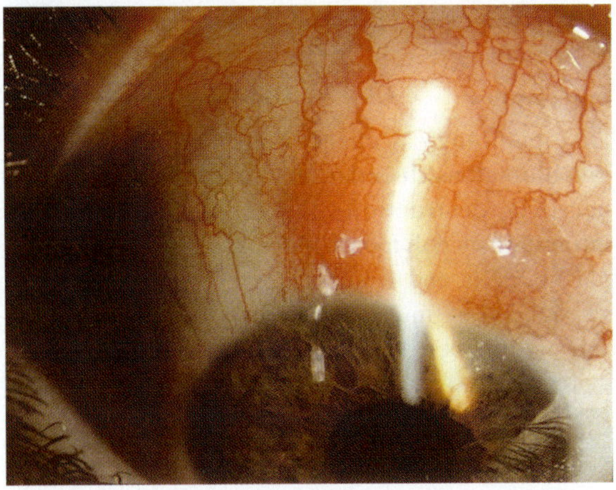

Fig. 6.4. Non-necrotizing anterior nodular scleritis.

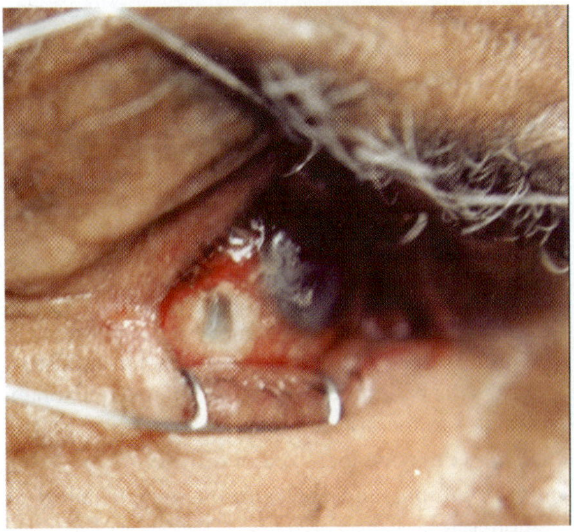

Fig. 6.5. Anterior necrotizing scleritis with inflammation.

Signs. The salient features of different clinical types of scleritis are as follows:

1. *Non-necrotizing anterior diffuse scleritis.* It is the commonest variety, characterised by widespread inflammation involving a quadrant or more of the anterior sclera. The involved area is raised and salmon pink to purple in colour (Fig. 6.3).

2. *Non-necrotizing anterior nodular scleritis.* It is characterised by one or two hard, purplish elevated immovable scleral nodules, usually situated near the limbus (Fig. 6.4). Sometimes, the nodules are arranged in a ring around the limbus (*annular scleritis*).

3. *Anterior necrotizing scleritis with inflammation.* It is an acute severe form of scleritis characterised by intense localised inflammation associated with areas of infarction due to vasculitis (Fig. 6.5). The affected necrosed area is thinned out and sclera becomes transparent and ectatic with uveal tissue shining through it. It is usually associated with anterior uveitis.

4. *Anterior necrotizing scleritis without inflammation* (scleromalacia perforans). This specific entity typically occurs in elderly females usually suffering from long-standing rheumatoid arthritis. It is characterised by development of yellowish patch of melting sclera (due to obliteration of arterial supply); which often together with the overlying episclera and conjunctiva completely separates from the surrounding normal sclera. This sequestrum of sclera becomes dead white in colour, which eventually absorbs leaving behind it a large punched out area of thin sclera through which the uveal tissue shines (Fig. 6.6). Spontaneous perforation is extremely rare.

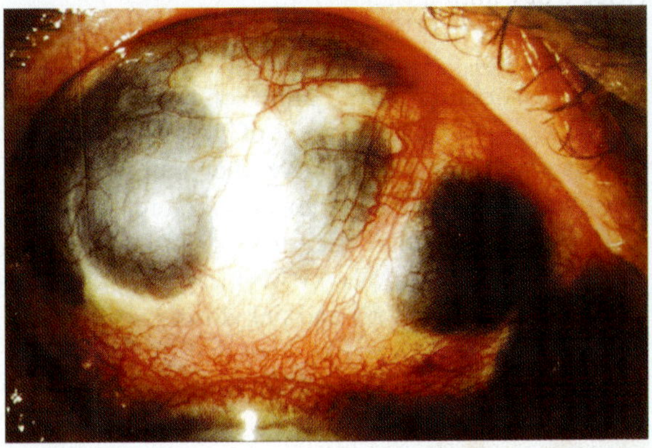

Fig. 6.6. Anterior necrotizing scleritis without inflammation (Scleromalacia perforans).

5. *Posterior scleritis.* It is an inflammation involving the sclera behind the equator. The condition is frequently misdiagnosed. It is characterised by features of associated inflammation of adjacent structures, which include: exudative retinal detachment, macular oedema, proptosis and limitation of ocular movements.

Complications

These are quite common with necrotizing scleritis and include sclerosing keratitis, keratolysis, complicated cataract and secondary glaucoma.

Investigations

Following laboratory studies may be helpful in identifying associated systemic diseases or in establishing the nature of immunologic reaction:

1. TLC, DLC and ESR.
2. Serum levels of complement (C3), immune complexes, rheumatoid factor, antinuclear antibodies and L.E cells for an immunological survey.
3. FTA - ABS, VDRL for syphilis.
4. Serum uric acid for gout.
5. Urine analysis.
6. Mantoux test.
7. X-rays of chest, paranasal sinuses, sacroiliac joint and orbit (to rule out foreign body especially in patients with nodular scleritis).

Treatment

Non-necrotising scleritis. It is treated by topical steroid eye drops and systemic indomethacin 75 mg twice a day until inflammation resolves.

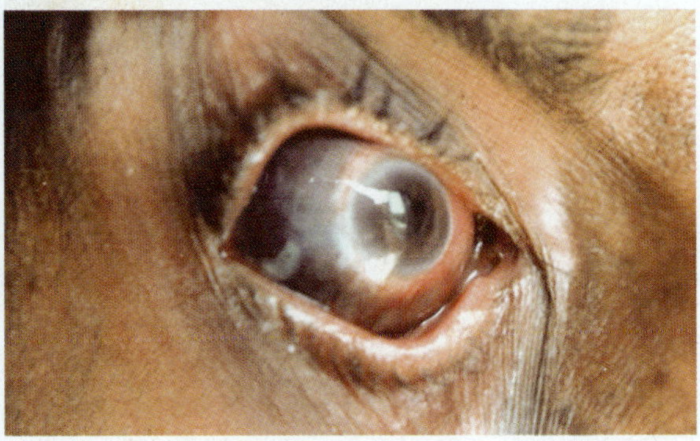

Fig. 6.7. Blue sclera.

Necrotising scleritis. It is treated by topical steroids and heavy doses of oral steroids tapered slowly. In non-responsive cases, immuno-suppressive agents like methotrexate or cyclophosphamide may be required. Subconjunctival steroids are contraindicated because they may lead to scleral thinning and perforation.

BLUE SCLERA

It is an asymptomatic condition characterised by marked, generalised blue discolouration of sclera due to thinning (Fig. 6.7). It is a typical association of osteogenesis imperfecta. Its other causes are Marfan's syndrome, Ehlers-Danlos syndrome, pseudoxanthoma elasticum, buphthalmos, high myopia and healed scleritis.

STAPHYLOMAS

Staphyloma refers to a localised bulging of weak and thin outer tunic of the eyeball (cornea or sclera), lined by uveal tissue which shines through the thinned out fibrous coat.

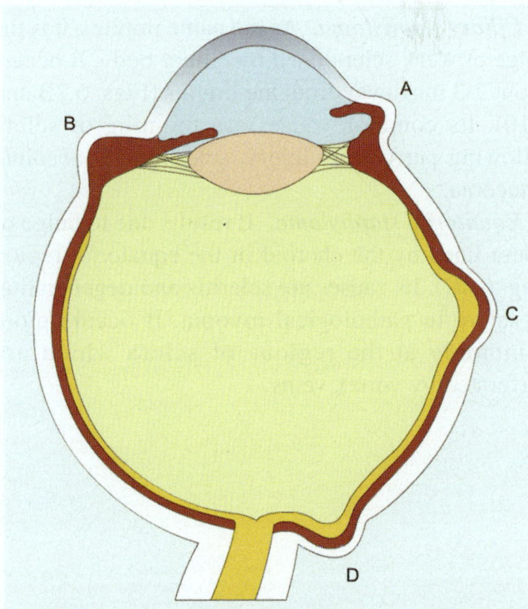

Fig. 6.8. Staphylomas (diagramatic depiction) : A, intercalary; B, ciliary; C, equatorial; D, posterior.

Types

Anatomically it can be divided into anterior, intercalary, ciliary, equatorial and posterior staphyloma (Fig. 6.8).

1. ***Anterior staphyloma.*** (see page 128)

2. ***Intercalary staphyloma.*** It is the name given to the localised bulge in limbal area lined by root of iris (Figs. 6.8A and 6.9). It results due to ectasia of weak scar tissue formed at the limbus, following healing of a perforating injury or a peripheral corneal ulcer. There may be associated secondary angle closure glaucoma, which may cause progression of bulge if not treated. Defective vision occurs due to marked corneal astigmatism.

Treatment consists of localised staphylectomy under heavy doses of oral steroids.

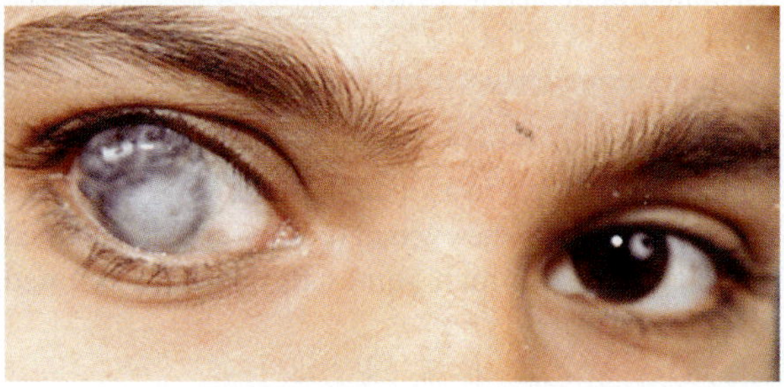

Fig. 6.9. Intercalary staphyloma.

3. ***Ciliary staphyloma.*** As the name implies, it is the bulge of weak sclera lined by ciliary body. It occurs about 2-3 mm away from the limbus (Figs. 6.8B and 6.10). Its common causes are thinning of sclera following perforating injury, scleritis and absolute glaucoma.

4. ***Equatorial staphyloma.*** It results due to bulge of sclera lined by the choroid in the equatorial region (Fig. 6.8C). Its causes are scleritis and degeneration of sclera in pathological myopia. It occurs more commonly at the regions of sclera which are perforated by vortex veins.

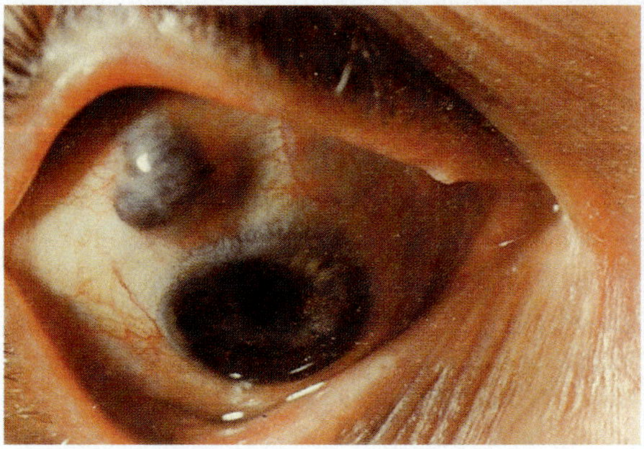

Fig. 6.10. Ciliary staphyloma.

5. ***Posterior staphyloma.*** It refers to bulge of weak sclera lined by the choroid behind the equator (Fig. 6.8D). Here again the common causes are pathological myopia, posterior scleritis and perforating injuries. It is diagnosed on ophthalmoscopy. The area is excavated with retinal vessels dipping in it (just like marked cupping of optic disc in glaucoma) (Fig. 6.11). Its floor is focussed with minus lenses in ophthalmoscope as compared to its margins.

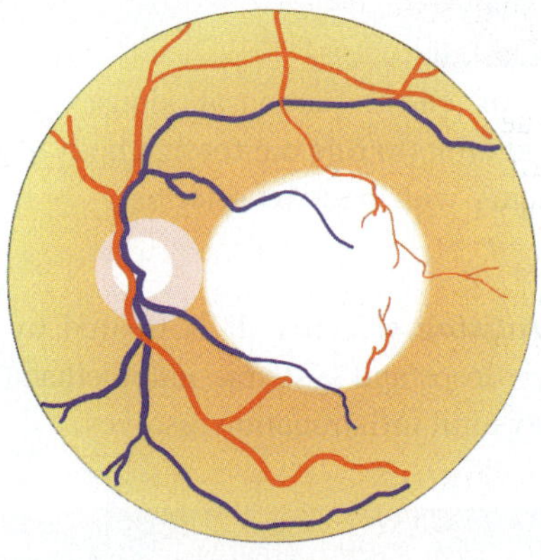

Fig. 6.11. Fundus photograph showing excavation of retinal tissue in posterior staphyloma.

7 CHAPTER

Diseases of the Uveal Tract

APPLIED ANATOMY

Uveal tissue constitutes the middle vascular coat of the eyeball. From anterior to posterior it can be divided into three parts, namely, *iris, ciliary body* and *choroid*. However, the entire uveal tract is developmentally, structurally and functionally one indivisible structure.

THE IRIS

Iris is the anterior most part of the uveal tract. It is a thin circular disc corresponding to the diaphragm of a camera. In its centre is an aperture of about 4 mm diameter called *pupil* which regulates the amount of light reaching the retina. At periphery, the iris is attached to the middle of anterior surface of the ciliary body. It divides the space between the cornea and lens into anterior and posterior chambers.

***Macroscopic appearance*.** Anterior surface of the iris can be divided into a ciliary zone and a pupillary zone by a zigzag line called *collarette* (Fig. 7.1).

1. *Ciliary zone.* It presents series of radial streaks due to underlying radial blood vessels and crypts which are depressions where superficial layer of iris is missing. Crypts are arranged in two rows —the peripheral present near the iris root and the central present near the collarette.
2. *Pupillary zone.* This part of the iris lies between the collarette and pigmented pupillary frill and is relatively smooth and flat.

Microscopic structure (Fig. 7.2) . The iris consists of four layers which from anterior to posterior are :

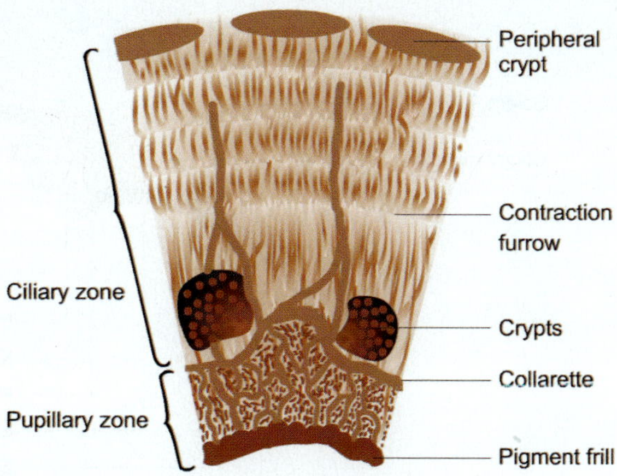

Fig. 7.1. Macroscopic appearance of anterior surface of iris.

1. *Anterior limiting layer.* It is the anterior most condensed part of the stroma. It consists of melanocytes and fibroblasts. Previously this layer was called endothelial layer of iris which was a misnomer. This layer is deficient in the areas of crypts. The definitive colour of the iris depends on this layer. In blue iris this layer is thin and contains few pigment cells. While in brown iris it is thick and densely pigmented.
2. *Iris stroma.* It consists of loosely arranged collagenous network in which are embedded the sphincter pupillae muscle, dilator pupillae muscle, vessels, nerves, pigment cells and other cells which include lymphocytes, fibroblasts, macrophages and mast cells.
   - *Sphincter pupillae muscle* forms one millimetre broad circular band in the pupillary part of the iris. It is supplied by parasympathetic fibres through third nerve. It constricts the pupil.
   - *Dilator pupillae muscle* lies in the posterior part of stroma of the ciliary zone of iris. Its myofilaments are located in the outer part of the cells of anterior pigment epithelial layer. It is supplied by cervical sympathetic nerves and dilates the pupil.
3. *Anterior epithelial layer.* It is anterior continuation of the pigment epithelium of retina and ciliary body. This layer gives rise to the dilator pupillae muscle.
4. *Posterior pigmented epithelial layer.* It is anterior continuation of the non-pigmented epithelium of ciliary body. At the pupillary margin it forms the pigmented frill and becomes continuous with the anterior pigmented epithelial layer.

CILIARY BODY

Ciliary body is forward continuation of the choroid at ora serrata. In cut-section, it is triangular in shape. The anterior side of the triangle forms the part of the angle of anterior and posterior chambers. In its middle the iris is attached. The outer side of the triangle lies against the sclera with a suprachoroidal space in between. The inner side of the triangle is divided into two parts. The anterior part (about 2 mm) having finger-like ciliary processes is called *pars plicata* and the posterior smooth part (about 4 mm) is called *pars plana* (Fig. 7.2).

Microscopic structure (Fig. 7.2). From without inwards ciliary body consists of following five layers:

1. *Supraciliary lamina.* It is the outermost condensed part of the stroma and consists of pigmented collagen fibres. Posteriorly, it is the continuation of suprachoroidal lamina and anteriorly it becomes continuous with the anterior limiting membrane of iris.
2. *Stroma of the ciliary body.* It consists of connective tissue of collagen and fibroblasts. Embedded in the stroma are ciliary muscle, vessels, nerves, pigment and other cells.

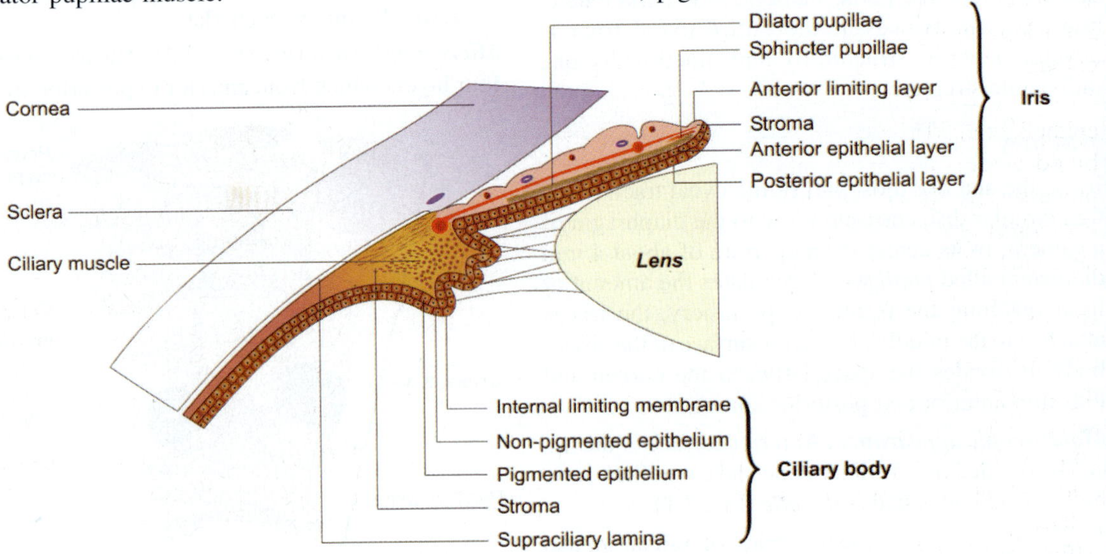

Fig. 7.2. Microscopic structure of iris and ciliary body.

Ciliary muscle occupies most of the outer part of ciliary body. In cut section it is triangular in shape. It is a non-striated muscle having three parts:

- Longitudinal or meridional fibres which help in aqueous outflow;
- Circular fibres which help in accommodation; and
- Radial or oblique fibres act in the same way as the longitudinal fibres.
- *Nerve supply*. Ciliary muscle is supplied by parasympathetic fibres through the short ciliary nerves.

3. *Layer of pigmented epithelium.* It is forward continuation of the retinal pigment epithelium. Anteriorly it is continuous with the anterior pigmented epithelium of the iris.
4. *Layer of non-pigmented epithelium.* It consists mainly of low columnar or cuboidal cells, and is the forward continuation of the sensory retina. It continues anteriorly as the posterior (internal) pigmented epithelium of the iris.
5. *Internal limiting membrane.* It is the forward continuation of the internal limiting membrane of the retina. It lines the non-pigmented epithelial layer.

Ciliary processes. These are finger-like projections from the pars plicata part of the ciliary body. These are about 70-80 in number. Each process is about 2 mm long and 0.5 mm in diameter. These are white in colour.

Structure. Each process is lined by two layers of epithelial cells. The core of the ciliary process contains blood vessels and loose connective tissue. These processes are the site of aqueous production.

Functions of ciliary body. (i) Formation of aqueous humour. (ii) Ciliary muscles help in accommodation.

CHOROID

Choroid is posterior most part of the vascular coat of the eyeball. It extends from optic disc to the ora serrata. Its inner surface is smooth, brown and lies in contact with pigment epithelium of the retina. The outer surface is rough and lies in contact with the sclera.

Microscopic structure (Fig. 7.3). From without inwards choroid consists of following three layers:

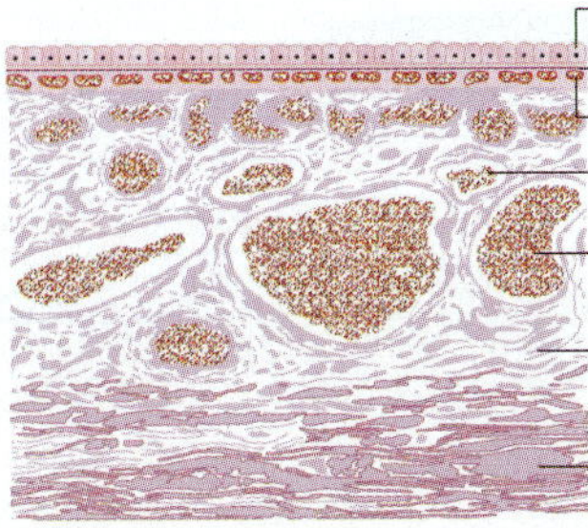

Fig. 7.3. Microscopic structure of the choroid.

1. *Suprachoroidal lamina.* It is a thin membrane of condensed collagen fibres, melanocytes and fibroblasts. It is continuous anteriorly with the supraciliary lamina. The potential space between the membrane and sclera is called *suprachoroidal space* which contains long and short posterior ciliary arteries and nerves.
2. *Stroma of the choroid.* It consists of loose collagenous tissue with some elastic and reticulum fibres. It also contains pigment cells and plasma cells. Its main bulk is formed by vessels which are arranged in three layers. From without inwards these are: (i) layer of large vessels (Haller's layer), (ii) layer of medium vessels (Sattler's layer) and (iii) layer of choriocapillaris which nourishes the outer layers of the retina.
3. *Basal lamina.* It is also called *Bruch's membrane* and lines the layer of choriocapillaris. It lies in approximation with pigment epithelium of the retina.

Blood supply of the uveal tract

Arterial supply. The uveal tract is supplied by three sets of arteries (Fig. 7.4):

1. *Short posterior ciliary arteries.* These arise as two trunks from the ophthalmic artery. Each trunk divides into 10-20 branches which pierce the sclera around the optic nerve and supply the choroid in a segmental manner.
2. *Long posterior ciliary arteries.* These are two in number, nasal and temporal. These pierce the sclera obliquely on medial and lateral side of the optic nerve and run forward in the suprachoroidal space to reach the ciliary muscle, without giving any branch. At the anterior end of ciliary muscle these anastomose with each other and with the anterior ciliary arteries and give rise to branches which supply the ciliary body.

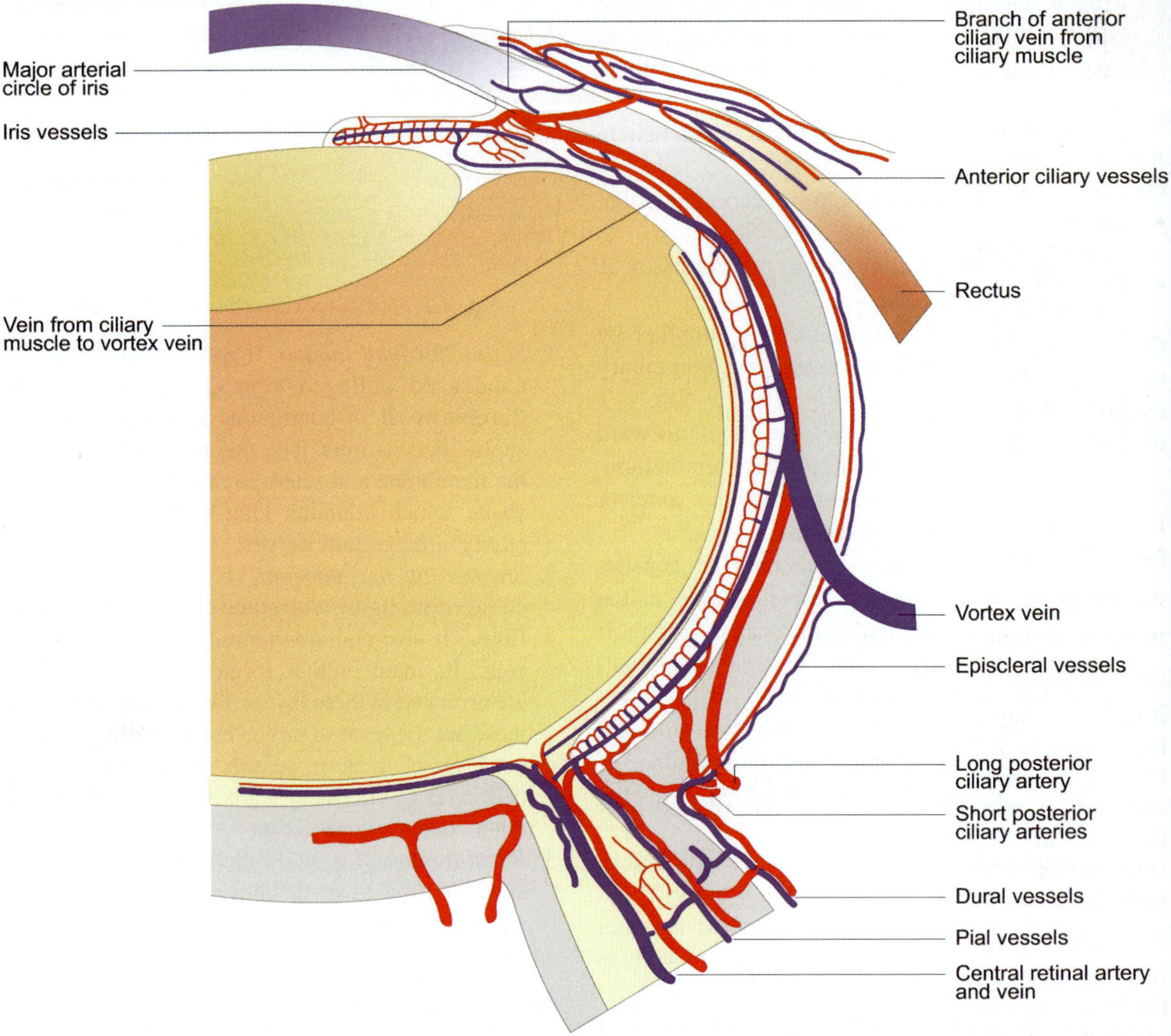

Fig. 7.4. Blood supply of the uveal tract.

3. *Anterior ciliary arteries.* These are derived from the muscular branches of ophthalmic artery. These are 7 in number i.e., 2 each from arteries of superior rectus, inferior rectus, and medial rectus muscle and one from that of lateral rectus muscle. These arteries pass anteriorly in the episclera, give branches to sclera, limbus and conjunctiva and ultimately pierce the sclera near the limbus to enter the ciliary muscle; where they anastomose with the two long posterior ciliary arteries to form the *circulus arteriosus major*, near the root of iris. Several branches arise from the circulus arteriosus major and supply the ciliary processes (one branch for each process). Similarly, many branches from this major arterial circle run radially through the iris towards pupillary margin, where they anastomose with each other to form *circulus arteriosus minor.*

Venous drainage. A series of small veins which drain blood from the iris, ciliary body and choroid join to form the vortex veins. The vortex veins are four in number–superior temporal, inferior temporal, superior nasal and inferior nasal. They pierce the sclera behind the equator and drain into superior and inferior ophthalmic veins which in turn drain into the cavernous sinus.

CONGENITAL ANOMALIES OF UVEAL TRACT

HETEROCHROMIA OF IRIS

It refers to variations in the iris colour and is a common congenital anomaly.

- *Heterochromia iridium*, colour of one iris differs from the other.
- *Heterochromia iridis*, one sector of the iris differs from the remainder of iris.

Congenital heterochromia must be differentiated from the acquired heterochromia as seen in heterochromic cyclitis, siderosis, Horner's syndrome and malignant melanoma of iris.

CORECTOPIA

It refers to abnormally eccentric placed pupil. Normally pupil is placed slightly nasal to the centre.

POLYCORIA

In this condition, there are more than one pupil.

CONGENITAL ANIRIDIA (IRIDREMIA)

It refers to congenital absence of iris. *True aniridia*, i.e., complete absence of the iris is extremely rare. Usually, a peripheral rim of iris is present and this condition is called '*Clinical aniridia*'. Zonules of the lens and ciliary processes are often visible. The condition is usually familial and may be associated with glaucoma due to angle anomalies.

PERSISTENT PUPILLARY MEMBRANE

It represents the remnants of the vascular sheath of the lens. It is characterised by stellate-shaped shreds of the pigmented tissue coming from anterior surface of the iris (attached at collarette) (Fig. 7.5). These float freely in the anterior chamber or may be attached to the anterior surface of the lens.

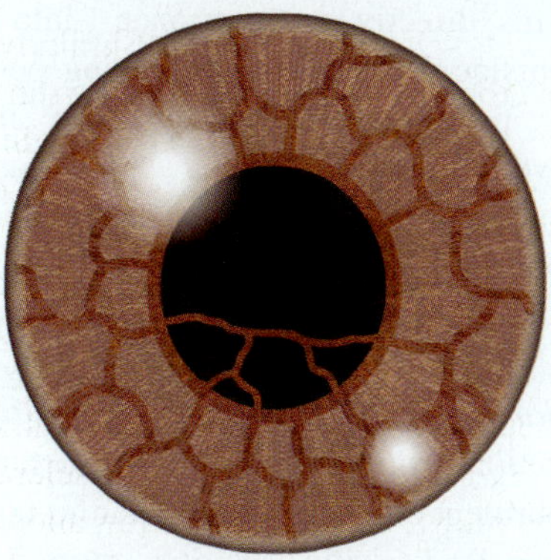

Fig. 7.5. Persistent pupillary membrane.

CONGENITAL COLOBOMA OF THE UVEAL TRACT

Congenital coloboma (absence of tissue) of iris (Fig. 7.6), ciliary body and choroid (Fig. 7.7) may be seen in association or independently. Coloboma may be typical or atypical.

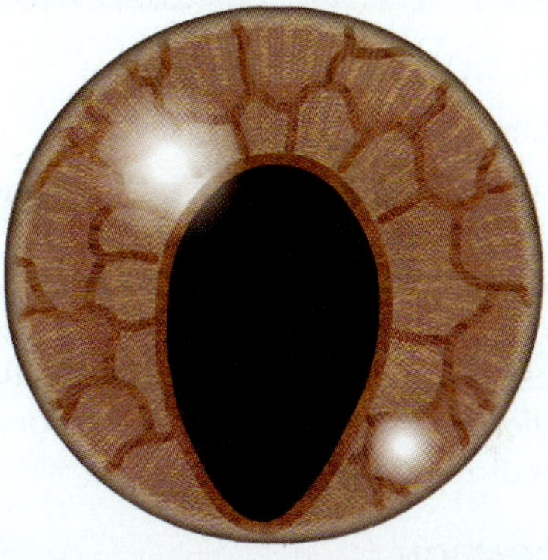

Fig. 7.6. Typical coloboma of the iris.

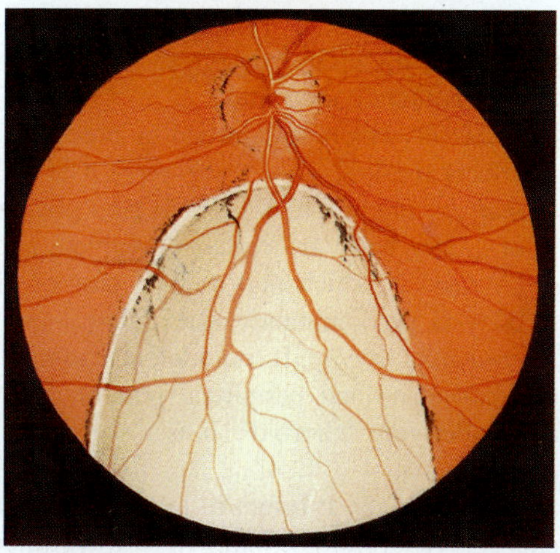

Fig. 7.7. Coloboma of the choroid.

Typical coloboma is seen in the inferonasal quadrant and occurs due to defective closure of the embryonic fissure. Typical coloboma may be complete or incomplete.

- *Complete coloboma* extends from pupil to the optic nerve, with a sector-shaped gap occupying about one-eighth of the circumference of the retina, choroid, ciliary body, iris and causes a corresponding indentation of the lens where the zonular fibres are missing.

- *Incomplete coloboma* may involve the iris alone, or iris and ciliary body (more common), or iris, ciliary body and part of choroid (i.e. stops short of optic nerve).

Atypical coloboma is occasionally found in other positions. It is usually incomplete.

UVEITIS

GENERAL CONSIDERATIONS

DEFINITION

The term uveitis strictly means inflammation of the uveal tissue only. However, clinically there is always some associated inflammation of the adjacent structures such as retina, vitreous, sclera and cornea. Due to close relationship of the anatomically distinct parts of the uveal tract, the inflammatory process usually tends to involve the uvea as a whole.

CLASSIFICATION

I. Anatomical Classification

1. *Anterior uveitis.* It is inflammation of the uveal tissue from iris up to pars plicata of ciliary body. It may be subdivided into:
   - *Iritis,* in which inflammation predominantly affects the iris.
   - *Iridocyctitis* in which iris and pars plicata part of ciliary body are equally involved, and
   - *Cyclitis,* in which pars plicata part of ciliary body is predominantly affected.
2. *Intermediate uveitis.* It includes inflammation of the pars plana and peripheral part of the retina and underlying 'choroid'. It is also called 'pars planitis'.
3. *Posterior uveitis.* It refers to inflammation of the choroid (choroiditis). Almost always there is associated inflammation of retina and hence the term '*chorioretinitis*' is used.
4. *Panuveitis.* It is inflammation of the whole uvea.

II. Clinical Classification

1. *Acute uveitis.* It has got a sudden symptomatic onset and the disease lasts for about six weeks to 3 months.
2. *Chronic uveitis.* It frequently has an insiduous and asymptomatic onset. It persists longer than 3 months to years and is usually diagnosed when it causes defective vision.
3. *Recurrent uveitis.* This is characterised by repeated episodes with inactive periods of ≥ 3 months of treatment.

III. Pathological Classification

1. Suppurative or purulent uveitis.
2. Non-suppurative uveitis. It has been further subdivided into two groups (Wood's classification).
   (i) Non-granulomatous uveitis, and
   (ii) Granulomatous uveitis

IV. Etiological (Duke Elder's) Classification

1. Infective uveitis
2. Immune-related uveitis
3. Toxic uveitis
4. Traumatic uveitis
5. Uveitis associated with non-infective systemic diseases
6. Idiopathic uveitis

ETIOLOGY

Despite a great deal of experimental research and many sophisticated methods of investigations, etiology and immunology of the uveitis is still largely not understood. Even today, the cause of many clinical conditions is disputed (remains presumptive) and in many others etiology is unknown. The etiological concepts of uveitis as proposed by Duke Elder, in general, are discussed here.

1. *Infective uveitis.* In this, inflammation of the uveal tissue is induced by invasion of the organisms. Uveal infections may be exogenous, secondary or endogenous.

i *Exogenous infection* wherein the infecting organisms directly gain entrance into the eye from outside. It can occur following penetrating injuries, perforation of corneal ulcer and post-operatively (after intraocular operations). Such infections usually result in an acute iridocyclitis of suppurative (purulent) nature, which soon turns into endophthalmitis or even panophthalmitis.

ii *Secondary infection* of the uvea occurs by spread of infection from neighbouring structures, e.g., acute purulent conjunctivitis. (pneumo-coccal and gonococcal), keratitis, scleritis, retinitis, orbital cellulitis and orbital thrombophlebitis.

iii *Endogenous infections* are caused by the entrance of organisms from some source situated elsewhere in the body, by way of the bloodstream. Endogenous infections play important role in the inflammations of uvea.

Types of infectious uveitis. Depending upon the causative organisms, the infectious uveitis may be classified as follows:

i. *Bacterial infections.* These may be granulomatous e.g., tubercular, leprotic, syphilitic, brucellosis or pyogenic such as streptococci, staphylococci, pneumococci and gonococcus.
ii. *Viral infections* associated with uveitis are herpes simplex, herpes zoster and cytomegalo inclusion virus (CMV).
iii. *Fungal uveitis* is rare and may accompany systemic aspergillosis, candidiasis and blastomycosis. It also includes presumed ocular histoplasmosis syndrome.
iv. *Parasitic uveitis* is known in toxoplasmosis, toxocariasis, onchocerciasis and amoebiasis.
v. *Rickettsial uveitis* may occur in scrub typhus and epidemic typhus.

2. *Immune related uveitis.* Immune related uveitis is of the commonest occurrence in clinical practice. The complex subject of immune linked inflammation of uveal tissue is still not clearly understood. It may be caused by the following ways:

i. *Microbial allergy.* In this, primary source of infection is somewhere else in the body and the escape of the organisms or their products into the bloodstream causes sensitisation of the uveal tissue with the formation of antibodies. At a later date a renewal of infection in the original focus may again cause dissemination of the organisms or their products (antigens); which on meeting the sensitised uveal tissue excite an allergic inflammatory response.

Primary focus of infection can be a minute tubercular lesion in the lymph nodes or lungs. Once it used to be the most common cause of uveitis worldwide, but now it is rare. However, in developing countries like India tubercular infections still play an important role. Other sources of primary focus are streptococcal and other infections in the teeth, paranasal sinuses, tonsils, prostate, genitals and urinary tract.

ii. *Anaphylactic uveitis.* It is said to accompany the systemic anaphylactic reactions like serum sickness and angioneurotic oedema.

iii. *Atopic uveitis.* It occurs due to airborne allergens and inhalants, e.g., seasonal iritis due to pollens. A similar reaction to such materials as danders of cats, chicken feather, house dust, egg albumin and beef proteins has also been noted.

iv. *Autoimmune uveitis.* It is found in association with autoimmune disorders such as Still's disease, rheumatoid arthritis, Wegener's granulomatosis, systemic lupus erythematosus, Reiter's disease and so on.

In phacoanaphytic endophthalmitis, lens proteins play role of autoantigens. Similarly, sympathetic ophthalmitis has been attributed to be an autoimmune reaction to uveal pigments, by some workers.

v. *HLA-associated uveitis:* Human leucocytic antigens (HLA) is the old name for the histocompatibility antigens. There are about 70 such antigens in human beings, on the basis of which an individual can be assigned to different HLA phenotypes. Recently, lot of stress is being laid on the role of HLA in uveitis, since a number of diseases associated with uveitis occur much more frequently in persons with certain specific HLA-phenotype. A few examples of HLA-associated diseases with uveitis are as follows:

- HLA-B27: Acute anterior uveitis associated with ankylosing spondylitis and also in Reiter's syndrome.
- HLA-B5: Uveitis in Behcet's disease.
- HLA-DR4 and DW15: Vogt Koyanagi Harada's disease.

3. *Toxic uveitis.* Toxins responsible for uveitis can be endotoxins, endocular toxins or exogenous toxins.

i. *Endotoxins* produced inside the body play a major role. These may be autotoxins or microbial toxins (produced by organisms involving the body tissues). Toxic uveitis seen in patients with acute pneumococcal or gonococcal conjunctivitis, and in patients with fungal corneal ulcer, is thought to be due to microbial toxins.

ii. *Endocular toxins* are produced from the ocular tissues. Uveitis seen in patients with blind eyes, long-standing retinal detachment and intraocular haemorrhages is said to be due to endocular toxins. Other examples are uveitis associated with intraocular tumours and phacotoxic uveitis.

iii. ***Exogenous toxins*** causing uveitis are irritant chemical substances of inorganic, animal or vegetative origin. Certain drugs producing uveitis (such as miotics and cytotoxic drugs) are other examples of exogenous toxins.

4. ***Traumatic uveitis.*** It is often seen in accidental or operative injuries to the uveal tissue. Different mechanisms which may produce uveitis following trauma include:

- Direct mechanical effects of trauma.
- Irritative effects of blood products after intraocular haemorrhage (haemophthalmitis).
- Microbial invasion.
- Chemical effects of retained intraocular foreign bodies; and
- Sympathetic ophthalmia in the other eye.

5. ***Uveitis associated with non-infective systemic diseases.*** Certain systemic diseases frequently complicated by uveitis include: sarocoidosis, collagen related diseases (polyarteritis nodosa (PAN), disseminated lupus erythematosus (DLE), rheumatic and rheumatoid arthritis), metabolic diseases (diabetes mellitus and gout), disease of the central nervous system (e.g., disseminated sclerosis) and diseases of skin (psoriasis, lichen planus, erythema nodosum, pemphigus and so on).

6. ***Idiopathic uveitis.*** It may be specific or non-specific.

i. ***Idiopathic specific uveitis entities*** include the conditions which have certain special characteristics of their own e.g., pars planitis, sympathetic ophthalmitis and Fuchs' hetero-chromic iridocyclitis.

ii. ***Nonspecific idiopathic uveitis entities*** include the condition which do not belong to any of the known etiological groups. About more than 25 percent cases of uveitis fall in this group.

PATHOLOGY OF UVEITIS

Inflammation of the uvea fundamentally has the same characteristics as any other tissue of the body, i.e., a vascular and a cellular response. However, due to extreme vascularity and looseness of the uveal tissue, the inflammatory responses are exaggerated and thus produces special results.

Pathologically, inflammations of the uveal tract may be divided into suppurative (purulent) and non-suppurative (non-purulent) varieties. Wood has further classified non-suppurative uveitis into a non-granulomatous and granulomatous types. Although morphologic description is still of some value, the rigid division of uveitis by Wood into these two categories has been questioned on both clinical and pathological grounds. Certain transitional forms of uveitis have also been recognised. Some of these (e.g., phacoanaphylactic endophthalmitis and sympathetic ophthalmia) showing pathological features of granulomatous uveitis are caused by hypersensitivity reactions. While uveitis due to tissue invasion by leptospirae presents the manifestation of non-granulomatous uveitis. Nonetheless, the classification is often useful in getting oriented towards the subject of uveitis, its workup and therapy. Therefore, it is worthwhile to describe the pathological features of these overlapping (both clinically and pathologically) conditions as distinct varieties.

1. ***Pathology of suppurative uveitis.*** Purulent inflammation of the uvea is usually a part of endophthalmitis or panophthalmitis occurring as a result of exogenous infection by pyogenic organisms which include *Staphylococcus*, *Streptococcus*, *Psuedomonas*, *Pneumococcus* and *Gonococcus*.

The pathological reaction is characterised by an outpouring of purulent exudate and infiltration by polymorphonuclear cells of uveal tissue, anterior chamber, posterior chamber and vitreous cavity. As a result, the whole uveal tissue is thickened and necrotic and the cavities of eye become filled with pus.

2. ***Pathology of non-granulomatous uveitis.*** Non-granulomatous uveitis may be an acute or chronic exudative inflammation of uveal tissue (predominantly iris and ciliary body), usually occurring either due to a physical and toxic insult to the tissue, or as a result of different hypersensitivity reactions.

The pathological alterations of the nongranulomatous reaction consists of marked dilatation and increased permeability of vessels, breakdown of blood aqueous barrier with an outpouring of fibrinous exudate and infiltration by lymphocytes, plasma cells and large macrophages of the uveal tissue, anterior chamber, posterior chamber and vitreous cavity. The inflammation is usually diffuse.

As a result of these pathological reactions iris becomes waterlogged, oedematous, muddy with blurring of crypts and furrows. As a consequence its mobility is reduced, pupil becomes small in size due to sphincter irritation and engorgement of radial vessels of iris. Exudates and lymphocytes poured into the anterior chamber result in aqueous flare and deposition of fine KPs at the back of cornea. Due to exudates in the posterior chamber, the posterior surface of iris adheres to the anterior capsule of lens leading to posterior synechiae formation. In severe inflammation, due to pouring of exudate from ciliary processes, behind the lens, an exudative membrane called *cyclitic membrane* may be formed.

After healing, pin-point areas of necrosis or atrophy are evident. Subsequent attacks lead to structural changes like atrophy, gliosis and fibrosis which cause adhesions, scarring and eventually destruction of eye.

3. *Pathology of granulomatous uveitis*. Granulomatous uveitis is a chronic inflammation of proliferative nature which typically occurs in response to anything which acts as an irritant foreign body, whether it be inorganic or organic material introduced from outside, a haemorrhage or necrotic tissue within the eye, or one of the certain specific organisms of non-pyogenic and relatively non-virulent character. The common organisms which excite this type of inflammation are those responsible for tuberculosis, leprosy, syphilis, brucellosis, leptospirosis, as well as most viral, mycotic, protozoal and helminthic infections. A typical granulomatous inflammation is also seen in sarcoidosis, sympathetic ophthalmitis and Vogt-Koyanagi-Harada's disease.

The pathological reaction in granulomatous uveitis is characterised by infiltration with lymphocytes, plasma cells and with mobilization and proliferation of large mononuclear cells which eventually become epithelioid and giant cells and aggregate into nodules. Iris nodules are usually formed near pupillary border (*Koeppe's nodules).* Similar nodular collection of the cells is deposited at the back of cornea in the form of mutton fat keratic precipitates and aqueous flare is minimal. Necrosis in the adjacent structures leads to a repairative process resulting in fibrosis and gliosis of the involved area.

NON-SUPPURATIVE UVEITIS

ANTERIOR UVEITIS (IRIDOCYCLITIS)

DEFINITION

(See page 146).

ETIOLOGY

(See page 146).

CLINICAL FEATURES

Though anterior uveitis, almost always present as a combined inflammation of iris and ciliary body (iridocyclitis), the reaction may be more marked in iris (iritis) or ciliary body (cyclitis). Clinically it may present as acute or chronic anterior uveitis. Main symptoms of *acute anterior uveitis* are pain, photophobia, redness, lacrimation and decreased vision. In *chronic uveitis,* however the eye may be white with minimal symptoms even in the presence of signs of severe inflammation.

Symptoms

1. *Pain.* It is dominating symptom of acute anterior uveitis. Patients usually complain of a dull aching throbbing sensation which is typically worse at night. The ocular pain is usually referred along the distribution of branches of fifth nerve, especially towards forehead and scalp.

2. *Redness.* It is due to circumcorneal congestion, which occurs as a result of active hyperaemia of anterior ciliary vessels due to the effect of toxins, histamine and histamine-like substances and axon reflex.

3. *Photophobia and blepharospasm* observed in patients with acute anterior uveitis is due to a reflex between sensory fibres of fifth nerve (which are irritated) and motor fibres of the seventh nerve, supplying the orbicularis oculi muscle.

4. *Lacrimation* occurs as a result of lacrimatory reflex mediated by fifth nerve (afferent) and secretomotor fibres of the seventh nerve (efferent).

5. *Defective vision* in a patient with iridocyclitis may vary from a slight blur in early phase to marked deterioration in late phase. Factors responsible for visual disturbance include induced myopia due to ciliary spasm, corneal haze (due to oedema and KPs), aqueous turbidity, pupillary block due to exudates, complicated cataract, vitreous haze, cyclitic membrane, associated macular oedema, papillitis or secondary glaucoma. One or more factors may contribute in different cases depending upon the severity and duration of the disease.

Signs

Slit lamp biomicroscopic examination is essential to elicit most of the signs of uveitis (Fig. 7.8).

I. *Lid oedema* usually mild, may accompany a severe attack of acute anterior uveitis.

II. *Circumcorneal congestion* is marked in acute iridocyclitis and minimal in chronic iridocyclitis. It must be differentiated from superficial congestion occurring in acute conjunctivitis (see page 154, Table 7.1).

III. *Corneal signs* include corneal oedema, KPs and posterior corneal opacities.

1. *Corneal oedema* is due to toxic endothelitis and raised intraocular pressure when present.

2. *Keratic precipitates (KPs)* are proteinaceous-cellular deposits occurring at the back of cornea.

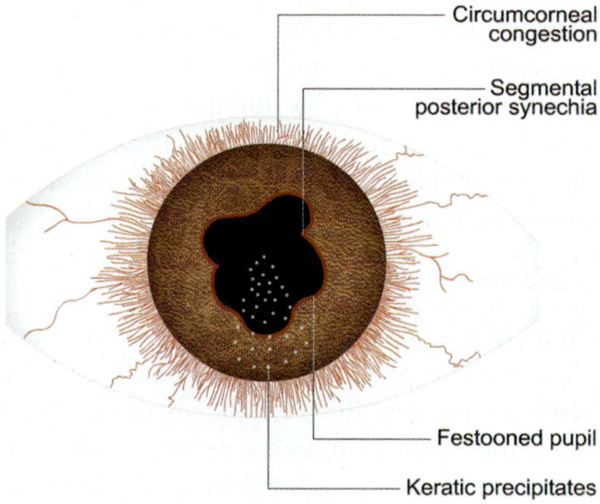

A

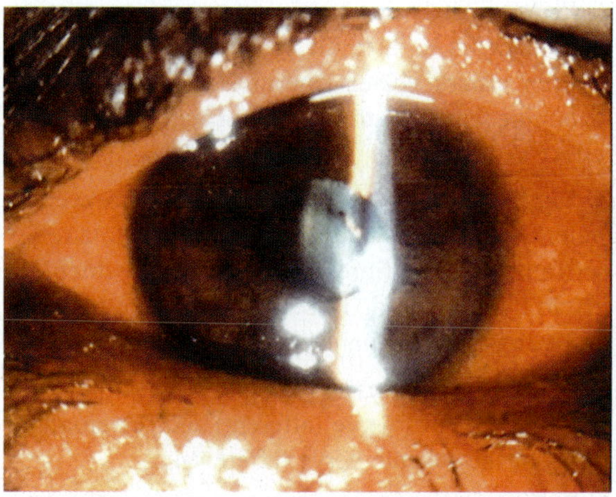

B

Fig. 7.8. Signs of anterior uveitis : A, diagrammatic depiction; B, clinical photograph of a patient with acute anterior uveitis.

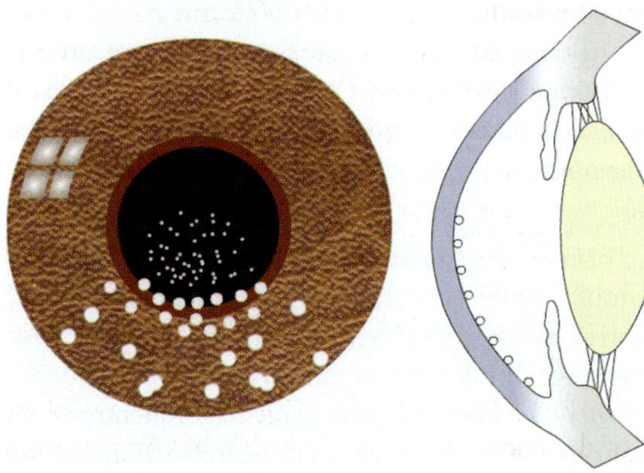

A

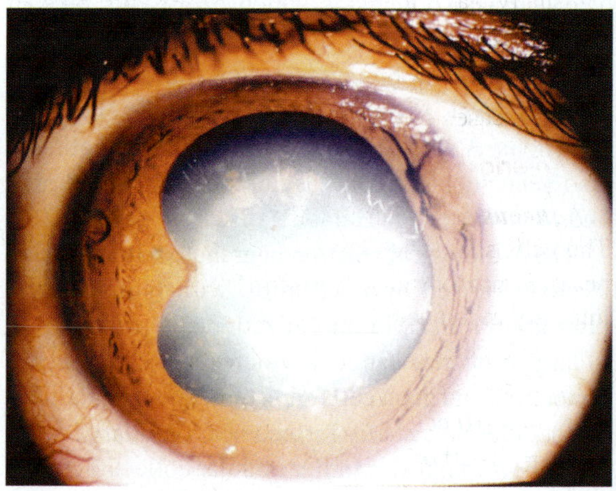

B

Fig. 7.9. Keratic precipitates (KPs); A, diagrammatic depiction; B, clinical photograph of a patient with granulomatous anterior uveitis showing mutton fat KPs and broad segmental synechiae.

Mostly, these are arranged in a triangular fashion occupying the centre and inferior part of cornea due to convection currents in the aqueous humour (Fig. 7.9). The composition and morphology of KPs varies with the severity, duration and type of uveitis. Following types of KPs may be seen:

i. *Mutton fat KPs.* These typically occur in granulomatous iridocyclitis and are composed of epithelioid cells and macrophages. They are large, thick, fluffy, lardaceous KPs, having a greasy or waxy appearance. Mutton fat KPs are usually a few (10 to 15) in number (Fig. 7.9B).
ii. *Small and medium KPs* (granular KPs). These are pathognomic of non-granulomatous uveitis and are composed of lymphocytes. These small, discrete, dirty white KPs are arranged irregularly at the back of cornea. Small KPs may be numerous.
iii. *Fine KPs*, also called as 'stellate' KPs, typically cover entire corneal endothelium and form the so called *endothelial dusting*. These are seen in Fuch's heterochromic iridocyclitis, herpetic iritis and CMV retinitis.
iv. *Old KPs.* These are sign of healed uveitis. Either of the above described KPs with healing process shrink, fade, become pigmented and irregular in shape (crenated margins). Old mutton fat KPs usually have a ground glass appearance due to hyalinization.

3. *Posterior corneal opacity* may be formed in long-standing cases of iridocyclitis.

IV. *Anterior chamber signs*

1.*Aqueous cells.* It is an early feature of iridocyclitis. The cells should be counted in an oblique slit-lamp beam, 3-mm long and 1-mm wide, with maximal light intensity and magnification, and graded as :

- – = 0 cells,
- ± = 1–5 cells,
- +1 = 6–10 cells,
- +2 = 11–20 cells,
- +3 = 21–50 cells, and
- +4 = over 50 cells

2. *Aqueous flare.* It is due to leakage of protein particles into the aqueous humour from damaged blood vessels. It is demonstrated on the slit lamp examination by a point beam of light passed obliquely to the plane of iris (Fig. 7.10). In the beam of light, protein particles are seen as suspended and moving dust particles. This is based on the 'Brownian movements' or 'Tyndal phenomenon'. Aqueous flare is usually marked in nongranulomatous and minimal in granulomatous uveitis. The flare is graded from 0 to +4. Grade :

- 0 = no aqueous flare.
- +1 = just detectable.
- +2 = moderate flare with clear iris details.
- +3 = marked flare (iris details not clear).
- +4 = intense flare (fixed coagulated aqueous with considerable fibrin).

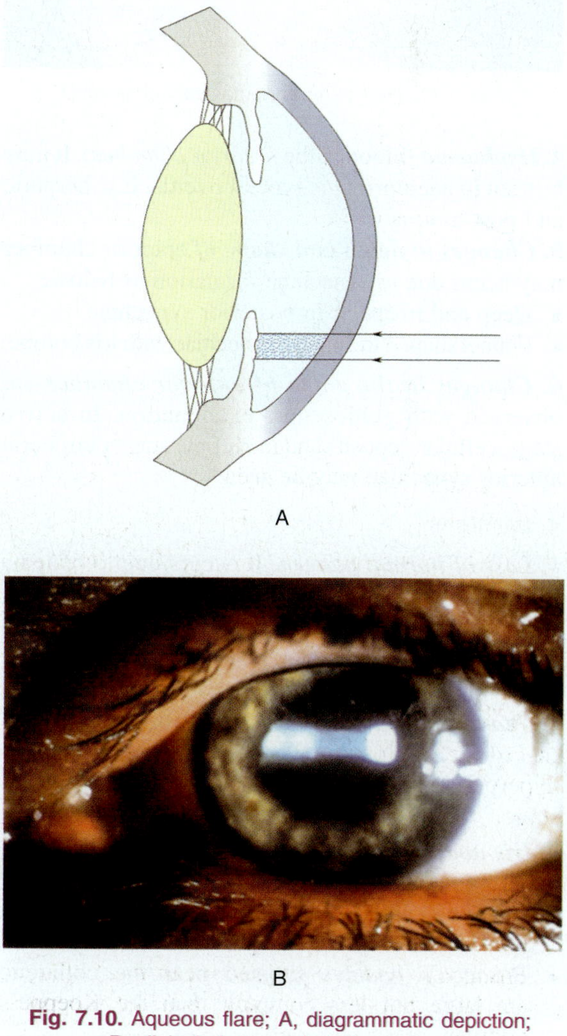

Fig. 7.10. Aqueous flare; A, diagrammatic depiction; B, clinical photograph of the patient.

3. ***Hypopyon.*** When exudates are heavy and thick, they settle down in lower part of the anterior chamber as hypopyon (sterile pus in the anterior chamber) (Fig. 7.11).

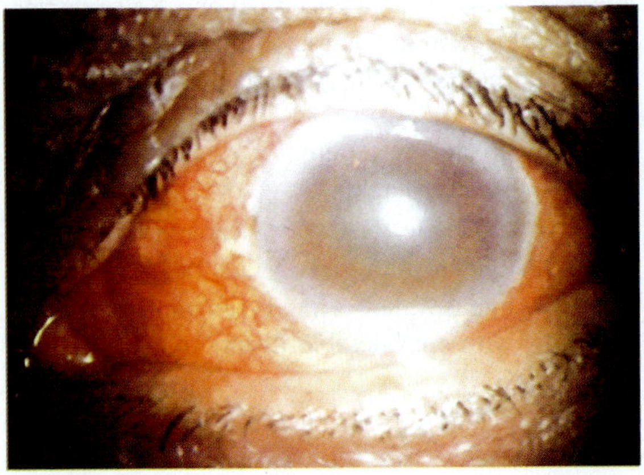

Fig. 7.11. Hypopyon in acute anterior uveitis.

4. ***Hyphaema*** (blood in the *anterior chamber*). It may be seen in haemorrhagic type of uveitis. E.g. herpetic and post traumatic.

5. ***Changes in depth and shape of*** anterior chamber may occur due to synechiae formation as below:

- Deep and irregular in posterior synechiae
- Funnel shaped in annular synechiae with iris bombe.

6. ***Changes in the angle of anterior chamber*** are observed with gonioscopic examination. In active stage, cellular deposits and in chronic stage peripheral anterior synechiae may be seen.

V. *Iris signs*

1. ***Loss of normal pattern.*** It occurs due to oedema and waterlogging of iris in active phase and due to atrophic changes in chronic phase. Iris atrophy is typically observed in Fuchs' heterochromic iridocyclitis.

2. ***Changes in iris colour.*** Iris usually becomes muddy in colour during active phase and may show hyperpigmented and depigmented areas in healed stage.

3. ***Iris nodules*** (Fig. 7.12). These occur typically in granulomatous uveitis.

- *Koeppe's nodules* are situated at the pupillary border and may initiate posterior synechia.
- *Busacca's nodules* situated near the collarette are large but less common than the Koeppe's nodules.

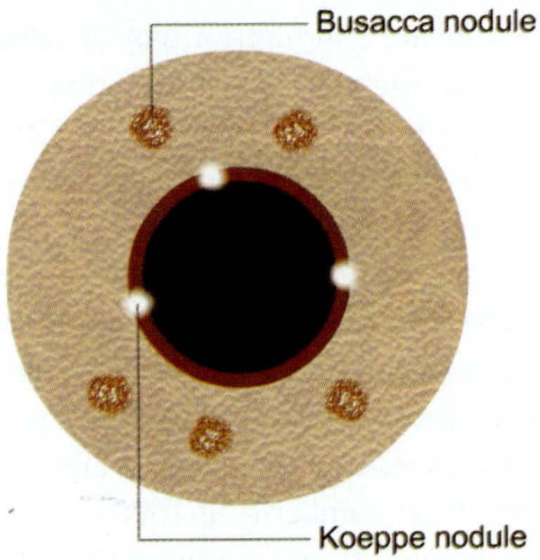

A

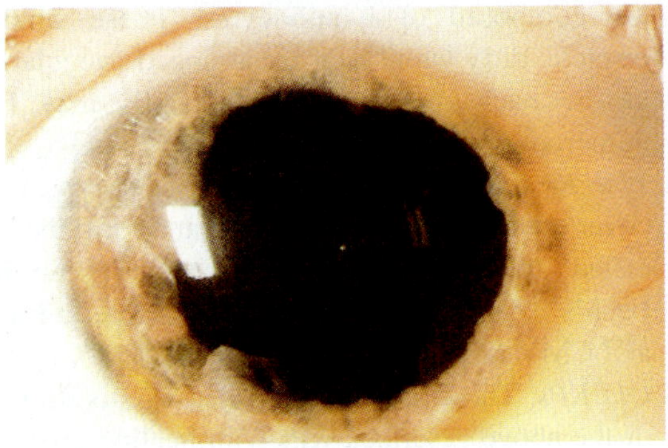

B

Fig. 7.12. Iris nodules: A, diagrammatic depiction; B, clinical photograph showing Koeppe's nodules at the pupillary margins in a patient with sarcoidosis.

4. ***Posterior synechiae.*** These are adhesions between the posterior surface of iris and anterior capsule of crystalline lens (or any other structure which may be artificial lens, after cataract, posterior capsule left after extracapsular cataract extraction) or anterior hyaloid face. These are formed due to organisation of the fibrin-rich exudates. Morphologically, posterior synechiae may be segmental, annular or total.

i. *Segmental posterior synechiae* refers to adhesions of iris to the lens at some points (Fig. 7.8).

ii. *Annular posterior synechiae* (ring synechiae) are 360° adhesions of pupillary margin to anterior capsule of lens. These prevent the circulation of aqueous humour from posterior chamber to anterior chamber (*seclusio pupillae*). Thus, the aqueous collects behind the iris and pushes it anteriorly (leading to *'iris-bombe'* formation)

(Fig. 7.13). This is usually followed by a rise in intraocular pressure.

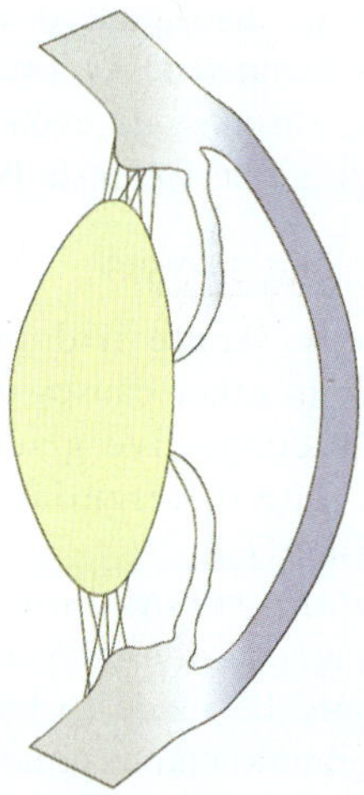

Fig. 7.13. Annular posterior synechiae.

iii. *Total posterior synechiae* due to plastering of total posterior surface of iris with the anterior capsule of lens are rarely formed in acute plastic type of uveitis. This results in deepening of anterior chamber (Fig. 7.14).

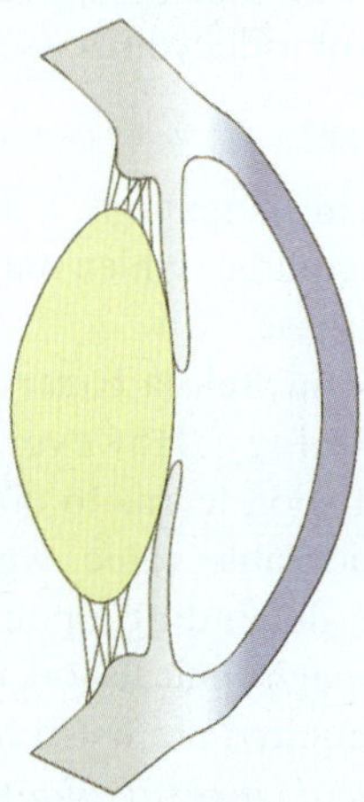

Fig. 7.14. Total posterior synechiae causing deep anterior chamber

5. ***Neovascularisation of iris*** (rubeosis iridis) develops in some eyes with chronic iridocyclitis and in Fuch's heterochromic iridocyclitis.

VI. *Pupillary signs*

1. ***Narrow pupil.*** It occurs in acute attack of iridocyclitis (Fig. 7.8B) due to irritation of sphincter pupillae by toxins. Iris oedema and engorged radial vessels of iris also contribute in making the pupil narrow.

2. ***Irregular pupil shape.*** It results from segmental posterior synechiae formation. Dilatation of pupil with mydriatics (e.g. atropine) at this stage results in *festooned pupil* (Fig. 7.8A and 7.15).

3. ***Ectropion pupillae*** (evertion of pupillary margin). It may develop due to contraction of fibrinous exudate on the anterior surface of the iris.

4. ***Pupillary reaction*** becomes sluggish or may even be absent due to oedema and hyperaemia of iris which hamper its movements.

5. ***Occlusio pupillae*** results when the pupil is completely occluded due to organisation of the exudates across the entire pupillary area.

VII. *Changes in the lens*

1. ***Pigment dispersal*** on the anterior capsule of lens is almost of universal occurrence in case of anterior uveitis.

2. ***Exudates*** may be deposited on the lens in cases with acute plastic iridocyclitis.

3. ***Complicated cataract*** may develop as a complication of persistent iridocyclitis. Typical features of a complicated cataract in early stage are '*polychromatic luster*' and '*bread-crumb*' appearance of the early posterior subcapsular opacities. In the presence of posterior synechiae, the complicated cataract progresses rapidly to maturity (Fig. 7.15).

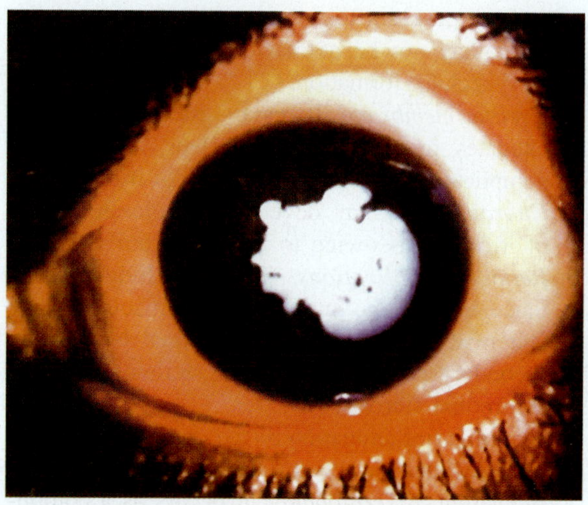

Fig. 7.15. Iridocyclitis with posterior synechiae, festooned pupil and complicated cataract.

VIII. *Changes in the vitreous and retina*

- *Exudates and inflammatory cells* may be seen in the anterior vitreous after an attack of acute iridocyclitis.
- *Cystoid macular edema* (CME) may occur, specially in chronic iridocyclitis.

IX. *Changes in the intraocular pressure.* IOP may be:

- Normal, or
- Increased (secondary glaucoma) or,
- Decreased (in acute iridocyclitis due to acute ciliary shock and in chronic, longstanding iridocyclitis due to atrophy of ciliary process ultimately leading to phthisis bulbi).

COMPLICATIONS AND SEQUELAE

1. *Complicated cataract.* It is a common complication of iridocyclitis as described above.
2. *Secondary glaucoma.* It may occur as an early or late complication of iridocyclitis.
   i. *Early glaucoma.* In active phase of the disease, presence of exudates and inflammatory cells in the anterior chamber may cause clogging of trabecular meshwork resulting in the decreased aqueous drainage and thus a rise in intraocular pressure (*hypertensive uveitis*).
   ii. *Late glaucoma in iridocyclitis* (post-inflammatory glaucoma) is the result of pupil block (seclusio pupillae due to ring synechiae formation, or occlusio pupillae due to organised exudates) not allowing the aqueous to flow from posterior to anterior chamber. There may or may not be associated peripheral anterior synechiae formation.
3. *Cyclitic membrane.* It results due to fibrosis of exudates present behind the lens. It is a late complication of acute plastic type of iridocyclitis.
4. *Choroiditis.* It may develop in prolonged cases of iridocyclitis owing to their continuity.
5. *Retinal complications.* These include cystoid macular oedema, macular scar, macular hole, epiretinal membrane, exudative retinal detachment, secondary periphlebitis retinae, retinal scars and sub-retinal fibrosis.
6. *Papillitis* (inflammation of the optic disc). It may be associated in severe cases of iridocyclitis.
7. *Band-shaped keratopathy.* It occurs as a complication of long-standing chronic uveitis (Fig. 5.17), especially in children having Still's disease.
8. *Phthisis bulbi.* It is the final stage end result of any form of chronic uveitis. In this condition, ciliary body is disorganised and so aqueous production is hampered. As a result of it the eye becomes soft, shrinks and eventually becomes a small atrophic globe (phthisis bulbi).

DIFFERENTIAL DIAGNOSIS

1. *Acute red eye.* Acute iridocyclitis must be differentiated from other causes of acute red eye, especially acute congestive glaucoma and acute conjunctivitis. The differentiating features are summarised in Table 7.1.

2. *Granulomatous versus non-granulomatous uveitis.* Once diagnosis of iridocyclitis is established, an attempt should be made to know whether the condition is of granulomatous or non-granulomatous type. The main clinical differences between the two are summarised in Table 7.2.

3. *Etiological differential diagnosis.* Efforts should also be made to distinguish between the different etiological varieties of iridocyclitis. This may be possible in some cases after thorough investigations and with a knowledge of special features of different clinical entities, which are described under the subject of 'special types of iridocyclitis' (see pages 160-167).

INVESTIGATIONS

Before ordering investigations, a thorough, systemic examination is required, which may provide clues to the underline disease.

Investigations include a battery of tests because of its varied etiology. However, an experienced ophthalmologist soon learns to order a few investigations of considerable value, which will differ in individual case depending upon the information gained from thorough clinical work up. A few common investigations required are listed here:

1. *Haematological investigations*
   - *TLC and DLC* to have a general information about inflammatory response of body.
   - *ESR* to ascertain existence of any chronic inflammatory condition in the body.
   - *Blood sugar levels* to rule out diabetes mellitus.
   - *Blood uric acid* in patients suspected of having gout.
   - *Serological tests* for syphilis, toxoplasmosis, and histoplasmosis.

Table 7.1. Distinguishing features between acute conjunctivitis, acute iridocyclitis and acute congestive glaucoma.

	Feature	*Acute conjunctivitis*	*Acute iridocyclitis*	*Acute congestive glaucoma*
1.	Onset	Gradual	Usually gradual	Sudden
2.	Pain	Mild discomfort	Moderate in eye and along the first division of trigeminal nerve	Severe in eye and the entire trigeminal area
3.	Discharge	Mucopurulent	Watery	Watery
4.	Coloured halos	May be present	Absent	Present
5.	Vision	Good	Slightly impaired	Markedly impaired
6.	Congestion	Superficial conjunctival	Deep ciliary	Deep ciliary
7.	Tenderness	Absent	Marked	Marked
8.	Pupil	Normal	Small and irregular	Large and vertically oval
9.	Media	Clear	Hazy due to KPs, aqueous flare and pupillary exudates	Hazy due to edematous cornea
10.	Anterior chamber	Normal	May be deep	Very shallow
11.	Iris	Normal	Muddy	Oedematous
12.	Intraocular pressure	Normal	Usually normal	Raised
13.	Constitutional symptoms	Absent	Little	Prostration and vomiting

Table 7.2. Differences between granulomatous and non-granulomatous uveitis.

	Feature	*Granulomatous*	*Non-granulomatous*
1.	Onset	Insidious	Acute
2.	Pain	Minimal	Marked
3.	Photophobia	Slight	Marked
4.	Ciliary congestion	Minimal	Marked
5.	Keratic precipitates (KPs)	Mutton fat	Small
6.	Aqueous flare	Mild	Marked
7.	Iris nodules	Usually present	Absent
8.	Posterior synechiae	Thick and broad based	Thin and tenuous
9.	Fundus	Nodular lesions	Diffuse involvement

- *Tests for* antinuclear antibodies, Rh factor, LE cells, C-reactive proteins and anti-streptolysin-0, ACE (for sarcoidosis).

2. *Urine examination* for WBCs, pus cells, RBCs and culture to rule out urinary tract infections.
3. *Stool examination* for cyst and ova to rule out parasitic infestations.
4. *Radiological investigations* include:
   - *X-rays* of chest, paranasal sinuses, sacroiliac joints and lumbar spine.
   - *CT scan* high resolution. CT scan of thorax should be considered for suspected sarcoidosis cases.
   - *MRI scan* of head for suspected sarcoidosis, demyelination and lymphomas.
5. *Skin tests.* These include tuberculin test, Kveim's test and toxoplasmin test.

TREATMENT OF IRIDOCYCLITIS

I. Non-specific treatment

(a) Local therapy

1. ***Cycloplegic drugs.*** These are very useful and most effective during acute phase of iridocyclitis. Commonly used drug is 1 percent *atropine sulfate* eye ointment or drops instilled 2-3 times a day. In case of atropine allergy, other cycloplegics like 2 percent *homatropine* or 1 percent *cyclopentolate* eyedrops may be instilled 3-4 times a day. Alternatively for more powerful cycloplegic effect a subconjunctival injection of 0.25 ml *mydricain* (a mixture of atropine, adrenaline and procaine) should be given. The cycloplegics should be continued for at least 2-3 weeks after the eye becomes quiet, otherwise relapse may occur.

Mode of action. In iridocyclitis, atropine (i) gives comfort and rest to the eye by relieving spasm of iris sphincter and ciliary muscle, (ii) prevents the formation of synechiae and may break the already formed synechiae, (iii) reduces exudation by decreasing hyperaemia and vascular permeability and (iv) increases the blood supply to anterior uvea by relieving pressure on the anterior ciliary arteries. As a result more antibodies reach the target tissues and more toxins are absorbed.

2. *Corticosteroids*, administered locally, are very effective in cases of iridocyclitis. They reduce inflammation by their anti-inflammatory effect; being anti-allergic, are of special use in allergic type of uveitis; and due to their antifibrotic activity, they reduce fibrosis and thus prevent disorganisation and destruction of the tissues. Commonly used steroidal preparations contain dexamethasone, betamethasone, hydrocortisone or prednisolone (see page 456).

Route of administration: Locally, steroids are used as (i) eye drops 4-6 times a day, (ii) eye ointment at bed time, and (iii) Anterior sub-Tenon injection is given in severe cases.

3. *Broad spectrum antibiotic drops,* though of no use in iridocyclitis, are usually prescribed with topical steroid preparations to provide an umbrella cover for them.

(b) *Systemic therapy*

1. *Corticosteroids.* When administered systemically they have a definite role in non-granulomatous iridocyclitis, where inflammation, most of the times, is due to antigen-antibody reaction. Even in other types of uveitis, the systemic steroids are helpful due to their potent non-specific anti-inflammatory and antifibrotic effects. Systemic corticosteroids are usually indicated in intractable anterior uveitis resistant to topical therapy.

Dosage schedules. A wide variety of steroids are available. Usually, treatment is started with high doses of prednisolone (60-100 mg) or equivalent quantities of other steroids (dexamethasone or betamethasone). *Daily therapy regime* is preferred for marked inflammatory activity for at least 2 weeks. In the absence of acute disease, *alternate day therapy regime* should be chosen. The dose of steroids is decreased by a week's interval and tapered completely in about 6-8 weeks in both the regimes.

Note: Steroids (both topical and systemic) may cause many ocular (e.g., steroid-induced glaucoma and cataract) and systemic side-effects. Hence, an eagle's eye watchfulness is required for it.

2. *Non-steroidal anti-inflammatory drugs* (NSAIDS) such as aspirin can be used where steroids are contraindicated. Phenylbutazone and oxyphenbutazone are potent anti-inflammatory drugs of particular value in uveitis associated with rheumatoid disease. Naproxen is useful in patients with ankylosing spondylitis.

3. *Immunosuppressive drugs.* These should be used only in desperate and extremely serious cases of uveitis, in which vigorous use of steroids have failed to resolve the inflammation and there is an imminent danger of blindness. These drugs are dangerous and should be used with great caution in the supervision of a haematologist and an oncologist. These drugs are specially useful in severe cases of Behcet's syndrome, sympathetic ophthalmia, pars planitis and VKH syndrome. A few available cytotoxic immunosuppressive drugs include cyclo-phosphamide, chlorambucil, azathioprine and methotrexate. Cyclosporin is a powerful anti-T-cell immunosuppressive drug which is effective in cases resistant to cytotoxic immunosuppressive agents, but it is a highly renal toxic drug.

4. *Azithromycin or tetracycline or erythromycin* should be considered to treat chlamydial infection in patients and their sexual partners in Reiter's syndrome having urethritis and iritis.

(c) *Physical measures*

1. *Hot fomentation.* It is very soothing, diminishes pain and increases circulation, and thus reduces the venous stasis. As a result more antibodies are brought and toxins are drained. Hot fomentation can be done by dry heat or wet heat.

2. *Dark goggles.* These give a feeling of comfort, especially when used in sunlight, by reducing photophobia, lacrimation and blepharospasm.

II. Specific treatment of the cause

The non-specific treatment described above is very effective and usually eats away the uveal inflammation, in most of the cases, but it does not cure the disease, resulting in relapses. Therefore, all possible efforts should be made to find out and treat the underlying cause. Unfortunately, in spite of the advanced diagnostic tests, still it is not possible to ascertain the cause in a large number of cases.

So, a full course of antitubercular drugs for underlying Koch's disease, adequate treatment for syphilis, toxoplasmosis etc., when detected should be carried out. When no cause is ascertained, a full course of broad spectrum antibiotics may be helpful by eradicating some masked focus of infection in patients with non-granulomatous uveitis.

III. Treatment of complications

1. *Inflammatory glaucoma* (hypertensive uveitis). In such cases, drugs to lower intraocular pressure such as 0.5 percent timolol maleate eyedrops twice a day and tablet acetazolamide (250 mg thrice a day) should be added, over and above the usual treatment of iridocyclitis. Pilocarpine and latanoprost eye drops are contraindicated in inflammatory glaucoma.

2. *Post-inflammatory glaucoma* due to ring synechiae is treated by laser iridotomy. Surgical iridectomy may be done when laser is not available. However, surgery should be performed in a quiet eye under high doses of corticosteroids.

3. *Complicated cataract* requires lens extraction with guarded prognosis in spite of all precautions. The presence of fresh KPs is considered a contraindication for intraocular surgery.

4. *Retinal detachment* of exudative type usually settles itself if uveitis is treated aggressively. A tractional detachment requires vitrectomy and management of complicated retinal detachment, with poor visual prognosis.

5. *Phthisis bulbi* especially when painful, requires removal by enucleation operation.

INTERMEDIATE UVEITIS

Intermediate uveitis refers to inflammation involving pars plana ciliaris, peripheral retina, choroid and vitreous base.

Epidemiology

- Accounts for 10% of all cases of uveitis and 20% of cases of uveitis in children,
- Bilateral in 80% of cases,
- Males and females are equally affected,
- Age: onset typically in 2nd and 4th decade (bimodal)

Etiology

- *Idiopathic* in about 85% cases. Immunogenic predisposition is reported with a positive correlation with HLA-DR2.
- *Known causes* (15% cases) include tuberculosis, syphilis, sarcoidosis, and Lyme disease.

Clinical features

Symptoms

- *Asymptomatic* in many cases,
- *Floaters of insidious* onset is common presentation,
- *Blurring of vision* and decreased vision may occur later,
- *Pain, photophobia and redness* are conspicuously absent.

Signs

Anterior segment signs. On cursory examination eye looks white and quiet. Anterior segment may or may not show signs of minimal activity in the form of:

- Low grade flare and cells,
- Few KPs due to spill-over anterior uveitis,
- Lens may show complicated cataract in late stages.

Posterior segment signs pathognomic of intermediate uveitis are:

- *Common vitreous signs* include: vitreous cells (+1 to +4), anterior vitreous condensation and snowball or cotton ball opacities (Ant's eggs).
- *Snowbanking* i.e. yellowish white exudates (posterior hypopyon) and collagen bands over the pars plana with or without associated peripheral retinal periphlebits form the hallmark of intermediate uveitis. These are best seen with indirect ophthalmoscopy and Goldman three mirror examination.
- *Severe vitreous opacification* obscuring retina and even presenting as leucocoria may occur rarely.

Course, prognosis and complications

Course and prognosis. Relatively good prognosis if well treated. Course is usually chronic with three distinct patterns:

- Single, mild self limiting episode (10%) cases,
- Prolonged course without exacerbations (60% cases)
- Chronic smoldering course with multiple subacute exacerbations (30% cases)

Complications include: Complicated cataract (42%), Cystoid macular oedema (28%), band keratopathy, secondary glaucoma, vitreous haemorrhage and tractional retinal detachment.

Treatment

Modified 4 step protocol of Kaplan is as below:

Step 1: Periocular and systemic steroids. Topical steroids are not of much use. *Posterior sub-tenon injection* of triamcinolone 40mg/3 weeks × 3 injections are indicated initially. *Systemic steroids* are given in unresponsive cases.

Step 2: Immunosuppressive drugs such as cyclosporine, azathioprime, methotrexate or cyclophosphamide should be given next with careful monitoring of effects and potential side effects.

Step 3: Cryotherapy or indirect laser photocoagulation should be tried in cases with snowbanking.

Step 4: Pars-plana vitrectomy is indicated in severe cases and when step 3 measures fail. It helps by removing inflammatory debris, antigenic load and possible traction on macula. Its role in tractional RD is unequivocal.

POSTERIOR UVEITIS

Posterior uveitis refers to inflammation of the choroid (*choroiditis*). Since the outer layers of retina are in close contact with the choroid and also depend on it for the nourishment, the choroidal inflammation almost always involves the adjoining retina, and the resultant lesion is called *chorioretinitis.*

Etiology and pathology

These are same as described for uveitis in general considerations.

Clinical types

Non-suppurative choroiditis may be non-granulomatous or granulomatous (more common). Non-suppurative choroidal inflammation is characterised by exudation and cellular infiltration, resulting in a greyish white lesion hiding the normal reddish hue of choroidal vessels.

Non-suppurative choroiditis is usually bilateral and morphologically (depending upon the number and location of lesions) can be classified into diffuse, disseminated and circumscribed (localised) choroiditis.

1. *Diffuse choroiditis.* It refers to large spreading lesions involving most of the choroidal tissue. It is usually tubercular or syphilitic in origin.

2. *Disseminated choroiditis*. It is characterised by multiple but small areas of inflammation scattered over the greater part of choroid (Fig. 7.16). Such a condition may be due to syphilis or tuberculosis, but in many cases the cause is obscure.

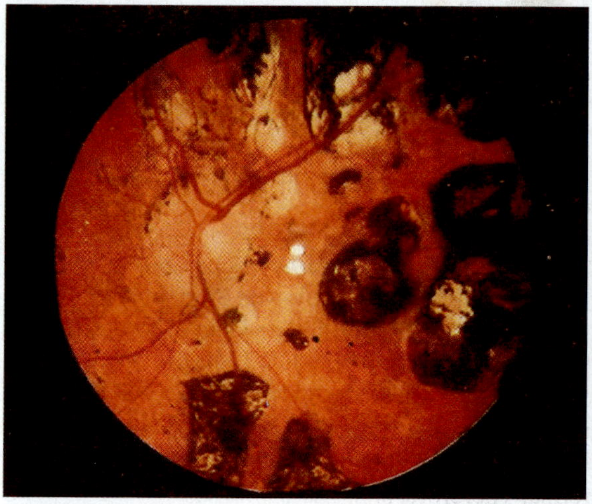

Fig. 7.16. Healed lesions of disseminated chorioretinitis.

3. *Circumscribed/localised/focal choroiditis.* It is characterised by a single patch or a few small patches of inflammation localised in a particular area. Such patches of choroiditis are described by a name depending upon the location of the lesion which are as follows:

i. *Central choroiditis.* As the name indicates it involves the macular area and may occur either alone (Fig. 7.17) or in combination with disseminated choroiditis. A typical patch of central choroiditis may occur in toxoplasmosis, histoplasmosis, tuberculosis, syphilis and rarely due to visceral larva migrans.

ii. *Juxtacaecal or juxtapapillary choroiditis.* It is the name given to a patch of choroiditis involving an area adjoining the optic disc. One example is *Jensen's choroiditis* which typically occurs in young persons.

iii. *Anterior peripheral choroiditis.* It implies occurrence of multiple small patches of choroiditis (similar to disseminated choroiditis) only in the peripheral part of choroid (anterior to equator). Such lesions are often syphilitic in origin.

iv. *Equatorial choroiditis.* It involves the choroid in the equatorial region only.

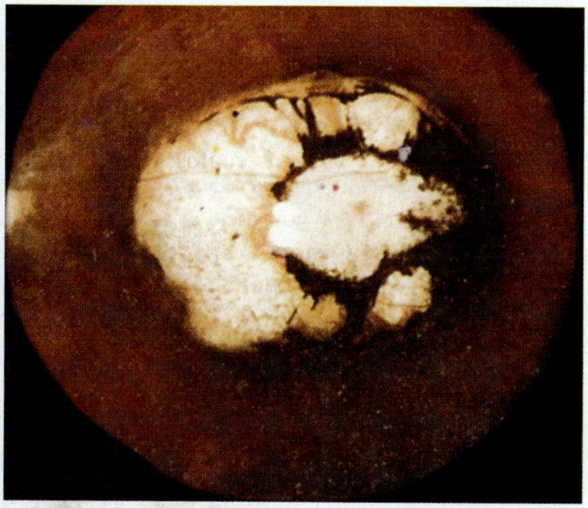

Fig. 7.17. A healed patch of central chorioretinitis.

Clinical picture

Symptoms. Choroiditis is a painless condition, usually characterised by visual symptoms due to associated vitreous haze and involvement of the retina. Therefore, small patches situated in periphery may be symptomless and are usually discovered as healed patches on routine fundus examination. On the contrary, a central patch produces marked symptoms which draw immediate attention. Various visual symptoms experienced by a patient of choroiditis are summarised below:

1. *Defective vision.* It is usually mild due to vitreous haze, but may be severe as in central choroiditis.
2. *Photopsia.* It is a subjective sensation of flashes of light resulting due to irritation of rods and cones.
3. *Black spots floating in front of the eyes.* It is a very common complaint of such patients. They occur due to large exudative clumps in the vitreous.
4. *Metamorphopsia.* Herein, patients perceive distorted images of the object. This results due to alteration in the retinal contour caused by a raised patch of choroiditis.
5. *Micropsia* which results due to separation of visual cells is a common complaint. In this the objects appear smaller than they are.
6. *Macropsia,* i.e., perception of the objects larger than they are, may occur due to crowding together of rods and cones.
7. *Positive scotoma,* i.e., perception of a fixed large spot in the field of vision, corresponding to the lesion may be noted by many patients.

Signs. Usually there are no external signs and the eye looks quiet. However, fine KPs may be seen on biomicroscopy due to associated cyclitis. Fundus examination may reveal following signs:

1. *Vitreous opacities* due to choroiditis are usually present in its middle or posterior part. These may be fine, coarse, stringy or snowball opacities.
2. *Features of a patch of choroiditis.*
   i. *Active patch of choriditis,* looks as a pale-yellow or dirty white raised area with ill-defined edges. This results due to exudation and cellular infiltration of the choroid which hide the choroidal vessels. The lesion is typically deeper to the retinal vessels. The overlying retina is often cloudy and oedematous.
   ii. *Healed patch of choriditis,* when active inflammation subsides, becomes more sharply defined and delineated from the rest of the normal area due to atrophy of choroidal tissue. The involved area shows white sclera below the atrophic choroid and black pigmented clumps at the periphery of the lesion (Figs. 7.16 and 7.17). A healed patch of chorioretinitis must be differentiated from the degenerative conditions such as pathological myopia and retinitis pigmentosa.

Complications

These include extension of the inflammation to anterior uvea, complicated cataract, vitreous degeneration, macular oedema, secondary periphlebitis retinae and retinal detachment.

Treatment

It is broadly on the lines of anterior uveitis.

1. *Non-specific therapy* consists of periocular and systemic corticosteroids. Posterior sub-tenon injections of depot corticosteroids are effective in checking the acute phase of posterior uveitis.

- Rarely, *immunosuppresive* agents may be required to check the inflammation.

2. *Specific treatment* is required for the causative disease such as toxoplasmosis, toxocariasis, tuberculosis, syphilis, etc.

SPECIFIC CLINICO-ETIOLOGICAL TYPES OF NON-SUPPURATIVE UVEITIS

The manifold forms of uveitis have been classified under various headings. Since the classical description of non-suppurative uveitis by Wood (1947) into two main groups *non-granulomatous* and *granulomatous,* most of the uveitis patients have been categorized according to their gross objective similarities. In spite of the many sophisticated methods of investigations, even today, the cause in many clinical conditions is disputed and in others it is unknown. However, with the background of present update knowledge, to some extent, it has been possible to assign a patient with uveitis to a particular group based either on the etiological or typical clinical presentation of the disease. Detailed description of each such clinical entity is beyond the scope of this chapter. However, classification and salient features of some 'specific clinico-etiological' types of uveitis are described here:

Classification

I. *Uveitis associated with chronic systemic bacterial infections:*
   1. Tubercular uveitis
   2. Syphilitic uveitis
   3. Leprotic uveitis

II. *Uveitis associated with non-infectious systemic diseases*
   1. Uveitis in sarcoidosis
   2. Behcet's disease.

III. *Uveitis associated with arthritis*
   1. Uveitis with Ankylosing spondylitis
   2. Reiter's syndrome
   3. Still's disease

IV. *Parasitic uveitis*
   1. Toxoplasmosis
   2. Toxocariasis
   3. Onchocerciasis
   4. Amoebiasis

V. *Fungal uveitis*
   1. Presumed ocular histoplasmosis syndrome
   2. Candidiasis

VI. *Viral uveitis*
   1. Herpes simplex uveitis
   2. Herpes zoster uveitis
   3. Acquired cytomegalovirus uveitis
   4. Uveitis in acquired immune deficiency syndrome (AIDS)

VII. *Lens induced uveitis*
   1. Phacotoxic uveitis
   2. Phacoanaphylactic endophthalmitis

VIII. *Traumatic uveitis*

IX. *Uveitis associated with malignant intraocular tumours*

X. *Idiopathic specific uveitis syndromes*
   1. Fuchs' uveitis syndrome
   2. Intermediate uveitis (see page 157)
   3. Sympathetic ophthalmitis (see page 441)
   4. Glaucomatocyclitic crisis.
   5. Vogt-Koyanagi-Harada's syndrome.
   6. Bird shot retinochoroidopathy.
   7. Acute multifocal placoid pigment epitheliopathy (AMPPE)
   8. Serpiginous choroidopathy.

I. UVEITIS IN CHRONIC SYSTEMIC BACTERIAL INFECTIONS

TUBERCULAR UVEITIS

Tuberculosis is a chronic granulomatous infection caused by bovine or human tubercle bacilli. It may cause both anterior and posterior uveitis. At one time very common, it is now becoming a rare cause. It accounts for 1% of uveitis in developed countries. However, in developing countries it still continues to be a common cause of uveitis.

CLINICAL PRESENTATIONS

1. *Tubercular anterior uveitis*. It may occur as acute non-granulomatous iridocyclitis or granulomatous anterior uveitis which in turn may be in the form of miliary tubercular iritis or conglomerate granuloma (solitary tuberculoma).

2. *Tubercular posterior uveitis*. It may occur as:

i. *Multiple miliary tubercles* in the choroid which appear as round yellow white nodules one-sixth to two and half disc diameter in size. These are usually associated with tubercular meningitis.

ii. *Diffuse or disseminated choroiditis* in chronic tuberculosis.

iii. *Choroidal granuloma* may occur rarely as a solitary lesion.

3. *Vasculitis*. (Eales' disease) (see page 268).

***Diagnosis*.** There is no specific clinical finding in tubercular uveitis. Diagnosis is made from positive skin test, associated findings of systemic tuberculosis, intractable uveitis unresponsive to steroid therapy, a positive response to isoniazid test (a dramatic response of iritis to isoniazid 300 mg OD for 3 weeks).

***Treatment*.** In addition to usual treatment of uveitis, chemotherapy with rifampicin and isoniazid should be given for 12 months. Systemic corticosteroids should be deferred.

ACQUIRED SYPHILITIC UVEITIS

Acquired syphilis is a chronic venereal infection caused by *Treponema pallidum* (spirochaete). It affects both the anterior and posterior uvea.

1. *Syphilitic anterior uveitis*. It may occur as acute plastic iritis or granulomatous iritis. *Acute plastic iritis* typically occurs in the secondary stage of syphilis and also as a Herxheimer reaction 24-48 hours after therapeutic dose of the penicillin.

Gummatous anterior uveitis occurs late in the secondary or rarely during the tertiary stage of syphilis. It is characterised by formation of yellowish red highly vascularised multiple nodules arranged near the pupillary border or ciliary border of iris.

2. *Syphilitic posterior uveitis*. It may occur as disseminated, peripheral or diffuse choroiditis.

***Diagnosis*.** Once suspected clinically, diagnosis is confirmed by FTA-ABS (fluorescent treponemal antibody absorption) blood test, which is specific and more sensitive than TPI (treponema pallidum immobilisation) test and VDRL tests.

***Treatment*.** In addition to local therapy of the uveitis, patient should be treated by systemic penicillin or other antisyphilitic drugs.

LEPROTIC UVEITIS

Leprosy (Hansen's disease) is caused by *Mycobacterium leprae* which is an acid-fast bacillus. The disease occurs in two principal forms: lepromatous and tuberculoid. Leprosy involves predominantly anterior uvea; more commonly in lepromatous than in the tuberculoid form of disease.

***Clinical types*.** Lepromatous uveitis may occur as acute iritis (non-granulomatous) or chronic iritis (granulomatous).

1. *Acute iritis.* It is caused by antigen-antibody deposition and is characterised by severe exudative reaction.
2. *Chronic granulomatous iritis.* It occurs due to direct organismal invasion and is characterised by presence of small glistening 'iris pearls' near the pupillary margin in a necklace form; small pearls enlarge and coalesce to form large pearls. Rarely, a nodular lepromata may be seen.

***Treatment*.** Besides usual local therapy of iridocyclitis antileprotic treatment with Dapsone 50-100 mg daily or other drugs should also be instituted.

II. UVEITIS IN NON-INFECTIOUS SYSTEMIC DISEASES

UVEITIS IN SARCOIDOSIS

Sarcoidosis is a granulomatous multi-system disease of unknown etiology, characterised by formation of non-caseating epithelioid cell granuloma in the affected tissue. The disease typically affects young adults (20-50 years), being more common in females than males, and more common in those of African heritage than Caucasians. It frequently presents with bilateral hilar lymphadenopathy, pulmonary infiltration, skin and ocular lesions.

Ocular lesions

Ocular lesions, occur in 20-50% patients with sarcoidosis and include sarcoid uveitis, conjunctival lesions and lacrimal gland.

I. *Sarcoid uveitis* accounts for 2% cases and may be anterior, intermediate, posterior or panuveitis.

1. *Anterior uveitis:* Typically presents as granulomatous iridocyclitis characterized by iris nodules, large mutton fat KPs (in a triangular distribution), anterior chamber cells flare, and posterior synechiae.

2. *Intermediate uveitis* is characterized by vitreous cells, snowball opacities and snowbanking.

3. *Posterior uveitis* lesions include choroidal and retinal granulomas, cystoid macular edema, periphlebitis retinae with sheathing, appearing as candle wax droppings. Peripheral multifocal chorioretinitis characterised by small, punched out atrophic spots, are highly suggestive of sarcoidosis.

Uveoparotid fever (Heerfordt's syndrome). It is characterised by bilateral granulomatous pan-uveitis, painful enlargement of parotid glands, cranial nerve palsies, skin rashes, fever and malaise.

Complications of sarcoid uveitis include complicated cataract , inflammatory glaucoma and cystoid macular edema.

II. *Other ocular lesions of sarcoidosis* include:

1. *Conjunctival lesions* include sarcoid nodules , and keratoconjunctivitis sicca.
2. *Lacrimal glands* may be enlarged. When associated with diffuse swelling of salivary glands, constitute the so called Mickulicz's syndrome.

Diagnosis and treatment

Diagnosis. Once suspected clinically, it is supported by positive Kveim test, abnormal X-ray chest (in 90 percent cases) and raised levels of serum angiotensin converting enzyme (ACE). *Confirmation* of the disease is made by histological proof from biopsy of the conjunctival nodule, skin lesions or enlarged lymph node.

Treatment of sarcoid uveitis is on general lines (see page 155). In short, topical, periocular and systemic steroids constitute the treatment of sarcoid uveitis, depending upon the severity.

BEHCET'S DISEASE

It is an idiopathic multisystem disease characterised by recurrent, non-granulomatous uveitis, aphthous ulceration, genital ulcerations and erythema multiforme.

Etiology. It is still unknown; the basic lesion is an obliterative vasculitis probably caused by circulating immune complexes. The disease typically affects the young men who are positive for HLA-B51.

Clinical features. *Uveitis seen in Behcet's disease* is typically bilateral, acute recurrent iridocyclitis associated with hypopyon. It may also be associated with posterior uveitis, vitritis, periphlebitis retinae and retinitis in the form of white necrotic infiltrates.

Treatment. No satisfactory treatment is available, and thus the disease has got comparatively poor visual prognosis.

- *Corticosteroids* may be helpful initially but ultimate response is poor.
- *Immunosupressive drugs* such as methotrexate, azathioprene and cyclosporin are needed in resistant cases and for an acute flare.

III. UVEITIS IN ARTHRITIS

UVEITIS WITH ANKYLOSING SPONDYLITIS

Ankylosing spondylitis is an idiopathic chronic inflammatory arthritis, usually involving the sacroiliac and posterior inter-vertebral joints. The disease affects young males (20-40 years) who are positive for HLA-B27. About 30 to 35 percent patients with ankylosing spondylitis develop uveitis.

Clinical features. Uveitis associated with ankylosing spondylitis is characteristically an acute, recurrent, non-granulomatous type of iridocyclitis. The disease usually affects one eye at a time.

Treatment. It is on the lines of usual treatment of anterior uveitis (see page 155). Long-term aspirin or indomethacin may decrease the recurrences.

REITER'S SYNDROME

It is characterised by a triad of urethritis, arthritis and conjunctivitis with or without iridocyclitis.

Etiology. It is not known exactly. The syndrome typically involves young males who are positive for HLA-B27. The disease occurs in three forms: postvenereal due to non-gonococcal arthritis, postdysenteric and articular form.

Ocular features. These include: (i) Acute mucopurulent conjunctivitis which may be associated with superifical punctate keratitis. (ii) Acute non-granulomatous type of iridocyclitis occurs in 20-30 percent cases of Reiter's syndrome.

Treatment. The iridocyclitis responds well to usual treatment (see page 155). A course of systemic tetracycline 250 mg QID for 10 days may be useful in post-venereal form suspected of being caused by Chlamydia infection.

JUVENILE IDIOPATHIC ARTHRITIS

Juvenile idiopathic arthritis (JIA) is a chronic inflammatory arthritis involving multiple joints (knee, elbow, ankle and interphalangeal joints) in children below the age of 16 years. The disease is also referred as *Juvenile rheumatoid arthritis,* though the patients are sero-negative for rheumatoid factor. In 30 percent cases, polyarthritis is associated with hepatosplenomegaly and other systemic features, and the condition is labelled as *Still's disease.*

Anterior uveitis associated with JIA is a bilateral (70%), chronic non-granulomatous disease, affecting female children more than the male (4:1). It usually develops before the age of 6 years. Nearly half of the patients are positive for HLA-DW5 and 75 percent are positive for antinuclear antibodies (ANA). The onset of uveitis is asymptomatic and the eye is white even in the presence of severe uveitis. Therefore, slit-lamp examination is mandatory in children suffering from JIA.

Complications like posterior synechiae, complicated cataract and band-shaped keratopathy are fairly common.

Treatment is on the usual lines (see page 155).

IV. PARASITIC UVEITIS

TOXOPLASMOSIS

It is a protozoan infestation caused by *Toxoplasma gondii,* derived from cats (definitive host). Humans and other animals (cattle, sheep and pigs) are intermediate hosts. The disease primarily affects central nervous system (brain and retina). Systemic lesions are more marked in immunocompromised patients (e.g. HIV+ patients) as compared to immunocompetent patients. Toxoplasmosis is the most common cause of posterior uveitis and accounts for approximately 90% of focal necrotizing retinitis. Systemic toxoplasmosis occurs in humans in three forms: congenital, acquired and recurrent.

1. *Congenital toxoplasmosis.* It is much more common than the acquired form, and the infestation is acquired by the foetus through transplacental route from the mother contracting acute infestation during pregnancy. When pregnant females catch disease, about 49 percent infants are born with the disease which may be active or inactive at birth.

The characteristic *triad of congenital toxoplasmosis* includes: convulsions, chorio-retinitis and intracranial calcification. In active stage the typical lesion is *necrotic granulomatous retinochoroiditis* involving the macular region associated with marked vitritis. Most of the infants are born with inactive disease, characterised by bilateral healed punched out heavily pigmented chorioretinal scars in the macular area (Fig. 7.17), which is usually discovered when the child is brought for defective vision or squint check up.

2. *Acquired toxoplasmosis.* In the past, acquired toxoplasmosis was considered of doubtful existence and most toxoplasmosis was thought to be congenital but acquired disease is increasingly recognized. The infestation is acquired by eating the under-cooked meat of intermediate host containing cyst form of the parasite. Most of the patients are subclinical (asymptomatic); and the typical chorioretinal lesion similar to congenital toxoplasmosis is discovered by chance. Other lesions include punctate outer retinal toxoplasmosis (PORT). More common in HIV+ patients.

3. *Recurrent toxoplasmic retinochoroiditis*

Pathogenesis. The parasites reaching the foetus through placenta involve its brain and retina, and also excite antibodies formation. After healing of the active retinal lesion (with which the infant is born), the parasites remain encysted there in inactive form. After about 10-40 years (average 25 years), the retinal cysts rupture and release hundreds of parasites, which by direct invasion cause a fresh lesion of focal necrotizing retinochoroidits, adjacent to the edge of old inactive pigmented scar. In addition to this lesion, an inflammation in the iris, choroid and retinal vessels is excited due to antigen-antibody reaction.

Clinical features. Recurrent toxoplasmic retinochoroiditis is a very common disease. It is characterised by a whitish-yellow, slightly raised area of infiltration located near the margin of old punched out scarred lesion in the macular region associated with severe vitritis. There may be associated non-granulomatous type of mild anterior uveitis.

Diagnosis. The clinically suspected lesion is confirmed by 'Indirect fluorescein antibody test', haemagglutination test or ELISA test. The old methylene blue dye test is obsolete.

Treatment. The active lesion of toxoplasmosis is treated by topical and systemic steroids along with a course of a antitoxoplasmic drug either spiramycin, clindamycin, sulfadiazine or pyremethamine.

TOXOCARIASIS

It is an infestation caused by an intestinal roundworm of dogs (*Toxocara canis*) and cats (*Toxocara catis*). The young children who play with dogs and cats or eat dirt are infested by ova of these worms. These ova develop into larva in the human gut, and then produce the condition visceral larva migrans (VLM).

Ocular toxocariasis. It is ocular infestation by these larva and is almost always unilateral. Clinically it can present as follows:

1. *Toxocara chronic endophthalmitis.* It usually presents with leucocoria due to marked vitreous clouding. The condition is seen in children between the age of 2-10 years and mimics retinoblastoma.
2. *Posterior pole granuloma.* It presents as a yellow-white, round, solitary, raised nodule, about 1-2 disc diameter in size, located either at the macula or in the centrocaecal area. The condition is usually seen in children between 5 and 15 years of age, presenting with unilateral loss of vision.
3. *Peripheral granuloma.* It is situated anterior to the equator and may be associated with vitreous band formation. It may present from 6 to 40 years of age.

Diagnosis is made on the basis of clinical picture and ELISA blood test.

Treatment. It consists of periocular (posterior sub-Tenon) injection of steroid and systemic steroids. Pars plana vitrectomy may be required in unresponsive patients with endophthalmitis and in patients with vitreous band formation.

V. FUNGAL UVEITIS

PRESUMED OCULAR HISTOPLASMOSIS SYNDROME (POHS)

Etiology. It is thought to be caused by the fungus *Histoplasma capsulatum* (though the fungus has not been isolated from the affected eyes); as the disease is more common in areas where histoplamosis is endemic (e.g., Mississippi-Ohio-Missouri river valley) and 90 percent of patients with POHS show positive histoplasmin skin test. POHS has also been reported from United Kingdom, suggesting that perhaps some other etiological agents are also capable of producing the disease.

Clinical features. POHS is characterised by following features:

1. *Histospots.* These are atrophic spots scattered in the mid-retinal periphery. They are roundish, yellowish-white lesions measuring 0.2 to 0.7 disc diameter in size. These begin to appear in early childhood and represent the scars of disseminated histoplasma choroiditis.
2. *Macular lesion.* It starts as atrophic macular scar (macular histospot); followed by a hole in the Bruch's membrane, which then allows ingrowth of capillaries leading to sub-retinal choroidal neovascularisation. Leakage of fluid from the neovascular membrane causes serous detachment, which when complicated by repeated haemorrhages constitutes haemorrhagic detachment. Ultimately, there develops fibrous disciform scar, which is associated with a marked permanent visual loss.

Diagnosis. The clinical diagnosis is supported but not confirmed by positive histoplasmin test, and complement fixation tests (negative in two thirds cases). Fluorescein angiography helps in early diagnosis of subretinal neovascular membrane.

Treatment. Active lesions at the macula are often treated with systemic corticosteroids. Early laser photocoagulation of subretinal neovascular membrane may prevent marked permanent visual loss which occurs due to fibrous disciform scars. For subfoveal membrane PDT should be considered. Emerging threapy include anti-VEGF treatment.

CANDIDIASIS

It is an opportunistic infection caused by *Candida albicans*. It occurs in immuno-compromised patients which include: patients suffering from AIDS, malignancies, those receiving long-term antibiotics, steroids or cytotoxic drugs. Patients with long-term indwelling intravenous catheter used for haemodialysis, and drug addicts are also prone to such infection.

Ocular candidiasis. It is not a common condition. It may occur as anterior uveitis, multifocal chorioretinitis, or endophthalmitis.

1. *Anterior uveitis* is associated with hypopyon.
2. *Multifocal chorioretinitis* is a more common lesion. It is characterised by occurrence of multiple

small, round, whitish areas, which may be associated with areas of haemorrhages with pale centre (Roth's spots).

3. *Candida endophthalmitis* is characterised by areas of severe retinal necrosis associated with vitreoretinal abscesses. Vitreous exudates present as 'puff ball' or 'cotton ball' colonies, which when joined by exudative strands form 'string of pearls'.

Treatment. It consists of :

- *Topical* cycloplegics, and antifungal drugs.
- *Systemic antifungal drugs* like ketoconazole, flucytosine or amphotericin-B are also needed.
- *Pars plana vitrectomy* is required for *Candida* endophthalmitis.

VI. VIRAL UVEITIS

UVEITIS IN HERPES ZOSTER OPHTHALMICUS

Herpes zoster ophthalmicus (HZO) is the involvement of ophthalmic division of fifth nerve by varicella zoster (described on page 104).

Anterior uveitis develops in 40-50 percent cases with HZO within 2 weeks of onset of the skin rashes. A typical HZO keratitis may be associated with mild iritis especially in patients with a vesicular eruption on the tip of nose. The iridocyclitis is *non-granulomatous* characterised by presence of small KPs, mild aqueous flare and occasional haemorrhagic hypopyon. Complications like *iris atrophy* and secondary glaucoma are not uncommon. Complicated cataract may also develop in late stages.

Treatment. Topical steroids and cycloplegics to be continued for several months. *Systemic acyclovir* helps in early control of lesions of HZO.

HERPES SIMPLEX UVEITIS

It is associated with keratitis in most of the cases. It may be seen in association with dendritic or geographical corneal ulceration or with disciform keratitis. Rarely, anterior uveitis may occur even without keratitis. It is a mild grade non-granulomatous iridocyclitis excited by hypersensitivity reaction.

Treatment. Keratitis is treated with antiviral drugs and cycloplegics. Steroids for iritis are contraindicated in the presence of active viral ulcers. Nonsteroidal anti-inflammatory drugs may be added in such cases.

CYTOMEGALOVIRUS RETINITIS

Cytomegalovirus (CMV) retinitis usually occurs in immunocompromised patients e.g., those suffering from AIDS, on cytotoxic chemotherapy, or long term immuno-suppression following renal transplantation. It is the most frequent (40% prevalance) ocular opportunistic infection in patients with AIDS. It occurs only when CD 4+ counts < 50 cells mm^3. However, since the advent of Highly Active Antiretroviral Therapy (HAART) there has occured a dramatic reduction in CMV retinitis.

Clinical features

Symptoms. Often asymptomatic, some patients may present with scotoma or decreased vision and/or floaters in one or both eyes.

Anterior segment signs are usually absent. Rarely few stellate KPs may be seen.

Posterior segment signs include:

- *Haemorrhagic retinitis* (see Fig.11.5) characterised by areas of necrosis (yellow white exudates) associated with areas of vasculitis (perivascular sheathing), retinal haemorrhages and loss of fundal details (pizza pie appearance) is a typical presentation in fulminant form of the disease. There occurs progressive retinal atrophy.
- *Grannular retinitis* characterised by peripheral granular opacities with occasional haemorrhage seen in indolent form of the disease.
- *Complications* include retinal detachment (up to 30%), retinal atrophy and optic nerve disease.

Treatment

- *HAART* is recommended to reduce retroviral load and to increase CD4+ count in patients with AIDS.
- *Specific anti-CMV treatment* includes: valaganciclovir, ganciclovir, foscarnet, and intravenous injections of cidofovir individually or in combination.

ACUTE RETINAL NECROSIS

Etiology

Acute retinal necrosis (ARN) is a rare clinical syndrome caused by any of the following viruses:

- *Varicella-zoster virus* (VZV). It is the commonest cause of ARN, particularly in older patients.

- *Herpes simplex virus* 1 and 2 (HSV 1 & 2) both cause ARN, typically in younger patients.
- *Cytomegalo virus* (CMV) can also cause ARN, very rarely.

Clinical features

Symptoms include decreased visual acuity, floaters, ocular discomfort, pain and photophobia.

Signs are as follows:

- *Anterior segment* may or may not show signs of inflammation in the anterior chamber.
- *Vitritis* is usually marked
- *Retinal lesions* include areas of focal, well demarcated peripheral necrotising retinitis, associated with occlusive arteritis. Posterior pole is typically spared.

Complications include: retinal detachment (rhegmatogenous or tractional), and ischaemic optic neuropathy.

Treatment consists of:

- *Systemic antiviral drugs* e.g. aciclovir i.v. 10 mg/kg body weight TID, for two weeks then PO dose for 6-12 weeks. Alternative drug is valaciclovir.
  Note: Lifelong antiviral cover is required in immunosuppressed patients.
- *Systemic steroids* are needed to control inflammation.
- *Aspirin* to prevent arterial occlusion.
- *Barrier laser photocoagulation* for retinal breaks.
- *Vitrectomy with silicon oil injection* for associated retinal detachment.

PROGRESSIVE OUTER RETINAL NECROSIS

Progressive outer retinal necrosis (PORN) is a very rare devastating necrotizing retinitis caused by a Varicella Zoster Virus (VZV) infection in immunocompromised patients (usually in patients suffering with AIDS with CD4+ T-cell counts < 50/mm^2.

Clinical features

- *Painless rapid loss of vision* in one or both eyes is the presenting symptom.
- *Retinal lesions* include rapidly coalescing white areas of outer retinal necrosis (often central as well as peripheral) but with minimal vasculitis, retinitis or viritis (cf ARN). Retinal detachment is an extremely common complication.

Treatment consists of intravenous injection of ganciclovir or foscarnet combined with intravitreal ganciclovir.

VII. LENS-INDUCED UVEITIS

PHACOANAPHYLACTIC UVEITIS

It is an immunologic response to lens proteins in the sensitized eyes presenting as severe granulomatous anterior uveitis. The disease may occur following extracapsular cataract extraction, trauma to lens or leak of proteins in hypermature cataract.

Clinical features. These include severe pain, loss of vision, marked congestion and signs of granulomatous iridocyclitis associated with presence of lens matter in the anterior chamber.

Treatment. It consists of removal of causative lens matter, topical steroids and cycloplegics. Visual prognosis is usually poor.

PHACOTOXIC UVEITIS

It is an ill-understood entity. This term is used to describe mild iridocyclitis associated with the presence of lens matter in the anterior chamber either following trauma or extracapsular cataract extraction or leak from hypermature cataracts. The uveal response due to direct toxic effect of lens matter or a mild form of allergic reaction is yet to be ascertained.

Treatment. It consists of removal of lens matter, topical steroids and cycloplegics.

VIII. TRAUMATIC UVEITIS

(See page 433)

IX. UVEITIS ASSOCIATED WITH INTRAOCULAR TUMOURS

(See pages 174 and 301)

X. IDIOPATHIC SPECIFIC UVEITIS SYNDROMES

FUCHS' UVEITIS SYNDROME (FUS)

Fuchs' 'heterochromic iridocyclitis' is a chronic non-granulomatous type of low grade anterior uveitis typically associated with ealy cataract formation. It typically occurs unilaterally in middle-aged persons. The disease is characterised by: (i) heterochromia of iris, (ii) diffuse stromal iris atrophy, (moth-eaten appearance), may cause transillumination defects, (iii) fine stelleta KPs at the back of cornea, (iv) faint aqueous flare, (v) absence of posterior synechiae, (vi) a fairly common rubeosis iridis, sometimes associated with neovascularisation of the angle of anterior chamber, and (vii) comparatively early development of compli- cated cataract and secondary glaucoma (usually open angle type).

Treatment. Topical corticosteroids are all that is required. Cycloplegics are not required as usually there are no posterior synechiae. Associated glaucoma should be treated as for POAG.

GLAUCOMATOCYCLITIC CRISIS

Posner Schlossman syndrome is characterised by: (i) recurrent unilateral attacks of acute rise of intraocular pressure (40-50 mm of Hg) without shallowing of anterior chamber associated with, (ii) fine KPs at the back of cornea, without any posterior synechiae, (iii) epithelial oedema of cornea, (iv) a dilated pupil, and (v) a white eye (no congestion).

The disease typically affects young adults, 40 percent of whom are positive for HLA-BW54.

Treatment. It includes medical treatment to lower intraocular pressure along with a short course of topical steroids.

SYMPATHETIC OPHTHALMITIS

It is a rare bilateral granulomatous panuveitis which is known to occur following penetrating ocular trauma usually associated with incarceration of uveal tissue in the wound. The injured eye is called 'exciting eye' and the fellow eye which also develops uveitis is called 'sympathising eye'. (For details see page 441).

VOGT-KOYANAGI-HARADA (VKH) SYNDROME

It is an idiopathic multisystem disorder which includes cutaneous, neurological and ocular lesions. The disease is comparatively more common in Japanese who are usually positive for HLA-DR4 and DW15.

Clinical features are as follows:

1. *Cutaneous lesions* include: alopecia, poliosis and vitiligo.
2. *Neurological lesions* are in the form of meningism, and encephalopathy.
3. *Auditory features*: tinnitus, vertigo and deafness.
4. *Ocular features include*:

i. *Anterior uveitis* is typically bilateral chronic granulomatous characterised by iris nodules, posterior synechiae.

ii. *Posterior uveitis* lesions include multifocal choroiditis leading to exudative retinal detachment, choroidal depigmentation (sunset glow fundus), Daln-Fuch's nodules and peripheral yellow-white choroidal granuloma.

Complications include: cataract, glaucoma and CNV membrane.

Treatments of uveitis is on general lines (see page 155).

- *Corticosteroids* administered topically, periocularly and systemically (in high doses) constitute the main stay of treatment.
- *Immunosuppressive drugs* such as methotrexate, azathioprine, and cyclosporine should be considered for resistant and recurrent cases.

ACUTE POSTERIOR MULTIFOCAL PLACOID PIGMENT EPITHELIOPATHY (APMPPE)

Clinical features. It is a rare idiopathic self-limiting disorder characterised by bilateral, deep, placoid, cream coloured or grey white chorioretinal lesions involving the posterior pole and post-equatorial part of the fundus. Visual loss, seen in early stage due to macular lesions, usually recovers within 2 weeks. After healing, multifocal areas of depigmentation and pigment clumping involving the retinal pigment epithelium are left.

Complications though rare include mild anterior uveitis, vascular sheathing, and exudative retinal detachment.

Treatment. No treatment is effective.

SERPIGINOUS GEOGRAPHICAL CHOROIDOPATHY

It is a rare, idiopathic, recurrent, bilaterally asymmetrical inflammation involving the choriocapillaris and pigment epithelium of the retina. The disease typically affects patients between 40 and 60 years of age and is characterised by cream coloured patches with hazy borders present around the optic disc which spread in a tongue fashion. After few weeks the lesions heal leaving behind punched out areas of retinal pigment epithelium and choroidal atrophy. No treatment is effective.

BIRD-SHOT RETINOCHOROIDOPATHY

It is a rare, idiopathic, bilaterally symmetrical chronic multifocal chorioretinitis characterised by numerous flat creamy-yellow spots due to focal chorioretinal hypopigmentation, resembling the pattern of 'bird-shot scatter from a shotgun'. The disease, more common in females than males, typically affects middle-aged healthy persons who are positive for HLA-A29. It runs a long chronic course of several years.

Treatment with corticosteroids is usually not effective.

PURULENT UVEITIS

Purulent uveitis is suppurative inflammation of the uveal tract occurring as a result of direct invasion by the pyogenic organisms. It may start as purulent anterior uveitis (iridocyclitis) or purulent posterior uveitis (choroiditis) which soon progresses to involve the retina and vitreous, resulting in purulent endophthalmitis and ultimately leading to panophthalmitis.

ENDOPHTHALMITIS

Endophthalmitis is defined as an inflammation of the inner structures of the eyeball i.e., uveal tissue and retina associated with pouring of exudates in the vitreous cavity, anterior chamber and posterior chamber.

Etiology

Etiologically endophthalmitis may be infectious or non-infectious (sterile).

A. *Infective endophthalmitis*

Modes of Infection

1. *Exogenous infections.* Purulent inflammations are generally caused by exogenous infections following perforating injuries, perforation of infected corneal ulcers or as postoperative infections following intraocular operations.
2. *Endogenous or metastatic endophthalmitis.* It may occur rarely through blood stream from some infected focus in the body such as caries teeth, generalised septicaemia and puerperal sepsis.
3. *Secondary infections from surrounding structures.* It is very rare. However, cases of purulent intraocular inflammation have been reported following extension of infection from orbital cellulitis, thrombophlebitis and infected corneal ulcers.

Causative organisms

1. *Bacterial endophthalmitis.* The most frequent pathogens causing acute bacterial endophthalmitis are gram positive cocci i.e., *Staphylococcus epidermidis* and *Staphylococcus aureus.* Other causative bacteria include *Streptococci, Pseudomonas, Pneumococci* and *Corynebacterium. Propionio* bacterium acnes and *Actinomyces* are gram-positive organisms capable of producing slow grade endophthalmitis.
2. *Fungal endophthalmitis* is comparatively rare. It is caused by *Aspergillus, Fusarium, Candida* etc.

B. *Non-infective (sterile) endophthalmitis*

Sterile endophthalmitis refers to inflammation of inner structures of eyeball caused by certain toxins/toxic substances. It occurs in following situations.

1. *Postoperative sterile endophthalmitis* may occur as toxic reaction to:
   - Chemicals adherent to intraocular lens (IOL) or
   - Chemicals adherent to instruments.

Severe reaction mainly confined to the anterior segment is also called 'Toxic anterior segment syndrome' (TASS).

2. *Post-traumatic sterile endophthalmitis* may occur as toxic reaction to retain intraocular foreign body, e.g., pure copper.
3. *Phacoanaphylactic endophthalmitis* may be induced by lens proteins in patients with Morgagnian cataract.
4. *Intraocular tumour necrosis* may present as sterile endophthalmitis (masquerade syndrome).

Note: Since postoperative acute bacterial endophthalmitis is most important, so clinical features and treatment described below pertain to this condition.

Clinical picture of acute bacterial endophthalmitis

Acute postoperative endophthalmitis is a catastrophic complication of intraocular surgery with an incidence of about 0.1%. Source of infection in most of the cases is thought to be patient's own periocular bacterial flora of the eyelids, conjunctiva, and lacrimal sac. Other potential sources of infection include contaminated solutions and instruments, and environmental flora including that of surgeon and operating room personnel.

Symptoms. Acute bacterial endophthalmitis usually occurs within 7 days of operation and is characterised by severe ocular pain, redness, lacrimation, photophobia and loss of vision.

Signs are as follows (Fig. 7.18):

1. *Lids* become red and swollen.
2. *Conjunctiva* shows chemosis and marked circumcorneal congestion.
3. *Cornea* is oedematous, cloudy and ring infiltration may be formed.
4. *Edges of wound* become yellow and necrotic and wound may gape (Fig. 7.19) in exogenous form.
5. *Anterior chamber* shows hypopyon; soon it becomes full of pus.
6. *Iris,* when visible, is oedematous and muddy.
7. *Pupil* shows yellow reflex due to purulent exudation in vitreous. When anterior chamber becomes full of pus, iris and pupil details are not seen.
8. *Vitreous exudation.* In metastatic forms and in cases with deep infections, vitreous cavity is filled with exudation and pus. Soon a yellowish white mass is seen through fixed dilated pupil. This sign is called *amaurotic cat's-eye reflex.*
9. *Intraocular pressure* is raised in early stages, but in severe cases, the ciliary processes are destroyed, and a fall in intraocular pressure may ultimately result in shrinkage of the globe.

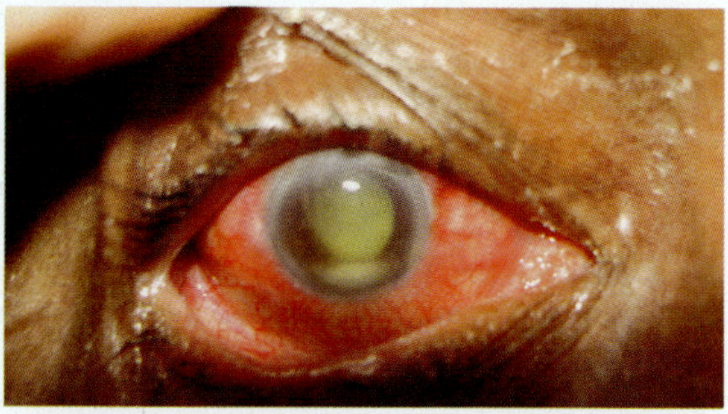

Fig. 7.18. Postoperative acute endophthalmitis.

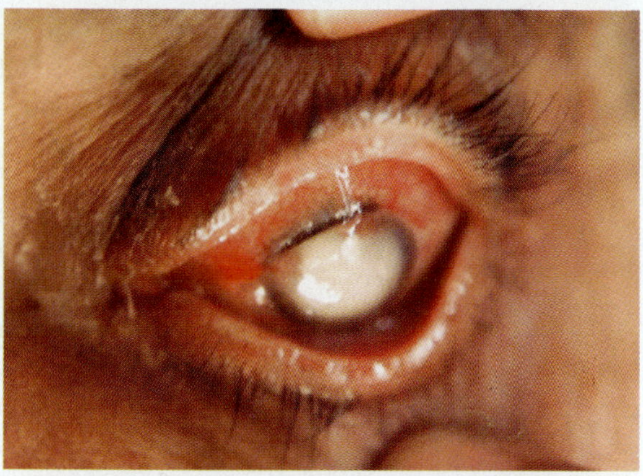

Fig. 7.19. Severe postoperative endophthalmitis with wound gape.

Treatment

An early diagnosis and vigorous therapy is the hallmark of the treatment of endophthalmitis. Following therapeutic regime is recommended for suspected bacterial endophthalmitis.

A. Antibiotic therapy

1. *Intravitreal antibiotics and diagnostic tap* should be made as early as possible. It is performed transconjunctivally under topical anaesthesia from the area of pars plana (4-5 mm from the limbus). The vitreous tap is made using 23-gauge needle followed by the intravitreal injection using a disposable tuberculin syringe and 30-gauge needle.

The main stay of treatment of acute bacterial endophthalmitis is intravitreal injection of antibiotics at the earliest possible. Usually a combination of two antibiotics – one effective against gram positive coagulase negative *Staphylococci* and the other against gram-negative *Bacilli* is used as below:

- *First choice:* Vancomycin 1 mg in 0.1 ml plus ceftazidime 2.25 mg in 0.1 ml.
- *Second choice:* Vancomycin 1 mg in 0.1 ml plus Amikacin 0.4 mg in 0.1 ml.

Note:

- Some surgeons prefer to add dexamethasone 0.4 mg in 0.1 ml to limit post-inflammatory consequences.
- Gentamycin is 4 times more retinotoxic (causes macular infarction) than amikacin. Preferably the aminoglycosides should be avoided.
- The aspirated fluid sample should be used for bacterial culture and smear examination. If vitreous aspirate is collected in an emergency when immediate facilities for culture are not available, it should be stored promptly in refrigerator at 4°C.
- If there is no improvement, a repeat intravitreal injection should be given after 48 hours taking into consideration the reports of bacteriological examination.

2. ***Topical concentrated antibiotics*** should be started immediately and used frequently (every 30 minute to 1 hourly). To begin with, a combination of two drugs should be preferred, one having a predominant effect on the gram-positive organisms and the other against gram-negative organisms as below:

- Vancomycin (50 mg/ml) or cefazoline (50 mg/ml) plus.
- Amikacin (20 mg/ml) or tobramycin (15 mg%).

3. ***Systemic antibiotics*** have limited role in the management of endophthalmitis, but most of the surgeons do use them.

- *Ciprofloxacin* intravenous infusion 200 mg BD for 3-4 days followed by orally 500 mg BD for 6-7 days, or
- *Vancomycin* 1 gm IV BD and *ceftazidime* 2 g IV 8 hourly, or
- *Cefazoline* 1.5 gm IV 6 hourly and *amikacin* 1 gm IV three times a day.

B. Steroid therapy

Steroids limit the tissue damage caused by inflammatory process. Most surgeons recommend their use after 24 to 48 hours of control of infection by intensive antibiotic therapy. However, some surgeons recommend their immediate use (controversial). Routes of administration and doses are:

- *Intravitreal injection* of dexamethasone 0.4 mg in 0.1 ml along with antibiotics.
- *Topical* dexamethasone (0.1%) or predacetate (1%) used frequently.
- *Systemic steroids.* Oral corticosteroids should preferably be started after 24 hours of intensive antibiotic therapy. A daily therapy regime with 60 mg prednisolone to be followed by 50, 40, 30, 20 and 10 mg for 2 days, each may be adopted.

C. Supportive therapy

1. *Cycloplegics.* Preferably 1% atropine or alternatively 2% homatropine eyedrops should be instilled TDS or QID.
2. *Antiglaucoma drugs.* In patients with raised intraocular pressure drugs such a oral acetazolamide (250 mg TDS) and timolol (0.5% BD) may be prescribed.

D. Vitrectomy operation should be performed if the patient does not improve with the above intensive therapy for 48 to 72 hours or when the patient presents with severe infection with visual acuity reduced to light perception. Vitrectomy helps in removal of infecting organisms, toxins and enzymes present in the infected vitreous mass.

PANOPHTHALMITIS

It is an intense purulent inflammation of the whole eyeball including the Tenon's capsule. The disease usually begins either as purulent anterior or purulent posterior uveitis; and soon a full-fledged picture of panophthalmitis develops, following through a very short stage of endophthalmitis.

Etiology

- *Panophthalmitis* is an acute bacterial infection.
- *Mode of infection* and *causative organisms* are same as described for infective bacterial endophthalmitis (page 150, 151).

Clinical picture

Symptoms. These include:

- Severe ocular pain and headache,
- Complete loss of vision,
- Profuse watering,
- Purulent discharge,
- Marked redness and swelling of the eyes, and
- Associated constitutional symptoms are malaise and fever.

Signs are as follows (Fig.7.20):

1. *Lids* show a marked oedema and hyperaemia.
2. *Eyeball* is slightly proptosed, ocular movements are limited and painful.

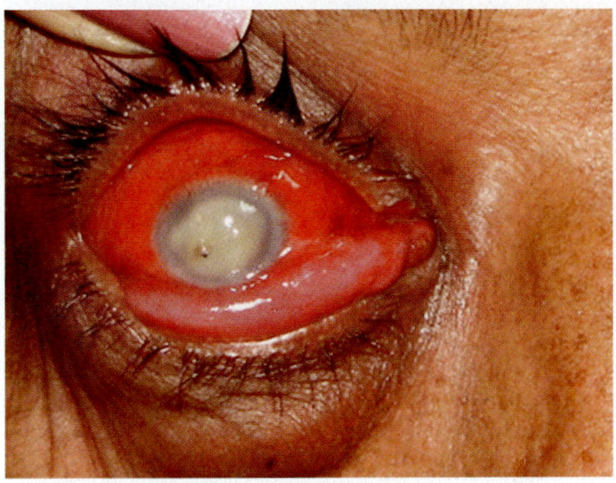

Fig. 7.20. Panophthalmitis.

3. *Conjunctiva* shows marked chemosis and ciliary as well as conjunctival congestion.
4. *Cornea* is cloudy and oedematous.
5. *Anterior chamber* is full of pus.
6. *Vision* is completely lost and perception of light is absent.
7. *Intraocular pressure* is markedly raised.
8. *Globe perforation* may occur at limbus, pus comes out and intraocular pressure falls.

Complications include:
- Orbital cellulitis
- Cavernous sinus thrombosis
- Meningitis or encephalitis

Treatment

There is little hope of saving such an eye and the pain and toxaemia lend an urgency to its removal.
1. *Anti-inflammatory and analgesics* should be started immediately to relieve pain.
2. *Broad spectrum antibiotics* should be administered to prevent further spread of infection in the surrounding structures.
3. *Evisceration* operation should be performed to avoid the risk of intracranial dissemination of infection.

EVISCERATION

It is the removal of the contents of the eyeball leaving behind the sclera. Frill evisceration is preferred over simple evisceration. In it, only about 3-mm frill of the sclera is left around the optic nerve.

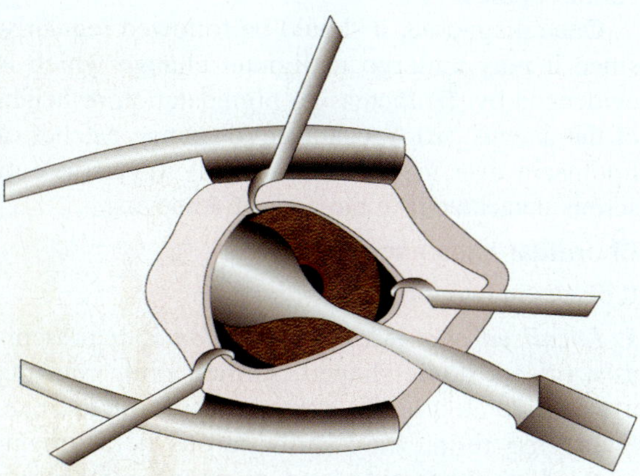

Fig. 7.21. Removal of intraocular contents in evisceration.

Indications. These include: panophthalmitis, expulsive choroidal haemorrhage and bleeding anterior staphyloma.

Surgical steps of frill evisceration (Fig. 7.21)
1. *Initial steps* upto separation of the conjunctiva and Tenon's capsule are similar to enucleation (see page 304).
2. *Removal of cornea.* A cut at the limbus is made with a razor blade fragment or with a No. 11 scalpel blade and then the cornea is excised with corneoscleral scissors.
3. *Removal of intraocular contents.* The uveal tissue is separated from the sclera with the help of an evisceration spatula and the contents are scooped out using the evisceration curette.
4. *Separation of extraocular muscles* is done as for enucleation.
5. *Removal of sclera.* Using curved scissors the sclera is excised leaving behind only a 3-mm frill around the optic nerve.
6. *Closure of Tenon's capsule and conjunctiva* and other final steps are similar to enucleation (see page 304).

DEGENERATIVE CONDITIONS OF THE UVEAL TRACT

(A) DEGENERATIONS OF THE IRIS

1. *Simple iris atrophy.* It is characterised by depigmentation with thinning of iris stroma. Small patches of depigmentation are usually seen near the pupillary margin. A patch of simple iris atrophy may be senile, post-inflammatory, glaucomatous or neurogenic due to lesions of the ciliary ganglion.

2. *Essential iris atrophy.* It is a rare idiopathic condition characterised by unilateral progressive atrophy of the iris. The condition typically affects young females 5 times more than the males. Initially there occurs displacement of pupil away from the atrophic zone. Slowly the iris tissue melts away at many places resulting in pseudopolycoria. In advanced cases, intractable glaucoma supervenes due to formation of dense anterior peripheral synechiae.

3. ***Iridoschisis.*** It is a rare bilateral atrophy occurring as a senile degeneration in patients over 65 years of age. It may also occur as a later effect of iris trauma. It is characterised by formation of a cleft between the anterior and posterior stroma of the iris. As a consequence the strands of anterior stroma float into the anterior chamber.

(B) DEGENERATIONS AND DYSTROPHIES OF THE CHOROID

I. Primary choroidal degenerations

1. ***Senile central choroidal atrophy.*** It is characterised by formation of multiple drusens (colloid bodies) which look as yellowish spots. These are scattered throughout the fundus, but more marked in the macular area.

2. ***Central areolar choroidal atrophy.*** It comprises bilateral punched out, circular atrophic lesion in the macular region. The lesion is characterised by white shining sclera, traversed by large ribbon-shaped choroidal vessels. Thus, there occurs atrophy of the choriocapillaris, retinal pigment epithelium and photoreceptors.

3. ***Essential gyrate atrophy.*** It is an inborn error of amino acid (ornithine) metabolism characterised by progressive patches of atrophy of choroid and retinal pigment epithelium (RPE). The disease begins in first decade of life with symptoms of night blindness and progresses slowly to involve the whole fundus by the age of 40-50 years with preservation of only macula.

4. ***Choroidremia.*** It is a hereditary choroidal dystrophy involving the males. The disease begins in first decade of life with symptoms of night blindness and fine whitish patches of choroidal and RPE atrophy. The lesions progress slowly and by the age of 40 years almost whole of the choroidal tissue and RPE disappear rendering the patient blind. At this age fundus picture is characterised by whitish sclera with overlying almost normal retinal vessels.

5. ***Myopic chorioretinal degeneration.*** (see page 35)

II. Secondary choroidal degeneration

It occurs following inflammatory lesions of the fundus. It is characterised by scattered area of chorioretinal atrophy and pigment clumping. Ophthalmoscopic picture resembles retinitis pigmentosa and hence also labelled sometimes as *'pseudoretinitis pigmentosa'*.

TUMOURS OF THE UVEAL TRACT

CLASSIFICATION

I. *Tumours of choroid*
- a) Benign
  1. Naevus
  2. Haemangioma
  3. Melanocytoma
  4. Choroidal osteoma
- b) Malignant
  1. Melanoma

II. *Tumours of ciliary body*
- a) Benign
  1. Hyperplasia
  2. Benign cyst
  3. Meduloepithelioma
- b) Malignant
  1. Melanoma

III. *Tumours of iris*
- a) Benign
  1. Naevus
  2. Benign cyst
  3. Naevoxanthoendothelioma
- b) Malignant
  1. Melanoma

TUMOURS OF THE CHOROID

Naevus

It is a commonly occurring asymptomatic lesion, usually diagnosed on routine fundus examination. It typically presents as a flat, dark grey lesion with feathered margins, usually associated with overlying colloid bodies.

Once diagnosed, it should be followed regularly, since it may undergo malignant change which is evidenced by: (i) Increasing pigmentation or height of the naevus. (ii) Appearance of orange patches of lipofuscin over the surface and (iii) Appearance of serous detachment in the area of a naevus.

Choroidal haemangioma

It occurs in two forms:

1. ***Localised choroidal haemangioma.*** It presents as a raised, dome-shaped, salmon pink swelling usually situated at the posterior pole of the eye. Overlying retina may show serous detachment, cystoid degeneration and pigment epithelium mottling. Fluorescein angiography is usually diagnostic.

2. *Diffuse choroidal haemangioma.* It is seen in association with Sturge-Weber syndrome and causes diffuse deep red discoloration of the fundus.

Melanocytoma

It is a rare tumour which presents as a jet black lesion around the optic disc.

Choroidal osteoma

It is a very rare benign tumour which presents as elevated, yellowish-orange lesion in the posterior pole. It typically affects the young women.

Malignant melanoma of choroid

It is the most common primary intraocular tumour of adults, usually seen between 40-70 years of age. It is rare in blacks and comparatively more common in whites. It arises from the neural crest derived pigment cells of the uvea as a solitary tumour and is usually unilateral.

Pathology

Gross pathology. The tumour may arise from a pre-existing naevus or *denovo* from the mature melanocytes present in the stroma. It may occur in two forms:

1. *Circumscribed (pedunculated) tumour:* Initially it appears as flat, slate-grey area, which becomes raised and pigmented with growth and eventually ruptures through the Bruch's membrane (Collar-Stud tumour). Further, growth of the tumour produces exudative retinal detachment.
2. *Diffuse (flat) malignant melanoma:* It spreads slowly throughout the uvea, without forming a tumour mass. It accounts for only 5 percent cases. In it symptoms occur late.

Histopathology. Microscopically uveal melanomas are of following four types (Modified Callender's classification):

1. *Spindle cell melanomas.* These are composed of spindle-shaped cells and make up 45% of all tumours. Such tumours have best prognosis (80 percent 10 year survival).
2. *Epithelioid cell melanomas.* These consist of large, oval or round, pleomorphic cells with larger nuclei and abundant acidophilic cytoplasm. This type of tumours have the worst prognosis (35 percent 10 year survival). These make up 5% of all tumours.
3. *Mixed cell melanomas.* These are composed of both spindle and epithelioid cells and thus carry an intermediate prognosis (45 percent 10 year survival). These make up 45% of all tumours.
4. *Necrotic melanomas.* These make up the remaining 5% of the all tumours. In these tumours the predominant cell type is unrecognizable.

Clinical picture

For the purpose of description only the clinical picture can be divided into four stages.

1. *Quiescent stage*. During this stage symptoms depend upon the location and size of tumour. Small tumour located in the periphery may not produce any symptom, while tumours arising from the posterior pole present with early visual loss. A large tumour associated with exudative retinal detachment may produce marked loss of vision.

Signs. Fundus examination during this stage may reveal following signs:

i. *A small tumour* limited to the choroid appears as an elevated pigmented oval mass (Fig. 7.22). Rarely the tumour may be amelanotic. The earliest pathognomic sign at this stage is appearance of orange patches in the pigment epithelium due to accumulation of the lipofuscin.

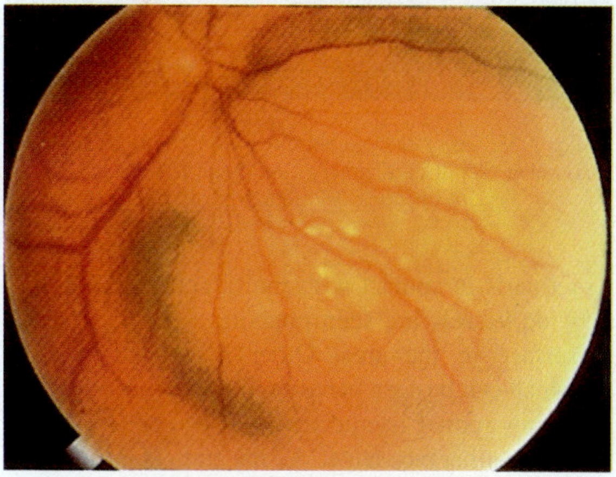

Fig. 7.22. Fundus photograph showing choroidal melanoma as raised pigmented subretinal mass.

ii. *A large tumour* which penetrates through the Bruch's membrane and grows in the subretinal space is characterised by a large exudative retinal detachment (Fig. 7.23). At the central summit, the

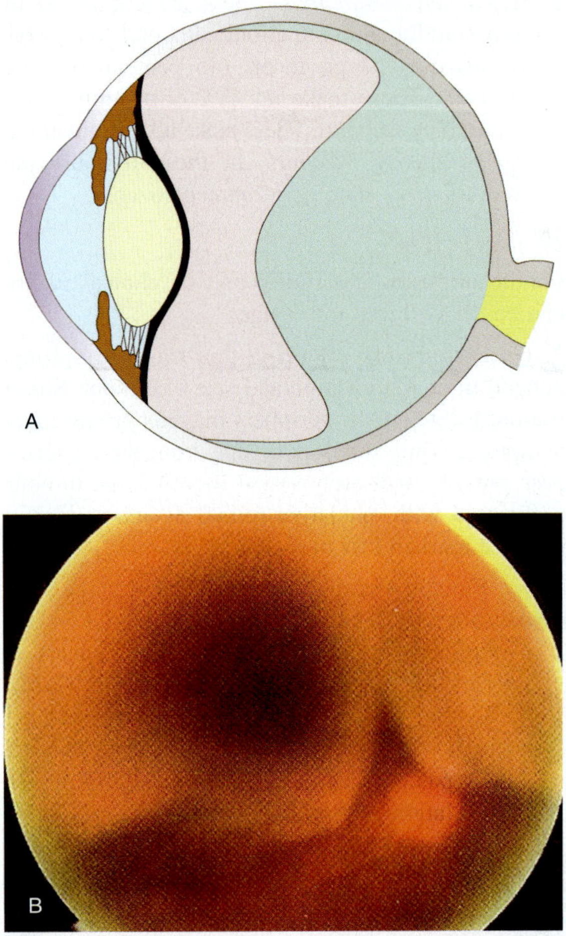

Fig. 7.23. Malignant melanoma of the choroid causing exudative retinal detachment : A; diagrammatic depiction in cut section ; B, fundus photograph.

retina is in contact with the tumour. Ribbon-like wide vessels are seen coursing over the tumour surface in the area. Other associated features which can be seen occasionally include subretinal or intraretinal haemorrhage, choroidal folds and vitreous haemorrhage. As the tumour grows, the exudative retinal detachment deepens and gradually the tumour fills the whole eye.

2. *Glaucomatous stage.* It develops when tumour is left untreated during the quiescent stage. Glaucoma may develop due to obstruction to the venous outflow by pressure on the vortex veins, blockage of the angle of anterior chamber by forward displacement of the lens iris diaphragm due to increasing growth of the tumour.

Symptoms. The patient complains of severe pain, redness and watering in an already blind eye.

Signs. (i) Conjunctiva is chemosed and congested. (ii) Cornea may show oedema. (iii) Anterior chamber is usually shallow. (iv) Pupil is fixed and dilated. (v) Lens is usually opaque, obstructing the back view. (vi) Intraocular pressure is raised, usually eye is stony hard. (vii) Sometimes features of iridocyclitis may be seen due to tumour-induced uveitis.

3. *Stage of extraocular extension.* Due to progressive growth the tumour may burst through sclera, usually at the limbus. The extraocular spread may occur even early along the perivascular spaces of the vortex veins or ciliary vessels. It is followed by rapid fungation and involvement of extraocular tissues resulting in marked proptosis (Fig. 7.24).

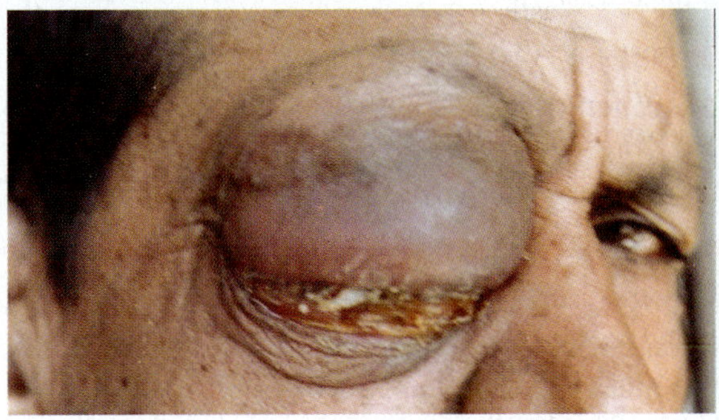

Fig. 7.24. Extensive malignant melanoma of the choroid involving orbit.

4. *Stage of distant metastasis*. Lymphatic spread is usually not known. Blood-borne metastasis usually occurs in liver and is the commonest cause of death.

Differential diagnosis

1. *During quiescent stage* differential diagnosis may be considered as below:
   i. A small tumour without an overlying exudative retinal detachment should be differentiated from a naevus, melanocytoma and hyperplasia of the pigment epithelium.
   ii. A tumour with overlying exudative retinal detachment should be differentiated from simple retinal detachment and other causes of exudative detachment especially choroidal haemangioma and secondary deposits.

2. *During glaucomatous stage* differentiation is to be made from other causes of acute glaucoma.

Investigations

1. *Indirect ophthalmoscopic examination.* It allows three-dimensional stereoscopic view of the lesion. It also depicts the presence of shifting fluid which is pathognomic of exudative retinal detachment.
2. *Transillumination test.* It indicates a tumour mass and thus helps to differentiate from choroidal detachment and simple retinal detachment.
3. *Ultrasonography.* Both A and B scan help to outline the tumour mass in the presence of hazy media.
4. *Fluorescein angiography* is of limited diagnostic value because there is no pathognomic pattern.
5. *Radioactive tracer.* It is based on the fact that the neoplastic tissue has an increased rate of phosphate (32p) uptake.
6. *MRI.* Choroidal melanomas are hyperintense in T1-weighted and hypointense in T2-weighted images.

Treatment

1. *Conservative treatment* to salvage the eyeball should be instituted when there is no doubt of diagnosis and the tumour is not very large. However, when the diagnosis is doubtful, *observation* is indicated especially for small asymptomatic lesions with absence of suspicious features (i.e. associated subretinal fluid/detachment, lipofuscin on the surface, thickness >2 mm). Methods used for conservative treatment and their indications are:

i. *Brachytherapy* using cobalt-60 or iodine-125 plaques surgically placed externally on the sclera is usually the treatment of choice in tumours less than 10 mm in elevation and less than 16 mm in basal diameter. Supplemental transpupillary thermotherapy may be required to enhance the results.

ii. *External beam radiotherapy* (EBR) with protons or helium ions is indicated in tumours unsuitable for brachytherapy either because of size or posterior location to within 4 mm of disc or fovea.

iii. *Transpupillary thermotherapy (TTT)* with diode laser is indicated in selected small tumours, particularly if pigmented and located near the fovea or optic disc. It can also be supplemented over brachytherapy to enhance results.

iv. *Trans-scleral local resection* is indicated in tumours that are too thick for radiotherapy and usually less than 16 mm in diameter. It is a very difficult procedure which is performed under systemic arterial hypotension.

v. *Stereostatic radiosurgery* is a new method indicated in large tumours. It involves single-session delivery of ionizing radiation to a stereotactically localized volume of tissue with the help of Gamma knife.

2. *Enucleation.* It is indicated for very larger tumours >16 mm basal diameter or >10 mm apical height in which conservative methods to salvage the eyeball are not effective.

3. *Exenteration or debulking* with chemotherapy and radiotherapy is required at the stage of extra-ocular spread.

4. *Palliative treatment* with chemotherapy and immunotherapy may be of some use in prolonging life of the patients with distant metastasis.

TUMOURS OF CILIARY BODY

Hyperplasia and benign cyst

These are insignificant lesions of the ciliary body.

Medulloepithelioma (diktyoma)

It is a rare congenital tumour arising from the non-pigmented epithelium of the ciliary body. It presents in the first decade of life.

Malignant melanoma

In the ciliary body it is usually diagnosed very late, due to its hidden location. It may extend anteriorly, posteriorly or grow circumferentially.

Clinical features

1. *Earliest features* of a localised melonoma include slight hypotony, unaccountable defective vision and localised 'sentinel' dilated episcleral veins in the quadrant containing tumour.
2. *An anterior spreading tumour* may present as follows:
   i. It may cause pressure on the lens resulting in anterior displacement, subluxation and cataract formation.
   ii. It may involve iris and is visible immediately. Soon it may involve the angle of anterior chamber resulting in secondary glaucoma.

iii. It may extend out through sclera along the vessels, presenting as an epibulbar mass.

3. *Posterior spreading tumour* may involve choroid and present as exudative retinal detachment.
4. *The tumour may extend circumferentially* involving whole of the ciliary body.

Pathological features

These are similar to that of choroidal melanoma.

Treatment

1. *Enucleation.* It is required for large ciliary body tumours extending anteriorly, posteriorly or circumferentially.
2. *Local resection.* Cyclectomy or irido-cyclectomy may be enough, if fortunately tumour is detected in early stage.

TUMOURS OF IRIS

Naevus

It is the most common lesion of the iris. It presents as a flat, pigmented, circumscribed lesion of variable size. Rarely malignant change may occur in it, so it should be observed.

Naevoxanthoendothelioma

It is a rare fleshy vascular lesion seen in babies. It may cause recurrent hyphaema. It is treated with X-rays or steroids.

Malignant melanoma

It presents as a single or multiple rapidly growing vascular nodules. It spreads in the angle producing secondary glaucoma. It may penetrate through limbus and present as epibulbar mass. Pathological features are similar to that of melanoma of the choroid.

Treatment

1. *Wide iridectomy.* It is performed for a tumour limited to the iris.
2. *Iridocyclectomy.* It is required for a tumour involving iris and ciliary body.
3. *Enucleation.* It should be performed when iris melanoma is associated with secondary glaucoma.

8

CHAPTER

Diseases of the Lens

ANATOMY AND PHYSIOLOGY
- Applied anatomy
- Applied physiology and biochemistry

CATARACT
- Congenital and developmental cataracts
- Acquired cataract
- Management of cataract in adults

SURGICAL TECHNIQUES FOR CATARACT EXTRACTION
- Intracapsular cataract extraction
- Conventional extracapsular cataract extraction
- Manual small incision cataract surgery
- Phacoemulsification
- Surgical techniques of extracapsular cataract extraction for childhood cataract
- Intraocular lens implantation
- Postoperative management after cataract operation
- Complications of cataract surgery and their management

DISPLACEMENTS OF THE LENS
- Clinico-etiological types
- Topographical types
  - Subluxation
  - Dislocation

CONGENITAL ANOMALIES OF THE LENS

ANATOMY AND PHYSIOLOGY

APPLIED ANATOMY

- The lens is a transparent, biconvex, crystalline structure placed between iris and the vitreous in a saucer shaped depression, the patellar fossa.
- Its diameter is 9-10 mm and thickness varies with age from 3.5 mm (at birth) to 5 mm (at extreme of age). Its weight varies from 135 mg (0-9 years) to 255 mg (40-80 years of age).
- It has got two surfaces: the anterior surface is less convex (radius of curvature 10 mm) than the posterior (radius of curvature 6 mm). These two surfaces meet at the equator.
- Its refractive index is 1.39 and total dioptric power is about 18 D (range 16-20 D).
- The accommodative power of lens varies with age, being 14-16 D (at birth); 7-8 D (at 25 years of age) and 1-2 D (at 50 years of age).

Structure (Fig. 8.1)

1. ***Lens capsule***. It is a thin, transparent, hyaline membrane surrounding the lens which is thicker over the anterior than the posterior surface. The lens capsule is thickest at pre-equator regions (14 μ) and thinnest at the posterior pole (3 μ).

2. ***Anterior epithelium.*** It is a single layer of cuboidal cells which lies deep to the anterior capsule. In the equatorial region these cells become columnar, are actively dividing and elongating to form new lens fibres throughout the life. There is no posterior epithelium, as these cells are used up in filling the central cavity of lens vesicle during development of the lens.

3. ***Lens fibres.*** The epithelial cells elongate to form lens fibres which have a complicated structural form. Mature lens fibres are cells which have lost their nuclei. As the lens fibres are formed throughout the life, these are arranged compactly as nucleus and cortex of the lens (Fig. 8.2).

i. *Nucleus.* It is the central part containing the oldest fibres. It consists of different zones, which are laid down successively as the development proceeds. In the beam of slit-lamp these are seen as zones of discontinuity. Depending upon the period of development, the different zones of the lens nucleus include:

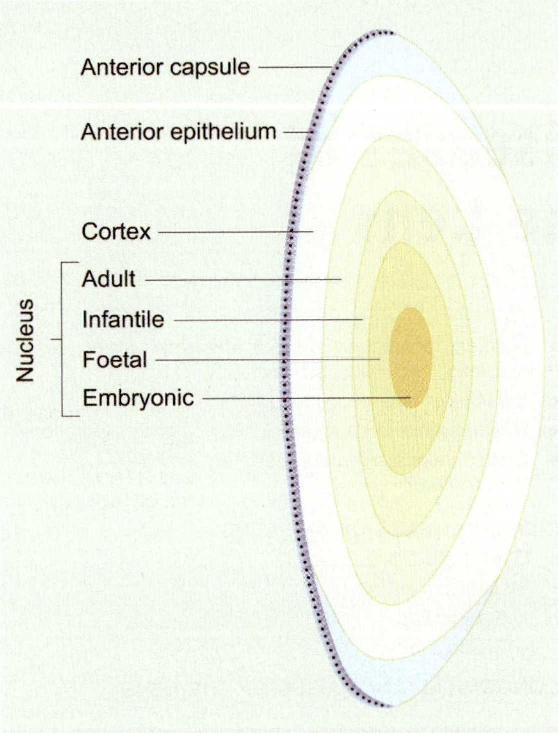

Fig. 8.1. Structure of the crystalline lens.

- *Embryonic nucleus.* It is the innermost part of nucleus which corresponds to the lens upto first 3 months of gestation. It consists of *primary lens fibres* which are formed by elongation of the cells of posterior wall of lens vesicle.
- *Fetal nucleus.* It lies around the embryonic nucleus and corresponds to the lens from 3 months of gestation till birth. Its fibres meet around sutures which are anteriorly Y-shaped and posteriorly inverted Y-shaped (Fig. 8.2).
- *Infantile nucleus* corresponds to the lens from birth to puberty, and
- *Adult nucleus* corresponds to the lens fibres formed after puberty to rest of the life.

ii. *Cortex.* It is the peripheral part which comprises the youngest lens fibres.

4. *Suspensory ligaments of lens* (Zonules of Zinn). Also called as *ciliary zonules,* these consist essentially of a series of fibres passing from ciliary body to the lens. These hold the lens in position and enable the ciliary muscle to act on it. These fibres are arranged in three groups:

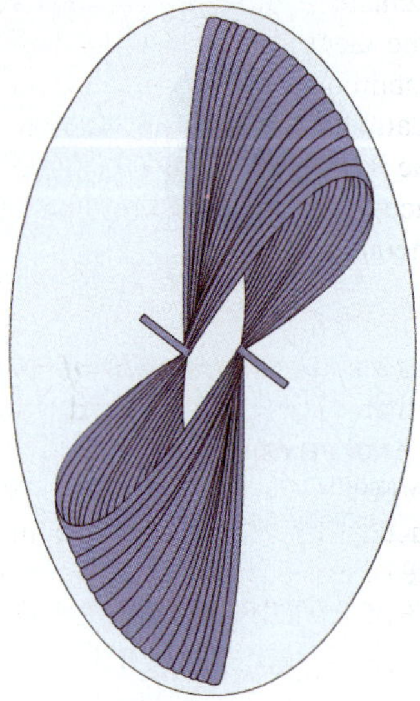

Fig. 8.2. Y-shaped sutures of the fetal nuclear fibres.

i. *Anterior fibres* originating from comparatively anteriorly placed ciliary processes pass posteriorly to be inserted posterior to the equator.
ii. *Middle group of fibres* passes from the summits of the ciliary processes almost directly inward to be inserted at the equator.
iii. *Posterior fibres* arising from pars plana and anterior part of ora serrata pass anteriorly to get inserted anterior to the equator.

APPLIED PHYSIOLOGY AND BIOCHEMISTRY

The crystalline lens is a transparent structure playing main role in the focussing mechanism for vision. Its physiological aspects include:

- Lens transparency,
- Metabolic activities of the lens, and
- Accommodation (see page 40)

Lens transparency

Factors that play significant role in maintaining outstanding clarity and transparency of lens are:

- Avascularity,
- Tightly-packed nature of lens cells,
- Narrow lens fibre membranes,
- Loss of organelles
- The arrangement of lens proteins,
- Semipermeable character of lens capsule,

- Pump mechanism of lens fibre membranes that regulate the electrolyte and water balance in the lens, maintaining relative dehydration and
- Auto-oxidation and high concentration of reduced glutathione in the lens maintains the lens proteins in a reduced state and ensures the integrity of the cell membrane pump.

Metabolism

Lens requires a continuous supply of energy (ATP) for active transport of ions and aminoacids, maintenance of lens dehydration, and for a continuous protein and GSH synthesis. Most of the energy produced is utilized in the epithelium which is the major site of all active transport processes. Only about 10-20% of the ATP generated is used for protein synthesis.

Source of nutrient supply. The crystalline lens, being an avascular structure is dependent for its metabolism on chemical exchanges with the aqueous humour. The chemical composition of the lens vis a vis aqueous humour and the chemical exchange between the two is depicted in Fig. 8.3.

Pathways of glucose metabolism. Glucose is very essential for the normal working of the lens. Metabolic activity of the lens is largely limited to epithelium, and cortex, while the nucleus is relatively inert. Pathways of glucose metabolism in the lens are as follows:

- *Glycolytic pathway.* In the lens, 80% glucose is metabolised anaerobically by this pathway.
- *Pentose, Hexose, Monophosphate (HMP) shunt* is responsible for metabolism of 15% of glucose.

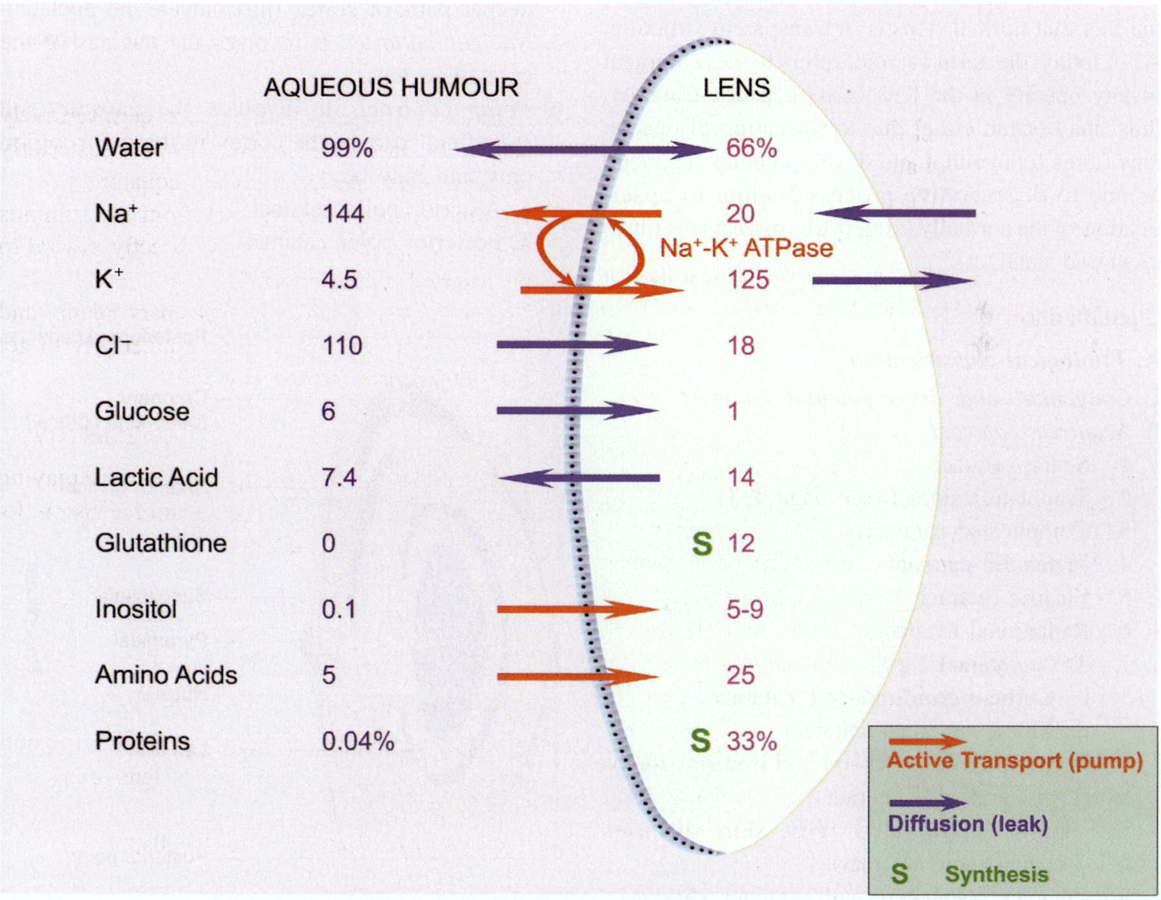

Fig. 8.3. Chemical composition of the lens vis-a-vis aqueous humour and the chemical exchange (pump-leak mechanism) between them. Values are in m moles/kg of lens water unless otherwise stated.

- *Kreb's citric acid cycle* metabolises only a small proportion by the oxidative process.
- *Sorbitol pathway* is relatively inconsequential in the normal lens; however, it is extremely important in the production of cataract in diabetic and galactosemic patients.

CATARACT

Definition

The word '*cataract*' dates from the Middle Ages and has been derived from the Greek word '*katarraktes*' which means '*waterfall*'. This term was coined assuming that an 'abnormal humour' developed and flowed in front of the lens to decrease the vision.
The present definition of cataract came much latter after the understanding of the lens anatomy and of the fact that normal lens is a transparent structure. As of today the term cataract refers to development of any opacity in the lens or its capsule. Cataract, thus may occur, either due to formation of opaque lens fibres (congenital and developmental cataracts) or due to degenerative process leading to opacification of the normally formed transparent lens fibres (acquired cataract).

Classification

A. *Etiological classification*

I. *Congenital and developmental cataract*

II. *Acquired cataract*

1. Senile cataract
2. Traumatic cataract (see page 433)
3. Complicated cataract
4. Metabolic cataract
5. Electric cataract
6. Radiational cataract
7. Toxic cataract e.g.,
   - i Corticosteroid-induced cataract
   - ii. Miotics-induced cataract
   - iii. Copper (in chalcosis) and iron (in siderosis) induced cataract.
8. Cataract associated with skin diseases (Dermatogenic cataract).
9. Cataract associated with osseous diseases.
10. Cataract with miscellaneous syndromes e.g.,
    - i. Dystrophica myotonica
    - ii. Down's syndrome.
    - iii. Lowe's syndrome
    - iv. Treacher - Collin's syndrome

B. *Morphological classification* (Fig. 8.4)

1. *Capsular cataract.* It involves the capsule and may be:
   - i. Anterior capsular cataract
   - ii. Posterior capsular cataract
2. *Subcapsular cataract.* It involves the superficial most part of the cortex (just below the capsule) and includes:
   - i. Anterior subcapsular cataract
   - ii. Posterior subcapsular cataract
3. *Cortical cataract.* It involves the major part of the cortex.
4. *Supranuclear cataract.* It involves only the deeper parts of cortex (just outside the nucleus).
5. *Nuclear cataract.* It involves the nucleus of the crystalline lens.
6. *Polar cataract.* It involves the capsule and superficial part of the cortex in the polar region only and may be:
   - i. Anterior polar cataract
   - ii. Posterior polar cataract

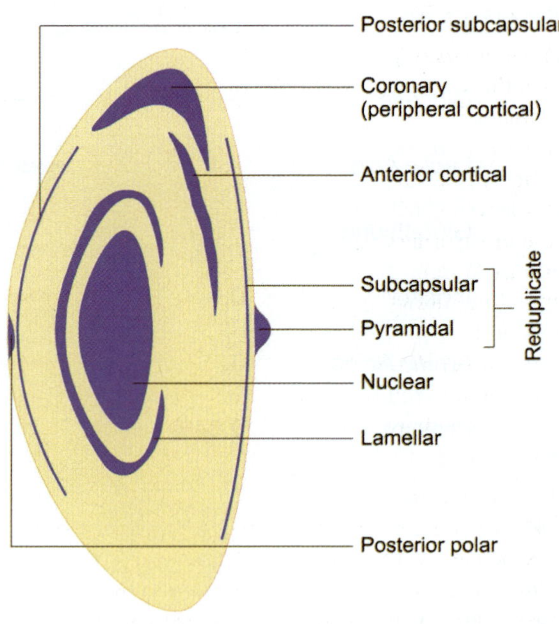

Fig. 8.4. Morphological shapes of cataract.

CONGENITAL AND DEVELOPMENTAL CATARACTS

Congenital and developmental cataracts occur due to some disturbance in the normal growth of the lens. When the disturbance occurs before birth, the child is born with a *congenital cataract.* Therefore, in congenital cataract the opacity is limited to either embryonic or foetal nucleus. *Developmental cataract* may occur from infancy to adolescence. Therefore, such opacities may involve infantile or adult nucleus, deeper parts of cortex or capsule. Developmental cataract typically affects the particular zone which is being formed when this process is disturbed. The fibres laid down previously and subsequently are often normally formed and remain clear. Congenital and developmental opacities assume most variegated appearance and minute opacities (without visual disturbance) are very common in normal population. These are detected with the beam of slit lamp under full mydriasis.

Etiology

About one third cases are idiopathic, one third are hereditary, and the rest one third due to other causes.

I. *Idiopathic.* About 33 percent cases are sporadic and of unknown etiology.

II. *Heredity.* About one-third of all congenital cataracts are hereditary.

Inherited cases without systemic disorders. In these cases the mode of inheritance is usually autosomal dominant.

Inherited cases with systemic disorders. These include the cataract occurring due to chromosomal disorders (e.g. trisomy 21), and those associated with skeletal disorders (e.g. Stickler syndrome), central nervous system disorders (e.g. cerebro-oculo-facial syndrome), renal system disorders (e.g. Lowe's syndrome)

Common familial cataracts. These include cataracta pulverulenta, zonular cataract (also occurs as non-familial), coronary cataract and total soft cataract (may also occur due to rubella).

III. *Maternal factors*

1. *Malnutrition* during pregnancy has been associated with non-familial zonular cataract.
2. *Infections.* Maternal infections like rubella are associated with cataract in 50 percent of cases. Other maternal infections associated with congenital cataract include *toxoplasmosis* and *cytomegalo-inclusion* disease.
3. *Drugs ingestion.* Congenital cataracts have also been reported in the children of mothers who have taken certain drugs during pregnancy (e.g., *thalidomide, corticosteroids).*
4. *Radiation.* Maternal exposure to radiation during pregnancy may cause congenital cataracts.

IV. *Foetal or infantile factors*

1. *Deficient oxygenation* (anoxia) owing to placental haemorrhage.
2. *Birth trauma,* may cause cataract.
3. *Metabolic disorders* of the foetus or infant such as galactosemia, galactokinase deficiency and neonatal hypoglycemia.
4. *Cataracts associated with other congenital anomalies* e.g., as seen in Lowe's syndrome, myotonia dystrophica and congenital icthyosis.
5. *Ocular diseases associated with developmental cataract* include persistent hyperplastic primary vitreous (PHPV), aniridia anterior chamber cleavage syndrome retinopathy of prematurity, lenticonus posterior and microopthalmos.
6. *Malnutrition* in early infancy may also cause developmental cataract.

Clinical types

Congenital and developmental cataracts have been variously classified. A simple morphological classification of congenital and developmental cataract is as under:

I. *Congenital capsular cataracts*
   1. Anterior capsular cataract
   2. Posterior capsular cataract

II. *Polar cataracts*
   1. Anterior polar cataract
   2. Posterior polar cataract

III. *Nuclear cataract*

IV. *Lamellar cataract*

V. *Sutural and axial cataracts*
   1. Floriform cataract
   2. Coralliform cataract
   3. Spear-shaped cataract
   4. Anterior axial embryonic cataract

VI. *Generalized cataracts*
   1. Coronary cataract
   2. Blue dot cataract
   3. Total congenital cataract
   4. Congenital membranous cataract

I. *Congenital capsular cataracts*

1. *Anterior capsular cataracts* are nonaxial, stationary and visually insignificant.

2. *Posterior capsular cataracts* are rare and can be associated with persistent hyaloid artery remnants.

II. *Polar cataracts*

1. *Anterior polar cataract.* It involves the central part of the anterior capsule and the adjoining superficial-most cortex. It may arise in the following ways:

i. *Due to delayed development of anterior chamber.* In this case the opacity is congenital usually bilateral, stationary and visually insignificant.

ii. *Due to corneal perforation.* Such cataracts may also be acquired in infantile stage and follow contact of the lens capsule with the back of cornea, usually after perforation due to ophthalmia neonatorum or any other cause.

Morphological types: Anterior polar cataracts may occur as any of the following morphological patterns:

i. *Thickened white plaque* in the centre of anterior capsule.

ii. *Anterior pyramidal cataract.* In this the thickened capsular opacity is cone-shaped with its apex towards cornea.

iii. *Reduplicated cataract* (double cataract). Sometimes along with thickening of central point of anterior capsule, lens fibres lying immediately beneath it also become opaque and are subsequently separated from the capsule by laying of transparent fibres in between. The burried opacity is called '*imprint*' and the two together constitute reduplicated cataract.

2. *Posterior polar cataract.* It is a very common lens anomaly and consists of a small circular circumscribed opacity involving the posterior pole.

Associations. Posterior polar cataract may be associated with:

- Persistent hyaloid artery remnants (Mittendorf dot),
- Posterior lenticonus, and
- Persistent hyperplastic primary vitreous (PHPV).

Types. Posterior polar cataract occurs in two forms:

- Stationary form and
- Progressive form which progresses after birth.

III. *Nuclear cataracts*

i. ***Cataracta centralis pulverulenta*** (Embryonic nuclear cataract). It has dominant genetic trait and occurs due to inhibition of the lens development at a very early stage and thus, involves the embryonic nucleus. The condition is bilateral and is characterised by a small rounded opacity lying exactly in the centre of the lens. The opacity has a powdery appearance (pulverulenta) and usually does not affect the vision.

ii. *Total nuclear cataract*. It usually involves the embryonic and fetal nucleus and sometimes infantile nucleus as well. It is characterized by a dense chalky white central opacity seriously impairing vision. The opacities are usually bilateral and non progressive.

IV. *Lamellar cataract*

Lamellar or Zonular cataract refer to the developmental cataract in which the opacity occupies a discrete zone in the lens. It is the most common type of congenital cataract presenting with visual impairment. It accounts for about 40 percent of the cases.

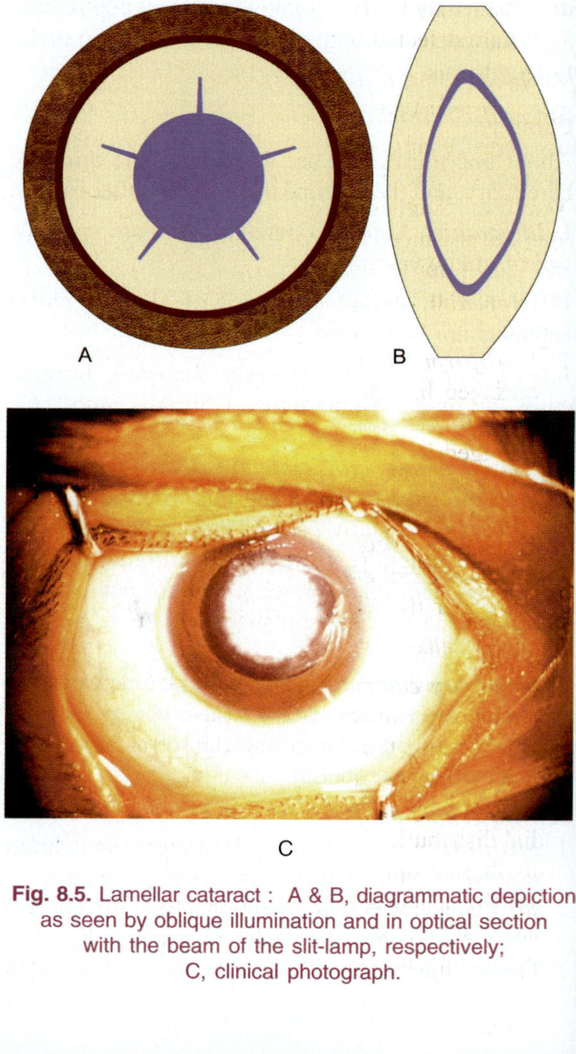

Fig. 8.5. Lamellar cataract : A & B, diagrammatic depiction as seen by oblique illumination and in optical section with the beam of the slit-lamp, respectively; C, clinical photograph.

Etiology. It may be either genetic or environmental in origin.

- *Genetic pattern* is usually of familial autosomal dominant variety.
- *Environmental form* is associated with:
  - vitamin D deficiency,
  - hypocalcemia
  - sometimes maternal rubella infection contracted between 7th and 8th week of gestation may also cause lamellar cataract.

Characteristic features. Typically, this cataract occurs in a zone of foetal nucleus surrounding the embryonic nucleus (Fig. 8.5).

- Occasionally two such rings of opacity are seen.
- The main mass of the lens internal and external to the zone of cataract is clear, except for small linear opacities like spokes of a wheel (riders) which may be seen towards the equator.
- It is usually bilateral and frequently causes severe visual defects.

V. *Sutural and axial cataracts*

Sutural cataracts are comparatively of common occurrence and consist of a series of *punctate opacities* scattered around the anterior and posterior Y-sutures. Such cataracts are usually static, bilateral and do not have much effect on the vision. The individual opacities vary in size and shape and have different patterns and thus are named accordingly as under:

1. *Floriform cataract.* Here the opacities are arranged like the petals of a flower.
2. *Coralliform cataract.* Here the opacities are arranged in the form of a coral.
3. *Spear-shaped cataract.* The lenticular opacities are in the form of scattered heaps of shining crystalline needles.
4. *Anterior axial embryonic cataract* occurs as fine dots near the anterior Y-suture of fetal nucleus.

VI. *Generalized cataracts*

1. *Coronary cataract* (Fig. 8.6). It is an extremely common form of developmental cataract occurring about puberty; thus involving either the adolescent nucleus or deeper layer of the cortex. The opacities are often many hundreds in number and have a regular radial distribution in the periphery of lens (corona of club-shaped opacities) encircling the central axis. Since the opacities are situated peripherally, vision is usually unaffected. Sometimes the associated large punctate opacities may marginally reduce the vision.

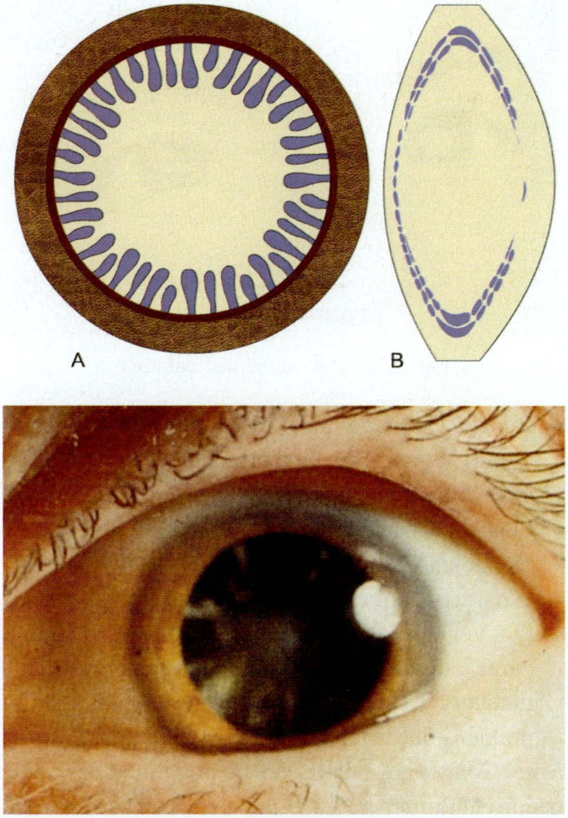

A B

C

Fig. 8.6. Coronary cataract : A & B as seen by oblique illumination and in optical section with the beam of the slit-lamp, respectively, C, clinical photograph.

2. *Blue dot cataract.* It is also called *cataracta-punctata-caerulea.* Perhaps this is the most common type of congenital cataract. It usually forms in the first two decades of life. The characteristic punctate opacities are in the form of rounded bluish dots situated in the peripheral part of adolescent nucleus and deeper layer of the cortex. Opacities are usually stationary and do not affect vision. However, large punctate opacities associated with coronary cataract may marginally reduce the vision.

3. *Total congenital cataract.* It is a common variety and may be unilateral or bilateral (Fig. 8.7). In many cases there may be hereditary character. Its other important cause is maternal rubella.

Rubella Cataract

- Maternal Rubella infection acquired during first trimester (second or third month) may cause rubella cataract.

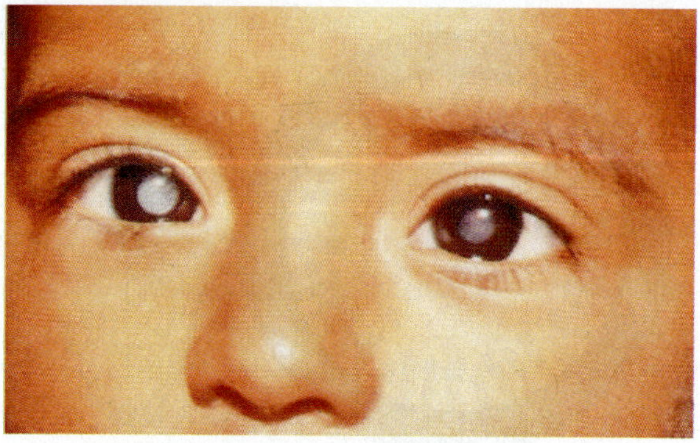

Fig. 8.7. Total congenital cataract.

- Rubella cataract-typically, the child is born with a 'pearly white' nuclear cataract. It is a progressive type of cataract.
- Lens matter may remain soft or may even liquify (congenital Morgagnian cataract).
- Cataractous nucleus may harbour the virus upto two years of age. Therefore, removal of such a cataract is usually followed by a severe inflammatory reaction (uveitis or even endophthalmitis) probably due to liberation of retained viruses.

Note: Congenital rubella can be prevented by vaccination of the mother. Since, the rubella vaccine is toxic to foetus, it must therefore, be administered atleast three months before the pregnancy.

Rubella Syndrome. Congenital rubella cataract may occur alone or as part of the classical rubella syndrome which consists of:

i. *Ocular defects* (Congenital cataract, salt and pepper chorioretinopathy, microphthalmos, cloudy cornea and poorly dilating pupil).
ii. *Ear defects* (Deafness due to destruction of organ of Corti).
iii. *Heart defects* (Patent ductus arteriosus, pulmonary stenosis and ventricular septal defects).

4. *Congenital membranous cataract.* Sometimes there may occur total or partial absorption of congenital cataract, leaving behind thin membranous cataract. Rarely there is complete disappearance of all the lens fibres and only a fine transparent lens capsule remains behind. Such a patient may be misdiagnosed as having congenital aphakia. This is associated with Hallermann-Streiff-Francois Syndrome.

Differential diagnosis

Congenital cataracts presenting with *leukocoria* need to be differentiated from various other conditions presenting with leukocoria such as retinoblastoma, retinopathy of prematurity, persistent hyperplastic primary vitreous (PHPV), etc. (also see page 302).

Management of congenital and developmental cataract

A. *Clinico-investigative work up.* A detailed clinico-investigative work up is most essential in the management of paediatric cataract. It should aim at knowing the prognostic factors and indications and timing of surgery.

1. *Ocular examination* should be carried out with special reference to:

- *Density and morphology of cataract.* Density is indicated by quality of red reflex seen on distant direct ophthalmoscopy before and after dilation of pupil. Cataract morphology may suggest underlying cause.
- *Assessment of visual function* is difficult in infants and small children. An idea may be made from the density and morphology of the cataract by oblique illumination examination and fundus examination. Special tests like fixation reflex, forced choice preferential looking test, visually evoked potential (VEP), optic-kinetic nystagmus (OKN) etc. also provide useful information.
- *Associated ocular defects* which need to be noted include microphthalmos, glaucoma, PHPV, foveal hypoplasia, optic nerve hypoplasia, and rubella retinopathy etc.

2. *Laboratory investigations* should be carried out to detect following systemic associations in non-hereditary cataracts:

- *Intrauterine infections* viz. toxoplasmosis, rubella, cytomegalo virus and herpes virus by TORCH test.
- *Galactosemia* by urine test for reducing substances, red blood cell transferase and glactokinase levels.
- *Lowe's syndrome* by urine chromatography for amino acids.
- *Hyperglycemia* by blood sugar level.

- *Hypocalcemia* by serum calcium and phosphate levels and X-ray skull.

B. *Prognostic factors* which need to be noted are:

- Density of cataract,
- Unilateral or bilateral cataract,
- Time of presentation,
- Associated ocular defects, and
- Associated systemic defects

C. *Indications and timing of paediatric cataract surgery,*

1. *Partial cataracts and small central cataracts* which are visually insignificant can safely be ignored and observed or may need non-surgical treatment with pupillary dilatation.
2. *Bilateral dense cataracts* should be removed early (within 6 weeks of birth) to prevent stimulus deprivation amblyopia. Second eye should be operated within a few days of the first eye.
3. *Unilateral dense cataract* should preferably be removed as early as possible (within days) after birth with optical correction in the first few weeks. However, it must be born in mind that visual prognosis in most of the unilateral cases is very poor even after timely operation, because correction of aphakia and prevention of amblyopia in infants is an uphill task.

D. *Surgical procedures.* Childhood cataracts, (congenital, developmental as well as acquired) can be dealt with anterior capsulorrhexis and irrigation aspiration of the lens matter or lensectomy. Surgical technique of these procedures is described on page 193.

Note. The *needling operation* (which was performed in the past) is now obsolete because of high rates of complications.

E. *Correction of paediatric aphakia*. It is still an unsolved query. Presently common views are as follows:

- *Children above the age of 2 years* can be corrected by implantation of posterior chamber intraocular lens during surgery.
- *Children below the age of 2 years* should preferably be treated by extended wear contact lens. Spectacles can be prescribed in bilateral cases. Later on secondary IOL implantation may be considered. Present trend is to do primary implantation at the earliest possible specially in unilateral cataract i.e. in all cases, because most surgeons have reported negative experiences in the compliance with glasses and contact lenses.

Paediatric IOL: size, design and power. The main concerns regarding the use of IOL in children are the growth of the eye, IOL power considerations, increased uveal reaction and long-term safety. Present recommendations are :

- *Size of IOL* above the age of 2 years may be standard 12 to 12.75 mm diameter for in the bag implantation.
- *Design of IOL* recommended has been one-piece PMMA with modified C-shaped haptics (preferably heparin coated). However, the capsular and inflammatory responses remain a problem. Presently most surgeon are prefering foldable IOLs made of hydrophobic acrylic material (e.g. Acrysof IOL, alcone lab, USA).
- *Power of IOL.* Most surgeons target emmetropia in older children (> 8 years). In children between 2-8 years of age 10% undercorrection and below 2 years an undercorrection by 20% is recommended from the calculated biometric power to counter the myopic shift.

F. *Correction of amblyopia*. It is the central theme around which management of childhood cataract and aphakia revolves. In spite of best efforts, it continues to be the main cause of ultimate low vision in these children. (For management see page 339).

ACQUIRED CATARACT

We have studied that congenital and developmental cataracts occur due to disturbance in the formation of the lens fibres, i.e., instead of clear, opaque lens fibres are produced. While, in acquired cataract, opacification occurs due to degeneration of the already formed normal fibres. A few common varieties of acquired cataract are described here.

AGE RELATED CATARACT

'Age-related cataract' also called as senile cataract is the commonest type of acquired cataract affecting equally persons of either sex usually above the age of 50 years. The condition is usually bilateral, but almost always one eye is affected earlier than the other.

Morphologically, the senile cataract occurs in two forms, the cortical (soft cataract) and the nuclear (hard cataract). The cortical senile cataract may start as cuneiform (more commonly) or cupuliform cataract.

It is very common to find nuclear and cortical senile cataracts co-existing in the same eye; and for this reason it is difficult to give an accurate assessment of their relative frequency. In general, the predominant form can be given as cuneiform 70 percent, nuclear 25 percent and cupuliform 5 percent.

Etiology

Senile cataract is essentially an ageing process. Though its precise etiopathogenesis is not clear, the various factors implicated are as follows:

A. *Risk Factors*

Risk factors affecting age of onset, type and maturation of senile cataract are as below:

1. ***Age.*** Age is the most important risk factor, i.e. why it is called age related cataract. As mentioned above it usually occurs after the age of 50 years. When it occur before 45 years of age, the term pre-senile cataract is used. By the age of 70 years, over 90% of the individuals develop senile cataract.

2. ***Sex.*** Without any doubt, the senile cataract affects both males as well as females. However, in many studies it is reported that prevalence of cataract is greater in females than males at all ages.

3. ***Heredity.*** It plays a considerable role in the incidence, age of onset and maturation of senile cataract in different families.

4. ***Ultraviolet irradiations.*** More exposure to UV irradiation from sunlight have been implicated for early onset and maturation of senile cataract in many epidemiological studies.

5. ***Dietary factors.*** Diet deficient in certain proteins, amino acids, vitamins (riboflavin, vitamin E, vitamin C), and essential elements have also been blamed for early onset and maturation of senile cataract.

6. ***Dehydrational crisis.*** An association with prior episode of severe dehydrational crisis (due to diarrhoea, cholera etc.) and age of onset and maturation of cataract is also suggested.

7. ***Smoking*** has also been reported to have some effect on the age of onset of senile cataract. In numerous studies worldwide smoking has consistently been associated with an increase in the frequency of nuclear cataract. Smoking causes accumulation of pigmented molecules—3 hydroxy-kynurinine and chromophores, which lead to yellowing. Cyanates in smoke causes carbamylation and protein denaturation.

B. Causes of presenile cataract. The term presenile cataract is used when the cataractous changes similar to senile cataract occur before 50 years of age. Its common causes are:

1. *Heredity.* As mentioned above because of influence of heredity, the cataractous changes may occur at an earlier age in successive generations.
2. *Diabetes mellitus.* Age-related cataract occurs earlier in diabetics. Nuclear cataract is more common and tends to progress rapidly.
3. *Myotonic dystrophy* is associated with posterior subcapsular type of presenile cataract.
4. *Atopic dermatitis* may be associated with presenile cataract (atopic cataract) in 10% of the cases.

C. *Concept of syn- and co-cataractogenic factors*

It has been conceptualized that cataract is the result of multiple subthreshold cataractogenic stresses acting in a concert. Age has been implicated as one of these cataractogenic stresses and that superimposition of other toxic stresses on the ageing lens may accelerated the rate of cataract formation. Conversely, the elimination of one or more subcataractogenic stresses may delay the cataract formation.

D. Mechanism of loss of transparency. It is basically different in nuclear and cortical senile cataracts.

1. ***Cortical senile cataract.*** Its main biochemical features are in decreased levels in the crystalline lens of total proteins, amino acids and potassium associated with increased concentration of sodium and marked hydration of the lens, followed by coagulation of lens proteins. The probable course of events leading to senile opacification of cortex is as shown in the Fig. 8.8.

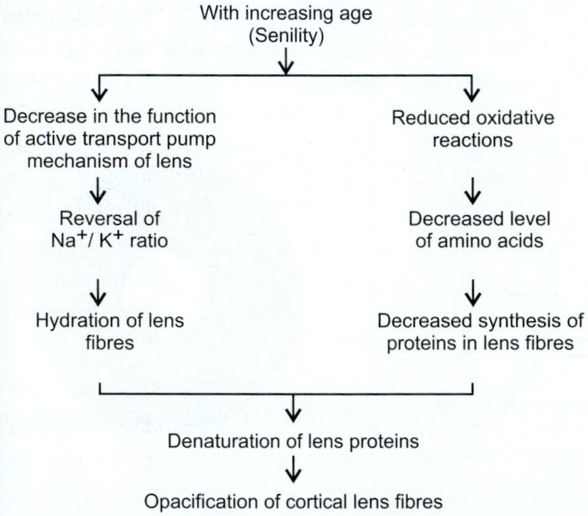

Fig. 8.8. Flow chart depicting probable course of events involved in occurence of cortical senile cataract.

2. *Nuclear senile cataract.* In this the usual degenerative changes are intensification of the age-related nuclear sclerosis associated with dehydration and compaction of the nucleus resulting in a hard cataract. It is accompanied by a significant increase in water insoluble proteins. However, the total protein content and distribution of cations remain normal. There may or may not be associated deposition of pigment urochrome and/or melanin derived from amino acids in the lens.

Stages of maturation

[A] *Maturation of the cortical type of senile cataract*

1. *Stage of lamellar separation.* The earliest senile change is demarcation of cortical fibres owing to their separation by fluid. This phenomenon of lamellar separation can be demonstrated by slit-lamp examination only. These changes are reversible.

2. *Stage of incipient cataract.* In this stage early detectable opacities with clear areas between them are seen. Two distinct types of senile cortical cataracts can be recognised at this stage:

(a) *Cuneiform senile cortical cataract.* It is characterised by wedge-shaped opacities with clear areas in between. These extend from equator towards centre and in early stages can only be demonstrated after dilatation of the pupil. They are first seen in the lower nasal quadrant. These opacities are present both in anterior and posterior cortex and their apices slowly progress towards the pupil. On oblique illumination these present a typical radial spoke-like pattern of greyish white opacities (Fig. 8.9). On distant direct ophthalmoscopy, these opacities appear as dark lines against the red fundal glow.

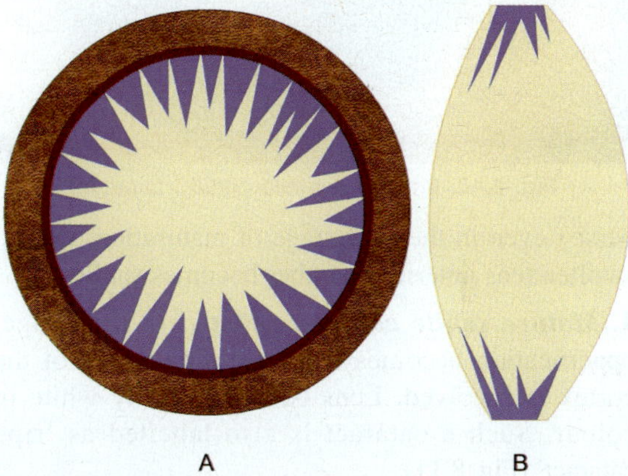

Fig. 8.9. Diagrammatic depiction of Immature senile cataract (cuneiform type): A, as seen by oblique illumination; B, in optical section with the beam of the slit-lamp.

Since the cuneiform cataract starts at periphery and extends centrally, the visual disturbances are noted at a comparatively late stage.

(b) *Cupuliform senile cortical cataract.* Here a saucer- shaped opacity develops just below the capsule usually in the central part of posterior cortex (*posterior subcapsular cataract*), which gradually extends outwards. There is usually a definite demarcation between the cataract and the surrounding clear cortex. Cupuliform cataract lies right in the pathway of the axial rays and thus causes an early loss of visual acuity.

3. *Immature senile cataract (ISC).* In this stage, opacification progresses further. The *cuneiform* (Fig. 8.9) or *cupuliform* patterns can be recognised till the advanced stage of ISC when opacification becomes more diffuse and irregular. The lens appears greyish white (Fig. 8.10) but clear cortex is still present and so iris shadow is visible.

In some patients, at this stage, lens may become swollen due to continued hydration. This condition is called '*intumescent cataract*'. Intumescence may

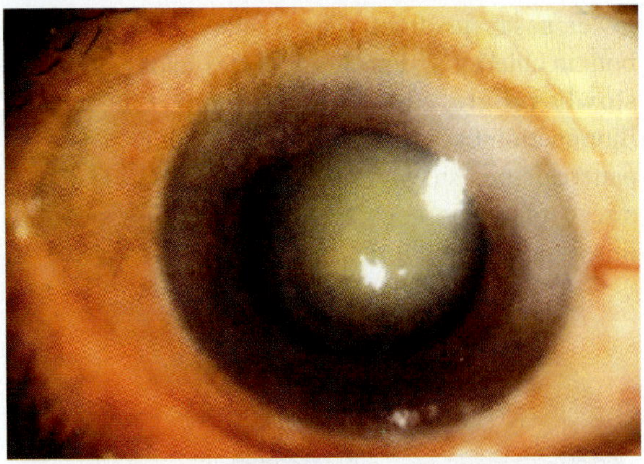

Fig. 8.10. Immature senile cortical cataract.

persist even in the next stage of maturation. Due to swollen lens anterior chamber becomes shallow.

4. *Mature senile cataract (MSC).* In this stage, opacification becomes complete, i.e., whole of the cortex is involved. Lens becomes pearly white in colour. Such a cataract is also labelled as 'ripe cataract' (Fig. 8.11).

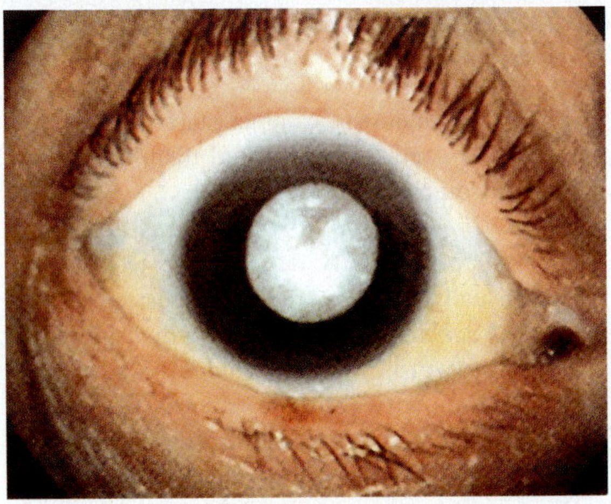

Fig. 8.11. Mature senile cortical cataract.

5. *Hypermature senile cataract (HMSC).* When the mature cataract is left in situ, the stage of hypermaturity sets in. The hypermature cataract may occur in any of the two forms:

(a) *Morgagnian hypermature cataract*: In some patients, after maturity the whole cortex liquefies and the lens is converted into a bag of milky fluid. The small brownish nucleus settles at the bottom, altering its position with change in the position of the head. Such a cataract is called *Morgagnian cataract* (Fig. 8.12). Sometimes in this stage, calcium deposits may also be seen on the lens capsule.

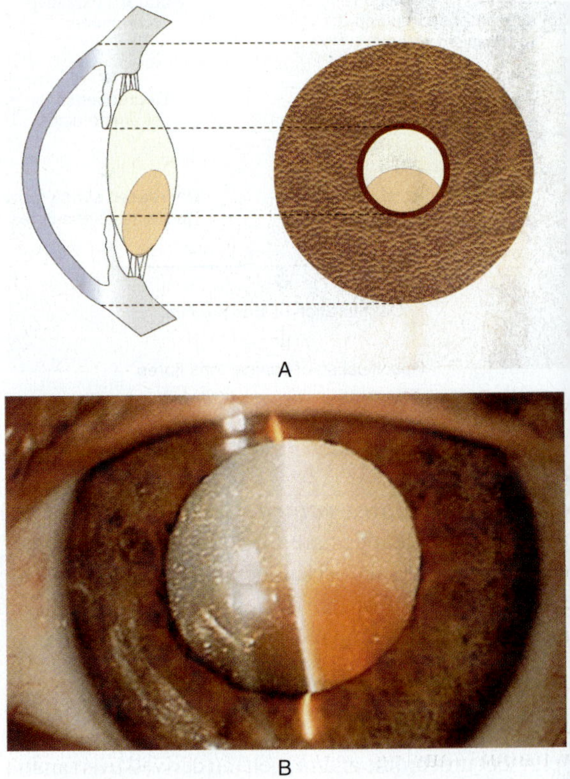

Fig. 8.12. Morgagnian hypermature senile cataract : A, diagrammatic depiction; B, clinical photograph.

(b) *Sclerotic type hypermature cataract:* Sometimes after the stage of maturity, the cortex becomes disintegrated and the lens becomes shrunken due to leakage of water. The anterior capsule is wrinkled and thickened due to proliferation of anterior cells and a dense white capsular cataract may be formed in the pupillary area. Due to shrinkage of lens, anterior chamber becomes deep and iris becomes tremulous (iridodonesis).

[B] *Maturation of nuclear senile cataract*

Progressive nuclear sclerotic process renders the lens inelastic and hard, decreases its ability to accommodate and obstructs the light rays. These changes begin centrally (Fig. 8.13) and spread slowly peripherally almost up to the capsule when it becomes mature; however, a very thin layer of clear cortex may remain unaffected.

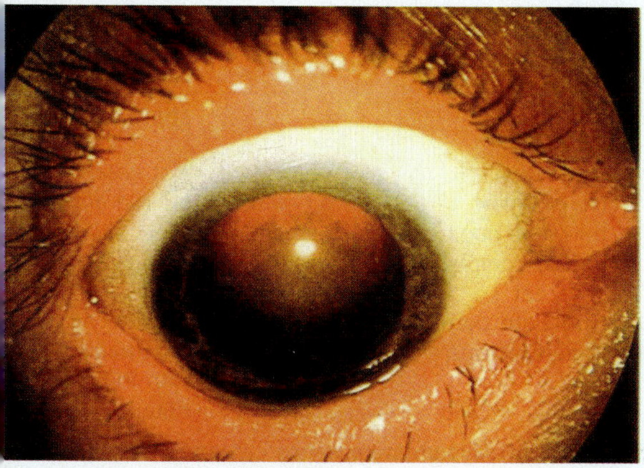

Fig. 8.13. Early nuclear senile cataract.

The nucleus may become diffusely cloudy (greyish) or tinted (yellow to black) due to deposition of pigments. In practice, the commonly observed pigmented nuclear cataracts are either amber, brown (*cataracta brunescens*) or black (*cataracta nigra*) and rarely reddish (*cataracta rubra*) in colour (Fig. 8.14).

Clinical features

Symptoms. An opacity of the lens may be present without causing any symptoms; and may be discovered on routine ocular examination. Common symptoms of cataract are as follows:

1. *Glare.* One of the earliest visual disturbances with the cataract is glare or intolerance of bright light; such as direct sunlight or the headlights of an oncoming motor vehicle. The amount of glare or dazzle will vary with the location and size of the opacity.
2. *Uniocular polyopia* (i.e., doubling or trebling of objects): It is also one of the early symptoms. It occurs due to irregular refraction by the lens owing to variable refractive index as a result of cataractous process.
3. *Coloured halos.* These may be perceived by some patients owing to breaking of white light into coloured spectrum due to presence of water droplets in the lens.
4. *Black spots in front of eyes.* Stationary black spots may be perceived by some patients.
5. *Image blur, distortion of images and misty vision* may occur in early stages of cataract.
6. *Loss of vision.* Visual deterioration due to senile cataract has some typical features. It is painless and gradually progressive in nature.

- Patients with central opacities (e.g., cupuliform cataract i.e. posterior subcapsular cataract) have early loss of vision. These patients see better when pupil is dilated due to dim light in the evening (*day blindness*).
- In patients with peripheral opacities (e.g. cuneiform cataract) visual loss is delayed and the vision improves in bright light when pupil is contracted.
- In patients with nuclear sclerosis, distant vision deteriorates due to progressive index myopia. Such patients may be able to read without presbyopic glasses. This improvement in near vision is referred to as '*second sight*'.

As opacification progresses, vision steadily diminishes, until only perception of light and accurate *projection of rays* remains in the stage of mature cataract.

Signs. Following examination should be carried out to look for different signs of cataract:

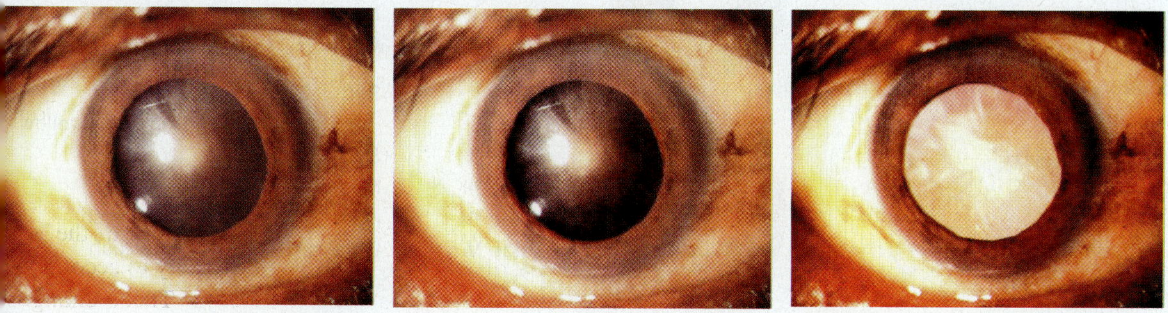

A B C

Fig. 8.14. Nuclear cataract: A, cataracta brunescens; B, cataracta nigra; and C, cataracta rubra.

Table 8.1. Signs of senile cataract

Examination	Nuclear cataract	ISC	MSC	HMSC(M)	HMSC(S)
1. Visual acuity	6/9 to PL+	6/9 to FC+	HM+ to PL+	PL+	PL+
2. Colour of lens	Grey, amber, brown, black or red	Greyish white	Pearly white with sinking brownish nucleus	Milky white	Dirty white with hyper-white spots
3. Iris shadow	Seen	Seen	Not seen	Not seen	Not seen
4. Distant direct ophthalmoscopy with dilated pupil	Central dark area against red fundal glow	Multiple dark areas against red fundal glow	No red glow but white pupil due to complete cataract	No red glow milky white pupil	No red glow
5. Slit-lamp examination	Nuclear opacity clear cortex	Areas of normal with cataractous cortex	Complete cortex is cataractous	Milky white sunken brownish nucleus	Shrunken cataractous lens with thickened anterior capsule

ISC: Immature senile cataract, MSC: Mature senile cataract, HMSC (M) Hypermature senile cataract (Morgagnian), HMSC (S): Hypermature senile cataract (Sclerotic), PL: Perception of light, HM: Hand movements, FC: Finger counting.

1. *Visual acuity testing.* Depending upon the location and maturation of cataract, the visual acuity may range from 6/9 to just PL + (Table 8.1).
2. *Oblique illumination examination.* It reveals colour of the lens in pupillary area which varies in different types of cataracts (Table 8.1).
3. *Test for iris shadow.* When an oblique beam of light is thrown on the pupil, a crescentric shadow of pupillary margin of the iris will be formed on the greyish opacity of the lens, as long as clear cortex is present between the opacity and the pupillary margin (Fig. 8.15). When lens is completely transparent or opaque, no iris shadow is formed. Hence, presence of iris shadow is a sign of immature cataract.

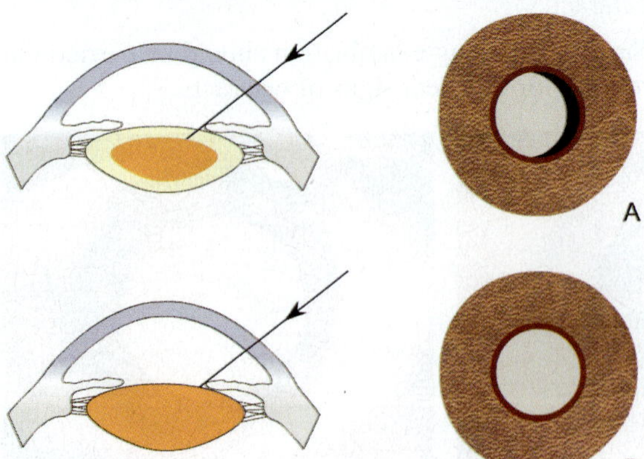

Fig. 8.15. Diagrammatic depiction of iris shadow in : immature cataract (A) and no iris shadow in mature cataract (B).

4. *Distant direct ophthalmoscopic examination* (for procedure see page 596). A reddish yellow fundal glow is observed in the absence of any opacity in the media. Partial cataractous lens shows black shadow against the red glow in the area of cataract. Complete cataractous lens does not even reveal red glow (Table 8.1).
5. *Slit-lamp examination* should be performed with a fully-dilated pupil. The examination reveals complete morphology of opacity (site, size, shape, colour pattern and hardness of the nucleus).

Grading of nucleus hardness in a cataractous lens is important for setting the parameters of machine in phacoemulsification technique of cataract extraction. The hardness of the nucleus, depending upon its colour on slit-lamp examination, can be graded as shown in Table 8.2 and Fig. 8.16:

Table 8.2. Grading of nucleus hardness on slit-lamp biomicroscopy.

Grade of hardness	Description of hardness	Colour of nucleus
Grade I	Soft	White or greenish yellow
Grade II	Soft-medium	Yellowish
Grade III	Medium-hard	Amber
Grade IV	Hard	Brownish
Grade V	Ultrahard (rock-hard)	Blackish

The signs observed on above examinations in different stages of senile cataract are shown in Table 8.1

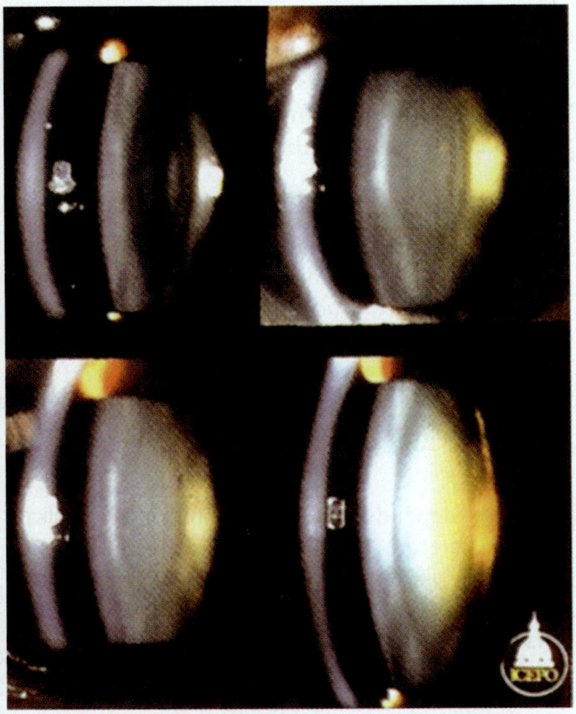

Fig. 8.16. Slit-lamp biomicroscopic grading of nucleus hardness in cataractous lens.

Differential diagnosis

1. *Immature senile cataract (ISC)* can be differentiated from the nuclear sclerosis without any cataract as shown in Table 8.3.

Table 8.3. Immature senile cataract versus nuclear sclerosis

ISC	*Nuclear sclerosis*
1. Painless progressive loss of vision	1. Painless progressive loss of vision
2. Greyish colour of lens on oblique illumination examination	2. Greyish colour of lens
3. Iris shadow is present	3. Iris shadow is absent
4. Black spots against red glow are observed on distant direct ophthalmoscopy	4. No black spots are seen against red glow
5. Slit-lamp examination reveals area of cataractous cortex	5. Slit-lamp examination reveals clear lens
6. Visual acuity does not improve on pin-hole testing	6. Visual acuity usually improves on pin-hole testing

II. *Mature senile cataract* can be differentiated from other causes of white pupillary reflex (leukocoria) as shown in Table 8.4.

Table 8.4. Differences between mature senile cataract and leukocoria

MSC	*Leukocoria*
1. White reflex in pupillary area	1. White reflex in pupillary area
2. Size of pupil usually normal	2. Pupil usually semidilated
3. Fourth Purkinje image is absent	3. Fourth Purkinje image is present
4. Slit-lamp examination shows cataractous lens	4. Slit-lamp examination shows transparent lens with white reflex behind the lens
5. Ultrasonography normal	5. Ultrasonography reveals opacity in the vitreous cavity

Complications

1. *Phacoanaphylactic uveitis.* A hypermature cataract may leak lens proteins into anterior chamber. These proteins may act as antigens and induce antigen-antibody reaction leading to phacoanaphylactic uveitis.

2. *Lens-induced glaucoma.* It may occur by different mechanisms e.g., due to intumescent lens *(phacomorphic glaucoma)* and leakage of proteins into the anterior chamber from a hypermature cataract *(phacolytic glaucoma)* (for detail see page 247).

3. *Subluxation or dislocation of lens.* It may occur due to degeneration of zonules in hypermature stage.

METABOLIC CATARACTS

These cataracts occur due to endocrine disorders and biochemical abnormalities. A few common varieties of metabolic cataracts are described here.

Diabetic cataract

Diabetes is associated with two types of cataracts:

1. *Senile cataract in diabetics* appears at an early age and progresses rapidly.

2. *True diabetic cataract.* The classical diabetic cataract is also called *'snowflake cataract'* or *'snowstorm cataract'*. It is a rare condition, usually occurring in young adults due to osmotic overhydration of the lens. Osmotic over hydration of the lens occurs due to accumulation of sorbitol, when glucose is metabolised by aldose reductase. Initially a large number of fluid vacuoles appear underneath the anterior and posterior capsules, which is soon followed by appearance of bilateral snowflake-like white opacities in the cortex. Such opacities may resolve spontaneously or mature within a few days.

Galactosaemic cataract

It is associated with inborn error of galactose metabolism. Galactosaemia occurs in two forms:

1. *Classical galactosaemia* occurs due to deficiency of galactose-1 phosphate uridyl-transferase (GPUT); and
2. A related disorder occurs due to *deficiency of galactokinase (GK).*

Characteristic features. Galactosaemia is frequently associated with the development of bilateral cataract (*oil droplet central lens opacities*). The lens changes may be reversible and occurrence of cataract may be prevented, if milk and milk products are eliminated from the diet when diagnosed at an early stage.

Hypocalcaemic (Tetanic) cataract

Cataractous changes may be associated with parathyroid tetany, which may occur due to atrophy or inadvertent removal (during thyroidectomy) of parathyroid glands. Multicoloured crystals or small discrete white flecks of opacities are formed in the cortex which seldom mature. In infants, hypocalcemia may produce zonular cataract, characterized by a thin opacified lamella deep in the infantile cortex.

Cataract due to error of copper metabolism

Inborn error of copper metabolism results in Wilson's disease (hepatolenticular degeneration). The green '*sunflower cataract*' characterised by yellowish brown dots may be observed rarely in such patients due to the deposition of cuprous oxide in the anterior lens capsule and subcapsular cortex in a stellate pattern. The more commonly observed ocular feature of Wilson's disease is golden 'Kayser-Fleischer ring' (KF ring) due to deposition in peripheral part of Descemet's membrane in the cornea.

Cataract in Lowe's syndrome

Lowe's (Oculo-cerebral-renal) syndrome is a rare inborn error of amino acid metabolism.

- *Ocular features* include congenital cataract, glaucoma and blue sclera.
- *Systemic features* of this syndrome are mental retardation, dwarfism, osteomalacia, muscular hypotonia and frontal prominence.

COMPLICATED CATARACT

It refers to opacification of the lens secondary to some other intraocular disease. Some authors use the term *secondary cataract* for the complicated cataract. Many authors use the term secondary cataract to denote after cataract. Therefore, to avoid confusion and controversy, preferably, the term secondary cataract should be discarded.

Etiology

The lens depends for its nutrition on intraocular fluids. Therefore, any condition in which the ocular circulation is disturbed or in which inflammatory toxins are formed, will disturb nutrition of the crystalline lens, resulting in development of complicated cataract. Some important ocular conditions giving rise to complicated cataract are listed here.

1. *Inflammatory conditions.* These include uveal inflammations (like iridocyclitis, parsplanitis, choroiditis), hypopyon corneal ulcer and endophthalmitis.
2. *Degenerative conditions* such as retinitis pigmentosa and other pigmentary retinal dystrophies and myopic chorioretinal degeneration.
3. *Retinal detachment.* Complicated cataract may occur in long-standing cases.
4. *Glaucoma (primary or secondary)* may sometimes result in complicated cataract. The underlying cause here is probably the embarrassment to the intraocular circulation, consequent to the raised pressure.
5. *Intraocular tumours* such as retinoblastoma or melanoma may give rise to complicated cataract in late stages.

Clinical features

Typically the complicated cataract starts as *posterior subcapsular cortical cataract.* The opacity is irregular in outline and variable in density. In the beam of slit-lamp the opacities have an appearance like '*bread-crumb*'. A very characteristic sign is the appearance of iridescent coloured particles the so-called '*polychromatic lustre*' of reds, greens and blues. A diffuse yellow-haze is seen in the adjoining cortex. Slowly the opacity spreads in the rest of the cortex, and finally the entire lens becomes opaque, giving chalky white appearance. Deposition of calcium is common in the later stages.

DRUG INDUCED CATARACTS

Corticosteroid-induced cataract

Posterior subcapsular opacities are associated with the use of topical as well as systemic steroids. The exact relationship between dose and duration of corticosteroid therapy with the development of cataract is still unclear. However, in general, prolonged use of steroids in high doses may result in cataract formation. Children are more susceptible than adults.

Therefore, it is recommended that all patients with diseases requiring prolonged corticosteroids therapy should be regularly examined on slit-lamp by an ophthalmologist. Further, intermittent regimes should be preferred over regular therapy and whenever possible steroids should be substituted by non-steroidal anti-inflammatory drugs (NSAIDs).

Miotics-induced cataract

Anterior subcapsular granular type of cataract may be associated with long-term use of miotics, particularly long acting cholinesterase inhibitors such as echothiophate, demecarium bromide, disopropyl fluorophosphate (DFP). Removal of the drug may stop progression and occasionally may cause reversal of cataract.

Other drug induced cataracts

Other drugs associated with fine toxic cataracts are amiodarone, chlorpromazine, busulphan, gold and allopurinol.

RADIATIONAL CATARACT

Exposure to almost all types of radiant energy is known to produce cataract by causing damage to the lens epithelium. Following types are known:

1. Infrared (heat) cataract

Prolonged exposure (over several years) to infra-red rays may cause discoid posterior subcapsular opacities and true exfoliation of the anterior capsule. It is typically seen in persons working in glass industries, so also called as '*glass-blower's* or *glass-worker's cataract*'.

2. Irradiation cataract

Exposure to X-rays, γ-rays or neutrons may be associated with irradiation cataract. There is usually a latent period ranging from 6 months to a few years between exposure and development of the cataract. People prone to get such cataracts are inadequately protected technicians, patients treated for malignant tumours and workers of atomic energy plants.

3. Ultraviolet radiation cataract

Long term exposure to ultraviolet radiation has been linked with senile cataract in many studies.

ELECTRIC CATARACT

It is known to occur after passage of powerful electric current through the body. The cataract usually starts as punctate subcapsular opacities which mature rapidly. The source of current can be a live electricity wire or a flash of lightning.

SYNDERMATOTIC CATARACT

Lens opacities associated with cutaneous disease are termed *syndermatotic cataracts*. Such cataracts are bilateral and occur at a young age. *Atopic dermatitis* is the most common cutaneous disease associated with cataract *(Atopic cataract)*. Other skin disorders associated with cataract include poikiloderma, vasculare atrophicus, scleroderma and keratotis follicularis.

MANAGEMENT OF CATARACT IN ADULTS

Treatment of cataract essentially consists of its surgical removal. However, certain non-surgical measures may be of help, in peculiar circumstances, till surgery is taken up.

A. Non-surgical measures

1. *Treatment of cause of cataract.* In acquired cataracts, thorough search should be made to find out the cause of cataract. Treatment of the causative disease, many a time, may stop progression and sometimes in early stages may cause even regression of cataractous changes and thus defer the surgical treatment. Some common examples include:

- Adequate control of diabetes mellitus, when discovered.
- Removal of cataractogenic drugs such as corticosteroids, phenothiazenes and strong miotics, may delay or prevent cataractogenesis.

- Removal of irradiation (infrared or X-rays) may also delay or prevent cataract formation.
- Early and adequate treatment of ocular diseases like uveitis may prevent occurrence of complicated cataract.

2. ***Measures to delay progression*** include:
- *Topical preparations containing iodide salts of calcium and potassium* are being prescribed in abundance in early stages of cataract (especially in senile cataract) in a bid to delay its progression. However, till date no conclusive results about their role are available.
- *Role of vitamin E* and *aspirin* in delaying the process of cataractogenesis is also mentioned.

3. ***Measures to improve vision in the presence of incipient and immature cataract*** may be of great solace to the patient. These include:
- *Refraction,* which often changes with considerable rapidity, should be corrected at frequent intervals.
- *Arrangement of illumination.* Patients with peripheral opacities (pupillary area still free), may be instructed to use brilliant illumination. Conversely, in the presence of central opacities, a dull light placed beside and slightly behind the patient's head will give the best result.
- *Use of dark goggles* in patients with central opacities is of great value and comfort when worn outdoors.
- *Mydriatics.* The patients with a small axial cataract, frequently may benefit from pupillary dilatation. This allows the clear paraxial lens to participate in light transmission, image formation and focussing. Mydriatics such as 5 percent phenylephrine or 1 percent tropicamide; 1 drop b.i.d. in the affected eye may clarify vision.

B. Surgical management

Indications

1. ***Visual improvement.*** This is by far the most common indication. When surgery should be advised for visual improvement varies from person to person depending upon the individual visual needs. So, an individual should be operated for cataract, when the visual handicap becomes a significant deterrent to the maintenance of his or her usual life-style.

2. ***Medical indications.*** Sometimes patients may be comfortable from the visual point (due to useful vision from the other eye or otherwise) but may be advised cataract surgery due to medical grounds such as
- Lens induced glaucoma,
- Phacoanaphylactic endophthalmitis and
- Retinal diseases like diabetic retinopathy or retinal detachment, treatment of which is being hampered by the presence of lens opacities.

3. ***Cosmetic indication.*** Sometimes patient with mature cataract may insist for cataract extraction (even with no hope of getting useful vision), in order to obtain a black pupil.

Preoperative evaluation and workup

Once it has been decided to operate for cataract, a thorough preoperative evaluation should be carried out before contemplating surgery. This should include:

I. ***General medical examination of the patient*** to exclude the presence of systemic diseases especially: diabetes mellitus; hypertension and cardiac problems; obstructive lung disorders and any potential source of infection in the body such as septic gums, urinary tract infection etc.

II. ***Ocular examination.*** A thorough examination of eyes including slit lamp biomicroscopy is desirable in all cases. The following useful information is essential before the patient is considered for surgery:

1. ***Visual status assessment*** should include:
- *Visual acuity* should be noted unaided, best corrected and with pin hole testing.
- *Perception of light* (PL) must be noted. Absence of PL indicates nil visual prognosis.
- *Projection of rays* (PR) It is a crude but an important and easy test for function of the peripheral retina. It is tested in a semi-dark room with the opposite eye covered. A thin beam of light is thrown in the patient's eye from four directions (up, down, medial and lateral) and the patient is asked to look straight ahead and point out the direction from which the light seems to come. Inaccurate PR may be due to old retinal detachment, visual pathway defects, advanced glaucoma, large area of chorio-retinal atrophy and indicates poor visual prognosis. However, sometimes in dense cataract PR may be inaccurate with good visual prognosis.
- *Potential visual acuity tests* which may be required in the presence of opaque media include:

– Laser interferometry (LI), and
– Potential acuity meter (PAM) test.

2. *Pupils* should be examined to check for:
- Light reactions and RAPD, and
- Ability of the pupils to dilate adequately before surgery.

3. *Anterior segment evaluation* by slit lamp biomicroscopy is must before cataract surgery.
- *Cornea* should be examined to note any scarring, endothelial status (guttata). In patients with suspicion of endothelial dystrophy, *specular microscopy examination* should be carried out for endothelial cell count and morphology. Normal cell count in elderly patients is 2000-2500 cell/mm^2. Special care is needed in patients with cell counts below 1500 cells/mm^2.
- *Keratic precipitates* (*K.Ps.*) noted at the back of cornea suggest management of subtle uveitis before the cataract surgery.
- *Cataractous lens* should be evaluated for morphology and maturity of cataract and for grade of nuclear sclerosis (especially important for planning phacoemulsification surgery. See page 190)
- *Other signs* to be particularly looked for include posterior synechiae, pseudoexfoliation, iridodonosis, pigments over the anterior lens capsule, and anterior chamber depth.

4. *Intraocular pressure* (IOP) should be measured in each case, preferably by applanation tonometry. Presence of a raised IOP needs a priority management.

5. *Examination of lids, conjunctiva and lacrimal apparatus*. Search for local source of infection should be made by ruling out conjunctival infections, meibomitis, blepharitis and lacrimal sac infection. Conjunctival swab culture and sensitivity should be carried out in doubtful cases. Lacrimal sac should receive special attention. Lacrimal syringing should be carried out in a patient with history of watering from the eyes. In cases where chronic dacryocystitis is discovered, either DCR (dacryocystorhinostomy) or DCT (dacryocystectomy) operation should be performed, before the cataract surgery.

6. *Fundus examination,* wherever possible, should be carried out with special attention on macula, to rule out other causes of decreased vision. Indirect ophthalmoscopy may be useful in hazy media.

7. *Macular function tests* are important to predict the visual potential in patients with very dense cataracts where fundus examination is not possible a few simple macular functions tests are as below:

i. *Projection of rays (PR).* It is a crude but an important and easy test for function of the peripheral retina. It is tested in a semi-dark room with the opposite eye covered. A thin beam of light is thrown in the patient's eye from four directions (up, down, medial and lateral) and the patient is asked to look straight ahead and point out the direction from which the light seems to come.

ii. *Two-light discrimination test.* The patient is asked to look through an opaque disc perforated with two pin-holes behind which a light is held. The holes are 2 inches apart and kept about 2 feet away from the eye. If the patient can perceive two lights, it indicates normal macular function.

iii. *Maddox rod test.* The patient is asked to look at a distant bright light through a Maddox rod. An accurate perception of red line indicates normal function.

iv. *Colour perception.* It indicates that some macular function is present and optic nerve is relatively normal.

v. *Entoptic visualisation.* It is evaluated by rubbing a point source of light (such as bare lighted bulb of torch) against the closed eyelids. If the patient perceives the retinal vascular pattern in black outline, it is favourable indication of retinal function. Being subjective in nature, the importance of negative test can be considered if the patient can perceive the pattern with the opposite eye.

8. *Objective test for evaluating retina* are required if some retinal pathology is suspected. These tests includes ultrasonic evaluation of posterior segment of the eye; electrophysiological studies such as ERG (electroretinogram), EOG (electrooculogram) and VER (visually-evoked response);

9. *Keratometry and biometry* to calculate power of intraocular lens (IOL) to be implanted are performed in each case to be taken up for cataract surgery (For details see page 208)

Preoperative medications and preparations

1. *Consent*, with detailed information about the procedure, risks involved and outcome expected, should be obtained from each patient.

2. *Scrub bath, care of hair and marking of the eye.* Each patient should be instructed to have a scrub bath including face and hair wash with soap and water. Male patients must get their beard cleaned and hair trimmed. Female patients should comb their hair properly. The eye to be operated should be marked.

3. *Preoperative antibiotics and disinfectants* are required to prevent postoperative endophthalmitis:

- *Topical antibiotics* such as fourth-generation fluoroquinolone (0.3% moxifloxacin or 0.3% gatifloxacin) may be used QID for 3 days before surgery to eradicate conjunctival bacterial flora.
- *Povidone-Iodine (10%) solution* should be used to paint the lids and facial skin 3 hours before surgery.
- *Povidonbe-Iodine (5%) solution* should be used to irrigate the conjunctival sac just before surgery.

4. *IOP lowering* is must for conventional extra-capsular cataract extraction (ECCE). A few surgeons also prefer to lower IOP in manual small incision cataract surgery (SICS) and phacoemulsification. It can be accomplished by mechanical pressure (digital massage or Honan balloon) and/or by IOP lowering drugs (I.V. mannitol or acetazolamide).

5. *Mydriasis*, sustained through out the procedure is required. It can be obtained by:

- *Topical tropicamide* 1% (or cyclopentolate)+ phenylephrine 2.5% instilled every 15 minutes 4 times before surgery.
- *Topical cyclooxygenase* inhibitor e.g. flurbiprofen 0.3% or, ketorolac 0.5%, or diclofenac 0.1 % instilled 3 times a day before the surgery and every 15 minutes, 4 times immediately before the surgery helps in maintaining mydriasis during the procedure.

Anaesthesia

Cataract extraction can be performed under general or local anaesthesia. Local anaesthesia is preferred whenever possible. Many surgeons prefer only topical anaesthesia for phacoemulsification (for details see page 603).

Types and choice of surgical techniques

I. *Intracapsular cataract extraction (ICCE)* . In this technique, the entire cataractous lens along with the intact capsule is removed. Therefore, weak and degenerated zonules are a pre-requisite for this method.

Indications. ICCE has stood the test of time and had been widely employed for about 50 years over the world. Now (for the last 30 years) it has been almost entirely replaced by planned extracapsular techniques. At present the only indications of ICCE is markedly subluxated and dislocated lens.

II. *Extracapsular cataract extraction techniques.* In these techniques, major portion of anterior capsule with epithelium, nucleus and cortex are removed; leaving behind intact posterior capsule.

Indications. Presently, extracapsular cataract extraction techniques are the surgery of choice for almost all types of adulthood as well as childhood cataracts unless contraindicated.

Contraindications. The only absolute contraindication for ECCE is markedly subluxated or dislocated lens.

Advantages of ECCE techniques over ICCE

1. ECCE is a universal operation and can be performed at all ages, except when zonules are not intact; whereas ICCE cannot be performed below 40 years of age.
2. Posterior chamber IOL can be implanted after ECCE, while it cannot be implanted after ICCE.
3. Postoperative vitreous related problems (such as herniation in anterior chamber, pupillary block and vitreous touch syndrome) associated with ICCE are not seen after ECCE.
4. Incidence of postoperative complications such as endophthalmitis, cystoid macular oedema and retinal detachment are much less after ECCE as compared to that after ICCE.
5. Postoperative astigmatism is less with ECCE techniques, as the incision is smaller.
6. Prognosis for subsequent glaucoma filtering or corneal transplantation (if required) is much improved with ECCE.
7. Incidence of secondary rubeosis in diabetics is reduced after ECCE.

Different techniques of extracapsular cataract extraction

The surgical techniques of ECCE presently in vogue are:

- Conventional extracapsular cataract extraction (ECCE),
- Manual small incision cataract surgery (SICS),
- Phacoemulsification

Conventional ECCE versus SICS

Conventional large incision ECCE, though still being performed by many surgeons, is being largely replaced by small incision cataract surgery (SICS) and phacoemulsification techniques.

Merits of conventional ECCE over SICS. The only merit of conventional ECCE over SICS is that it is a simple technique to master with short learning curve.

Demerits of conventional ECCE over SICS include:

- Long incision (10 to 12 mm).
- Multiple sutures are required.
- Open chamber surgery with high risk of vitreous prolapse, operative hard eye and expulsive choroidal haemorrhage.
- High incidence of post-operative astigmatism.
- Postoperative suture-related problems like irritation and suture abscess etc.
- Postoperative wound-related problems such as wound leak, shallowing of anterior chamber and iris prolapse.
- Needs suture removal, during which infection may occur.

Merits of manual SICS over phacoemulsification

1. *Universal applicability* i.e., all types of cataracts including hard cataracts (grade IV and V) can be operated by this technique.
2. *Learning curve.* This procedure is much easier to learn as compared to phacoemulsification.
3. *Not machine dependent.* The biggest advantage of manual SICS is that it is not machine dependent and thus can be practised anywhere.
4. *Less surgical complications.* Disastrous complication like nuclear drop into vitreous cavity is much less than phacoemulsification technique.
5. *Operating time* in manual SICS is less than that of phocoemulsification, especially in hard cataract. Therefore, it is ideal for mass surgery.
6. *Cost effective.* With manual SICS, the expenses are vastly reduced as compared to considerable expenses in acquiring and maintaining phaco machine. There is no need to spend on consumable items like the phacotip, sleeves, tubing and probe. Further, in SICS non-foldable (PMMA) IOLs are used which are much cheaper than foldable IOLs.

Demerits of manual SICS over phacoemulsification

1. *Conjunctival congestion* persists for 5-7 days at the site of conjunctival flap.
2. *Mild tenderness* sometime may be present owing to scleral incision.
3. *Postoperative hyphema* may be noted sometimes.
4. *Surgical induced astigmatism* is more as the incision in SICS is large (about 6 mm) as compared to phacoemulsification (about 3.2 mm).

Merits of phacoemulsification over manual SICS

1. *Topical anaesthesia* may be sufficient for phacoemulsification in expert hands.
2. *Postoperative congestion* is minimal after phacoemulsification, as phaco is usually performed through a clear corneal incision.
3. *Small incision.* The chief advantage of phacoemulsification over manual SICS is that it can be performed through a smaller (3.2 mm) incision.
4. *Less corneal complications.* Phacoemulsification can be performed in the posterior chamber without prolapsing the nucleus into the anterior chamber, thereby minimising the risk of corneal complications.
5. *Visual rehabilitation* is comparatively quicker in phacoemulsification as compared to manual SICS.
6. *Postoperative astigmatism* is comparatively less when foldable IOLs are implanted through a smaller incision (3.2 mm).

Demerits of phacoemulsification vis-a-vis manual SICS

1. *Learning curve* for phacoemulsification is more painful both for the surgeons and patients.
2. *Complications* encountered during phacoemulsification like nuclear drop are unforgiving.
3. *Machine dependent.* This procedure is solely machine dependent and in the event of an unfortunate machine failure in the middle of surgery one has to shift to conventional ECCE.
4. *High cost.* Cost of this technique is very high because of expensive machine, accessories and maintenance.
5. *Limitations.* It is very difficult to deal with hard cataracts (grade IV and V) with this technique, and also there is high risk of serious corneal complications due to more use of phaco energy in such cases.

Conclusion. Inspite of the demerits listed above the phacoemulsification has become the preferred method of cataract extraction world wide because the complication rate in the expert hands is minimal and the technique provides an almost quiet eye early postoperatively and an early visual rehabilitation.

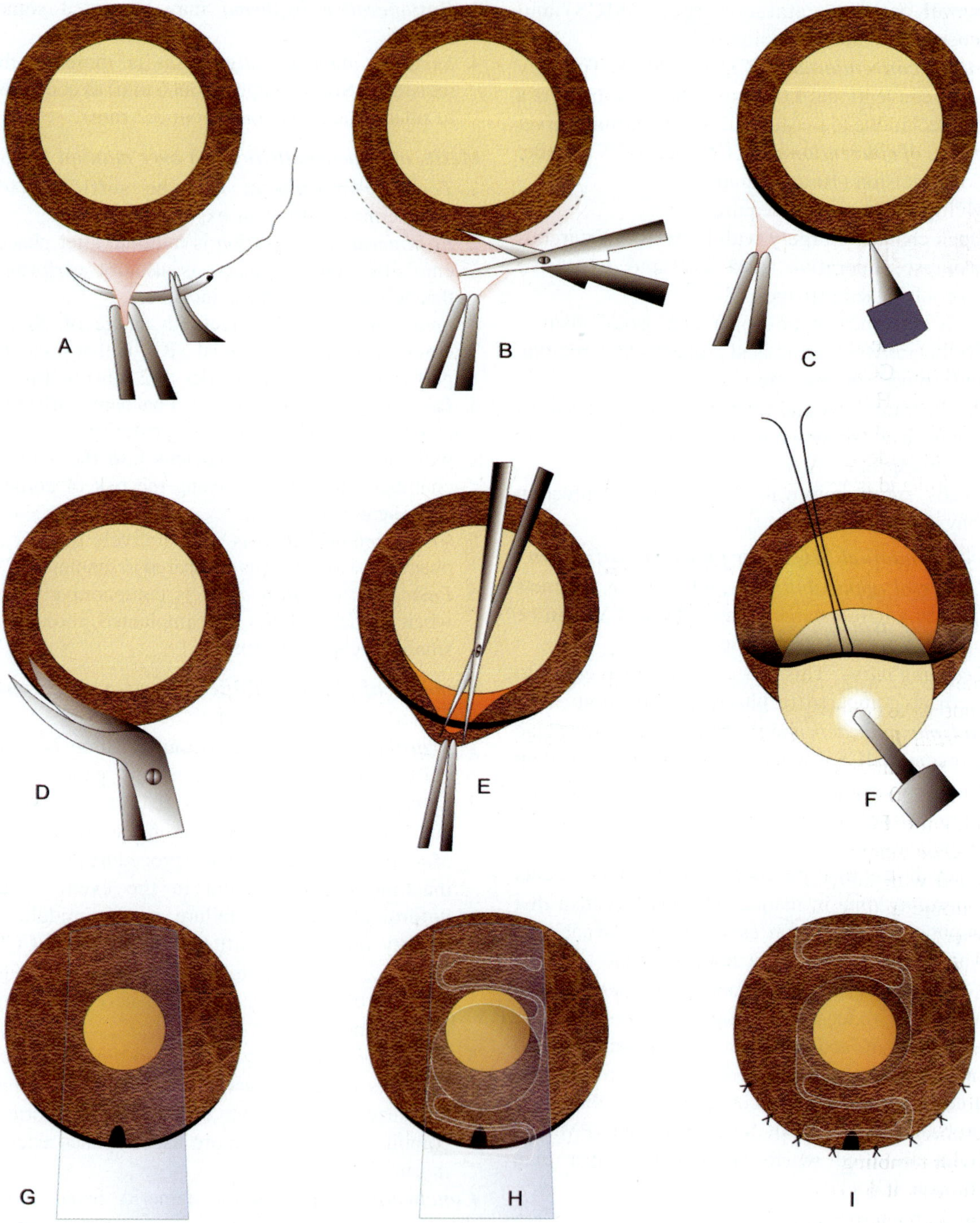

Fig. 8.17. Surgical steps of intracapsular cataract extraction with anterior chamber intraocular lens implantation: A, passing of superior rectus suture; B, fornix based conjunctival flap; C, partial thickness groove; D, completion of corneo-scleral section; E, peripheral iridectomy; F, cryolens extraction; G&H, insertion of Kelman multiflex intraocular lens in anterior chamber; I, corneo-scleral suturing.

However, for the masses, especially in developing countries, the manual SICS offers the advantages of sutureless cataract surgery as a low cost alternative to phacoemulsification with the added advantages of having wider applicability and an easier learning curve.

SURGICAL TECHNIQUES FOR CATARACT EXTRACTION

INTRACAPSULAR CATARACT EXTRACTION

Presently, the technique of intracapsular cataract extraction (ICCE) is obsolete and sparingly performed world wide. However, the surgical steps are described in detail as a mark of respect to the technique which has been widely employed for about 50 years over the world and is an important landmark in the history of cataract surgery.

Surgical steps of the ICCE technique are as follows:

1. ***Superior rectus (bridle) suture*** is passed to fix the eye in downward gaze (Fig. 8.17A).

2. ***Conjunctival flap*** (fornix based) is prepared to expose the limbus (Fig. 8.17B) and *haemostasis* is achieved by wet field or heat cautery. All surgeons do not make conjunctival flap.

3. ***Partial thickness groove or gutter*** is made through about two-thirds depth of anterior limbal area from 9.30 to 2.30 O'clock (150°) with the help of a razor blade knife (Fig. 8.17C).

4. ***Corneoscleral section.*** The anterior chamber is opened with the razor blade knife or with 3.2 mm keratome and section is completed using sclerocorneal scissors (Fig. 8.17D).

5. ***Iridectomy*** (Fig. 8.17E). A peripheral iridectomy may be performed by using iris forceps and de Wecker's scissors to prevent postoperative pupil block glaucoma.

6. ***Methods of lens delivery.*** In ICCE the lens can be delivered by any of the following methods:

i. *Indian Smith method.* Here the lens is delivered with tumbling technique by applying pressure on limbus at 6 O'clock position with lens expressor and counterpressure at 12 O'clock with the lens spatula. With this method lower pole is delivered first.

ii. *Cryoextraction.* In this technique, cornea is lifted up, lens surface is dried with a swab, iris is retracted up and tip of the cryoprobe is applied on the anterior surface of the lens in the upper quadrant. Freezing is activated (–40°C) to create adhesions between the lens and the probe. The zonules are ruptured by gentle rotatory movements and the lens is then extracted out by sliding movements. In this technique, upper pole of the lens is delivered first (Fig. 8.17F).

iii. *Capsule forceps method.* The Arruga's capsule holding forceps is introduced close into the anterior chamber and the anterior capsule of the lens is caught at 6 O'clock position. The lens is lifted slightly and its zonules are ruptured by gentle sideways movements. Then the lens is extracted with gentle sliding movements by the forceps assisted by a pressure at 6 O'clock position on the limbus by the lens expressor.

iv. *Irisophake method.* This technique is obsolete and thus not in much use.

v. *Wire vectis method.* It is employed in cases with subluxated or dislocated lens only. In this method the loop of the wire vectis is slide gently below the subluxated lens, which is then lifted out of the eye.

7. ***Formation of anterior chamber.*** After the delivery of lens, iris is reposited into the anterior chamber with the help of iris repositor and chamber is formed by injecting sterile air or balanced salt solution.

8. ***Implantation of anterior chamber (ACIOL)*** (Figs. 8.17 G and H). (For details see page 208).

9. ***Closure of incision*** is done with 5 to 7 interrupted sutures (8-0, 9-0 or 10-0 nylon) (Fig. 8.17I).

10. ***Conjunctival flap*** is reposited and secured by wet-field cautery.

11. ***Subconjunctival injection*** of dexamethasone 0.25 ml and gentamicin 0.5 ml is given.

12. ***Patching of eye*** is done with a pad and sticking plaster or a bandage is applied.

SURGICAL TECHNIQUES OF EXTRA CAPSULAR CATARACT EXTRACTION FOR ADULTHOOD CATARACTS

The surgical techniques of ECCE can be described separately for adulthood cataracts and childhood cataracts. The surgical techniques of ECCE presently in vogue for adulthood cataracts include:

- Conventional, extracapsular cataract extraction (ECCE),
- Manual small incision cataract surgery (SICS), and
- Phacoemulsification.

CONVENTIONAL EXTRACAPSULAR CATARACT EXTRACTION

Surgical steps of conventional ECCE are :

1. ***Superior rectus (bridle) suture*** is passed to fix the eye in downward gaze (Fig. 8.17A).

2. ***Conjunctival flap*** (fornix based) is prepared to expose the limbus (Fig. 8.17B) and *haemostasis* is achieved by wet field cautery. Many surgeons do not make conjunctival flap.

3. ***Partial thickness groove or gutter*** is made through about two-thirds depth of anterior limbal area from 10 to 2 O'clock (120°) with the help of a razor blade knife (Fig. 8.17C).

4. ***Entry into anterior chamber.*** The anterior chamber is entered with the razor blade knife or with 3.2 mm keratome.

5. ***Injection of viscoelastic substance in anterior chamber.*** A viscoelastic substance such as 2% methylcellulose or 1% sodium hyaluronate is injected into the anterior chamber. This maintains the anterior chamber and protects the endothelium (For details see page 458).

6. ***Anterior capsulotomy.*** It can be performed by any of the following methods:

i. *Can-opener's technique.* In this an irrigating cystitome (or simply a 26 gauge needle, bent at its tip) is introduced into the anterior chamber and multiple small radial cuts are made in the anterior capsule for 360° (Fig. 8.18A).

ii. *Linear capsulotomy* (Envelope technique). Here a straight incision is made in the anterior capsule (in the upper part) from 2-10 O' clock position. The rest of the capsulotomy is completed in the end after removal of nucleus and cortex.

iii. *Continuous circular capsulorrhexis* (CCC). Recently this is the most commonly performed procedure. In this the anterior capsule is torn in a circular fashion either with the help of an irrigating bent-needle cystitome or with a capsulorrhexis forceps (Fig. 8.20B).

7. ***Removal of anterior capsule.*** It is removed with the help of a Kelman-McPherson forceps (Fig. 8.18B).

8. ***Completion of corneoscleral section.*** It is completed from 10 to 2 O'clock position either with the help of corneo-scleral section enlarging scissors or 5.2 mm blunt keratome (Fig. 8.18C).

9. ***Hydrodissection.*** After the anterior capsulotomy, the balanced salt solution (BSS) is injected under the peripheral part of the anterior capsule. This manoeuvre separates the corticonuclear mass from the capsule.

10. ***Removal of nucleus.*** After hydrodissection the nucleus can be removed by any of the following techniques:

i. *Pressure and counter-pressure method.* In it the posterior pressure is applied at 12 O'clock position with corneal forceps or lens spatula and the nucleus is expressed out by counter-pressure exerted at 6 O'clock position with a lens hook (Fig. 8.18D).

ii. *Irrigating wire vectis technique.* In this method, loop of an irrigating wire vectis is gently passed below the nucleus, which is then lifted out of the eye.

11. ***Aspiration of the cortex.*** The remaining cortex is aspirated out using a two-way irrigation and aspiration cannula (Fig. 8.18E).

12. ***Implantation of IOL.*** The PMMA posterior chamber IOL is implanted in the capsular bag after inflating the bag with viscoelastic substance (Figs. 8.18 G and H).

13. ***Closure of the incision*** is done by a total of 3 to 5 interrupted or continuous 10-0 nylon sutures (Fig. 8.18I).

14. ***Removal of viscoelastic substance.*** Before tying the last suture the visco-elastic material is aspirated out with 2-way cannula and anterior chamber is filled with BSS.

15. ***Conjunctival flap*** is reposited and secured by wet field cautery.

16. ***Subconjunctival injection*** of dexamethasone 0.25 ml and gentamicin 0.5 ml is given.

17. ***Patching of eye*** is done with a pad and sticking plaster or a bandage is applied.

MANUAL SMALL INCISION CATARACT SURGERY

Manual small incision cataract surgery (SICS) has become very popular because of its merits over

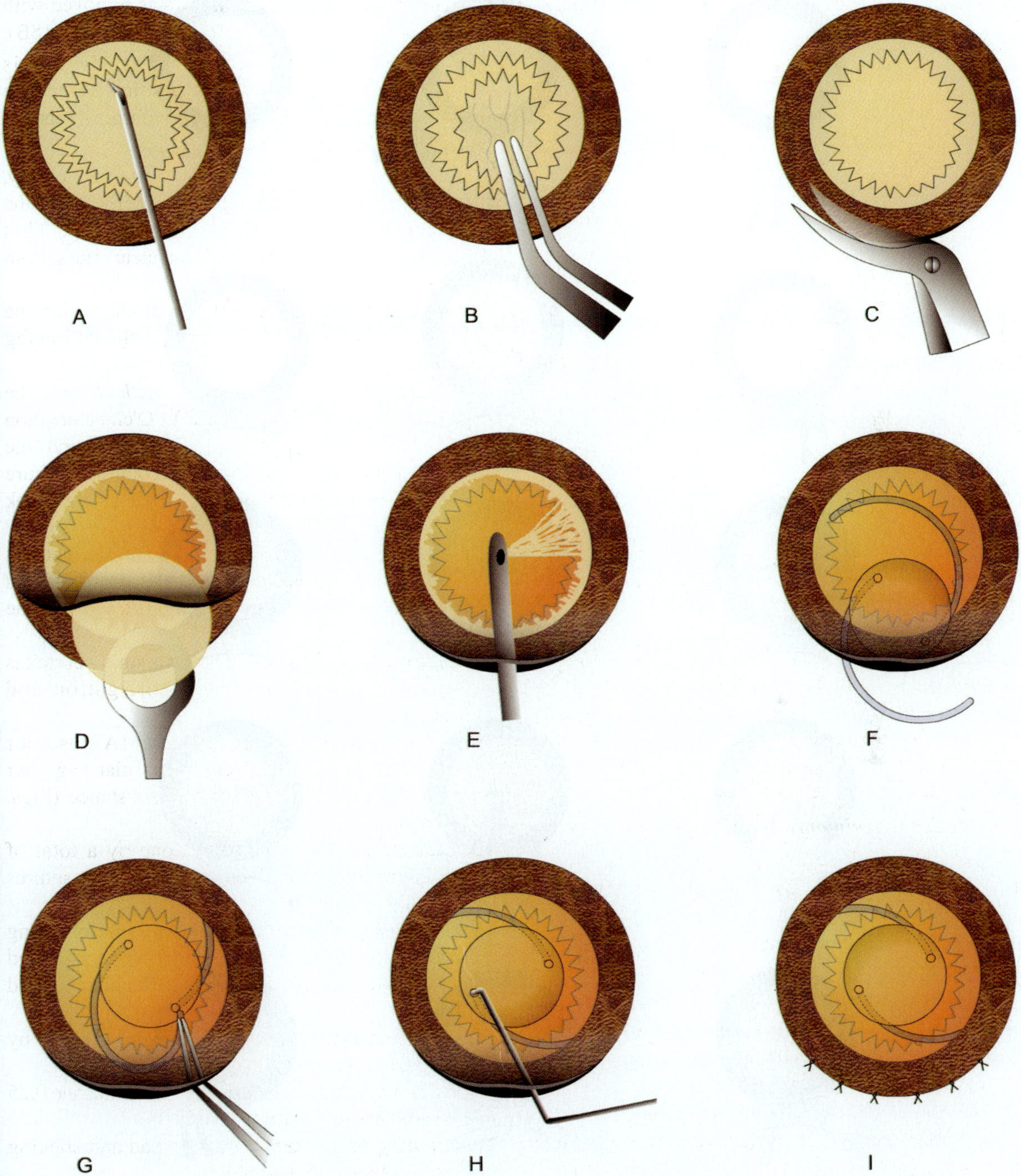

Fig. 8.18. Surgical steps of conventional extracapsular cataract extraction with posterior chamber intraocular lens implantation: A, anterior capsulotomy can-opener's technique; B, removal of anterior capsule; C, completion of corneo-scleral section; D, removal of nucleus (pressure and counter-pressure method); E, aspiration of cortex; F, insertion of inferior haptic of posterior chamber IOL; G, insertion of superior haptic of PCIOL; H, dialing of the IOL; I, corneo-scleral suturing.

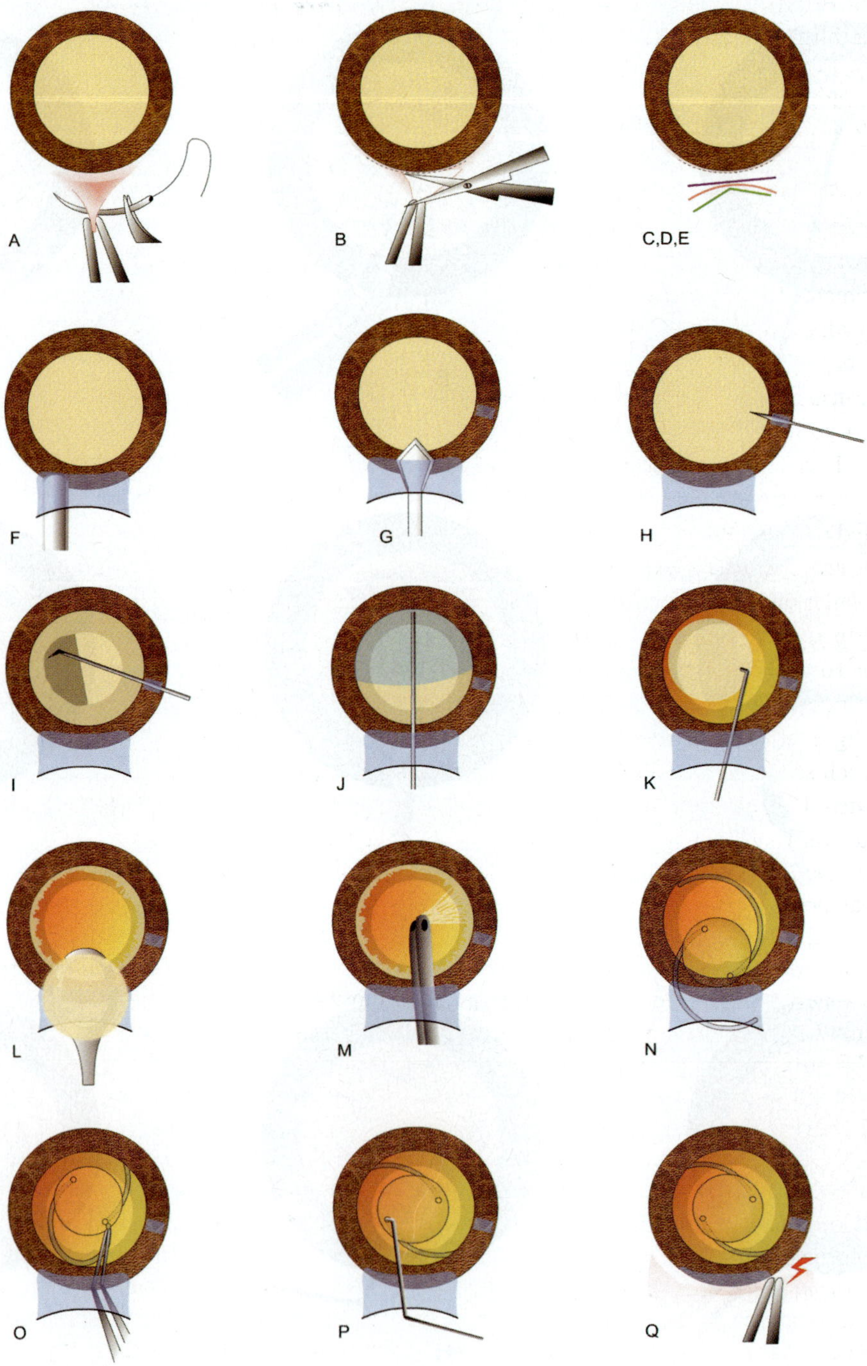

Fig. 8.19. Surgical steps of manual small incision cataract surgery (SICS): A, superior rectus bridle suture; B, conjunctival flap and exposure of sclera; C, D & E, external scleral incisions (straight, frown shaped, and chevron, respectively) part of tunnel incision; F, sclero-corneal tunnel with crescent knife; G, internal corneal incision; H, side port entry; I, large CCC; J, hydrodissection; K, prolapse of nucleus into anterior chamber; L, nucleus delivery with irrigating wire vectis; M, aspiration of cortex; N, insertion of inferior haptic of posterior chamber IOL; O, insertion of superior haptic of PCIOL; P, dialing of the IOL, Q, reposition and anchoring of conjunctival flap.

conventional ECCE as well as phacoemulsification technique highlighted earlier (see pages 196-197). In this technique ECCE with intraocular lens implantation is performed through a sutureless self-sealing valvular sclero - corneo tunnel incision.

Surgical steps of manual SICS are (Fig. 8.19) :

1. *Superior rectus (bridle) suture* is passed to fix the eye in downward gaze (Fig. 8.19A). This is specifically important in manual SICS where in addition to fixation of globe, it also provides a countertraction force during delivery of nucleus and epinucleus.

Note. SICs can also be performed from temporal side, especially in patients with against the rule (ATR) astigmatism. In this situation bridle suture is passed through the lateral rectus muscle and all the next steps are performed on the temporal quadrant.

2. *Conjunctival flap and exposure of sclera* (Fig. 8.19B). A small fornix based conjunctival flap is made with the help of sharp-tipped scissors along the limbus from 10 to 2 O'clock positions. Conjunctiva and the Tenon's capsule are dissected, separated from the underlying sclera and retracted to expose about 4 mm strip of sclera along the entire incision length.

3. *Haemostasis* is achieved by applying gentle and just adequate wet field cautery.

4. *Sclero-corneal tunnel incision.* A self-sealing sclero-corneal tunnel incision is made in manual SICS. It consists of following components:

i. *External scleral incision.* A one-third to half-thickness external scleral groove is made about 1.5 to 2 mm behind the limbus. It varies from 5.5 mm to 7.5 mm in length depending upon the hardness of nucleus. It may be straight, frown shaped or chevron in configuration (Figs. 18.19C, D and E).

ii. *Sclero-corneal tunnel.* It is made with the help of a crescent knife. It usually extends 1-1.5 mm into the clear cornea (Fig. 8.19F).

iii. *Internal corneal incision.* It is made with the help of a sharp 3.2 mm angled keratome (Fig. 8.19G).

5. *Side-port entry* of about 1.5-mm valvular corneal incision is made at 9 O'clock position (Fig. 8.19H). This helps in aspiration of the sub-incisional cortex and deepening the anterior chamber at the end of surgery.

6. *Anterior capsulotomy.* As described in conventional ECCE, the capsulotomy in manual SICS can be either a canopner, or envelope or CCC. However, a large sized CCC is preferred (Fig. 8.19I).

7. *Hydrodissection.* As described in ECCE hydrodissection (Fig. 8.19J) is essential to separate corticonuclear mass from the posterior capsule in SICS.

8. *Nuclear management.* It consists of following manoeuvres :

i. *Prolapse of nucleus* out of the capsular bag into the anterior chamber is usually initiated during hydrodissection and completed by rotating the nucleus with Sinskey's hook (Fig. 8.19K).

ii. *Delivery of the nucleus outside* through the corneo-scleral tunnel can be done by any of the following methods:
   - Irrigating wire vectis method (Fig. 8.19L). (It is the most commonly used method).
   - Blumenthal's technique,
   - Phacosandwitch technique,
   - Phacofracture technique, and
   - Fishhook technique.

9. *Aspiration of cortex.* The remaining cortex is aspirated out using a two-way irrigation and aspiration cannula (Fig. 8.19M) from the main incision and/or side port entry.

10. *IOL implantation.* A posterior chamber IOL is implanted in the capsular bag after filling the bag with viscoelastic substance (Figs. 8.19N, O and P).

11. *Removal of viscoelastic material* is done thoroughly from the anterior chamber and capsular bag with the help of two-way irrigation aspiration cannula. Excessive left out viscoelastic material may cause secondary glaucoma.

12. *Wound closure.* The anterior chamber is deepened with balanced salt solution / Ringer's lactate solution injected through side port entry. This leads to self sealing of the sclero-corneal tunnel incision due to valve effect. Rarely a single infinity suture may be required to seal the wound. The conjunctival flap is reposited back and is anchored with the help of wet field cautery (Fig. 8.19Q).

PHACOEMULSIFICATION

It is presently the most popular method of extracapsular cataract extraction. It differs from the conventional ECCE and manual SICS as follows:

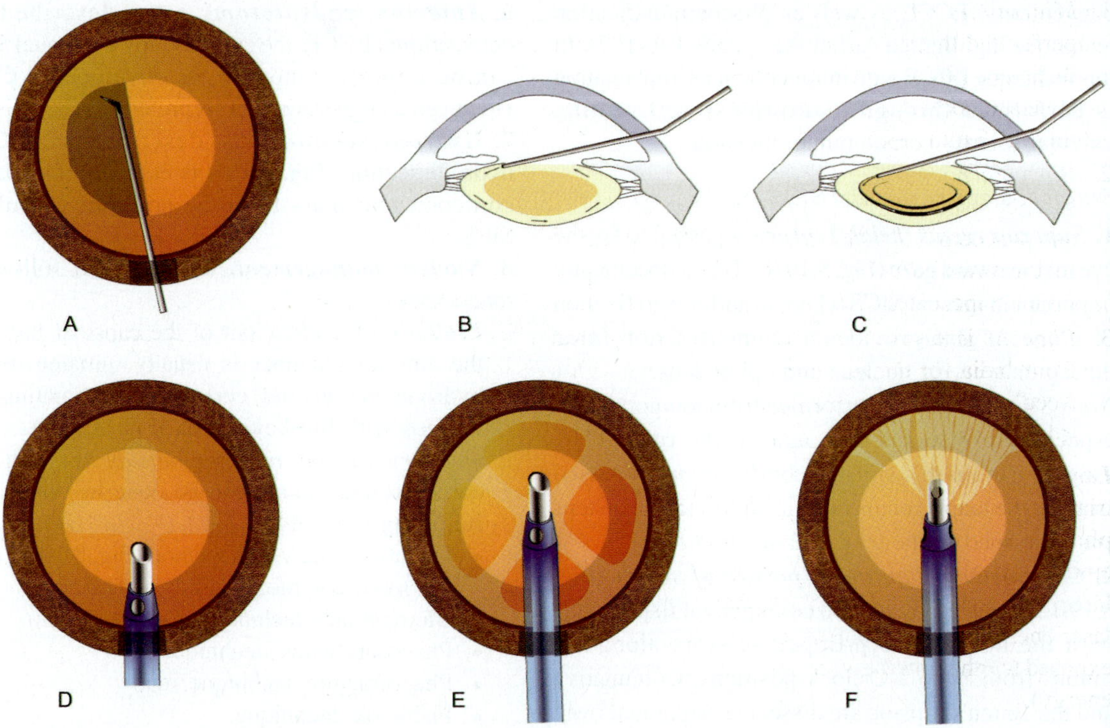

Fig. 8.20. Surgical steps of phacoemulsification : A, continuous curvilinear capsulorrhexis; B, hydrodissection; C, hydrodelineation; D&E; nucleus emulsification by divide and conquer technique (four quadrant cracking); F, aspiration of cortex.

1. *Corneoscleral incision* required is very small (3 mm). Therefore, sutureless surgery is possible with self-sealing scleral tunnel or clear corneal incision made with a 3 mm keratome.
2. *Continuous curvilinear capsulorrhexis* (CCC) of 4-6 mm is preferred over other methods of anterior capsulotomy (Fig. 8.20A).
3. *Hydrodissection* i.e., separation of capsule from the cortex by injecting fluid exactly between the two (Fig. 8.20B) is must for phacoemulsification in SICS. This procedure facilitates nucleus rotation and manipulation during phacoemulsification. Some surgeons also perform hydrodelineation (Fig. 8.20C).
4. *Nucleus is emulsified* and aspirated by phacoemulsifier. Phacoemulsifier basically acts through a hollow 1-mm titanium needle which vibrates by piezoelectric crystal in its longitudinal axis at an ultrasonic speed of 40000 times a second and thus emulsifies the nucleus. Many different techniques are being used to accomplish nucleotomy. A few common names are:
   - 'Chip and flip technique',
   - 'Divide and conquer technique' (Figs. 8.20 D and E)
   - 'Stop and chop' technique and
   - 'Phaco chop technique'.
5. *Remaining cortical lens matter is aspirated* with the help of an irrigation-aspiration technique (Fig. 8.20F).
6. *IOL implantation.* Foldable IOL is most ideal with phacoemulsification technique (see page 208). However, phacoprofile (5.25 optic size) rigid (PMMA) IOL can also be implanted after enlarging the incision.
7. *Next steps* i.e., removal of viscoelastic substance and wound closure are similar to that of SICS.

Microincision cataract surgery

Microincision cataract surgery (MICS) refers to the phacoemulsification techniques which can be performed through a microincision (< 2 mm). These techniques offer almost no surgically induced astigmatism. Various MICS techniques have been developed. A few to mention are:

1. *Microincision coaxial phacoemulsification* performed through around 2 mm incision with a dedicated phacomachine is essentially similar to standard coaxial phacoemulsification performed through 3 mm incision.
2. *Bimanual microphacoemulsification* (B-MICS) in essence uses separate hand piece for irrigation and phacoemulsification aspiration. The technique requires two limbal incision of 1.2×1.4 mm made with a trapezoidal blade.
3. *Phaconit* is the term used by Prof. Amar Agarwal from India for the bimanual *Phaco* done with a *N*eedle *I*ncision *T*echnique through an incision < 1 mm in size.

Laser phacoemulsification. This technique is under trial and perhaps may soon replace the conventional phacoemulsification. In it the lens nucleus is emulsified utilizing laser energy (Er:YAG or Nd:YAG laser). The advantage of this technique is that the laser energy used to emulsify cataractous lens is not exposed to other intraocular structures (c.f. ultrasonic energy).

SURGICAL TECHNIQUES OF EXTRACAPSULAR CATARACT EXTRACTION FOR CHILDHOOD CATARACT

Surgical techniques employed for childhood cataract are essentially of two types:

- Irrigation and aspiration of lens matter, and
- Lensectomy

1. Irrigation and aspiration of lens matter

Irrigation and aspiration of lens matter is preferably done by corneo-scleral tunnel techniques which include:

- Manual Irrigation-aspiration technique, and
- Phaco-aspiration technique

The corneo-scleral tunnel techniques (closed chamber surgery) as described for phacoemulsification is preferred over the conventional ECCE technique (open chamber surgery).

Surgical steps of irrigation and aspiration of lens matter by corneo-scleral tunnel incision techniques are as follows :

1 to 5 initial steps upto making of side port entry are similar as described for manual SICS in adults except that size of the tunnel incision is 3-4 mm (page 191 Figs. 8.19A to H).

6. *Anterior capsulorhexis* of about 5 mm size is made as described on page 189 (Figs. 8.20A). In children the anterior capsule is more elastic than in adults and therefore, the capsulorhexis may be difficult due to tendency to run outwards.

7. *Irrigation and aspiration of lens matter* (which is soft in children) can be done by any of the following methods:

- Manually with a two-way irrigation and aspiration Simcoe cannula (Fig. 8.19M) or,
- With a phacoprobe (phaco-aspiration) (Fig. 8.20F)

8. *Posterior capsulorhexis* of about 3-4 mm size is recomnended in younger children to avoid the problem of posterior capsule opacification.

9. *Anterior vitrectomy* of limited amount should be performed with a vitrector in very young children.

10. *Implantation of IOL* is done in the capsular bag after inflating it with viscoelastic substance (Figs. 8.19N, O and P). Foldable acrylic IOLs are preferred in children. It has been postulated that acrylic IOLs induce less cellular reaction and are more adhesive to the capsular bag than PMMA IOLs. Some surgeons prefer to capture the lens optic through posterior capsulorhexis.

Note: Steps 8, 9 and 10 (the lens material choice and optic capture as described in step 10) are measures to prevent formation of after cataract, the incidence of which is very high in children.

11. *Removal of viscoelastic material* is done with the help of two-way cannula or irrigation–aspiration probe of phaco machine.

12. *Wound closure*. Though a well constructed corneo-scleral tunnel often does not require a suture in adults. However, it is mandatory to close the wound in children to ensure wound stability and reduce postoperative astigmatism. The absorbable suture (10 – 0 vicryl is adequate for closure of the wound keeping in mind the rapid healing characteristic and difficulty of removing sutures in children.

2. Lensectomy

In this operation most of the lens including anterior and posterior capsule along with anterior vitreous are removed with the help of a vitreous cutter, infusion and suction machine (Fig. 8.21). Childhood cataracts, both congenital/developmental and acquired, being soft are easily dealt with this procedure especially in

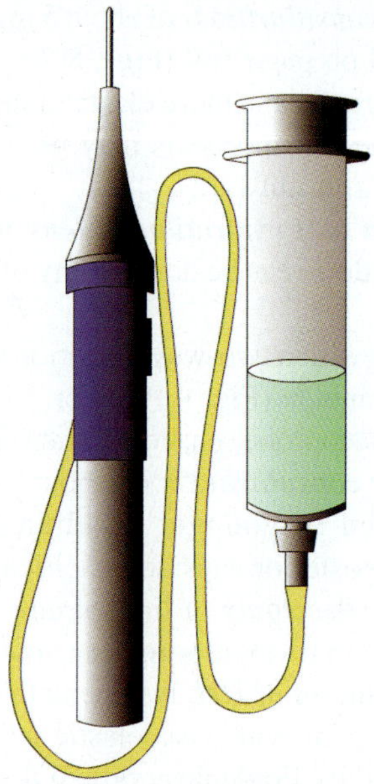

Fig. 8.21. Kaufman's vitrector.

very young children (less than 2 years of age) in which primary IOL implantation is not planned. Lensectomy in children is performed under general anaesthesia. Either pars plana or limbal approach may be adopted. In pars plana approach, the lens is punctured at its equator and stirred with the help of a Ziegler's or any other needle-knife introduced through the sclera and ciliary body, from a point about 3.5-4 mm behind the limbus. The cutter (ocutome) of the vitrectomy machine is introduced after enlarging the sclerotomy (Fig. 8.22) and lensectomy along with anterior vitrectomy is completed using cutting, irrigation and aspiration mechanisms. The aim of modern lensectomy is to leave in situ a peripheral rim of capsule as an alternative to complete lensectomy. Secondary IOL implantation can be planned at a later date.

INTRAOCULAR LENS IMPLANTATION

Presently, intraocular lens (IOL) implantation is the method of choice for correcting aphakia. Its advantages and disadvantages over spectacles and contact lenses are described in aphakia (see page 32).

The IOL implant history had its beginning on November 29, 1949, when Harold Ridley, a British ophthalmologist, performed his first case. Since then history of IOLs has always been exciting, often frustrating and finally rewarding and now highly developed.

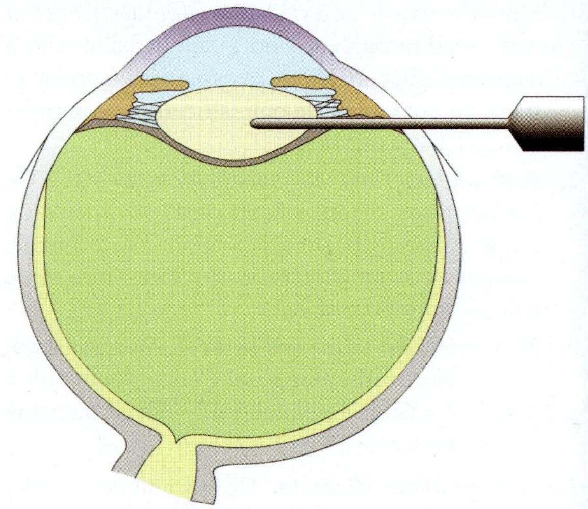

Fig. 8.22. Pars plana lensectomy.

Types of intraocular lenses

During the last two decades a large number of different types and styles of lenses have been developed.

A. ***Based on the method of fixation in the eye***, the major classes of IOLs are as follows:

1. *Anterior chamber IOL.* These are not very popular due to comparatively higher incidence of bullous keratopathy. When indicated, 'Kelman multiflex' (Fig. 8.23A) type of ACIOL is used commonly. These lenses lie entirely in front of the iris and are supported in the angle of anterior chamber (Fig. 8.24). ACIOL can be inserted after ICCE or ECCE.

2. *Iris-supported lenses.* These lenses are fixed on the iris with the help of sutures, loops or claws. These lenses are also not very popular due to high incidence of postoperative complications. Example of iris supported lens is Singh and Worst's iris claw lens (Figs. 8.23B and 8.25).

3. *Posterior chamber lenses.* PCIOLs rest entirely behind the iris (Fig. 8.26). They may be supported by the ciliary sulcus or the capsular bag. Recent trend is towards 'in-the-bag-fixation'. Commonly used model of PCIOLs is modified C-loop (Fig. 8.23C).

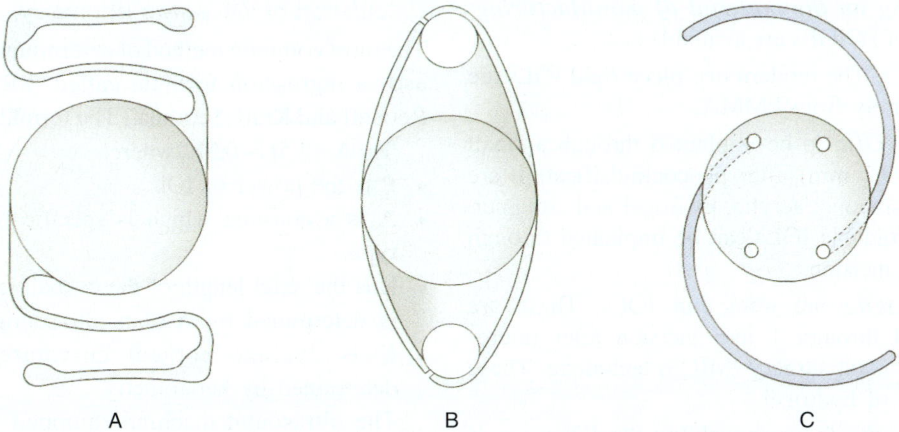

Fig. 8.23. Types of intraocular lenses based on methods of fixation: A, Kelman multiflex (an anterior chamber IOL); B, Singh and Worst's iris claw lens; C, posterior chamber IOL – modified C-loop type.

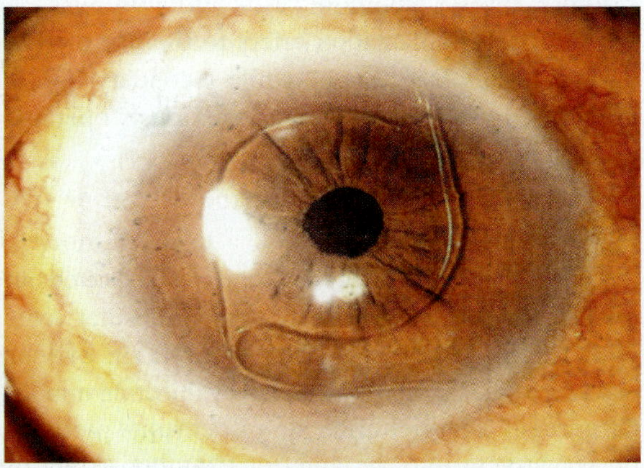

Fig. 8.24. Pseudophakia with Kelman Multiflex anterior chamber intraocular lens implant.

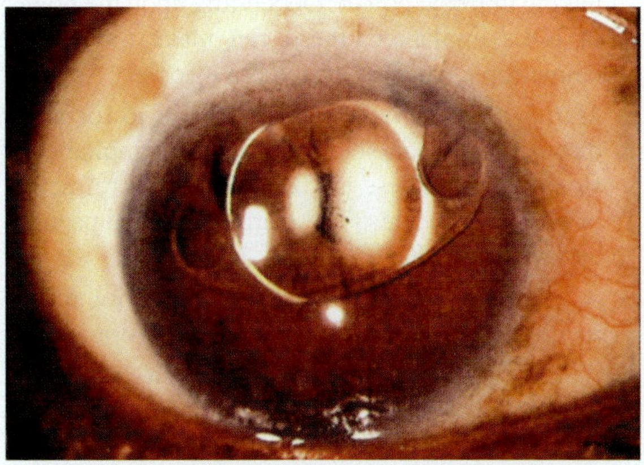

Fig. 8.25. Pseudophakia with iris claw intraocular lens implant.

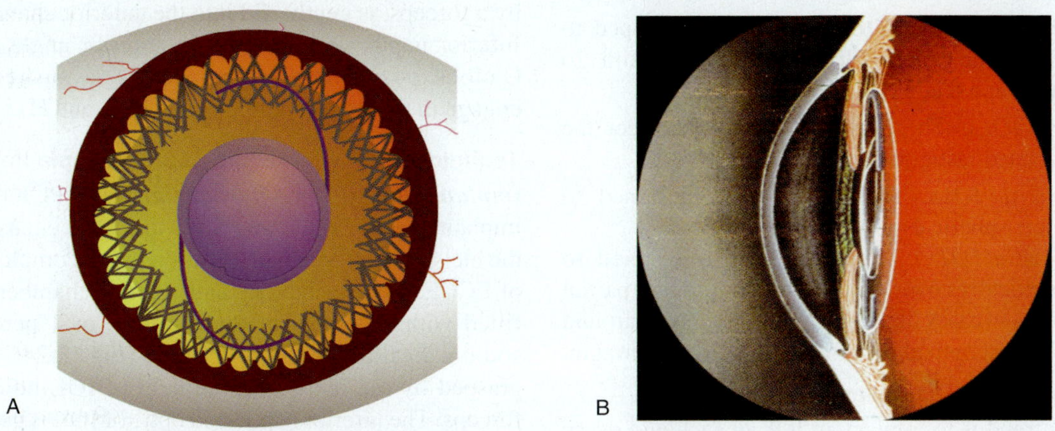

Fig. 8.26. Pseudophakia with posterior chamber intraocular lens A : as seen on retroillumination with slit-lamp; B, diagrammatic depiction of PCIOL implanted in the capsular bag.

B. ***Depending on the material of manufacturing***, three types of PCIOLs are available :

1. *Rigid IOLs.* The modern one piece rigid IOLs are made entirely from PMMA.
2. *Foldable IOLs,* to be implanted through a small incision (3.2 mm) after phacoemulsification are made of silicone, acrylic, hydrogel and collamer. Thinner foldable IOLs can be implanted through 2-2.2 mm incision.
3. *Rollable IOLs* are ultra thin IOLs. These are implanted through 1 mm incision after micro-incision catarat surgery (MICS) technique. These are made of hydrogel.

C. ***Based on the focussing ability*** the IOLs are of following types:

1. *Unifocal IOLs* are the most commonly used ones having unifocal power. Depending upon the power of IOLs implanted, these can make the patient emmetropic, myopic or hypermetropic.
2. *Multifocal IOLs* have separate optics to focus for distance and near, so also known as simultaneous vision lenses. These are based on either refractive or diffractive optics. These are also called pseudo-accomodative IOLs.
3. *Accomodative IOLs* exhibit some anterior movement of optic to improve the near vision.

D. ***Aphakic versus phakic refractive IOLs.*** In addition to the aphakic IOLs which are implanted after lens extraction, special phakic IOLs have been developed to correct the refractive errors. These are also called implantable contact lenses (ICLs) and are of three types (For details see page 48).

E. ***Special function IOLs.*** These are developed to provide some special function in addition to correcting aphakia. Examples are:

1. *Toric IOLs.* These are designed to correct the associated astigmatism.
2. *Aspheric IOLs.* These have been designed to reduce spherical abberations.
3. *Aniridia IOLs.* These lenses are devised to cosmetically cover the defects of aniridia or partial iris loss in cases like trauma. In these lenses around the central optical part, there is a black diaphragm.

Indications of IOL implantation

Recent trend is to implant an IOL in each and every case being operated for cataract; unless it is contraindicated.

Calculation of IOL power (Biometry)

The most common method of determining IOL power uses a regression formula called 'SRK (Sanders, Retzlaff and Kraff) formula'. The formula is :

$P = A - 2.5L - 0.9K$, where:

- P is the power of IOL,
- A is a constant which is specific for each lens type.
- L is the axial length of the eyeball in mm, which is determined by A-scan ultrasonography.
- K is average corneal curvature, which is determined by keratometry.

The ultrasound machine equipped with A-scan and IOL power calculation software is called '*Biometer*'.

Primary versus secondary IOL implantation

Primary IOL implantation refers to the use of IOL during surgery for cataract, while secondary IOL is implanted to correct aphakia in a previously operated eye.

Surgical technique of anterior chamber IOL implantation

Anterior chamber IOL implantation can be carried out after ICCE and after large posterior capsular rents with ECCE techniques. After completion of lens extraction, the pupil is constricted by injecting miotics (1 percent acetylcholine or pilocarpine without preservatives) into the anterior chamber. Anterior chamber is filled with 2 percent methylcellulose or 1 percent sodium hyaluronate (Healon). The IOL, held by a forceps, is gently slid into the anterior chamber. Inferior haptic is pushed in the inferior angle at 6 O'clock position and upper haptic is pushed to engage in the upper angle (Figs. 8.17 G and H).

Technique of posterior chamber IOL implantation

Implantation of rigid intraocular lens. PCIOL is implanted after ECCE and SICS and after enlarging the incision in phacoemulsification. After completion of ECCE, the capsular bag and anterior chamber are filled with 2 percent methylcellulose or 1 percent sodium hyaluronate. The PCIOL (Fig. 8.24C), is grasped by the optic with the help of IOL holding forceps. The inferior haptic and optic of IOL is gently inserted into the capsular bag behind the iris at 6 O'clock position (Fig. 8.18F). The superior haptic is grasped by its tip, and is gently pushed down and then released to slide in the upper part of the capsular bag behind the iris (Fig. 8.18G). The IOL is then dialled into the horizontal position (Fig. 8.18H).

Implantation of foldable IOLs is made either with the help of holder-folder forceps or the foldable IOL injector.

Scleral fixation of posterior chamber IOL is done as an alternative to anterior chamber IOL (ACIOL). Posterior chamber IOL can be fixated to the sclera in the ciliary sulcus region with the help of sutures or a biological glue (glued IOLs).

POSTOPERATIVE MANAGEMENT AFTER CATARACT OPERATION

1. The patient is asked to lie quietly upon the back for about 2-3 hours and advised to take nil orally.
2. For mild to moderate postoperative pain injection diclofenac sodium may be given.
3. Next morning bandage/eye patch is removed and eye is inspected for any postoperative complication.
4. Antibiotic-steroid eyedrops are used for four times, three times, two times and then once a day for 2 weeks each.
5. After 6-8 weeks of operation corneoscleral sutures are removed (when applied). *Now a days most surgeons are doing sutureless cataract surgery.*
6. Final spectacles are prescribed after about 8 weeks of operation.

COMPLICATIONS OF CATARACT SURGERY AND THEIR MANAGEMENT

Now-a-days cataract surgery is being performed largely by extracapsular cataract extraction technique. Therefore, complications encountered during these techniques are described in general. Wherever necessary a specific reference of the technique viz. conventional ECCE, manual SICS and phacoemulsification in relation to the particular complication is highlighted.

Complications encountered during surgical management of cataract can be enumerated under the following heads:

(A) Preoperative complications
(B) Operative complications
(C) Early postoperative complications
(D) Delayed (late) postoperative complications
(E) IOL-related complications

[A] Preoperative complications

1. *Anxiety.* Some patients may develop anxiety, on the eve of operation due to fear and apprehension of operation. Anxiolytic drugs such as diazepam 2 to 5 mg at bed time usually alleviate such symptoms.

2. *Nausea and gastritis.* A few patients may develop nausea and gastritis due to preoperative medicines such as acetazolamide and/or glycerol. Oral antacids and omission of further dose of such medicines usually relieve the symptoms.

3. *Irritative or allergic conjunctivitis* may occur in some patients due to preoperative topical antibiotic drops. Postponing the operation for 2 days along with withdrawal of such drugs is required.

4. *Corneal abrasion* may develop due to inadvertent injury during Schiotz tonometry. Patching with antibiotic ointment for a day and postponement of operation for 2 days is required.

5. *Complications due to local anaesthesia*

- *Retrobulbar haemorrhage* may occur due to retrobulbar block. Immediate pressure bandage after instilling one drop of 2% pilocarpine and postponement of operation for a week is advised. Since, presently most cases are done under peribulbar or topical anaesthesia, so incidence of retrobulbar haemorrhage has decreased drastically.
- *Oculocardiac reflex,* which manifests as bradycardia and/or cardiac arrhythmia, has also been observed due to retrobulbar/peribulbar block. An intravenous injection of atropine is helpful.
- *Perforation of globe* may also occur sometimes. To prevent such catastrophy, gentle injection with blunt-tipped needle is recommended. Further, peribulbar anaesthesia may be preferred over retrobulbar block.
- *Subconjunctival haemorrhage* is a minor complication observed frequently, and does not need much attention.
- *Spontaneous dislocation of lens* in vitreous has also been reported (in patients with weak and degenerated zonules especially with hypermature cataract) during vigorous ocular massage after retrobulbar block. The operation should be postponed and further management is on the lines of posterior dislocation of lens (page 204).

[B] Operative complications

1. *Superior rectus muscle laceration* and/or haematoma, may occur while applying the bridle suture. Usually no treatment is required.

2. *Excessive bleeding* may be encountered during the preparation of conjunctival flap or during incision into the anterior chamber. Bleeding vessels may be gently cauterised.

3. *Incision related complications* depend upon the type of cataract surgery being performed.

i. *In conventional ECCE* there may occur *irregular incision.* Irregular incision leading to defective coaptation of wound may occur due to blunt cutting instruments.

ii. *In manual SICS and phacoemulsification* following complications may occur while making the self-sealing tunnel incision.
   - *Button holing of anterior wall of tunnel* can occur because of superficial dissection of the scleral flap (Fig. 8.27B). As a remedy, abandon this dissection and re-enter at a deeper plane from the other side of the external incision.
   - *Premature entry into the anterior chamber* can occur because of deep dissection (Fig. 8.27C). Once this is detected, dissection in that area should be stopped and a new dissection started at a lesser depth at the other end of the tunnel.
   - *Scleral disinsertion* can occur due to very deep groove incision. In it there occurs complete separation of inferior sclera from the sclera superior to the incision (Fig. 8.27D). Scleral disinsertion needs to be managed by radial sutures.

4. *Injury to the cornea (Descemet's detachment), iris and lens* may occur when anterior chamber is entered with a sharp-tipped instrument such as keratome or a piece of razor blade. A gentle handling with proper hypotony reduces the incidence of such inadvertent injuries.

5. *Iris injury and iridodialysis* (tear of iris from root) may occur inadvertently during intraocular manipulation.

6. *Complications related to anterior capsulorhexis.* Continuous curvilinear capsulorhexis (CCC) is the preferred technique for opening the anterior capsule for SICS and phacoemulsification. Following complications may occur:

- *Escaping capsulorhexis* i.e., capsulorhexis moves peripherally and may extend to the equator or posterior capsule.
- *Small capsulorhexis.* It predisposes to posterior capsular tear and nuclear drop during hydrodissection. It also predisposes to occurrence of zonular dehiscence. Therefore, a small sized capsulorhexis should always be enlarged by 2 or 3 relaxing incisions before proceeding further.
- *Very large capsulorhexis* may cause problems for in the bag placement of IOL.
- *Eccentric capsulorhexis* can lead to IOL decentration at a later stage.

7. *Posterior capsular rupture (PCR).* It is a dreaded complication during extracapsular cataract extraction. In manual SICS and phacoemulsification PCR is even more feared because it can lead to nuclear drop into the vitreous. The PCR can occur in following situations:

- During forceful hydrodissection,
- By direct injury with some instrument such as Sinskey's hook, chopper or phacotip, and
- During cortex aspiration (accidental PCR)

8. *Zonular dehiscence* may occur in all techniques of ECCE but is especially common during nucleus prolapse into the anterior chamber in manual SICS.

9. *Vitreous loss:* It is the most serious complication which may occur following accidental rupture of posterior capsule during any technique of ECCE. Therefore, adequate measures as described below should be taken to prevent vitreous loss (especially useful in conventional ECCE).

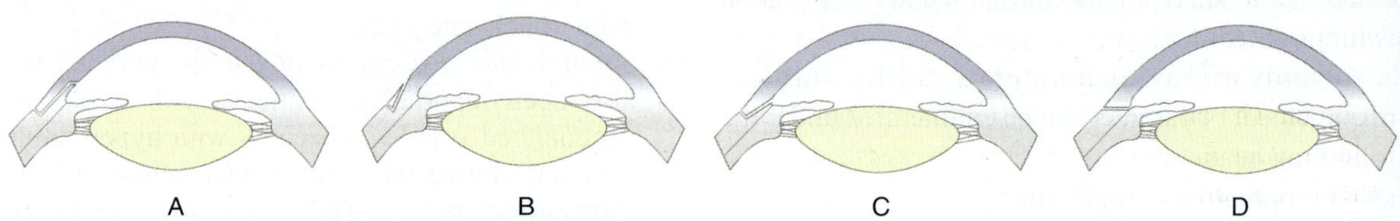

Fig. 8.27. Configuration of sclerocorneal tunnel incision: A, correct incision; B, buttonholing of anterior wall of the tunnel; C, premature entry into the anterior chamber; and D, scleral disinsertion.

- To *decrease vitreous volume:* Preoperative use of hyperosmotic agents like 20 percent mannitol or oral glycerol is suggested.
- *To decrease aqueous volume:* Preoperatively acetazolamide 500 mg orally should be used and adequate ocular massage should be carried out digitally after injecting local anaesthesia.
- *To decrease orbital volume:* adequate ocular massage and orbital compression by use of superpinky, Honan's ball, or 30 mm of Hg pressure by paediatric sphygmomanometer should be carried out.
- *Better ocular akinesia* and anaesthesia decrease the chances of pressure from eye muscle.
- *Minimising the external pressure* on eyeball by not using eye speculum, reducing pull on bridle suture and overall gentle handling during surgery.
- *Use of Flieringa ring* to prevent collapse of sclera especially in myopic patients decreases the incidence of vitreous loss.
- *When IOP is high* in spite of all above measures and operation cannot be postponed, in that situation a planned posterior-sclerotomy with drainage of vitreous from pars plana will prevent rupture of the anterior hyaloid face and vitreous loss.

Management of vitreous loss. Once the vitreous loss has occurred, the aim should be to clear it from the anterior chamber and incision site. This can be achieved by performing partial anterior vitrectomy, with the use of automated vitrectors.

A meticulously performed partial anterior vitrectomy will reduce the incidence of postoperative problems associated with vitreous loss such as updrawn pupil, iris prolapse and vitreous touch syndrome.

10. *Nucleus drop into the vitreous cavity.* It occurs more frequently with phacoemulsification, less frequently with manual SICS and sparingly with conventional ECCE. It is a dreadful complication which occurs due to sudden and large PCR.

Management. Once the nucleus has dropped into the vitreous cavity, no attempt should be made to fish it out. The case must be referred to vitreoretinal surgeon after a thorough anterior vitrectomy and cortical clean up.

11. *Posterior loss of lens fragments* into the vitreous cavity may occur after PCR or zonular dehiscence during phacoemulsification. It is potentially serious because it may result in glaucoma, chronic uveitis, chronic CME and even retinal detachment.

Management. The case should be managed by vitreoretinal surgeon by performing pars plana vitrectomy and removal of nuclear fragments.

12. *Expulsive choroidal haemorrhage.* It is one of the most dramatic and serious complications of cataract surgery. It usually occurs in hypertensives and patients with arteriosclerotic changes. It may occur during operation or during immediate postoperative period. Its incidence was high in ICCE and conventional ECCE but has decreased markedly with valvular incision of manual SICS and phacoemulsification technique.

It is *characterised* by spontaneous gaping of the wound followed by expulsion of the lens, vitreous, retina, uvea and finally a gush of bright red blood. Although *treatment* is unsatisfactory, the surgeon should attempt to drain subchoroidal blood by performing an equatorial sclerotomy. Most of the time eye is lost so evisceration operation has to be performed.

[C] Early postoperative complications

1. *Hyphaema.* Collection of blood in the anterior chamber may occur from conjunctival or scleral vessels and rarely from the root of the iris.

Treatment. Most hyphaemas absorb spontaneously and thus need no treatment. Sometimes hyphaema may be large and associated with rise in IOP. In such cases, IOP should be lowered by acetazolamide and hyperosmotic agents. If the blood does not get absorbed in a week's time, then a paracentesis should be done to drain the blood.

2. *Iris prolapse.* It is usually caused by inadequate suturing of the incision after ICCE and conventional ECCE and occurs during first or second postoperative day. This complication is not known with manual SICS and phacoemulsification technique.

Management: A small prolapse of less than 24 hours duration may be reposited back and wound sutured. A large prolapse of long duration needs abscission and suturing of wound.

3. *Striate keratopathy.* Characterised by mild corneal oedema with Descemet's folds is a common complication observed during immediate postoperative period. This occurs due to endothelial damage during surgery.

Management. Mild striate keratopathy usually disappears spontaneously within a week. Moderate to severe keratopathy may be treated by instillation of hypertonic saline drops (5% sodium chloride) along with steroids.

4. *Flat (shallow or nonformed) anterior chamber.* It has become a relatively rare complication due to improved wound closure. It may be due to wound leak, *ciliochoroidal detachment* or pupil block.

i. *Flat anterior chamber with wound leak* is associated with hypotony. It is diagnosed by Seidel's test. In this test, a drop of fluorescein is instilled into the lower fornix and patient is asked to blink to spread the dye evenly. The incision is then examined with slit lamp using cobalt-blue filter. At the site of leakage, fluorescein will be diluted by aqueous. In most cases wound leak is cured within 4 days with pressure bandage and oral acetazolamide. If the condition persists, injection of air in the anterior chamber and resuturing of the leaking wound should be carried out.

ii. *Ciliochoroidal detachment.* It may or may not be associated with wound leak. Detached cilio-choroid presents as a convex brownish mass in the involved quadrant with shallow anterior chamber. In most cases choroidal detachment is cured within 4 days with pressure bandage and use of oral acetazolamide. If the condition persists, suprachoroidal drainage with injection of air in the anterior chamber is indicated.

iii. *Pupil block due to vitreous bulge* (after ICCE or due to adhesions with IOL more common with AC-IOLs) leads to formation of iris bombe and shallowing of anterior chamber. If the condition persists for 5-7 days, permanent peripheral anterior synechiae (PAS) may be formed leading to secondary angle closure glaucoma.

Pupil block is managed initially with mydriatic, hyperosmotic agents (e.g., 20% mannitol) and acetazolamide. If not relieved, then laser or surgical peripheral iridectomy should be performed to bypass the pupillary block.

5. *Postoperative anterior uveitis* can be induced by instrumental trauma, undue handling of uveal tissue, reaction to residual cortex or chemical reaction induced by viscoelastics, pilocarpine etc.

Management includes more aggressive use of topical steroids, cycloplegics and NSAIDs. Rarely systemic steroids may be required in cases with severe fibrinous reaction.

6. *Toxic anterior segment syndrome (TASS)* (see page 168)

7. *Bacterial endophthalmitis.* This is one of the most dreaded complications with an incidence of 0.2 to 0.5 percent. The principal sources of infection are contaminated solutions, instruments, surgeon's hands, patient's own flora from conjunctiva, eyelids and air-borne bacteria.

Symptoms and signs of bacterial endophthalmitis are generally present between 48 and 72 hours after surgery and include: ocular pain, diminshed vision, lid oedema, conjunctival chemosis and marked circumciliary congestion, corneal oedema, exudates in pupillary area, hypopyon and diminished or absent red pupillary glow.

Management. It is an emergency and should be managed energetically (see page 169).

[D] Late postoperative complications

These complications may occur after weeks, months or years of cataract surgery.

1. *Cystoid macular oedema (CME).* Collection of fluid in the form of cystic loculi in the Henle's layer of macula is a frequent complication of cataract surgery. However, in most cases it is clinically insignificant, does not produce any visual problem and undergoes spontaneous regression. In few cases, a significant CME typically produces visual diminution one to three months after cataract extraction. On funduscopy it gives *honeycomb appearance*. On fluorescein angiography it depicts typical *flower petal pattern* (see Fig. 11.25) due to leakage of dye from perifoveal capillaries.

In most cases it is associated with vitreous incarceration in the wound and mild iritis. Role of some prostaglandins is being widely considered in its etiopathogenesis. Therefore, immediate preoperative and postoperative use of antiprostaglandins (indomethacin or flurbiprofen or ketorolac) eyedrops is recommended as prophylaxis of CME.

In cases of CME with vitreous incarceration, anterior vitrectomy along with steroids and antiprostaglandins may improve visual acuity and decrease the amount of discomfort.

2. *Delayed chronic postoperative endophthalmitis* is caused when an organism of low virulence (propionobacterium acne or staph epidermidis) becomes trapped within the capsular bag. It has an onset ranging from 4 weeks to years (mean 9 months) postoperatively and typically follows an uneventful cataract extraction with a PCIOL in the bag.

3. ***Pseudophakic bullous keratopathy (PBK)*** is usually a continuation of postoperative corneal oedema produced by surgical or chemical insult to a healthy or compromised corneal endothelium. PBK is becoming a common indication of penetrating keratoplasty (PK).

4. ***Retinal detachment (RD).*** Incidence of retinal detachment is higher in aphakic patients as compared to phakics. It has been noted that retinal detachment is more common after ICCE than after ECCE. Other risk factors for aphakic retinal detachment include vitreous loss during operation, associated myopia and lattice degeneration of the retina.

5. ***Epithelial ingrowth.*** Rarely conjunctival epithelial cells may invade the anterior chamber through a defect in the incision. This abnormal epithelial membrane slowly grows and lines the back of cornea and trabecular meshwork leading to intractable glaucoma. In late stages, the epithelial membrane extends on the iris and anterior part of the vitreous.

6. ***Fibrous downgrowth*** into the anterior chamber may occur very rarely when the cataract wound apposition is not perfect. It may cause secondary glaucoma, disorganisation of anterior segment and ultimately phthisis bulbi.

7. ***After cataract.*** It is also known as 'secondary cataract'. It is the opacity which persists or develops after extracapsular lens extraction.

Causes. (i) *Residual opaque lens matter* may persist as after cataract when it is imprisoned between the remains of the anterior and posterior capsule, surrounded by fibrin (following iritis) or blood (following hyphaema). (ii) *Proliferative type* of after cataract may develop from the left-out anterior epithelial cells. The proliferative hyaline bands may sweep across the whole posterior capsule.

Clinical types. After cataract may present as thickened posterior capsule, or dense membranous after cataract (Fig. 8.28A) or *Soemmering's ring* which refers to a thick ring of after cataract formed behind the iris, enclosed between the two layers of capsule (Fig. 8.28B) or *Elschnig's pearls* in which the vacuolated subcapsular epithelial cells are clustered like soap bubbles along the posterior capsule (Fig. 8.28C).

Treatment is as follows:

i. Thin membranous after cataract and thickened posterior capsule are best treated by YAG-laser capsulotomy or discission with cystitome or Zeigler's knife.
ii. Dense membranous after cataract needs surgical membranectomy.
iii. Soemmering's ring after cataract with clean central posterior capsule needs no treatment.
iv. Elschnig's pearls involving the central part of the posterior capsule can be treated by YAG-laser capsulotomy or discission with cystitome.

7. ***Glaucoma-in-aphakia and pseudophakia*** (see page 250).

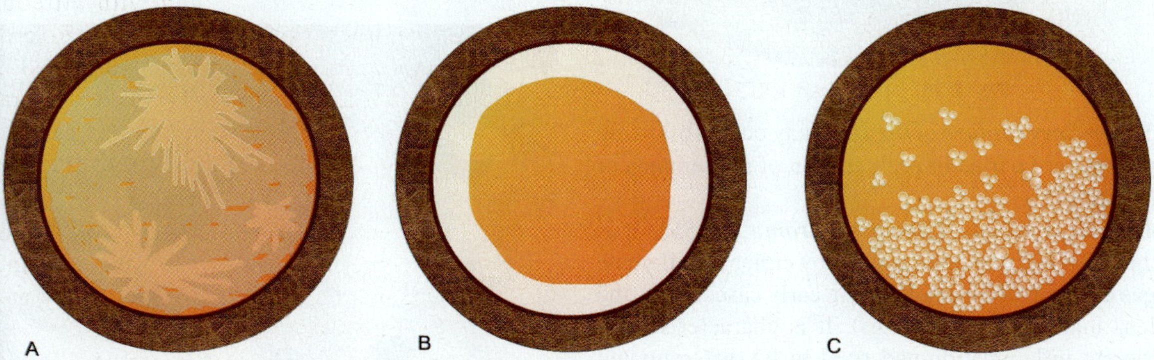

Fig. 8.28. Types of after cataract : A, dense membranous; B, Soemmering's ring; C, Elschnig's pearls.

[E] IOL-related complications

In addition to the complications of cataract surgery, following IOL-related complications may be seen:

1. *Complications like* cystoid macular oedema, corneal endothelial damage, uveitis and secondary glaucoma are seen more frequently with IOL implantation, especially with anterior chamber and iris supported IOLs.

UGH syndrome refers to concurrent occurrence of uveitis, glaucoma and hyphaema. It used to occur commonly with rigid anterior chamber IOLs, which are not used now-a-days.

2. *Malpositions of IOL* (Fig. 8.29). These may be in the form of decentration, subluxation and dislocation. The fancy names attached to various malpositions of IOL are:

- *Sun-set syndrome* (Inferior subluxation of IOL).
- *Sun-rise syndrome* (Superior subluxation of IOL).
- *Lost lens syndrome* refers to complete dislocation of an IOL into the vitreous cavity.
- *Windshield wiper syndrome.* It results when a very small IOL is placed vertically in the sulcus. In this the superior loop moves to the left and right, with movements of the head.

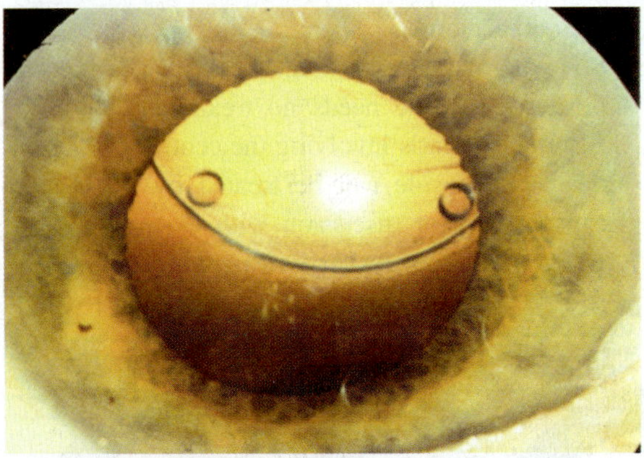

Fig. 8.29. Decentered IOL.

3. *Pupillary capture of the IOL* may occur following postoperative iritis or proliferation of the remains of lens fibres.

4. *Toxic anterior segment syndrome (TASS).* It is the uveal inflammation excited by either the ethylene gas used for sterilising IOLs (in early cases) or by the lens material (in late cases). It is characterised by violent inflammation and need to be differentiated from endophthalmitis.

DISPLACEMENTS OF THE LENS

Displacement of the lens from its normal position (in patellar fossa) results from partial or complete rupture of the lens zonules.

CLINICO-ETIOLOGICAL TYPES

I. Congenital displacements

These may occur in the following forms:

(a) *Simple ectopia lentis.* In this condition displacement is bilaterally symmetrical and usually upwards. It is transmitted by autosomal dominant inheritance.

(b) *Ectopia lentis et pupillae.* It is an autosomal recessive disorder, characterised by displacement of the lens associated with slit-shaped pupil which is displaced in the opposite direction. *Other associations* may be cataract, glaucoma, axial myopia macrocornea, abnormal iris transillumination and retinal detachment.

(c) *Ectopia lentis with systemic anomalies.* Salient features of some common conditions are as follows:

1. *Marfan's syndrome.* It is an autosomal dominant mesodermal dysplasia. In this condition lens is displaced upwards and temporally (bilaterally symmetrical) (Fig. 8.30). Systemic anomalies include arachnodactyly (spider fingers), long extremities, hyperextensibility of joints, high arched palate and dissecting aortic aneurysm.

2. *Homocystinuria.* It is an autosomal recessive, inborn error of metabolism. In it the lens is usually subluxated downwards and nasally.

- *Systemic features* are fair complexion, malar flush, mental retardation, fits and poor motor control.

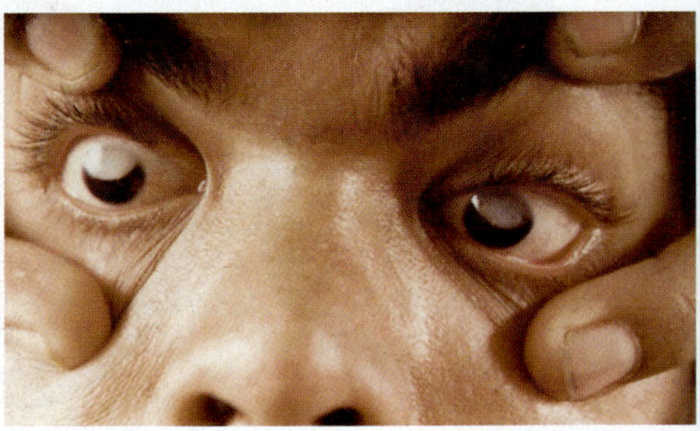

Fig. 8.30. Subluxated IOL in Marfan's syndrome.

- *Diagnosis* is established by detecting homocystine in urine by sodium nitro-prusside test.

3. *Weil-Marchesani syndrome.* It is condition of autosomal recessive mesodermal dysplasia. *Ocular features* are spherophakia, and forward subluxation of lens which may cause pupil block glaucoma. *Systemic features* are short stature, stubby fingers and mental retardation.

4. *Ehlers-Danlos syndrome.* In it the *ocular features* are subluxation of lens and blue sclera. The *systemic features* include hyperextensibility of joints and loose skin with folds.

5. *Hyperlysinaemia.* It is an autsomal recessive inborne error of metabolism occurring due to deficiency of the enzyme lysin alphaketoglutarate reductase. It is an extremely rare condition occasionally associated with ectopia lentis. *Systemic features* include lax ligaments, hypotonic muscles, seizures and mental handicap.

6. *Stickler syndrome.* Ectopia lentis is occasionally associated in this condition (for details see page 287).

7. *Sulphite oxidase deficiency.* It is a very rare autosomal recessive disorder of sulphur metabolism. Ectopia lentis is a universal *ocular feature*. The *systemic features* include progressive muscular rigidity, decerebrate posture, and mental handicap. It is a fatal disease, death usually occurs before 5 years of age.

II. Traumatic displacement of the lens

It is usually associated with concussion injuries. *Couching* is an iatrogenic posterior dislocation of lens performed as a *treatment of cataract* in olden days.

III. Consecutive or spontaneous displacement

It results from intraocular diseases giving rise to mechanical stretching, inflammatory disintegration or degeneration of the zonules. A few common conditions associated with consecutive displacements are: hypermature cataract, buphthalmos, high myopia, staphyloma, intraocular tumours and uveitis.

TOPOGRAPHICAL TYPES

Topographically, displacements of the lens may be classified as subluxation and luxation or dislocation.

I. Subluxation

It is partial displacement in which lens is moved sideways (up, down, medially or laterally), but remains behind the pupil. It results from partial rupture or unequal stretching of the zonules (Figs. 8.30 and 8.31A).

Clinical features are as follows:

- *Defective vision* occurs due to marked astigmatism or lenticular myopia.
- *Uniocular diplopia* may result from partial aphakia.
- *Anterior chamber* becomes deep and irregular.
- *Iridodonesis* is usually present.
- *Dark edge* of the subluxated lens is seen on distant direct ophthalmoscopy.

Complications of subluxated lens include:

- Complete dislocation,
- Cataractous changes,

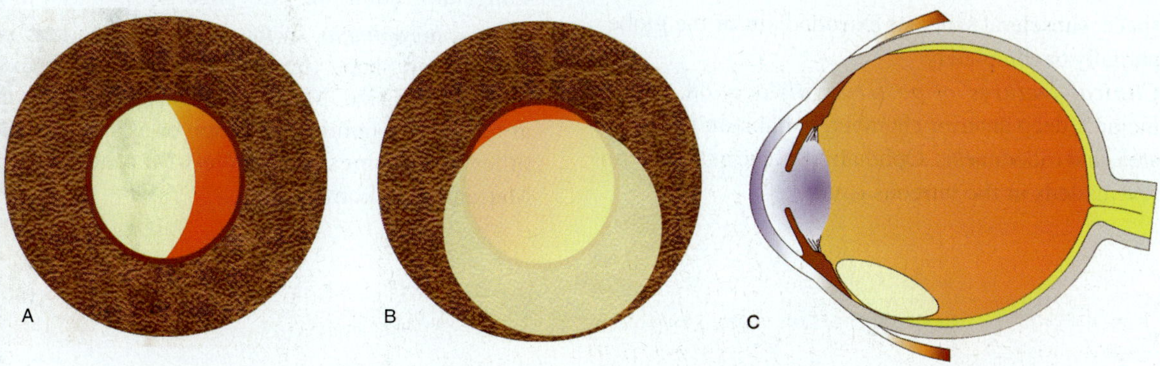

Fig. 8.31. Displacements of lens: A, subluxation; B, anterior dislocation; C, posterior dislocation.

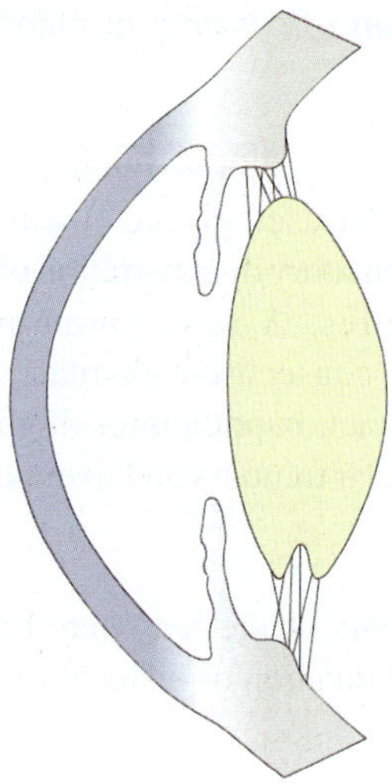

Fig. 8.32.
Coloboma of the lens.

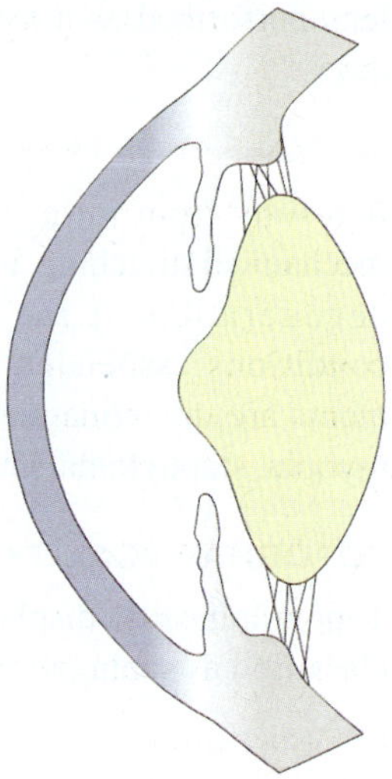

Fig. 8.33.
Lenticonus anterior.

- Uveitis and
- Secondary glaucoma.

Management. *Spectacles or contact lens* correction for phakic or aphakic area (whichever is better) is helpful in many cases. *Surgery* is controversial and usually associated with high risk of retinal detachment. Lensectomy with anterior vitrectomy may be performed in desperate cases.

II. Dislocation or luxation of the lens

In it all the zonules are severed from the lens. A dislocated lens may be incarcerated into the pupil or present in the anterior chamber (Fig. 8.31B), the vitreous (Fig. 8.31C) (where it may be floating – *lens nutans;* or fixed to retina – *lens fixata),* sub-retinal space, subscleral space or extruded out of the globe, partially or completely.

Clinical features *of posterior dislocation.* These include: deep anterior chamber, aphakia in pupillary area, and iridodonesis. Ophthalmoscopic examination reveals lens in the vitreous cavity.

Clinical features of anterior dislocation are deep anterior chamber and presence of lens in the anterior chamber. Clear lens looks like an oil drop in the aqueous.

Complications associated with dislocated lens are *uveitis* and *secondary glaucoma.*

Management. A lens dislocated in the anterior chamber and that incarcerated in the pupil should be removed as early as possible. A dislocated lens from the vitreous cavity should be removed only if it is causing uveitis or glaucoma. From the vitreous cavity lens can be removed after total vitrectomy, either with the help of an insulated vitreous cryoprobe or by aspiration facility of vitrectomy probe (only soft cataract).

CONGENITAL ANOMALIES OF THE LENS

1. *Coloboma of the lens.* It is seen as a notch in the lower quadrant of the equator (Fig. 8.32). It is usually unilateral and often hereditary.
2. *Congenital ectopia lentis* (see lens displacement page 202).
3. *Lenticonus.* It refers to cone-shaped elevation of the anterior pole (lenticonus anterior, Fig. 8.33) or posterior pole (lenticonus posterior) of the lens. Lenticonus anterior may occur in Alport's syndrome and lenticonus posterior in Lowe's syndrome. On distant direct ophthalmoscopy, both present as an oil globule lying in the centre of the red reflex. Slit-lamp examination confirms the diagnosis.
4. *Congenital cataract.* (see page 180).
5. *Microspherophakia.* In this condition, the lens is spherical in shape (instead of normal biconvex) and small in size. Microspherophakia may occur as an isolated familial condition or as a feature of other syndromes e.g., Weil-Marchesani or Marfan's syndrome.

CHAPTER

9 Glaucoma

ANATOMY AND PHYSIOLOGY
- Applied anatomy
- Applied physiology

GENERAL CONSIDERATIONS
- Definition and classification of glaucoma
- Pathogenesis of glaucomatous ocular damage

CONGENITAL/DEVELOPMENTAL GLAUCOMAS
- Terminology
- Primary congenital/Developmental glaucoma
- Developmental glaucomas with associated anomalies

PRIMARY OPEN-ANGLE GLAUCOMA AND RELATED CONDITIONS
- Primary open-angle glaucoma
- Ocular hypertension
- Normal tension glaucoma

PRIMARY ANGLE-CLOSURE GLAUCOMA
- Epidemiology
- Etiopathogenesis
- Classification and clinical presentation
  - Primary angle closure suspect
  - Primary angle closure
  - Pimary angle closure glaucoma

SECONDARY GLAUCOMAS

SURGICAL PROCEDURES FOR GLAUCOMA

ANATOMY AND PHYSIOLOGY

APPLIED ANATOMY

Pathophysiology of glaucoma revolves around the aqueous humour dynamics. The principal ocular structures concerned with it are ciliary body, angle of anterior chamber and the aqueous outflow system.

Ciliary body

It is the seat of aqueous production. Applied aspects of its anatomy have been described on page 142.

Angle of anterior chamber

Angle of anterior chamber plays an important role in the process of aqueous drainage. It is formed by root of iris, anterior-most part of ciliary body, scleral spur, trabecular meshwork and *Schwalbe's line* (prominent end of Descemet's membrane of cornea) (Fig. 9.1). The angle width varies in different individuals and plays a vital role in the pathomechanism of different types of glaucoma. Clinically the angle structures can be visualised by gonioscopic examination (see page 578).

Gonioscopic grading of the angle width. Various systems have been suggested to grade angle width. The most commonly used Shaffer's system of grading the angle is given in Table 9.1 and is shown in Fig. 9.2.

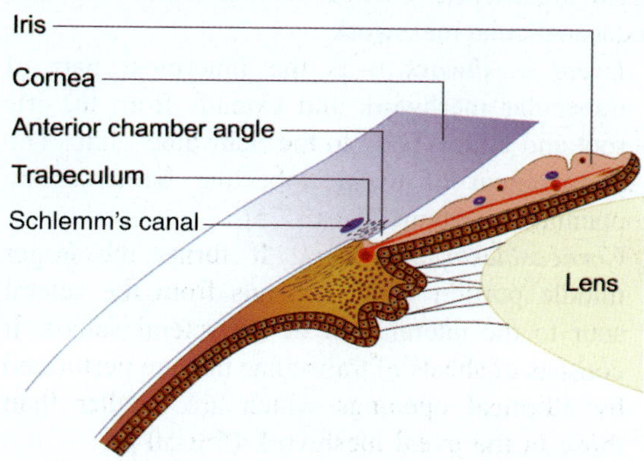

Fig. 9.1. Section of the anterior ocular structures showing region of the anterior chamber.

Table 9.1. Shaffer's system of grading the angle width

Grade	*Angle width*	*Configuration*	*Risk of closure*	*Structures visible on gonioscopy*
4	40°	Wide open	Closure impossible	SL, TM, SS, CBB
3	30°	Open angle	Closure impossible	SL, TM, SS
2	20°	Moderately narrow	Closure possible	SL, TM
1	10°	Very narrow	High risk of closure	SL only
S	< 10°	Slit angle	Closure imminent	No angle structures seen
0	0°	Closed	Closed	None of the angle structures visible

SL = Schwalbe's line, TM = Trabecular meshwork, SS = Scleral spur, CBB = Ciliary body band

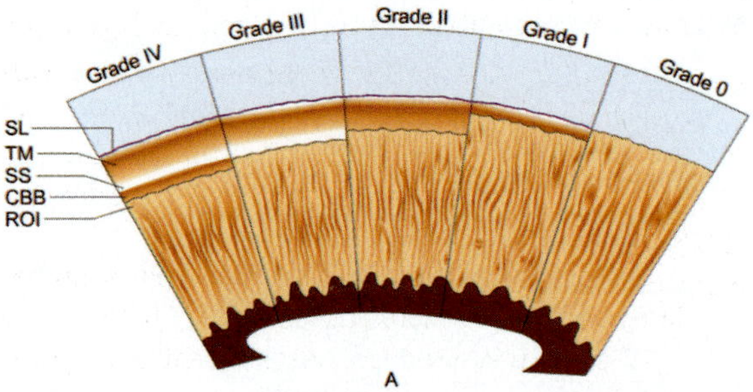

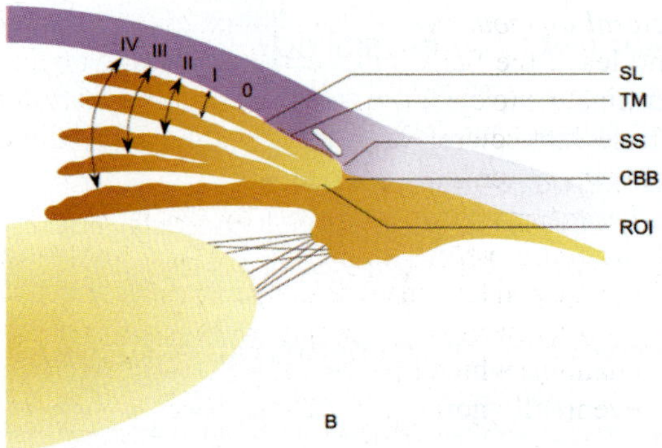

Fig. 9.2. Diagrammatic depiction of various angle structures (SL, Schwalbe's line; TM, trabecular meshwork; SS, scleral spur; CBB, ciliary body band; ROI, root of iris) as seen in different grades of angle width (Schaffer's grading system): A, gonioscopic view; B, configuration of the angle in cross section of the anterior chamber.

Aqueous outflow system

It includes the trabecular meshwork, Schlemm's canal, collector channels, aqueous veins and the episcleral veins (Fig. 9.3A).

1. *Trabecular meshwork.* It is a sieve-like structure through which aqueous humour leaves the eye. It consists of three layers, which from inside out are uveal meshwork, corneo scleral meshwork and juxtacanalicular meshwork.

i. *Uveal meshwork.* It is the innermost part of trabecular meshwork and extends from the iris root and ciliary body to the Schwalbe's line. The arrangement of uveal trabecular bands create openings of about 25μ to 75μ.

ii. *Corneoscleral meshwork.* It forms the larger middle portion which extends from the scleral spur to the lateral wall of the scleral sulcus. It consists of sheets of trabeculae that are perforated by elliptical openings which are smaller than those in the uveal meshwork (5 μ-50 μ).

iii *Juxtacanalicular (endothelial) meshwork.* It forms the outermost portion of trabecular meshwork and consists of juxtacanalicular space (filled with ground substance) and cells. The juxtacanalicular cell cytoplasmic processes attach externally to the processes arising from the innerwall endothelium of Schlemm's canal and internally to the processes arising from the cells of corneoscleral meshwork. Thus, this narrow

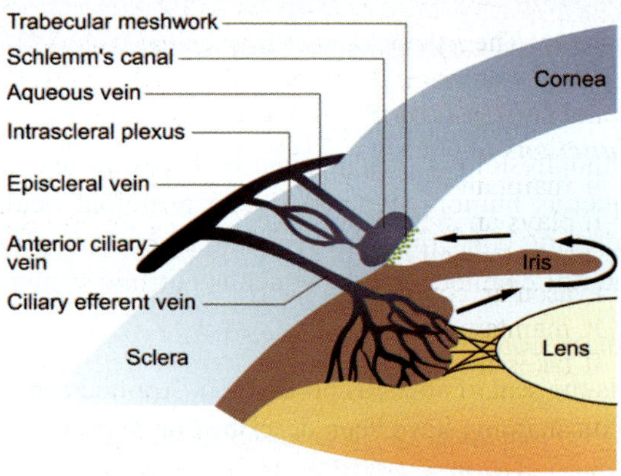

Fig. 9.3.A The aqueous outflow system.

part of trabeculum connects the corneoscleral meshwork with Schlemm's canal. This part of trabecular meshwork mainly offers normal resistance to the aqueous outflow.

2. *Schlemm's canal.* This is an endothelial lined oval channel present circumferentially in the scleral sulcus. The endothelial cells of its inner wall are irregular, spindle-shaped and contain giant vacuoles. The outer wall of the canal is lined by smooth flat cells and contains the openings of collector channels.

3. *Collector channels.* These, also called *intra-scleral aqueous vessels,* are about 25-35 in number and leave the Schlemm's canal at oblique angles to terminate into episcleral veins in a laminated fashion. These intrascleral aqueous vessels can be divided into two systems (Fig. 9.3A):

- *Direct system.* It is formed by the larger vessels *(aqueous veins)* which run a short intrascleral course and terminate directly into episcleral veins.
- *Indirect system.* It is formed by the smaller collector channels which form an intrascleral plexus before eventually going into episcleral veins.

APPLIED PHYSIOLOGY

The physiological processes concerned with the dynamics of aqueous humour are its production, drainage and maintenance of intraocular pressure.

Aqueous humour and its production

Volume. The aqueous humour is a clear watery fluid filling the anterior chamber (0.25 ml) and posterior chamber (0.06 ml) of the eyeball.

Functions of aqueous humour are:

- It maintains a proper intraocular pressure.
- It plays an important metabolic role by providing substrates and by removing metabolites from the avascular cornea and lens.
- It maintains optical transparency.
- It takes the place of lymph that is absent within the eyeball.

Refractive index of aqueous humour is 1.336.

Composition. Constituents of normal aqueous humour are:

- *Water* 99.9% and *solids* 0.1% (given below).
- *Proteins* (colloid content). Because of blood aqueous barrier the protein content of aqueous humour (5-16 mg%) is much less than that of plasma (6-7 gm%). However, in inflammation of uvea (iridocyclitis) the blood-aqueous barrier is broken and the protein content of aqueous is increased (plasmoid aqueous).
- *Amino acid constituent* of aqueous humour is about 5 mg/kg water.
- *Non-colloid constituents* in millimols/kg water are glucose (6.0), urea (7), ascorbate (0.9), lactic acid (7.4), inositol (0.1), Na^+ (144), K^+ (4.5), Cl^- (10), and HCO_3^- (34).
- *Oxygen* is present in the aqueous humour in dissolved state.

***Note*:** Thus, composition of aqueous is similar to plasma except that it has:

- High concentrations of ascorbate, pyruvate and lactate; and
- Low concentration of protein, urea and glucose.

Aqueous humour: anterior chamber versus posterior chamber. The composition of aqeuous humour in anterior chamber differs from that of the aqueous humour in posterior chamber because of metabolic interchange. The main differences are:

- HCO_3^- in posterior chamber aqueous is higher than in the anterior chamber.
- Cl^- concentration in posterior chamber is lower than in the anterior chamber.
- Ascorbate concentration of posterior aqueous is slightly higher than that of anterior chamber aqueous.

Production. Aqueous humour is derived from plasma within the capillary network of ciliary processes. The normal aqueous production rate is 2.3 μl/min. The three mechanisms *diffusion, ultrafiltration and secretion* (active transport) play a part in its production at different levels. The steps involved in the process of production are summarized below:

1. *Ultrafiltration.* First of all, by ultrafiltration, most of the plasma substances pass out from the capillary wall and loose connective tissue. Thus, the plasma filtrate (dialysate) accumulates behind the pigmented and non-pigmented epithelium of ciliary processes.
2. *Secretion.* First the dialysate from the plasma is transported into the pigment epithelium. Paired Na^+/H^+ and Cl^-/HCO_3^- antiports actively transports Na^+ and Cl^- from the stroma into the cells. Intercellular gap junctions also play critical rule. The tight junctions between the cells of the non-pigment epithelium create part of blood aqueous barrier. Certain substances are actively transported (secreted) across this barrier into the posterior chamber. The active transport is brought about by Na^+-K^+ activated ATPase pump, calcium

and voltage gated ion channels and carbonic anhydrase enzyme system. Substances that are actively transported include sodium, chlorides, potassium, ascorbic acid, amino acids and bicarbonates.

3. *Diffusion.* Active transport of these substances across the non-pigmented ciliary epithelium results in an osmotic gradient leading to the movement of other plasma constituents into the posterior chamber by ultrafiltration and diffusion. Sodium is primarily responsible for the movement of water into the posterior chamber. As the aqueous humour passes from the posterior chamber to Schlemm's canal, there occurs sufficient diffusional exchange with the surrounding structures (ciliary body, iris lens, cornea and trabecular meshwork). As a result the anterior chamber aqueous resembles plasma more closely than does the posterior chamber aqueous humour.

Control of aqueous formation. The diurnal variation in intraocular pressure certainly indicates that some endogenous factors do influence the aqueous formation. The exact role of such factors is yet to be clearly understood. Vasopressin and adenyl-cyclase have been described to affect aqueous formation by influencing active transport of sodium.

Ultrafiltration and diffusion, which primarily operate against concentration gradient, the passive mechanisms of aqueous formation, are dependent on the level of blood pressure in the ciliary capillaries, the plasma osmotic pressure and the level of intra-ocular pressure.

Drainage of aqueous humour

Aqueous humour flows from the posterior chamber into the anterior chamber through the pupil against slight physiologic resistance. From the anterior chamber the aqueous is drained out by two routes (Fig. 9.3B):

1. *Trabecular (conventional) outflow*. Trabecular meshwork is the main outlet for aqueous from the anterior chamber. Approximately 70 to 80 percent of the total aqueous is drained out via this route.

Free flow of aqueous occurs from trabecular meshwork up to inner wall of Schlemm's canal which appears to provide some resistance to outflow.

Mechanism of aqueous transport across inner wall of Schlemm's canal. It is partially understood. *Vacuolation theory* is the most accepted view. According to it, transcellular spaces exist in the endothelial cells forming inner wall of Schlemm's canal. These open as a system of vacuoles and pores, primarily in response to pressure, and transport the aqueous from the juxtacanalicular connective tissue to Schlemm's canal (Fig. 9.4).

From Schlemm's canal the aqueous is transported via 25-35 external collector channels into the episcleral veins by direct and indirect systems (Fig. 9.3A). A pressure gradient between intraocular pressure and intrascleral venous pressure (about 10 mm of Hg) is responsible for unidirectional flow of aqueous.

Aqueous outflow system: A passive filter versus dynamic mechanical pump.

Aqueous flow through the aqueous outflow system has long been considered a *passive filter mechanism* against the pressure gradient. However, recently it has been reported that aqueous outflow system acts as a *biomechanical pump* which operates through oscillatory pressure transients caused by the ocular pulse, blinking and eye movements.

2. *Uveoscleral (unconventional) outflow*. It is responsible for about 20 to 30 percent of the total

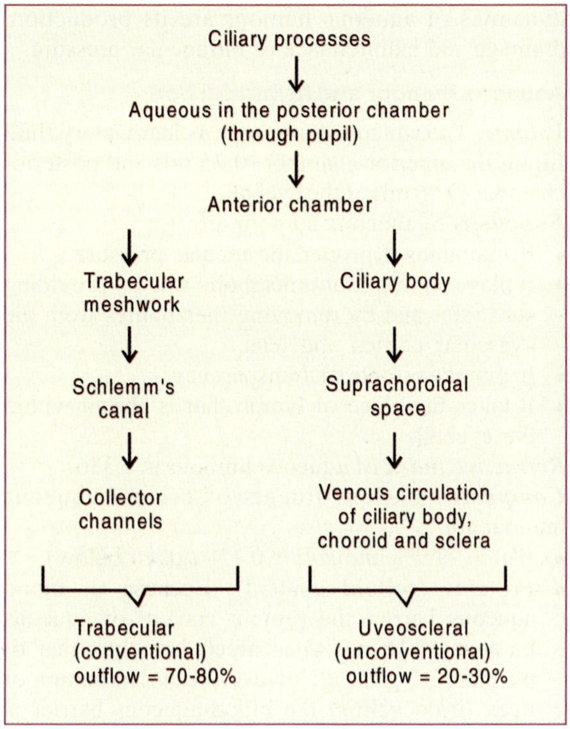

Fig. 9.3.B Flow chart depicting drainage of aqueous humour

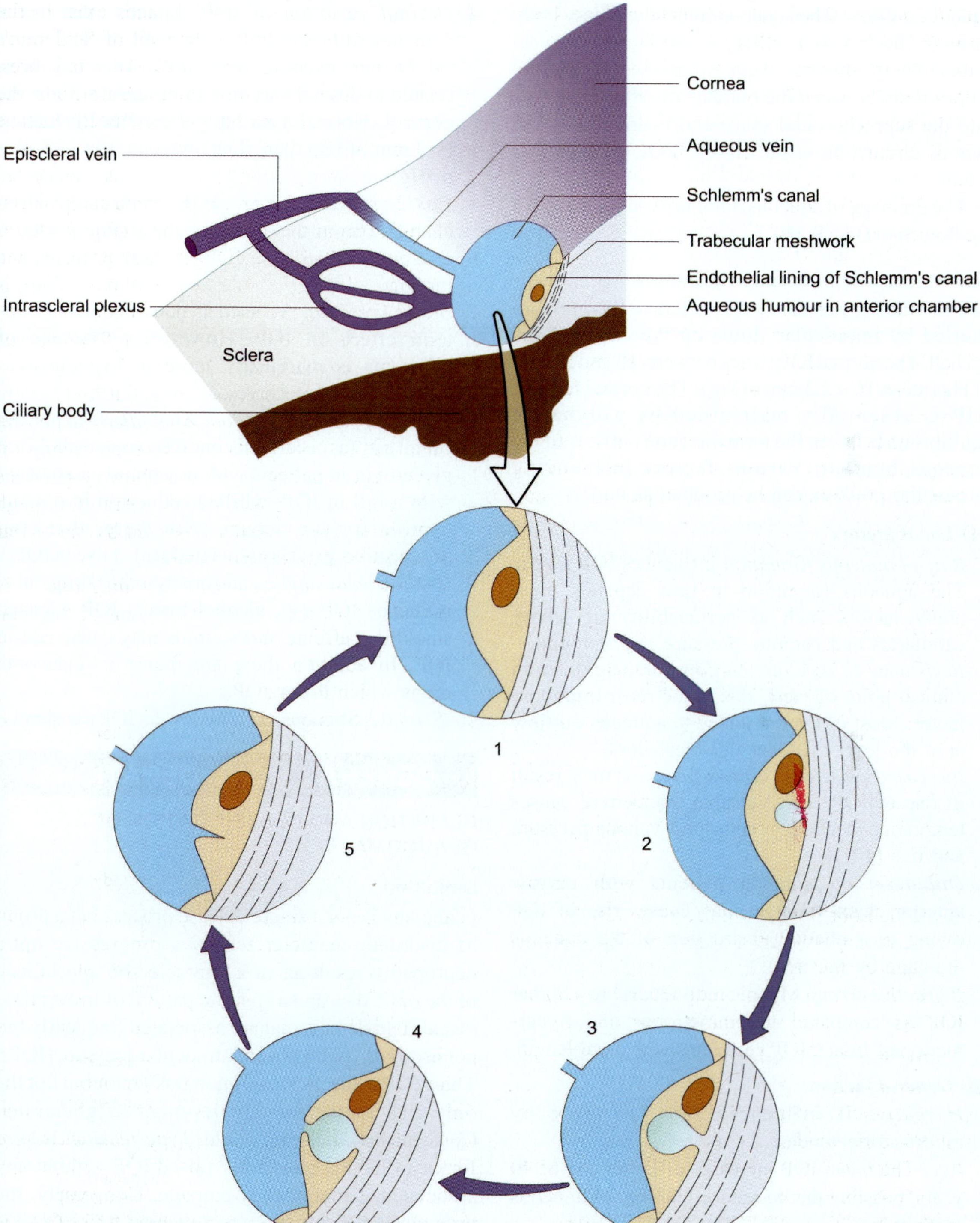

Fig. 9.4. Vaculation theory of aqueous transport across the inner wall of the Schlemm's canal: 1. Non-vacuolated stage; 2. Stage of early infolding of basal surface of the endothelial cell; 3. Stage of macrovacuolar structure formation; 4. Stage of vacuolar transcellular channel formation; 5.Stage of occlusion of the basal infolding.

aqueous outflow. The aqueous enters the ciliary body through the iris root, ciliary body face and uveal trabecular meshwork. Aqueous passes across the ciliary body between the bundles of ciliary muscles into the suprachoroidal space and is drained by the venous circulation of the ciliary body, choroid and sclera.

The drainage of aqueous humour is summarized in the flowchart (Fig. 9.3B).

Maintenance of intraocular pressure

The intraocular pressure (IOP) refers to the pressure exerted by intraocular fluids on the coats of the eyeball. The normal IOP varies between 10 and 21 mm of Hg (mean 16 ± 2.5 mm of Hg). The normal level of IOP is essentially maintained by a dynamic equilibrium between the formation and outflow of the aqueous humour. Various factors influencing intraocular pressure can be grouped as under:

(A) Local factors

1. *Rate of aqueous formation* influences IOP levels. The aqueous formation in turn depends upon many factors such as permeability of ciliary capillaries and osmotic pressure of the blood.
2. *Resistance to aqueous outflow* (drainage). From clinical point of view, this is the most important factor. Most of the resistance to aqueous outflow is at the level of trabecular meshwork.
3. *Increased episcleral venous pressure* may result in rise of IOP. The Valsalva manoeuvre causes temporary increase in episcleral venous pressure and rise in IOP.
4. *Dilatation of pupil* in patients with narrow anterior chamber angle may cause rise of IOP owing to a relative obstruction of the aqeuous drainage by the iris.
5. *Refractive errors.* Myopic individuals have higher IOP as compared to emmetropes and hypermetropes. Infact, IOP correlates with axial length.

(B) General factors

1. *Heredity.* It influences IOP, possibly by multifactorial modes.
2. *Age.* The mean IOP increases after the age of 40 years, possibly due to reduced facility of aqueous outflow.
3. *Sex.* IOP is equal between the sexes in ages 20-40 years. In older age groups increase in mean IOP with age is greater in females.
4. *Diurnal variation of IOP.* Usually, there is a tendency of higher IOP in the morning and lower in the late evening (Fig. 9.8). This has been related to diurnal variation in the levels of plasma cortisol. Normal eyes have a smaller fluctuation (< 5 mm of Hg) than glaucomatous eyes (> 8 mm of Hg).
5. *Postural variations.* IOP increases when changing from the sitting to the supine position.
6. *Seasonal variations.* IOP is higher in winter months.
7. *Blood pressure.* As such it does not have long-term effect on IOP. However, prevalence of glaucoma is marginally more in hypertensives than the normotensives.
8. *Osmotic pressure of blood.* An increase in plasma osmolarity (as occurs after intravenous mannitol, oral glycerol or in patients with uraemia) is associated with a fall in IOP, while a reduction in plasma osmolarity (as occurs with water drinking provocative tests) is associated with a rise in IOP.
9. *General anaesthetics* and many other drugs also influence IOP e.g., alcohol lowers IOP, tobacco smoking, caffeine and steroids may cause rise in IOP. In addition there are many antiglaucoma drugs which lower IOP.
10. *Exercise.* Strenous exercise lowers IOP transiently.

GENERAL CONSIDERATIONS

DEFINITION AND CLASSIFICATION OF GLAUCOMA

Definition

Glaucoma is not a single disease process but a group of disorders characterized by a progressive optic neuropathy resulting in a characterstic appearance of the optic disc and a specific pattern of irreversible visual field defects that are associated frequently but not invariably with raised intraocular pressure (IOP). Thus, IOP is the most common risk factor but not the only risk factor for development of glaucoma. Consequently the term '*ocular hypertension*' is used for cases having constantly raised IOP without any associated glaucomatous damage. Conversely, the term *normal* or *low tension glaucoma (NTG/LTG)* is suggested for the typical cupping of the disc and/or visual field defects associated with a normal or low IOP.

Classification

Clinico-etiologically glaucoma may be classified as follows:

(A) *Congenital/developmental glaucomas*

1. Primary congenital glaucoma (without associated anomalies).
2. Developmental glaucoma (with associated anomalies).

(B) *Primary adult glaucomas*

1. Primary open angle glaucomas (POAG)
2. Primary angle closure glaucoma (PACG)
3. Primary mixed mechanism glaucoma

(C) *Secondary glaucomas*

PATHOGENESIS OF GLAUCOMATOUS OCULAR DAMAGE

As mentioned in definition, all glaucomas (classified above and described later) are characterized by a progressive optic neuropathy. It has now been recognized that progressive optic neuropathy results from the death of retinal ganglion cells (RGCs) in a typical pattern which results in characteristic optic disc appearance and specific visual field defects.

Pathogenesis of retinal ganglion cell death

Retinal ganglion cell (RGC) death is initiated when some pathologic event blocks the transport of growth factors (neurotrophins) from the brain to the RGCs. The blockage of these neurotrophins initiate a damaging cascade, and the cell is unable to maintain its normal function. The RGCs losing their ability to maintain normal function undergo apoptosis and also trigger apoptosis of adjacent cells. Apoptosis is a genetically controlled cell suicide programme whereby irreversibly damaged cells die, and are subsequently engulfed by neighbouring cells, without eliciting any inflammatory response.

Retinal ganglion cell death is, of course, associated with loss of retinal nerve fibres. As the loss of nerve fibres extends beyond the normal physiological overlap of functional zones, the characteristic optic disc changes and specific visual field defects become apparent over the time.

Etiological factors

Factors involved in the etiology of retinal ganglion cell death and thus in the etiology of glaucomatous optic neuropathy can be grouped as below:

A. *Primary insults*

1. *Raised intraocular pressure* (*Mechanical theory*). Raised intraocular pressure causes mechanical stretch on the lamina cribrosa leading to axonal deformation and ischaemia by altering capillary blood flow. As a result of this, neurotrophins (growth factors) are not able to reach the retinal ganglion cell bodies in sufficient amount needed for their survival.

2. *Pressure independent factors* (*Vascular insufficiency theory*). Factors affecting vascular perfusion of optic nerve head in the absence of raised IOP have been implicated in the glaucomatous optic neuropathy in patients with normal tension glaucoma (NTG). However, these may be the additional factors in cases of raised IOP as well. These factors include:

i. *Failure of autoregulatory mechanism of blood flow.* The retina and optic nerve share a peculiar mechanism of autoregulation of blood flow with rest of the central nervous system. Once the autoregulatory mechanisms are compromised, blood flow may not be adequate beyond some critical range of IOP (which may be raised or in normal range).

ii. *Vasospasm* is another mechanism affecting vascular perfusion of optic nerve head. This hypothesis gets credence from the convincing association between NTG and vasospastic disorders (migranous headache and Raynaud's phenomenon).

iii. *Systemic hypotension*, particularly nocturnal dips in patients with night time administration of antihypertensive drugs, has been implicated for low vascular perfusion of optic nerve head resulting in NTG and progression of damage in POAG.

iv. *Other factors* such as acute blood loss and abnormal coagulability profile have also been associated with NTG.

B. *Secondary insults (Excitotoxicity theory)*

Neuronal degeneration is believed to be driven by toxic factors such as glutamate (excitatory toxin), oxygen free radicals, or nitric oxide which are released when RGCs undergo death due to primary insults. In this way the secondary insult leads to continued damage mediated apoptosis, even after the primary insult has been controlled.

CONGENITAL / DEVELOPMENTAL GLAUCOMAS

TERMINOLOGY

The congenital glaucomas are a group of diverse disorders in which abnormal high intraocular pressure results due to developmental abnormalities of the angle of anterior chamber obstructing the drainage of aqueous humour. Sometimes glaucoma may not occur until several years after birth; therefore, the term *developmental glaucoma* is preferred to describe such disorders.

Types

1. Primary developmental/congenital glaucoma.
2. Developmental glaucoma with associated specific ocular or systemic congenital anomalies.

PRIMARY DEVELOPMENTAL/CONGENITAL GLAUCOMA

It refers to abnormally high IOP which results due to developmental anomaly of the angle of the anterior chamber, not associated with any other ocular or systemic anomaly. Depending upon the age of onset the developmental glaucomas are termed as follows:

1. ***New born glaucoma,*** also called as *true congenital glaucoma*, is labelled when IOP is raised during intrauterine life and child is born with ocular enlargement. It accounts for about 25 percent of cases.

2. ***Infantile glaucoma*** is labelled when the disease manifests prior to the child's third birthday. It accounts for about 65 percent of cases.

3. ***Juvenile glaucoma*** is labelled in the rest 10 percent of cases who develop pressure rise after 3 years but before adulthood.

When the disease manifests prior to age of 3 years, the eyeball enlarges and so the term '*buphthalmos*' (bull-like eyes) is used. As it results due to retention of aqueous humour (watery solution), the term '*hydrophthalmos*, has also been suggested.

Prevalence and genetic pattern

- *Sporadic occurrence* is seen in most cases 90%.
- *Autosomal recessive* inheritance with incomplete penetrance is seen in about 10 percent cases.
- *Genes* inplicated are GLC3A, GLC3B and GLC3C.
- *Sex linkage* is not common in inheritance although over 65 percent of the patients are boys.
- *Bilateral* occurence is seen in 70 percent cases, though the involvement may be asymmetric.
- *Prevalence* of the disease is only 1 child in 10,000 births.

Pathogenesis

Maldevelopment, from neural crest derived cells, of trabeculum including the iridotrabecular junction *(trabeculodysgenesis)* is responsible for impaired aqueous outflow resulting in raised IOP. In primary congenital glaucoma the trabeculodysgenesis is not associated with any other major ocular anomalies. Clinically, trabeculodys-genesis is characterized by absence of the angle recess with iris having a flat or concave direct insertion into the surface of trabeculum as follows:

- *Flat iris insertion* is more common than the concave iris insertion. In it the iris inserts flatly and abruptly into the thickened trabeculum either at or anterior to scleral spur (more often) or posterior to scleral spur. It is often possible to visualize a portion of ciliary body and scleral spur.
- *Concave iris insertion* is less common. In it the superficial iris tissue sweeps over the irido-trabecular junction and the trabeculum and thus, obscures the scleral spur and ciliary body.

Clinical features

1. ***Lacrimation, photophobia and blepharospasm*** often occur together and form the *classic triad* of symptoms of congenital glaucoma. Often there is *history of rubbing* of the eyes. These are thought to be caused by irritation of corneal nerves, which occurs as a result of the elevated IOP. Photophobia is usually the initial sign, but is not enough by itself to arouse suspicion in most cases.

2. ***Corneal signs***. Corneal signs include its oedema, enlargement and Descemet's breaks.

i. *Corneal oedema.* It is frequently the first sign which arouses suspicion. At first it is epithelial, but later there is stromal involvement and permanent opacities may occur.

ii. *Corneal enlargement.* It occurs alongwith enlargement of globe-buphthalmos (Fig. 9.5), especially when the onset is before the age of 3 years. Normal infant cornea measures 10.5 mm. A diameter of more than 13 mm confirms enlargement. Prognosis is usually poor in infants with corneal diameter of more than 16 mm.

iii. *Tears and breaks in Descemet's membrane* (Haab's striae). These occur because Descemet's membrane is less elastic than the corneal stroma. Tears are usually peripheral and concentric with the limbus.

3. *Sclera* becomes thin and appears blue due to underlying uveal tissue.

4. *Anterior chamber* becomes deep.

5. *Iris* may show iridodonesis and atrophic patches in late stage.

6. *Lens* becomes flat due to stretching of zonules and may even subluxate.

7. *Optic disc* may show variable cupping and atrophy especially after third year.

8. *IOP* is raised which is neither marked nor acute.

9. *Axial myopia* may occur because of increase in axial length which may give rise to anisometropic amblyopia.

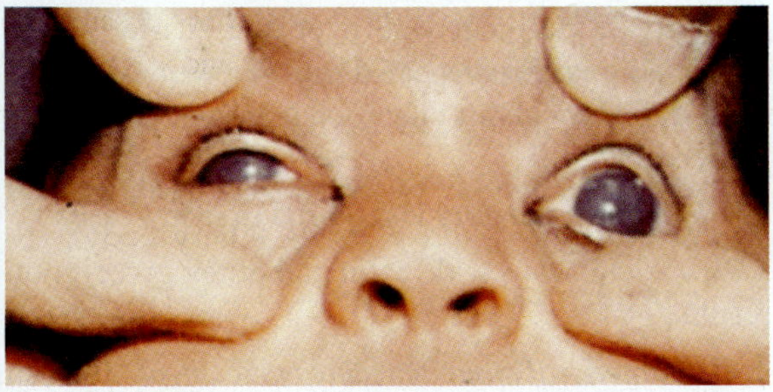

Fig. 9.5. A child with congenital glaucoma.

Examination (Evaluation)

A complete examination under general anaesthesia (EUA) should be performed on each child suspected of having congenital glaucoma. The examination should include following:

1. *Measurement of IOP* with Schiotz or preferably hand held Perkin's applanation tonometer since scleral rigidity is very low in children. IOP measurement under GA is unpredictably altered.
2. *Measurement of corneal diameter* by callipers.
3. *Slit lamp examination* should be carried out with portable slit lamp.
4. *Ophthalmoscopy* to evaluate optic disc.
5. *Gonioscopic examination* of angle of anterior chamber reveals trabeculodysgenesis with either flat or concave iris insertion as described in pathogenesis.

Differential diagnosis

It is to be considered for different presenting signs as follows:

1. *Cloudy cornea.* In unilateral cases the commonest cause is trauma with rupture of Descemet's membrane (forceps injury). In bilateral cases causes may be trauma, mucopolysaccharidosis, interstitial keratitis and corneal endothelial dystrophy.
2. *Large cornea* due to buphthalmos should be differentiated from megalocornea, sclerocornea and high myopia.
3. *Lacrimation* in an infant is usually considered to be due to congenital nasolacrimal duct blockage and thus early diagnosis of congenital glaucoma may be missed. Other causes of watering in small child include corneal abrasion, Meesman's corneal dystrophy and Reis-Buckler dystrophy.
4. *Photophobia* may be due to keratitis or uveitis.
5. *Raised IOP in infants* may also be associated with retinoblastoma, retinopathy of prematurity, persistent primary hyperplastic vitreous, traumatic glaucoma and secondary congenital glaucoma seen in rubella, aniridia and Sturge-Weber syndrome.
6. *Optic disc changes* need to be differentiated from congenital anomalies of the disc such as pit, coloboma, hypoplasia, tilted disc and large physiological cup.

Treatment

Medical Treatment

Treatment of congenital glaucoma is primarily surgical. However, IOP must be lowered by medical treatment with hyperosmotic agents, acetazolamide and beta-blockers till surgery is taken up. Miotics are not used in such cases because they paradoxically increase IOP. Alpha-2 agonist (brimonidine) causes CNS depression in children and is contraindicated.

Surgical procedures for congenital glaucoma

I. *Incisional angle surgery,* which can be performed by the internal approach (goniotomy) or by external approach (trabeculectomy).

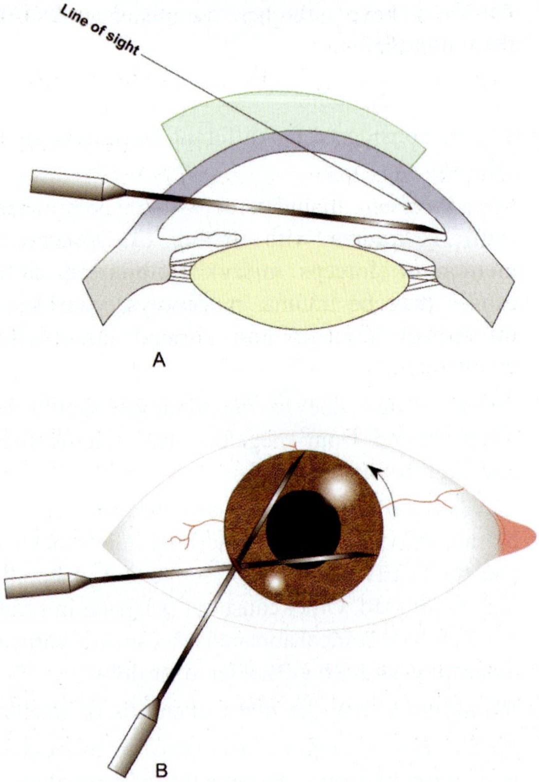

Fig. 9.6. Technique of goniotomy : A, showing position of goniotomy knife in the angle under direct visualization; B, showing procedure of sweeping the knife in the angle.

1. *Goniotomy* (Fig. 9.6). In this procedure a Barkan's goniotomy knife is passed through the limbus on the temporal side. Under gonioscopic control the knife is passed across the anterior chamber to the nasal part of the angle. An incision is made in the angle approximately midway between root of the iris and Schwalbe's ring through approximately 75°. The knife is then withdrawn. Although the procedure may have to be repeated, the eventual success rate is about 85 percent.

2. *Trabeculotomy.* This is useful when corneal clouding prevents visualization of the angle or in cases where goniotomy has failed. In this, canal of Schlemm is exposed at about 12 O'clock position by a vertical scleral incision after making a conjunctival flap and partial thickness scleral flap. The lower prong of Harm's trabeculotome is passed along the Schlemm's canal on one side and the upper prong is used as a guide (Fig. 9.7). Then the trabeculotome is rotated so as to break the inner wall over one quarter of the canal. This is then repeated on the other side. The main difficulty in this operation is localization of the Schlemm's canal.

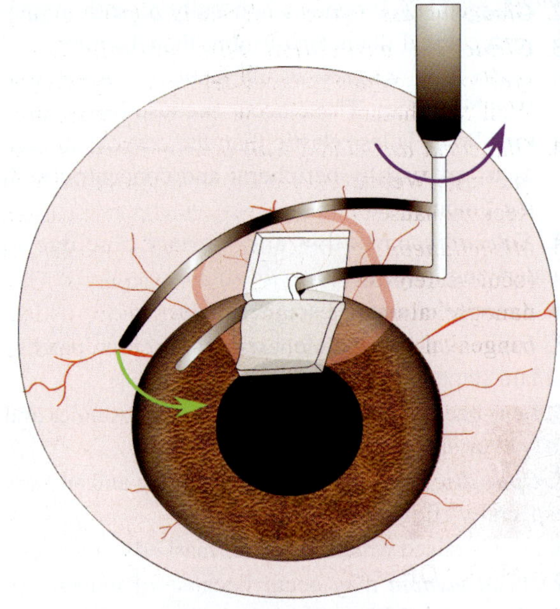

Fig. 9.7. Technique of trabeculotomy.

II. *Filteration surgery* is required in many cases:

1. *Trabeculotomy* with antimetabolites gives good results.

2. *Combined trabeculotomy and trabeculectomy* with anti-metabolites has been accepted as the standard procedure.

III. *Glaucoma drainage devices* (GDD) are required in incalcitrant cases.

DEVELOPMENTAL GLAUCOMAS WITH ASSOCIATED ANOMALIES

A wide variety of systemic and/or ocular anomalies have an associated raised IOP, usually due to developmental defects of the anterior chamber angle. Some of the associations are as follows:

1. *Glaucoma associated with iridocorneal dysgenesis.* These include: posterior embryotoxon characterised by a prominent Schwalbe's ring (Axenfeld anomaly), Rieger anomaly, Rieger syndrome, Peter's anomaly and combined Rieger syndrome and Peter's anomaly.

2. *Glaucoma associated with aniridia* (50% cases).
3. *Glaucoma associated with ectopia lentis syndromes,* which include Marfan's syndrome, Weil-Marchesani syndrome and homocystinuria.
4. *Glaucoma associated with phakomatosis* is seen in Sturge-Weber syndrome (50% cases) and Von Recklinghausen's neurofibromatosis (25% cases).
5. *Miscellaneous conditions.* Lowe's syndrome (oculo-cerebro-renal syndrome), naevus of Ota, nanophthalmos, congenital ectropion uveae, congenital microcornea and rubella syndrome.

PRIMARY OPEN-ANGLE GLAUCOMA AND RELATED CONDITIONS

PRIMARY OPEN-ANGLE GLAUCOMA

As the name implies, it is a type of primary glaucoma, where there is no obvious systemic or ocular cause of rise in the intraocular pressure. Primary open angle glaucoma (POAG), also known as chronic simple glaucoma of adult onset, is typically characterised by:

- Slowly progressive raised intraocular pressure (>21 mm Hg recorded on at least few occasions) associated with,
- Open normal appearing anterior chamber angle,
- Characteristic optic disc cupping, and
- Specific visual field defects.

ETIOPATHOGENESIS

Etiopathogenesis of POAG is not known exactly. Some of the known facts are as follows:

A. ***Predisposing and risk factors.*** These include the following:

1. *Heredity.* POAG has a polygenic inheritance. The approximate risk of getting disease is 10% in the siblings, and 4% in the offspring of patients with POAG.
2. *Age.* The risk increases with increasing age. The POAG is more commonly seen in elders between 5th and 7th decades.
3. *Race.* POAG is significantly more common, develops earlier and is more severe in black people than in white.
4. *Myopes* are more predisposed than the normals.
5. *Diabetics* have a higher prevalence of POAG than non-diabetics.
6. *Cigarette smoking* is also thought to increase its risk.
7. *High blood pressure* is not the cause of rise in IOP, however the prevalence of POAG is more in hypertensives than the normotensives. Most meaningful blood pressure variable related to glaucoma is diastolic perfusion pressure (diastolic blood pressure–IOP). A diastolic perfusion pressure of <55 mm Hg is an important risk factor for glaucoma.
8. *Thyrotoxicosis* is also not the cause of rise in IOP, but the prevalence of POAG is more in patients suffering from Graves' ophthalmic disease than the normals.
9. *Corticosteroid responsiveness.* Patients with POAG and their offspring and sibilings are more likely to respond to six weeks topical steroid therapy with a significant rise of IOP.

B. *Pathogenesis of rise in IOP.* It is certain that rise in IOP occurs due to decrease in the aqueous outflow facility due to increased resistance to aqueous outflow caused by:

- Thickening and sclerosis of trabecular meshwork with faulty collagen tissue.
- Narrowing of intertrabecular spaces.
- Deposition of amorphous material in the juxta-canalicular space.
- Collapse of Schlemm's canal and absence of giant vacuoles in the cells lining it.

The exact cause of these changes is uncertain. Detection of increased gammaglobulin and plasma cells in trabecular meshwork on immunohisto- chemistry and positive antinuclear antibody reaction in some cases support an *immunogenic mechanism* in POAG.

C. *Pathogenesis of optic neuropathy.* (See page 223)

EPIDEMIOLOGY OF POAG

Prevalence of POAG varies in different populations. In general, it affects about 1 in 100 of the general population (of either sex) above the age of 40 years. It forms about one-third cases of all glaucomas.

CLINICAL FEATURES

Symptoms

1. *Asymptomatic.* The disease is insidious and usually asymptomatic, until it has caused a significant loss

of visual field. Therefore, periodic eye examination is required after middle age.
2. *Headache and eye ache* of mild intensity may be experienced in the course of the disease.
3. *Scotoma* (defect in the visual field) may be noticed occasionally by some observant patients.
4. *Difficulty in reading and close work*, often persistently increasing, is experienced by most patients. This occurs due to increasing accommodative failure as a result of constant pressure on the ciliary muscle and its nerve supply. Therefore, patients usually complain of *frequent changes in presbyopic glasses.*
5. *Delayed dark adaptation* may develop, a disability which becomes increasingly disturbing in the late stages.
6. *Significant loss of vision and blindness* is the end result of untreated cases of POAG.

Signs

I. *Anterior segment signs.* Ocular examination including slit-lamp biomicroscopy may reveal normal anterior segment. In late stages pupil reflex becomes sluggish and cornea may show slight haze. A low (<555 μm) central corneal thickness (CCT) is a significant risk factor for POAG.

II. *Intraocular pressure changes.* In the initial stages the IOP may not be raised permanently, but there is an exaggeration of the normal diurnal variation. Therefore, repeated observations of IOP (every 3-4 hour), for 24 hours is required during this stage (*Diurnal variation test*). In most patients IOP falls during the evening, contrary to what happens in angle-closure glaucoma. Different patterns of diurnal variation of IOP shown in Fig. 9.8 are:

- Morning rise in IOP-20% of cases
- Afternoon rise in IOP-25% of cases
- Biphasic rise in IOP-55% of cases

A variation in IOP of over 5 mm Hg (Schiotz) is suspicious and over 8 mm of Hg is diagnostic of glaucoma. In later stages, IOP is permanently raised above 21 mm of Hg and ranges between 30 and 45 mm of Hg.

III. *Optic disc changes.* Optic disc changes, usually observed on routine fundus examination, provide an important clue for suspecting POAG. These are typically progressive, asymmetric and present a variety of characteristic clinical patterns. It is essential, therefore, to record the appearance of the nerve head in such a way that will accurately reveal subtle glaucomatous changes over the course of follow-up evaluation.

Examination techniques. Careful assessment of disc changes can be made by direct ophthalmoscopy, slit-lamp biomicroscopy using a + 90D lens, Hruby lens

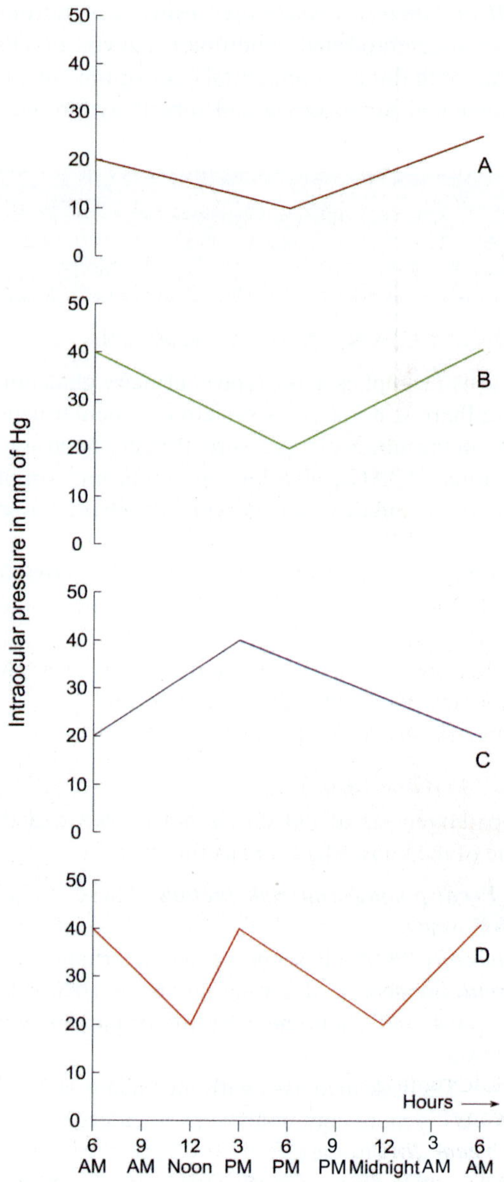

Fig. 9.8. Patterns of diurnal variations of IOP: A, normal slight morning rise; B, morning rise seen in 20% cases of POAG; C, afternoon rise seen in 25% cases of POAG; D, biphasic variation seen in 55% cases of POAG.

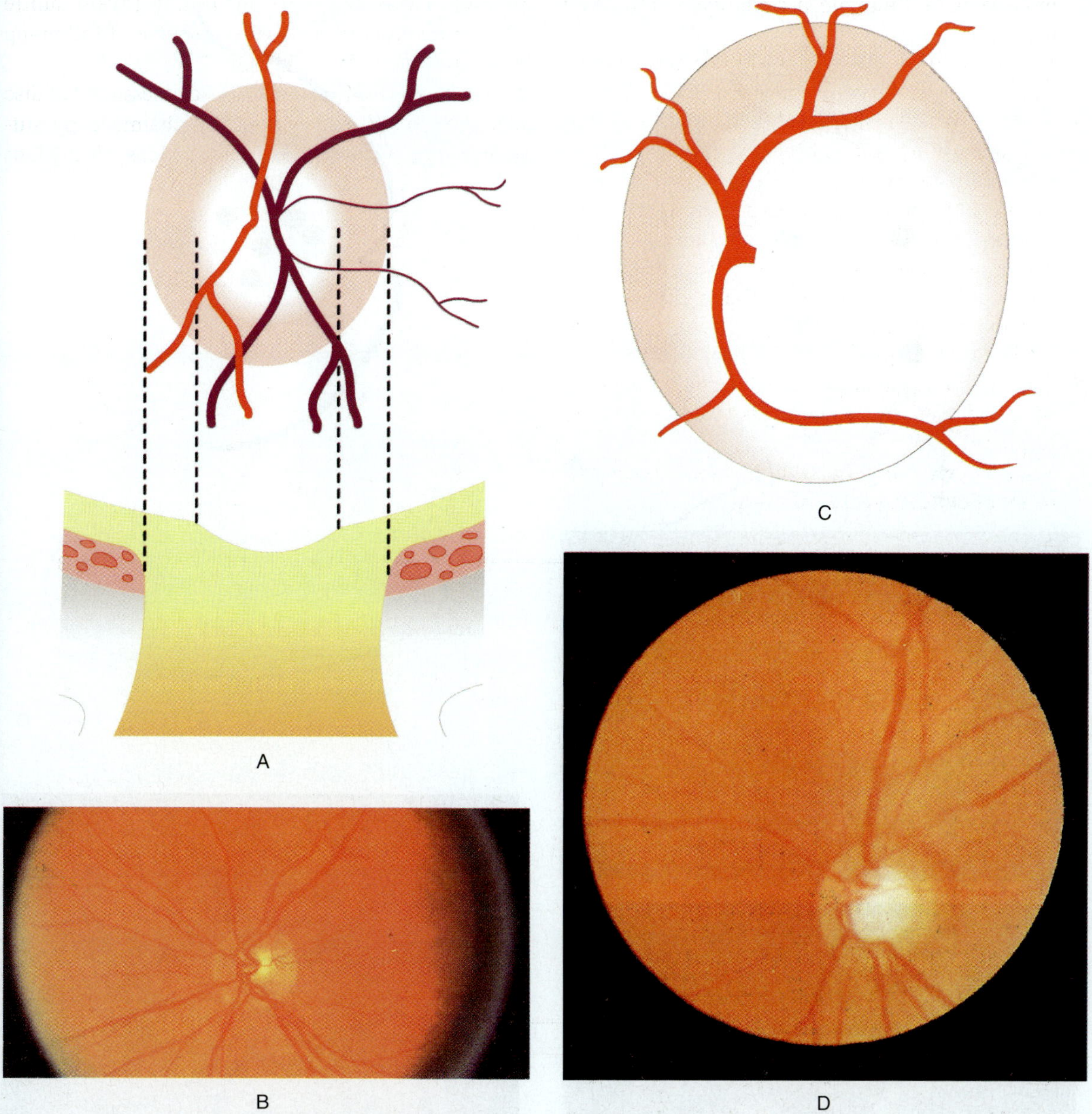

Fig. 9.9. Normal optic disc (A, diagrammatic depiction; B, fundus photograph) and optic disc showing early glaucomatous changes (C, diagrammatic depiction; D, fundus photograph).

or Goldmann contact lens and indirect ophthalmoscopy.

The recording and documentation techniques include serial drawings, photography and photogrammetry. Confocal scanning laser topography (CSLT) i.e., Heidelberg retinal tomograph (HRT) is an accurate and sensitive method for this purpose. Other advanced imaging techniques include optical coherence tomography (OCT) and scanning laser polarimetry i.e., Nerve fibre analyser (NFA).

Glaucomatous changes in the optic disc can be described as early changes, advanced changes and glaucomatous optic atrophy. Figures 9.9A and B show normal disc configuration.

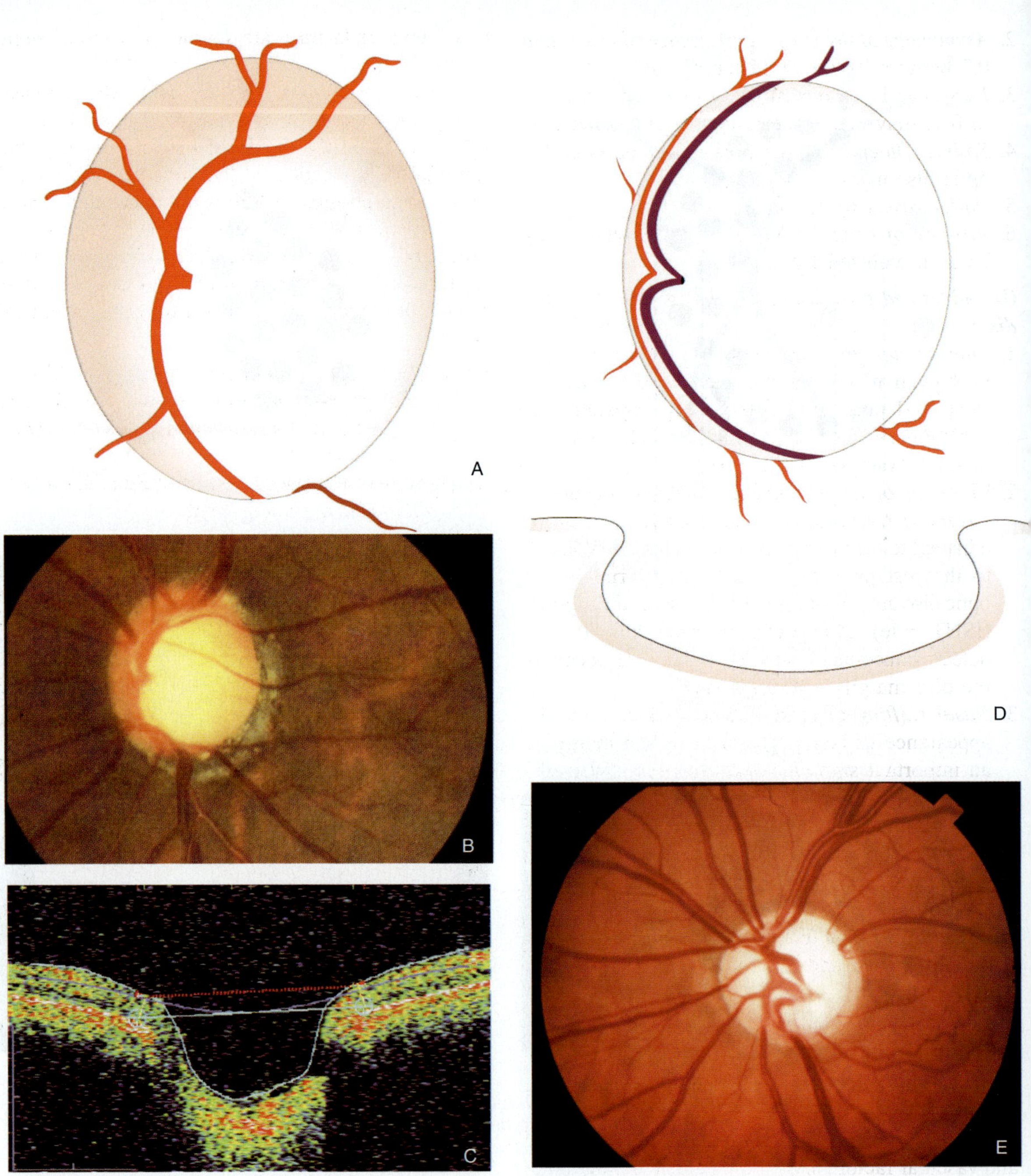

Fig. 9.10. Optic disc showing advanced glaucomatous changes (A, diagramatic depiction; B, fundus photograph; C, OCt Pictures) and glaucomotous optic atrophy (D, diagramatic depiction; E, fundus photograph);

(a) ***Early glaucomatous changes*** (Figs. 9.9C and D) should be suspected to exist if fundus examination reveals one or more of the following signs:

1. *Vertically oval cup* due to selective loss of neural rim tissue in the inferior and superior poles.

2. *Asymmetry of the cups.* A difference of more than 0.2 between two eyes is significant.
3. *Large cup* i.e., 0.6 or more (normal cup size is 0.3 to 0.4) may occur due to concentric expansion.
4. *Splinter haemorrhages* present on or near the optic disc margin.
5. *Pallor areas* on the disc.
6. *Atrophy of retinal nerve fibre layer* which may be seen with red free light.

(b) *Advanced glaucomatous changes in the optic disc*:

1. *Marked cupping* (cup size 0.7 to 0.9), excavation may even reach the disc margin, the sides are steep and not shelving (c.f. deep physiological cup) (Figs. 9.10A and B) which are well delineated on OCT examination Fig. 9.10C).
2. *Thinning of neuroretinal rim* which occurs in advanced cases is seen as a crescentric shadow adjacent to the disc margin. Normally, the thickest to thinnest parts of the neuroretinal rim of the optic disc are inferior, superior, nasal and temporal. (ISNT rule). Any variation from this help to detect glaucoma. Notching of the rim specially the disc margin is pathognomic.
3. *Nasal shifting* of retinal vessels which have the appearance of being broken off at the margin is an important sign (*Bayonetting sign*). When the edges overhang, the course of the vessels as they climb the sides of the cup is hidden.
4. *Pulsations of the retinal arterioles* may be seen at the disc margin (a pathognomic sign of glaucoma), when IOP is very high.
5. *Lamellar dot sign* the pores in the lamina cribrosa are slit-shaped and are visible up to the margin of the disc.

(c) *Glaucomatous optic atrophy*. As the damage progresses, all the neural tissue of the disc is destroyed and the optic nerve head appears white and deeply excavated (Figs. 9.10 C and D).

***Pathophysiology of disc changes*.** Both mechanical and vascular factors play a role in the cupping of the disc.

- *Mechanical effect* of raised IOP forces the lamina cribrosa backwards and squeezes the nerve fibres within its meshes to disturb axoplasmic flow.
- *Vascular factors* contribute in ischaemic atrophy of the nerve fibres without corresponding increase of supporting glial tissue. As a result, large caverns or lacunae are formed (*cavernous optic atrophy*).

IV. *Visual field defects.* Visual field defects appear only after about 40% of axons have been damaged and subsequently the field defects usually run parallel to the changes at the optic nerve head and continue to progress if IOP is not controlled. These can be described as early and late field defects.

***Anatomical basis of field defects*.** For better understanding of the actual field defects, it is mandatory to have a knowledge of their anatomical basis.

(A) *Distribution of retinal nerve fibres* (Fig. 9.11).

1. Fibres from nasal half of the retina come directly to the optic disc as superior and inferior *radiating fibres* (srf and irf).
2. Those from the macular area come horizontally as *papillomacular bundle* (pmb).
3. Fibres from the temporal retina arch above and below the macula and papillomacular bundle as superior and inferior *arcuate fibres* with a horizontal raphe in between (saf and iaf).

(B) *Arrangement of nerve fibres within optic nerve head* (Fig. 9.12): Those from the peripheral part of the

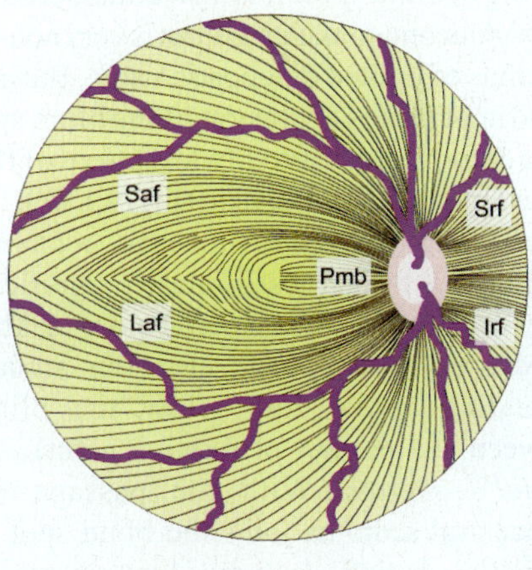

Fig. 9.11. Distribution of retinal nerve fibres.

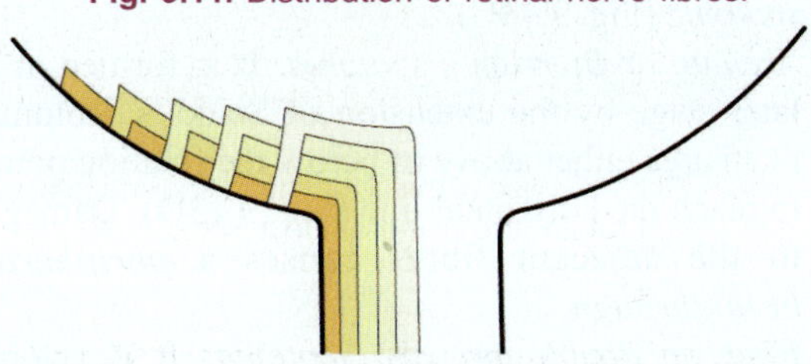

Fig. 9.12. Arrangement of nerve fibres within optic nerve head.

retina lie deep in the retina but occupy the most peripheral (superficial) part of the optic disc. While fibres originating closer to the nerve head lie superficially in the retina and occupy a more central (deep) portion of the disc.

The arcuate nerve fibres occupy the superior and inferior temporal portions of optic nerve head and are most sensitive to glaucomatous damage; accounting for the early loss in the corresponding regions of the visual field. Macular fibres are most resistant to the glaucomatous damage and explain the retention of the central vision till end.

Progression of field defects. Visual field defects in glaucoma are initially observed in Bjerrum's area (10-25 degree from fixation) and correlate with optic disc changes. The natural history of the progressive glaucomatous field loss, more or less, takes the following sequence:

1. *Isopter contraction.* It refers to mild generalised constriction of central as well as peripheral field. It is the earliest visual field defect occurring in glaucoma. However, it is of limited diagnostic value, as it may also occur in many other conditions.
2. *Baring of blind spot.* It is also considered to be an early glaucomatous change, but is very non-specific and thus of limited diagnostic value. Baring of the blind spot means exclusion of the blind spot from the central field due to inward curve of the outer boundary of 30° central field (Fig. 9.13A).
3. *Small wing-shaped paracentral scotoma* (Fig. 9.13B). It is the earliest clinically significant field defect. It may appear either below or above the blind spot in Bjerrum's area (an arcuate area extending above and below the blind spot between 10° and 20° of fixation point).
4. *Seidel's scotoma.* With the passage of time paracentral scotoma joins the blind spot to form a sickle shaped scotoma known as *Seidel's scotoma* (Fig. 9.13C).
5. *Arcuate or Bjerrum's scotoma.* It is formed at a later stage by the extension of Seidel's scotoma in an area either above or below the fixation point to reach the horizontal line (Fig. 9.13D). Damage to the adjacent fibres causes a *peripheral breakthrough.*
6. *Ring or double arcuate scotoma.* It develops when the two arcuate scotomas join together (Fig. 9.13E).

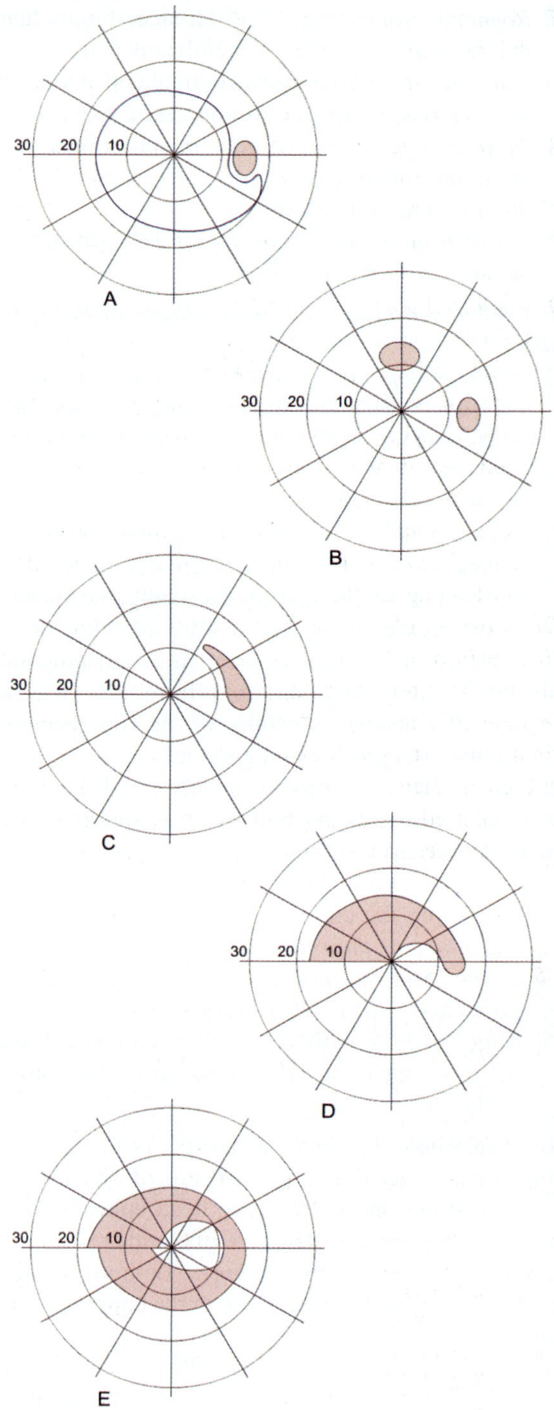

Fig. 9.13. Field defects in POAG: A, Baring of blind spot; B, Superior paracentral scotoma; C, Seidel's scotoma; D, Bjerrum's scotoma; E, Double arcuate scotoma and Roenne's central nasal step.

7. *Roenne's central nasal step.* It is created when the two arcuate scotomas run in different arcs and meet to form a sharp right-angled defect at the horizontal meridian (Fig. 9.13E).
8. *Peripheral field defects.* These appear sometimes at an early stage and sometimes only late in the disease. The *peripheral nasal step of Roenne's* results from unequal contraction of the peripheral isopter.
9. *Advanced glaucomatous field defects.* The visual field loss gradually spreads centrally as well as peripherally, and eventually only a small island of central vision *(tubular vision)* and an accompanying temporal island are left. With the continued damage, these islands of vision also progressively diminish in size until the tiny central island is totally extinguished. The *temporal island of the vision* is more resistant and is lost in the end leaving the patient with no light perception.

Diagnosis of glaucoma field defects on HFA single field printout. Glaucomatous field defects should always be interpreted in conjunction with clinical features (IOP and optic disc changes). Further, before final interpretation, the fields must be tested twice, as there is often a significant improvement in the field when plotted second time (because patients become more familiar with the machine and test process).

Criteria to grade glaucomatous field defects. The criteria to label early, moderate and severe glaucomatous field defect from the HFA central 30-2 test, single printout is depicted in Table 9.2.

Note. For proper understanding of Table 9.2, evaluation of the Humphrey single field printout described on page 485 should be revised.

Ocular associations

POAG may sometimes be associated with high myopia, Fuchs' endothelial dystrophy, retinitis pigmentosa, central retinal vein occlusion and primary retinal detachment.

INVESTIGATIONS

1. *Tonometry.* Applanation tonometry should be preferred over Schiotz tonometry (see page 510).
2. *Central corneal thickness* (CCT) measurement is essential in the work-up for glaucoma since a thinner cornea underestimates and a thicker cornea overestimates the IOP on applanation tonometry. A low CCT (< 545 microns) is an independent risk factor for conversion of ocular hypertension to POAG. It has been suggested that a correction factor should be applied to the 10P readings in patients with CCT less than 545 microns and more than 600 microns.

Table 9.2. Criteria to diagnose early, moderate and severe glaucomatous field defects from HFA: 30-2- test.

Sr. no.	*Parameter*	*Criteria for glaucomatous field defects*		
		Early defects	*Moderate defects*	*Severe defects*
1.	Mean deviation (MD)	< – 6 dB	– 6dB – 12 dB	> – 12dB
2.	Corrected pattern standard deviation (CPSD)	Depressed to p < 5%	Depressed to p < 5%	Depressed to the p < 5%
3.	Pattern deviation plot			
	• Points depressed below the p < 5% or	< 18 (25%)	< 37 (50%)	> 37 (>50%)
	• Points depressed below the p < 1%	< 10	< 20	> 20
4.	Glaucoma Hemifield Test (GHT)	Outside normal limits	Outside normal limits	Outside normal limits
5.	Sensitivity in central 5 degree	No point < 15dB	One hemifield may have point with sensitivity <15dB No point has 0 dB	Both hemifield have points with sensitivity <15dB Any point has 0 dB

3. *Diurnal variation test* is especially useful in detection of early cases (see page 228).
4. *Gonioscopy.* It reveals a wide open angle of anterior chamber. Its primary importance in POAG is to rule out other forms of glaucoma. (For details see pages 217 and 578).
5. *Documentation of optic disc changes* is of utmost importance (see pages 228-229).
6. *Slit-lamp examination* of anterior segment to rule out causes of secondary open angle glaucoma.
7. *Perimetry* to detect the visual field defects.
8. *Nerve fibre layer analyzer* (NFLA) is a recently introduced device which helps in detecting the glaucomatous damage to the retinal nerve fibres before the appearance of actual visual field changes and/or optic disc changes.
9. *Provocative tests* are required in border-line cases. The test commonly performed is water drinking test. Other provocative tests not frequently performed include combined water drinking and tonography, bulbar pressure test, prescoline test and caffeine test.

Water drinking test. It is based on the theory that glaucomatous eyes have a greater response to water drinking. In it after an 8 hours fast, baseline IOP is noted and the patient is asked to drink one litre of water, following which IOP is noted every 15 min. for 1 hour. The maximum rise in IOP occurs in 15-30 min. and returns to baseline level after 60 minutes in both normal and the glaucomatous eyes. A rise of 8 mm of Hg or more is said to be diagnostic of POAG.

DIAGNOSIS

Depending upon the level of intraocular pressure (IOP), glaucomatous cupping of the optic disc and the visual field changes (Fig. 9.14) the patients are assigned to one of the following diagnostic entities:

1. *Primary open angle glaucoma (POAG).* Characteristically POAG is labelled when raised IOP (>21 mm of Hg) is associated with definite glaucomatous optic disc cupping and visual field changes.

However, patients with raised IOP and either typical field defects or disc changes are also labelled as having POAG.

2. *Ocular hypertension.* This term is used when a patient has an IOP constantly more than 21 mm of Hg

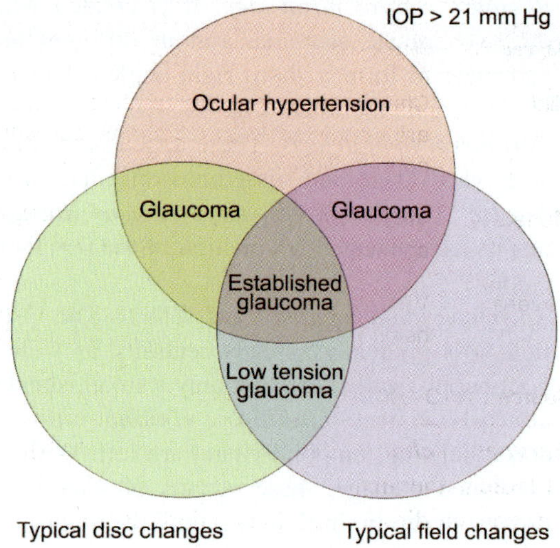

Fig. 9.14. Triad of abnormalities in disc, field and intraocular pressure (IOP) for the diagnosis of glaucoma.

but no optic disc and visual field changes (for details see page 237).

3. *Normal tension glaucoma (NTG) or low tension glaucoma (LTG)* is diagnosed when typical glaucomatous disc cupping with or without visual field changes is associated with an intraocular pressure constantly below 21 mm of Hg (For details see page 237).

MANAGEMENT

General considerations

Baseline evaluation and grading of severity of glaucoma. The aim of treatment is to lower intraocular pressure to a level where (further) visual loss does not occur. The management thus requires careful and regular periodic supervision by an ophthalmologist. Therefore, it is important to perform a good baseline examination with which future progress can be compared. The initial data should include: visual acuity, slit-lamp examination of anterior segment, tonometry (preferably with applanation tonometer); measurement of central corneal thickness, optic disc evaluation (preferably with fundus photography), gonioscopy and visual field charting.

American Academy of Ophthalmology (AAO) grades severity of glaucoma damage into mild, moderate and severe (Table 9.3).

Table 9.3. Severity of glaucoma damage

Degree	*Description*
Mild	Characteristic optic-nerve abnormalities are consistent with glaucoma but with normal visual field.
Moderate	Visual-field abnormalities in one hemi-field and not within 5 degrees of fixation.
Severe	Visual-field abnormalities in both hemifields and within 5 degrees of fixation.

Source : AAO 2000a

Therapeutic choices include:

- Medical therapy,
- Argon or diode laser trabeculoplasty, and
- Filteration surgery.

A. Medical therapy

The initial therapy of POAG is still medical, with surgery as the last resort.

Antiglaucoma drugs available are described in detail on pages 423-427.

Basic principles of medical therapy of POAG

1. *Identification of target pressure.* From the baseline evaluation data a 'target pressure' (below which glaucomatous damage is not likely to progress) should be identified for each patient. The target pressure is identified taking into account the severity of existing damage, the level of IOP, age, and general health of the patient. Although it is not possible to predict the safe level of IOP, however, progression is uncommon if IOP is maintained at less than 16 to 18 mm of Hg in patients having mild to moderate damage. Lower target pressures (12-14 mm Hg) are required in patients with severe damage.
2. *Single drug therapy.* One topically instilled antiglaucoma drug should be chosen after due consideration to the patient's personal and medical factors. If the initial drug chosen is ineffective or intolerable, it should be replaced by the drug of second choice.
3. *Combination therapy.* If one drug is not sufficient to control IOP then a combination therapy with two or more drugs should be tried.
4. *Monitoring of therapy* by disc changes and field changes and tonometry is most essential on regular follow-up. In the event of progress of glaucomatous damage the target pressure is reset at a lower level.

Treatment regimes

There are no clear-cut prescribed treatment regimens for medical therapy of POAG. However, at present considerations are as follows:

I. *Single drug therapy.* *Antiglaucoma drugs used are:*

1. *Topical beta-blockers* are being recommended as the *first drug of choice* for medical therapy of POAG in poor and average income patients. These lower IOP by reducing the aqueous secretion due to their effect on beta 2-receptors in the ciliary processes.

Preparations. In terms of effectiveness, there is little difference between various beta-blockers. However, each offers a slight advantage over the other, which may help in choosing the particular medication as follows:

- *Timolol maleate*, a non-selective beta blocker (0.25, 0.5% : 1-2 times/day), is most popular as initial therapy. However, it should not be used in patients having associated bronchial asthma and/ or heart blocks.
- *Betaxolol* (0.25% : 2 times/day). Being a selective beta-1 blocker it is preferred as initial therapy in patients with asthma and other pulmonary problems.
- *Levobunolol* (0.25, 0.5% : 1-2 times/day). Its action lasts the longest and so is more reliable for once a day use than timolol.
- *Carteolol* (1%: 1-2 times/day). It raises triglycerides and lowers high density lipoproteins the least. Therefore, it is the best choice in patients with POAG having associated hyperlipidemias or atherosclerotic cardiovascular disease.

2. *Prostaglandin analogus*. These decrease the IOP by increasing the uveo-scleral outflow of aqueous. Presently, a prostaglandin analogue is being considered the drug of first choice for the treatment of POAG (provided patient can afford to buy it). Further, these form a very good adjunctive drug to beta-blockers, dorzolamide and even pilocarpine when additional therapy is indicated. The available preparations include:

- *Latanoprost* (0.005%) to be used HS,
- *Travoprost* (0.004%) to be used HS,

- *Bimatoprost* (0.03%, a prostamide) to be used HS, and
- *Unoprostone* (0.15%) to be used BID.

3. ***Adrenergic drugs.*** Role in POAG is as follows:

i. *Epinephrine hydrochloride* (0.5, 1, 2%: 1-2 times/day) and *dipivefrine hydrochloride* (0.1%: 1-2 times/day). These drugs lower the IOP by increasing aqueous outflow by stimulating alpha receptors in the aqueous outflow system. These are characterized by a high allergic reaction rate. Their long-term use has also been recognized as a risk factor for failure of filtration glaucoma surgery. For these reasons, epinephrine compounds are no longer being used as first line or second line drug. However, dipivefrine may be combined with beta-blockers in patients where other drugs are contraindicated.

ii. *Brimonidine* (0.2% : 2 times/day). It is a selective alpha-2-adrenergic agonist and lowers IOP by decreasing aqueous production and also by increasing uveo-scleral outflow. Because of increased allergic reactions and tachyphylaxis rates it is not considered the drug of first choice in POAG. It is used as second drug of choice and also for combination therapy with other drugs.

4. ***Dorzolamide*** (2%: 2-3 times/day). It is a recently introduced topical carbonic anhydrase inhibitor which lowers IOP by decreasing aqueous production by altering ion transport along the ciliary process epithelium. It has replaced pilocarpine as the second line of drug and even as an adjunct drug.

5. ***Pilocarpine*** (1, 2, 4%: 3-4 times/day). It is a very effective drug and had remained as the sheet anchor in the medical management of POAG for a long time. However, presently it is not being preferred as the first drug of choice or even as second choice. It is because of the fact that in younger patients it causes problems due to spasm of accommodation and miosis. Most, but not all, older patients tolerate pilocarpine very well; however, axial lenticular opacities when present preclude its use in many such patients. Therefore, presently pilocarpine is being considered only as an adjunctive therapy where other combinations fail and as second choice in poor patients.

Mechanism of action. Pilocarpine contracts longitudinal muscle of ciliary body and opens spaces in trabecular meshwork, thereby mechanically increasing aqueous outflow.

II. *Combination topical therapy.* If one drug is not effective, then a combination of two drugs—one drug which decreases aqueous production (timolol or other betablocker, or brimonidine or dorzolamide) and other drug which increase aqueous outflow (latanoprost or brimonidine or pilocarpine) may be used.

III. *Role of oral carbonic anhydrase inhibitors in POAG.* Acetazolamide and methazolamide are not recommended for long-term use because of their side-effects. However, acetazolamide 250 mg-tds may be added to control IOP for short term.

IV. *Hyperosmotic agents* like mannitol 1-2 gm/kg body weight may be used initially when patients present with very high IOP (>30 mm Hg)

V. *Neuroprotective agents.* Neuroprotection is an IOP independent method of treating the retinal ganglion cells (RGCs) that are damaged in glaucoma. Some currently available neuroprotective agents have shown effects *in vitro* and in animal models, however, results in human clinical trials are either lacking or inconclusive.

B. Laser trabeculoplasty

Laser trabeculoplasty can be done using argon laser (ALT), or diode laser (DLT) and selective laser trabeculoplasty (SLT).

It should be considered in patients where IOP is uncontrolled despite maximal tolerated medical therapy. It can also be considered as primary therapy where there is non-compliance to medical therapy.

Technique and role of argon (ALT) or diode laser trabeculoplasty (DLT) in POAG. It has an additive effect to medical therapy. Its hypotensive effect is caused by increasing outflow facility, possibly by producing collagen shrinkage on the inner aspect of the trabecular meshwork and opening the intratrabecular spaces. It has been shown to lower IOP by 8-10 mm of Hg in patients on medical therapy and by 12-16 mm in patients who are not receiving medical treatment.

Treatment regime usually employed consists of 50 spots on the anterior half of the trabecular meshwork over 180°.

Complications. These include transient acute rise of IOP, which can be prevented by pretreatment with apraclonidine (an alpha agonist) and/or acetazolamide; and inflammation which can be lessened by use of topical steroids for 3-4 days. Less commonly haemorrhage, uveitis, peripheral anterior synechiae and reduced accommodation may occur.

Selective laser trabeculoplasty (SLT), based on the principle of selective photothermolysis, targets selectively pigmented trabecular meshwork (TM) cells without causing thermal or collateral damage to non-pigmented cells or structures unlike ALT or DLT. SLT is performed using Q-switched frequency doubled 532 nm ND:YAG laser with a pulse duration of 3 ms, a spot size of 400 microns and energy setting of 0.8 mJ. Pressure lowering effect of SLT is similar to ALT with the advantage of not causing scarring and damage to TM. Further, SLT can be used in patients treated with ALT.

C. Surgical therapy

Indications

1. Uncontrolled glaucoma despite maximal medical therapy and laser trabeculoplasty.
2. Non-compliance of medical therapy and non-availability of ALT/SLT.
3. Failure of medical therapy and unsuitable for ALT either due to lack of cooperation or inability to visualize the trabeculum.
4. Eyes with advanced disease i.e., having very high IOP, advanced cupping and advanced field loss should be treated with filtration surgery as primary line of management.

Types of surgery

Surgical treatment of POAG primarily consists of a fistulizing (filtration) surgery which provides a new channel for aqueous outflow and successfully controls the IOP (below 21 mm of Hg). Trabeculectomy is the most frequently performed filtration surgery now-a-days. The details of filtration operations are described on page 237.

OCULAR HYPERTENSION

Ocular hypertension or glaucoma suspect, either of these terms is used when a patient has an IOP constantly more than 21 mm of Hg but no optic disc and visual field changes. These patients should be carefully monitored by an ophthalmologist and should be treated as cases of POAG in the presence of high risk factors

High risk factors include:

- Significant diurnal variation, i.e., a difference of more than 8 mm of Hg between the lowest and the highest values of IOP.
- Significantly positive water drinking provocative test.
- When associated with splinter haemorrhages over or near the optic disc.
- IOP constantly more than 28 mm of Hg.
- Retinal nerve fibre large defects.
- Parapapillary changes.
- Central corneal thickness < 555 µm.
- Greater PSD on Humphery's field analysis.

Other risk factors include:

- Significant asymmetry in the cup size of the two eyes, i.e., a difference of more than 0.2.
- Strong family history of glaucoma.
- When associated with high myopia, diabetes or pigmentary changes in the anterior chamber.

Treatment

- *Patients with high-risk factors* should be treated on the lines of POAG (see page 235). The aim should be to reduce IOP by 20%.
- *Patients with no high risk factors* should be annually followed by examination of optic disc, perimetry and record of IOP. Treatment is not required till glaucomatous damage is documented.

NORMAL TENSION GLAUCOMA

Definition and prevalence

The term normal tension glaucoma (NTG), also referred to as low tension glaucoma is labelled when typical glaucomatous disc changes and visual field defects are associated with an intraocular pressure (IOP) constantly below 21 mm of Hg. Characteristically the angle of anterior chamber is open on gonioscopy and there is no secondary cause for glaucomatous disc changes. NTG is variant of POAG which accounts for 16% of all cases of POAG and its prevalence above the age of 40 years is 0.2%.

Etiopathogenesis

It is believed to result from chronic low vascular perfusion, which makes the optic nerve head susceptible to normal IOP. This view is supported by following association which are more common in NTG than in POAG:

- Raynaud phenomenon i.e., peripheral vascular spasm on cooling,
- Migraine,
- Nocturnal systemic hypotension and overtreated systemic hypertension.
- Reduced blood flow velocity in the ophthalmic artery (as revealed on transcranial Doppler ultrasonography).

Clinical features

As described in definition the clinical features of NTG (disc changes and visual field defects) are similar to POAG, but the IOP is consistently below 21 mm Hg. Other characteristic features of NTG are some associations mentioned in the etiopathogenesis.

Differential diagnosis

1. *POAG.* In early stages POAG may present with normal IOP because of a wide diurnal variation. Diurnal variation test usually depicts IOP higher than 21 mm of Hg at some hours of the day in patients with POAG.

2. *Congenital optic disc anomalies* such as large optic disc pits or colobomas may be mistaken for acquired glaucomatous damage. A careful examination should help in differentiation.

Treatment

1. *Medical treatment to lower IOP.* The aim of the treatment is to lower IOP by 30% i.e., to achieve IOP levels of about 12-14 mm of Hg. Some important facts about medical treatment of NTG are:

- *Betaxolol* may be considered the drug of choice because in addition to lowering IOP it also increases optic nerve blood flow.
- *Other beta blockers and adrenergic drugs* (such as dipivefrine) should better be avoided (as these cause nocturnal systemic hypotension and are likely to affect adversely the optic nerve perfusion).
- *Drugs with neuroprotective effect* like brimonidine may be preferred.
- *Prostaglandin analogues,* e.g., latanoprost tend to have a greater ocular hypotensive effect in eyes with normal IOP.

2. *Trabeculectomy* may be considered when progressive field loss occurs despite IOP in lower teens.

3. *Systemic calcium channel blockers* (e.g., nifedipine) may be useful in patients with confirmed peripheral vasospasm.

4. *Monitoring of systemic blood pressure* should be done for 24 hours. If nocturnal dip is detected, it may be necessary to avoid night dose of anti-hypertensive medication.

PRIMARY ANGLE-CLOSURE GLAUCOMA

Note: Since in the new classification, described of 'Association of International Glaucoma Societies' (AIGS), in 2006, the word glaucoma is used only when the optic disc and visual field changes are present, so the term '*primary angle closure disease*' should replace the term '*primary angle closure glaucoma*'. ***Primary angle closure disease***, is characterised by apposition of peripheral iris against the trabecular meshwork (TM) resulting in obstruction of aqueous outflow by closure of an already narrow angle of the anterior chamber. The condition is not associated with any other ocular and systemic abnormalities.

EPIDEMIOLOGY

Salient points regarding epidemiology of primary angle closure disease as per International Society of Geographical and Epidemiological Ophthalmology (ISGEO) are as below:

1. *For every 10 occludable angles (PAC suspects) seen there is only one case of PACG.* Thus most occludable eyes do not get glaucoma; and so does not justify prophylactic Laser P.I. in all such cases.
2. *Chronic PACG (asymptomatic) is more common than acute PACG* (symptomatic) (3:1); meaning thereby that most patients do not know they have disease; justifying need for glaucoma screening.
3. *There is great ethnic variability in the prevalence of PACG*. The ratio of POAG versus PACG reported for different ethnic groups is as below:

   Ethnic group — *POAG : PACG*
   - Europeans, and Africans and Hispanics: 5 : 1
   - Urban Chinese : 1 : 2
   - Mongolian : 1 : 3
   - Indian : 1 : 1
4. *Major cause of world glaucoma blindness* is PACG.

ETIOPATHOGENESIS

Etiopathogenesis of primary angle closure disease can be discussed as below:

A. Predisposing risk factors

B. Pathogenesis of rise in IOP

A. Predisposing risk factors

I. Demographic risk factors

1. *Age.* PACG with pupillary block occurs with greatest frequency in 6th and 7th decades of life
2. *Gender.* Male to Female ratio is 1:3
3. *Heredity.* Most cases of PACG with pupillary block are sporadic in nature. However, predisposing anatomical factors, i.e., shallow anterior chamber and narrow angles have been reported as more common in first degree relatives of the patients.
4. *Race.* In Caucasians, PACG accounts for about 6% of all glaucomas and was present in sixth to seventh decade. It is more common in South-East Asians, Chinese and Eskimos but uncommon in Blacks. In Asians it was present in 5th to 6th decade and accounts for 50% of primary adult glaucomas in this ethnic group.

II. ***Anatomical and ocular risk factors***

Eyes anatomically predisposed to develop primary angle-closure glaucoma (PACG) include:

- Hypermetropic eyes with shallow anterior chamber and short axial length.
- Eyes in which iris-lens diaphragm is placed anteriorly.
- Eyes with narrow angle of anterior chamber, which may be due to small eyeball, relatively large size of the lens and smaller diameter of the cornea or bigger size of the ciliary body or more anterior insertion of the iris on the ciliary body.
- Plateau iris configuration.

B. Pathomechanisms of rise in intraocular pressure

Three pathomechanisms implicated in the causation of rise in IOP of the eyes at risk of PACG are:

- Pupillary block mechanism,
- Plateau iris configuration and syndrome and
- Phacomorphic mechanism

1. Pupillary block mechanism. Pupillary block mechanism is responsible for causation of rise in IOP in most (70%) of the predisposed patients.

Precipitating factors. In a predisposed patient with occludable angles the pupillary block causing angle closure is precipitated by the following factors:

- *Physiological mydriasis* e.g. while reading in dim illumination, watching television or cinema in a darkened room, during anxiety and emotional stress (sympathetic overactivity)
- *Pharmacological mydriasis* is well documented to precipitate an attack of acute angle closure. Medications other than topical mydriatics (e.g. phenylephrine, tropicamide, cylopentolate, homatropine and atropine) reported to precipitate the attack include tranquilizers, bronchodilators, antidepressants, vasoconstrictors including common nasal decongestants, antimalaria agents and antispasmodics.
- *Pharmacological miosis* induced by drugs like echothiophate and pilocarpine is also reported to precipitate an attack of acute PAC.

Mechanism of rise in IOP after mydriasis. The probable sequence of events resulting in rise of IOP in an anatomically predisposed eye is as follows:

First of all due to the effect of precipitating factors there occurs *mid dilatation* of the pupil which increases the amount of apposition between iris and anteriorly placed lens with a considerable pressure resulting in *relative pupil block* (Fig. 9.15A). Consequently the aqueous collects in the posterior

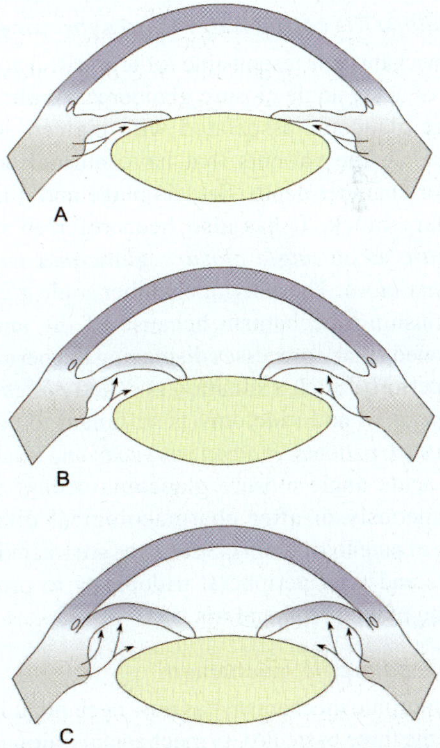

Fig. 9.15. Mechanism of angle closure glaucoma: A, relative pupil block; B, iris bombe formation; C, appositional angle closure.

chamber and pushes the peripheral flaccid iris anteriorly (*Iris bombe)* (Fig. 9.15B), resulting in *appositional angle closure* due to iridocorneal contact (Fig. 9.15C). Eventually there occurs rise in IOP which is transient to begin with. But slowly the appositional angle closure is converted into *synechial angle closure* (due to formation of peripheral anterior synechiae) and an attack of rise in IOP may last long.

In some cases a mechanical occlusion of the angle by the iris is sufficient to block the drainage of aqueous. For this reason the instillation of atropine in an eye with a narrow angle is dangerous, since it may precipitate an attack of raised IOP.

Mechanism of rise in IOP after miosis. The drugs that constrict pupil are also reported to increase pupillary block. Further these drugs also contract the ciliary muscles allowing the zonules to relax and the lens to move forward. Because of this reason, it is advisable to avoid miotics such as pilocarpine in the prevention of PACG in predisposed eyes (e.g. fellow eye of patient with acute attack).

2. *Plateau iris configuration and syndrome*

This mechanism is responsible for few (10%) atypical cases of acute angle closure glaucoma. Acute angle closure glaucoma associated with plateau iris is atypical in the patients that have normal central anterior chamber depth, flat iris plane and minimal pupillary block. It has also been referred in the literature as an *angle closure glaucoma without pupillary block*. The anterior chamber angle is closed by a pushing mechanism because of the anterior positioned ciliary processes displacing the peripheral iris anteriorly. Such a situation is called *plateau iris configuration* and iridotomy is sufficient to control IOP in such patients. *Plateau iris syndrome* is labeled when acute angle closure glaucoma occurs either spontaneously or after pharmacological dilation, inspite of patent iridotomy. Such eyes are treated with miotics and laser peripheral iridoplasty to produce thinning of the peripheral iris.

3. *Phacomorphic mechanism*

Phacomorphic mechanism has now been included as one of the three basic PACG mechanisms, along with pupillary block and plateau iris. The abnormal lens may contribute by either causing pupillary block or by pushing the peripheral iris forward into the angle structures. Though the term phacomorphic glaucoma refers to an acute secondary angle closure glaucoma caused by the intumescent or other lens morphological abnormalities; but now UBM and OCT studies have shown that phacomorphic mechanism may be responsible for initiating acute primary angle closure glaucoma in predisposed patients (having occludable angle). This also forms the base of lens extraction as a treatment modality for acute primary angle closure glaucoma.

***Note*:** In addition to meticulous gonioscopic examination, the high resolution ultrasonic biomicroscopy (UBM) examination and Anterior Segment OCT (AS-OCT) are very useful in understanding the pathogenesis of primary angle closure disease. These investigations are particularly useful in the documentation of plateau iris configuration, plateau iris syndrome, phacomorphic mechanism and post peripheral iridectomy angle dynamics. Further , these investigations are also helpful in differentiating primary and secondary angle closure glaucoma.

CLASSIFICATION AND CLINICAL PRESENTATIONS

World glaucoma experts under the auspices of the "Association of International Glaucoma Societies" (AIGS) in 2006 have proposed following twenty first century consensus classification based on IOP measurements, gonioscopy, disc and visual field evaluation:

1. Primary Angle Closure Suspect (PACS)
2. Primary Angle Closure (PAC)
3. Primary Angle Closure Glaucoma (PACG)

In this newer classification the word glaucoma is used only when the optic disc changes and field changes are present. Further, this classification is based only on the signs and has not taken into consideration the presenting symptoms. Therefore, the clinical presentations described here have been taken from the old ***clinical classification*** which includes following types:

- Latent primary angle-closure glaucoma,
- Subacute (intermittent) primary angle-closure glaucoma,
- Acute primary angle-closure glaucoma.
- Chronic primary angle closure glaucoma.

I. PRIMARY ANGLE CLOSURE SUSPECT

Primary angle-closure suspect (PACS), can be considered to replace the term 'latent primary angle-closure glaucoma' of clinical classification.

Clinical features and diagnostic criteria

Symptoms are absent in this stage

Presenting situations of diagnosis include:

- Suspicious clinical signs on routine ocular examination in patients coming for some other complaints.
- Fellow eye of the patients presenting with acute attack of PAC.
- Glaucoma screening programme

Suspicious clinical signs noted on routine ocular examination include:

1. *Eclipse sign.* Eclipse sign, which indicates decreased axial anterior chamber depth, can be elicited by shining a penlight across the anterior chamber from the temporal side and noting a shadow on the nasal side (Fig. 9.16).

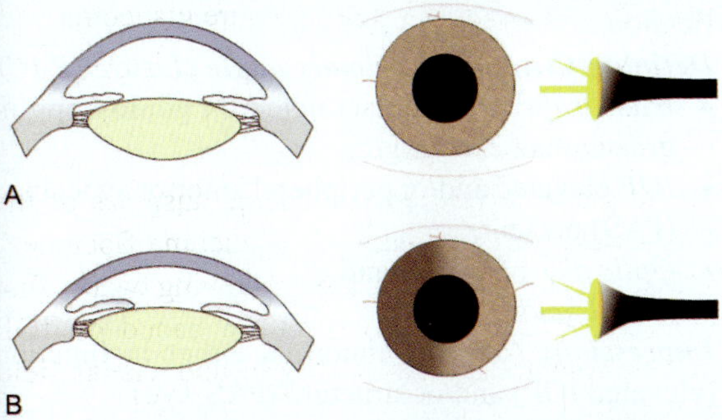

Fig. 9.16. Estimation of anterior chamber depth by oblique illumination: A, normal; B, shallow.

2. *Slit-lamp biomicroscopic signs* include:
   - Decreased axial anterior chamber depth,
   - Convex shaped iris lens diaphragm, and
   - Close proximity of the iris to cornea in the periphery.
3. *Van Herick slit-lamp grading of the angle* may be used with a fair accuracy. Here, the peripheral anterior chamber depth (PACD) is compared to the adjacent corneal thickness (CT) and the presumed angle width is graded as follows (Fig. 9.17):
   - Grade 4 (Wide open angle): PACD = $^3/_4$ to 1 CT
   - Grade 3 (Mild narrow angle): PACD = ¼ to ½ CT

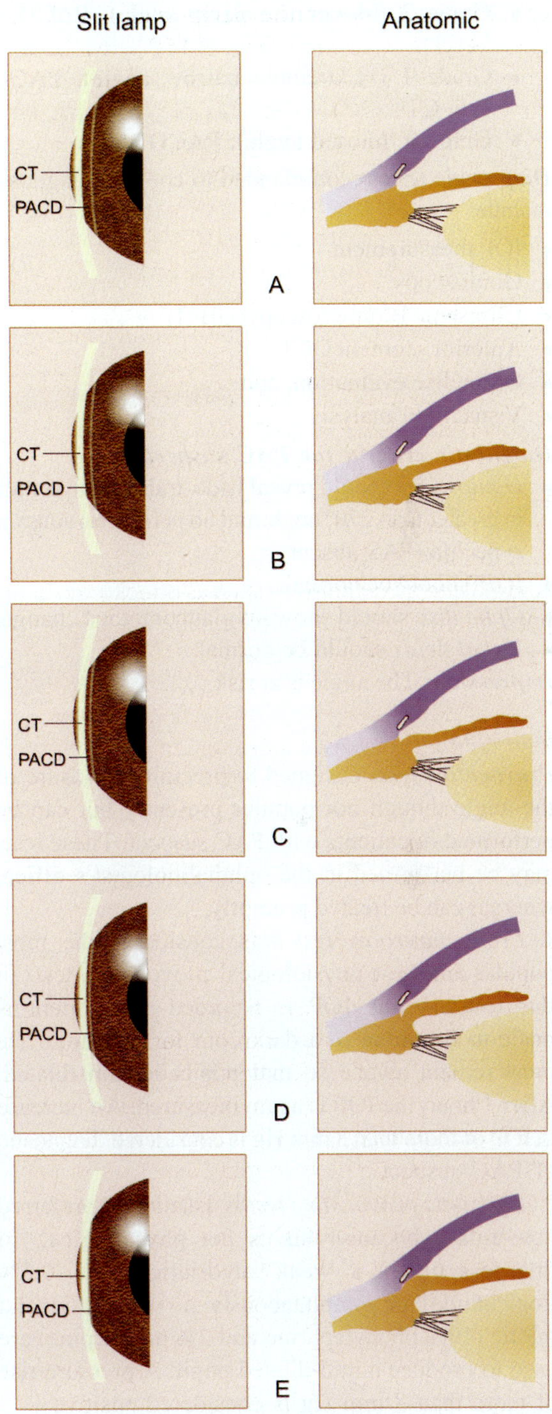

Fig. 9.17. Van Herick method of slit-lamp grading of angle width: A, Grade IV; B, Grade III; C, Grade II; and D, Grade I, and E Grade 0. PACD = Peripheral anterior chamber depth; CT = Corneal thickeners

- Grade 2 (Moderate narrow angle): PACD = ¼ CT
- Grade 1 (Extremely narrow angle): PACD < ¼ CT
- Grade 0 (closed angle): PACD = Nil

Diagnostic tests recommended to confirm diagnosis include:

- IOP measurement
- Gonioscopy
- Ultrasonic Biomicroscopy(UBM)
- Anterior segment OCT
- Optic disc evaluation, and
- Visual field analysis

Diagnostic criteria for PAC suspect:

- *Gonioscopy* should reveal irido-trabecular contact in greater than 270° angle and no peripheral anterior synechia (PAS absent).
- *IOP* should be normal.
- *Optic disc* should show no glaucomatous change.
- *Visual fields* should be normal.

***Impression*:** The angle is at risk.

Management

Provocative tests designed to precipitate closure of the angle though not popular presently but can be performed in patients with PAC suspect. These tests may be performed in the ophthalmologist's office, where it can be treated promptly.

1. *Prone-darkroom test* was considered the most popular and best physiological provocative test. In this test baseline IOP is recorded and patient is made to lie prone in a darkroom for one hour. He must remain awake so that pupils remain dilated. After 1 hour, the IOP is again measured. An increase in IOP of more than 8 mm Hg is considered diagnostic of PAC suspect.

2. *Mydriatic provocative test* is usually not preferred now-a-days because this is not physiological. In this test either a weak mydriatic (e.g., 0.5% tropicamide) or simultaneously a mydriatic and miotic (10% phenylephrine and 2% pilocarpine) are used to produce a mid-dilated pupil. A pressure rise of more than 8 mm Hg is considered positive.

Inferences from provocative tests

- *A positive provocative test* indicates that angle is capable of spontaneous closure.
- *A negative provocative test* in the presence of occludable angles on gonioscopy does not rule out a possibility of spontaneous closure. So, patient should be warned of possible symptoms of an acute attack of PAC.

Treatment

- *Prophylactic laser iridotomy* is warranted if more than 270^0 of oppositional iridotrabecular contact is seen on gonioscopy in the fellow eye of all patients presenting with acute PAC or PACG in one eye. If untreated, the risk of conversion to PACG during the next 5 years is about 50%.
- *Periodic follow up.* Patients with PAC suspect in both eyes need to be followed periodically and educated about the symptoms of the disease.

II. PRIMARY ANGLE CLOSURE

Note: Primary angle closure (PAC) can be considered to replace the terms 'subacute (intermittent) primary angle-closure glaucoma', and 'acute primary angle-closure glaucoma' included in the clinical classification.

Defining Criteria for primary angle closure (PAC)

- *Irido-trabecular* contact noted on gonioscopy in greater than 270° angle,
- *IOP* elevated and/or peripheral anterior synechiae (PAS) present,
- *Optic disc* : Normal, and
- *Visual fields* : Normal

***Impression*:** Angle is abnormal either in function (elevated IOP) and/or structure (PAS +ve)

Clinical course

Eyes with PAC may follow any of the following clinical courses:

- May manifest as subacute or acute primary angle closure.
- May remain asymptomatic (quescent PAC) and convert to PACG .

Subacute primary angle-closure

In subacute primary angle-closure (*Subacute PAC*) there occurs an attack of transient rise of IOP (40-50 mm Hg) which may last for few minutes to 1-2 hours. Such an attack in a patient with PAC is usually precipitated by:

- *Physiological mydriasis* e.g., while reading in dim illumination, watching television or cinema in a darkened room, or during anxiety (sympathetic overactivity); or

- *Physiological shallowing of anterior chamber* after lying in prone position.
- *Pharmacological mydriasis* following use of pupil dilating drugs for fundus examination.

Clinical features

Symptoms

- *The episode of subacute PAC* is marked by experience of unilateral transient blurring of vision, coloured halos around light, headache, browache and eyeache on the affected side.
- *Self-termination of the attack* occurs possibly due to physiological miosis induced by bright light, sleep or otherwise.
- *Recurrent attacks* of such episodes are not uncommon. Between the recurrent attacks the eyes are free of symptoms.

Signs. Usually, during examination the eye is white and not congested. However, all the signs described above in the definition of primary angle-closure (PAC) should be elicited to lable PAC.

Diagnosis and treatment

Same as described for primary angle-closure suspect (see page 227).

Differential diagnosis of coloured halos in PAC. Coloured halos during intermittent attacks of raised 10P in PAC occur due to accumulation of fluid in the corneal epithelium and alteration in the refractive condition of the corneal lamellae. Patient typically gives history of seeing colours distributed as in the spectrum of rainbow (red being outside and violet innermost) while watching on a lighted bulb or the moon.

The coloured halos in glaucoma must be differentiated from those found in acute purulent conjunctivitis and early cataractous changes. In conjunctivits, halos can be eliminated by irrigating the discharge. The halos of glaucoma and immature cataract may be differentiated by Fincham's test in which a stenopaeic slit is passed across the pupil. During this test glaucomatous halo remains intact, while a halo due to cataract is broken up into segments (Fig. 9.18).

Acute primary angle-closure

An attack of acute rise in IOP in patients with primary angle closure (PAC) may occur due to pupillary block causing sudden closure of the angle. It usually does not terminate of its own and thus if not treated lasts for many days. This is sight threatening emergency.

Clinical features

Symptoms

- *Pain.* Typically acute attack is characterised by sudden onset of very severe pain in the eye which radiates along the branches of 5th nerve.
- *Nausea, vomiting and prostrations* are frequently associated with pain.
- *Rapidly progressive impairment of vision*, redness, photophobia and lacrimation develop in all cases.

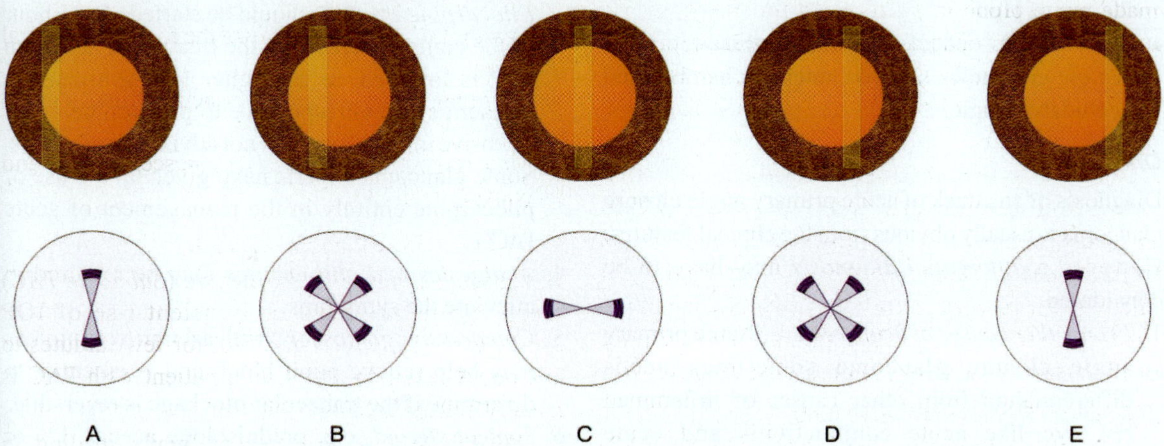

Fig. 9.18. Emsley-Fincham stenopaeic-slit test demonstrating breaking up of halos due to immature cataract into different segments.

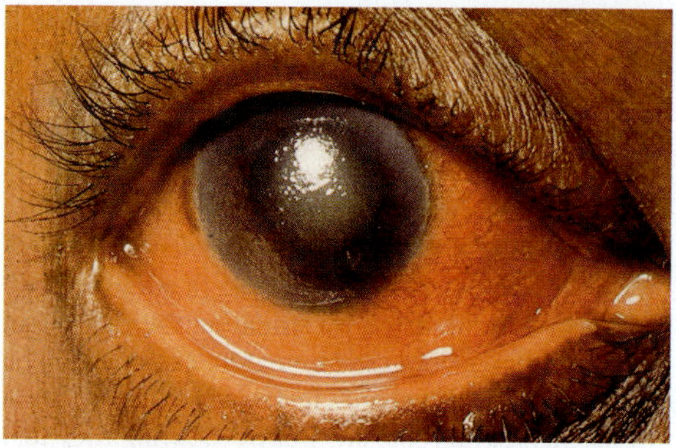

Fig. 9.19. Clinical photograph of a patient with acute congestive glaucoma. Note ciliary congestion, corneal oedema and middilated pupil.

- *Past history.* About 5 percent patients give history of typical previous intermittent attacks of subacute angle-closure.

Signs (Fig. 9.19)

- *Lids* may be oedematous,
- *Conjunctiva* is chemosed, and congested, (both conjunctival and ciliary vessels are congested),
- *Cornea* becomes oedematous and insensitive,
- *Anterior chamber* is very shallow. Aqueous flare or cells may be seen in anterior chamber,
- *Angle of anterior chamber* is completely closed as seen on gonioscopy (shaffer grade 0),
- *Iris* may be discoloured,
- *Pupil* is semidilated, vertically oval and fixed. It is non-reactive to both light and accommodation,
- *IOP* is markedly elevated, usually between 40 and 70 mm of Hg,
- *Optic disc* is oedematous and hyperaemic,
- *Fellow eye* shows shallow anterior chamber and occludable angle.

Diagnosis

Diagnosis of an attack of acute primary angle closure glaucoma is usually obvious from the clinical features. However, a *differential diagnosis* may have to be considered:

1. *From other causes of acute red eye.* Acute primary angle closure glaucoma sometimes needs differentiation from other causes of inflammed red eye like acute conjunctivitis and acute iridocyclitis (see pages 154-155).
2. *From secondary acute glaucomas* such as:
   - Phacomorphic glaucoma (see page 247),
   - Acute neovascular glaucoma (see page 249) and
   - Glaucomatocyclitic crisis (see page 167).

Management

Acute angle closure is a *serious ocular emergency* condition and needs to be managed aggressively as below:

- Immediate medical therapy to lower IOP,
- Definitive treatment,
- Prophylaxis of the fellow eye, and
- Long term glaucoma surveillance and IOP management of both eyes

A. Immediate medical therapy to lower IOP

1. *Systemic hyperosmotic agents* are required initially if IOP is more than 40 mm Hg.
   - *Intravenous mannitol* (1gm/kg body weight) should be preferred in the presence of nausea and vomiting.
   - *Oral hyperosmotics* e.g. glycerol 1gm/kg body weight of 50% solution in lemon juice may be given if well tolerated and not contraindicated (as in diabetes mellitus).
2. *Systemic carbonic anhydrase inhibitors* e.g. acetazolamide 500 mg i/v stat followed by 250 mg tablet 3 times a day.
3. *Topical anti-glaucoma drugs* to be instilled immediately include:
   - *Beta blocker* e.g. 0.5% timolol or 0.5% betaxolol
   - *Alpha adrenergic agonists* e.g. brimonidine 0.1-0.2%.
   - *Prostaglandin analogue* e.g. latanoprost 0.005%.

   Role of miotic therapy:
   - *Pilocarpine* 2% QID should be started after 1 hour of the commencement of the treatment, i.e. when IOP is lowered, as at higher IOP sphincter is ischaemic and unresponsive to pilocarpine.
   - Intensive miotic therapy is not advised now-a-days. Some glaucoma experts have given up the use of pilocarpine entirely in the management of acute PACG.
4. *Analgesics and anti-emetics* may be required to alleviate the symptoms.
5. *Compressive gonioscopy* with a 4 mirror goniolens may help relieve pupil block and is essential to determine if the trabecular blockage is reversible.
6. *Topical steroid*, e.g. prednisolone acetate 1% or dexamethasone eye drops administered 3-4 times a day reduces the inflammation.

3. *Definitive therapy*

1. *Laser Peripheral Iridotomy* (PI). Gonioscopy should be performed as soon as cornea becomes clear. Laser PI should be performed if PAS are seen in <270° angle. PI re-establishes communication between posterior and anterior chamber, so it bypasses the pupillary block and immediately relieves the crowding of the angle
   - *Laser iridotomy* (with Nd:YAG laser or Argon Laser) should always be preferred over surgical PI. However, if lasers are not available surgical PI should be done (see page 252 for technique).
2. *Filtration surgery*, i.e. trabeculectomy should be performed in cases where IOP is not controlled with the maximum medical therapy following an attack of acute PAC or when gonioscopy reveals PAS >270° angle and also when peripheral iridotomy is not effective.
   Mechanism: Filtration surgery provides an alternative to the angle for drainage of aqueous from anterior chamber into subconjunctival space.
   Surgical technique. (See page 253).
3. *Clear lens extraction* by phacoemulsification with intraocular lens implantation has recently been recommended by some workers, especially in the presence of cataract.

C. *Prophylactic treatment in the normal fellow eye*

Prophylactic laser iridotomy (preferably) or surgical peripheral iridectomy should be performed on the fellow asymptomatic eye as early as possible as chances of acute attack are 50% in such eyes.

D. *Long term glaucoma surveillance and IOP management in both eyes*

Long term glaucoma surveillance and IOP management in both eyes of a patient with acute PAC is must to ultimately prevent glaucomatous blindness

- *Eyes treated with PI* (both affected and fellow eye) may develop PACG at any time. So it should be treated as and when required.
- *Filtration surgery* may fail anytime during the course and hence need to be repeated with antimetabolites.

Sequelae of acute PAC

The clinical status of the eye after an attack of acute PAC with or without treatment is considered a sequelae of acute PAC. It may be seen as clinical settings:

1. *Postsurgical acute PAC.* This refers to the clinical status of the eye after laser peripheral iridotomy (PI) treatment for an attack of acute PAC. It may occur in two clinical settings:

i. With normalized IOP after successful laser PI, the eye usually quitens after sometime with or without marks of an acute attack (i.e., Vogt's triad, see below).

ii. With raised IOP after unsuccessful laser PI, which needs to be treated by trabeculectomy operation.

2. *Spontaneous angle reopening* may occur very rarely in some cases and the attack of acute PAC may subside itself without treatment.

Treatment of such cases is similar to that of subacute primary angle-closure (PAC).

3. *Ciliary body shut down.* It refers to the temporary cessation of aqueous humour secretion due to ischaemic damage to the ciliary epithelium after an attack of acute PAC.

Clinical features in this stage are similar to acute PAC except that the IOP is low and pain is markedly reduced. Subsequent recovery of ciliary function may lead to chronic elevation of IOP with cupping and visual field defects i.e., PACG.

Treatment includes:

- *Topical steroid drops* to reduce inflammation.
- *Laser iridotomy* should be performed when cornea becomes clear and IOP should be monitored.
- *Trabeculectomy* is required when IOP rises constantly.

4. *Vogt's triad.* It may be seen in both treated and non- treated cases after an attack of acute PAC. It is characterized by:

- Glaukomflecken (anterior subcapsular lenticular opacity),
- Patches of iris atrophy, and
- Slightly dilated non-reacting pupil (due to sphincter atrophy).

III. PRIMARY ANGLE CLOSURE GLAUCOMA

Note: Primary angle closure glaucoma (PACG) can be considered to replace the term 'chronic primary angle closure glaucoma' used in the clinical classification.

Defining criteria for primary angle closure glaucoma is:

- *Irido-trabecular contact* is noted on gonioscopy in greater than 270° of angle,
- *PAS* are formed,
- *IOP* is elevated,
- *Optic disc* shows glaucomatous damage, and
- *Visual fields* show typical glaucomatous defects.

Impression: Angle is abnormal in function (elevated IOP) and structure (PAS + ve) with optic neuropathy.

Note: In circumstances where advanced PACG disease with compromised media prohibits disc and visual field testing, e.g. cataract or corneal disease, a coarser definition holds for PACG whereby an IOP > 24 mm Hg and visual acuity of < 3/60 or a history of prior glaucoma surgery, will suffice.

Pathogenesis

Primary angle-closure glaucoma (PACG) results from gradual synechial closure of the angle of anterior chamber. Untreated patients with PAC may over the period covert to PACG with or without history of subacute or acute attack of PAC.

Clinical features

Clinical features given below are similar to POAG except that angle is narrow:

- *Intraocular pressure* (IOP) remains constantly raised.
- *Eyeball* remains white (no congestion) and painless, except in post acute angle closure cases where the eye may be congested and irritable.
- *Optic disc* shows glaucomatous cupping,
- *Visual field defects* similar to POAG occur (see page 232).
- *Gonioscopy* reveals more than 270 degree of angle closure along with peripheral anterior synechiae (PAS). The gonioscopic findings provide the only differentiating feature between POAG and chronic PACG.

Treatment

- *Laser iridotomy* alone or alongwith medical therapy similar to POAG (see page 235) should be tried first.
- *Trabeculectomy* (filtration surgery) is needed when the above treatment fails to control IOP.
- *Prophylactic laser iridotomy* in fellow eye must also be performed.

Absolute primary angle-closure glaucoma

Primary angle closure glaucoma, if untreated, gradually passes into the final phase of absolute glaucoma.

Clinical features

- *Painful blind eye.* The eye is painful, irritable and completely blind (no light perception).
- *Perilimbal reddish blue zone* i.e., a slight ciliary flush around the cornea due to dilated anterior ciliary veins.
- *Caput medusae* i.e., a few prominent and enlarged vessels are seen in long standing cases.
- *Cornea* in early cases is clear but insensitive. Slowly it becomes hazy and may develop epithelial bullae (*bullous keratopathy)* or filaments (*filamentary keratitis)*.
- *Anterior chamber* is very shallow.
- *Iris* becomes atrophic.
- *Pupil* becomes fixed and dilated and gives a greenish hue.
- *Optic disc* shows glaucomatous optic atrophy.
- *Intraocular pressure* is high; eyeball becomes stony hard.

Management of absolute glaucoma

1. *Retrobulbar alcohol injection:* It may be given to relieve pain. First, 1 ml of 2 percent xylocaine is injected followed after about 5-10 minutes by 1 ml of 80 percent alcohol. It destroys the ciliary ganglion.
2. *Destruction of secretory ciliary epithelium* to lower the IOP may be carried out by *cyclo-cryotherapy* (see page 256) or *cyclodiathermy* or *cyclophotocoagulation*.
3. *Enucleation of eyeball.* It may be considered when pain is not relieved by conservative methods. The frequency with which a painful blind eye with high IOP contains a malignant growth, justifies its removal. (For surgical technique of enucleation see page 304).

Complications. If not treated, due to prolonged high IOP following complications may occur:

1. *Corneal ulceration.* It results from prolonged epithelial oedema and insensitivity. Sometimes, corneal ulcer may even perforate.
2. *Staphyloma formation.* As a result of continued high IOP, sclera becomes very thin and atrophic and ultimately bulges out either in the ciliary region (ciliary staphyloma) or equatorial region (equatorial staphyloma).
3. *Atrophic bulbi.* Ultimately the ciliary body degenerates, IOP falls and the eyeball shrinks.

SECONDARY GLAUCOMAS

Secondary glaucoma *per se* is not a disease entity, but a group of disorders in which rise of intraocular pressure is associated with some primary ocular or systemic disease. Therefore, clinical features comprise that of primary disease and that due to effects of raised intraocular pressure.

Classification

(A) *Depending upon the mechanism of rise in IOP*

1. *Secondary open angle glaucomas* in which aqueous outflow may be blocked by a pretrabecular membrane, trabecular clogging, oedema and scarring or elevated episcleral venous pressure.
2. *Secondary angle closure glaucomas* which may or may not be associated with pupil block.

(B) *Depending upon the causative primary disease,* secondary glaucomas are named as follows:

1. Lens-induced (phacogenic) glaucomas.
2. Inflammatory glaucoma (glaucoma due to intraocular inflammation).
3. Pigmentary glaucoma.
4. Neovascular glaucoma.
5. Glaucomas associated with irido-corneal endothelial syndromes.
6. Pseudoexfoliative glaucoma.
7. Glaucomas associated with intraocular haemorrhage.
8. Steroid-induced glaucoma.
9. Traumatic glaucoma.
10. Glaucoma-in-aphakia.
11. Glaucoma associated with intraocular tumours.

LENS-INDUCED (PHACOGENIC) GLAUCOMAS

In this group IOP is raised secondary to some disorder of the crystalline lens. Lens induced glaucoma can be classified as below:

Lens induced secondary angle closure glaucoma

- Phacomorphic glaucoma (due to swollen lens)
- Phacotopic glaucoma (due to anterior lens displacement)

Lens induced secondary open angle glaucoma

- Phacolytic glaucoma
- Lens particle glaucoma
- Phacoanaphylactic glaucoma

1. Phacomorphic glaucoma

Causes. Phacomorphic glaucoma is an acute secondary angle-closure glaucoma caused by:

- *Intumescent lens* i.e., swollen cataractous lens due to rapid maturation of cataract or sometimes following traumatic rupture of capsule is the main cause of phacomorphic glaucoma.
- *Anterior subluxation or dislocation of the lens and spherophakia* (congenital small spherical lens) are causes of phacotopic (a variant of phacomorphic) glaucoma.

Pathogenesis. The swollen lens pushes the iris forward and oblitrates the angle resulting in *secondary acute angle closure-glaucoma.* Further, the increased iridolenticular contact also causes potential pupillary block and iris bombe formation.

Clinical presentation. Phacomorphic glaucoma presents as acute congestive glaucoma with features almost similar to acute primary angle-closure (see page 243) except that the lens is always cataractous and swollen (Fig. 9.20). Demonstration of deep anterior chamber and open angle in the fellow eye helps in differentiating from the acute primary angle closure glaucoma.

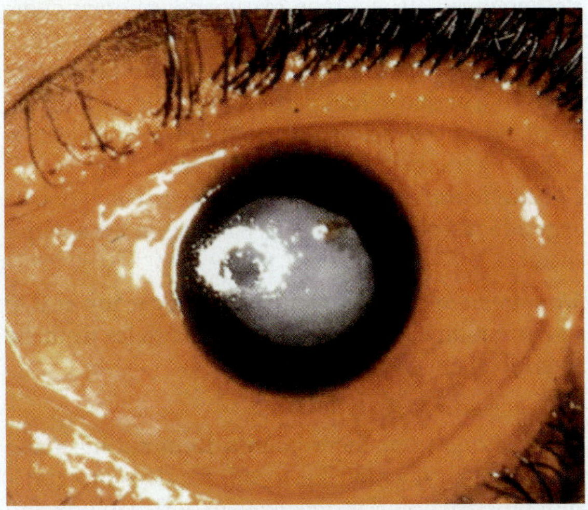

Fig. 9.20. Phacomorphic glaucoma. Note ciliary congestion, dilated pupil and intumescent senile cataractous lens.

Treatment should be immediate and consists of:

- *Medical treatment* to control IOP by i.v. mannitol, systemic acetazolamide and topical betablockers.
- *Laser iridotomy* may be effective in breaking the angle closure attack.

- *Cataract extraction* with implantation of PCIOL (which is the main treatment of phacomorphic glaucoma) should be performed once the eye becomes quiet.

2. Phacolytic glaucoma (Lens protein glaucoma)

Pathogenesis. It is a type of *secondary open angle glaucoma*, in which trabecular meshwork is clogged by the lens proteins, macrophages which have phagocytosed the lens proteins, and inflammatory debris. Leakage of the lens proteins occurs through an intact capsule in the hypermature (Morgagnian) cataractous lens.

Clinical features. The condition is characterised by:
- *Features of congestive glaucoma* due to an acute rise of IOP in an eye having hypermature cataract.
- *Anterior chamber* may become deep and aqueous may contain fine white protein particles, which settle down as pseudohypopyon.
- *Anterior chamber angle* is open on gonioscopy.

Management. It consists of medical therapy to lower the IOP (see page 235) followed by extraction of the hypermature cataractous lens with PCIOL implantation.

3. Lens particle glaucoma

Pathogenesis. It is a type of *secondary open angle glaucoma*, in which trabecular meshwork is blocked by the lens particles floating in the aqueous humour. It may occur due to lens particles left after accidental or planned extracapsular cataract extraction or following traumatic rupture of the lens.

Clinical features. Symptoms of acute rise in IOP (see page 243) associated with lens particles in the anterior chamber.

Management includes medical therapy to lower IOP and irrigation-aspiration of the lens particles from the anterior chamber.

4. Phacoantigenic glaucoma

In this condition, there occurs fulminating acute inflammatory reaction due to antigen (lens protein) – antibody reaction. The mechanism of rise in IOP and its management is similar to that of acute inflammatory glaucoma. Typical finding is a granulomatous inflamma- tion in the involved eye after it goes surgical trauma.

Pathogenesis. As in the case of lens particle glaucoma, there is usually a preceding disruption of lens capsule by extracapsular cataract extraction, penetrating injury, or leak of proteins from the capsule. Distinguishing feature is a latent period during which sensitization to the lens proteins occurs. IOP is then raised due to inflammatory reaction of the uveal tissue excited by the lens matter. Basically, it is also a type of secondary open angle glaucoma where trabecular meshwork is clogged by both inflammatory cells and the lens particles.

Management consists of medical therapy to lower IOP, treatment of iridocyclitis with steroids and cycloplegics. Irrigation-aspiration of the lens matter from anterior chamber (if required) should always be done after proper control of inflammation.

GLAUCOMAS DUE TO UVEITIS

The IOP can be raised by varied mechanisms in inflammations of the uveal tissue (iridocyclitis). Even in other ocular inflammations such as keratitis and scleritis, the rise in IOP is usually due to secondary involvement of the anterior uveal tract.

Types. I. Non specific inflammatory glaucomas, and II. Specific hypertensive uveitis syndromes

I. Non specific inflammatory glaucoma

Based on the mechanism of rise in IOP the inflammatory glaucoma can be :
- Open-angle inflammatory glaucoma,
- Angle-closure inflammatory glaucoma, and

1. Open-angle inflammatory glaucoma

Clinically the open-angle inflammatory glaucoma may manifest as acute or chronic entity .

i. *Acute open-angle inflammatory glaucoma*

Mechanisms of rise in IOP. The acute open-angle glaucoma occurs due to trabecular clogging (by inflammatory cells, exudates and turbid aqueous humour), trabecular oedema (due to associated trabeculitis), and prostaglandin–induced rise in IOP.

Clinical features. It is characterized by features of acute iridocyclitis associated with raised IOP with open-angle of anterior chamber. IOP usually returns to normal after the acute episode of inflammation.

Management. It includes treatment of iridocyclitis and medical therapy to lower IOP by use of hyperosmotic agents, acetazolamide and beta-blocker eye drops (timolol or betaxolol).

ii. *Chronic open angle inflammatory glaucoma*

Mechanism of rise in IOP includes chronic trabeculitis, and trabecular scarring.

Clinical features include raised IOP, open angle, no active inflammation but signs of previous episode of uveitis are often present. Some chronic cases may also have signs of glaucomatous disc changes and field defects.

Treatment consist of:

- *Medical therapy* with topical beta blockers, and / or carbonic anhydrase inhibitors and alpha agonist may be useful. Preferably avoid pilocarpine and prostaglandin agonists.
- *Trabeculectomy*, under cover of steroids, may be tried , if medical treatment fails. The results are usually poorer than POAG, but can be improved by augmented trabeculectomy or tube procedures.
- *Cyclodestructive procedures (e.g.* cyclodiode) may need to be considered if surgical treatment fails.

2. Angle-closure inflammatory glaucoma

When uveitis is not treated, over the period PAS are formed causing synechiae angle closure.

Mechanisms of rise in IOP include:

- *Secondary angle-closure with pupil block.* Pupillary block due to *annular synechiae* or occlusio pupillae leads to iris bombe formation followed by angle closure.
- *Secondary angle-closure without pupil block* occurs due to organisation of the inflammatory debris in the angle, which on contraction pulls the iris over the trabeculum. It is followed by gradual and progressive synechial angle closure with eventual elevation of IOP.

Clinical features include raised IOP, seclusio papillae, iris bombe, shallow anterior chamber.

Management. It includes prophylaxis and curative treatment.

1. *Prophylaxis.* Acute iridocyclitis should be treated energetically with local steroids and atropine to prevent formation of synechiae.
2. *Curative treatment.* It consists of medical therapy to lower IOP (miotics are contraindicated). Surgical or laser *iridotomy* may be useful in pupil block without angle closure. *Filtration surgery* may be performed (with guarded results) in the presence of angle closure.

II. Specific hypertensive uveitis syndromes

These include:

- Fuchs' uveitis syndrome (see page 166) and
- Glaucomatocyclitic crisis (see page 167).

PIGMENTARY GLAUCOMA

It is a type of *secondary open-angle glaucoma* wherein clogging up of the trabecular meshwork occurs by the pigment particles. About 50% of patients with the *Pigment Dispersion Syndrome* (PDS) develop glaucoma.

Pathogenesis. Exact mechanism of pigment shedding is not known. It is believed that, perhaps, pigment release is caused by mechanical rubbing of the posterior pigment layer of iris with the zonular fibrils.

Clinical features. The condition typically occurs in young myopic males. Characteristic glaucomatous features are similar to primary open angle glaucoma (POAG), associated with deposition of pigment granules in the anterior segment structures such as iris, posterior surface of the cornea (*Krukenberg's spindle),* trabecular meshwork, ciliary zonules and the crystalline lens. Gonioscopy shows pigment accumulation along the Schwalbe's line especially inferiorly (*Sampaolesi's line*). Iris transillumination shows radial slit-like transillumination defects in the mid periphery (pathognomic feature).

Treatment. It is exactly on the lines of primary open angle glaucoma.

NEOVASCULAR GLAUCOMA (NVG)

It is an intractable glaucoma which results due to formation of neovascular membrane involving the angle of anterior chamber.

Etiology. It is usually associated with neovascularization of iris (rubeosis iridis). Neovascularization develops following retinal ischaemia, which is a common feature of :

- Proliferative diabetic retinopathy,
- Central retinal vein occlusion,
- Sickle-cell retinopathy and
- Eales' disease.
- Other rare causes are chronic intraocular inflammations, intraocular tumours, long-standing retinal detachment and central retinal artery occlusion.

Clinical profile. NVG occurs in three stages:

1. *Pre-glaucomatous stage* (stage of rubeosis iridis);
2. *Open-angle glaucoma stage*— due to formation of a pretrabecular neovascular membrane; and
3. *Secondary angle closure glaucoma*—due to goniosynechiae resulting from contracture of the neovascular membrane (zipper-angle closure).

Treatment of NVG is usually frustrating.

- *Panretinal photocoagulation* may be carried out to prevent further neovascularization.

- *Medical therapy and conventional filtration surgery* are usually not effective in controlling the IOP.
- *Artificial filtration shunt* (Seton operation) may control the IOP.

GLAUCOMA ASSOCIATED WITH INTRAOCULAR TUMOURS

Secondary glaucoma due to intraocular tumours such as malignant melanoma (of iris, choroid, ciliary body) and retinoblastoma may occur by one or more of the following *mechanisms:*

- *Trabecular block* due to clogging by tumour cells or direct invasion by tumour seedlings.
- *Neovascularization* of the angle.
- *Venous stasis* following obstruction of the vortex veins.
- *Angle closure* due to forward displacement of iris-lens diaphragm by increasing tumour mass.

Treatment. Enucleation of the eyeball should be carried out as early as possible.

PSEUDOEXFOLIATIVE GLAUCOMA (GLAUCOMA CAPSULARE)

Pseudoexfoliation syndrome (PES) is characterised by deposition of an amorphous grey dandruff-like material on the pupillary border, anterior lens surface, posterior surface of iris, zonules and ciliary processes. The exact source of the exfoliative material is still not known. The condition is associated with *secondary open-angle glaucoma* in about 50 per cent of the cases. Exact *mechanism* of rise of IOP is also not clear. Trabecular blockage by the exfoliative material is considered as the probable cause. *Clinically* the glaucoma behaves like POAG and is thus managed on the same lines.

GLAUCOMAS-IN-APHAKIA/PSEUDOPHAKIA

It is the term used to replace the old term 'aphakic glaucoma'. It implies association of glaucoma with aphakia or pseudophakia. It includes following conditions:

1. *Raised IOP with deep anterior chamber in early postoperative period:* It may be due to hyphaema, inflammation, retained cortical matter or vitreous filling the anterior chamber.
2. *Secondary angle-closure glaucoma due to flat anterior chamber.* It may occur following long-standing wound leak.
3. *Secondary angle-closure glaucoma due to pupil block.* It may occur following formation of annular synechiae or vitreous herniation.
4. *Undiagnosed pre-existing primary open-angle glaucoma* may be associated with aphakia/ pseudophakia.
5. *Steroid-induced glaucoma.* It may develop in patients operated for cataract due to postoperative treatment with steroids.
6. *Epithelial ingrowth* may cause an intractable glaucoma in late postoperative period by invading the trabeculum and the anterior segment structures.
7. *Aphakic/pseudophakic malignant glaucoma* (see page 251).

STEROID-INDUCED GLAUCOMA

It is a type of secondary open-angle glaucoma which develops following topical, and sometimes systemic steroid therapy.

Etiopathogenesis. It has been postulated that the response of IOP to steroids is genetically determined. Roughly, 5 percent of general population is high steroid responder (develop marked rise of IOP after about 6 weeks of steroid therapy), 35 percent are moderate and 60 percent are non-responders. The precise mechanism responsible for the obstruction to aqueous outflow is unknown. Following theories have been put forward:

- *Glycosaminoglycans (GAG) theory.* Corticosteroids inhibit the release of hydrolases (by stabilizing lysosomal membrane). Consequently the GAGs present in the trabecular meshwork cannot depolymerize and they retain water in the extracellular space. This leads to narrowing of trabecular spaces and decrease in aqueous outflow.
- *Endothelial cell theory.* Under normal circumstances the endothelial cells lining the trabecular meshwork act as phagocytes and phagocytose the debris from the aqueous humour. Corticosteroids are known to suppress the phagocytic activity of endothelial cells leading to collection of debris in the trabecular meshwork and decreasing the aqueous outflow.
- *Prostaglandin theory.* Prostaglandin E and F (PGE and PGF) are known to increase the aqueous outflow facility. Corticosteroids can inhibit the synthesis of PGE and PGF leading to decrease in aqueous outflow facility and increase in IOP.

Clinical features. Steroid-induced glaucoma typically resembles POAG (page 215). It usually develops following weeks of topical therapy with strong steroids and months of therapy with weak steroids.

Management. It can be *prevented* by a judicious use of steroids and a regular monitoring of IOP when steroid therapy is a must. Its *treatment* consists of:

- Discontinuation of steroids. IOP may normalise within 10 days to 4 weeks in 98 percent of cases.
- Medical therapy with 0.5% timolol maleate is effective during the normalisation period.
- Filtration surgery is required occasionally in intractable cases.

TRAUMATIC GLAUCOMA

A secondary glaucoma may complicate perforating as well as blunt injuries.

Mechanisms. Traumatic glaucoma may develop by one or more of the following mechanisms:

- *Inflammatory glaucoma* due to iridocyclitis (see page 248).
- *Glaucoma* due to intraocular haemorrhage (see page 252).
- *Lens-induced glaucoma* due to ruptured, swollen or dislocated lens (see page 247).
- *Angle-closure* due to peripheral anterior synechiae formation following perforating corneal injury producing adherant leucoma.
- *Epithelial or fibrous in growth*, may involve trabeculum.
- *Angle recession (cleavage) glaucoma.* Angle recession refers to rupture in the ciliary body face (between scleral spur and iris root). Unilateral open angle glaucoma usually occurs after years (may be 10 years) of blunt trauma. Angle recession is not the cause of glaucoma but just indicator of old trauma. Glaucoma occurs due to slowly induced fibrosis of trabecular meshwork.

Management. It consists of medical therapy with topical 0.5 percent timolol and oral acetazolamide, treatment of associated causative mechanism (e.g., atropine and steroids for control of inflammation) and surgical intervention according to the situation.

CILIARY BLOCK GLAUCOMA

Ciliary block glaucoma (originally termed as *malignant glaucoma)* is a rare condition which may occur as a complication of any intraocular operation. It classically occurs in patients with primary angle closure glaucoma operated for peripheral iridectomy or filtration (e.g. trabeculectomy) surgery. It is characterised by a markedly raised IOP associated with shallow or absent anterior chamber.

Mechanism of rise in IOP. It is believed that, rarely following intraocular operation, the tips of ciliary processes rotate forward and press against the equator of the lens in phakic eyes (*cilio-lenticular block*) or against the intraocular lens in pseudophakic eyes (*cilio-IOL block*) or against the anterior hyaloid phase of vitreous in aphakic eyes (*cilio-vitreal block*) and thus block the forward flow of aqueous humour, which is diverted posteriorly and collects as aqueous pockets in the vitreous (Fig. 9.21). As a consequence of this the iris lens diaphragm is pushed forward, IOP is raised and anterior chamber becomes flat.

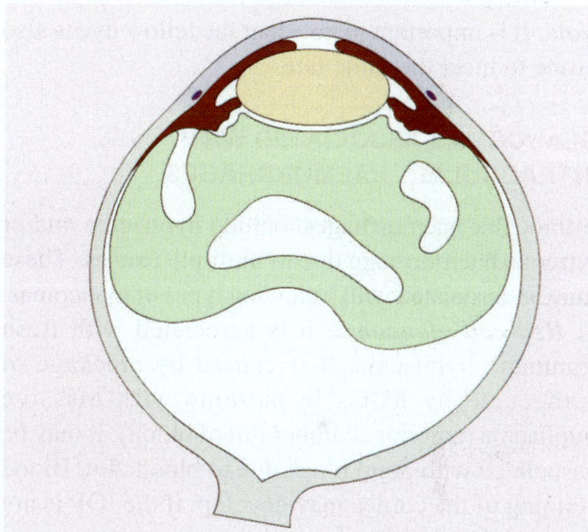

Fig. 9.21. Pockets of aqueous humour in the vitreous in patients with ciliary-block glaucoma.

Clinical features. Patient develops severe pain and blurring of vision following any intraocular operation (usually after peripheral iridectomy, filtering surgery or trabeculectomy in patients with primary angle-closure glaucoma). On examination the main features of the ciliary block glaucoma noted are

- Persistent *flat anterior chamber* following any intraocular operation,
- *Markedly raised IOP* in early postoperative period,
- *Negative Seidel's* test and
- Unresponsiveness or even aggravation by miotics.
- Malignant glaucoma may be phakic, aphakic or pseudophakic.

Management. *Medical therapy* consists of 1 percent atropine drops or ointment to dilate ciliary ring and break the cilio-lenticular or cilio-vitreal contact, acetazolamide 250 mg QID and 0.5 percent timolol maleate eyedrops to decrease aqueous production, and intravenous mannitol to cause deturgescence of the vitreous gel. *YAG laser hyaloidotomy* can be undertaken in aphakic and pseudophakic patients. If the condition does not respond to medical therapy in 4-5 days, *surgical therapy* in the form of pars plana vitrectomy with or without lensectomy (as the case may be) is required when the above measures fail. It is usually effective, but sometimes the condition tends to recur.

Note: It is important to note that the fellow eye is also prone to meet the same fate.

GLAUCOMAS ASSOCIATED WITH INTRAOCULAR HAEMORRHAGES

Intraocular haemorrhages include hyphaema and/or vitreous haemorrhage due to multiple causes. These may be associated with following types of glaucomas:

1. *Red cell glaucoma.* It is associated with fresh traumatic hyphaema. It is caused by blockage of trabeculae by RBCs in patients with massive hyphaema (anterior chamber full of blood). It may be associated with pupil block due to blood clot. Blood staining of the cornea may develop, if the IOP is not lowered within a few days.

2. *Haemolytic glaucoma.* It is an acute secondary open angle glaucoma due to the obstruction (clogging) of the trabecular meshwork caused by macrophages laden with lysed RBC debris.

3. *Ghost cell glaucoma.* It is a type of secondary open angle glaucoma which occurs in aphakic or pseudophakic eyes with vitreous haemorrhage. After about 2 weeks of haemorrhage the RBCs degenerate, lose their pliability and become *khaki*-coloured cells (ghost cells) which pass from the vitreous into the anterior chamber, and block the pores of trabeculae leading to rise in IOP.

4. *Hemosiderotic glaucoma.* It is a rare variety of secondary glaucoma occurring due to sclerotic changes in trabecular meshwork caused by the iron from the phagocytosed haemoglobin by the endothelial cells of trabeculum.

GLAUCOMAS ASSOCIATED WITH IRIDOCORNEAL ENDOTHELIAL SYNDROMES

Iridocorneal endothelial (ICE) syndromes include three clinical entities:

- *Progressive iris atrophy,*
- *Chandler's syndrome, and*
- *Cogan-Reese syndrome.*

Pathogenesis. The common feature of the ICE syndromes is the presence of abnormal corneal endothelial cells which proliferate to form an endothelial membrane in the angle of anterior chamber. Glaucoma is caused by secondary synechial angle-closure as a result of contraction of this endothelial membrane.

Clinical features. The ICE syndromes typically affect middle-aged women. The raised IOP is associated with characteristic features of the causative condition.

- In *'progressive iris atrophy'*, iris features predominate with marked corectopia, atrophy and hole formation.
- While in *Chandler's syndrome,* changes in iris are mild to absent and the corneal oedema even at normal IOP predominates.
- Hallmark of *Cogan-Reese syndrome* is nodular or diffuse pigmented lesions of the iris (therefore also called as *iris naevus syndrome*) which may or may not be associated with corneal changes.

Treatment is usually frustating:

- *Medical treatment* is often ineffective
- *Trabeculectomy operation* usually fails,
- *Artificial filteration shunt* may control the IOP.

SURGICAL PROCEDURES FOR GLAUCOMA

PERIPHERAL IRIDECTOMY

Indications

1. Treatment of all stages of primary angle-closure glaucoma.
2. Prophylaxis in the fellow eye.

Note. Laser iridotomy should always be perferred over surgical iridectomy.

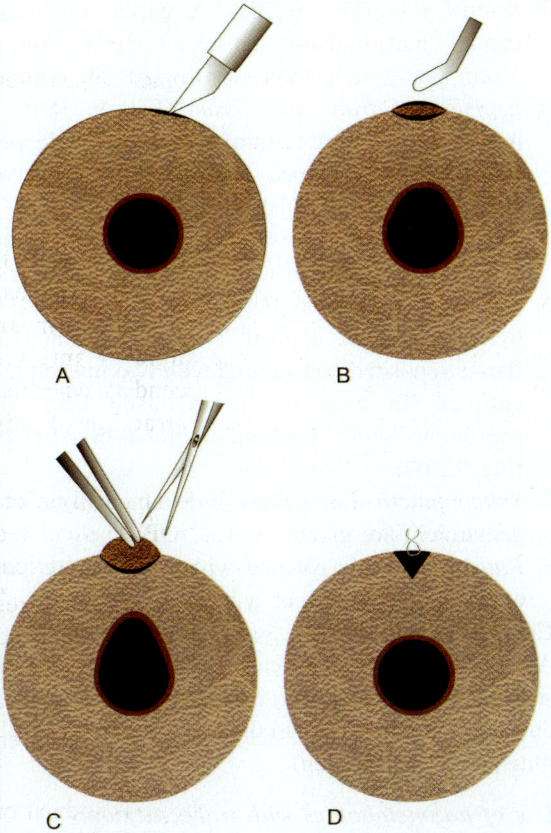

Fig. 9.22. Technique of peripheral iridectomy: A, anterior limbal incision to open the anterior chamber; B, prolapse of peripheral iris by pressure at the posterior lip of the incision; C, excision of the prolapsed knuckle of the iris by de Wecker's scissors; D, suturing the wound.

Surgical technique (Fig. 9.22)

1. *Incision.* A 4 mm limbal or preferably corneal incision is made with the help of razor blade fragment.
2. *Iris prolapsed.* The posterior lip of the wound is depressed so that the iris prolapses. If the iris does not prolapse, it is grasped at the periphery with iris forceps.
3. *Iridectomy.* A small full thickness piece of iris is excised by de Wecker's scissors.
4. *Reposition of iris.* Iris is reposited back into the anterior chamber by stroking the lips of the wound or with iris repositors.
5. *Wound closure* is done with one or two 10-0 nylon sutures with buried knots.
6. *Subconjunctival injection of* dexamethasone 0.25 ml and gentamicin 0.5 ml is given.
7. *Patching of eye* is done with a sterile eye pad and sticking plaster.

GONIOTOMY AND TRABECULOTOMY

These operations are indicated in congenital and developmental glaucomas (For details, see page 226).

FILTERING OPERATIONS

Filtering operations provide a new channel for aqueous outflow and successfully control the IOP (below 21 mm of Hg). Fistulizing operations can be divided into three groups:

1. *Free-filtering operations* (Full thickness fistula). These are no longer performed now-a-days, because of high rate of postoperative complications. Their names are mentioned only for historical interest. These operations included Elliot's sclero-corneal trephining, punch sclerectomy, Scheie's thermosclerostomy and iridencleisis.
2. *Guarded filtering surgery* (Partial thickness fistula e.g., trabeculectomy).
3. *Non-penetrating filtration surgery* e.g., deep sclerectomy and viscocanalostomy.

Trabeculectomy

Trabeculectomy, first described by *Carain* in 1980 is the most frequently performed partial thickness filtering surgery till date.

Indications

1. Primary angle-closure glaucoma with peripheral anterior synechial involving more than 270° angle or where PI and medical treatment fail.
2. Primary open-angle glaucoma not controlled with medical treatment.
3. Congenital and developmental glaucomas where trabeculotomy and goniotomy fail.
4. Secondary glaucomas where medical therapy is not effective.

Mechanisms of filtration

1. A new channel (fistula) is created around the margin of scleral flap, through which aqueous flows from anterior chamber into the subconjunctival space.

2. If the tissue is dissected posterior to the scleral spur, a cyclodialysis may be produced leading to increased uveoscleral outflow.
3. When trabeculectomy was introduced, it was thought that aqueous flows through the cut ends of Schlemm's canal. However, now it is established that this mechanism has a negligible role.

Surgical technique of trabeculectomy (Fig. 9.23)

1. *Initial steps* of anaesthesia, cleansing, draping, exposure of eyeball and fixation with superior rectus suture are similar to cataract operation (see page 199).
2. *Conjunctival flap* (Fig. 9.23A). A fornix-based or limbal-based conjunctival flap is fashioned and the underlying sclera is exposed. The Tenon's capsule is cleared away using a Tooke's knife, and haemostasis is achieved with cautery.

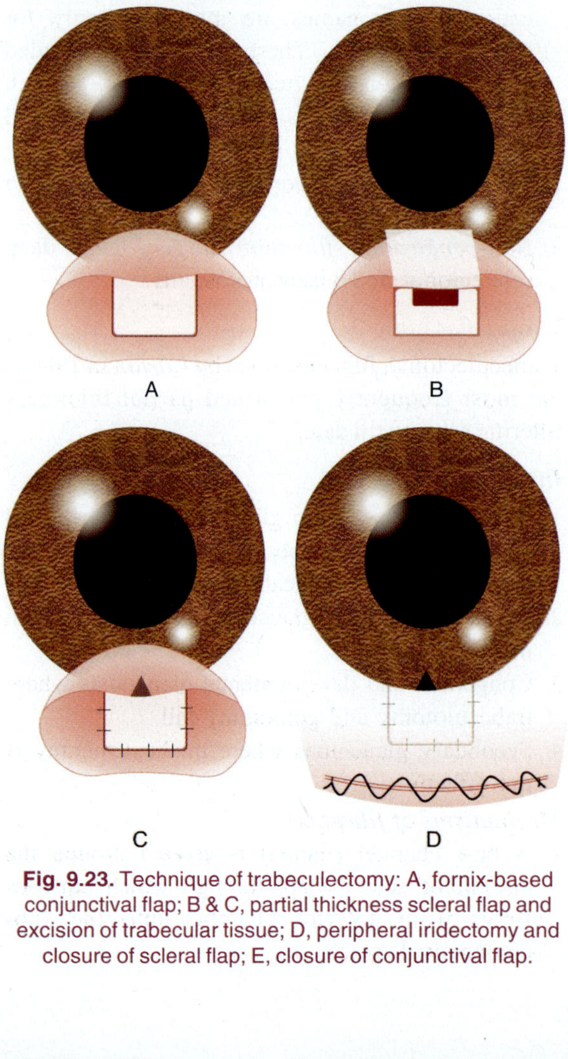

A B C D

Fig. 9.23. Technique of trabeculectomy: A, fornix-based conjunctival flap; B & C, partial thickness scleral flap and excision of trabecular tissue; D, peripheral iridectomy and closure of scleral flap; E, closure of conjunctival flap.

3. *Scleral flap* (Fig. 9.23B). A partial thickness (usually half) limbal-based scleral flap of 5 mm × 5 mm size is reflected down towards the cornea.
4. *Excision of trabecular tissue* (Fig. 9.23B): A narrow strip (4 mm × 2 mm) of the exposed deeper sclera near the cornea containing the canal of Schlemm and trabecular meshwork is excised.
5. *Peripheral iridectomy* (Fig. 9.23C) is performed at 12 O'clock position with de Wecker's scissors.
6. *Closure.* The scleral flap is replaced and 10-0 nylon sutures are applied. Then the conjunctival flap is reposited and sutured with two interrupted sutures (in case of fornix-based flap) or continuous suture (in case of limbal-based flap) (Fig. 9.23D).
7. *Subconjunctival injections* of dexamethasone and gentamicin are given.
8. *Patching.* Eye is patched with a sterile eye pad and sticking plaster or a bandage.

Complications

A few common complications are postoperative shallow anterior chamber, hyphaema, iritis, cataract due to accidental injury to the lens, and endophthalmitis (not very common).

Use of antimetabolites with trabeculectomy

It is recommended that antimetabolites should be used for wound modulation, when any of the following risk factors for the failure of conventional trabeculectomy are present :

1. Previous failed filtration surgery.
2. Glaucoma-in-aphakia.
3. Certain secondary glaucomas e.g. inflammatory glaucoma, post-traumatic angle recession glaucoma, neovascular glaucoma and glaucomas associated with ICE syndrome.
4. Patients treated with topical antiglaucoma medications (particularly sympathomimetics) for over three years.
5. Chronic cicatrizing conjunctival inflammation.

Antimetabolite agents. Either 5-fluorouracil (5-FU) or mitomycin-C can be used. Mitomycin-C is only used at the time of surgery. A sponge soaked in 0.02% (2 mg in 10 ml) solution of mitomycin-C is placed at the site of filtration between the scleral and Tenon's capsule for 2 minutes, followed by a thorough irrigation with balanced salt solution.

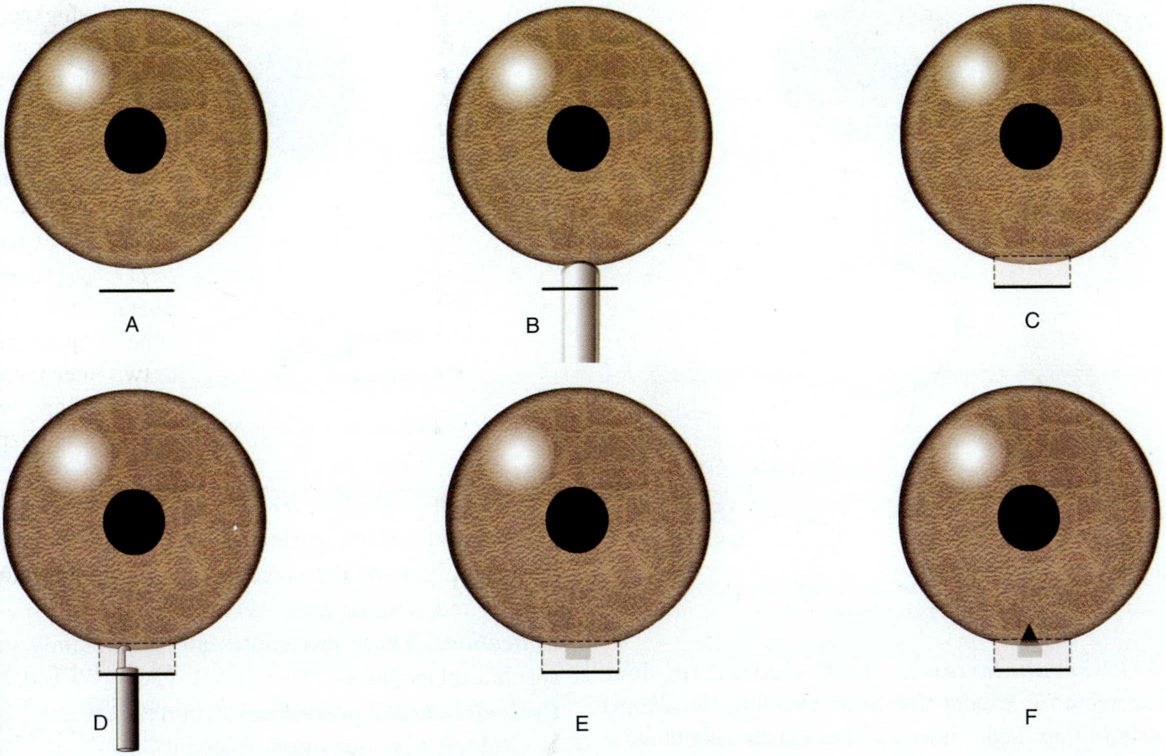

Fig. 9.24. Sutureless trabeculectomy.

Sutureless trabeculectomy

1. *Initial steps* and
2. *Conjuctival flap* fashioning is similaar to conventional trabeculectomy.
3. *Sclero-corneal valvular tunnel*, 4 mm × 4 mm in size, is made by first making 4 mm partial thickness scleral groove about 2.5 mm away from the superior limbus with the help of a razor blade fragment (Fig. 9.24A). A 4 mm wide sclero-corneal tunnel which extends about 1.5 mm in the clear cornea is then made with the help of a crescent knife (Fig. 9.24B).
4. *Entry into the anterior chamber* is made with the help of a sharp 3.2 mm angled keratome (Fig. 9.24C).
5. *Punching of posterior lip of the anterior chamber entry site*. (Fig. 9.24D) is then performed with the help of a Kelly's punch (Fig. 24.61) to make a sclerostomy of about 2 mm × 2 mm in size.
6. *Peripheral iridectomy* (Fig. 9.24F) is performed at 12 O'clock position with the help of de Wecker's or Vanna's scissors.
7. *Closure*. Anterior chamber is filled with balanced salt solution (BSS) or air to close the valvular sclero-corneal tunnel incision. Conjunctival flap is reposited and anchored with wet field cautry.

Non-penetrating filteration surgery

Recently some techniques of non-penetrating filteration surgery (in which anterior chamber is not entered) have been advocated to reduce the incidence of post-operative endophthalmitis, overfiltration and hypotony. Main disadvantage of non-penetrating filteration surgery is inferior IOP control as compared to conventional trabeculectomy. The two currently used procedures are:

1. *Deep sclerectomy.* In this procedure, after making a partial thickness scleral flap, (as in conventional trabeculectomy, Fig.9.23A), a second deep partial-thickness scleral flap is fashioned and excised leaving behind a thin membrane consisting of very thin sclera, trabeculum and Descemet's membrane (through which aqueous diffuses out). The superficial scleral flap is loosely approximated and conjunctival incision is closed.

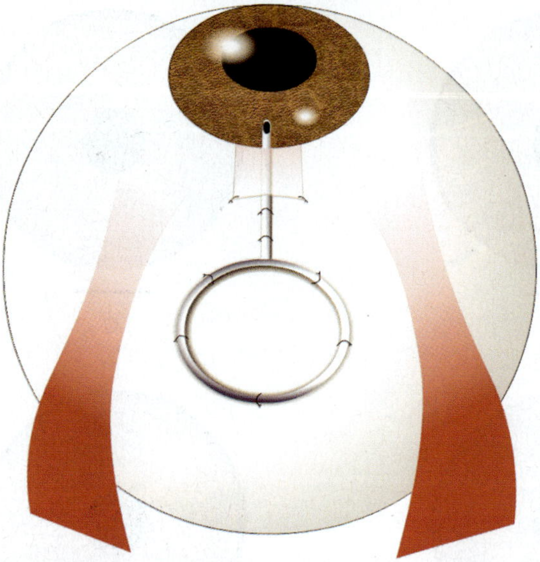

Fig. 9.25. Artificial drainage shunt operation using Molteno implant.

2. *Viscocanalostomy.* It is similar to deep sclerectomy, except that after excising the deeper scleral flap, high viscosity viscoelastic substance is injected into the Schlemm's canal with a special cannula.

ARTIFICIAL DRAINAGE SHUNT OPERATIONS

Artificial drainage shunts or the so called glaucoma valve implants are plastic devices which allow aqueous outflow by creating a communication between the anterior chamber and sub-Tenon's space. The operation using glaucoma valve implant is also known as *Seton operation.*

Glaucoma valve implants commonly used include Molteno (Fig. 9.25) Krupin-Denver and AGV.

Indications of artificial drainage shunts include :

- Neovascular glaucoma;
- Glaucoma with aniridia; and
- Intractable cases of primary and secondary glaucoma where even trabeculectomy with adjunct antimetabolite therapy fails.

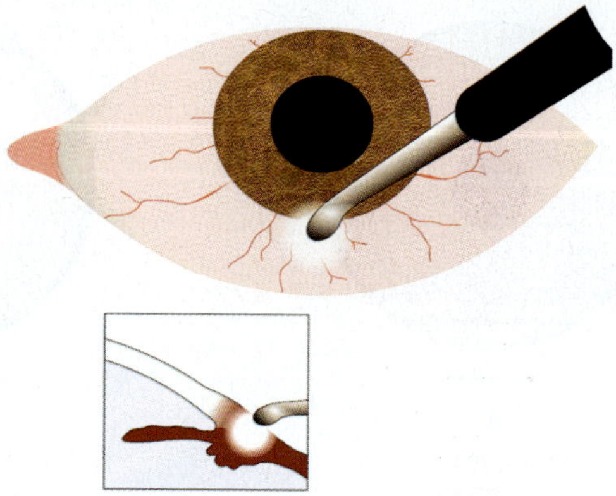

Fig. 9.26. Site of cyclocryopexy.

CYCLO-DESTRUCTIVE PROCEDURES

Cyclo-destructive procedures lower IOP by destroying part of the secretory ciliary epithelium thereby reducing aqueous secretion.

Indications. These procedures are used mainly in absolute glaucomas.

Cyclo-destructive procedures in current use are:

1. Cyclocryotherapy (most frequent),
2. Nd: Yag laser cyclodestruction, and
3. Diode laser cyclophotocoagulation.

Technique of cyclocryopexy

1. *Anaesthesia.* Topical and peribulbar block anaesthesia is given.
2. *Lids separation* is done with eye speculum.
3. *Cryoapplications.* Cryo is applied with a retinal probe placed 3 mm from the limbus. A freezing at –80°C for 1 minute is done in an area of 180° of the globe (Fig. 9.26).

If ineffective, the procedure may be repeated in the same area after 3 weeks. If still ineffective, then the remaining 180° should be treated.

Mechanism. IOP is lowered due to destruction of the secretory ciliary epithelium. The cells are destroyed by intracellular freezing.

10 CHAPTER

Diseases of the Vitreous

APPLIED ANATOMY

Vitreous humour is an inert, transparent, jelly-like structure that fills the posterior four-fifth of the cavity of eyeball and is about 4 ml in volume. It is a hydrophilic gel that mainly serves the optical functions. In addition, it mechanically stabilizes the volume of the globe and is a pathway for nutrients to reach the lens and retina.

Structure.

The normal youthful vitreous gel is composed of a network of randomly-oriented collagen fibrils interspersed with numerous spheroidal macromolecules of hyaluronic acid. The collapse of this structure with age or otherwise leads to conversion of the gel into sol. The vitreous body can be divided into two parts: the cortex and the nucleus (the main vitreous body) (Fig. 10.1).

1. *Cortical vitreous*. It lies adjacent to the retina posteriorly and ciliary body, zonules and lens anteriorly. The density of collagen fibrils is greater in this peripheral part. The condensation of these fibrils form a false anatomic membrane which is called as *anterior hyaloid membrane* anterior to ora serrata and *posterior hyaloid membrane* posterior to ora. The attachment of the anterior hyaloid membrane to the posterior lens surface is firm in young and weak in elders whereas posterior hyaloid membrane remains loosely attached to the internal limiting membrane of the retina throughout life. These membranes cannot be discerned in a normal eye unless the lens has been extracted and posterior vitreous detachment has occurred.

2. *The main vitreous body (nucleus)*. It has a less dense fibrillar structure and is a true biological gel. It is here where liquefactions of the vitreous gel start first. Microscopically the vitreous body is homogenous, but exhibits wavy lines as of watered silk in the slit-lamp beams. Running down the centre of the vitreous body from the optic disc to the posterior pole of the lens is the *hyaloid canal* (Cloquet's canal) of doubtful existence in adults. Down this canal ran the hyaloid artery of the foetus.

Attachments.

The part of the vitreous about 4 mm across the ora serrata is called as *vitreous base,* where the attachment of the vitreous is strongest. The other firm attachments are around the margins of the optic disc, foveal region and back of the crystalline lens by hyaloidocapsular ligament of Wiegert.

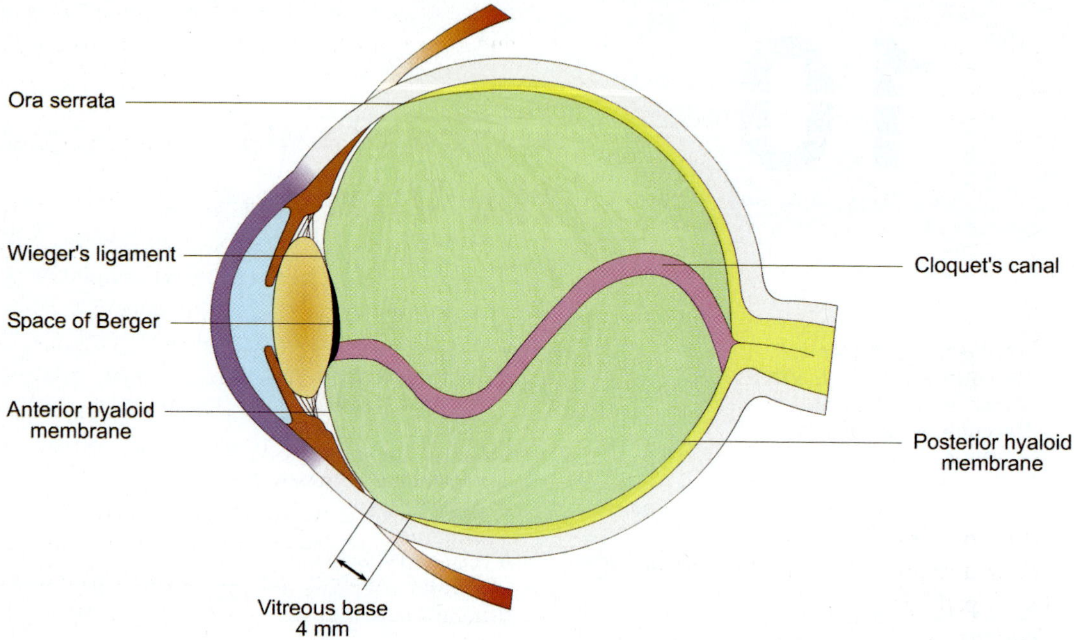

Fig. 10.1. Gross anatomy of the vitreous.

DISORDERS OF THE VITREOUS

VITREOUS LIQUEFACTION

Vitreous liquefaction (synchysis) is the most common degenerative change in the vitreous.

Causes of liquefaction include:

1. *Degenerations* such as senile, myopic, and that associated with retinitis pigmentosa.
2. *Post-inflammatory,* particularly following uveitis.
3. *Trauma to the vitreous* which may be mechanical (blunt as well as perforating).
4. *Thermal effects* on vitreous following diathermy, photocoagulation and cryocoagulation.
5. *Radiation effects* may also cause liquefaction.

Clinical features. On slit-lamp biomicroscopy the vitreous liquefaction (synchysis) is characterised by the absence of normal fine fibrillar structure and visible pockets of liquefaction associated with appearance of coarse aggregate material which moves freely in free vitreous. Liquefaction is usually associated with collapse (synersis) and opacities in the vitreous which may be seen subjectively as black floaters in front of the eye.

VITREOUS DETACHMENTS

1. Posterior vitreous detachment (PVD)

It refers to the separation of the cortical vitreous from the retina anywhere posterior to vitreous base (3-4 mm wide area of attachment of vitreous to the ora serrata).

PVD with vitreous liquefaction (synchysis) and collapse (synersis) is of common occurrence in majority of the normal subjects above the age of 65 years (Fig. 10.2). It occurs in eyes with senile liquefaction, developing a hole in the posterior hyaloid membrane. The synchytic fluid collects between the posterior hyaloid membrane and the internal limiting membrane of the retina, and leads to PVD up to the base along with collapse of the remaining vitreous gel (synersis). These changes occur more frequently in the aphakics than the phakics and in the myopes than the emmetropes.

Clinical features. PVD may be associated with flashes of light and floaters. Biomicroscopic examination of the vitreous reveals a collapsed vitreous (synersis) behind the lens and an optically clear space between the detached posterior hyaloid phase and the retina.

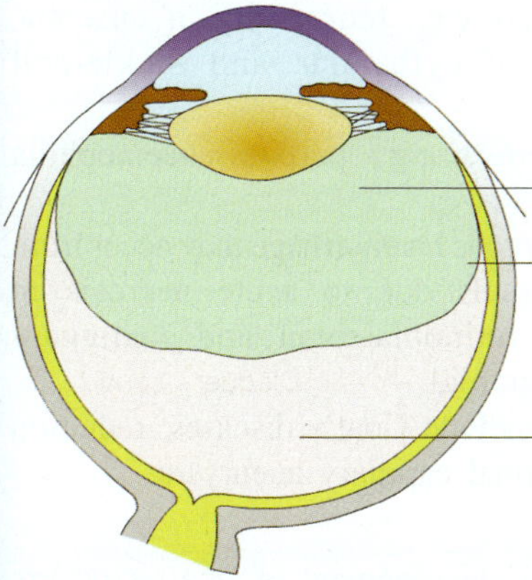

Fig. 10.2. Posterior vitreous detachment with synchysis and synersis.

A ring-like opacity (Weiss ring or Fuchs ring), representing a ring of attachment of vitreous to the optic disc, is pathognomic of PVD.

Complications of PVD. These include retinal breaks, vitreous haemorrhage, retinal haemorrhages and cystoid maculopathy.

Management:

- *Uncomplicated PVD requires no treatment.* Just reassure but give 'retinal detachment warning' i.e. to report immediately on noticing an increase in floaters, or flashing lights or the appearance of persistent curtain or shadow in the field of vision.
- *Retinal tear complicating* PVD may need to be treated by laser photocoagulation.
- *Vitreous haemorrhage complicating* PVD needs to be managed (see page 260)
- *Retinal detachment complicating* PVD requires urgent treatment (see page 296)

2. Detachment of the vitreous base and the anterior vitreous

It usually occurs following blunt trauma. It may be associated with vitreous haemorrhage, anterior retinal dialysis and dislocation of crystalline lens.

VITREOUS OPACITIES

Since vitreous is a transparent structure, any relatively non-transparent structure present in it will form an opacity and cause symptoms of floaters. Common conditions associated with vitreous opacities are described below.

Muscae volitantes. These are physiological opacities and represent the residues of primitive hyaloid vasculature. Patient perceives them as fine dots and filaments, which often drift in and out of the visual field, against a bright background (e.g., clear blue sky).

Persistent hyperplastic primary vitreous (PHPV) results from failure of the primary vitreous structure to regress combined with the hypoplasia of the posterior portion of vascular meshwork.

Clinically it is characterized by a white pupillary reflex (leucocoria) seen shortly after birth. Associated anomalies include congenital cataract, glaucoma, long and extended ciliary processes, microphthalmos and vitreous haemorrhage.

Differential diagnosis needs to be made from other causes of leucocoria especially retinoblastoma, congenital cataract and retinopathy of prematurity. Computerised tomography (CT) scanning helps in diagnosis.

Treatment consists of pars plana lensectomy and excision of the membranes with anterior vitrectomy provided the diagnosis is made early. Visual prognosis is often poor.

Inflammatory vitreous opacities. These consist of exudates poured into the vitreous in patients with anterior uveitis (iridocyclitis), posterior uveitis (choroiditis), pars planitis, pan uveitis and endophthalmitis.

Vitreous aggregates and condensation with liquefaction. It is the commonest cause of vitreous opacities. Condensation of the collagen fibrillar network is a feature of the vitreous degeneration which may be senile, myopic, post-traumatic or post-inflammatory in origin.

Amyloid degeneration. It is a rare condition in which amorphous amyloid material is deposited in the vitreous as a part of the generalised amyloidosis. These vitreous opacities are linear with footplate attachments to the retina and the posterior lens surface.

Asteroid hyalosis. It is characterised by small, white rounded bodies suspended in the vitreous gel. These are formed due to accumulation of calcium containing lipids. Asteroid hyalosis is a unilateral, asymptomatic condition usually seen in old patients with healthy vitreous. There is a genetic relationship between this condition, diabetes and hypercholesterolaemia. The genesis is unknown and there is no effective treatment.

Synchysis scintillans. In this condition, vitreous is laden with small white angular and crystalline bodies formed of cholesterol. It affects the damaged eyes which have suffered from trauma, vitreous haemorrhage or inflammatory disease in the past. In this condition vitreous is liquid and so, the crystals sink to the bottom, but are stirred up with every movement to settle down again with every pause. This phenomenon appears as a beautiful shower of golden rain on ophthalmoscopic examination. Since the condition occurs in a damaged eye, it may occur at any age. The condition is generally symptomless, and untreatable.

Red cell opacities. These are caused by small vitreous haemorrhages or leftouts of the massive vitreous haemorrhage.

Tumour cells opacities. These may be seen as free-floating opacities in some patients with retinoblastoma, and reticulum cell sarcoma.

VITREOUS HAEMORRHAGE

Vitreous haemorrhage usually occurs from the retinal vessels and may present as pre-retinal (sub-hyaloid) or an intragel haemorrhage. The intragel haemorrhage may involve anterior, middle, posterior or the whole vitreous body.

Causes

Causes of vitreous haemorrhage are as follows:

1. *Retinal tear*, *PVD* and *RD* may have associated vitreous haemorrhage.
2. *Trauma to eye,* which may be blunt or perforating (with or without retained intraocular foreign body) in nature.
3. *Inflammatory diseases* such as erosion of the vessels in acute chorioretinitis and periphlebitis retinae primary (eale's disease) or secondary to uveitis.
4. *Vascular disorders e.g.,* hypertensive retinopathy, and central retinal vein occlusion.
5. *Metabolic diseases* such as diabetic retinopathy.
6. *Exudative age related macular degeneration* usually high CNVM, may have vitreous haemorrhage.
7. *Blood dyscrasias* e.g., retinopathy of anaemia, leukaemias, polycythemias and sickle-cell retinopathy.
8. *Bleeding disorders* e.g., purpura, haemophilia and scurvy.
9. *Neoplasms.* Vitreous haemorrhage may occur from rupture of vessels due to acute necrosis in tumours like retinoblastoma and malignant melanoma of choroid.
10. *Other causes* include Coat's diseases, radiation retinopathy, retinal capillary aneurysm.

Clinical features

Symptoms. Sudden development of floaters occurs when the vitreous haemorrhage is small. In massive vitreous haemorrhage, patient develops sudden painless loss of vision.

Signs

- *Distant direct ophthalmoscopy* reveals black shadows against the red glow in small haemorrhages and no red glow in a large haemorrhage.
- *Direct and indirect ophthalmoscopy* may show presence of blood in the vitreous cavity.
- *Ultrasonography* with B-scan is particularly helpful in diagnosing vitreous haemorrhage.

Fate of vitreous haemorrhage

1. *Complete absorption* may occur without organization and the vitreous becomes clear within 4-8 weeks.
2. *Organization* of haemorrhage with formation of a yellowish-white debris occurs in persistent or recurrent bleeding.
3. *Complications* like vitreous liquefaction, degeneration and khaki cell glaucoma (in aphakia) may occur.
4. *Retinitis proliferans* may occur which may be complicated by tractional retinal detachment.

Treatment

1. *Conservative treatment* consists of bed rest and elevation of patient's head. This will allow the blood to settle down.
2. *Treatment of the cause.* Once the blood settles down, indirect ophthalmoscopy should be performed to locate and further manage the causative lesion such as a retinal break, phlebitis, proliferative retinopathy, etc.

3. *Vitrectomy* by pars plana route should be considered to clear the vitreous, if the haemorrhage is not absorbed after 3 months. Early vitrectomy may be required when associated with retinal detachment.

VITREO-RETINAL DEGENERATIONS

See page 286.

VITRECTOMY

Vitrectomy i.e., surgical removal of the vitreous is now a frequently performed procedure. Common terms used in relation to vitrectomy are:

- *Anterior vitrectomy.* It refers to removal of anterior part of the vitreous.
- *Core vitrectomy.* It refers to removal of the central bulk of the vitreous. It is usually indicated in endophthalmitis.
- *Subtotal and total vitrectomy.* In this almost whole of the vitreous is removed.

TECHNIQUES

Open-sky vitrectomy

This technique is employed to perform only anterior vitrectomy.

Indications

- Vitreous loss during cataract extraction.
- Aphakic keratoplasty.
- Anterior chamber reconstruction after perforating trauma with vitreous loss.
- Removal of subluxated and anteriorly dislocated lens.

Surgical technique.
Open sky vitrectomy is performed through the primary wound to manage the disturbed vitreous during cataract surgery or aphakic keratoplasty. It should be performed using an automated vitrectomy machine. However, if the vitrectomy machine is not available, it can be performed with the help of a triangular cellulose sponge and de Wecker's scissors (*sponge vitrectomy*).

Closed vitrectomy (Pars plana vitrectomy)

Pars plana approach is employed to perform anterior vitrectomy, core vitrectomy, subtotal and total vitrectomy.

Indications

- Endophthalmitis with vitreous abscess.
- Vitreous haemorrhage.
- Proliferative retinopathies such as those associated with diabetes, Eales' disease, retinopathy of prematurity and retinitis proliferans.
- Complicated cases of retinal detachment such as those associated with giant retinal tears, retinal dialysis and massive vitreous traction.
- Removal of intraocular foreign bodies.
- Removal of dropped nucleus or intraocular lens from the vitreous cavity.

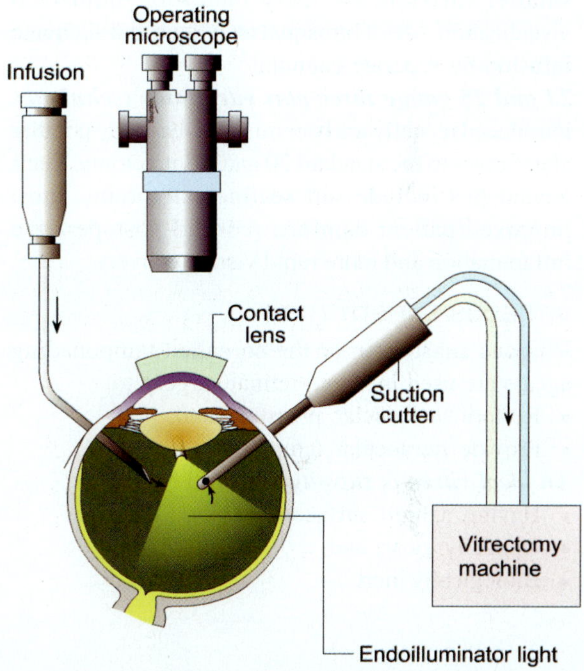

Fig. 10.3. Three-port pars plana vitrectomy using divided system approach

- Persistent primary hyperplastic vitreous.
- Vitreous membranes and bands.
- Macular pathology like macular hole, and epiretinal membrane.

Surgical techniques

Pars plana vitrectomy is a highly sophisticated microsurgery which can be performed by using two type of systems:

1. ***Full function system vitrectomy*** is now-a-days not used. It employs a multifunction system that comprises vitreous infusion, suction, cutter and illumination (VISC), all in one.

2. *Divided system approach* is the most commonly employed technique in modern vitrectomy. In this technique three separate incisions are given in pars plana region. That is why the procedure is also called *three-port pars plana vitrectomy*. The cutting and aspiration functions are contained in one probe, illumination is provided by a separate fiberoptic probe and infusion is provided by a cannula introduced through the third pars plana incision (Fig. 10.3).

Advantages of divided system approach include smaller instruments, easy handling, improved visualization, use of bimanual technique and adequate infusion by separate cannula.

23 and 25 gauge three-port vitrectomy techniques introduced recently are becoming increasingly popular alternatives to the standard 20 gauge vitrectomy. Their advantages include self sealing sclerotomy sites, improved patient comfort, reduced postoperative inflammation and more rapid visual recovery.

VITREOUS SUBSTITUTES

Vitreous substitutes or the so called tamponading agents are used in vitreo-retinal surgery to:

- Restore intraocular pressure, and
- Provide intraocular tamponade.

An ideal vitreous substitute should be:

- Having a high surface tension,
- Optically clear, and
- Biologically inert.

Currently used vitreous substitutes in the absence of an ideal substitute are:

1. *Air* is commonly used internal tamponade in uncomplicated cases. It is absorbed within 3 days.
2. *Physiological solutions* such as Ringer's lactate or balanced salt solution (BSS) can be used as substitute after vitrectomy for endophthalmitis or uncomplicated vitreous haemorrhage.
3. *Expanding gases* are preferred over air in complex cases requiring prolonged intraocular tamponade. They are used as 40% mixture with air. Examples are:
   - *Sulphur hexafluoride* (SF_6). It doubles its volume and lasts for 10 days.
   - *Perfluoropropane* (C_3F_8). It quadruples its volume and lasts for 28 days.
4. *Perfluorocarbon liquids* (PFCL) are heavy liquids which are mainly used:
   - To remove dropped nucleus or IOL from the vitreous cavity,
   - To unfold a giant retinal tear, and
   - To stabilize the posterior retina during peeling of the epiretinal membrane.

   Agent most commonly used is perfluoro-n-octane.
5. *Silicone oil* allows more controlled retinal manipulation during operation and can be used for prolonged intraocular tamponade after retinal detachment surgery.

11

CHAPTER

Diseases of the Retina

APPLIED ANATOMY

Retina, the innermost tunic of the eyeball, is a thin, delicate and transparent membrane. It is the most highly-developed tissue of the eye. It appears purplish-red due to the visual purple of the rods and underlying vascular choroid.

Gross anatomy

Retina extends from the optic disc to the ora serrata. Grossly it can be divided into two distinct regions: posterior pole and peripheral retina separated by the so called retinal equator.

Retinal equator is an imaginary line which is considered to lie in line with the exit of the four vena verticose.

Posterior pole refers to the area of the retina posterior to the retinal equator. The posterior pole of the retina includes two distinct areas: the optic disc and macula lutea (Fig. 11.1). Posterior pole of the retina is best examined by slit-lamp indirect biomicroscopy using +78D and +90D lens and direct ophthalmoscopy.

Optic disc. It is a pink coloured, well-defined circular area of 1.5-mm diameter. At the optic disc all the retinal layers terminate except the nerve fibres, which pass through the lamina cribrosa to run into the optic nerve. A depression seen in the disc is called the *physiological cup*. The central retinal artery and vein emerge through the centre of this cup.

Macula lutea. It is also called the *yellow spot*. It is comparatively deeper red than the surrounding fundus and is situated at the posterior pole temporal to the optic disc. It is about 5.5 mm in diameter. *Fovea centralis* is the central depressed part of the macula. It is about 1.5 mm in diameter and is the most sensitive part of the retina. In its centre is a shining pit called *foveola* (0.35-mm diameter) which is situated about 2 disc diameters (3 mm) away from the temporal margin of the disc and about 1 mm below the horizontal meridian. An area about 0.8 mm in diameter (including foveola and some surrounding area) does not contain any retinal capillaries and is called foveal avascular zone (FAZ). Surrounding the fovea are the parafoveal and perifoveal areas.

Peripheral retina refers to the area bounded posteriorly by the retinal equator and anteriorly by the ora serrata. Peripheral retina is best examined with indirect ophthalmoscopy and by the use of Goldman three mirror contact lens.

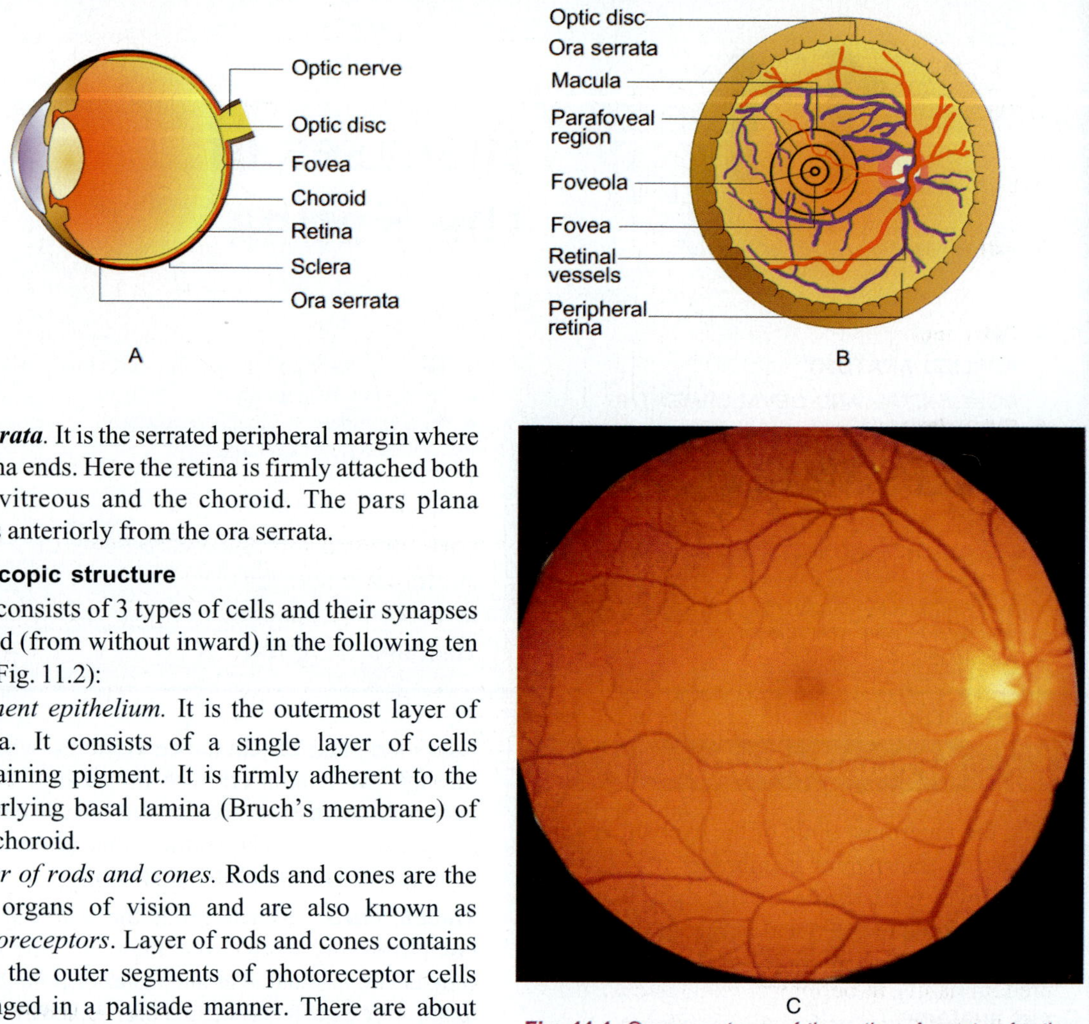

Fig. 11.1. Gross anatomy of the retina: A, parts of retina in horizontal section at the level of fovea; B, diagrammatic fundus view; C, fundus photograph.

Ora serrata. It is the serrated peripheral margin where the retina ends. Here the retina is firmly attached both to the vitreous and the choroid. The pars plana extends anteriorly from the ora serrata.

Microscopic structure

Retina consists of 3 types of cells and their synapses arranged (from without inward) in the following ten layers (Fig. 11.2):

1. *Pigment epithelium.* It is the outermost layer of retina. It consists of a single layer of cells containing pigment. It is firmly adherent to the underlying basal lamina (Bruch's membrane) of the choroid.
2. *Layer of rods and cones.* Rods and cones are the end organs of vision and are also known as *photoreceptors*. Layer of rods and cones contains only the outer segments of photoreceptor cells arranged in a palisade manner. There are about 120 millions rods and 6.5 millions cones. *Rods* contain a photosensitive substance visual purple *(rhodopsin)* and subserve the peripheral vision and vision of low illumination (*scotopic vision). Cones* also contain a photosensitive substance and are primarily responsible for highly discriminatory central vision (*photopic vision*) and colour vision.
3. *External limiting membrane.* It is a fenestrated membrane, through which pass processes of the rods and cones.
4. *Outer nuclear layer.* It consists of nuclei of rods and cones.
5. *Outer plexiform layer.* It consists of connections of rod spherules and cone pedicles with the dendrites of bipolar cells and horizontal cells.
6. *Inner nuclear layer.* It mainly consists of cell bodies of bipolar cells. It also contains cell bodies of horizontal, amacrine and Muller's cells and capillaries of central artery of retina. The bipolar cells constitute the first order neurons.
7. *Inner plexiform layer.* It essentially consists of connections between the axons of bipolar cells dendrites of the ganglion cells, and processes of amacrine cells.
8. *Ganglion cell layer.* It mainly contains the cell bodies of ganglion cells (the second order neurons of visual pathway). There are two types of ganglion cells. The *midget ganglion cells* are

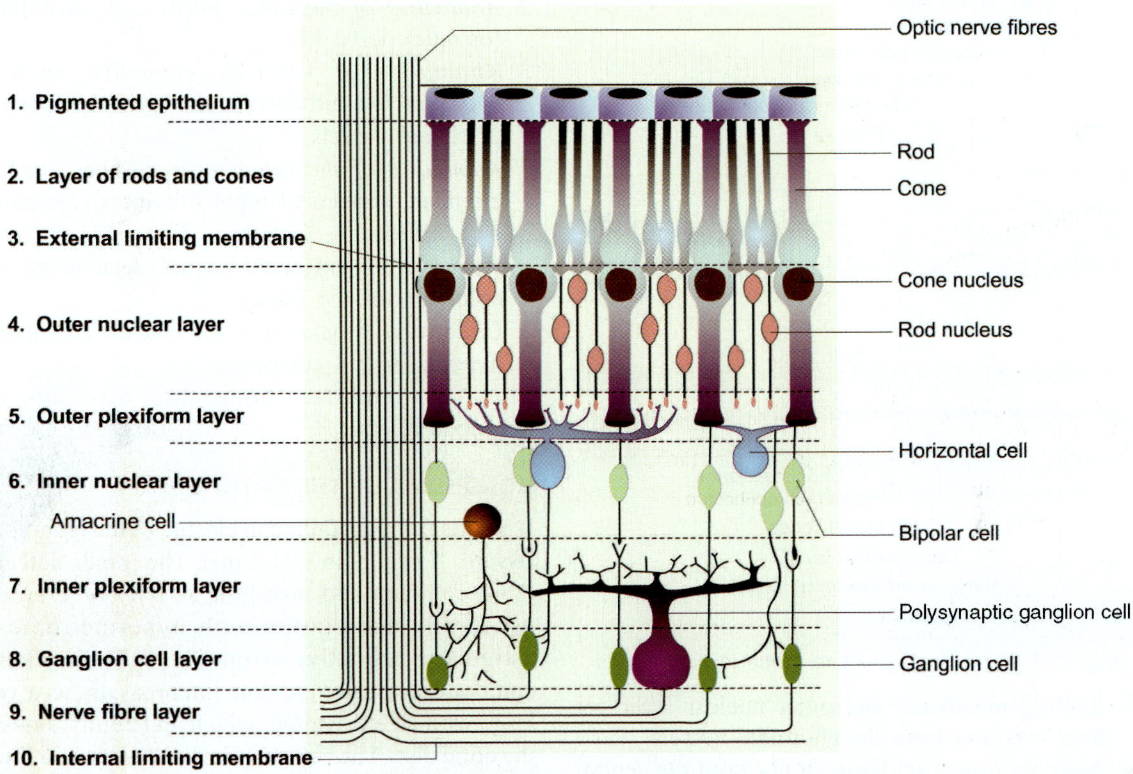

Fig. 11.2. Microscopic structure of the retina.

present in the macular region and the dendrite of each such cell synapses with the axon of single bipolar cell. *Polysynaptic ganglion* cells lie predominantly in peripheral retina and each such cell may synapse with up to a hundred bipolar cells.

9. *Nerve fibre layer* (stratum opticum) consists of axons of the ganglion cells, which pass through the lamina cribrosa to form the optic nerve. For distribution and arrangement of retinal nerve fibres see Figs. 9.11 and 9.12, respectively and page 216.
10. *Internal limiting membrane.* It is the innermost layer and separates the retina from vitreous. It is formed by the union of terminal expansions of the Muller's fibres, and is essentially a basement membrane.

Structure of fovea centralis

In this area (Fig. 11.3), there are no rods, cones are tightly packed and other layers of retina are very thin. Its central part (foveola) largely consists of cones and their nuclei covered by a thin internal limiting membrane. All other retinal layers are absent in this region. In the foveal region surrounding the foveola, the cone axons are arranged obliquely (Henle's layer) to reach the margin of the fovea.

Functional divisions of retina

Functionally retina can be divided into *temporal retina* and *nasal retina* by a line drawn vertically through the centre of fovea. Nerve fibres arising from temporal retina pass through the optic nerve and optic tract of the same side to terminate in the ipsilateral geniculate body while the nerve fibres originating from the nasal retina after passing through the optic nerve cross in the optic chiasma and travel through the contralateral optic tract to terminate in the contralateral geniculate body.

Blood supply

- *Outer four layers of the retina*, viz, pigment epithelium, layer of rods and cones, external

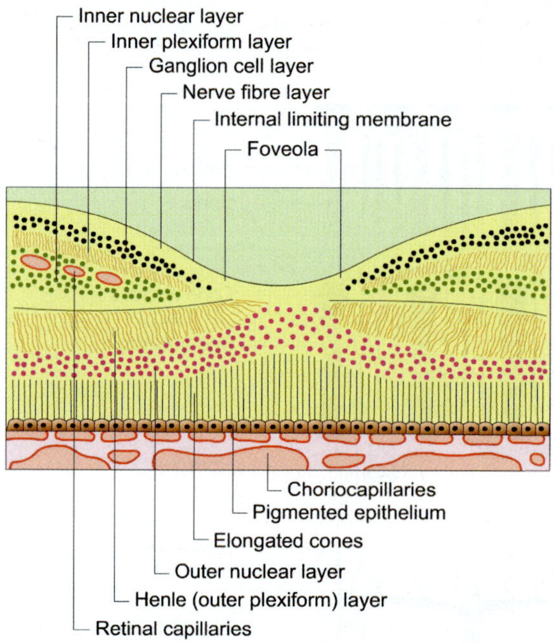

Fig. 11.3. Microscopic structure of the fovea centralis.

limiting membrane and outer nuclear layer get their nutrition from the choroidal vessels.

- *Inner six layers* get their supply from the central retinal artery, which is a branch of the ophthalmic artery.
- *Central retinal artery* emerges from centre of the physiological cup of the optic disc and divides into four branches, namely the superior-nasal, superior-temporal, inferior-nasal and inferior-temporal. These are end arteries i.e., they do not anastomose with each other.
- *The retinal veins.* These follow the pattern of the retinal arteries. The central retinal vein drains into the cavernous sinus directly or through the superior ophthalmic vein. The only place where the retinal system anastomosis with ciliary system is in the region of lamina cribrosa.

CONGENITAL AND DEVELOPMENTAL DISORDERS

CLASSIFICATION

1. *Anomalies of the optic disc.* These include crescents, situs inversus, congenital pigmentation, coloboma, drusen and hypoplasia of the optic disc.
2. *Anomalies of the nerve fibres* e.g., medullated (opaque) nerve fibres.
3. *Anomalies of vascular elements,* such as persistent hyaloid artery and congenital tortuosity of retinal vessels.
4. *Anomalies of the retina proper.* These include albinism, congenital night blindness, congenital day blindness, Oguchi's disease, congenital retinal cyst, congenital retinal detachment and coloboma of the fundus.
5. *Congenital anomalies of the macula* are aplasia, hypoplasia and coloboma.

A few important congenital disorders are described briefly.

COLOBOMA OF THE OPTIC DISC

It results from the failure in closure of the embryonic fissure. It occurs in two forms. The minor defect is more common and manifests as *inferior crescent,* usually in association with hypermetropic or astigmatic refractive error. The fully-developed coloboma typically presents inferonasally as a very large whitish excavation, which apparently looks as the optic disc. The actual optic disc is seen as a linear horizontal pinkish band confined to a small superior wedge. Defective vision and a superior visual field defect is usually associated.

DRUSEN OF THE OPTIC DISC

Drusens are intrapapillary refractile bodies, which usually lie deep beneath the surface of the disc tissue in childhood and emerge out by the early teens. Thus, in children they present as pseudo-papilloedema and by teens they can be recognised ophthalmoscopically as waxy pea-like irregular refractile bodies.

HYPOPLASIA OF OPTIC DISC

Hypoplasia of the optic nerve may occur as an isolated anomaly or in association with other anomalies of central nervous system. The condition is bilateral in 60 per cent of cases. It is associated with maternal alcohol use, diabetes and intake of certain drugs in pregnancy. It forms a significant cause of blindness at birth in developed countries. Diagnosis of mild cases presents little difficulty. In typical cases the disc is small and surrounded by a yellowish and a pigmented ring; referred to as 'double ring sign'.

MEDULLATED NERVE FIBRES

These, also known as *opaque nerve fibres*, represent myelination of nerve fibres of the retina. Normally, the medullation of optic nerve proceeds from brain downwards to the eyeball and stops at the level of lamina cribrosa. Occasionally the process of myelination continues after birth for an invariable distance in the nerve fibre layer of retina beyond the optic disc on ophthalmoscopic examination. These appear as a whitish patch with feathery margins, usually present adjoining the disc margin. The traversing retinal vessels are partially concealed by the opaque nerve fibres (Fig. 11.4). Such a lesion, characteristically, exhibits *enlargement of blind spot* on visual field charting. The medullary sheaths disappear in demyelinating disorders and optic atrophy (due to any cause) and thus no trace of this abnormality is left behind.

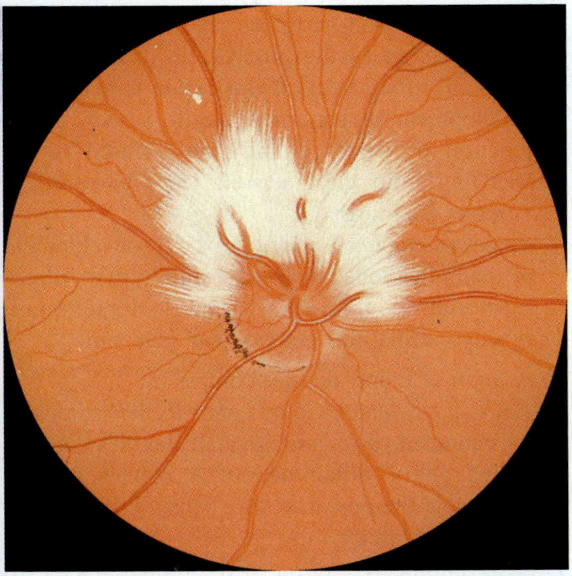

Fig. 11.4. Opaque nerve fibres.

PERSISTENT HYALOID ARTERY

Congenital remnants of the hyaloid arterial system may persist in different forms.

Bergmester's papilla refers to the flake of glial tissue projecting from the optic disc. It is the commonest congenital anomaly of the hyaloid system.

Vascular loop or a thread of obliterated vessel may sometimes be seen running forward into the vitreous. It may even be reaching up to the back of the lens.

Mittendorf dot represents remnant of the anterior end of hyaloid artery, attached to the posterior lens capsule. It is usually associated with a posterior polar cataract.

INFLAMMATORY DISORDERS OF THE RETINA

These may present as retinitis (pure retinal inflammation), chorioretinitis (inflammation of retina and choroid), neuroretinitis (inflammation of optic disc and surrounding retina), or retinal vasculitis (inflammation of the retinal vessels).

RETINITIS

I. *Non-specific retinitis*. It is caused by pyogenic organisms and may be either acute or subacute.

1. *Acute purulent retinitis.* It occurs as metastatic infection in patients with pyaemia. The infection usually involves the surrounding structures and soon converts into metastatic endophthalmitis or even panophthalmitis.
2. *Subacute retinitis of Roth.* It typically occurs in patients suffering from subacute bacterial endocarditis (SABE). It is characterised by multiple superficial retinal haemorrhages, involving posterior part of the fundus. Most of the haemorrhages have a white spot in the centre (Roth's spots). Vision may be blurred due to involvement of the macular region or due to associated papillitis.

II. *Specific retinitis*. It may be bacterial (tuberculosis, leprosy, syphilis and actinomycosis), viral (cytomegalic inclusion disease, rubella, herpes zoster), mycotic, rickettsial or parasitic in origin.

Cytomegalo virus (CMV) retinitis (Fig. 11.5), zoster retinitis, progressive outer retinal necrosis (PORN) caused by an aggressive variant of varicella zoster virus, and acute retinal necrosis (ARN) caused by herpes simplex virus II (in patients under the age of 15 years) and by varicella zoster virus and herpes simplex virus-I (in older individuals) have become more conspicuous in patients with AIDS (HIV infection).

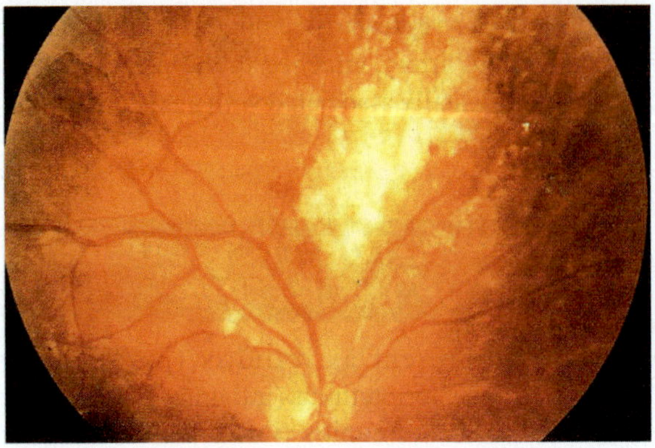

Fig. 11.5. Fundus photograph showing typical cytomegalovirus (CMV) retinitis in a patient with AIDS. Note white necrotic retina associated with retinal haemorrhages.

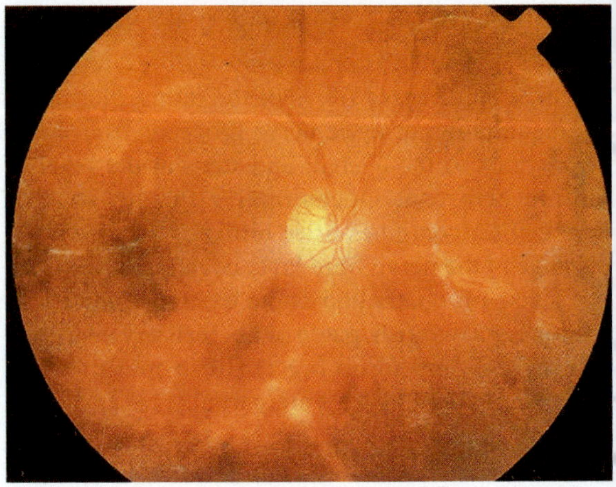

Fig. 11.6. Fundus photograph of a patient with Eales' disease (stage of inflammation). Note venous congestion, perivascular exudates and sheets of haemorrhages present near the affected veins.

RETINAL VASCULITIS

Inflammation of the retinal vessels may be primary (Eales' disease) or secondary to uveitis.

Eales' disease

It is an idiopathic inflammation of the peripheral retinal veins. It is characterised by recurrent vitreous haemorrhage; so also referred to as primary vitreous haemorrhage. The disease is rare in Caucasians but is an important cause of visual morbidity in young Asian males.

Etiology. It is not known exactly. Many workers consider it to be a hypersensitivity reaction to tubercular proteins.

Clinical features. It is a bilateral disease, typically affecting young adult males. The common presenting symptoms are sudden appearance of floaters (black spots) in front of the eye or painless loss of vision due to vitreous haemorrhage. The haemorrhage clears up but recurrences are very common.

Clinical course of the Eales' disease can be described in four stages:

1. *Stage of inflammation* (Fig. 11.6). The affected peripheral veins are congested and perivascular exudates and sheathing are seen along their surface. Superficial haemorrhages ranging from flame-shaped to sheets of haemorrhages may be present near the affected veins.
2. *Stage of ischaemia* is characterized by obliteration of the involved vessels and development of areas of capillary non-perfusion in the periphery as evidenced on fundus fluorescein angiography.
3. *Stage of retinal neovascularization* is marked by development of abnormal fragile vessels at the junction of perfused and non-perfused retina. Bleeding from these vessels leads to recurrent vitreous haemorrhage.
4. *Stage of sequelae* is characterized by development of complications such as proliferative vitreoretinopathy, tractional retinal detachment, rubeosis iridis and neovascular glaucoma.

Treatment of Eales' disease comprises:

1. *Medical treatment*. Course of *oral corticosteroids* for extended periods is the mainstay of treatment during active inflammation. A course of antitubercular therapy has also been recommended in selective cases.
2. *Laser photocoagulation* of the retina either PRP or feeder vessel photocoagulation is indicated in stage of neovascularizion.
3. *Vitreoretinal surgery* is required for nonresolving vitreous haemorrhage and tractional retinal detachment.

VASCULAR DISORDERS OF RETINA

Common vascular disorders of retina include: retinal artery occlusions, retinal vein occlusions, diabetic retinopathy, hypertensive retinopathy, sickle cell retinopathy, retinopathy of prematurity and retinal telangiectasia.

RETINAL ARTERY OCCLUSIONS

Etiology

Occlusive disorders of retinal vessels are more common in patients suffering from hypertension and other cardiovascular diseases. Common causes of retinal artery occlusion are:

- *Atherosclerosis-related thrombosis* at the level of lamina cribrosa is the most common cause (75%) of CRAO.
- *Emboli* from the carotid artery and those of cardiac origin account for about 20% cases of CRAO. Three types of *emboli* are known:
  - *Cholesterol emboli* (Hollenhorst plaque) are refractile and orange and seen at retinal vessel bifurcation. These arise from atheromas in the carotid artery.
  - *Calcium emboli* are white in colour and arise from the cardiac valves.
  - *Platelet fibrin emboli* are dull white in colour and arise from atheromas in the carotid artery. They may cause retinal ischaemic attacks (TIA).
- *Retinal arteritis with obliteration* (associated with giant cell arteritis) and periarteritis (associated with polyarteritis nodosa, systemic lupus erythematosus, Wegner's granulomatosis and scleroderma) are other causes of CRAO.
- *Angiospasm* is a rare cause of retinal artery occlusion. It is commonly associated with amaurosis.
- *Raised intraocular pressure* may occasionally be associated with obstruction of retinal arteries for example due to tight encirclage in retinal detachment surgery.
- *Thrombophilic disorders* such as inherited defects of anticoagulants may occasionally be associated with CRAO in young individuals.
- *Other rare causes* are retinal migrain, sickling haemoglobinopathies and hypercoagulation disorders such as oral contraceptives, polycythemia, and antiphospholipid syndrome.

Clinical features

Clinically retinal artery occlusion may present as central retinal artery occlusion or branch artery occlusion. It is more common in males than females. It is usually unilateral but rarely may be bilateral (1 to 2% cases).

1. *Central retinal artery occlusion (CRAO)*. It occurs due to obstruction at the level of lamina cribrosa.

Symptoms. Patient complains of sudden painless loss of vision occuring over seconds. Patient may give history of transient visual loss (amaurosis fugax) in the past.

Signs of CRAO are as below:

1. *Visual acuity* is markedly reduced except in a few cases with cilioretinal artery supplying the macula (Fig.11.7).
2. *Direct pupillary reflex* is absent, i.e. afferent pupillary defect (APD) is profound and total (amaurotic pupil).
3. *Fundus examination* shows (Fig. 11.7):

- *Marked narrowing of retinal arteries* and mild narrowing of retinal veins.
- *Retina becomes milky white* due to ischaemic odema in eyes with cilioretinal artery part of macula remains normal in colour (Fig 11.7).
- *Cherry red spot* is seen in the center of macula due to vascular choroid shining through the thin retina in foveal region, in contrast to the surrounding pale retina.
- *Cattle tracking*, i.e. segmentation of blood column is seen in the retinal vein.

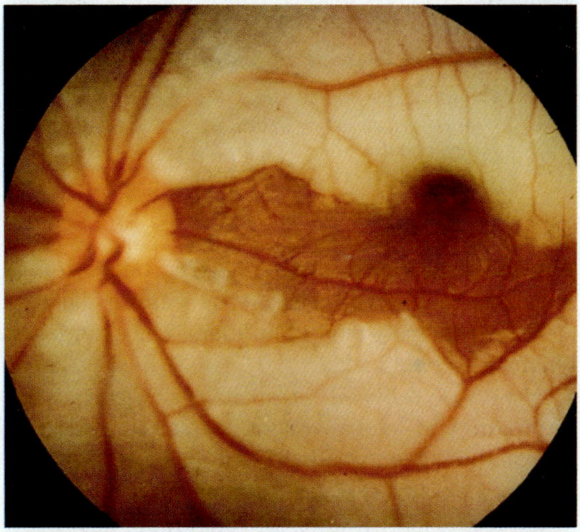

Fig. 11.7. Fundus photograph showing marked retinal pallor in acute central retinal artery occlusion (CRAO) with sparing of the territory supplied by cilioretinal artery.

- *Atrophic changes* in the form of grossly attenuated thread like arteries and consecutive opticatrophy occur in long standing cases (see Fig 12.12B)

4. *Fundus fluorescein angiography* (FFA) shows delay in arterial filing (cilioretinal artery when present will fill in early phase) and masking of choroidal vasculature due to retinal odema.

2. *Branch retinal artery occlusion (BRAO)*. It usually occurs following lodgement of embolus at a bifurcation. Retina distal to occlusion becomes oedematous with narrowed arterioles (Fig. 11.8). Later on the involved area is atrophied leading to permanent sectoral visual field defect.

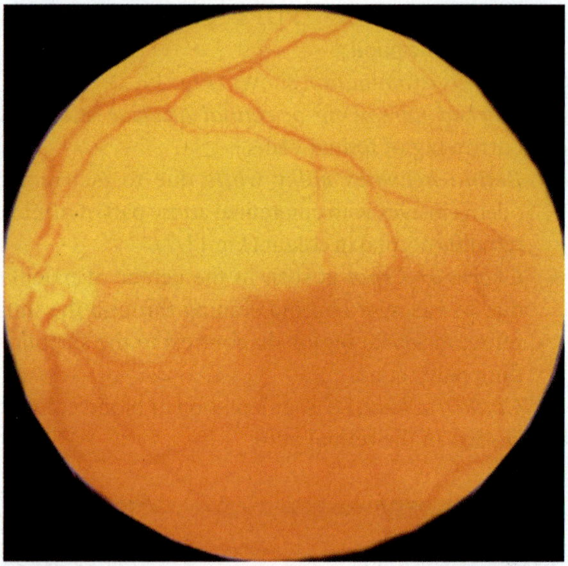

Fig. 11.8. Superotemporal branch retinal artery occlusion (BRAO). Note retinal pallor in superotemporal area and whitish emboli on the optic disc and in superior temporal branch of retinal artery.

Management

Treatment of central retinal artery occlusion is unsatisfactory, as retinal tissue cannot survive ischaemia for more than a few hours. The emergency treatment should include:

1. *Immediate lowering of intraocular pressure* by intermittent ocular massage and intravenous mannitol. It may aid the arterial perfusion and also help in dislodging the embolus. Even paracentesis of anterior chamber has been recommended for this purpose.
2. *Vasodilators and inhalation of a mixture* of 5 percent carbon dioxide and 95 percent oxygen (practically patient should be asked to breathe in a polythene bag) may help by relieving element of angiospasm.
3. *Anterior chamber paracentesis* should be considered.
4. *Intravenous acetazolamide* 500 mg should be given immediately.
5. *Anticoagulants* may be helpful in some cases.
6. *Intravenous steroids* are indicated in patients with giant cell arteritis.

Complications

In some cases 'neovascular glaucoma' with incidence varying from 1% to 5%, may occur as a delayed complication of central retinal artery occlusion.

RETINAL VEIN OCCLUSIONS

Retinal vein occlusions are more common than the artery occlusions. These typically affect elderly patients in sixth or seventh decade of life.

Etiology

1. *Pressure on the vein by an atherosclerotic retinal artery* where the two share a common adventitia (e.g., just behind the lamina cribrosa and at arteriovenous crossings), secondarily induces thrombosis in the lumen of vein.
2. *Hypertension and diabetes mellitus* are common predisposing factors.
3. *Hyperviscosity of blood* as in polycythemia, hyperlipidemia, macroglobulinemia, leukemia, multiple myeloma, cryoglobulinemia.
4. *Periphlebitis retinae* which can be central or peripheral associated with sarcoidosis, syphillis, and SLE.
5. *Raised introcular pressure.* Central retinal vein occlusion is more common in patients with primary open-angle glaucoma.
6. *Local causes* are orbital cellulitis, orbital tumors, facial erysipelas and cavernous sinus thrombosis.

Classification

1. *Central retinal vein occlusion* (CRVO). It may be non-ischaemic CRVO (venous stasis retinopathy) or ischaemic CRVO (haemorrhagic retinopathy).
2. *Branch retinal vein occlusion* (BRVO).

Non-ischaemic CRVO

Non-ischaemic CRVO (venous stasis retinopathy) is the most common clinical variety (75%). It is

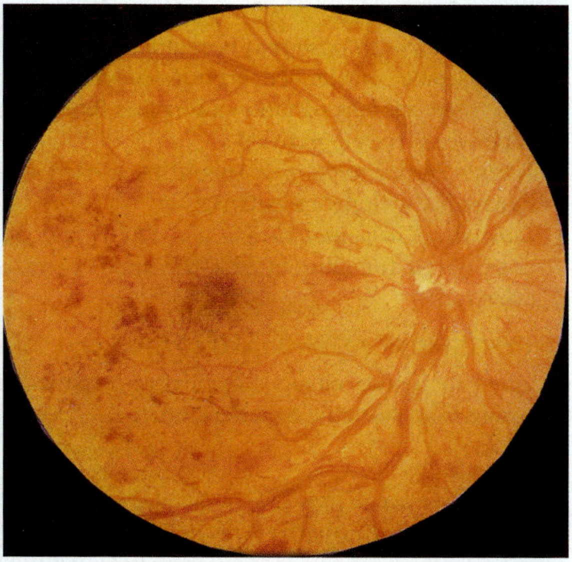

Fig. 11.9. Central retinal vein occlusion (non-ischaemic).

characterised by mild to moderate visual loss and no RAPD.

- *Early cases* on fundus examination (Fig. 11.9) reveal mild venous congestion and tortuosity, a few superficial flame-shaped haemorrhages more in the peripheral than the posterior retina, mild papilloedema and mild or no macular oedema.
- *In late stages* (after 6-9 months), there appears sheathing around the main veins, and a few cilioretinal collaterals around the disc. Retinal haemorrhages are partly absorbed. Macula may show chronic cystoid oedema in moderate cases or may be normal in mild cases.

Treatment is usually not required.

- The condition resolves with almost normal vision in about 50 percent cases.
- Visual loss in rest of the cases is due to chronic cystoid macular oedema, for which intravitreal triamcinolone acetonide may be given with good initial results. However, recurrences are common.
- *Treatment of associations* such as hypertension and others is most important.

Note : About 15% cases of non-ischaemic CRVO are converted to ischaemic CRVO in four months and about 30% in 3 years.

Ischaemic CRVO

Ischaemic CRVO (Haemorrhagic retinopathy) refers to acute (sudden) complete occlusion of central retinal

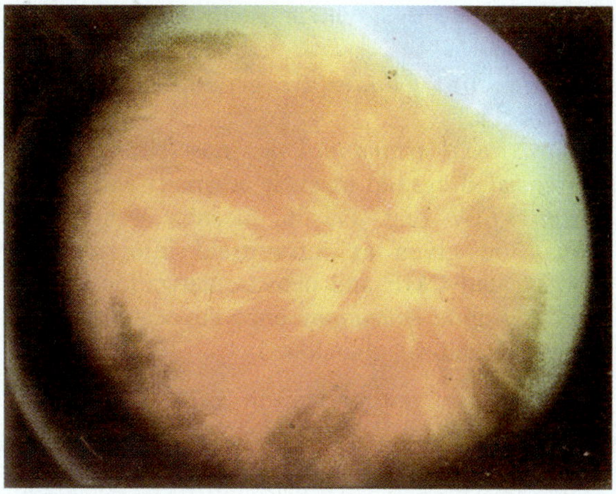

Fig. 11.10. Central retinal vein occlusion (ischaemic).

vein. It is characterised by marked sudden visual loss and RAPD.

- *Early cases* on fundus examination (Fig. 11.10) reveal massive engorgement, congestion and tortuousity of retinal veins, massive retinal haemorrhages (almost whole fundus is full of haemorrhages giving a 'splashed-tomato' appearance), numerous cotton wool spots (usually more than 6 to 10) and disc edema and hyperaemia. Macular area is full of haemorrhages and is severely oedematous.
- In *late stages*, marked sheathing around veins and collaterals is seen around the disc. Neovascularisation may be seen at the disc (NVD) or in the periphery (NVE). *Macula* shows marked pigmentary changes and chronic cystoid oedema.

Pathognomic features for ischaemic CRVO differentiating it from non-ischaemic CRVO are:

- Presence of relative afferent pupillary defect (RAPD),
- Visual field defects, and
- Reduced amplitude of b-wave of electroretinogram.

Complications. Rubeosis iridis and neovascular glaucoma (NVG) occurs in about 20 per cent cases within 3 months (so also called as 90 days glaucoma), A few cases develop vitreous haemorrhage and proliferative retinopathy.

Treatment is as below:

- *Panretinal photocoagulation* (PRP) or cryoapplication, if the media is hazy, may be required to prevent neovascular glaucoma in patients with widespread capillary occlusion. Photocoagulation should be carried out when most of the intraretinal blood is absorbed, which usually takes about 3-4 months.

- *Treatment of under lying conditions* by the physician.
- *Intravitreal triamcinolone* may be given for associated cystoid macular edema (CME).
- *Anti VEGF* (e.g. avastin, lucentis or macugen) may be given as intravitreal injections for associated CME and neovascularization.
- *Radial optic neurotomy* once advocated has lost ground and so abandoned.

Branch retinal vein occlusion (BRVO)

It is more common than the central retinal vein occlusion. It may occur as:

- *Hemispheric occlusion* due to occlusion in the main branch at the disc.
- *Quadrantic occlusion* due to occlusion at the level of A-V crossing, and
- *Small branch occlusion* either as macular branch occlusion or peripheral branch occlusion.

Features of BRVO are as below:

- *Retinal oedema* and *haemorrhages* are limited to the area drained by the affected vein (Fig. 11.11).
- *Vision* is affected only when the macular area is involved.
- *Secondary glaucoma* occurs rarely in these cases.
- *Chronic macular oedema* and neovascularisation may occur as complications of BRVO in about one third cases.

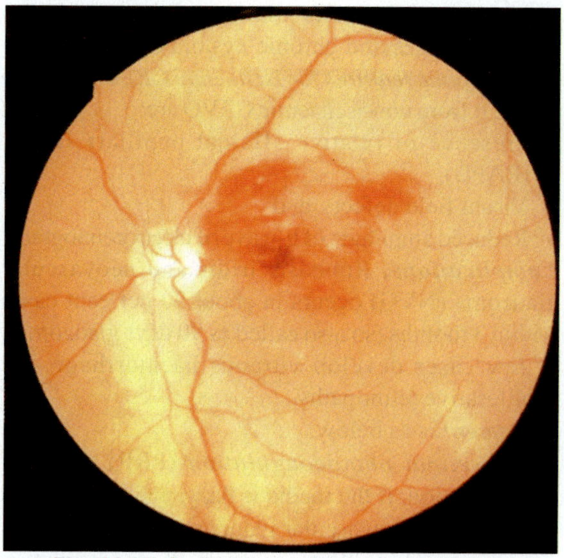

Fig. 11.11. Superotemporal branch retinal vein occlusion (BRVO).

Treatment is as below:

- *Grid photocoagulation* may be required in patients with chronic macular oedema provided the vision after three months of follow up is less than 6/12 and macula is well perfused.
- *Scatter photocoagulation* should be carried out in patients with neovascularisation.
- *Intravitreal trimcinolone* and *anti VEGF* may be considered for associated CME and neovascularization.

HYPERTENSIVE RETINOPATHY

It refers to fundus changes occurring in patients suffering from systemic hypertension.

Pathogenesis

Three factors which play role in the pathogenesis of hypertensive retinopathy are vasoconstriction, arteriosclerosis and increased vascular permeability.

1. *Vasoconstriction.* Primary response of the retinal arterioles to raised blood pressure is narrowing (vasoconstriction) and is related to the *severity of hypertension*. It occurs in the pure form in young individuals, but is affected by the pre-existing involutional sclerosis in older patients.

2. *Arteriosclerotic changes* which manifest as changes in arteriolar reflex and A-V nipping result from thickening of the vessel wall and are a reflection of the *duration of hypertension*. In older patients arteriosclerotic changes may preexist due to involutional sclerosis.

3. *Increased vascular permeability* results from hypoxia and is responsible for haemorrhages, exudates and focal retinal oedema.

Grading of hypertensive retinopathy

Keith and Wegner (1939) have classified hypertensive retinopathy changes into following four grades:

- *Grade I* (Fig. 11.12A). It consists of mild generalized arteriolar attenuation, particularly of small branches, with broadening of the arteriolar light reflex and vein concealment.
- *Grade II* (Fig. 11.12B). It comprises marked generalized narrowing and focal attenuation of arterioles associated with deflection of veins at arteriovenous crossings (Salus' sign).
- *Grade III* (Fig. 11.12C). This consists of Grade II changes plus copper-wiring of arterioles, banking

of veins distal to arteriovenous crossings (Bonnet sign), tapering of veins on either side of the crossings (Gunn sign) and right-angle deflection of veins (Salu's sign). Flame-shaped haemorrhages, cotton-wool spots and hard exudates are also present.

- *Grade IV* (Fig. 11.12D). This consists of all changes of Grade III plus silver-wiring of arterioles and papilloedema.

Clinical types

Clinically, hypertensive retinopathy may occur in four circumstances:

1. *Hypertension with involutionary (senile) sclerosis.* When hypertension occurs in elderly patients (after the age of 50 years) in the presence of involutionary sclerosis the fundus changes comprise augmented arteriosclerotic retinopathy.

2. *Hypertension without sclerosis.* It occurs in young people, where elastic retinal arterioles are exposed to raised blood pressure for a short duration. There are few retinal signs. The arterioles are constricted, pale and straight with acute-angled branching. There are minimal signs of arteriovenous crossing. Occasionally small haemorrhages may be found. Exudates and papilloedema are never seen.

3. *Hypertension with compensatory arteriolar sclerosis.* This condition is seen in young patients with prolonged benign hypertension usually associated with benign nephrosclerosis. The young arterioles respond by proliferative and fibrous changes in the tunica media (compensatory arteriolar sclerosis). Advanced fundus changes in these patients have been described as 'albuminuric or renal retinopathy'.

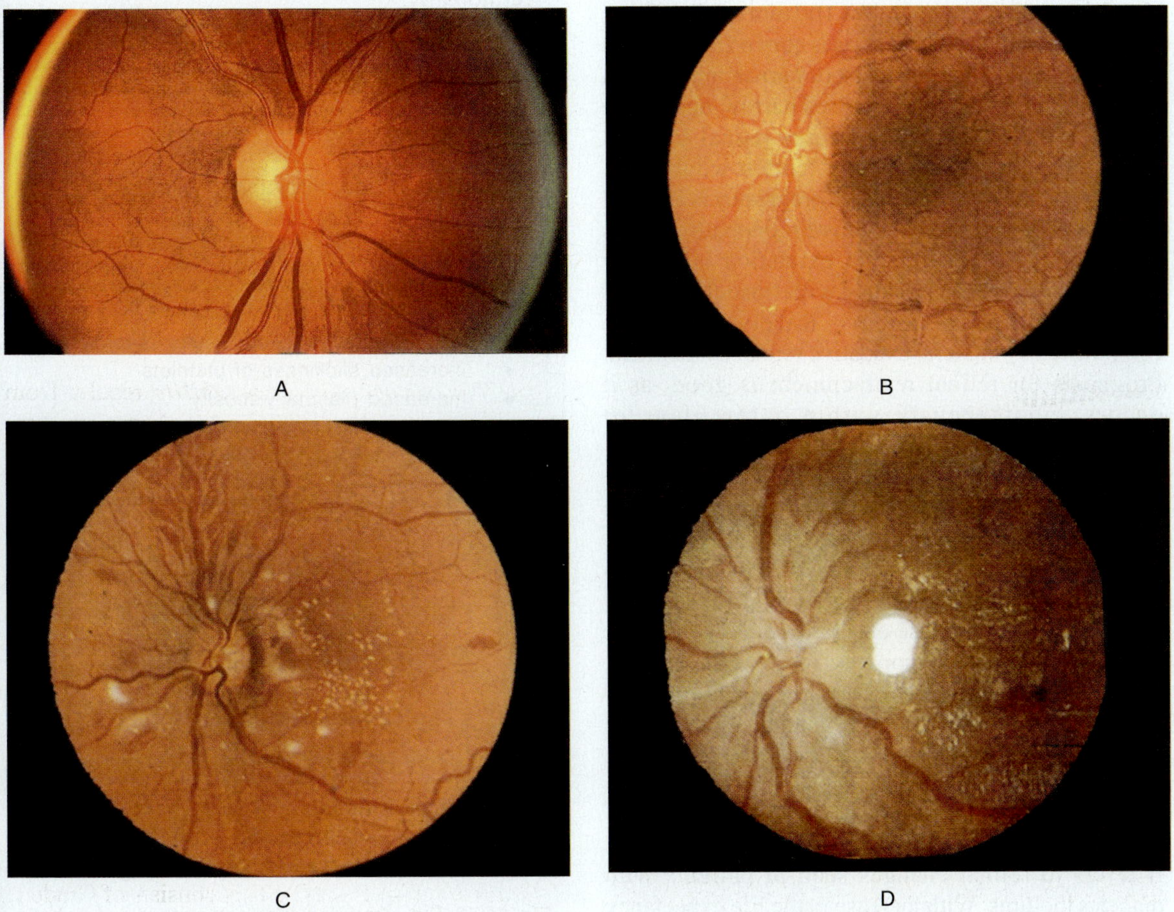

Fig. 11.12. Hypertensive retinopathy: A, grade I, B, grade II, C, grade III; D, grade IV.

4. *Malignant hypertension.* It is not a separate variety of hypertension, but is an expression of its rapid progression to a serious degree in a patient with relatively young arterioles undefended by fibrosis. The fundus picture is characterised by marked arteriolar narrowing, papilloedema (an essential feature of malignant hypertension), retinal oedema over the posterior pole, clusters of superficial flame-shaped haemorrhages and an abundance of cotton wool spots.

RETINOPATHY IN PREGNANCY-INDUCED HYPERTENSION

Pregnancy-induced hypertension (PIH), previously known as 'toxaemia of pregnancy', is a disease of unknown etiology characterised by raised blood pressure, proteinuria and generalised oedema. Retinal changes are liable to occur in this condition when blood pressure rises above 160/100 mm of Hg and are marked when blood pressure rises above 200/130 mm of Hg. Earliest changes consist of narrowing of nasal arterioles, followed by generalised narrowing. Severe persistent spasm of vessels causes retinal hypoxia characterised by appearance of 'cotton wool spots' and superficial haemorrhages. If pregnancy is allowed to continue, further progression of retinopathy occurs rapidly. Retinal oedema and exudation is usually marked and may be associated with 'macular star' or 'flat macular detachment'. Rarely it may be complicated by bilateral exudative retinal detachment. Prognosis for retinal reattachment is good, as it occurs spontaneously within a few days of termination of pregnancy.

Management. Changes of retinopathy are reversible and disappear after the delivery, unless organic vascular disease is established. Therefore, in pre-organic stage when patient responds well to conservative treatment, the pregnancy may justifiably be continued under close observation. However, the advent of hypoxic retinopathy (cotton wool spots, retinal oedema and haemorrhages) should be considered an indication for termination of pregnancy; otherwise, permanent visual loss or even loss of life (of both mother and foetus) may occur.

DIABETIC RETINOPATHY

It refers to retinal changes seen in patients with diabetes mellitus. With increase in the life expectancy of diabetics, the incidence of diabetic retinopathy (DR) has increased. In Western countries, it is the leading cause of blindness.

Etiopathogenesis

Risk factors

1. *Duration of diabetes* is the most important determining factor. Roughly 50 percent of patients develop DR after 10 years, 70 percent after 20 years and 90 percent after 30 years of onset of the disease.
2. *Sex.* Incidence is more in females than males (4:3).
3. *Poor metabolic control* is less important than duration, but is nevertheless relevant to the development and progression of DR.
4. *Heredity.* It is transmitted as a recessive trait without sex linkage. The effect of heredity is more on the proliferative retinopathy.
5. *Pregnancy* may accelerate the changes of diabetic retinopathy.
6. *Hypertension,* when associated, may also accentuate the changes of diabetic retinopathy.
7. *Other risk factors* include smoking, obesity, anaemia and hyperlipidemia.

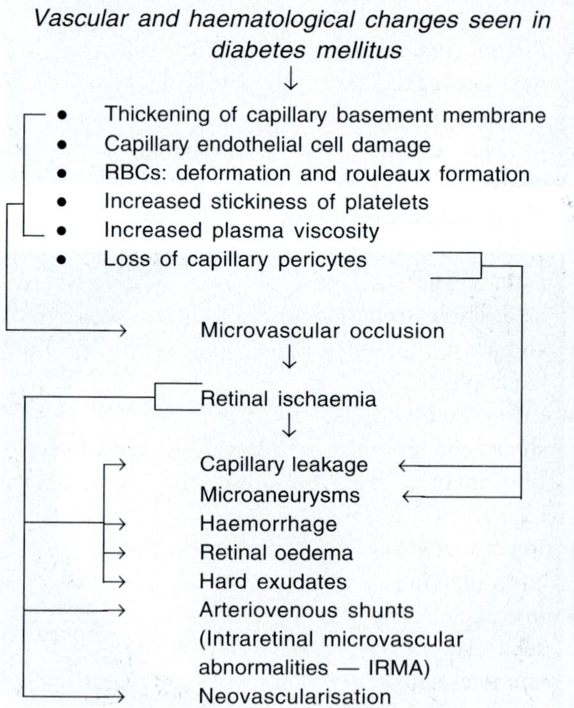

Fig. 11.13. Flowchart depicting pathogenesis of diabetic retinopathy.

Pathogenesis. Essentially, it is a microangiopathy affecting retinal precapillary arterioles, capillaries and venules. The speculative pathogenesis is depicted in the flow-chart (Fig. 11.13).

Classification

Diabetic retinopathy has been variously classified. Presently followed classification is as follows:

I. Non-proliferative diabetic retinopathy (NPDR)
  - Mild NPDR
  - Moderate NPDR
  - Severe NPDR
  - Very severe NPDR

II. Proliferative diabetic retinopathy (PDR)

III. Diabetic maculopathy

IV. Advanced diabetic eye disease (ADED)

I. Non-proliferative diabetic retinopathy (NPDR)

Ophthalmoscopic features of NPDR include:

- *Microaneurysms* are seen in the macular area (the earliest detectable lesion) and elsewhere in relation to area of capillary non-perfusion. These are formed due to focal dilation of capillary wall following loss of pericytes.
- *Retinal haemorrhages*, both deep (dot and blot haemorrhages) and superficial haemorrhages (flame-shaped), occur from capillary leakage.
- *Oedema* characterized by retinal thickening is caused by capillary leakage.
- *Hard exudates*–yellowish-white waxy-looking patches are arranged in clumps or in circinate pattern. These are commonly seen in the macular area. These occur due to chronic localised oedema and are composed of lipoprotein and lipid filled macrophages.
- *Cotton-wool spots*, are small whitish fluffy superficial lesions. These represent areas of nerve fibre infarcts. If cotton-wool spots > 8, there is high risk of developing PDR.
- *Venous abnormalities*, include beading, looping and dilatation.
- *Intraretinal microvascular abnormalities* (IRMA) seen as fine irregular red lines connecting arterioles with venules, represent arteriolar–venular shunts.
- *Dark-blot haemorrhages* representing haemorrhagic retinal infarcts.

ETDRS study classification:

On the basis of severity of the above findings the NPDR has been further classified as under:

1. *Mild NPDR* (Fig. 11.14A).
   - At least one microaneurysm or intraretinal haemorrhage.
   - Hard/soft exudates may or may not be present.
2. *Moderate NPDR* (Fig. 11.14B)
   - Microaneurysms/intraretinal haemorrhage in 2 or 3 quadrants.
   - Early mild IRMA.
   - Hard/soft exudates may or may not present.
3. *Severe NPDR*. Any one of the following (4-2-1 Rule) (Fig. 11.14C):
   - Four quadrants of severe microaneurysms/ intraretinal haemorrhages.
   - Two quadrants of venous beading.
   - One quadrant of IRMA changes.
4. *Very severe NPDR*. Any two of the following (4-2-1 Rule) (Fig. 11.14D):
   - Four quadrants of severe microaneurysms/ intraretinal haemorrhages.
   - Two quadrants of venous beading.
   - One quadrant of IRMA changes.

II. Proliferative diabetic retinopathy (PDR)

Proliferative diabetic retinopathy (Figs. 11.14 E and F) develops in more than 50 percent of cases after about 25 years of the onset of disease. Therefore, it is more common in patients with juvenile onset diabetes. The hallmark of PDR is the occurrence of neovascularisation over the changes of very severe non-proliferative diabetic retinopathy. It is characterised by proliferation of new vessels from the capillaries, in the form of neovascularisation at the optic disc (NVD) and/or elsewhere (NVE) in the fundus, usually along the course of the major temporal retinal vessels. These new vessels may proliferate in the plane of retina or spread into the vitreous as vascular fronds. Later on condensation of connective tissue around the new vessels results in formation of fibrovascular epiretinal membrane. Vitreous detachment and vitreous haemorrhage may occur in this stage.

Types. On the basis of high risk characteristics (HRCs) described by diabetic retinopathy study (DRS) group, the PDR can be further classified as below:

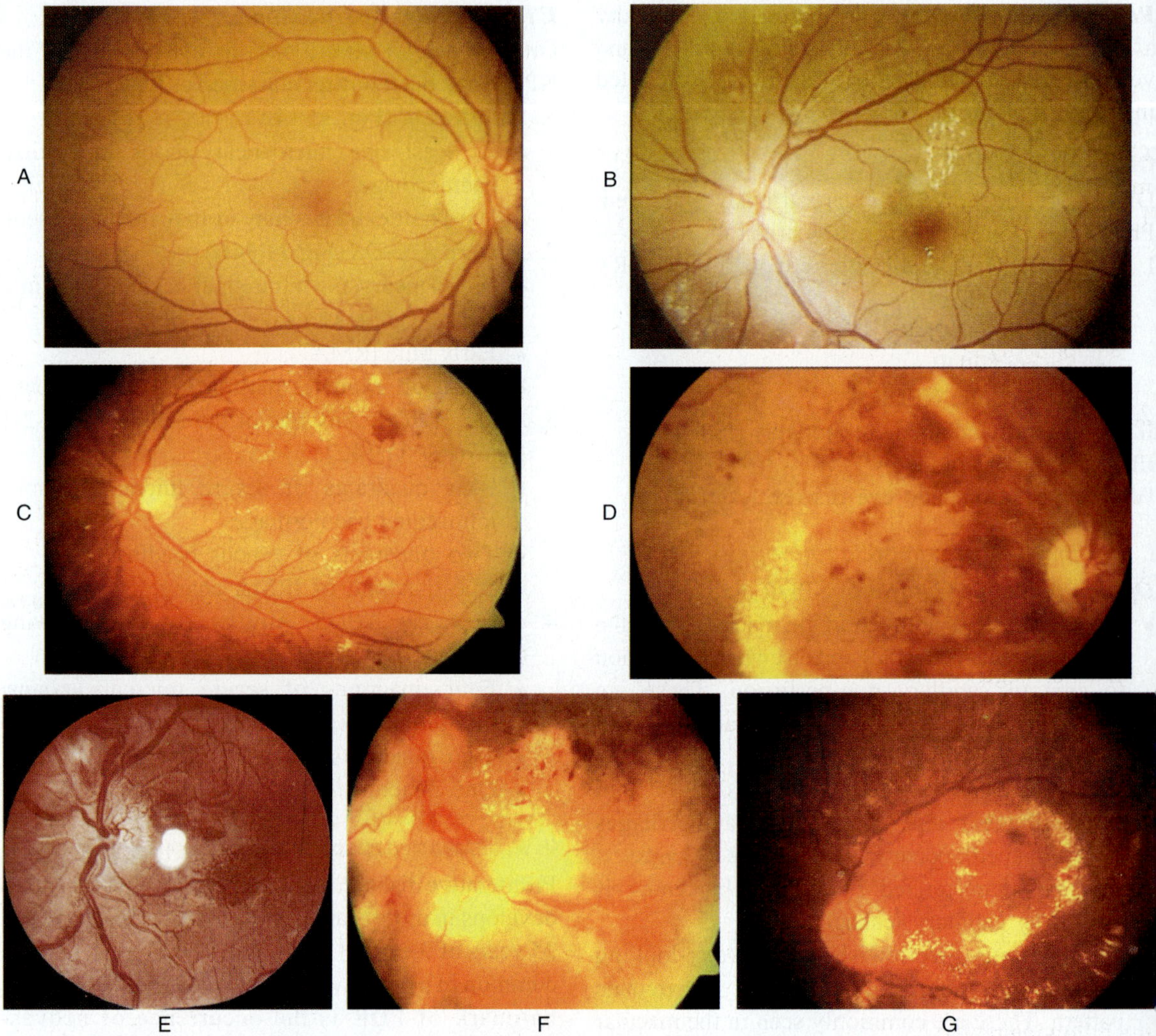

Fig. 11.14. Diabetic retinopathy: A, mild NPDR; B, moderate NPDR; C, severe NPDR; D, very severe NPDR; E, early PDR; F, high risk PDR; G, exudative diabetic maculopathy.

1. *PDR without HRCs (Early PDR)* (Fig. 11.14E), and
2. *PDR with HRCs (Advanced PDR)*. High risk characteristics (HRC) of PDR are as follows (Fig. 11.14F):
   - NVD 1/4 to 1/3 of disc area with or without vitreous haemorrhage (VH) or pre-retinal haemorrhage (PRH)
   - NVD < 1/4 disc area with VH or PRH
   - NVE > 1/2 disc area with VH or PRH

III. *Diabetic maculopathy*

Changes in macular region need special mention, due to their effect on vision. These changes may be associated with non-proliferative diabetic retinopathy (NPDR) or proliferative diabetic retinopathy (PDR). The diabetic macular edema occurs due to increased permeability of the retinal capillaries.

Clinically significant macular edema (CSME) is diagnosed if one of the following three criteria are present on slit-lamp examination with 90D lens:

- *Thickening of the retina* at or within 500 micron of the centre of the fovea.
- *Hard exudates* at or within 500 micron of the centre of fovea associated with adjacent retinal thickening.

- *Development of a zone of retinal thickening* one disc diameter or larger in size, at least a part of which is within one disc diameter of the foveal centre.

Clinico-angiographic classification of diabetic maculopathy is as below:

1. *Focal exudative maculopathy* (Fig. 11.14G). It is characterised by microaneurysms, haemorrhages, macular oedema and hard exudates which are usually arranged in a circinate pattern. Fluorescein angiography reveals focal leakage with adequate macular perfusion.
2. *Diffuse exudative maculopathy.* It is characterised by diffuse retinal oedema and thickening throughout the posterior pole, with relatively few hard exudates. Fluorescein angiography reveals diffuse leakage at the posterior pole.
3. *Ischaemic maculopathy.* It occurs due to microvascular blockage. Clinically it is characterised by marked visual loss with microaneurysms, haemorrhages, mild or no macular oedema and a few hard exudates. Fluorescein angiography shows areas of non-perfusion which in early cases are in the form of enlargement of foveal avascular zone (FAZ), later on areas of capillary dropouts are seen and in advanced cases precapillary arterioles are blocked.
4. *Mixed maculopathy.* In it combined features of ischaemic and exudative maculopathy are present.

OCT classification of diabetic macular oedema. OCT in diabetic macular oedema may show any of the following patterns:

- Sponge like thickening of retinal layers due to accumulation of fluid.
- Large cystoid spaces involving variable depth of retina with intervening septa.
- Serous detachment of retina.
- Tractional detachment of fovea.
- Taut posterior hyaloid membrane.

IV. *Advanced diabetic eye disease*

It is the end result of uncontrolled proliferative diabetic retinopathy. It is marked by complications such as:

- Persistent vitreous haemorrhage,
- Tractional retinal detachment and
- Neovascular glaucoma.

Investigations

- Urine examination,
- Blood sugar estimation.
- 24 hour urinary protein
- Renal function tests
- Lipid profile
- Haemogram
- Glycosylated haemoglobin (HbA1C)
- Fundus fluorescein angiography should be carried out to elucidate areas of neovascularisation, leakage and capillary nonperfusion.
- Optical Coherence Tomography (OCT) to study detailed structural changes in diabetic maculopathy.

Management

I. *Screening for diabetic retinopathy.* To prevent visual loss occurring from diabetic retinopathy a periodic follow-up is very important for a timely intervention. The recommendations for periodic fundus examination are as follows:

- *Every year,* till there is no diabetic retinopathy or there is mild NPDR.
- *Every 6 months,* in moderate NPDR.
- Every 3 months, in severe NPDR.
- Every 2 months, in PDR with no high risk characteristic.

II. *Medical treatment*. Besides laser and surgery to the eyes (as indicated and described below), the medical treatment also plays an essential role. Medical treatment for diabetic retinopathy can be discussed as:

1. *Control of systemic risk factors* is known to influence the occurrence, progression and effect of laser treatment on DR. The systemic risk factors which need attention are:

- Strict metabolic control of blood sugar,
- Control of associated hypertension
- Correction of dyslipidemia
- Control of associated anaemia, and
- Control of associated hypoproteinemia

2. *Role of pharmacological modulation.* Pharmacological inhibition of certain biochemical pathways involved in the pathogenesis of retinal changes in diabetes can be done by:

- Anti-vascular endothelial growth factors (Anti-VEGF) (role is well established) (see page 459)
- Other factors where role is still being evaluated include:

– Protein kinase C (PKC) inhbitors,
– Aldose reductase and ACE inhibitors, and
– Antioxidants such as vitamin E

3. *Role of intravitreal steroids* in reducing diabetic macular oedema is also being recommended by following modes of administration:

- Flucinolone acetonide intravitreal implant, and
- Intravitreal injection of triamcinolone (2 to 4 mg)

III. *Photocoagulation.* It remains the mainstay in the treatment of diabetic retinopathy and maculopathy. Double frequency YAG laser 532 nm is preferred. The protocol of laser application is different for macula and rest of the retina is as follows (Fig. 11.15):

i. Macular photocoagulation. Macula is treated by laser only if there is clinically significant macular oedema (CSME). Laser treatment is contraindicated in ischaemic diabetic maculopathy. In patients with PDR associated with CSME, macular photocoagulation should be considered first i.e., before PRP since the latter may worsen macular oedema. Macular photocoagulation includes two techniques:

- *Focal treatment* (Fig. 11.15A) is carried out for all focal lesions (microaneurysms, IRMA or short capillary segments) 500-3000 microns from the centre of the macula, believed to be leaking and causing CSME. Spot size of 100 μm of 0.1 second duration is used.
- *Grid treatment.* Grid pattern laser burns are applied in the macular area for diffuse diabetic macular oedema (Fig. 11.15B).

ii. Panretinal photocoagulation (PRP) or scatter laser consists of 1200-1600 spots, each 500 μm in size and 0.1 sec. duration. Laser burns are applied outside the temporal arcades and on nasal side one disc diameter from the disc upto the equator. The burns should be one burn width apart (Fig. 11.15C). In PRP inferior quadrant of retina is first coagulated. PRP produces destruction of hypoxic retina which is responsible for the production of vasoformative factors.

Indications for PRP are:

- PDR with HRCs,
- Neovascularization of iris (NVI),
- Severe NPDR associated with:
  – Poor compliance for follow up,
  – Before cataract surgery/YAG capsulotomy,
  – Renal failure,

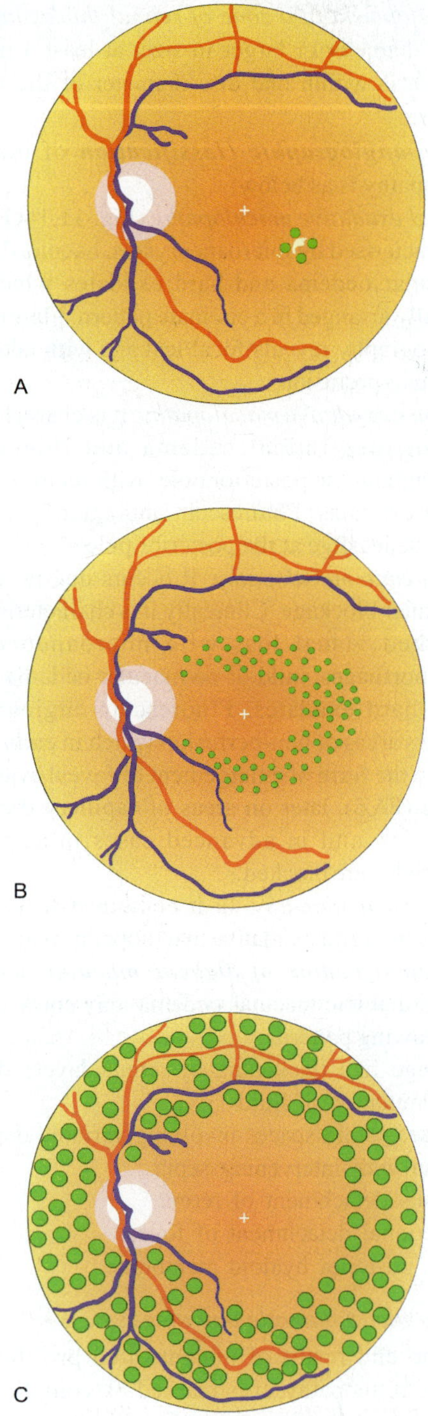

Fig. 11.15. Protocols of laser application in diabetic retinopathy: A, focal treatment; B, grid treatment and; C. panretinal photocoagulation

– One-eyed patient, and
– Pregnancy

IV. ***Surgical treatment.*** It is required in advanced cases of PDR. *Pars plana vitrectomy* is indicated for dense persistent vitreous haemorrhage, tractional retinal detachment, and epiretinal membranes. Associated retinal detachment also needs surgical repair.

SICKLE-CELL RETINOPATHY

Retinal changes in patients suffering from sickle cell haemoglobinopathies (abnormal haemoglobins) are primarily caused by retinal hypoxia; which results from blockage of small blood vessels by the abnormal-shaped rigid red blood cells.

Clinical features

Sickle-cell retinopathy can be divided into five self-explanatory stages as follows:

1. Stage of peripheral arteriolar occlusion and ischaemia.
2. Stage of peripheral arteriovenous anastomoses.
3. Stage of neovascularisation.
4. Stage of vitreous haemorrhage.
5. Stage of vitreoretinal traction bands and tractional retinal detachment.

Treatment

- *Panretinal photocoagulation (PRP)* is effective in regressing the neovascularisation.
- *Pars plana vitrectomy* is required for vitreoretinal tractional bands. It should be followed by repair of the retinal detachment, when present.

RETINOPATHIES OF BLOOD DYSCRASIAS

These are seen in patients suffering from anaemias, leukaemias and polycythemias.

Anaemic retinopathy

In anaemia, retinal changes are liable to occur when haemoglobin level falls by 50 percent and are consistently present when it is below 35 percent (5 gm%). Duration and type of anaemia do not influence the occurrence of retinopathy.

Characteristc features of anaemic retinopathy are as below:

- *Fundus background* becomes pale
- *Retinal arterioles* are also pale
- *Retinal veins* are tortuous and dilated
- *Retinal haemorrhages*, superficial flame shaped and preretinal (subhyaloid) may be seen in the posterior half of fundus
- *Roth spots*, i.e. haemorrhages with white center and
- *Cotton wool spots* may also be seen especially in patients with coexisting thrombocytopenia in aplastic anaemia.

Leukaemic retinopathy

Ocular involvement is more common with acute than chronic leukemia.

Characteristic features of leukaemic retinopathy include:

- *Fundus background* is pale and orangish
- *Retinal veins* are tortuous and dilated
- *Retinal arterioles* become pale and narrow
- *Perivascular leukemic infiltrates*, seen as grayish white lines along the course of veins, are seen in latter stages
- *Roth spots*, i.e. retinal haemorrhages with typical white center are very common
- *Sub hyaloid* i.e. large preretinal haemorrhages may also be seen.

Other ocular changes in leukemia include:

- *Orbital infiltration*, particularly in children presenting as proptosis
- *Ocular haemorrhages* in the form of subconjunctival haemorrhage and hyphaema (bleeding in anterior chamber)
- *Iris changes* in the form of iris thickening and irits
- *Pseudohypopyon*, i.e. collection of white cells in the anterior chamber.

RETINOPATHY OF PREMATURITY

Retinopathy of prematurity (ROP) is a bilateral proliferative retinopathy, occurring in premature infants with low birth weight who often have been exposed to high concentration of oxygen. Earlier this disease was known as *retrolental fibroplasia*.

Etiopathogenesis

Risk factors include:

- Low gestation age, especially < 32 weeks
- Low birth weight (< 1500 g, especially < 1250 g) and
- Supplemental oxygen therapy

Pathogenesis. In the normal development of retina, the vessels reach the nasal periphery after 8 months of gestation and temporal periphery about 1 month after delivery, by the effect of VEGF.

In premature birth, the production of VEGF is downregulated and vessel migration is halted. However, with growing age, because of increased metabolic demands, VEGFs are produced in excess resulting in neovascularization and fibrous proliferation progressively resulting in different stages of retinopathy of prematurity described below.

Clinical features

The condition has been divided into active ROP and cicatricial ROP. Clinically the evolution of the active ROP has been divided into five stages (Fig. 11.16):

***Stage* 1.** It is characterised by formation of a *demarcation line* seen at the edge of vessels, dividing the vascular from the avascular retina.

***Stage* 2.** The line structure of stage 1 acquires a volume to form a *ridge* with height and width.

***Stage* 3.** It is characterised by a *ridge with extra-retinal fibrovascular proliferation* into the vitreous. This stage is further subdivided into mild, moderate and severe, depending on the amount of fibrovascular proliferation.

***Stage* 4a.** It includes *subtotal retinal detachment not involving the macula.* It occurs as a result of exudation from incompetent blood vessels or traction from the fibrous (cicatricial) tissue.

***Stage* 4b.** It includes *subtotal retinal detachment involving the macula.*

***Stage* 5.** It is marked by total retinal detachment which is always funnel-shaped.

Location (zones of involvement) of ROP

The retina is divided into 3 zones. The centre of the retinal map for ROP is the optic disc not the macula as in other retinal charts (Fig. 11.17).

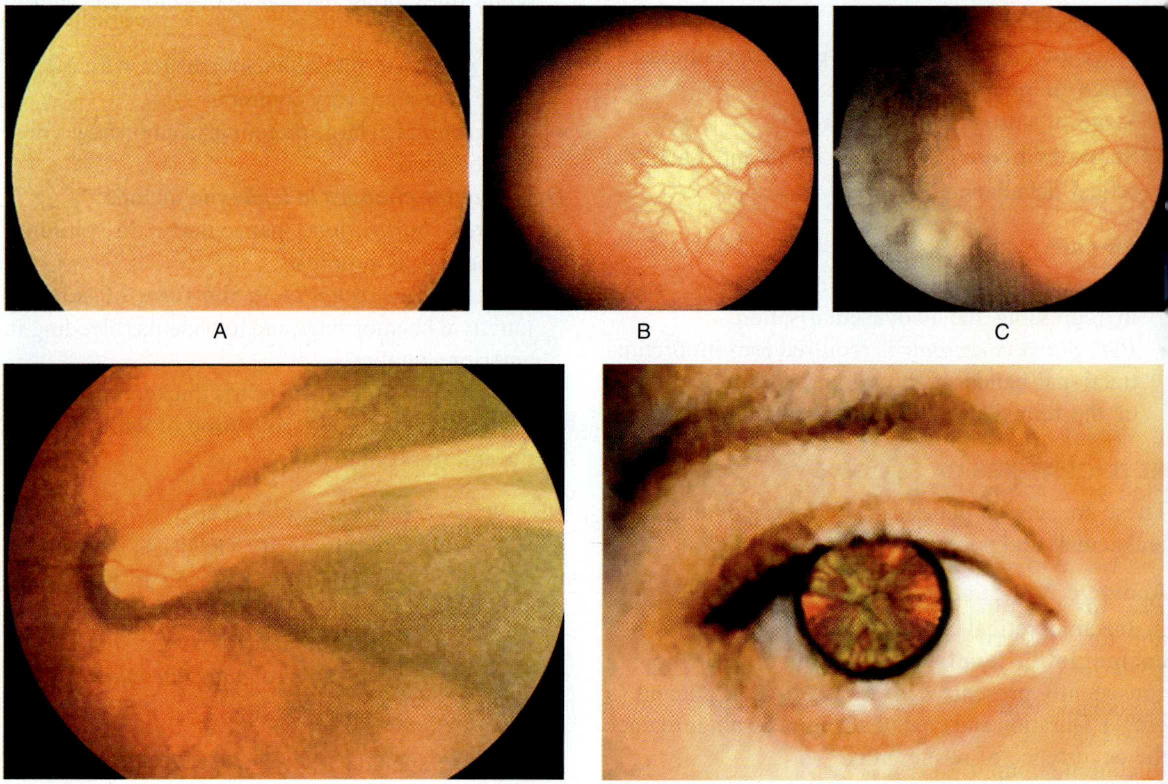

Fig. 11.16. Stages of retinopathy of prematurity (ROP) : A, stage 1. demarcation line; B, stage 2-demarcation ridge; C, stage 3 - extraretinal neovascularization and proliferation; D, stage 4b - subtotal retinal detachment involving macula; E, stage 5 - total retinal detachment.

Zone **I.** A circle drawn on the posterior pole, with the optic disc as the centre and twice the distance from the centre of disc to fovea as the radius, constitutes zone I. Any ROP in this zone is usually very severe because of a large peripheral area of avascular retina.

Zone **II.** A circle is drawn with the optic disc as the centre and the distance from the centre of disc to nasal ora serrata as the radius. The area between zone I and this boundary constitutes zone II.

Zone **III.** The temporal arc of retina left beyond the radius of zone II is zone III.

Extent of involvement

Extent of involvement is denoted by the clock hours of retinal involvement in the particular zone (Fig. 11.17).

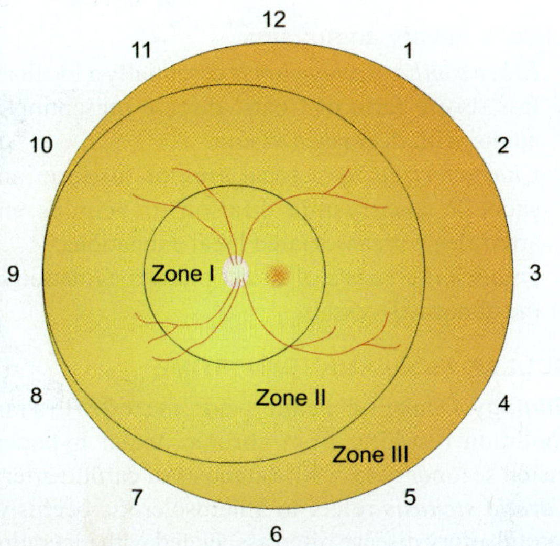

Fig. 11.17. Division of retina into zones (I,II,III) and clock hour positions to depict involvement in retinopathy of prematurity.

Other features

Plus disease refers to presence of engorged veins and tortuous arteries in at least two quadrants at posterior pole with any stage of ROP.

Associated with it is the engorgment and dilatation of iris vessels, which result in poor pharmacological dilatation of pupil. Plus diseases signifies a tendency to progression.

Pre-plus disease is labelled when venous dilation and arterial tortuosity is more than normal but insufficient to be defined as plus disease.

Rush-disease refers to the ROP located in Zone I with plus disease out of proportion to the peripheral retinopathy (since it may progress rapidly to Stage 5 ROP without passing through the other stages).

Prethreshold disease is defined as ROP in:

- Zone I, any stage, or
- Zone II, stage 2 with plus component, or
- Zone II or III, stage 3 with plus component but not reaching threshold clock hours.

Note: Pretheshold ROP needs very close observation as it can rapidly progress to threshold, which needs prompt treatment.

Threshold disease refers to stage 3 ROP with plus disease located in Zone I or II and involving 5 continuous or 8 discontinuous clock hours. This stage needs laser or cryotherapy in less than 72 hours.

Differential diagnosis

- *ROP* needs to be differentiated from familial exudative vitreoretinopathy (FEVR) and incontinentia pigmenti in girls.
- *Advanced retrolental fibroplasia* needs to be differentiated from other causes of *leukocoria* (see page 302).

Screening and management

Treatment of well-established disease is unsatisfactory. *Prophylaxis* is thus very important. To prevent ROP, the premature newborns should not be placed in incubator with an O_2 concentration of more than 30 percent and efforts should be made to avoid infection and attacks of apnoea. Further, a regular screening is very important.

All premature babies born at less than or equal to 32 weeks of gestational age and those weighing 1500g or less (for indian scenario < 1800 gm) should be screened for ROP. The first examination by indirect ophthalmosocpy should be done between 6 and 7 weeks post-natal age or 34 weeks post-conceptual age (whichever is earlier). The further line of action will depend upon the overall status of the eye as below:

I. ***Mature retina*** is labelled when the vessels have reached within one disc diameter of both nasal and temporal ora-serrata. Infants with mature retina does not require further follow-up.

II. *Immature retina* is labelled when the vessels are short of one disc diameter of the nasal or temporal ora but ROP is not developed yet. Such infants require further follow-up weekly.

III. *Retinopathy of prematurity.* When ROP is detected following measures should be taken:

- *Stage* 1 and 2. Since spontaneous regression of disease occurs in 80 to 90% of cases, so only a weekly examination is recommended.
- *Stage* 3, threshold disease should be treated by cryo or laser to prevent progression and to achieve regression.
- *Stage* 4a. Lens sparing vitrectomy is recommended in addition to cryo or laser therapy.
- *Stage* 4b and 5. Vitrectomy needs to be carried out in this stage.

Prognosis is poor in stage 4b and 5.

PRIMARY RETINAL TELANGIECTASIA

Primary Retinal Telangiectasia refer to idiopathic congenital or acquired retinal vascular malformations. Characterized by irregular dilation of capillary bed and segmental dilation of neighboring venules and arterioles. Primary retinal telangiectasia include:

- Idiopathic juxtafoveolar retinal telangiectasia,
- Coats' disease, and
- Leber's miliary aneurysm

Idiopathic juxtafoveolar retinal telangiectasia

This condition, also known as '*idiopathic macular telangiectasia*' is a rare condition presenting with mild decrease in visual acuity due to exudation from the juxtafoeal telangiactc retinal capillaries. This condition has been divided into three groups: 1 (A and B), 2 and 3, depending on the characteristics of lesion.

Coats disease

Coats' disease, also known as exudative retinopathy of Coats, is a severe form of retinal telangiectasia (idiopathic congenital vascular malformation).

Characteristic features of Coats' disease are:

- Typically affects one eye of boys in their first decade of life.
- In early stages it is characterised by large areas of intra and subretinal yellowish exudates and haemorrhages associated with overlying dilated and tortuous retinal blood vessels and a number of small aneurysms near the posterior pole and around the disc.
- It may present with visual loss, strabismus or leukocoria (whitish pupillary reflex) and thus needs to be differentiated from retinoblastoma.
- The condition usually progresses to produce exudative retinal detachment and a retrolental mass.
- In late stages complicated cataract, uveitis and secondary glaucoma occur, which eventually end in phthisis bulbi.
- FFA highlights abnormal vessels, leakage and areas of capillary drop out.

Treatment is as below:

- *Photocoagulation* or *cryotherapy* may check progression of the disease if applied in the early stage.
- However, once the retina is detached the treatment becomes increasingly difficult and success rate declines to 33 percent.

Leber's miliary aneurysms

- *Leber's miliary aneurysm is* essentially a localised less severe form of Coats' disease presenting in adults with decreased vision.
- *Characterized* by a local area of fusiform and saccular aneurysmic dilation of venules and arterioles with associated local exudation.
- *Treatment* consists of direct photocoagulation of the abnormal vessels.

OCULAR ISCHAEMIC SYNDROME

Etiology. Ocular ischaemic syndrome refers to a rare condition resulting from chronic ocular hypoperfusion secondary to > 90% stenosis of carotid artery.

Carotid stenosis refers to atherosclerotic occlusive carotid artery disease often associated with ulceration at the bifurcation of common carotid artery.

Risk factors for carotid stenosis include male gender, old age (60-90 years), smoking, hypertension, diabetes mellitus and hyperlipidaemia.

Manifestations of carotid occlusive disease include:

- Amaurosis fugax (transient retinal ischaemic attack),
- Retinal artery occlusion (due to embolus),
- Transient cerebral ischaemic attacks (TIA),
- Stroke, and
- Ocular ischaemic syndrome

Clinical features. Ocular ischaemic syndrome is usually unilateral (80%), affecting elder males more commonly than females (2:1).

Symptoms include:
- *Loss of vision,* which usually progresses gradually over several weeks or months.
- *Transient black outs* (amaurosis fugax) may be noted by some patients.
- *Pain*—ocular or periorbital may be complained by some patients.
- *Delayed dark adaptation* may be noted by few patients.

Signs include:
- *Cornea* may show oedema and striae.
- *Anterior chamber* may reveal faint aqueous flare with few, if any, cells (ischaemic pseudoiritis).
- *Pupil* may be mid dilated and poorly reacting.
- *Iris* shows rubeosis iridis (in 66% cases) and atrophic patches.
- *Cataract* may occur as a complication in advanced cases.
- *Neovascular glaucoma* is a frequent sequelae to anterior segment neovascularization.
- *Fundus examination* may reveal:
  - *Venous dilatation* with irregular caliber but no or only mild tortuosity.
  - *Retinal arterial* narrowing is present.
  - *Retina shows* midperipheral dot and blot haemorrhages, microaneurysms and cotton wool spots.
  - *Retinal neovascularization* is noted in 37% cases, which may be in the form of NVD and occasionally NVE.
  - *Macular oedema* is a common complication.

Differential diagnosis. Ocular ischaemic syndrome needs to be differentiated from non-ischaemic CRVO, diabetic retinopathy, hypertensive retinopathy and aortic arch disease caused by Takayasu arteritis, aortoarteritis, atherosclerosis and syphilis. (Table 11.1)

Investigations. In suspected cases the carotid stenosis can be confirmed by Doppler ultrasound and magnetic resonance angiography.

Treatment of ocular ischaemic syndrome includes:
- Treatment of neovascular glaucoma (see page 249).
- Treatment of proliferative retinopathy by pan-retinal photocoagulation (PRP) (see page 278).
- Treatment of pseudoiritis with topical steroid eye drops.
- Treatment of carotid stenosis is medical (antiplatelet therapy, oral anticoagulants) and surgical (carotid endarterectomy).

DYSTROPHIES AND DEGENERATIONS OF RETINA

A wide variety of dystrophies and degenerations of the retina have been described and variously classified. These lesions are beyond the scope of this chapter, only a common retinal dystrophy (retinitis pigmentosa), a few peripheral retinal degenerations and some of the vitreoretinal degenerations are described here.

Table 11.1. Differential diagnosis of ocular ischaemic syndrome

Condition	*Similarities*	*Differences*
1. Non-ischaemic CRVO	Unilateral retinal haemorrhages, venous dilatation and cotton wool spots	Veins are more tortuous, haemorrhages are more numerous, normal retinal arteriolar perfusion, disc oedema, and sometimes opticociliary shunt vessels can be seen on the disc
2. Diabetic retinopathy	Microaneurysms, dot and blot haemorrhages, venous dilatation, NVD and NVE, cotton wool spots	Usually bilateral, with characteristic hard exudates
3. Hypertensive retinopathy	Arteriolar narrowing and focal constriction, retinal haemorrhages and cotton wool spots	Usually bilateral, no marked venous changes, and NVD and NVE.
4. Aortic arch disease	Arteriolar narrowing, retinal haemorrhages, cotton wool spots, NVD and NVE	Usually bilateral, absent arm and neck pulses, cold hands, and spasm of arm muscles with excercise.

RETINITIS PIGMENTOSA

This primary pigmentary retinal dystrophy is a hereditary disorder predominantly affecting the rods more than the cones.

Inheritance

Retinitis pigmentosa (RP) may occur as:

1. ***Sporadic disorder***, isolated without family history due to mutation of rhodopsin gene (38%), or

2. ***Inherited disorder*** as below:

- *Autosomal recessive* (AR), most common (25%), intermediate severity
- *Autosomal dominant* (AD), next common (20%), least severe
- *X-linked* (XL), least common (9%), most severe

3. ***Undetermined inheritence*** accounts for 8% of cases.

Prevalence and demography

- *Prevalence.* It occurs in 1 person per 5000 of the world population.
- *Age.* It appears in the childhood and progresses slowly, often resulting in blindness in advanced middle age.
- *Race.* No race is known to be exempt or prone to it.
- *Sex.* Males are more commonly affected than females in a ratio of 3:2.
- *Laterality.* Disease is almost invariably bilateral and both eyes are equally affected.

Clinical features

A. ***Visual symptoms***

1. *Night blindness.* It is the characteristic feature and may present several years before the visible changes in the retina appear. It occurs due to degeneration of the rods.
2. *Dark adaptation.* Light threshold of the peripheral retina is increased; though the process of dark adaptation itself is not affected until very late.
3. *Tubular vision* occurs in advanced cases.

B. ***Fundus changes*** (Fig. 11.18)

1. *Retinal pigmentary changes.* These are typically perivascular and resemble bone corpuscles in shape. Initially, these changes are found in the equatorial region only and later spread both anteriorly and posteriorly.
2. *Retinal arterioles* are attenuated (narrowed) and may become thread-like in late stages.

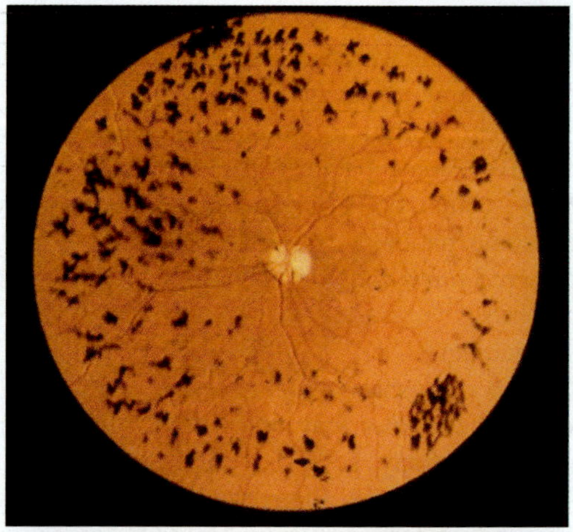

Fig. 11.18. Fundus picture of retinitis pigmentosa.

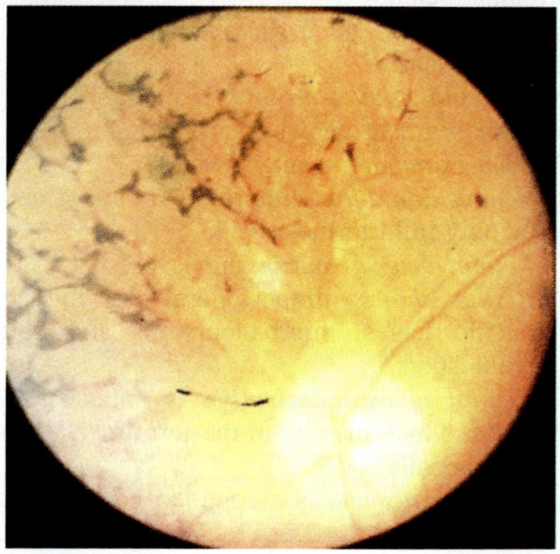

Fig. 11.19. Consecutive optic atrophy in retinitis pigmentosa.

3. *Optic disc* becomes pale and waxy in later stages and ultimately consecutive optic atrophy occurs (Fig. 11.19).
4. *Other associated changes* which may be seen are colloid bodies, choroidal sclerosis, cystoid macular oedema, atrophic or cellophane maculopathy.

C. ***Visual field changes*** (Fig. 11.20)

Annular or ring-shaped scotoma is a typical feature which corresponds to the degenerated equatorial zone of retina. As the disease progresses, scotoma increases anteriorly and posteriorly and ultimately only central vision is left (*tubular vision*). Eventually even this is also lost and the patient becomes blind.

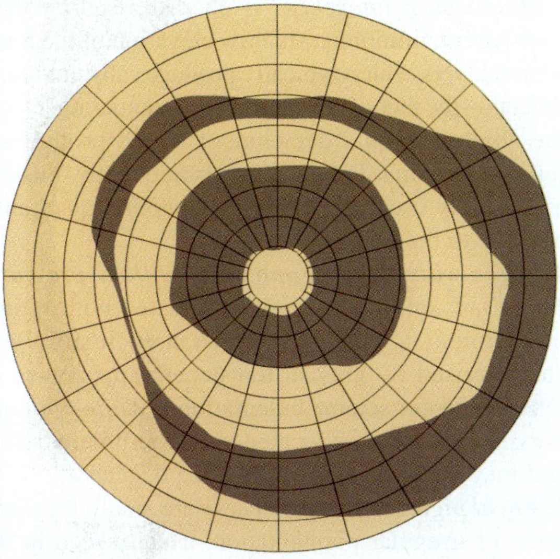

Fig. 11.20. Field changes in retinitis pigmentosa.

D. *Electrophysiological changes*

Typical electrophysiological changes appear early in the disease before the subjective symptoms or the objective signs (fundus changes) appear.

1. *Electro-retinogram* (ERG) is initially subnormal (scotopic affected before photopic; b-wave affected before a wave) and eventually extinguished.
2. *Electro-oculogram* (EOG) is subnormal with an absence of light peak.

Associations of retinitis pigmentosa

I. *Ocular associations*. These include myopia, primary open angle glaucoma, microphthalmos, conical cornea and posterior subcapsular cataract.

II. *Systemic associations*. Most cases of retinitis trigmentose (RP) are isolated (i.e. with no systemic features), but about 25% have associated systemic diseases. A number of specific syndromes are described:

1. *Laurence-Moon-Biedl syndrome.* It is characterised by retinitis pigmentosa, obesity, hypogenitalism, polydactyly and mental deficiency.
2. *Cockayne's syndrome.* It comprises retinitis pigmentosa, progressive infantile deafness, dwarfism, mental retardation, nystagmus and ataxia.
3. *Refsum's syndrome.* It is characterised by retinitis pigmentosa, peripheral neuropathy and cerebellar ataxia.
4. *Usher's syndrome.* It includes retinitis pigmentosa and labyrinthine deafness.
5. *Hallgren's syndrome.* It comprises retinitis pigmentosa, vestibulo-cerebellar ataxia, congenital deafness and mental deficiency.

Atypical forms of retinitis pigmentosa

1. *Retinitis pigmentosa sine pigmento.* It is characterised by all the clinical features of typical retinitis pigmentosa, except that there are no visible pigmentary changes in the fundus.
2. *Sectorial retinitis pigmentosa.* It is characterised by involvement of only one sector of the retina.
3. *Pericentric retinitis pigmentosa.* In this condition all the clinical features are similar to typical retinitis pigmentosa except that pigmentary changes are confined to an area, immediately around the macula.
4. *Retinitis punctata albescens.* It is characterised by the presence of innumerable discrete white dots scattered over the fundus without pigmentary changes. Other features are narrowing of arterioles, night blindness and constriction of visual fields.

Treatment

It is most unsatisfactory; rather we can say that till date there is no effective treatment for the disease.

1. *Measures to stop progression,* which have been tried from time to time, without any breakthrough include: vasodilators, placental extracts, transplantation of rectus muscles into suprachoroidal space, light exclusion therapy, ultrasonic therapy and acupuncture therapy.

   Recently *vitamin A* (15000 IU, PO, qd of palmitate form) has been recommended to check its progression.
2. *Correct any refractive error*, prescribe glasses.
3. *Systemic acetazolamide* (500 mg po) for associated cystoid macular oedema.
4. *Low vision aids (LVA)* in the form of 'magnifying glasses' and 'night vision device' may be of some help.
5. *Rehabilitation* of the patient should be carried out as per his socio-economic background.
6. *Prophylaxis.* Genetic counselling for no consanguinous marriages may help to reduce the

incidence of disease. Further, affected individuals should be advised not to produce children.

PERIPHERAL RETINAL DEGENERATIONS

1. Lattice degeneration. It is the most important degeneration associated with retinal detachment. Its incidence is 6 to 10% in general population and 15 to 20% in myopic patients. It is characterised by white arborizing lines arranged in a lattice pattern along with areas of retinal thinning and abnormal pigmentation (Fig. 11.21A). Small round retinal holes are frequently present in it. The typical lesion is spindle-shaped, located between the ora serrata and the equator with its long axis being circumferentially oriented. It involves more frequently the temporal than the nasal, and is superior than the inferior halves of the fundus.

2. Snail tract degeneration. It is a variant of lattice degeneration in which white lines are replaced by snow-flake areas which give the retina a white frost-like appearance (Fig. 11.21B).

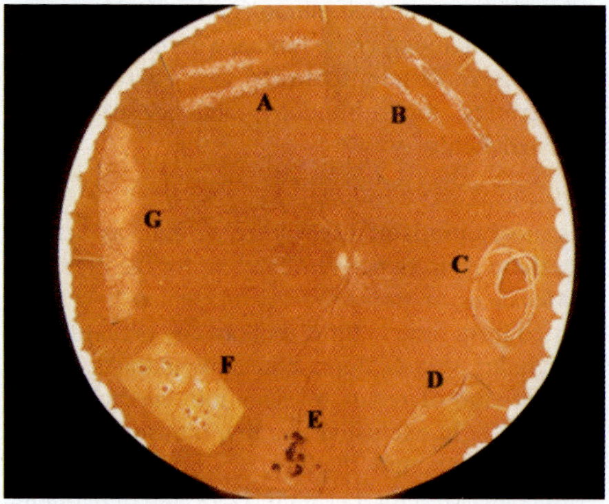

Fig. 11.21. Peripheral retinal degenerations: A, lattice degeneration, B, snail track degeneration: C, acquired retinoschisis; D, white-with-pressure; E, focal pigment clumps; F, diffuse chorioretinal degeneration; and G, peripheral cystoid degeneration.

3. Acquired retinoschisis. The term *retinoschisis* refers to splitting of the sensory retina into two layers at the level of the inner nuclear and outer plexiform layers. It occurs in two forms — the congenital and acquired. The latter, also called as *senile retinoschisis,* may rarely act as predisposing factor for primary retinal detachment.

Acquired retinoschisis is characterised by thin transparent, immobile, shallow elevation of the inner retinal layers which typically produces absolute field defects—the fact which helps in differentiating it from the shallow retinal detachment which produces a relative scotoma. The condition is frequently bilateral and usually involves the lower temporal quadrants anterior to the equator.

4. White-with-pressure and white-without pressure. These are not uncommonly associated with retinal detachment. *'White-with-pressure'* lesions are characterised by greyish translucent appearance of retina seen on scleral indentation. *'White-without-pressure'* lesions are located in the peripheral retina and may be associated with lattice degeneration.

5. Focal pigment clumps. These are small, localised areas of irregular pigmentation, usually seen in the equatorial region. These may be associated with posterior vitreous detachment and/or retinal tear.

6. Diffuse chorioretinal degeneration. It is characterised by diffuse areas of retinal thinning and depigmentation of underlying choroid. It commonly involves equatorial region of highly myopic eyes.

7. Peripheral cystoid retinal degeneration. It is a common degeneration seen in the eyes of old people. It may predispose to retinal detachment in some very old people.

VITREORETINAL DEGENERATIONS

Vitreoretinal degenerations or vitreoretinopathies include:

- Wagner's syndrome,
- Stickler syndrome,
- Favre-Goldmann syndrome,
- Familial exudative vitreoretinopathy,
- Erosive vitreoretinopathy,
- Dominant neovascular inflammatory vitreoretinopathy
- Dominant vitreoretinochoroidopathy.

Note: Characteristic features of some conditions are mentioned here.

Wagner's syndrome

Wagner's syndrome has an autosomal dominant (AD) inheritance with following features:

- *Vitreous* is liquified with condensed membranes.
- *Retina* shows narrow and sheathed vessels, and pigmented spots in the periphery.

- *Choroid* may be atrophied.
- *Cataract* may develop as late complication.

Stickler syndrome

Stickler syndrome, also known as *hereditary arthro-ophthalmopathy,* is an autosomal dominant connective tissue disorder characterized by following features:

Ocular features

- *Vitreous* is liquified and shows syneresis giving appearance of an optically-empty vitreous cavity.
- *Progressive myopia* is very common.
- *Radial lattice like degeneration* associated with pigmentary changes and vascular sheathing.
- *Bilateral retinal detachment* may occur in 30% cases (commonest inherited cause of retinal detachment in children).
- *Ectopia lentis* is occasionally associated.
- *Pre-senile cataract* occurs in 50% cases.

Orofacial abnormalities include flattered nasal bridge, maxillary hypoplasia, cleft palate and high arched palate.

Arthropathy is characterized by stiff, painful, prominent and hyperextensible large joints.

Other features include deafness and mitral valve prolapse.

Favre-Goldmann syndrome

It is an autosomal recessive condition presenting in childhood with nyctalopia. Characteristic features are:

- *Vitreous* shows syneresis but the cavity is not optically empty.
- *Retinoschisis,* both central (affecting macula) and peripheral, is present, although macular findings are more subtle.
- *Pigmentary changes* similar to retinitis pigmentosa are marked
- *ERG* is subnormal.

MACULAR DISORDERS

Macula, being concerned with vision, has attracted the attention of many retina specialists. Consequently, many disorders have been defined and variously classified. A simple, *etiological classification* for a broad overview of the macular lesions is as follows:

A. *Congenital anomalies.* These include aplasia, hypoplasia and coloboma.

B. *Hereditary dystrophies.* These include Best's disease, Stargardt's disease, butterfly-shaped dystrophy, bull's eye dystrophy and central areolar dystrophy.

C. *Acquired maculopathies* include:

1. *Traumatic lesions.* These include traumatic macular oedema, traumatic macular degeneration, macular haemorrhage and macular hole (see page 434).
2. *Inflammations* i.e., central chorioretinitis (see page 158).
3. *Solar retinopathy* i.e., photoretinitis.
4. *Degenerations.* Important conditions are age related macular degeneration (ARMD), and myopic degeneration.
5. *Metabolic disorders* include: diabetic maculopathy and sphingolipidosis.
6. *Toxic maculopathies.* These are chloroquine and phenothiazine-induced maculopathy.
7. *Miscellaneous acquired maculopathies.* A few common conditions are:

- Central serous chorio retinopathy (CSCR),
- Cystoid macular oedema (CME),
- Macular hole,
- Macular epiretinal membrane,
- Vitreomacular traction syndrome, and
- Idiopathic choroidal neovascularisation.

Note: Only a few macular disorders are described.

SOLAR RETINOPATHY

Solar retinopathy also known as *photoretinitis*, or *eclipse retinopathy*, refers to retinal injury induced by direct or indirect sun viewing. Solar retinopathy is associated with religious sun gazing, solar eclipse observing, telescopic solar viewing, sun bathing and sun watching in psychiatric disorders.

Causes of photic retinopathy, other than solar retinopathy, are:

- Welding arc exposure,
- Lightening retinopathy, and
- Retinal phototoxicity from ophthalmic instruments like operating microscope.

Pathogenesis

Solar radiations damage the retina through:

- *Photochemical effects* produced by UV and visible blue light, and
- *Thermal effects* may enhance the photochemical effects. The long visible wavelength and infra-red rays from the sun are absorbed by the pigment epithelium producing a thermal effect. Therefore, severity of lesion varies directly with the degree of pigmentation of the fundus, duration of exposure and the climatic conditions during exposure.

Clinical features

Symptoms. These include persistence of negative after-image of the sun, progressing later into a positive scotoma and metamorphopsia. Unilateral or bilateral decreased vision (6/12–6/60) which develops within 1 to 4 hours after solar exposure, usually improves to 6/6 –6/12 within six months.

Signs. Initially the fundus may appear normal. Shortly after exposure a small yellow spot with gray margin may be noted in the foveolar and parafoveolar region. The typical lesion, which appears later, consists of a central burnt-out hole in the pigment epithelium surrounded by aggregation of mottled pigment. Ophthalmoscopically, it appears as a bean-or kidney-shaped pigmented spot with yellowish white centre in the foveal region. In worst cases, typical macular hole may appear.

Treatment

There is no effective treatment for photoretinitis, so emphasis should be on prevention. Eclipse viewing should be discouraged unless there is proper use of protective eye wear filters (which absorb UV and infrared wave lengths).

Prognosis is guarded, since some scotoma and loss in visual acuity by one or two lines mostly persists.

CENTRAL SEROUS CHORIO RETINOPATHY

Central serous chorio retinopathy (CSCR) is characterised by spontaneous serous detachment of neurosensory retina in the macular region, with or without retinal pigment epithelium detachment.

Etiopathogenesis

Risk factors include:

- *Age and sex.* The disease affects typically young adult (20-50 yrs), males more than females,
- *Personality.* Type A personality individuals are more prone,
- *Emotional stress*,
- *Steroid* intake,
- *Hypertension*,
- *Pregnancy* (usually 3rd trimester), and
- *Cushing's disease*.

Pathogenesis is not known exactly. It is now believed that an increase in choroidal hyperpermeability causes a breach in the outer blood retinal barrier (a small opening or blow out of RPE). Leakage of fluid across this area results in development of localized serous detachment of neurosensory retina. What triggers the choroidal hyperpermeability is poorly understood. It is being suggested that an imbalance between the sympathetic parasympathetic drive that maintains autoregulation within the choroidal vasculature may be defective in patients with CSR.

Clinical features

Symptoms. Patient presents with a sudden onset of painless loss of vision (6/9-6/24) associated with relative positive scotoma, micropsia and metamorphopsia.

Signs. Ophthalmoscopic examination reveals:

- *Mild elevation of macular area*, demarcated by a circular ring-reflex.
- *Small yellow-grey elevations* may be seen due to RPE detachment.
- *Foveal reflex* is absent or distorted (Fig. 11.22).

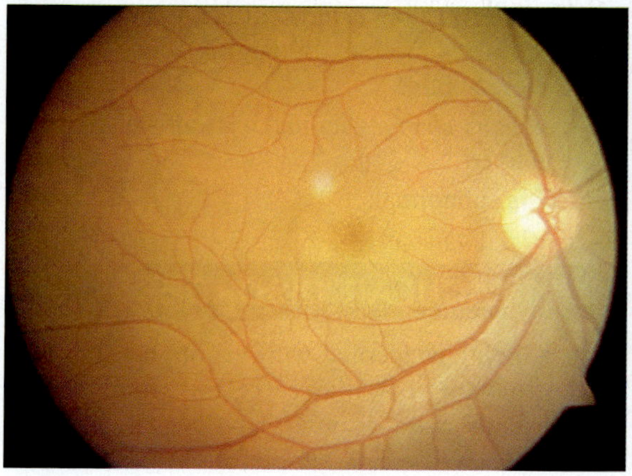

Fig. 11.22. Fundus photograph showing central serous retinopathy.

- *Multi-focal* pigmentary changes suggest chronicity.

Clinical course

CSR is usually self limiting but often recurrent. Three patterns are known:

- *Short clinical course* is characterized by spontaneous resolution within 3-6 months with near normal visual recovery. Recurrences are known in 30–50 % of all the cases.
- *Prolonged clinical course* (occurring in some patients) is labeled when resolution occurs between 6 to 12 months with persistent mild visual discomfort.
- *Chronic clinical course*, seen in very few cases (especially those above 50 yrs) is labeled when resolution occurs after 12 months. Such cases are characterized by permanent visual impairment due to progressive RPE changes.

Investigations

1. ***Fundus fluorescein angiography*** helps in confirming the diagnosis. Two patterns of progressive leakage and pooling from one or more points seen are:

- *Ink-blot pattern.* It consists of small hyperfluorescent spot which gradually increases in size (Fig. 11.23A).
- *Smoke-stack pattern.* It consists of a small hyperfluorescent spot which ascends vertically like a smoke-stack and gradually spreads laterally to take a mushroom or umbrella configuration (Fig. 11.23B).

2. ***ICG*** shows multiple areas of hyperfluorescence due to choroidal hyperpermeability.

3. ***OCT*** shows neuro sensory retinal detachment and accompanying small detachments of the RPE. (Fig. 11.23C)

Differential Diagnosis

Differential diagnosis of CSR includes other entities which may produce serous detachment of sensory retina in macular area. These include optic pit, idiopathic polypoidal choroidal vasculopathy, macular hole with serous detachment, choroidal tumors and pigment epithelial defect (PED).

Treatment

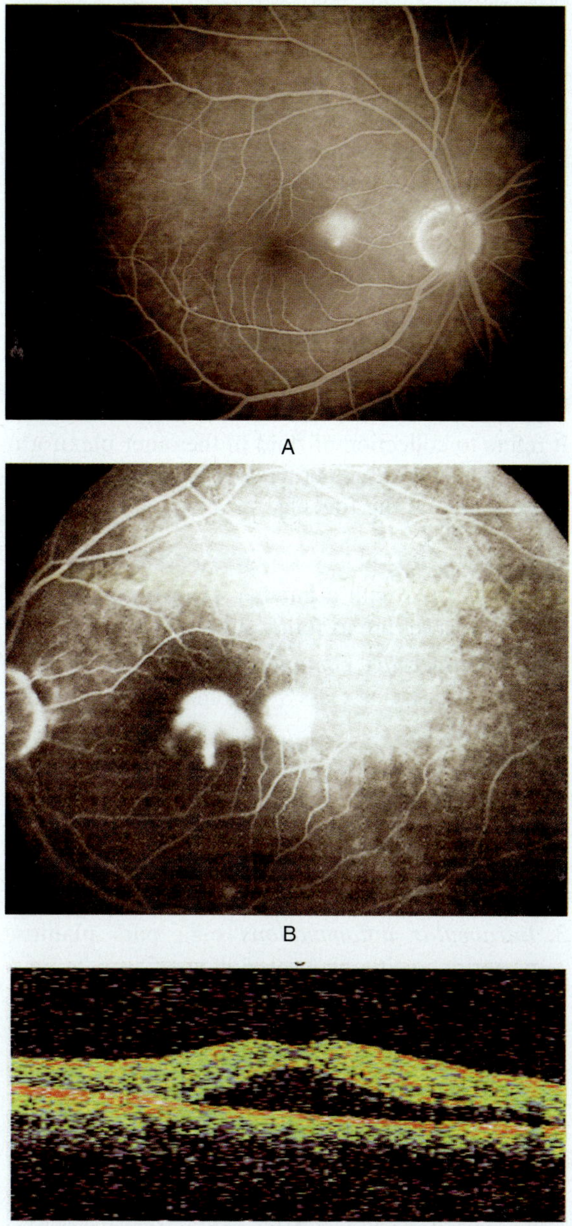

Fig. 11.23. Fundus fluorescein angiogram showing ink-blot pattern (A) and smoke-stack pattern (B) of hyperfluorescence in central serous retinopathy and (C) OCT picture of CSR

1. *Reassurance* is the only treatment required in majority of the cases, since CSR undergoes spontaneous resolution in 80 to 90 percent cases. Visual acuity returns to normal or near normal within 3 to 6 months.
2. *Laser photocoagulation* is indicated in following cases:

- Long-standing cases (more than 6 months).
- Patients having recurrent CSR with visual loss.
- Patients having permanent loss of vision in the other eye due to this condition.

  Contraindications include the cases having leak near or within the FAZ.

3. *Photodynamic therapy* (PDT) may be beneficial for those with severe disease not amenable to conventional laser treatment, e.g. with sub foveal leaks and chronic cases.
4. *Anti VEGF* can be considered if CNV develops.

CYSTOID MACULAR EDEMA (CME)

It refers to collection of fluid in the outer plexiform (Henle's layer) and inner nuclear layer of the retina, centred around the foveola.

Etiology

It is associated with a number of disorders. A few common causes are as follows:

1. *As postoperative complication* following cataract extraction (Irvine-Gass Syndrome) and penetrating keratoplasty.
2. *Retinal vascular disorders* e.g., diabetic retinopathy and central retinal vein occlusion (CRVO), branch retinal vein occlusion (BRVO), retinal telangiectasia (e.g. Coats' disease), periphlebitis retinae (Eales disease), and hypertensive retinopathy.
3. *Intraocular inflammations* e.g., pars planitis, posterior uveitis and anterior uveitis.
4. *Side-effect of topical drops* e.g., epinephrine, dipivefrine and prostaglandin analogues, especially in patients who have undergone cataract surgery.
5. *Retinal dystrophies* e.g., retinitis pigmentosa.
6. *Vitreo macular traction*
7. *Miscellaneous causes* include: macular epiretinal membrane (ERM), intraocular tumors, choroidal neovascularization (CNV) and collagen vascular diseases.

Pathogenesis

CME develops due to leakage of fluid following breakdown of inner blood-retinal barrier (i.e., leakage from the retinal capillaries).

Clinical features

1. *Visual loss.* Initially there is minimal to moderate loss of vision, unassociated with other symptoms. If oedema persists, there may occur permanent decrease in vision.
2. *Ophthalmoscopy* reveals loss of foveal contour, retinal thickening, a yellow spot at the center of fovea and in clinically established cases a typical '*Honey-comb appearance*' of macula (due to multiple cystoid oval spaces) (Fig. 11.24). CME is best examined with a fundus contact lens on slit-lamp or +90D lens. Associated features depend on the underlying cause, e.g. CRVO etc.

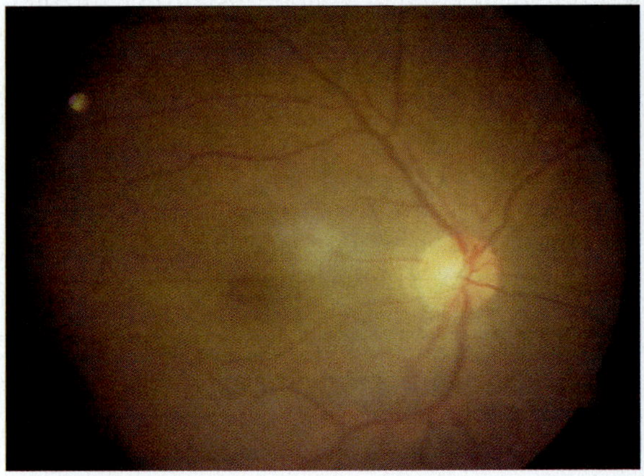

Fig. 11.24. Fundus photograph showing honey-comb appearance in cystoid macular edema (CME).

3. *Fundus fluorescein angiography* demonstrates leakage and accumulation of dye in the macular region which in a well-established case presents a '*flower petal appearance*' in late frames (Fig. 11.25A).
4. *Optical Coherence Tomography* (OCT) reveals loss of foveal depression, intraretinal area of decreased reflectivity with round optically clear regions (cystoid spaces) and over all retinal thicknening (Fig. 11.25 B). Detection rate on OCT is similar to FFA. It can also detect associated specific pathology e.g. vitreomacular traction.

Complications

Long-standing CME may end in lamellar macular hole.

Treatment

1. *Treatment of the causative factor,* e.g., photocoagulation for diabetic CSME; cessation of causative topical 2% adrenaline eye drops and so on.
2. *Topical antiprostaglandin* (NSAID) drops like ketorolac, diclofenac or profenac when used pre and post-operatively, prevent the occurrence of

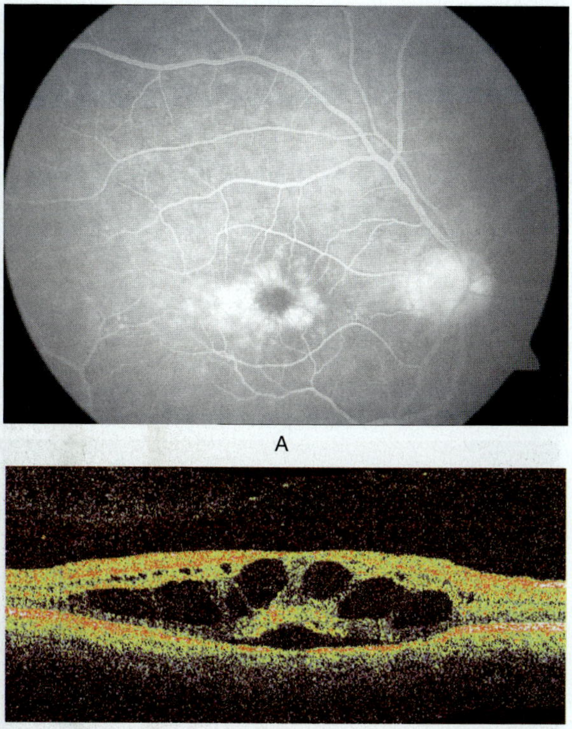

Fig. 11.25. Cystoid macular oedema: A, Fundus fluorescein angiogram showing flower petal appearance and B, OCT pictures showing cystoid spaces

CME associated with intraocular surgery these are also useful in the treatment of most CMEs when given for 3 to 4 months.

3. *Topical and systemic steroids* may be of some use in established cases.
4. *Systemic carbonic anhydrase inhibitors (CAIs)* e.g., oral acetazolamide may be beneficial in some cases of CME e.g. in retinitis pigmentosa.

AGE-RELATED MACULAR DEGENERATION

Age-related macular degeneration (ARMD), also called *senile macular degeneration,* is a bilateral disease of persons over 50 years of age. It is a leading cause of blindness in developed countries, in population above the age of 65 years. It is of two types non-exudative and exudative.

Etiopathogenesis

ARMD is an age-related disease of worldwide prevalence. Certain *risk factors* which may affect the age of onset and/or progression include heredity, nutrition, smoking, hypertension, exposure to sun light, hyperopia, blue eyes and cataract particularly nuclear opacity. The disease is most prevalent in Caucasians.

Clinical types

1. *Non-exudative or atrophic ARMD.* It is also called *dry* or *geographic ARMD* and is responsible for 90 percent cases.

Symptoms. It typically causes mild to moderate, gradual loss of vision. Patients may complain of distorted vision and difficulty in reading due to central shadowing.

Signs. Ophthalmoscopically, lesions of non exudative ARMD can be described as below (Fig. 11.26A):

- *Early cases* are characterized by occurrence of macular drusens, focal hyperpigmentation and pale area of retinal pigment atrophy (RPE atrophy). Macular drusens are well defined, yellowish white, slightly elevated spots. In early cases less than 20 small to medium sized drusens are seen.
- *Intermediate cases* show sharply circumscribed circular areas of RPE atrophy with variable loss of choriocapilaries along with drusens (1 large drusen > 125 μm and/or > 20 medium drusens (60-125 μm)). Large drusens are soft drusens with less sharply defined edges, tend to enlarge or coalesce.
- *Advanced cases* show enlargement of atrophic areas within which the larger choroidal vessels may become visible and pre existing drusen disappear (*Geographical atrophy*).

2. *Exudative ARMD.* It is also called *wet* or *neovascular ARMD*. It is responsible for only 10 percent cases of ARMD but is associated with comparatively rapidly progressive marked loss of vision.

Typical lesions of exudative ARMD seen in chronological order are as below:

- *Drusens with retinal pigment epithelial detachment* (PED) seen as sharply circumscribed dome shaped elevation.
- *Choroidal Neovascularization* (CNV) proliferating in sub RPE space (Type 1) is seen as grayish green or pinkish yellow raised lesion (Fig 11.26B). The CNV proliferating in sub retinal space (type 2) is seen as sub retinal halo or pigment plaque.

- *Haemorrhagic pigment epithelial detachment* (PED). It appears as dark elevated mount.
- *Haemorrhagic detachment of neurosensory retina* which assumes diffuse outline and a lighter red colour around and adjacent to the PED.
- *Disciform sub retinal scarring* in the macular region may result from gradual organization of blood with further fibrovascular ingrowth.

Early versus late ARMD

Early ARMD includes drusens, and areas of RPE hyperpigmentation and/or depigmentation.

Late ARMD includes geographic atrophy of RPE with visible underlying choroidal vessels, pigment epithelium detachment (PED) with or without neurosensory retinal detachment, subretinal or sub-RPE neovascularization, haemorrhage and disciform scars.

Diagnosis

Clinical diagnosis is made from the typical signs described above, which are best elucidated on examination of the macula by slit-lamp biomicroscopy with a +90D/+78D non-contact lens or Mainster contact lens.

Fundus fluorescein angiography and ***indocyanine green angiography*** help in detecting choroidal neovascularization (CNV) in relation to foveal avascular zone. CNV may be classical or occult:

- *Classical CNVM* is seen as lacy hyperfluorescence with progressive leakage (Fig. 11.26 C). It may be subfoveal, juxtafoveal or extrafoveal in location.
- *Occult CNVM* is seen as stippled hyperfluorescence (Type I) or as late leakage of undetermined source. (Type II).

Optical coherence tomography **(OCT)** reveals sub-retinal fluid, intraretinal thickening and choroidal neovascularization and haemorrages in exudative ARMD (Fig. 11.26 D).

Treatment

Non-exudative ARMD. There is no effective treatment. Measures to be tried include:

- *Dietary supplements and antioxidants.* The age-related eye disease study (AREDS) has suggested that use of certain specific antioxidants, vitamins and minerals (vitamin C and E, beta carotene, zinc

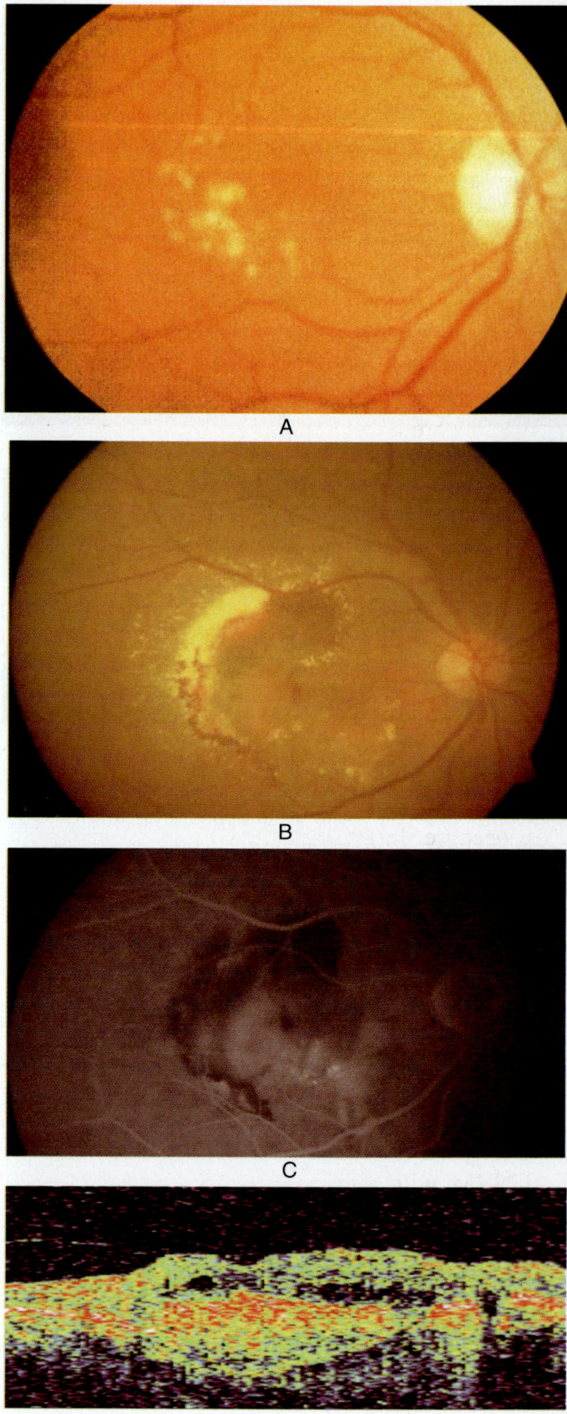

Fig. 11.26. Age-related macular degeneration: A, nonexudative; B, exudative; C, FFA showing leakage and lacy pattern in CNVM; D, OCT picture of CNVM.

and copper) could possibly prevent or delay the progression of ARMD.

- *Smoking cessation* may slow down the progress.
- *Amsler grid* used regular allows the patients to detect new or progressive metamorphopsia prompting them to seek ophthalmic advice.
- *Refraction* with increased near add maybe helpful in early cases.
- *Low vision aid* may be needed in advance cases.

Treatment modalities available for exudative (neovascular) ARMD are:

- *Intravitreal anti-VEGF therapy* has become the treatment of first choice for all CNV lesions Anti-VEGFs are injected intravitreally. These include:
  - Bevacizumab (Avastin), dose: 1.25 mg, or
  - Ranibizumab (Lucentis), dose: 0.5 mg/0.05 ml, or
  - Pegaptanib (Macugen), dose: 0.3 mg in 90 µl (For detail see page 459).

  Results of anti-VEGF are encouraging in the sense that they improve the vision in 30-40% of cases and stabilize the vision in rest of the cases. However, the effect is short lasting and repeated injections are required at an interval of 1-3 months.

  Note: Although anti-VEGF therapy is the preferred strategy for the treatment of CNV, some patients may choose not to undergo an intravitreal procedure. In these cases, options include PDT, TPT, argon laser photocoagulation.
- *Photodynamic therapy (PDT)* is the treatment of choice after anti-VEGF injections for subfoveal and juxtafoveal classic CNVM. In PDT, vertiporfin, a photosensitizer or light activated dye is injected intravenously. The area of CNVM is then exposed to light from a diode laser source at a wavelength (689 nm) that corresponds to absorption peak of the dye. The light-activated dye then causes disruption of cellular structures and occlusion of CNVM with minimum damage to the adjacent RPE, photoreceptors and capillaries.
- *Transpupillary thermotherapy (TTT)* with a diode laser (810 nm) may be considered for subfoveal occult CNVM. PDT is definitely better than TTT but is very expensive.
- *Double frequency YAG* 532nm photocoagulation may be used for extrafoveal choroidal neovascular membrane (CNVM).
- *Surgical treatment.* Submacular surgery to remove CNVM and macular translocation surgery are being evaluated.

MACULAR HOLE

Macular hole refers to a partial thickness of full thickness hole in the neurosensory retina in the foveal region.

Causes

1. *Senile* or *idiopathic* (83%), more common in females aged 60-80 years than males (F: M, 3:1).
2. *Traumatic* (5%)
3. *Other causes* include: cystoid mascular oedema, vitreomacular traction, post-surgical, myopia, post laser treatment, epiretinal membrane traction and post-inflammatory.

Pathogenesis: Senile macular holes are caused by tractional forces associated with early PVD.

Clinical features

Symptoms include:

- *Decreased vision*, typically around 6/60 level for a full thickness hole and better for a partial hole.
- *Metamorphopsia* or distortion of vision may be there.
- *Central scotoma* may be reported by some patients.

Signs. Based on the fundus appearance (best examined with 78/90D slit-lamp examination), the macular hole can be classified into four stages (Fig. 11.27):

- *Stage 1 or impending hole.* It is characterized by absent foveal reflex and a yellow spot (Stage 1A, Fig. 11.27A) or a yellow ring (Stage 1B) in the foveal region. *OCT examination* reveals a pseudocyst with a vitreous detachment in stage 1A (Fig. 11.27B), and progression of the pseudocyst with a break in the outer foveal layer in stage 1B.
- *Stage 2.* A small full thickness hole (Fig. 11.27C) in seen either in the center of the ring (central) or at the margin of the ring (eccentric). *OCT examination* shows a full thickness hole less than 400 µm in size. (Fig. 11.27D).
- *Stage 3.* A full thickness hole is seen as round reddish spot surrounded by a gray halo (cuff of sub retinal fluid (SRF)), but no PVD (Fig. 11.27E). *OCT examination* shows a full thickness macular hole more than 400 µm in size with partial vitreo macular adhesion/traction. (Fig. 11.27F).
- *Stage 4.* Full thickness hole with SRF cuff and complete PVD, i.e. posterior vitreous detachment (seen as Weiss ring) (Fig. 11.27G). *OCT examina-*

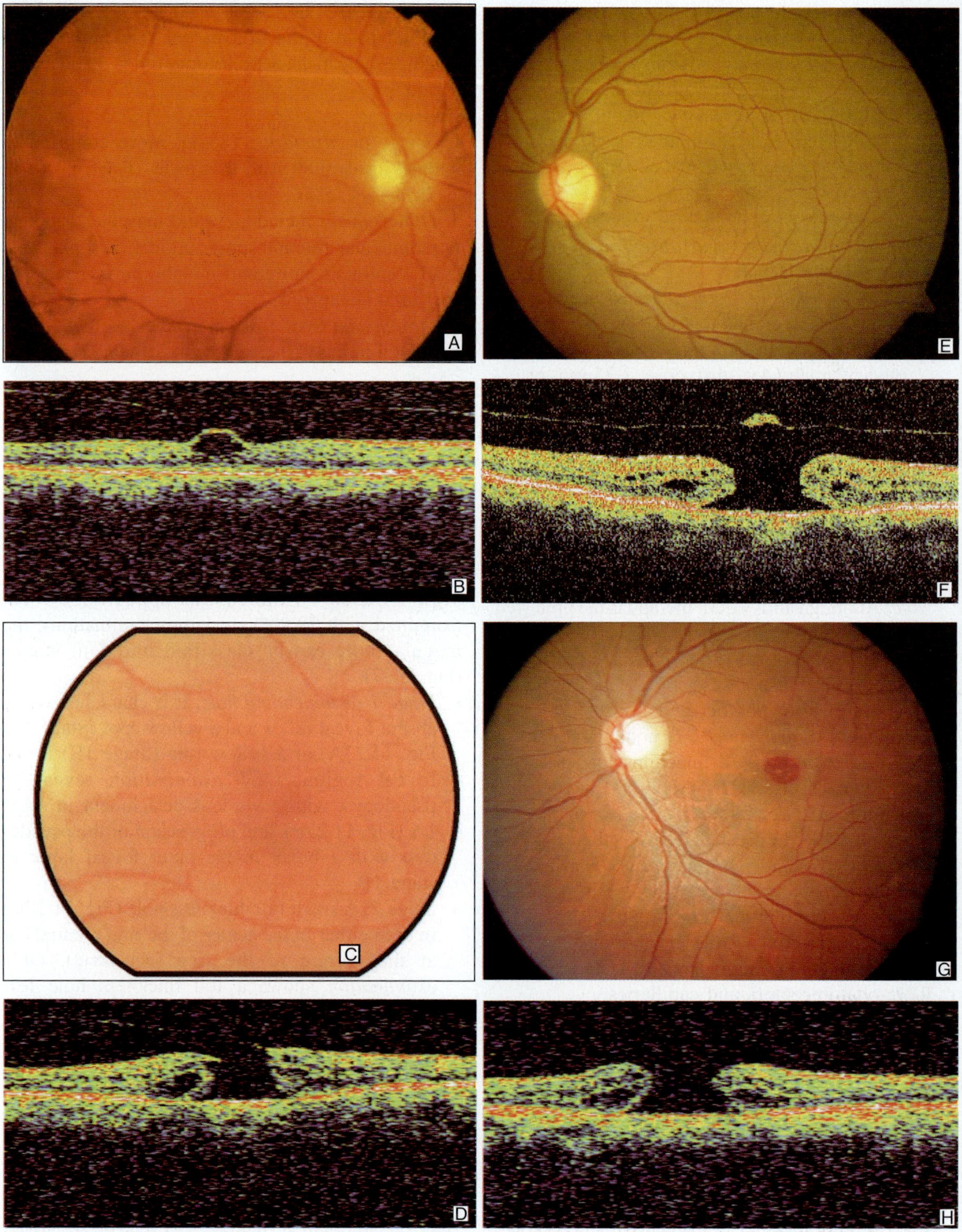

Fig 11.27. Macular hole stages 1,2,3,4: Fundus appearance (A,C,E,G) and OCT pictures (B,D,F,H), respectively.

tion confirms a large full thickness hole with posterior vitreous detached from the disc and macula. (Fig. 11.27H).

Management

Differential diagnosis of fundus appearance include:

- Macular pucker (epiretinal membrane) with pseudohole,
- Solar retinopathy,
- Intraretinal cyst (e.g., chronic CME with prominent central cyst) and
- Vitreomacular traction syndrome.

Investigations

1. *Fundus fluorescein angiography* reveals early foveal hyperfluorescence without leak in the late phase in patients with stage 2 to 4 macular holes.
2. *Optical Coherence Tomography* (OCT) (Fig. 11.27) is useful for:

- Differentiating true holes from the lamellar holes and cysts,
- Staging of the macular hole,
- Determining the degree of traction from the epiretinal membrane, and
- Planning the surgery.

Treatment

- *Stage 1.* Treatment is not recommended as spontaneous hole closure can occur. But close follow up and observation is required as 50% cases do progress.
- *Stage 2 to 4* holes of recent onset (<1 year) with reduced visual acuity (<6/24) should be treated with pars plana vitrectomy with posterior hyaloid removal, internal limiting (ILM) peeling and gas or silicon oil tamponade with strict post-operative face down position for 7-14 days.

Prognosis. Anatomical closure is reported in 60-85% of cases. Visual improvement is reported in 70% cases with recent onset holes.

Complications of surgery. A comparatively common complication is occurrence or progression of cataract. Other reported complications include: retinal breaks, retinal detachment, late reopening of the hole, RPE loss under the hole, photo-toxicity and endophthalmitis.

RETINAL DETACHMENT

Retinal detachment is the separation of neurosensory retina proper from the pigment epithelium. Normally these two layers are loosely attached to each other with a potential space in between. Hence, actually speaking the term retinal detachment is a misnomer and it should be retinal separation.

Classification

Clinico-etiologically retinal detachment can be classified into three types:

1. Rhegmatogenous or primary retinal detachment.
2. Tractional retinal detachment and
3. Exudative retinal detachment

RHEGMATOGENOUS OR PRIMARY RETINAL DETACHMENT

It is usually associated with a retinal break (hole or tear) through which subretinal fluid (SRF) seeps and separates the sensory retina from the pigmentary epithelium.

Etiology

It is still not clear exactly. The predisposing factors and the proposed pathogenesis is as follows:

A. *Predisposing factors* include:

1. *Age.* The condition is most common in 40-60 years. However, age is no bar.
2. *Sex.* More common in males (M:F—3:2).
3. *Myopia.* About 40 percent cases of rhegmatogenous retinal detachment are myopic.
4. *Aphakia.* The condition is more common in aphakes than phakes.
5. *Retinal degenerations* predisposed to retinal detachment are as follows:
   - Lattice degeneration
   - Snail track degeneration.
   - White-with-pressure and white-without-or occult pressure.
   - Acquired retinoschisis.
   - Focal pigment clumps.
6. *Trauma.* It may also act as a predisposing factor.
7. *Senile posterior vitreous detachment (PVD).* It is associated with retinal detachment in about 10% cases.

B. *Pathogenesis*

Pathogenesis of rhegmatogenous retinal detachment (RRD) is summarized in Fig. 11.28. The retinal breaks responsible for RRD are caused by the interplay between the *dynamic vitreoretinal traction* and predisposing degeneration in the peripheral retina. Dynamic vitreoretinal traction is induced by rapid eye movements especially in the presence of PVD, vitreous syneresis, aphakia and myopia. Once the retinal break is formed, the liquified vitreous may seep through it separating the sensory retina from the pigment epithelium. As the subretinal fluid (SRF) accumulates, it tends to gravitate downwards. The final shape and position of RD is determined by location of retinal break (*Lincoff's rule*) and the anatomical limits of optic disc and ora serrata.

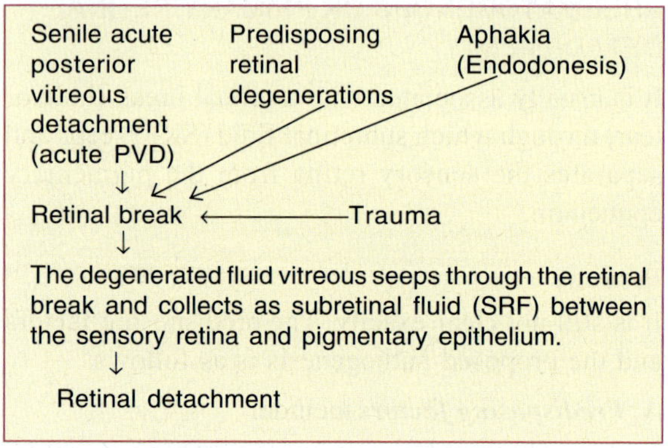

Fig. 11.28. Flow chart depicting pathogenesis of rhegmatogenous retinal detachment.

Clinical features

Prodromal symptoms. These include:

- *Dark spots* (floaters) in front of the eye (due to rapid vitreous degeneration), and
- *Photopsia,* i.e., sensation of flashes of light (due to irritation of retina by vitreous movements).

Symptoms of detached retina are as follows:

1. *Localised relative loss in the field of vision* (of detached retina) is noticed by the patient in early stage which progresses to a total loss when peripheral detachment proceeds gradually towards the macular area.
2. *Sudden painless loss of vision* occurs when the detachment is large and central. Such patients usually complain of sudden appearance of a dark cloud or veil in front of the eye.

Signs. These are elicited on following examinations:

1. *External examination,* eye is usually normal.
2. *Intraocular pressure* is usually slightly lower or may be normal.
3. *Marcus Gunn pupil* (relative afferent pupillary defect) is present in eyes with extensive RD.
4. *Plane mirror examination* or *Distant Direct Opthalmoscopy* reveals an altered red reflex in the pupillary area (i.e., greyish reflex in the quadrant of detached retina).
5. *Ophthalmoscopy* should be carried out both by direct and indirect techniques. Retinal detachment is best examined by indirect ophthalmoscopy using scleral indentation (to enhance visualization of the peripheral retina anterior to equator).
   - *Freshly-detached retina* gives grey reflex instead of normal pink reflex and is raised anteriorly (convex configuration). It is thrown into folds which oscillate with the movements of the eye. These may be small or may assume the shape of balloons in large bullous retinal detachment. In total detachment retina becomes funnel-shaped, being attached only at the disc and ora serrata. Retinal vessels appear as dark tortuous cords oscillating with the movement of detached retina.
   - *Retinal breaks* associated with rhegmatogenous detachment are located with difficulty. These look reddish in colour and vary in shape. These may be round, horse-shoe shaped, slit-like or in the form of a large anterior dialysis (Fig. 11.29). Retinal breaks are most frequently found in the periphery (commonest in the upper temporal quadrant). Associated retinal degenerations, pigmentation and haemorrhages may be discovered.
   - *Old retinal detachment* is characterized by retinal thinning (due to atrophy), formation of subretinal demarcation line (high water marks) due to proliferation of RPE cells at the junction of flat detachment and formation of secondary intraretinal cysts (in very old RD).
6. *Visual field charting* reveals scotomas corresponding to the area of detached retina, which are relative to begin with but become absolute in long-standing cases.
7. *Electroretinography (ERG)* is subnormal or absent.
8. *Ultrasonography* confirms the diagnosis. It is of particular value in patients with hazy media especially in the presence of dense cataracts and vitreous haemorrhage.

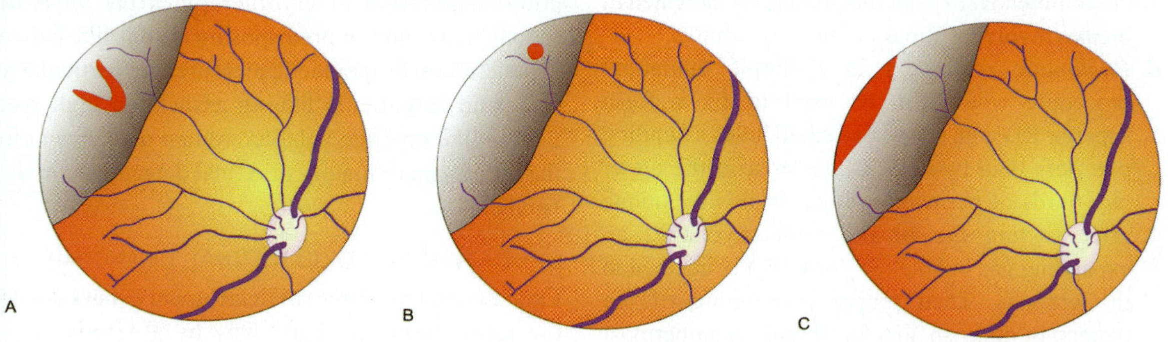

Fig. 11.29. Retinal detachment associated with: A, horse-shoe tear; B, round retinal hole; C, anterior dialysis.

Complications

These usually occur in long-standing cases and include proliferative vitreoretinopathy (PVR), complicated cataract, uveitis and phthisis bulbi.

Treatment

Basic principles and steps of RD surgery are:

1. ***Sealing of retinal breaks.*** All the retinal breaks should be detected, accurately localised and sealed by producing aseptic chorioretinitis, with cryocoagulation, or photocoagulation or diathermy. Cryocoagulation is more frequently utilised (Fig. 11.30).

2. ***SRF drainage.*** It allows immediate apposition between sensory retina and RPE. SRF drainage is done very carefully by inserting a fine needle through the sclera and choroid into the subretinal space and allowing SRF to drain away. SRF drainage may not be required in some cases.

3. ***To maintain chorioretinal apposition*** *for at least a couple of weeks.* This can be accomplished by either of the following procedures depending upon the clinical condition of the eye:

i. ***Scleral buckling*** i.e., inward indentation of sclera to provide *external tamponade* is still widely used to achieve the above mentioned goal successfully in simple cases of primary RD. Scleral buckling is achieved by inserting an explant (silicone sponge or solid silicone band) with the help of mattress type sutures applied in the sclera (Fig. 11.31). Radially oriented explant is most effective in sealing an isolated hole, and

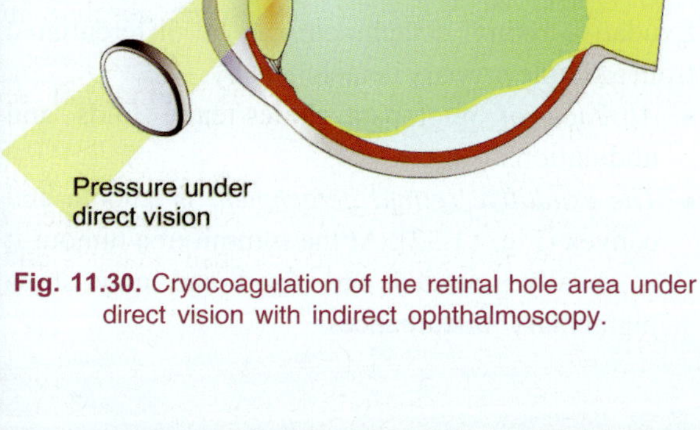

Fig. 11.30. Cryocoagulation of the retinal hole area under direct vision with indirect ophthalmoscopy.

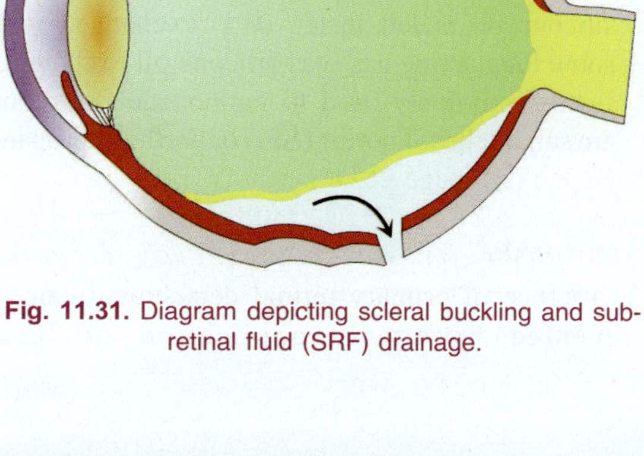

Fig. 11.31. Diagram depicting scleral buckling and subretinal fluid (SRF) drainage.

circumferential explant (encirclage) is indicated in breaks involving three or more quadrants.

ii. ***Pneumatic retinopexy*** is a simple outpatient procedure which can be used to fix a fresh superior RD with one or two small holes extending over less than two clock hour area in the upper two thirds of peripheral retina. In this technique after sealing the breaks with cryopaxy, an expanding gas bubble (SF_6 or C_3F_8) is injected in the vitreous. Then proper positioning of the patient is done so that the break is uppermost and the gas bubble remains in contact with the tear for 5-7 days.

iii. ***Parsplana vitrectomy, endolaser photocoagulation and internal tamponade.*** This procedure is indicated in:
   - All complicated primary RDs, and
   - All tractional RDs.
   - Presently, even in uncomplicated primary RDs (where scleral buckling is successful), the primary vitrectomy is being used with increasing frequency by the experts in a bid to provide better resutls.

Main steps of this procedure are:

- *Pars plana,3-port vitrectomy* (see page 261) is done to remove all membranes and vitreous and to clean the edges of retinal breaks.
- *Internal drainage of SRF* through existing retinal breaks using a fine needle or through a posterior retinotomy is done.
- *Flattening of the retina* is done by injecting silicone oil or perflurocarbon liquid.
- *Endolaser* is then applied around the area of posterior retinotomy, retinal tears, and holes to create chorioretinal adhesions.
- *To tamponade the retina internally* either silicone oil is left inside or is exchanged with some long acting gas (gas-silicone oil exchange). Gases commonly used to tamponade the retina are sulphur hexafluoride (SF_6) or perfluoropropane (C_3F_8) (see page 262).

Prophylaxis

Occurrence of primary retinal detachment can be prevented by timely application of laser photocoagulation or cryotherapy in the areas of retinal breaks and/or predisposing lesions like lattice degeneration. Prophylactic measures are particularly indicated in patients having associated high risk factors like myopia, aphakia, retinal detachment in the fellow eye or history of retinal detachment in the family.

EXUDATIVE OR SOLID RETINAL DETACHMENT

Exudative (serous) retinal detachment occurs due to the retina being pushed away by a neoplasm or accumulation of fluid beneath the retina following inflammatory or vascular lesions.

Etiology

Common causes of exudative retinal detachment can be grouped as under:

1. ***Systemic diseases.*** These include: toxaemia of pregnancy, renal hypertension, blood dyscrasias and polyarteritis nodosa.
2. ***Ocular diseases.*** These include:
   i. *Congenital abnormalities* such as nanophthalmos, optic pit, choroidal coloboma and familial exudative vitreoretinopathy (FEVR).
   ii. *Inflammations* such as Harada's disease, sympathetic ophthalmia, posterior scleritis, and orbital cellulitis;
   iii. *Vascular diseases* such as central serous retinopathy and exudative retinopathy of Coats;
   iv. *Neoplasms* e.g., malignant melanoma of choroid and retinoblastoma (exophytic type);
   v. *Sudden hypotony* due to perforation of globe and intraocular operations.
   vi. *Uveal effusion syndrome* is characterised by bilateral detachment of the peripheral choroid, ciliary body and retina.

Clinical features

Exudative retinal detachment can be differentiated from a simple primary detachment by:

- *Absence of* photopsia, holes/tears, folds and undulations.
- *The exudative retinal detachment* is smooth and convex (Fig. 11.32). At the summit of a tumour it is usually rounded and fixed and may show pigmentary disturbances.

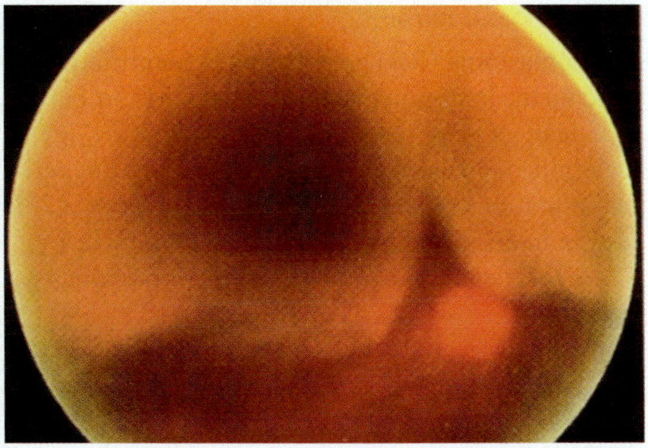

Fig. 11.32. Exudative retinal detachment in a patient with malignant melanoma of choroid.

- *Pattern of retinal vessels* may be disturbed occasionally, due to presence of neovascularisation on the tumour summit.
- *Shifting fluid* characterised by changing position of the detached area with gravity is the hallmark of exudative retinal detachment.
- *On transillumination test* a simple detachment appears transparent while solid detachment is opaque.

Investigations

1. *Ocular and systemic examination* should be carried out thoroughly.
2. *B-scan ultrasonography* may help delineate the underlying cause.
3. *FFA* may show source of fluid.
4. *CT Scan* and/or MRI is useful, specially in cases of intraocular tumours.

Treatment

- *Treatment of the cause* is required in most of the cases, as the exudative retinal detachment due to transudate, exudate and haemorrhage may undergo spontaneous regression following absorption of the fluid. Thus, the treatment should be for the causative disease.
- *Enucleation* is usually required in the presence of intraocular tumours.

TRACTIONAL RETINAL DETACHMENT

Tractional retinal detachment (TRD) occurs due to retina being mechanically pulled away from its bed by the contraction of fibrous tissue in the vitreous (vitreoretinal tractional bands).

Etiology

TRD is associated with the following conditions:

- Post-traumatic retraction of scar tissue especially following penetrating injury.
- Proliferative diabetic retinopathy.
- Post-haemorrhagic retinitis proliferans.
- Retinopathy of prematurity.
- Plastic cyclitis.
- Sickle cell retinopathy.
- Proliferative retinopathy in Eales' disease.
- Vitreo macular traction syndrome
- Incontinentia pigmenti
- Retinal dysplasia, and
- Toxocarisis

Clinical features

- Tractional retinal detachment (Fig. 11.33) is characterised by presence of vitreoretinal bands with lesions of the causative disease.
- Retinal breaks are usually absent and configuration of the detached area is concave.
- The highest elevation of the retina occurs at sites of vitreoretinal traction.
- Retinal mobility is severely reduced and shifting fluid is absent.

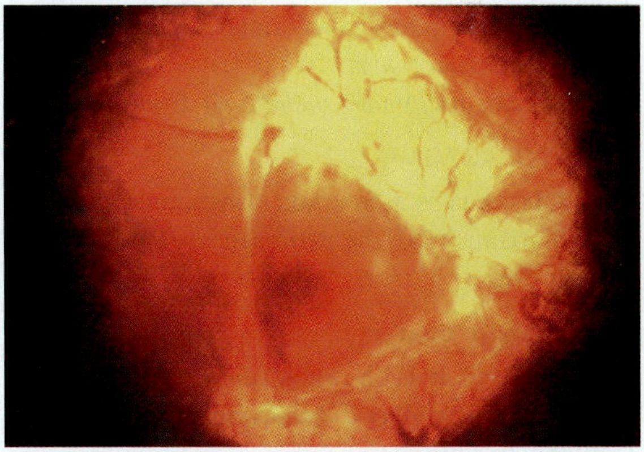

Fig. 11.33. Tractional retinal detachment in a patient with advanced diabetic retinopathy.

Treatment

- *Surgery* is difficult and requires pars plana vitrectomy to cut the vitreoretinal tractional bands and internal tamponade with either a long acting gas or silicon oil.
- *Prognosis* in such cases is usually not so good.

TUMOURS OF RETINA

Tumours of retina have become a subject of increasing interest to clinical ophthalmologists as well as ocular pathologists. Their classification is given here and only a few which are commonly seen are described.

Classification

A. *Primary tumours*

1. *Neuroblastic tumours.* These arise from sensory retina (retinoblastoma and astrocytoma) and pigment epithelium (benign epithelioma and melanotic malignant tumours).
2. *Mesodermal angiomata* e.g., cavernous haemangioma.
3. *Phakomatoses.* These include: angiomatosis retinae (von Hippel-Lindau disease), tuberous sclerosis (Bourneville's disease), neurofibromatosis (von Recklinghausen's disease and encephalo-trigeminal angiomatosis (Sturge-Weber syndrome).

B. *Secondary tumours*

1. *Direct extension* e.g., from malignant melanoma of the choroid.
2. *Metastatic carcinomas* from the gastrointestinal tract, genitourinary tract, lungs, and pancreas.
3. *Metastatic sarcomas.*
4. *Metastatic malignant melanoma* from the skin.

RETINOBLASTOMA

Retinoblastoma is a common congenital malignant tumour arising from the neurosensory retina in one or both eyes.

Demographic data

1. *Prevalence.* It is the most common intraocular tumour of childhood occurring 1 in 15,000 to 20,000 live births.
2. *Age.* Though congenital, it is not recognised at birth, and is usually seen between 1 and 2 years of age.
3. *Sex.* There is no sex predisposition.
4. *Race.* It is rarer in Negroes than Whites.
5. *Bilaterality.* In 25-30 percent cases, there is bilateral involvement, although one eye is affected more extensively and earlier than the other.

Genetics and heredity

Retinoblastoma (RB) gene has been identified as 14 band on the long-arm of chromosome 13 (13q 14) and is a 'cancer suppressor' or 'antioncogenic' gene. Deletion or inactivation of this protective gene by two mutations (*Knudson's two hit hypothesis, 1971*) results in occurrence of retinoblastoma.

Some facts about occurrence of Retinoblastoma are as below:

- *Of all cases*, only 10% are familial (inherited by autosomal dominant mode) and the rest about 90% occur sporadically.
- *Of sporadic cases*, about two third (i.e. 60% of all cases) occur by somatic mutation and one third (i.e. 30% of all cases) occur by germline mutation.
- Thus, the retinoblastoma either occurs as heritable (germline) cases (40%) or non-heritable somatic cases (60%).

1. *Heritable or germline cases.* In such cases first hit (mutation) occurs in one of the two alleles of retinoblastoma gene on the germ cells (gametes), before fertilization. This occurs either due to inheritence from the affected parent (10% cases) or sporadically in one of the gametes (30% cases). This means mutation will occur in all the somatic cells (predisposing to develop even non ocular tumors). Second hit (mutation) occurs late in the postzygote phase and affects second allele of one or more retinal cells, resulting in multifocal and usually bilateral tumour formation. About 15% of heritable cases are unilateral. Some heritable cases have trilateral retinoblastoma (i.e. having associated pinealoblastoma). Heritable case can transmit the disease by autosomal dominant way to 50% of offsprings. However, due to variable penetrance only 40% are affected.

2. *Non-heritable or somatic cases.* About 60% of retinoblastoma cases occur sporadically by both hits (mutations) occurring in the same retinal cell in the embryo after fertilization. These mutations generally result in unifocal and unilateral tumors which cannot be passed on to the offsprings.

Pathology

Origin. Retinoblastoma arises as malignant proliferation of the immature retinal neural cells called, *retinoblasts,* which have lost both antioncogenic genes.

Histopathology. The tumour chiefly consists of small round cells with large nuclei, resembling the cells of the nuclear layer of retina. These cells may present as a highly undifferentiated or well-differentiated tumour. Microscopic features of a well differentiated tumour include Flexner-Wintersteiner rosettes, (highly specific of retinoblastoma), Homer-Wright rosettes, pseudorosettes and fleurettes formation (Fig. 11.34). Other histologic features are presence of areas of necrosis and calcification.

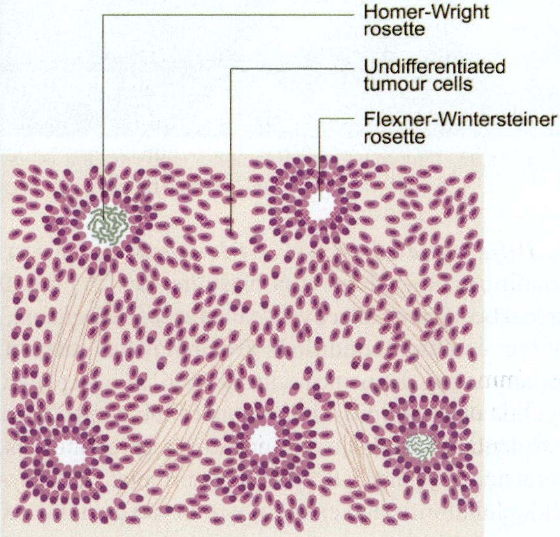

Fig. 11.34. Histopathological picture of retinoblastoma.

Clinical picture

It may be divided into four stages:

I. *Quiescent stage.* It lasts for about 6 months to one year. During this stage, child may have any of the following presenting features:

1. *Leukocoria or yellowish-white pupillary reflex* (also called as *amaurotic cat's eye appearance*) is the commonest presenting feature (60%). (Fig. 11.35)
2. *Squint,* usually convergent, is the second commonest mode of presentation.
3. *Nystagmus* is a rare feature, noticed in bilateral cases.
4. *Defective vision.* Very rarely, when the tumour arises late (3-5 years of age), the child may complain of defective vision.
5. *Ophthalmoscopic features of the tumour.* In the early stages, before the appearance of leukocoria, fundus examination after full mydriasis may reveal the growth. Ophthalmoscopic signs in two types of retinoblastoma are as follows:

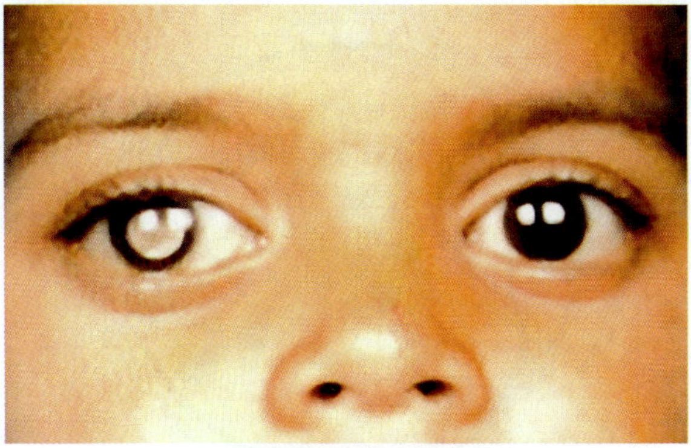

Fig. 11.35. Leukocoria right eye in a patient with retinoblastoma.

   i. *Endophytic retinoblastoma* (Fig. 11.36A): It grows inwards from the retina into the vitreous cavity. On ophthalmoscopic examination, the tumour looks like a well circumscribed polypoidal mass of white or pearly pink colour. Fine blood vessels and sometimes a haemorrhage may be present on its surface. In the presence of calcification, it gives the typical 'cottage cheese' appearance. There may be multiple growths projecting into the vitreous.
   ii. *Exophytic retinoblastoma* (Fig. 11.36B). It grows outwards and separates the retina from the choroid. On fundus examination it gives appearance of exudative retinal detachment (see page 298).

II. *Glaucomatous/inflammatory stage*. When retinoblastoma is left untreated during the quiescent stage, some patients may present with severe pain, redness, and watering. These symptoms occur either due to acute secondary glaucoma or apparent intra-ocular inflammation.

- *Acute secondary glaucoma* may occur either due to tumour pushing the lens-iris diaphragm forward or tumour cells clogging the trabecular mesh work. In this stage eyeball is enlarged (buphthalmos) with apparent proptosis, conjunctiva is congested, cornea become hazy, intraocular pressure is raised.
- *Apparent intra-ocular inflammation*. Occasionally, picture simulating severe, acute uveitis usually

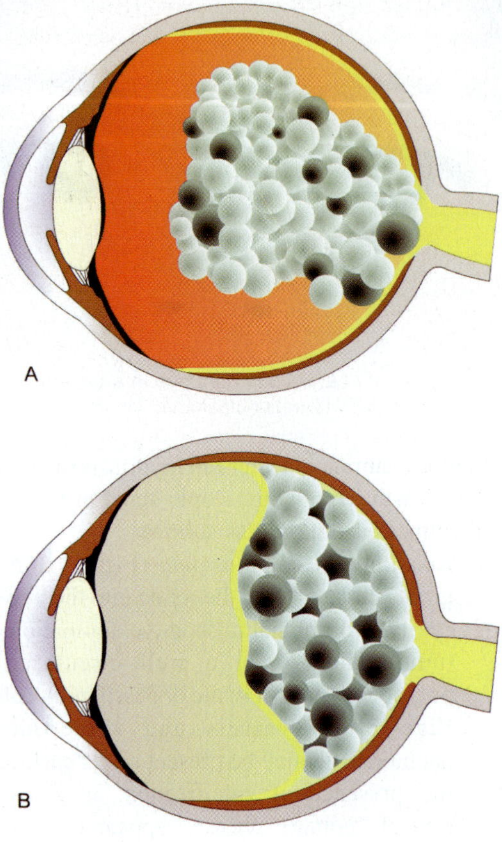

Fig. 11.36. Drawing of the cross-section of the eyeball showing: A, endophytic retinoblastoma; B, exophytic retinoblastoma.

associated with pseudohypopyon and/or hyphaema may be the presenting mode (retinoblastoma masquerading as iridocyclitis).

III. *Stage of extraocular extension*. Due to progressive enlargement of tumour the globe bursts through the sclera, usually near the limbus or near the optic disc. It is followed by rapid fungation and involvement of extraocular tissues resulting in marked proptosis (Fig. 11.37).

IV. *Stage of distant metastasis*. It is characterised by the involvement of distant structures as follows:

1. *Lymphatic spread* first occurs in the preauricular and neighbouring lymph nodes.
2. *Direct extension* by continuity to the optic nerve and brain is common.
3. *Metastasis by bloodstream* involves cranial and other bones. Metastasis in other organs, usually the liver, is relatively rare.

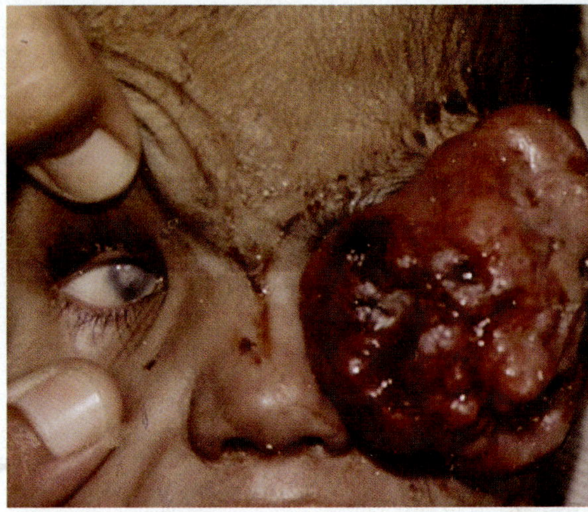

Fig. 11.37. Fungating retinoblastoma involving the orbit.

Differential diagnosis

1. *Differential diagnosis of leukocoria.* Various conditions other than retinoblastoma, which present as leukocoria are collectively called as '*pseudoglioma*'. A few common conditions are congenital cataract, inflammatory deposits in vitreous following a plastic cyclitis or choroiditis, coloboma of the choroid, the retrolental fibroplasia (retinopathy of prematurity), persistent hyperplastic primary vitreous, toxocara endophthalmitis and exudative retinopathy of Coats.

2. *Endophytic retinoblastoma* discovered on fundus examination should be differentiated from *retinal tumours* in tuberous sclerosis and neurofibromatosis, astrocytoma and a patch of exudative choroiditis.

3. *Exophytic retinoblastoma* should be differentiated from other causes of exudative retinal detachment in children such as: Coats' disease (see pages 282 and 298).

Diagnosis

1. *Examination under anaesthesia:* It should be performed in all clinically suspected cases. It should include fundus examination of both eyes after full mydriasis with atropine (direct as well as indirect ophthalmoscopy), measurement of intraocular pressure and corneal diameter.
2. *Plain X-rays of orbit* may show calcification which occurs in 75 percent cases of retinoblastoma.
3. *Lactic dehydrogenase (LDH)* level is raised in aqueous humour.

4. *Ultrasonography and CT scanning* are very useful in the diagnosis. CT also demonstrates extension to optic nerve, orbit and CNS, if any (Fig. 11.38). However, CT should be used sparingly because of potential risk of radiation sarcomas.

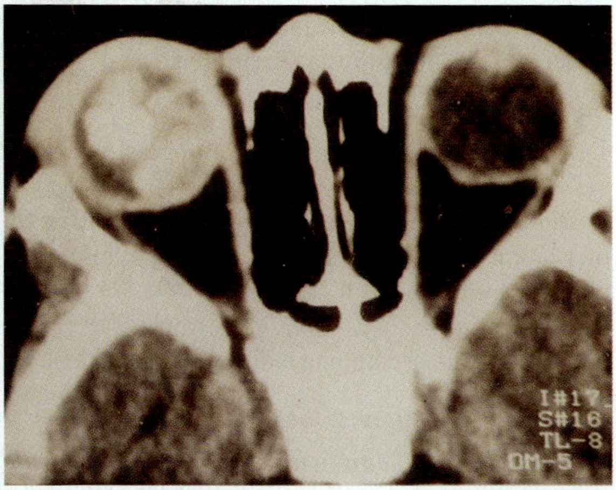

Fig. 11.38. CT Scan showing retinoblastoma.

Treatment

1. *Tumour destructive therapy.* When tumour is diagnosed at an early stage I i.e., when tumour involves less than half of retina and optic nerve is not involved (usually in the second eye of bilateral cases), it may be treated conservatively. Present recommendations for the treatment are primary systemic chemotherapy (for chemoreduction) followed by local therapy (for consolidation).

Chemotherapy recommended by most of the workers consists of vincristne, carboplatin and etoposide.

Local therapy. Depending upon the location and size of the tumour, therapy can be chosen from the following modalities:

- *Cryotherapy* is indicated for a small tumour located anterior to equator.
- *Laser photocoagulation* is used for a small tumour located posterior to equator.
- *Thermotherapy* with diode laser is used for a small tumour located posterior to equator away from macula.
- *Plaque radiotherapy* is very effective against localised viterous disease and for elevated tumours when laser is ineffective.
- *External beam radiotherapy* (EBR), once the main stay of treatment, is now reserved for diffuse disease in the only remaining eye.

However, if the above modalities are not available, the eyeball should be enucleated without hesitation.

2. *Enucleation.* It is the treatment of choice when:

- Tumour involves more than half of the retina.
- Optic nerve is involved.
- Glaucoma is present and anterior chamber is involved.

The eyeball should be enucleated along with maximum length of the optic nerve taking special care not to perforate the eyeball.

If optic nerve shows invasion, postoperative treatment should include:

- *Radiotherapy* (5000 rads) should be applied to the orbital apex.
- *Chemotherapy*, consisting of vincristine, carboplatin, and etoposide which may be combined with cyclosporin should be supplemented.

3. *Palliative therapy* is given in following cases where prognosis for life is dismal in spite of aggressive treatment:

- Retinoblastoma with orbital extension,
- Retinoblastoma with intracranial extension, and
- Retinoblastoma with distant metastasis.

Palliative therapy should include combination of:

- Chemotherapy,
- Surgical debulking of the orbit or orbital exentration, and
- External beam radiotherapy (EBRT)

Note: Exentration of the orbit (a mutilating surgery commonly performed in the past) is now not preferred by many surgeons.

Prognosis

If untreated the prognosis is almost always bad and the patient invariably dies. Rarely *spontaneous regression* with resultant cure and shrinkage of the eyeball may occur due to necrosis followed by calcification; suggesting role of some *immunological phenomenon.*

If the eyeball is enucleated before the occurrence of extraocular extension. Prognosis is fair (survival rate 70-85%).

Poor prognostic factors are: Optic nerve involvement, undifferentiated tumour cells and massive choroidal invasion.

Reese-Ellsworth classification to predict survival of the eye with retinoblastoma (not survival of patient) is as below:

Group 1: Very Favourable

A. Solitary tumour less than 4 disc diameters (DD) in size, at or behind the equator.

B. Multiple tumours, none over 4 DD in size, all at or behind the equator.

Group 2: Favourable

A. Solitary tumour 4–10 DD in size, at or behind the equator.

B. Multiple tumours, 4–10 DD in size, behind the equator.

Group 3: Doubtful

A. Any tumour anterior to the equator.

B. Solitary tumour, larger than 10 DD, behind the equator.

Group 4: Unfavourable

A. Multiple tumours, some larger than 10 DD in size.

B. Any lesion extending anteiorly to the ora serrata.

Group 5: Very Unfavourable

A. Massive tumours involving over half the retina.

B. Vitreous seedling.

ENUCLEATION

Enucleation is excision of the eyeball. It can be performed under local anaesthesia in adults and under general anaesthesia in children.

Indications

1. *Absolute indications* are retinoblastoma and malignant melanoma.

2. *Relative indications* are painful blind eye, mutilating ocular injuries, anterior staphyloma and phthisis bulbi.

3. *Indication for eye donation* from cadaver is presently the most common indication for enucleation.

Surgical techniques (Fig. 11.39)

1. *Separation of conjunctiva and Tenon's capsule* (Fig. 11.39A): Conjunctiva is incised all around the limbus with the help of spring scissors. Undermining

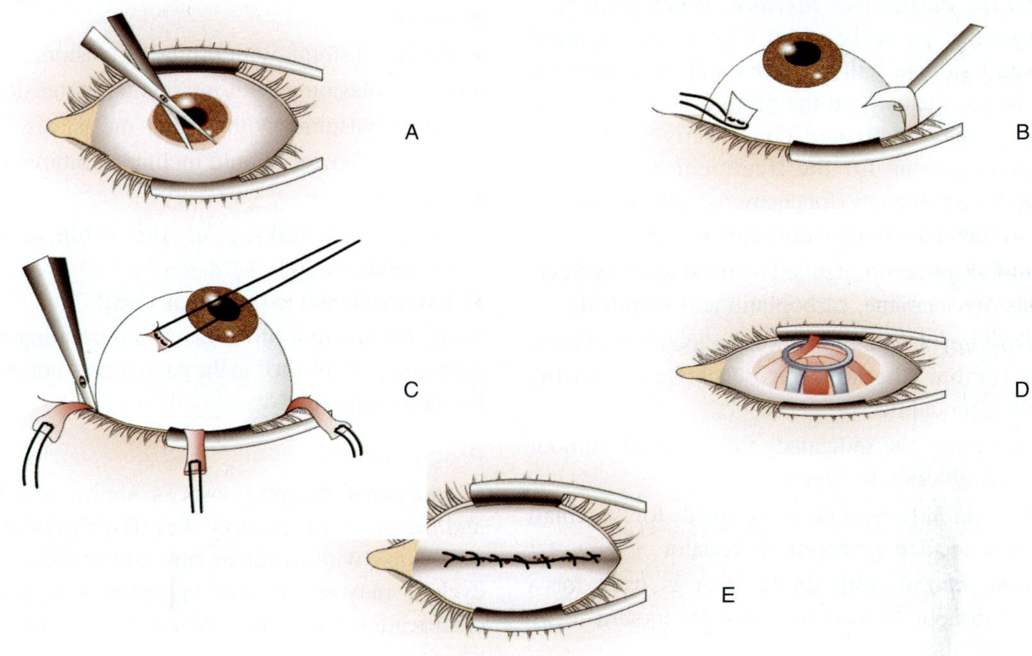

Fig. 11.39. Surgical steps of enucleation operation: A, separation of conjunctiva and Tenon's capsule; B, separation of extraocular muscles; C, cutting of optic nerve and removal of eyeball; D, insertion of an orbital implant; and E, closure of the conjunctiva.

of the conjunctiva and Tenon's capsule is done combinedly, all around up to the equator, using blunt-tipped curved scissors. This manoeuvre exposes the extraocular muscles.

2. *Separation of extraocular muscles* (Fig. 11.39B): The rectus muscles are pulled out one by one with the help of a muscle hook and a 3-0 silk suture is passed near the insertion of each muscle. The muscle is then cut with the help of tenotomy scissors leaving behind a small stump carrying the suture. The inferior and superior oblique muscles are hooked out and cut near the globe.

3. *Cutting of optic nerve* (Fig. 11.39C): The eyeball is prolapsed out by stretching and pushing down the eye speculum. The eyeball is pulled out with the help of sutures passed through the muscle stumps. The enucleation scissors is then introduced along the medial wall up to the posterior aspect of the eyeball. Optic nerve is felt and then cut with the scissors while maintaining a constant pull on the eyeball.

4. *Removal of eyeball.* The eyeball is pulled out of the orbit by incising the remaining tissue adherent to it and *haemostasis* is achieved by packing the orbital cavity with a wet pack and pressing it back.

5. *Inserting an orbital implant* (Fig. 11.39D): Preferably an orbital implant (made up of PMMA Medpor or hydroxyapatite) of appropriate size should be inserted into the orbit and sutured with the rectus muscles.

6. *Closure of conjunctiva and Tenon's capsule* is done separately. Tenon's capsule is sutured horizontally with 6-0 vicryl or chromic catgut. Conjunctiva is sutured vertically so that conjunctival fornies are retained deep with 6-0 silk sutures (Fig. 11.39 E) which are removed after 8-10 days. After completion of surgery, antibiotic ointment is applied, lids are closed and dressing is done with firm pressure using sterile eye pads and a bandage.

Fitting of artificial prosthetic eye

Conformer may be used postoperatively so that the conjuctival fornices are retained deep. A proper sized prosthetic eye can be inserted for good cosmetic appearance (Fig. 11.40) after 6 weeks when healing of the enucleated socket is complete.

PHACOMATOSES

Phacomatoses or neurocutaneous syndromes refer to a group of familial conditions (having autosomal dominant transmission) which are characterised by development of neoplasms in eye, skin and central nervous system. Phacomatoses includes the following conditions:

1. *Angiomatosis retinae (Von Hippel Lindau's syndrome).* This is a rare condition affecting males more often than females, in the third and fourth decade of life. The angiomatosis involves retina, brain, spinal cord, kidneys and adrenals. The usual clinical course of angiomatosis retinae comprises vascular dilatation, tortuosity and formation of aneurysms which vary from small and miliary to balloon-like angiomas, followed by appearance of haemorrhages and exudates, resembling eventually the exudative retinopathy of Coats. Massive exudation is frequently complicated by retinal detachment which may be prevented by an early destruction of angiomas with cryopexy or photocoagulation.

2. *Tuberous sclerosis (Bourneville disease).* It is characterised by a classic diagnostic triad of adenoma sebaceum, mental retardation and epilepsy associated with hamartomas of the brain, retina and viscera. The name tuberous sclerosis is derived from the potato-like appearance of the tumours in the cerebrum and

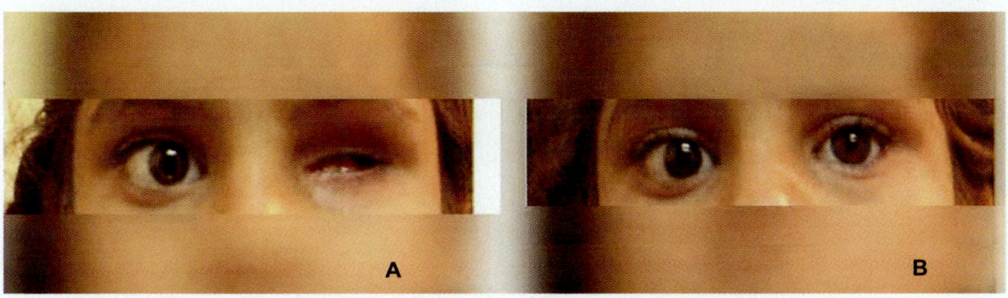

Fig. 11.40. Photographs of a patient without (A) and with (B) artificial eye.

other organs. Two types of hamartomas found in the retina are: (1) relatively flat and soft appearing white or grey lesions usually seen in the posterior pole; and (2) large nodular tumours having predilection for the region of the optic disc.

3. *Neurofibromatosis (von Recklinghausen's disease).* It is characterised by multiple tumours in the skin, nervous system and other organs. Cutaneous manifestations are very characteristic and vary from cafe-au-lait spots to neurofibromata. Ocular manifestations include neurofibromas of the lids and orbit, glioma of optic nerve and congenital glaucoma.

4. *Encephalofacial angiomatosis (Sturge-Weber syndrome).* It is characterised by angiomatosis in the form of port-wine stain (naevus flammeus), involving one side of the face which may be associated with choroidal haemangioma, leptomeningeal angioma and congenital glaucoma on the affected side.

12 CHAPTER

Neuro-opthalmology

ANATOMY AND PHYSIOLOGY

ANATOMY OF THE VISUAL PATHWAY

The visual pathway starting from retina consists of optic nerves, optic chiasma, optic tracts, lateral geniculate bodies, optic radiations and the visual cortex (Fig. 12.1).

Optic nerve

Each optic nerve (second cranial nerve) starts from the optic disc and extends up to optic chiasma, where the two nerves meet. It is the backward continuation of the nerve fibre layer of the retina, which consists of the axons originating from the ganglion cells. It also contains the afferent fibres of the pupillary light reflex.

Morphologically and embryologically, the optic nerve is comparable to a sensory tract. Unlike peripheral nerves it is not covered by neurilemma (so it does not regenerate when cut). The fibres of optic nerve, numbering about a million, are very fine (2-10 μm in diameter as compared to 20 μm of sensory nerves).

Parts of optic nerve. The optic nerve is about 47-50 mm in length, and can be divided into 4 parts: intraocular (1 mm), intraorbital (30 mm), intracanalicular (6-9 mm) and intracranial (10 mm).

1. *Intraocular part* starts from the optic disc (see page 263), pierces the choroid and sclera (converting it into a sieve-like structure—the lamina cribrosa). At the back of eyeball it becomes continuous with the intraorbital part.
2. *Intraorbital part* extends from back of the eyeball to the optic foramina. This part is slightly sinuous to give play for the eye movements. Posteriorly, near the optic foramina, it is closely surrounded by the annulus of Zinn and the

origin of the four rectus muscles. Some fibres of superior rectus muscle are adherent to its sheath here, and accounts for the painful ocular movements seen in retrobulbar neuritis. Anteriorly, the nerve is separated from the ocular muscles by the orbital fat.

3. *Intracanalicular part* is closely related to the ophthalmic artery which lies inferolateral to it and crosses obliquely over it, as it enters the orbit, to lie on its medial side. Sphenoid and posterior ethmoidal sinuses lie medial to it and are separated by a thin bony lamina. This relation accounts for retrobulbar neuritis following infection of the sinuses.
4. *Intracranial part* of the optic nerve lies above the cavernous sinus and converges with its fellow (over the diaphragma sellae) to form the optic chiasma.

Meningeal sheaths. Pia mater, arachnoid and dura covering the brain are continuous over the optic nerves. In the optic canal the dura is firmly adherent with the surrounding bone. The subarachnoid and subdural spaces around the optic nerve are also continuous with those of the brain.

Optic chiasma

It is a flattened structure measuring 12 mm (horizontally) and 8 mm (anterioposteriorly). It lies over the tuberculum and diaphragma sellae. Fibres originating from the nasal halves of the retina decussate at the chiasma (Fig. 12.1).

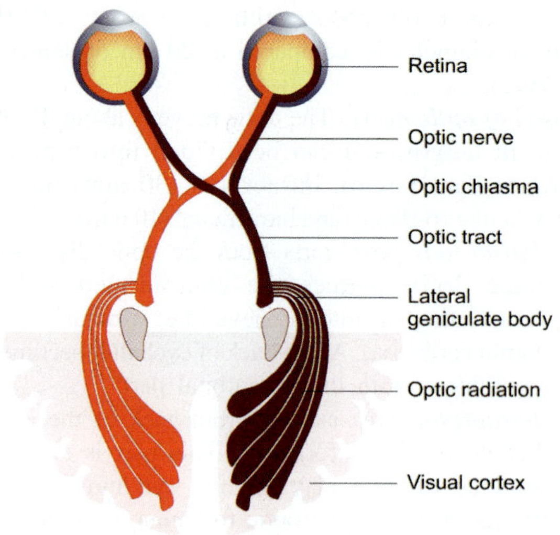

Fig. 12.1. Components of the visual pathway.

Optic tracts

These are cylindrical bundles of nerve fibres running outwards and backwards from the posterolateral aspect of the optic chiasma. Each optic tract consists of fibres from the temporal half of the retina of the same eye and the nasal half of the opposite eye. Posteriorly each optic tract ends in the lateral geniculate body (Fig. 12.1). The pupillary reflex fibres pass on to pretectal nucleus in the midbrain through the superior brachium. Some fibres terminate in the superior colliculus (see Fig. 12.6).

Lateral geniculate bodies

These are oval structures situated at the posterior termination of the optic tracts. Each geniculate body consists of six layers of neurons (grey matter) alternating with white matter (formed by optic fibres). The fibres of second-order neurons coming via optic tracts relay in these neurons.

Optic radiations

These extend from the lateral geniculate bodies to the visual cortex and consist of the axons of third-order neurons of visual pathway (Fig. 12.1).

Visual cortex

It is located on the medial aspect of the occipital lobe, above and below the calcarine fissure. It is subdivided into the visuosensory area (striate area 17) that receives the fibres of the radiations, and the surrounding visuopsychic area (peristriate area 18 and parastriate area 19).

Blood supply of the visual pathway

The visual pathway is mainly supplied by pial network of vessels except the orbital part of optic nerve which is also supplied by an axial system derived from the central artery of retina. The pial plexus around different parts of the visual pathway gets contribution from different arteries as shown in Fig. 12.2.

Blood supply of the optic nerve head (Fig. 12.3) needs special mention.

- *Surface layer* of the optic disc is supplied by capillaries derived from the retinal arterioles.
- *Prelaminar region* is mainly supplied by centripetal branches of the peripapillary choroid with some contribution from the vessels of lamina cribrosa.

- *Lamina cribrosa* is supplied by branches from the posterior ciliary arteries and arterial circle of Zinn.
- *Retrolaminar part* of the optic nerve is supplied by centrifugal branches from central retinal artery and centripetal branches from pial plexus formed by branches from the choroidal arteries, circle of Zinn, central retinal artery and ophthalmic artery.

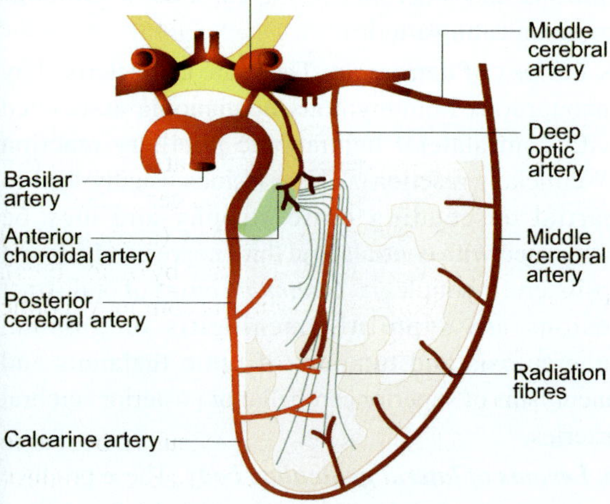

Fig. 12.2. Blood supply of posterior visual pathway.

PATHWAY OF VISUAL SENSATIONS VERSUS SOMATIC SENSATIONS

The pathway of somatic as well as visual sensations consists of three neurons (Fig. 12.4). The corresponding parts of the pathway of these sensations are shown in Table 12.1.

Table 12.1. Somatic vs. visual sensations

Feature	*Somatic sensation*	*Visual sensation*
1. Sensory end organ	Nerve endings in the skin	Rods and cones
2. Neurons of first order	Lie in posterior root ganglion	Lie in bipolar cell layer of the retina
3. Neurons of second order	Lie in nucleus gracilis or cuneatus	Lie in ganglion cells of the retina
4. Neurons of third order	Lie in thalamus	Lie in geniculate body

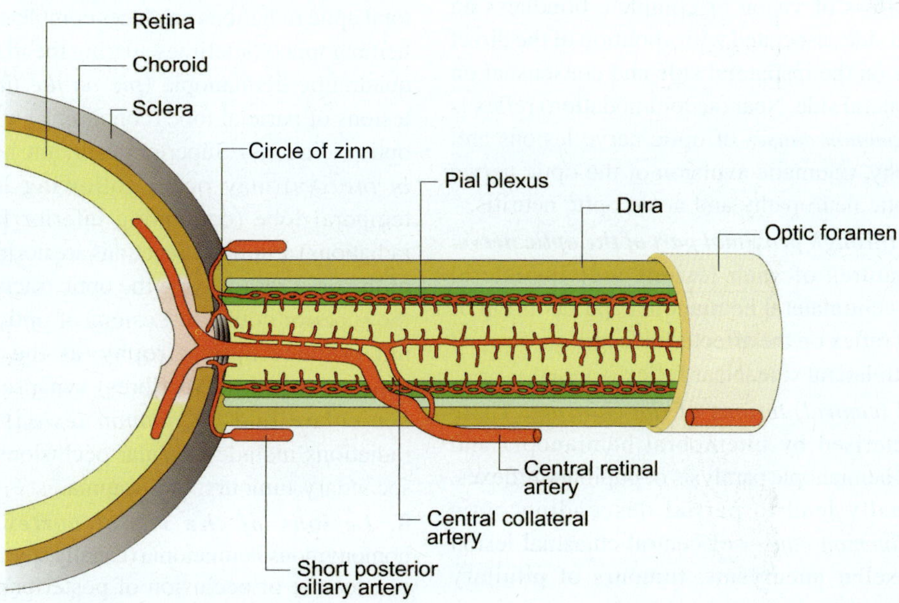

Fig. 12.3. Blood supply of the optic nerve.

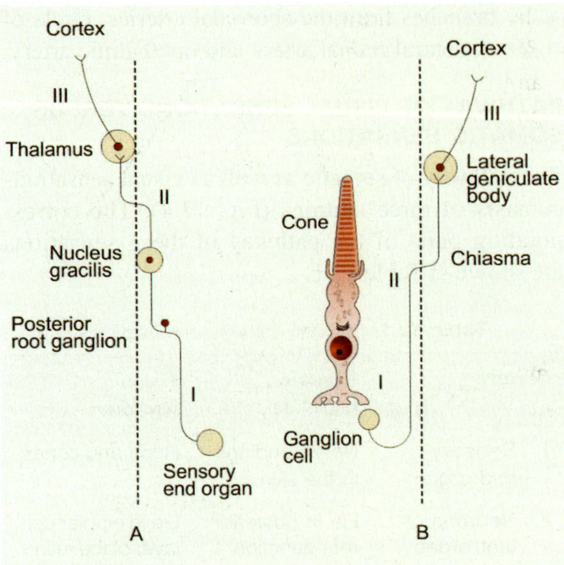

Fig. 12.4. Pathway of visual sensations (B) versus somatic sensations (A).

LESIONS OF THE VISUAL PATHWAY

Salient features and important causes of lesions of the visual pathway at different levels (Fig. 12.5) are as follows:

1. ***Lesions of the optic nerve.*** These are characterised by marked loss of vision or complete blindness on the affected side associated with abolition of the direct light reflex on the ipsilateral side and consensual on the contralateral side. Near (accommodation) reflex is present. *Common causes* of optic nerve lesions are: optic atrophy, traumatic avulsion of the optic nerve, indirect optic neuropathy and acute optic neuritis.

2. ***Lesions through proximal part of the optic nerve.*** Salient features of such lesions are: Ipsilateral blindness, contralateral hemianopia and abolition of direct light reflex on the affected side and consensual on the contralateral side. Near reflex is intact.

3. ***Sagittal (central) lesions of the chiasma.*** These are characterised by bitemporal hemianopia and bitemporal hemianopic paralysis of pupillary reflexes. These usually lead to partial descending optic atrophy. *Common causes* of central chiasmal lesion are: suprasellar aneurysms, tumours of pituitary gland, craniopharyngioma, suprasellar meningioma and glioma of third ventricle, third ventricular dilatation due to obstructive hydrocephalus and chronic chiasmal arachnoiditis.

4. ***Lateral chiasmal lesions.*** Salient features of such lesions are binasal hemianopia associated with binasal hemianopic paralysis of the pupillary reflexes. These usually lead to partial descending optic atrophy. *Common causes* of such lesions are distension of third ventricle causing pressure on each side of the chiasma and atheroma of the carotids or posterior communicating arteries.

5. ***Lesions of optic tract.*** These are characterised by incongruous homonymous hemianopia associated with contralateral hemianopic pupillary reaction (Wernicke's reaction). These lesions usually lead to partial descending optic atrophy and may be associated with contralateral third nerve paralysis and ipsilateral hemiplegia. *Common causes* of optic tract lesions are syphilitic meningitis or gumma, tuberculosis and tumours of optic thalamus and aneurysms of superior cerebellar or posterior cerebral arteries.

6. ***Lesions of lateral geniculate body.*** These produce homonymous hemianopia with sparing of pupillary reflexes, and may end in partial optic atrophy.

7. ***Lesions of optic radiations.*** Their features vary depending upon the site of lesion. Involvement of total optic radiations produces complete homonymous hemianopia (sometimes sparing the macula). Inferior quadrantic hemianopia (*pie on the floor*) occurs in lesions of parietal lobe (containing superior fibres of optic radiations). Superior quadrantic hemianopia (*pie in the sky*) may occur following lesions of the temporal lobe (containing inferior fibres of optic radiations). Pupillary reactions are normal as the fibres of the light reflex leave the optic tracts to synapse in the superior colliculi. Lesions of optic radiations do not produce optic atrophy, as the second order neurons (optic nerve fibres) synapse in the lateral geniculate body. *Common lesions* of the optic radiations include vascular occlusions, primary and secondary tumours, and trauma.

8. ***Lesions of the visual cortex.*** Congruous homonymous hemianopia (usually sparing the macula) is a feature of occlusion of posterior cerebral artery supplying the anterior part of occipital cortex. Congruous homonymous macular defect occurs in

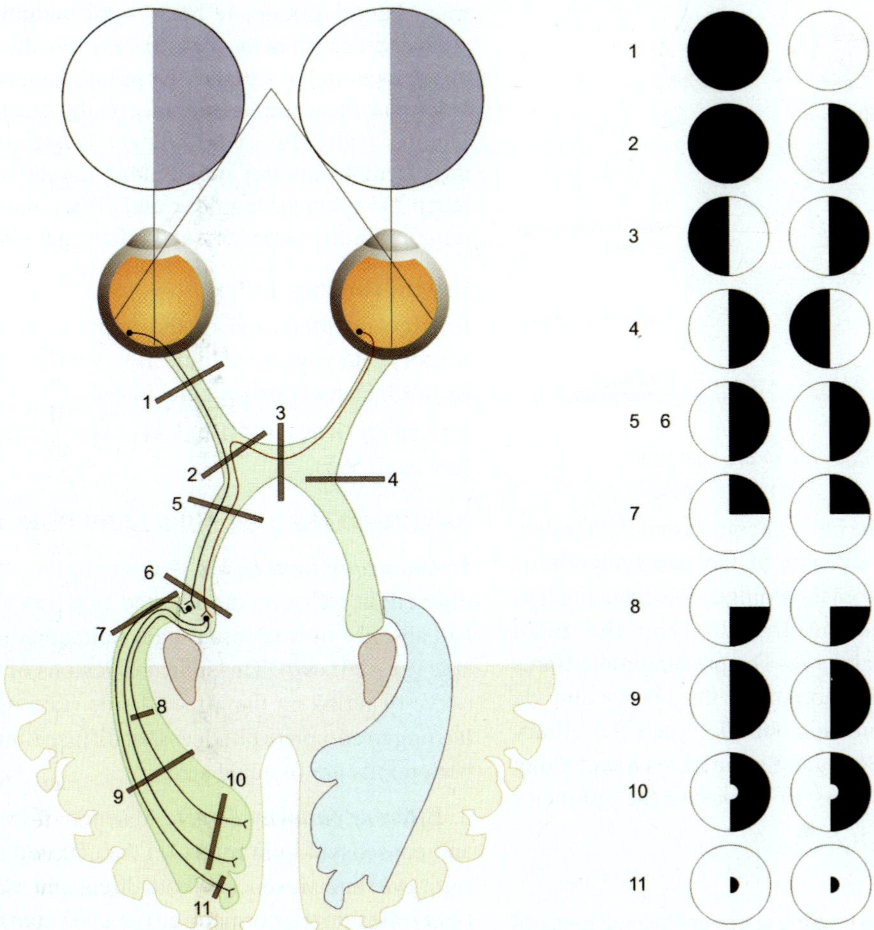

Fig. 12.5. Lesions of the visual pathways at the level of: 1. optic nerve; 2. proximal part of optic nerve; 3. central chiasma; 4. lateral chiasma (both sides); 5. optic tract; 6. geniculate body; 7. part of optic radiations in temporal lobe; 8. part of optic radiations in parietal lobe; 9. optic radiations; 10. visual cortex sparing the macula; 11. visual cortex, only macula.

lesions of the tip of the occipital cortex following head injury or gun shot injuries. Pupillary light reflexes are normal and optic atrophy does not occur following visual cortex lesions.

PUPILLARY REFLEXES AND THEIR ABNORMALITIES

PUPILLARY REFLEXES

Light reflex

When light is shone in one eye, both the pupils constrict. Constriction of the pupil to which light is shone is called *direct light reflex* and that of the other pupil is called *consensual (indirect) light reflex*. Light reflex is initiated by rods and cones.

Pathway of light reflex (Fig. 12.6). The *afferent fibres* extend from retina to the pretectal nucleus in the mid-brain. These travel along the optic nerve to the optic chiasma where fibres from the nasal retina decussate and travel along the opposite optic tract to terminate in the contralateral pretectal nucleus. While the fibres from the temporal retina remain uncrossed and travel along the optic tract of the same side to terminate in the ipsilateral pretectal nucleus.

Internuncial fibres connect each pretectal nucleus with Edinger-Westphal nuclei of both sides. This

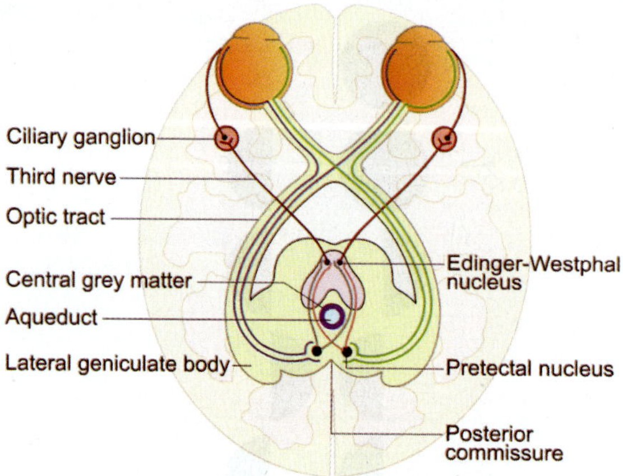

Fig. 12.6. Pathway of the light reflex.

connection forms the basis of consensual light reflex. *Efferent pathway* consists of the parasympathetic fibres which arise from the Edinger-Westphal nucleus in the mid-brain and travel along the third (oculomotor) cranial nerve. The preganglionic fibres enter the inferior division of the third nerve and via the nerve to the inferior oblique reach the ciliary ganglion to relay. Post-ganglionic fibres travel along the short ciliary nerves to innervate the sphincter pupillae.

Near reflex

Near reflex occurs on looking at a near object. It consists of two components: (a) convergence reflex, i.e., contraction of pupil on convergence; and (b) accommodation reflex, i.e., contraction of pupil associated with accommodation.

Pathway of convergence reflex (Fig. 12.7). Its afferent pathway is still not elucidated. It is assumed that the afferents from the medial recti travel centrally via the third nerve to the mesencephalic nucleus of the fifth nerve, to a presumptive convergence centre in the tectal or pretectal region. From this the impulse is relayed to the Edinger-Westphal nucleus and the subsequent efferent pathway of near reflex is along the 3rd nerve. The efferent fibres relay in the accessory ganglion before reaching the sphincter pupillae.

Pathway of accommodation reflex (Fig. 12.7). The afferent impulses extend from the retina to the parastriate cortex via the optic nerve, chiasma, optic tract, lateral geniculate body, optic radiations, and striate cortex. From the parastriate cortex the impulses are relayed to the Edinger-Westphal nucleus of both sides via the occipito-mesencephalic tract and the pontine centre. From the Edinger-Westphal nucleus the efferent impulses travel along the 3rd nerve and reach the sphincter pupillae and ciliary muscle after relaying in the accessory and ciliary ganglions.

Psychosensory reflex

It refers to dilatation of the pupil in response to sensory and psychic stimuli. It is very complex and its mechanism is still not elucidated.

EXAMINATION OF PUPILLARY REFLEXES

(see page 505)

ABNORMALITIES OF PUPILLARY REACTIONS

1. *Amaurotic light reflex.* It refers to the absence of direct light reflex on the affected side (say right eye) and absence of consensual light reflex on the normal side (i.e., left eye). This indicates lesions of the optic nerve or retina on the affected side (i.e., right eye), leading to complete blindness. In diffuse illumination both pupils are of equal size.

2. *Efferent pathway defect.* Absence of both direct and consensual light reflex on the affected side (say right eye) and presence of both direct and consensual light reflex on the normal side (i.e., left eye) indicates efferent pathway defect (sphincter paralysis). Near reflex is also absent on the affected side. Its causes include: effect of parasympatholytic drugs (e.g., atropine, homatropine), internal ophthalmoplegia, and third nerve paralysis.

3. *Wernicke's hemianopic pupil.* It indicates lesion of the optic tract. In this condition light reflex (ipsilateral direct and contralateral consensual) is absent when light is thrown on the temporal half of the retina of the affected side and nasal half of the opposite side; while it is present when the light is thrown on the nasal half of the affected side and temporal half of the opposite side.

4. *Marcus Gunn pupil.* It is the paradoxical response of a pupil to light in the presence of a relative afferent pathway defect (RAPD). It is tested by swinging flash light test. (For details see page 505).

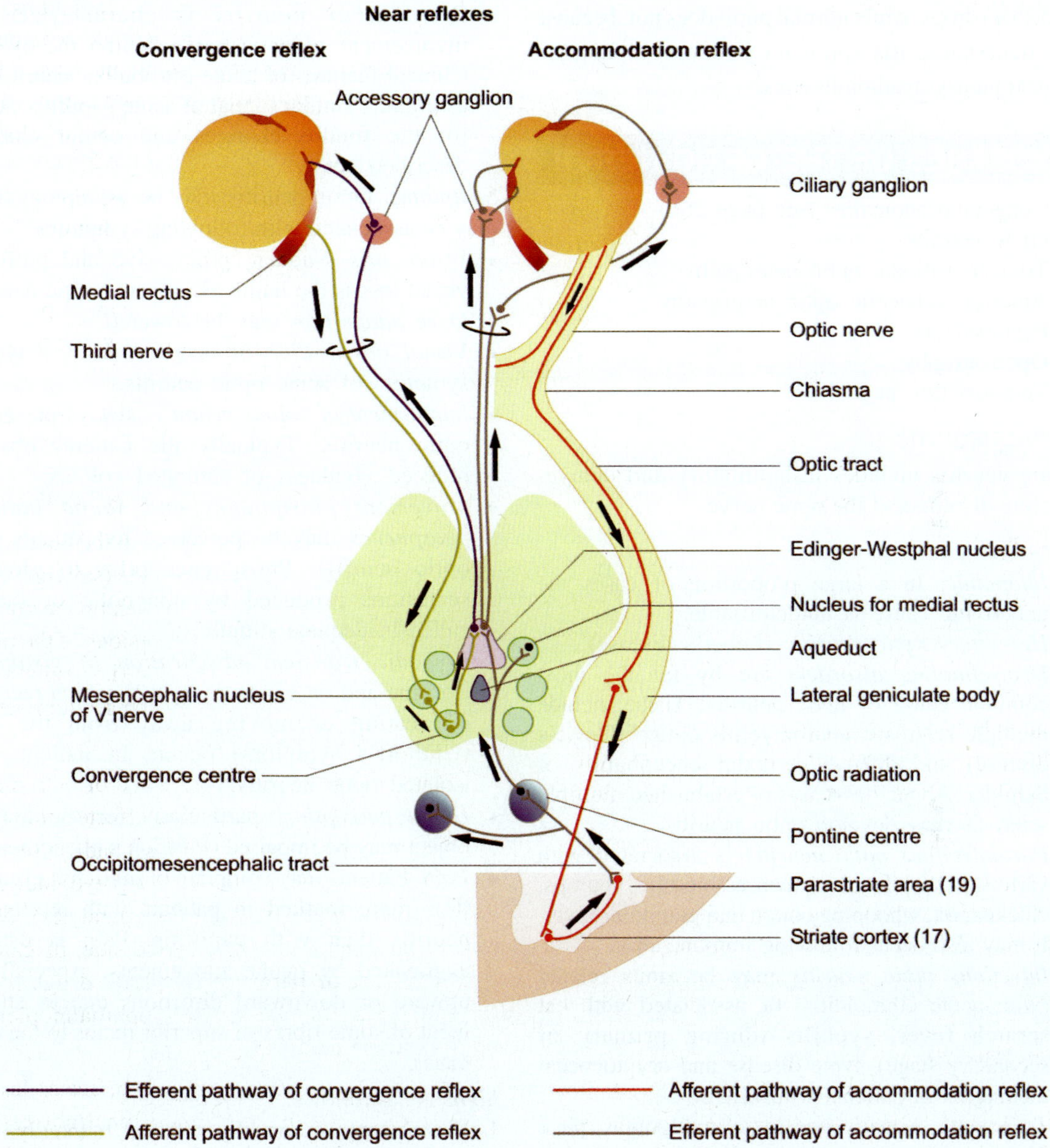

Fig. 12.7. Pathway of the near reflex.

5. *Argyll Robertson pupil (ARP)* . Here the pupil is slightly small in size and reaction to near reflex is present but light reflex is absent, i.e., there is light near dissociation (to remember, the acronym ARP may stand for 'accommodation reflex present'). Both pupils are involved and dilate poorly with mydriatics. It is caused by a lesion (usually neurosyphilis) in the region of tectum.

6. *The Adie's tonic pupil.* In this condition reaction to light is absent and to near reflex is very slow and tonic. The affected pupil is larger (anisocoria). It is caused by post ganglionic parasympathetic pupillo-motor damage. It is usually unilateral, associated with absent knee jerk and occurs more often in young women. Adie's pupil constricts with weak pilocarpine

(0.125%) drops, while normal pupil does not, because the denervated iris sphincter is supersensitive to topical parasympathomimetics.

DISEASES OF THE OPTIC NERVE

- Congenital anomalies (see page 266).
- Optic neuritis
- Toxic/nutritional optic neuropathy
- Anterior ischaemic optic neuropathy
- Papilloedema
- Optic atrophy
- Tumours (see page 421).

OPTIC NEURITIS

Optic neuritis includes inflammatory and demyelinating disorders of the optic nerve.

Etiology

1. *Idiopathic.* In a large proportion of cases the underlying cause is unidentifiable.
2. *Hereditary optic neuritis* (Leber's disease)
3. *Demyelinating disorders* are by far the most common cause of optic neuritis. These include multiple sclerosis, neuromyelitis optica (Devic's disease) and diffuse periaxial encephalitis of Schilder. About 70% cases of established multiple sclerosis may develop optic neuritis.
4. *Parainfectious optic neuritis* is associated with various viral infections such as measles, mumps, chickenpox, whooping cough and glandular fever. It may also occur following immunization.
5. *Infectious optic neuritis* may be sinus related (with acute ethmoiditis) or associated with cat scratch fever, syphilis (during primary or secondary stage), lyme disease and cryptococcal meningitis in patients with AIDS.
6. *Toxic optic neuritis* (see toxic amblyopias, page 316).

Clinical profile

Anatomical types. Optic neuritis can be classified into three anatomical types:

- *Papillitis.* It refers to involvement of the optic disc in inflammatory and demyelinating disorders. This condition is usually unilateral but sometimes may be bilateral.
- *Neuroretinitis* refers to combined involvement of optic disc and surrounding retina in the macular area.
- *Retrobulbar neuritis* is characterized by involvement of optic nerve behind the eyeball. Clinical features of acute retrobulbar neuritis are essentially similar to that of acute papillitis except for the fundus changes and ocular changes described below.

Symptoms. Optic neuritis may be asymptomatic or may be associated with following symptoms:

- *Visual loss.* Sudden, progressive and profound visual loss is the hallmark of acute optic neuritis.
- *Dark adaptation* may be lowered.
- *Visual obscuration in bright light* is a typical symptom of acute optic neuritis.
- *Impairment of colour vision* is always present in optic neuritis. Typically the patients observe reduced vividness of saturated colours.
- *Movement phosphenes and sound induced phosphenes* may be perceived by patients with optic neuritis. Phosphenes refer to glowing sensations produced by nonphotic or the so called inadequate stimuli.
- *Episodic transient obscuration of vision* on exertion and on exposure to heat, which recovers on resting or moving away from the heat (Uhthoff's symptom) occurs in patient with isolated optic neuritis.
- *Depth perception,* particularly for the moving object may be impaired (Pulfrich's phenomenon).
- *Pain.* Patients may complain of mild dull eyeache. It is more marked in patients with retrobulbar neuritis than with papillitis. Pain is usually aggravated by ocular movements, especially in upward or downward directions due to attachment of some fibres of superior rectus to the dura mater.

Signs are as follows:

1. *Visual acuity* is usually reduced markedly.
2. *Colour vision* is often severely impaired.
3. *Pupil* shows ill-sustained constriction to light. Marcus Gunn pupil which indicates relative afferent pupillary defect (RAPD) is a diagnostic sign. It is detected by the swinging flash light test (see page 505).
4. *Ophthalmoscopic features.* Papillitis is characterised by hyperaemia of the disc and blurring of the margins. Disc becomes oedematous and physiological cup is obliterated. Retinal veins are congested and tortuous. Splinter haemorrh-

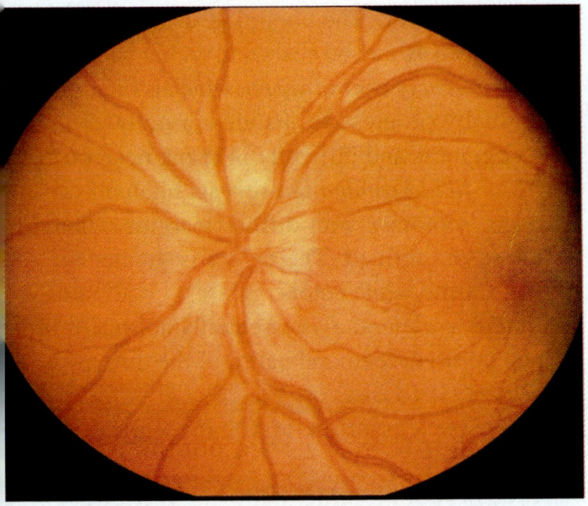

Fig. 12.8. Fundus photograph showing papillitis/neuroretinitis.

ages and fine exudates may be seen on the disc. Slit-lamp examination may reveal inflammatory cells in the vitreous. Inflammatory signs may also be present in the surrounding retina when papillitis is associated with macular star formation and the condition is labelled as '*neuroretinitis*' (Fig. 12.8). In majority of the cases with retrobulbar neuritis fundus appears normal and the condition is typically defined as a disease where neither the ophthalmologist nor the patient sees anything. Occasionally temporal pallor of the disc may be seen.

5. *Visual field changes.* The most common field defect in optic neuritis is a relative central or centrocaecal scotoma. Other field defects noted rarely include: paracentral nerve fibre bundle defect, a nerve fibre bundle defect extending up to periphery and a nerve fibre bundle defect involving fixation point and periphery. The field defects are more marked to red colour than the white.
6. *Contrast sensitivity* is impaired.
7. *Visually evoked response* (VER) shows reduced amplitude and delay in the transmission time.

Differential diagnosis

- *Papillitis* should be differentiated from papilloedema, ischaemic optic neuropathy, anterior orbital compressive neuropathy and pseudo-papilloedema (see Table 12.2).
- *Acute retrobulbar neuritis.* It must be differentiated from malingering, hysterical blindness, cortical blindness and indirect optic neuropathy.

Evolution, recovery and complications

In optic neuritis, typically, the visual acuity and colour vision is lost progressively over 2-5 days. The rate of visual recovery is slower than the rate of visual loss and usually starts within 2 weeks and takes between 4 and 6 weeks. About 75 to 90 percent cases get good visual recovery. However, recurrent attacks of acute retrobulbar neuritis are followed by primary optic atrophy and recurrent attack of papillitis are followed by postneuritic optic atrophy leading to complete blindness.

Treatment

Efforts should be made to find out and treat the underlying cause. There is no effective treatment for idiopathic and hereditary optic neuritis and that associated with demyelinating disorders. *Corticosteroid therapy* may shorten the period of visual loss, but will not influence the ultimate level of visual recovery in patients with optic neuritis. *Optic neuritis treatment trial* (ONTT) group has made following recommendations for the use of corticosteroids:

1. Oral prednisolone therapy alone is contraindicated in the treatment of acute optic neuritis, since, it did not improve visual outcome and was associated with a significant increase in the risk of new attacks of optic neuritis.
2. A patient presenting with acute optic neuritis should have brain MRI scan. If the brain shows lesions supportive of multiple sclerosis (MS), regardless of the severity of visual loss, each patient should receive immediate intravenous methylprednisolone (1 gm daily) for 3 days followed by oral prednisolone (1 mg/kg/day) for 11 days. Then taper prednisolone over 4 days. This therapy will delay conversion to clinical MS over the next 2 years.
3. Indications for intravenous methylprednisolone in acute optic neuritis patients with a normal brain MRI scan are:
   - Visual loss in both eyes simultaneously or subsequently within hours or days of each other.
   - When the only good eye is affected.
   - When the slow progressive visual loss continues to occur.

Leber's Hereditary Optic Neuropathy

Leber's hereditary optic neuropathy (LHON) is a type of hereditary optic neuritis which primarily affects males around the age of 20 years. It is transmitted by the female carriers. The condition is characterised by progressive visual failure. The fundus is initially normal or in the acute stage disc may be mildly hyperaemic with telangiectatic microangiopathy. Eventually bilateral primary optic atrophy ensues.

TOXIC/NUTRITIONAL OPTIC NEUROPATHY

Toxic/nutritional optic neuropathy also known as toxic amblyopia include those conditions wherein visual loss results from damage to the optic nerve fibres due to the effects of exogenous (commonly) or endogenous (rarely) poisons.

Varieties of toxic amblyopia described here include:

- Tobacco amblyopia,
- Ethyl alcohol amblyopia,
- Methyl alcohol amblyopia,
- Quinine amblyopia, and
- Ethambutol amblyopia

Tobacco amblyopia

Tobacco amblyopia typically occurs in men who are generally pipe smokers, heavy drinkers and have a diet deficient in proteins and vitamin B complex; and hence also labelled as 'tobacco-alcohol-amblyopia'.

Pathogenesis. The toxic agent involved is cyanide found in tobacco. The pathogenesis is summarised in Fig. 12.9.

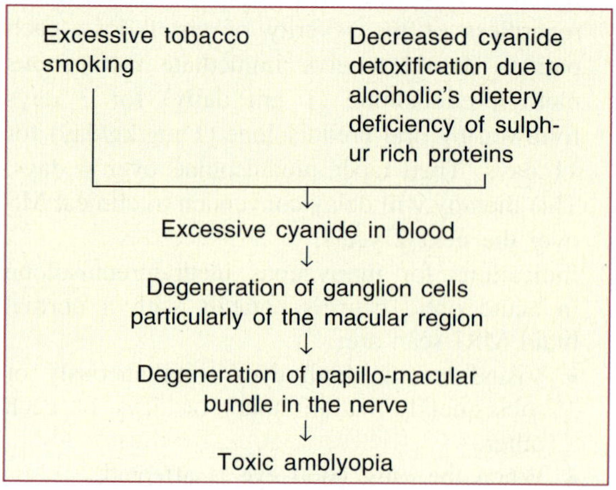

Fig. 12.9. Flow chart depicting pathogenesis of tobacco amblyopia.

Clinical features. The condition usually occurs in men between 40 and 60 years and is characterised by:

- *Impairment of central vision*, which is bilateral and gradually progressive. Patients usually complain of fogginess and difficulty in doing near work.
- *Visual field examination* reveals bilateral centro-caecal scotomas with diffuse margins which are not easily defined. The defect is greater for red than for the white colour.
- *Fundus examination* is essentially normal or there may be slight temporal pallor of the disc.

Treatment. It consists of:

- Complete cessation of tobacco and alcohol consumption,
- Hydroxycobalamine 1000 μg intramuscular injections weekly for 10 weeks
- Care of general health and nutrition.
- Vasodilators have also been tried.

Prognosis. It is good, if complete abstinence from tobacco and alcohol is maintained. Visual recovery is slow and may take several weeks to months.

Ethyl alcohol amblyopia

It usually occurs in association with tobacco amblyopia. However, it may also occur in non-smokers, who are heavy drinkers suffering from chronic gastritis. The optic neuritis occurs along with the peripheral neuritis of chronic and debilitated alcoholics.

Clinical picture and treatment is similar to tobacco amblyopia, but the prognosis is not so good.

Methyl alcohol amblyopia

Unlike ethyl alcohol (which produces chronic amblyopia), poisoning by methyl alcohol (methanol) is typically acute, usually resulting in optic atrophy and permanent blindness.

Etiology. It usually occurs due to intake of wood alcohol or methylated spirit in cheap adulterated or fortified beverages. Sometimes, it may also be absorbed by inhalation of fumes in industries, where methyl alcohol is used as a solvent. Rarely it may also be absorbed from the skin following prolonged daily use of liniments.

Pathogenesis. Methyl alcohol is metabolised very slowly and thus stays for a longer period in the body. It is oxidised into formic acid and formaldehyde in the tissues. These toxic agents cause oedema followed by degeneration of the ganglion cells of the retina, resulting in complete blindness due to optic atrophy.

Clinical features. *General symptoms of acute poisoning* are headache, dizziness, nausea, vomiting, abdominal pain, delirium, stupor and even death. *Presence of a characteristic odour* due to excretion of formaldehyde in the breath or sweat is a helpful diagnostic sign.

Ocular features. Patients are usually brought with almost complete blindness, which is noticed after 2-3 days, when stupor weans off. *Fundus examination* in early cases reveals mild disc oedema and markedly narrowed blood vessels. Finally bilateral primary optic atrophy ensues.

Treatment

1. *Gastric lavage to* wash away the methyl alcohol should be carried out immediately and at intervals during the first few days, as the alcohol in the system is continuously returned to stomach.
2. *Administration of alkali* to overcome acidosis should be done in early stages. Soda bicarb may be given orally or intravenously (500 ml of 5% solution).
3. *Ethyl alcohol.* It should also be given in early stages. It competes with the methyl alcohol for the enzyme alcohol dehydrogenase, thus preventing the oxidation of methanol to formaldehyde. It should be given in small frequent doses, 90 cc every 3 hours for 3 days.
4. *Eliminative treatment* by diaphoresis in the form of peritoneal dialysis is also helpful by washing the alcohol and formaldehyde from the system.
5. *Prognosis* is usually poor; death may occur due to acute poisoning. Blindness often occurs in those who survive.

Quinine amblyopia

It may occur even with small doses of the drug in susceptible individuals.

Clinical features. Patient may develop near total blindness. Deafness and tinnitus may be associated. The pupils are fixed and dilated. *Fundus examination* reveals retinal oedema, marked pallor of the disc and extreme attenuation of retinal vessels. *Visual fields* are markedly contracted.

Ethambutol amblyopia

Ethambutol is a frequently used antitubercular drug. It is used in the doses of 15 mg/kg per day. Sometimes, it may cause toxic optic neuropathy. Ethambutol toxicity usually occurs in patients who have associated alcoholism and diabetes.

Clinical features. There may occur optic neuritis with typical central scotoma. Involvement of optic chiasma may result in a true bitemporal hemianopia. Patients usually complain of reduced vision or impairment of colour vision during the course of antitubercular treatment. *Fundus examination* may reveal signs of papillitis. In most of the cases recovery occurs following cessation of the intake of drug.

ANTERIOR ISCHAEMIC OPTIC NEUROPATHY (AION)

Anterior Ischaemic Optic Neuropathy (AION) refers to ischaemic damage to the optic nerve head from occlusion of the short posterior ciliary arteries. It is of two types:

- Arteretic anterior ischaemic optic neuropathy (AAION), and
- Non arteretic anterior ischaemic optic neuropathy (NAAION)

Arteretic anterior ischaemic optic neuropathy

Etiology

Arteretic anterior ischaemic optic neuropathy (AAION), results from inflammatory and thrombic occlusion of short posterior ciliary arteries caused by Giant Cell Arteritis (GCA). It usually occurs in older patients (mean age 70 years) and accounts for only 5-10 % cases of AION.

Clinical features

Systemic and/or other ocular features of Giant Cell Arteritis (GCA) may also be associated with AAION.

Systemic features of GCA include:

- *Headache and tenderness* of the temporal arteries and scalp.
- *Jaw claudication*, characterized by pain on speaking or chewing , is pathogenomic of GCA. It is caused by ischaemia of masseter muscle.
- *Other symptoms* include fever, malaise, anorexia, weight loss, night sweats and joint and muscle pain.

Ocular presentations of GCA, other than AAION, include:

- *Transient Ischaemic Attacks* (TIA) i.e. amaurosis fugax, may precede AAION by several weeks.
- *Central retinal artery occlusion* (CRAO), or cilioretinal artery occlusion may sometimes be associated with AAION.
- *Ocular Ischaemic Syndrome* (see page 282) due to involvement of ophthalmic artery, is comparatively rare association of AAION.
- *Diplopia* may occur due to ischaemic paresis of extraocular muscles.

Features of AAION are as follows:

- *Visual loss* is usually marked (visual acuity < 6/60) and sudden, may be preceeded by TIA and general features of GCA.
- *RAPD* is present.
- *Optic disc edema* in AAION is typically pale as compared to NAION and may be associated with cotton wool spots and splinter haemorrhages.
- *Peripapillary pallor and edema deep to retina* may occur due to accompanying choroidal ischaemia.
- *Temporal arteries* loose pulsation and become tender.

Investigations

- *Fundus fluoroscein angiography* reveals delayed choroidal filling, an important differentiating sign of AAION from NAION.
- *Visual fields* show typical altitudinal hemianopia involving the inferior (commonly) or superior half (Fig. 12.10).

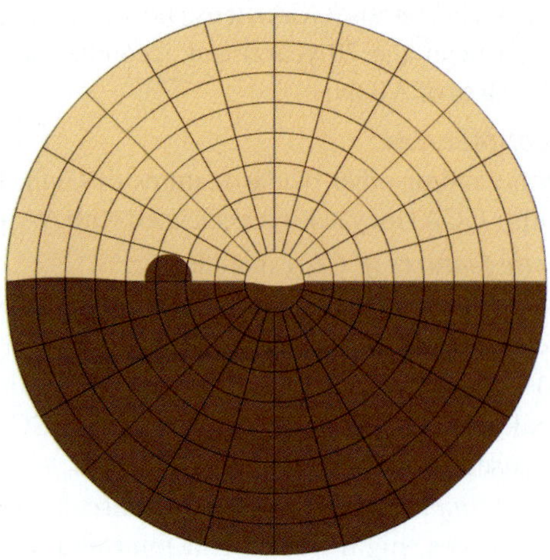

Fig. 12.10. Altitudinal hemianopia in AION.

- *ESR and C-reactive protein levels* are raised in patients with giant cell arteritis.
- *Temporal artery biopsy* is required for confirmation of diagnosis.

Treatment

Goal of treatment is to prevent visual loss in the fellow eye, apart from avoiding systemic vascular complications .

Corticosteroids, started immediately, as follows, constitute the main treatment.

- *Methylprednisolone* 1g/ day, intravenously for 3-5 days followed by
- *Prednisolone* per oral 80 mg/day to be tapered every week by 10mg. Daily maintenance therapy of 10 mg may have to be continued for 1-2 years.

Note: since treatment lasts long, special care has to be taken for side effects of steroids.

Non arteretic anterior ischaemic neuropathy

Non arteretic anterior ischaemic optic neuropathy (NAION) accounts for 90-95% cases of AION.

Etiology

Exact etiology of occlusion of posterior ciliary arteries causing infarction of the retrolaminar portion of the disc in this condition is not known.

Risk factors associated with NAION may be ocular or systemic.

- *Ocular risk factors* are disc at risk, i.e. structural crowding of the disc with a small cup, and cataract surgery.
- *Systemic risk factors* include hypertension, diabetes (particularly in young patients) smoking, hyperlipidemia, collagen vascular disease, hyperhomocystinemia, and sudden hypotensive events.
- *Drugs*, such as sildenafil (Viagra), presumably because of its hypotensive effect, may be associated with NAION.

Clinical features

Clinical features of NAION vis-à-vis AAION can be summarized as below:

- *Age of presentation* is slightly younger, i.e. mean age is 60 years as compared to 70 years in AAION.
- *Sex.* NAION is equally common in males and females while AAION is more common in females than males.

- *Associated symptoms* such as headache, scalp tenderness, jaw claudication and amaurosis fugax seen with AAION and absent in NAION.
- *Visual loss* with NAION is comparatively less marked.
- *Optic disc edema* is hyperaemic as compared to pale edema noted with AAION (Fig. 12.9)
- *ESR* as compared to AAION (mean 70 mm after 1st hour) is less raised in NAION (mean 20-40 mm after 1st hour).
- *C- reactive proteins* are normal in NAION, while they are raised in AAION.
- *FFA reveals* only disc delay in NAION, while in AAION both disc delay and choroidal delay are noted.

Differential diagnosis

NAION also need to be differentiated from optic neuritis, infiltrative optic neuropathy, anterior orbital compressive optic neuropathy and other forms of optic disc edema including diabetic papillopathy.

Treatment

No proven benefit of any treatment measures including steroids is reported.

- *Adressing the systemic risk factors* may probably reduce the incidence.
- *Aspirin* has a proven effect in reducing the incidence of stroke in patients at risk, but its role in reducing involvement of other eye is not clear.

PAPILLOEDEMA

The terms papilloedema and disc oedema look alike and per se mean swelling of the optic disc. However, arbitrarily the term '*papilloedema*' has been reserved for the passive disc swelling associated with increased intracranial pressure which is almost always bilateral although it may be asymmetrical. The term '*disc oedema* or *disc swelling*' includes all causes of active or passive oedematous swelling of the optic disc other than the causes of papilloedema.

Causes of disc oedema

1. *Inflammations* such as papillitis, neuroretinitis, papillophlebitis, and uveitis.
2. *Ocular hypotony* due to any cause.
3. *Vascular causes* include CRVO, diabetic papillopathy, uremia, anterior ischaemic optic neuropathy (AION).
4. *Orbital causes* are: tumours, Graves' orbitopathy, and orbital cellulitis.
5. *Infiltrative* condition include leukaemias, and lymphomas.

Etiopathogenesis of papilloedema

Causes. As discussed above, papilloedema occurs secondary to raised intracranial pressure which may be associated with following conditions:

1. *Congenital conditions* include aqueductal stenosis and craniosynostosis.
2. *Intracranial space-occupying lesions (ICSOLs).* These include brain tumours, abscess, tuberculoma, gumma, subdural haematoma and aneurysms. The ICSOLs in any position excepting medulla oblongata may induce papilloedema. Papilloedema is most frequently associated with tumours arising in posterior fossa, which obstruct aqueduct of Sylvius and least with pituitary tumours. Thus, the ICSOLs of cerebellum, midbrain and parieto-occipital region produce papilloedema more rapidly than the mass lesions of other areas. Further, the fast progressing lesions produce papilloedema more frequently and acutely than the slow growing lesions.
3. *Intracranial infections* such as meningitis and encephalitis may be associated with papilloedema.
4. *Intracranial haemorrhages.* Cerebral as well as subarachnoid haemorrhage can give rise to papilloedema which is frequent and considerable in extent.
5. *Obstruction of CSF absorption* via arachnoid villi which have been damaged previously.
6. *Tumours of spinal cord* occasionally give rise to papilloedema.
7. *Idiopathic intracranial hypertension (IIH)* also known as pseudotumour cerebri, is an important cause of raised intracranial pressure. It is a poorly understood condition, usually found in young obese women. It is characterised by chronic headache and bilateral papilloedema without any ICSOLs or enlargement of the ventricles due to hydrocephalus.

8. *Systemic conditions* include malignant hypertension, pregnancy induced hypertension (PIH), cardiopulmonary insufficiency, blood dyscrasias and nephritis.
9. *Diffuse cerebral oedema* from blunt head trauma may causes papilloedema.
10. *Cerebral venous sinus thrombosis* may also cause papilloedema.

Unilateral versus bilateral papilloedema. Disc swelling due to ocular and orbital lesions is usually unilateral. In majority of the cases with raised intracranial pressure, papilloedema is bilateral. However, unilateral cases as well as of unequal change do occur with raised intracranial pressure. A few such conditions are as follows:

1. *Foster-Kennedy syndrome.* It is associated with olfactory or sphenoidal meningiomata and frontal lobe tumours. In this condition, there occurs pressure optic atrophy on the side of lesion and papilloedema on the other side (due to raised intracranial pressure).
2. *Pseudo-Foster-Kennedy syndrome.* It is characterised by occurrence of unilateral papilloedema associated with raised intracranial pressure (due to any cause) and a pre-existing optic atrophy (due to any cause) on the other side.

Pathogenesis. Till date, Hayreh's theory is the most accepted one. It states that, 'papilloedema develops as a result of stasis of axoplasm in the prelaminar region of optic disc, due to an alteration in the pressure gradient across the lamina cribrosa.'

Increased intracranial pressure, malignant hypertension and orbital lesions produce disturbance in the pressure gradient by increasing the tissue pressure within the retrolaminar region. While, ocular hypotony alters it by lowering the tissue pressure within the prelaminar area.

Thus the axonal swelling in prelaminar region is the initial structural alteration, which in turn produces venous congestion and ultimately the extracellular oedema. This theory discards the old view that the papilloedema results due to compression of the central retinal vein by the raised cerebrospinal fluid pressure around the optic nerve.

Evolution and recovery. Papilloedema usually develops quickly, appearing within 1-5 days of raised intracranial pressure.

In cases with acute subarachnoid haemorrhage it may develop even more rapidly (within 2-8 hours). However, recovery from fully developed papilloedema is rather slow. It takes about 6-8 weeks to subside after the intracranial pressure is normalised.

Clinical features

[A] *General features.* Patients usually present to general physicians with general features of raised intracranial pressure. These include headache, nausea, projectile vomiting and diplopia. Focal neurological deficit may be associated.

[B] *Ocular features.* Patients may give history of recurrent attacks of transient blackout of vision (amaurosis fugax). *Visual acuity and pupillary reactions* usually remain fairly normal until the late stages of diseases when optic atrophy sets in.

Clinical features of papilloedema can be described under four stages: early, fully developed, chronic and atrophic.

1. *Early (incipient) papilloedema*

- *Symptoms* are usually absent and visual acuity is normal.
- *Pupillary reactions* are normal.
- *Ophthalmoscopic features* of early papilloedema are (Fig. 12.11A): (i) Obscuration of the disc margins (nasal margins are involved first followed by the superior, inferior and temporal) (ii) Blurring of peripapillary nerve fibre layer. (iii) Absence of spontaneous venous pulsation at the disc (appreciated in 80% of the normal individuals). (iv) Mild hyperaemia of the disc. (v) Splinter haemorrhages in the peripapillary region may be present.
- *Visual fields* are fairly normal.

2. *Established (fully developed) papilloedema*

- *Symptoms.* Patient may give history of transient visual obscurations in one or both eyes, lasting a few seconds, after standing. Visual acuity is usually normal,
- *Pupillary reaction* remain fairly normal,
- *Ophthalmoscopic features* (Fig. 12.11B): (i) Apparent optic disc oedema is seen as its forward elevation above the plane of retina; usually up to 1-2 mm (1 mm elevation is equivalent to +3 dioptres). (ii) Physiological cup of the optic disc is obliterated. (iii) Disc becomes markedly hyperaemic and blurring of the margin is present

all-around. (iv) Multiple cotton wool spots and superficial haemorrhages may be seen near the disc. (v) Veins becomes tortuous and engorged. (vi) In advanced cases, the disc appears to be enlarged and circumferential greyish white folds may develop due to separation of nerve fibres by the oedema. (vii) Rarely, hard exudates may radiate from the fovea in the form of an incomplete star.

- *Visual fields* show enlargement of blind spot.

3. *Chronic or long standing (vintage) papilloedema*

- *Symptoms.* Visual acuity is variably reduced depending upon the duration of the papilloedema.
- *Pupillary reactions* are usually normal.
- *Ophthalmoscopic features* (Fig. 12.11C). In this stage, acute haemorrhages and cotton wool spots resolve, and peripapillary oedema is resorbed. The optic disc gives appearance of the dome of a *champagne cork.* The central cup remains obliterated. Small drusen like crystalline deposits (corpora amylacea) may appear on the disc surface.
- *Visual fields.* Blind spot is enlarged and the visual fields begin to constrict.

4. *Atrophic papilloedema*

- *Symptoms.* Atrophic papilloedema develops after 6-9 months of chronic papilloedema and is characterized by severely impaired visual acuity.
- *Pupillary reaction.* Light reflex is impaired.
- *Ophthalmoscopic features* (Fig. 12.11D). It is characterised by greyish white discoloration and pallor of the disc due to atrophy of the neurons and associated gliosis. Prominence of the disc decreases in spite of persistent raised intracranial pressure. Retinal arterioles are narrowed and veins become less congested. Whitish sheathing develops around the vessels.
- *Visual fields.* Concentric contraction of peripheral fields becomes apparent as atrophy sets in.

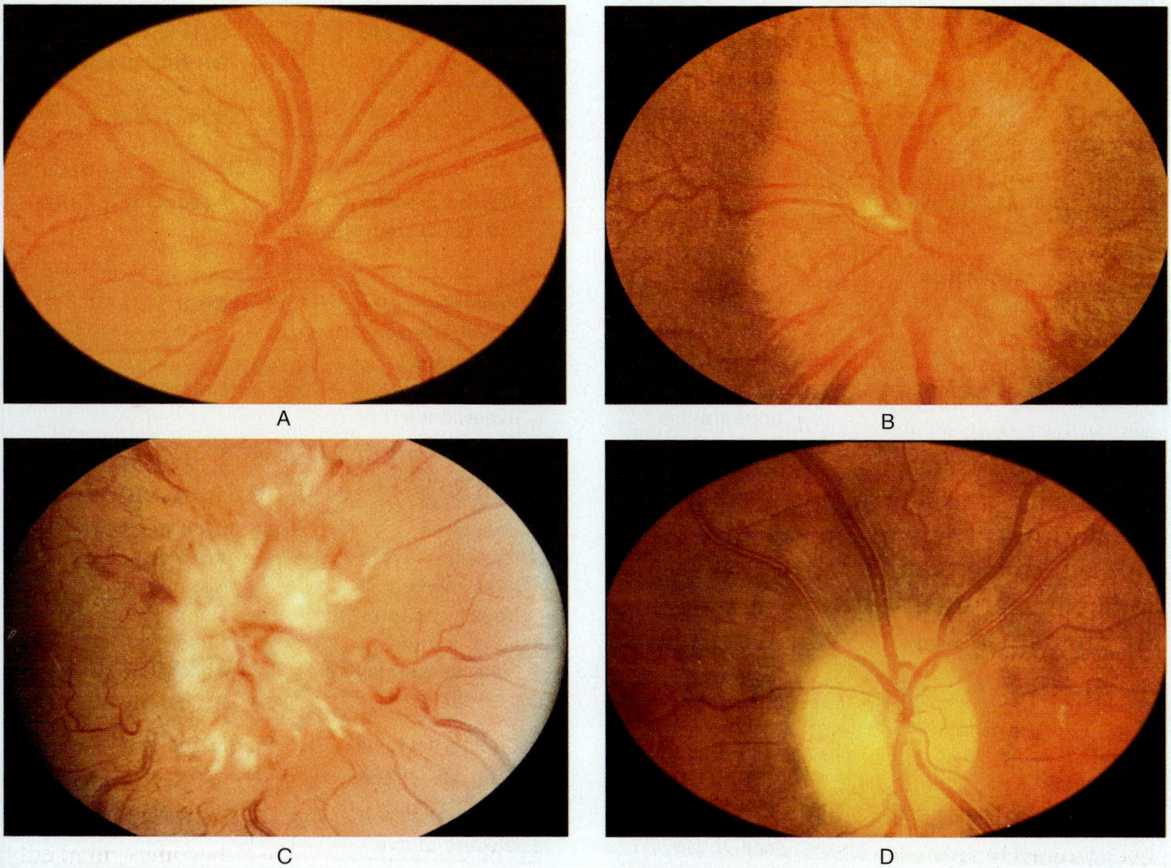

Fig. 12.11. Fundus photograph showing papilloedema: A, early; B, established; C, chronic; D, atrophic.

Differential diagnosis

Papilloedema should be differentiated from pseudopapilloedema and papillitis. *Pseudopapilloedema* is a non-specific term used to describe elevation of the disc similar to papilloedema, in conditions such as optic disc drusen, hypermetropia, and persistent hyaloid tissue. The differentiating points between papilloedema, papillitis and pseudopapilloedema (pseudopapillitis) due to hypermetropia are enumerated in Table 12.2.

Treatment and prognosis

Papilloedema is a neurological emergency and requires immediate hospitalisation. Urgent neuro imaging (CT scan or preferably MRI with a gladolinium enhancement) may reveal primary pathology. As a rule unless the causative disease is treatable or cerebral decompression is done, the course of papilloedema is chronic and ultimate visual prognosis is bad.

OPTIC ATROPHY

Optic atrophy refers to degeneration of the optic nerve, which occurs as an end result of any pathologic process that damages axons in the anterior visual system, i.e. from retinal ganglion cells to the lateral geniculate body.

Table 12.2. Differentiating features of papilloedema, papillitis and pseudopapillitis

Feature	*Papilloedema*	*Papillitis*	*Pseudopapillitis*
1. Laterality	Usually bilateral	Usually unilateral	May be unilateral or bilateral
2. Symptoms			
(i) Visual acuity	Transient attacks of blurred vision Later vision decreases due to optic atrophy	Marked loss of vision of sudden onset	Defective vision depending upon the degree of refractive error
(ii) Pain and tenderness	Absent	May be present with ocular movements	Absent
3. Fundus examination			
(i) Media	Clear	Posterior vitreous haze is common	Clear
(ii) Disc colour	Red and juicy appearance	Marked hyperaemia	Reddish
Disc margins	Blurred	Blurred	Not well defined
Disc swelling	2-6 dioptres	Usually not more than 3 dioptres	Depending upon the degree of hypermetropia
(iii) Peripapillary oedema	Present	Present	Absent
(iv) Venous engorgement	More marked	Less marked	Not present
(v) Retinal haemorrhages	Marked	Usually not present	Not present
(vi) Retinal exudates	More marked	Less marked	Absent
(vii) Macula	Macular star may be present	Macular fan may be present	Absent
4. Fields	Enlarged blind spot	Central scotoma more for colours	No defect
5. Fluorescein angiography	Vertical oval pool of dye due to leakage	Minimal leakage of dye	No leakage of dye

Classification

A. ***Primary versus secondary optic atrophy.*** It is customary to divide the optic atrophy into primary and secondary.

- *Primary optic atrophy* refers to the simple degeneration of the nerve fibres without any complicating process within the eye e.g., syphilitic optic atrophy of tabes dorsalis.
- *Secondary optic atrophy* occurs following any pathologic process which produces optic neuritis or papilloedema.

Recently, most of the authors have discarded the use of this time-honoured but non-informative classification. Further, such a classification is misleading since identical lesion at disc (e.g. papillitis in multiple sclerosis) will produce secondary optic atrophy and when involving optic nerve a little distance up (e.g. retrobulbar neuritis in multiple sclerosis) will produce an apparently primary optic atrophy.

B. ***Ophthalmoscopic classification.*** It is more useful to classify optic atrophy based on its ophthalmoscopic appearance. Common types are as follows:

1. Primary (simple) optic atrophy
2. Consecutive optic atrophy
3. Glaucomatous optic atrophy
4. Post-neuritic optic atrophy
5. Vascular (ischaemic) optic atrophy.

The etiology and salient features of each type will be considered separately.

C. ***Ascending versus descending optic atrophy.***

- *Ascending optic atrophy follows* damage to ganglion cells or nerve fibre layer due to diseases of the retina or optic disc. In it the nerve fibre degeneration progresses (ascends) from the eyeball towards the geniculate body.
- *Descending or retrograde optic atrophy proceeds* from the region of the optic tract, chiasma or posterior portion of the optic nerve towards the optic disc.

Pathological features

Degeneration of the optic nerve fibres is associated with attempted but unsuccessful regeneration which is characterised by proliferation of astrocytes and glial tissue. Ophthalmoscopic appearance of the atrophic optic disc depends upon the balance between loss of nerve tissue and gliosis. Following three situations may occur:

1. *Degeneration of the nerve fibres may be associated with excessive gliosis.* These changes are pathological features of the consecutive and postneuritic optic atrophy.
2. *Degeneration and gliosis may be orderly* and the proliferating astrocytes arrange themselves in longitudinal columns replacing the nerve fibres (columnar gliosis). Such pathological features are seen in primary optic atrophy.
3. *Degenration of the nerve fibres may be associated with negligible gliosis.* It occurs due to progressive decrease in blood supply. Such pathological changes are labelled as cavernous optic atrophy and are features of glaucomatous and ischaemic (vascular) optic atrophy.

Etiology

1. *Primary (simple) optic atrophy.* It results from the lesions proximal to the optic disc without antecedent papilloedema. Its common causes are: multiple sclerosis, retrobulbar neuritis (idiopathic), Leber's and other hereditary optic atrophies, intracranial tumours pressing directly on the anterior visual pathway (e.g. pituitary tumour), traumatic severance or avulsion of the optic nerve, toxic amblyopias (chronic retrobulbar neuritis) and tabes dorsalis.
2. *Consecutive optic atrophy.* It occurs following destruction of ganglion cells secondary to degenerative or inflammatory lesions of the choroid and/or retina. Its common causes are: diffuse chorioretinitis, retinal pigmentary dystrophies such as retinitis pigmentosa, pathological myopia and occlusion of central retinal artery.
3. *Postneuritic optic atrophy.* It develops as a sequelae to long-standing papilloedema or papillitis.
4. *Glaucomatous optic atrophy.* It results from the effect of long standing raised intraocular pressure.
5. *Vascular (ischaemic) optic atrophy.* It results from the conditions (other than glaucoma) producing disc ischaemia. These include: giant cell arteritis, severe haemorrhage, severe anaemia and quinine poisoning.

Clinical features of optic atrophy

1. *Loss of vision,* may be of sudden or gradual onset (depending upon the cause of optic

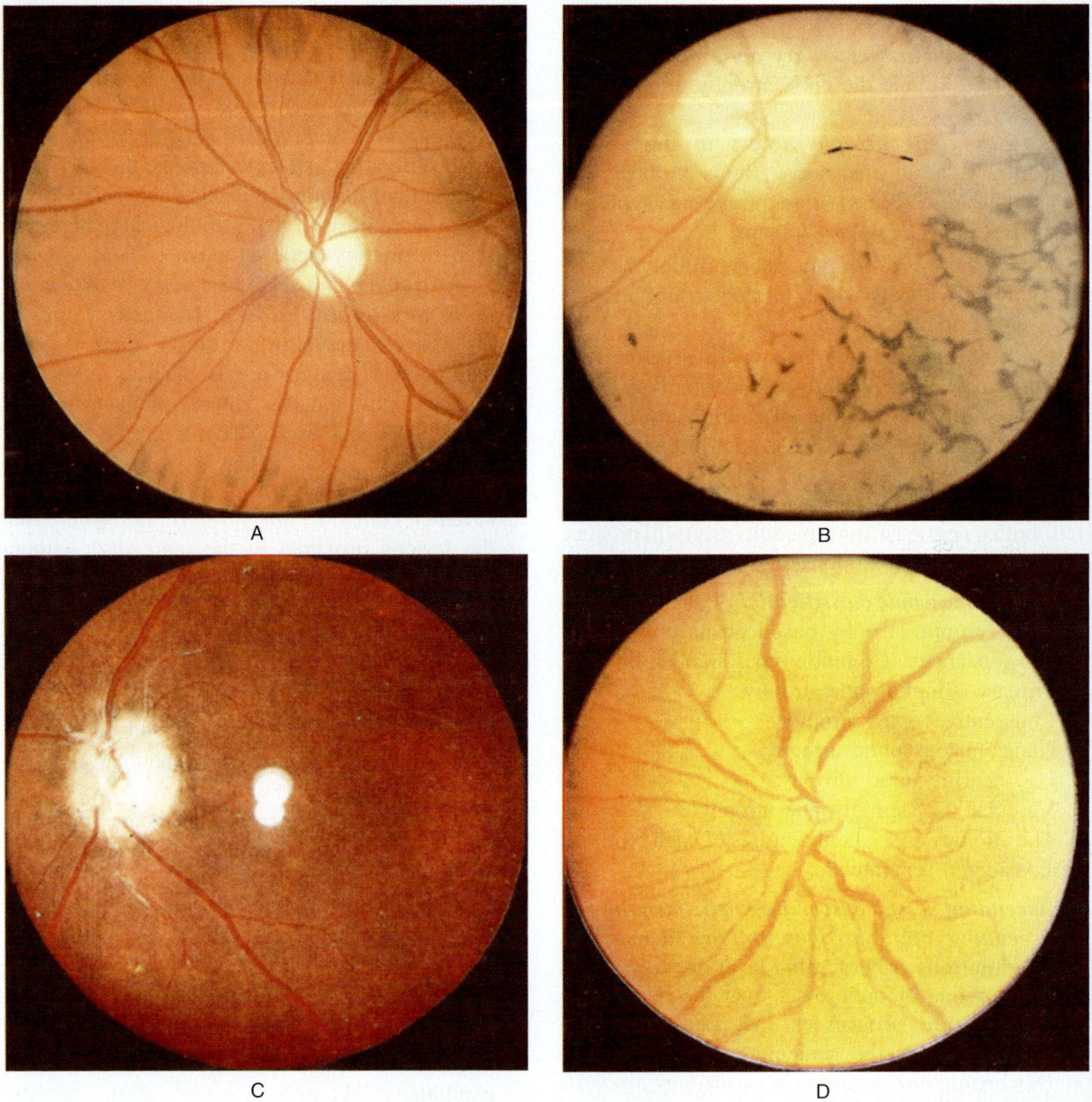

Fig. 12.12. Optic atrophy : A, primary; B, consecutive (in a patient with retinitis pigmentosa); C, postneuritic; D, ischaemic.

atrophy) and partial or total (depending upon the degree of atrophy). It is important to note that ophthalmoscopic signs cannot be correlated with the amount of vision.

2. *Pupil* is semidilated and direct light reflex is very sluggish or absent. Swinging flash light test depicts Marcus Gunn pupil (RAPD).
3. *Visual field loss* will vary with the distribution of the fibres that have been damaged. In general the field loss is peripheral in systemic infections, central in focal optic neuritis and eccentric when the nerve or tracts are compressed.
4. *Ophthalmoscopic appearance* of the disc will vary with the type of optic atrophy. However, ophthalmoscopic features of optic atrophy in general are pallor of the disc and decrease in the number of small blood vessels (Kastenbaum index). The pallor is not due to atrophy of the

nerve fibres but to loss of vasculature. Ophthalmoscopic features of different types of optic atrophy are as described below:

i. *Primary optic atrophy* (Fig. 12.12A). Colour of the disc is chalky white or white with bluish hue. Its edges (margins) are sharply outlined. Slight recession of the entire optic disc occurs in total atrophy. Lamina cribrosa is clearly seen at the bottom of the physiological cup. Major retinal vessels and surrounding retina are normal.
ii. *Consecutive optic atrophy* (Fig. 12.12B). Disc appears yellow waxy. Its edges are not so sharply defined as in primary optic atrophy. Retinal vessels are attenuated.
iii. *Post-neuritic optic atrophy* (Fig. 12.12C). Optic disc looks dirty white in colour. Due to gliosis its edges are blurred, physiological cup is obliterated and lamina cribrosa is not visible. Retinal vessels are attenuated and perivascular sheathing is often present.
iv. *Glaucomatous optic atrophy.* It is characterised by deep and wide cupping of the optic disc and nasal shift of the blood vessels (for details see page 231 and Fig. 9.10).
v. *Ischaemic optic atrophy.* Ophthalmoscopic features are pallor of the optic disc associated with marked attenuation of the vessels (Fig. 12.12D).

Differential diagnosis

Pallor of optic disc seen in partial optic atrophy must be differentiated from other causes of pallor disc which may be non-pathological and pathological.

1. *Non-pathological pallor of optic disc* is seen in: axial myopia, infants, and elderly people with sclerotic changes. Temporal pallor is associated with large physiological cup.
2. *Pathological causes of pallor disc* (other than optic atrophy) include hypoplasia, congenital pit, and coloboma.

Treatment

The underlying cause when treated may help in preserving some vision in patients with partial optic atrophy. However, once complete atrophy has set in, the vision cannot be recovered.

SYMPTOMATIC DISTURBANCES OF THE VISION

NIGHT BLINDNESS (NYCTALOPIA)

Night (scotopic) vision is a function of rods. Therefore, the conditions in which functioning of these nerve endings is deranged will result in night blindness. These include vitamin A deficiency, tapetoretinal degenerations (e.g., retinitis pigmentosa), congenital high myopia, familial congenital night blindness and Oguchi's disease. It may also develop in conditions of the ocular media interfering with the light rays in dim light (i.e. with dilated pupils). These include paracentral lenticular and corneal opacities. In advanced cases of primary open angle glaucoma, dark adaptation may be so much delayed that patient gives history of night blindness.

DAY BLINDNESS (HAMARLOPIA)

It is a symptomatic disturbance of the vision, in which the patient is able to see better in dimlight as compared to bright light of the day. Its causes are:

- Congenital deficiency of cones
- Central lenticular opacities (polar cataracts) and
- Central corneal opacities.

COLOUR BLINDNESS

An individual with normal colour vision is known as *trichromate*. In colour blindness, mechanism to appreciate one or more primary colours is either defective (anomalous) or absent (anopia). It may be congenital or acquired.

A. Congenital Colour Blindness.

It is an inherited condition affecting males more (3-4%) than females (0.4%). It may be of the following types:

- Dyschromatopsia
- Achromatopsia

1. Dyschromatopsia

Dyschromatopsia, literally means colour confusion due to deficiency of mechanism to perceive colours. It can be classified into:

- Anomalous trichromatsy
- Dichromatsy

- Blue cone monochromatism

a. ***Anomalous trichromatic colour vision.*** Here the mechanism to appreciate all the three primary colours is present but is defective for one or two of them. It may be of following types:

- *Protanomalous.* It refers to defective red colour appreciation.
- *Deuteranomalous.* It means defective green colour appreciation.
- *Tritanomalous.* It implies defective blue colour appreciation.

b. ***Dichromatic colour vision.*** In this conditon faculty to perceive one of the three primary colours is completely absent. Such individuals are called *dichromates* and may have one of the following types of defects:

- *Protanopia,* i.e., complete red colour defect.
- *Deuteranopia,* i.e., complete defect for green colour.
- *Tritanopia,* i.e., absence of blue colour appreciation.

Red-green deficiency (protanomalous, protanopia, deuteranomalous and deuteranopia) is more common. Such a defect is a source of danger in certain occupations such as drivers, sailors and traffic police. Blue deficiency (tritanomalous and tritanopia) is comparatively rare.

c. ***Blue cone monochromatism*** (BCM). It is a condition of complete absence of red and green cone function. It is characterised by:

- Poor day vision but normal night vision,
- Colour vision severely limited, only differences in blue hues are detectable,
- Reduced visual acuity (6/24 to 6/6),
- Small amplitude nystagmus, and
- Photosensitivity.

2. Achromatopsia

It is an extremely rare condition presenting as rod monochromatism.

Rod monochromatism may be complete or incomplete. It is inherited as an autosomal recessive trait affecting both sexes equally. It is characterized by:

- Total colour blindness,
- Day blindness (visual acuity is about 6/60),
- Nystagmus,
- Fundus is usually normal.

B. Acquired Colour Blindness.

It may follow damage to macula or optic nerve, Usually, it is associated with a central scotoma or decreased visual acuity.

- *Blue-yellow impairment* is seen in retinal lesions such as CSR, macular oedema and shallow retinal detachment.
- *Red-green deficiency* is seen in optic nerve lesions such as optic neuritis, Leber's optic atrophy and compression of the optic nerve.
- *Acquired blue colour defect* (blue blindness) may occur in old age due to increased sclerosis of the crystalline lens. It is owing to the physical absorption of the blue rays by the increased amber coloured pigment in the nucleus.

Tests for Colour Vision

These tests are designed for : (1) Screening defective colour vision from normal; (2) Qualitative classification of colour blindness i.e., protans, deuteran and tritan; and (3) Quantitative analysis of degree of deficiency i.e., mild, moderate or marked.

Commonly employed colour vision tests are as follows:

1. *Pseudo-isochromatic charts.* It is the most commonly employed test using Ishihara's plates (Fig. 12.13). In this there are patterns of coloured and grey dots which reveal one pattern to the normal individuals and another to the colour deficients. It is a quick method of screening colour blinds from the normals. Another test based on the same principle are:

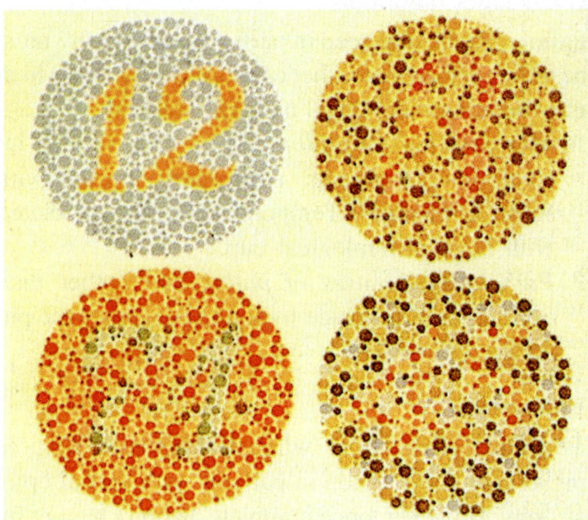

Fig. 12.13. Ishihara's pseudo-isochromatic chart.

- Hardy-Rand-Rittler plates (HRR), and
- American optical colour plate test

2. *Edridge-Green lantern test.* In this test the subject has to name the various colours shown to him by a lantern and the judgement is made by the mistake he makes.
3. *Farnsworth-Munsell 100 hue test.* It is a spectroscopic test in which subject has to arrange the coloured chips in ascending order. The colour vision is judged by the error score, i.e. greater the score poorer the colour vision.
4. *City university colour vision test.* It is also a spectroscopic test where a central coloured plate is to be matched to its closest hue from four surrounding colour plates.
5. *Nagel's anomaloscope.* In this test the observer is asked to mix red and green colour in such a proportion that the mixture should match the given yellow coloured disc. The judgement about the defect is made from the relative amount of red and green colours and the brightness setting used by the observer.
6. *Holmgren's wools test.* In this the subject is asked to make a series of colour-matches from a selection of skeins of coloured wools.

AMAUROSIS

It implies complete loss of sight in one or both eyes, in the absence of ophthalmoscopic or other marked objective signs.

1. Amaurosis fugax

It refers to a sudden, temporary and painless monocular visual loss occurring due to a transient failure of retinal circulation.

Common causes of amaurosis fugax are: carotid transient ischaemic attacks (TIA), embolization of retinal circulation, papilloedema, giant cell arteritis, Raynaud's disease, migraine, as a prodromal symptom of central retinal artery or carotid artery occlusion, hypertensive retinopathy, and venous stasis retinopathy. An attack of amaurosis fugax is typically described by the patients as a curtain that descends from above or ascends from below to occupy the upper or lower halves of their visual fields.

Clinical characteristics. The attack lasts for two to five minutes and resolves in the reverse pattern of progression, leaving no residual deficit. Due to brief duration of the attack, it is rarely possible to observe the fundus. When observed shortly after an attack, the fundus may either be normal or reveal signs of retinal ischaemia such as retinal oedema and small superficial haemorrhages. In some cases, retinal emboli in the form of white plugs (fibrin-platelet aggregates) may be seen.

2. Uraemic amaurosis

It is a sudden, bilateral, complete loss of sight occurring probably due to the effect of certain toxic materials upon the cells of the visual centre in patients suffering from acute nephritis, eclampsia of pregnancy and renal failure. The visual loss is associated with dilated pupils which generally react to light. The fundi are usually normal except for the coincidental findings of hypertensive retinopathy, when associated. Usually, the vision recovers in 12-48 hours.

AMBLYOPIA

It implies a partial loss of sight in one or both eyes, in the absence of ophthalmoscopic or other marked objective signs. It may be either congenital or acquired. Acquired amblyopia may be organic (toxic amblyopia; page 316) or functional.

Functional amblyopia results from the psychical suppression of the retinal image. It may be anisometropic, strabismic or due to stimulus deprivation (amblyopia ex anopsia) (see page 339).

CORTICAL BLINDNESS

Cortical blindness (visual cortex disease) is produced by bilateral occipital lobe lesions. Unilateral occipital lobe lesions typically produce contralateral macular sparing congruous homonymous hemianopia.

Causes of cortical blindness include:

- *Vascular lesions* producing bilateral occipital infarction are the commonest cause of cortical blindness (e.g., embolisation of posterior cerebral arteries).
- *Head injury* involving bilateral occipital lobes is the second common cause.
- *Tumours,* primary (e.g., falcotentorial meningiomas, bilateral gliomas) or metastatic are rare causes.
- *Other rare causes* of cortical blindness are migraine, hypoxic encephalopathy, Schilder's disease and other leukodystrophies.

Clinical features. Cortical blindness is characterized by:

- Bilateral loss of vision,
- Normal pupillary light reflexes,
- Visual imagination and visual imagery in dream are preserved
- *Anton syndrome* i.e., denial of blindness by the patients who obviously cannot see.
- *Riddoch phenomenon* i.e., ability to perceive kinetic but not static targets.

Management. A thorough neurological and cardiovascular investigative workup including MRI and MRI angiography should be carried out. Treatment depends upon the underlying cause. Partial or complete recovery may occur in patients with stroke progressing from cortical blindness through visual agnosia, and partially impaired perceptual function to recovery.

MALINGERING

In malingering a person poses to be visually defective, while he is not. The person may do so to gain some undue advantage or compensation. Usually, one eye is said to be blind which does not show any objective sign. Rarely, a person pretends to be completely blind. In such cases, a constant watch over the behaviour may settle the issue.

Differential diagnosis

Before diagnosing malingering following conditions (which produce visual loss with apparantly normal anterior segment and a normal fundus) should be ruled out:

1. *Amblyopia.* Many a time an individual may suddenly notice poor vision in one eye though the onset is usually in early childhood. It is important to identify an amblyogenic factor (see page 339).

2. *Cortical blindness* must be ruled out from its characteristic features (see page 327).

3. *Retrobulbar neuritis* a common cause of visual loss with normal fundus. Presence of a definite or relative afferent pupillary defect (RAPD) and VER are diagnostic.

4. *Cone rod dystrophy* is characterized by a positive family history, photophobia in bright light, abnormal dark adaptation and abnormal cone dystrophy electroretinogram.

5. *Chiasmal tumours* may sometimes present with visual loss and normal fundus (before the onset of optic atrophy). Sluggish pupillary reactions to light with characteristic visual field defects may be noted.

Tests for malingering

1. *Convex lens test.* Place a low convex or concave lens (0.25 D) before the blind eye and a high convex lens (+10 D) before the good eye. If the patient can read distant words, malingering is proved.
2. *Prism base down test.* Place a prism with its base downwards before the good eye and tell the person to look at a light source. If the patient admits seeing two lights, it confirms malingering.
3. *Prism base out test.* Ask the patient to look at a light source. Then a prism of 10 D is placed before the alleged blind eye with its base outwards. If the eye moves inwards (to eliminate diplopia) malingering is proved.
4. *Snellen's coloured types test.* It has letters printed in red and green. Place a red glass before the good eye. If the person can read all the letters, it confirms malingering because, normally one can see only red letters through red glass.

HYSTERICAL BLINDNESS

It is a form of psychoneurosis, commonly seen in attention-seeking personalities, especially females. ***Characteristic features*** include:

- *Sudden bilateral* loss of vision (cf. malingering). The patient otherwise shows little concern for the symptoms and negotiates well with the surroundings (c.f. malingering).
- *Blepharospasm* and lacrimation may be associated.
- *Pupillary responses* are essentially normal and so is the blink response.
- *Optokinetic nystagmus* is intact.
- *Visual fields* are concentrically contracted. One can commonly find spiral fields as the target moves closer to the fixation point.

Treatment includes psychological support and reassurance. Placebo tablets may also be helpful. A psychiatrist's help should be sought for, if these fail.

DISORDERS OF HIGHER VISUAL FUNCTIONS

Visual agnosia

Definition. Visual agnosia refers to a rare disorder in which ability to recognise the objects by sight (despite adequate visual acuity) is impaired while the ability to recognize by touch, smell or sound is retained.

Types of visual agnosia include:

- *Prosopagnosia.* In this patient cannot recognize familiar faces.
- *Object agnosia.* In this patient is not able to name and indicate the use of a seen object by spoken or written words or by gestures.

Site of lesion in visual agnosia is bilateral inferior (ventromedial) occipitotemporal junction.

Associated features include:

- *Bilateral homonymous hemianopia.*
- *Dyschromatopsia (disturbance of colour vision).*

Visual hallucinations

Visual hallucinations refer to the conditions in which patient alleges of seeing something that is not evident to others in the same environment.

Types. Visual hallucinations are of two types:

- *Elementary (unformed) hallucinations* include flashes of light, colours, luminous points, stars, multiple lights and geometric forms. They may be stationary or moving.
- *Complex (formed) hallucinations* include objects, persons or animals.

Causes of visual hallucinations include:

- *Occipital and temporal lobe lesions.* Elementary hallucinations are considered to have their origin in the occipital cortex and complex ones in the temporal cortex.
- *Drug induced.* Many drugs acting on the CNS in high doses are hallucinogenic.
- *Bilateral visual loss* in elderly individuals may be associated with formed hallucinations (Charles Bonnet syndrome).
- *Migraine* is a common cause of unformed hallucinations.
- *Optic nerve diseases* and *vitreous traction* are reported to produce unformed hallucinations.
- *Psychiatric disorders* are not the causes of isolated visual hallucinations.

Alexia and agraphia

Alexia means the inability to read (despite good vision). It is commonly associated with *agraphia* (inability to write).

Causes. *Alexia associated with agraphia* is produced by lesions of the angulate gyrus of the dominant hemisphere.

Alexia without agraphia is usually caused by lesions that destroy the visual pathway in the left occipital lobe and also interrupt the association fibres from the right occipital lobe that have crossed in the splenium of corpus callosum.

Visual illusions

In visual illusions patients perceive distortions in form, size, movement or colour of the objects seen. Some of the visual illusions are:

- *Palinopsia* (visual perservation) is an illusion whereby the patient continues to perceive an image after the actual object is no longer in view.
- *Optic anaesthesia* refers to false orientation of objects in space.
- *Cerebral dyschromotopsia* may occur as disappearance of colour (achromatopsia) or illusional colouring (e.g., erythropsia).
- *Cerebral diplopia or polyopia* are also reported to occur as rare symptoms of central nervous system disease.

Causes. Visual illusions are reported to occur in lesions of the occipital, occipitoparietal or occipitotemporal regions, and right hemisphere appears to be involved more often than the left.

OCULAR MANIFESTATIONS OF DISEASES OF CENTRAL NERVOUS SYSTEM

Ocular involvement in diseases of the central nervous system is not infrequent. A few common ocular lesions of these diseases are mentioned here.

INTRACRANIAL INFECTIONS

These include meningitis, encephalitis, brain abscess and neurosyphilis.

1. *Meningitis.* It may be complicated by papillitis, and paralysis of third, fourth and sixth cranial nerves. Chronic chiasmal arachnoiditis may produce bilateral optic atrophy. Tuberculous meningitis may be associated with choroidal tubercles.
2. *Encephalitis.* It may be complicated by papillitis and/or papilloedema. Cranial nerve palsies are

usually incomplete. Diplopia and ptosis are often present.

3. *Brain abscess.* It is frequently associated with papilloedema. Focal signs depend upon the site of the abscess, and are thus similar to tumours.
4. *Neurosyphilis.* Ocular involvement is quite frequent. Gummatous meningitis may be associated with papillitis, papilloedema or postneuritic optic atrophy and cranial nerve palsies. Third nerve is paralysed in nearly 30 per cent cases, less frequently the fifth and sixth, and least frequently the fourth. Tabes dorsalis and generalised paralysis of insane may be associated with primary optic atrophy, Argyll Robertson pupil, and internal and/or external ophthalmoplegia.

INTRACRANIAL ANEURYSMS

Intracranial aneurysms associated with ocular manifestations are located around the circle of Willis Intracranial aneurysms may produce complications by following mechanisms:

1. *Pressure effects* are as follows:

i. *Aneurysms of circle of Willis and internal carotid artery* (supraclenoid, infraclenoid i.e., intracavernous, and anterior communicating artery) may produce following pressure effects:

- *Central and peripheral visual loss* due to pressure on intracranial part of optic nerve and chiasma.
- *Slowly progressive ophthalmoplegia*, due to pressure, on motor nerves in the cavernous sinus.
- *Facial pain and paraesthesia* associated with corneal anaesthesia due to pressure on the branches of trigeminal nerve.
- *Horner's syndrome* due to pressure on sympathetic fibres along the carotid artery.

ii. *Posterior communicating artery aneurysm* typically presents with isolated painful third nerve palsy.

iii. *Vertebrobasilar artery aneurysms* may also be associated with third nerve palsy.

2. *Production of arteriolar venous fistula.* Carotid-cavernous fistula may be produced by rupture of a giant aneurysm of the intracavernous part of the internal carotid artery. *Pulsating exophthalmos* is a typical presentation of carotid-cavernous fistula.

3. *Subarachnoid haemorrhage.* Subarachnoid haemorrhage is a life-threatening complication associated with sudden rupture of aneurysm of the circle of Willis. It is characterized by:

- Sudden violent headache.
- Third nerve palsy with pupillary dilatation.
- Photophobia, signs of meningial irritation, vomiting and unconsiousness.
- *Terson syndrome* refers to the combination of bilateral intraocular haemorrhages (intraretinal, subhyaloid and vitreous haemorrhage) and subarachnoid haemorrhage due to aneurysmal rupture.

INTRACRANIAL HAEMORRHAGES

Ophthalmic signs of *intracerebral haemorrhage* are tonic conjugate and dysconjugate deviations. *Subarachnoid haemorrhage* may produce retinal haemorrhages (especially subhyaloid haemorrhage of the posterior pole), papilloedema, and ocular palsies.

INTRACRANIAL SPACE-OCCUPYING LESIONS (ICSOLS)

These include primary and secondary brain tumours, haematomas, granulomatous inflammations and parasitic cysts. Clinical features of the ICSOLs may be described under three heads:

I. *General effects of raised intracranial pressure*. These include headache, vomiting, papilloedema, drowsiness, giddiness, slowing of pulse rate and rise in blood pressure.

II. *False localising signs.* These occur due to the effect of raised intracranial pressure and displacement or distortion of the brain tissue. False localising signs of ophthalmological interest are as follows:

1. *Diplopia:* It occurs due to pressure palsy of the sixth nerve.
2. *Sluggish pupillary reflexes and unilateral mydriasis* may occur due to pressure on the 3rd nerve.
3. *Bitemporal hemianopia:* It results from downward pressure of the distended third ventricle on the chiasma.
4. *Homonymous hemianopia:* It may result from occipital herniation through the tentorium cerebelli with compression of the posterior cerebral artery.

III. *Focal signs of intracranial mass lesions.* These depend upon the site of the lesion. Focal signs of ophthalmological interest are as follows:

1. *Prefrontal tumours,* particularly meningioma of the olfactory groove, are associated with a pressure atrophy of the optic nerve on the side of lesion and papilloedema on the other side due to raised intracranial pressure (Foster-Kennedy syndrome).
2. *Temporal lobe tumours.* These may produce incongruous *crossed upper quadrantanopia* due to pressure on the optic radiations. *Visual hallucinations* may occur owing to irritation of the visuo-psychic area. Third and fifth cranial nerves may be involved due to downward pressure. Impairment of convergence and of superior conjugate movements may occur in late stages due to prolapse of the uncus through the tentorium cerebelli into the posterior fossa, with resulting distortion of the ventral part of midbrain.
3. *Parietal lobe tumours.* These are associated with crossed lower homonymous quadrantanopia due to involvement of the upper fibres of the optic radiations. Other lesions include visual and auditory hallucinations, conjugate deviations of the eyes and optokinetic nystagmus.
4. *Occipital lobe tumours.* These may produce crossed homonymous quadrantic or hemianopic defect involving the fixation point. Visual agnosia may also be associated.
5. *Mid-brain tumours.* These may be associated with homonymous hemianopia due to pressure on the optic tracts. Other signs depending upon the site of involvement are as follows:
   i. *Tumours of the upper part* produce spasmodic contraction of the upper lid followed by ptosis and loss of upward conjugate movements. In about 25 percent cases, an upper motor neuron facial paralysis and ipsilateral hemiplegia may also develop.
   ii. *Tumours of the intermediate level* may be associated with the following syndromes: (i) *Weber's syndrome.* It is characterised by ipsilateral third nerve palsy, contralateral hemiplegia and facial palsy of upper motor neuron type. (ii) *Benedikt's syndrome.* It is characterised by ipsilateral third nerve palsy associated with tremors and jerky movements of the contralateral side which occur due to involvement of the red nucleus.
6. *Tumours of the pons.* Lesions in the upper part are characterised by ipsilateral third nerve palsy, contralateral hemiplegia and upper motor neuron type facial palsy. While the lesions in the lower part of the pons produce *Millard-Gubler syndrome* which consists of ipsilateral sixth nerve palsy, contralateral hemiplegia and ipsilateral facial palsy; or *Foville's syndrome* is which sixth nerve paralysis is replaced by a loss of conjugate movements to the same side.
7. *Cerebellar tumours.* Those arising from the cerebellopontine angle produce *corneal anaesthesia* due to involvement of fifth nerve, early deafness and tinnitis of one side, sixth and seventh cranial nerve paralysis, cerebellar symptoms such as ataxia and vertigo, marked papilloedema and nystagmus.
8. *Chiasmal and pituitary tumours.* These include: pituitary adenomas, craniopharyngiomas and suprasellar meningiomas. These tumours typically produce *chiasmal syndrome* which is characterised by bitemporal visual field defects, optic atrophy and sometimes endocrinal disturbances.

DEMYELINATING DISEASES

These include multiple sclerosis, neuromyelitis optica and diffuse sclerosis. Ocular involvement may occur in all these conditions. Their salient features are as follows:

Multiple sclerosis

It is a demyelinating disorder of unknown etiology, affecting women more often than men, usually in the 15-50 years age group. Pathologically, the condition is characterised by a patchy destruction of the myelin sheaths throughout the central nervous system. Clinical course of the condition is marked by remissions and relapses. In this condition, optic neuritis is usually unilateral (see page 314). Other ocular lesions include internuclear ophthalmoplegia and vestibular or cerebellar nystagmus.

Neuromyelitis optica (Devic's disease)

It is characterised by bilateral optic neuritis associated with ascending myelitis, entailing a progressive quadriplegia and anaesthesia. Unlike multiple sclerosis, this condition is not characterised by remissions and is not associated with ocular palsies and nystagmus.

Diffuse sclerosis (Schilder's disease)
It typically affects children and adolescents and is characterised by progressive demyelination of the entire white matter of the cerebral hemispheres. *Ocular lesions* include: optic neuritis (papillitis or retrobulbar neuritis), cortical blindness (due to destruction of the visual centres and optic radiations), ophthalmoplegia and nystagmus.

OCULAR SIGNS IN HEAD INJURY

Ocular signs related only to the intracranial damage are described here. However, direct trauma to the eyeball and/or orbit is frequently associated with the head injury. Lesions of direct ocular trauma are described in the chapter on ocular injuries (pages 401-414).

A. Concussion injuries to the brain

These are usually associated with subdural haemorrhage and unconsciousness which may produce the following ocular signs:

1. *Hutchinson's pupil.* It is characterised by initial ipsilateral miosis followed by dilatation with no light reflex due to raised intracranial pressure. If the pressure rises still further, similar changes occur in the contralateral pupil. Therefore, presence of bilateral fixed and dilated pupils is an indication of immediate cerebral decompression.

2. *Papilloedema.* When it appears within 48 hours of the trauma, it indicates extra or intracerebral haemorrhage and is an indication for immediate surgical measures. While the papilloedema appearing after a week of head injury is usually due to cerebral oedema.

B. Fractures of the base of skull

Associated ocular signs are as follows:
1. *Cranial nerve palsies.* These are often seen with fractures of the base of the skull; most common being the ipsilateral facial paralysis of the lower motor neuron type. Extraocular muscle palsies due to involvement of sixth, third and fourth cranial nerves may also be seen.
2. *Optic nerve injury.* It may be injured directly, indirectly or compressed by the haemorrhage. Primary optic atrophy may appear in 2-4 weeks following injury. Presence of papilloedema suggests haemorrhage into the nerve sheath.
3. *Subconjunctival haemorrhage.* It may be seen when fracture of the base of skull is associated with fractures of the orbital roof. The subconjunctival haemorrhage is usually more marked in the upper quadrant and its posterior limit cannot be reached.
4. *Pupillary signs.* These are inconsistent and thus not pathognomic. However, usually pupil is dilated on the affected side.

13

CHAPTER

Disorders of Ocular Motility

ANATOMY AND PHYSIOLOGY OF THE OCULAR MOTILITY SYSTEM

EXTRAOCULAR MUSCLES

A set of six extraocular muscles (4 recti and 2 obliques) control the movements of each eye (Fig. 13.1). Rectus muscles are superior (SR), inferior (IR), medial (MR) and lateral (LR). The oblique muscles include superior (SO) and inferior (IO).

Origin and insertion

The rectus muscles originate from a common tendinous ring (the annulus of Zinn), which is attached at the apex of the orbit, encircling the optic foramina and medial part of the superior orbital fissure (Fig. 13.2). Medial rectus arises from the medial part of the ring, superior rectus from the superior part and also the adjoining dura covering the optic nerve, inferior rectus from the inferior part and lateral rectus from the lateral part by two heads which join in a 'V' form.

All the four recti run forward around the eyeball and are inserted into the sclera, by flat tendons (about 10-mm broad) at different distances from the limbus as under (Fig. 13.3):

- Medial rectus : 5.5 mm
- Inferior rectus : 6.5 mm
- Lateral rectus : 6.9 mm
- Superior rectus : 7.7 mm

The superior oblique muscle arises from the bone above and medial to the optic foramina. It runs forward and turns around a pulley — '*the trochlea*' (present in the anterior part of the superomedial angle of the orbit) and is inserted in the upper and outer part of the sclera behind the equator (Fig. 13.3C).

The inferior oblique muscle arises by a rounded tendon from the orbital plate of maxilla just lateral to the orifice of the nasolacrimal duct. It passes laterally and backward to be inserted into the lower and outer part of the sclera behind the equator (Fig. 13.3C).

Nerve supply

The extraocular muscles are supplied by third, fourth and sixth cranial nerves.

- *Third cranial nerve* (oculomotor) supplies the superior, medial and inferior recti and inferior oblique muscles.
- *Fourth cranial nerve* (trochlear) supplies the superior oblique, and

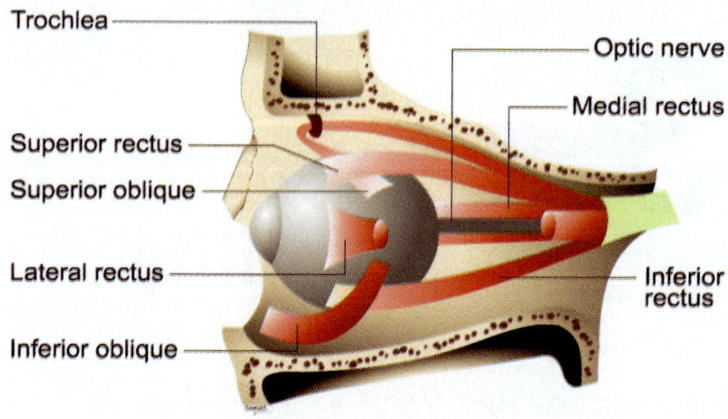

Fig. 13.1. Extraocular muscles.

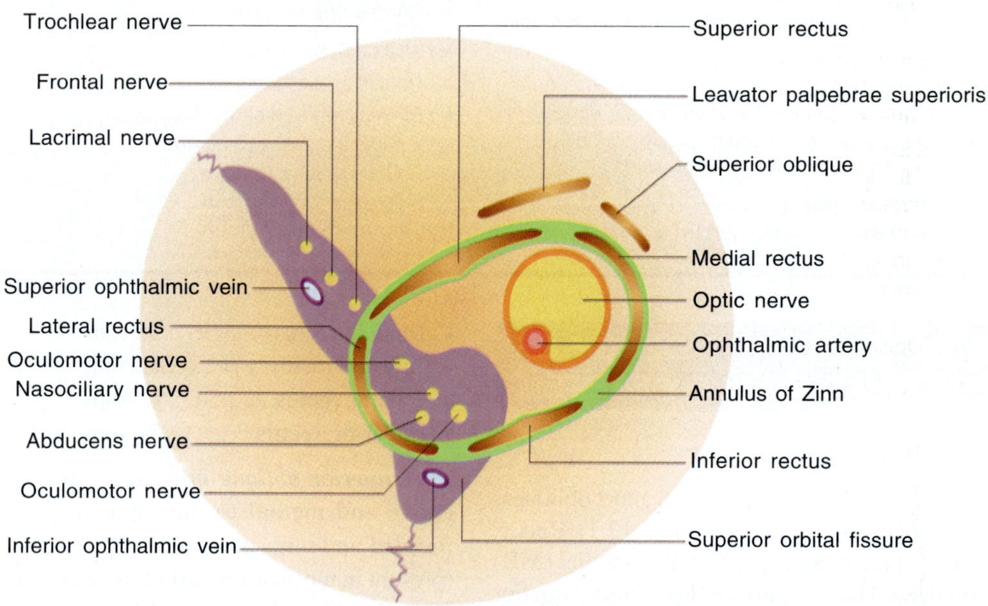

Fig. 13.2. Origin of the rectus muscles and the superior oblique muscle.

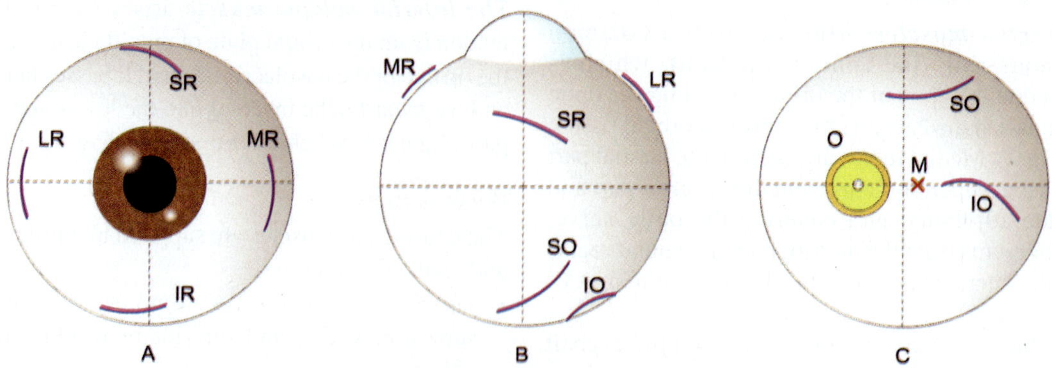

Fig. 13.3. Insertion lines of the extraocular muscles on the sclera as seen from: A, front; B, above; C, behind. SR, superior rectus; MR, medial rectus; IR, inferior rectus; LR, lateral rectus; SO, superior oblique; IO, inferior oblique.

- *Sixth nerve* (abducent) supplies the lateral rectus muscle.

Actions

The extraocular muscles rotate the eyeball around vertical, horizontal and antero-posterior axes. Medial and lateral rectus muscles are almost parallel to the optical axis of the eyeball; so they have got only the main action. While superior and inferior rectus muscles make an angle of 23° (Fig. 13.4) and reflected tendons of the superior and inferior oblique muscles of 51° (Fig. 13.5) with the optical axis in the primary position; so they have subsidiary actions in addition to the main action. Actions of each muscle (Fig. 13.6) are shown in Table 13.1.

Table 13.1. Actions of extraocular muscles

Muscle	*Primary action*	*Secondary action*	*Tertiary action*
MR	Adduction	—	—
LR	Abduction	—	—
SR	Elevation	Intorsion	Adduction
IR	Depression	Extorsion	Adduction
SO	Intorsion	Depression	Abduction
IO	Extorsion	Elevation	Abduction

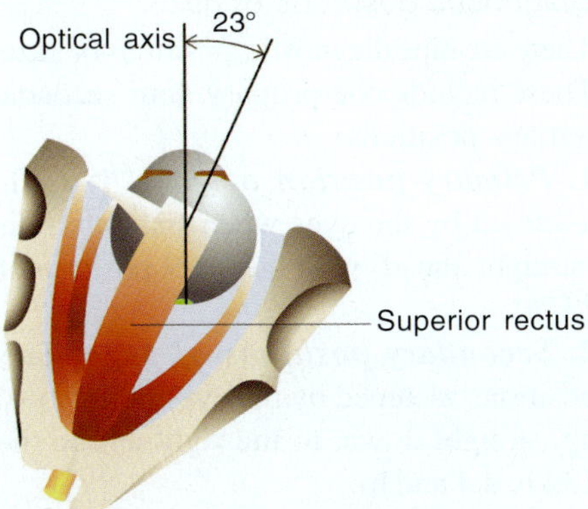

Fig. 13.4. Relation of the superior and inferior rectus muscles with the optical axis in primary position.

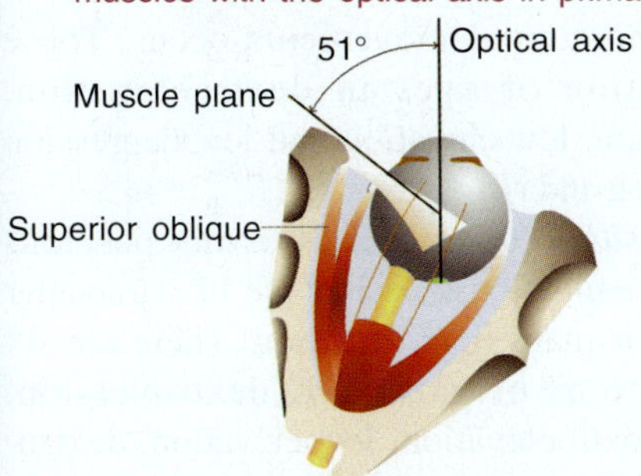

Fig. 13.5. Relation of the superior and inferior oblique muscles with the optical axis in primary position.

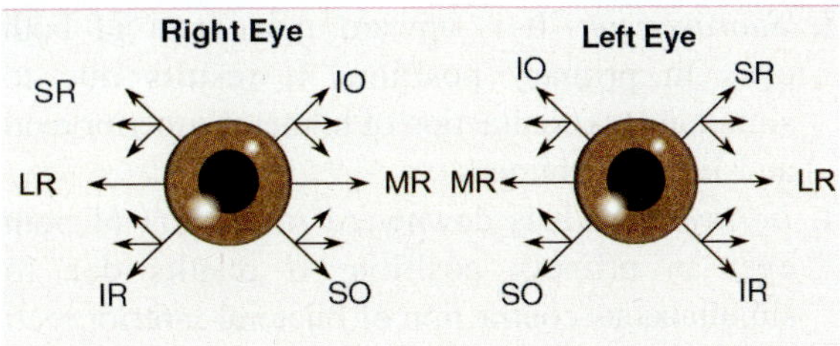

Fig. 13.6. Action of the extraocular muscles, SR (superior rectus); MR (medial rectus); IR (inferior rectus); SO (superior oblique); LR (lateral rectus); IO (inferior oblique).

OCULAR MOTILITY

Types of ocular movements

A. *Uniocular movements* are called 'ductions' and include the following:

1. *Adduction.* It is inward movement (medial rotation) along the vertical axis.
2. *Abduction.* It is outward movement (lateral rotation) along the vertical axis.
3. *Supraduction.* It is upward movement (elevation) along the horizontal axis.
4. *Infraduction.* It is downward movement (depression) along the horizontal axis.
5. *Incycloduction* (intorsion). It is a rotatory movement along the anteroposterior axis in which superior pole of the cornea (12 O'clock point) moves medially.
6. *Excycloduction* (extorsion). It is a rotatory movement along the anteroposterior axis in which superior pole of the cornea (12 O'clock point) moves laterally.

B. *Binocular movements*. These are of two types: versions and vergences.

a. *Versions,* also known as *conjugate movements*, are synchronous (simultaneous) symmetric movements of both eyes in the same direction. These include:

1. *Dextroversion.* It is the movement of both eyes to the right. It results due to simultaneous contraction of right lateral rectus and left medial rectus.
2. *Levoversion.* It refers to movement of both eyes to the left. It is produced by simultaneous contraction of left lateral rectus and right medial rectus.

3. *Supraversion.* It is upward movement of both eyes in primary position. It results due to simultaneous contraction of bilateral superior recti and inferior obliques.
4. *Infraversion.* It is downward movement of both eyes in primary position. It results due to simultaneous contraction of bilateral inferior recti and superior obliques.
5. *Dextrocycloversion.* It is rotational movement around the anteroposterior axis, in which superior pole of cornea of both the eyes tilts towards the right.
6. *Levocycloversion.* It is just the reverse of dextro-cycloversion. In this superior pole of cornea of both the eyes tilts towards the left.

b. *Vergences,* also called *disjugate movements*, are synchronous and symmetric movements of both eyes in opposite directions e.g.:

1. *Convergence.* It is simultaneous inward movement of both eyes which results from contraction of the medial recti.
2. *Divergence.* It is simultaneous outward movement of both eyes produced by contraction of the lateral recti.

Synergists, antagonists and yoke muscles

1. *Synergists.* It refers to the muscles having similar primary action in the same eye; e.g., superior rectus and inferior oblique of the same eye act as synergistic elevators.

2. *Antagonists.* These are the muscles having opposite actions in the same eye. For example, medial and lateral recti, superior and inferior recti and superior and inferior obliques are antagonists to each other in the same eye.

3. *Yoke muscles* (contralateral synergists). It refers to the pair of muscles (one from each eye) which contract simultaneously during version movements. For example, right lateral rectus and left medial rectus act as yoke muscles for dextroversion movements. Other pairs of yoke muscles are: right MR and left LR, right LR and left MR, right SR and left IO, right IR and left SO, right SO and left IR and right IO and left SR.

4. *Contralateral antagonists.* These are a pair of muscles (one from each eye) having opposite action; for example, right LR and left LR, right MR and left MR.

Laws governing ocular movements

1. *Hering's law of equal innervation.* According to law an equal and simultaneous innervation flows from the brain to a pair of muscles which contract simultaneously (yoke muscles) in different binocular movements, e.g.:

i) *During dextroversion*: right lateral rectus and left medial rectus muscles receive an equal and simultaneous flow of innervation.
ii) *During convergence*, both medial recti get equal innervation.
iii) *During dextroelevation*, right superior rectus and left inferior oblique receive equal and simultaneous innervation.

2. *Sherrington's law of reciprocal innervation*. According to it, during ocular motility increased flow of innervation to the contracting muscle is accompanied by decreased flow of innervation to the relaxing antagonist muscle. For example, during dextroversion, an increased innervation flow to the right LR and left MR is accompanied by decreased flow to the right MR and left LR muscles.

Diagnostic positions of gaze

There are nine diagnostic positions of gaze (Fig. 13.7). These include one primary, four secondary and four tertiary positions.

1. *Primary position of gaze.* It is the position assumed by the eyes when fixating a distant object (straight ahead) with the erect position of head (Fig. 13.7e).

2. *Secondary positions of gaze.* These are the positions assumed by the eyes while looking straight up, straight down, to the right and to the left (Figs. 13.7b, d, f and h).

3. *Tertiary positions of gaze.* These describe the positions assumed by the eyes when combination of vertical and horizontal movements occur. These include position of eyes in dextroelevation, dextrodepression, levoelevation and levodepression (Figs. 13.7a, c, g and i).

4. *Cardinal positions of gaze.* These are the positions which allow examination of each of the 12 extraocular muscles in their main field of action. There are six cardinal positions of gaze, viz, dextroversion, levoversion, dextroelevation, levoelevation, dextro-depression and levodepression (Figs. 13.7 a, c, d, f, g and i).

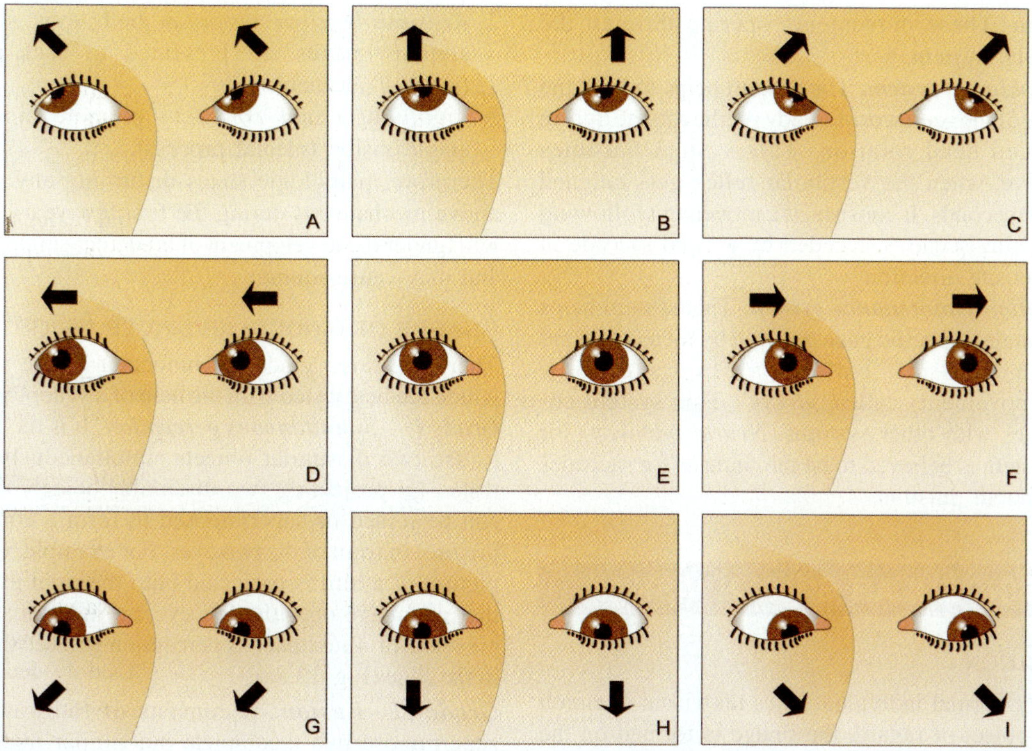

Fig. 13.7. Diagnostic positions of gaze: primary position (e); secondary positions (b, d, f, h); tertiary positions (a, c, g, i); cardinal positions (a, c, d, f, g, i).

SUPRANUCLEAR CONTROL OF EYE MOVEMENTS

There exists a highly accurate, still not fully elucidated, supranuclear control of eye movements which keeps the two eyes yoked together so that the image of the object of interest is simultaneously held on both fovea despite movement of the perceived object or the observer's head and/or body.

Supranuclear eye movement systems include:

1. Saccadic system
2. Smooth pursuit system
3. Vergence system
4. Vestibular system
5. Optokinetic system
6. Position maintenance system

All these systems perform specific functions and each one is controlled by a different neural system but share the same final common path the motor neurons that supply the extraocular muscles.

1. *Saccadic system.* Saccades are sudden, jerky conjugate eye movements, that occur as the gaze shifts from one object to another. Thus, they are performed to bring the image of an object quickly on the fovea. Though normally voluntary, saccades may be involuntarily aroused by peripheral, visual or auditory stimuli.

2. *Smooth pursuit eye movement system.* Smooth pursuit movements are tracking movements of the eye as they follow moving objects. These occur voluntarily when the eyes track moving objects but take place involuntarily if a repetitive visual pattern is displayed continuously. When the velocity of the moving object is more, the smooth pursuit movement is replaced by *small saccades (catchup saccades).*

3. *Vergence movement system.* Vergence movements allow focussing of an object which moves away from or towards the observer or when visual fixation shifts from one object to another at a different distance. Vergence movements are very slow disjugate movements.

4. *Vestibular eye movement system.* Vestibular movements are usually effective in compensating for the effects of head movements in disturbing visual fixation. These movements operate through the vestibular system.

5. *Optokinetic system.* The system helps to hold the images of the seen world steady on the retinae during sustained head rotation. This system becomes operative, when the vestibular reflex gets fatigued after 30 seconds. It consists of a movement following the moving scene, succeeded by a rapid saccade in the opposite direction.

6. *Position maintenance system.* This system helps to maintain a specific gaze position by means of rapid micromovements called *'flicks'* and slow micromovements called *'drifts'*. This system co-ordinates with other systems. *Neural pathway* for this system is believed to be the same as for saccades and smooth pursuits.

BINOCULAR SINGLE VISION

DEFINITION

When a normal individual fixes his visual attention on an object of regard, the image is formed on the fovea of both the eyes separately; but the individual perceives a single image. This state is called *binocular single vision.*

DEVELOPMENT OF BINOCULAR SINGLE VISION

Binocular single vision is a conditioned reflex which is not present since birth but is acquired during first 6 months and is completed during first few years. The process of its development is complex and partially understood.

Important mile stones in the visual development are:

- *At birth* there is no central fixation and the eyes move randomly.
- *By the first month* of life fixation reflex starts developing and becomes established by 6 months.
- *By 6 months* the macular stereopsis and accommodation reflex is fully developed.
- *By 6 years of age* full visual acuity (6/6) is attained and binocular single vision is well developed.

Prerequisites for development of binocular single vision

1. *Straight eyes* starting from the neonatal period, with precise coordination for all directions of gaze (motor mechanism).
2. *Reasonably clear vision* in both eyes so that similar images are presented to each retina (sensory mechanism).
3. *Ability of visual cortex* to promote binocular single vision (mental process).

Therefore, pathologic states disturbing any of the above mechanisms during the first few years of life will hinder the development of binocular single vision and may cause squint.

GRADES OF BINOCULAR SINGLE VISION

There are three grades of binocular single vision, which are best tested with the help of a synoptophore.

Grade I — Simultaneous perception. It is the power to see two dissimilar objects simultaneously. It is tested by projecting two dissimilar objects (which can be joined or superimposed to form a complete picture) in front of the two eyes. For example, when a picture of a bird is projected onto the right eye and that of a cage onto the left eye, an individual with presence of simultaneous perception will see the bird in the cage (Fig. 13.8a).

Grade II—Fusion. It consists of the power to superimpose two incomplete but similar images to form one complete image (Fig. 13.8b).

The ability of the subject to continue to see one complete picture when his eyes are made to converge or diverge a few degrees, gives the positive and negative fusion range, respectively.

Grade III— Stereopsis. It consists of the ability to perceive the third dimension (depth perception). It can be tested with stereopsis slides in synoptophore (Fig. 13.8c).

ANOMALIES OF BINOCULAR VISION

Anomalies of binocular vision include suppression, amblyopia, abnormal retinal correspondence (ARC), confusion and diplopia.

Suppression

It is a temporary active cortical inhibition of the image of an object formed on the retina of the squinting eye. This phenomenon occurs only during binocular vision (with both eyes open). However, when the fixating eye is covered, the squinting eye fixes (i.e., suppression disappears).

Tests to detect suppression include Worth's 4-dot test, four dioptre base out prism test, red glass test and synoptophore test (see pages 348-350).

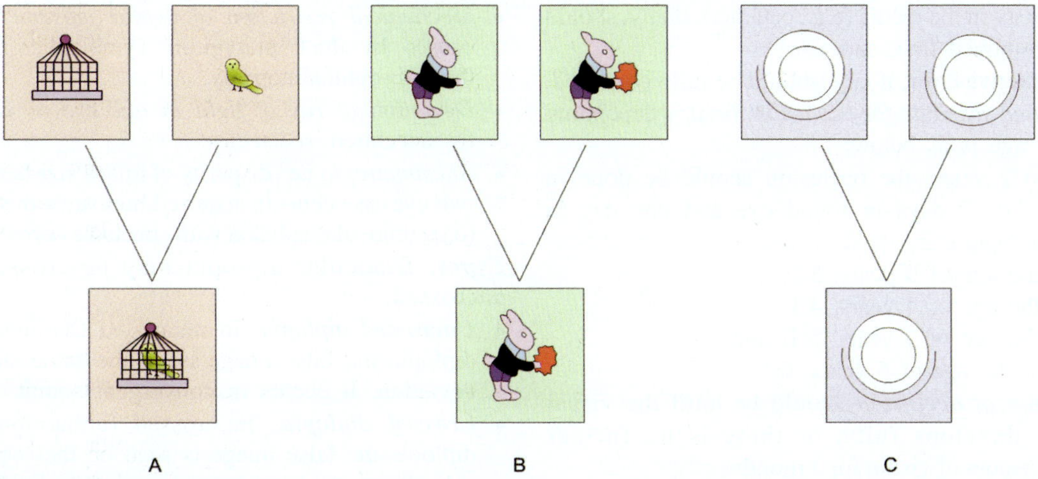

Fig. 13.8. Slides for testing three grades of binocular vision : A, simultaneous perception; B, fusion; C, stereopsis.

Amblyopia

Definition. Amblyopia, by definition, refers to a partial loss of vision in one or both eyes, in the absence of any organic disease of ocular media, retina and visual pathway.

Pathogenesis. Amblyopia is produced by certain amblyogenic factors operating during the critical period of visual development (birth to 6 years of age). The most sensitive period for development of amblyopia is first six months of life and it usually does not develop after the age of 6 years.

Amblyogenic factors include:

- Visual (form sense) deprivation as occurs in anisometropia,
- Light deprivation e.g., due to congenital cataract, and
- Abnormal binocular interaction e.g., in strabismus.

Types. Depending upon the cause, amblyopia is of following types:

1. *Strabismic amblyopia* results from prolonged uniocular suppression in children with unilateral constant squint who fixate with normal eye.
2. *Stimulus deprivation amblyopia* (old term: amblyopia ex anopsia) develops when one eye is totally excluded from seeing early in life as, in congenital or traumatic cataract, complete ptosis and dense central corneal opacity.
3. *Anisometropic amblyopia* occurs in an eye having higher degree of refractive error than the fellow eye. It is more common in aniso-hypermetropic than the anisomyopic children. Even 1-2 D hypermetropic anisometropia may cause amblyopia while upto 3D myopic anisometropia usually does not cause amblyopia.
4. *Isoametropic amblyopia* is bilateral amblyopia occurring in children with bilateral uncorrected high refractive error.
5. *Meridional amblyopia* occurs in children with uncorrected astigmatic refractive error. It is a selective amblyopia for a specific visual meridian.

Clinical characteristics of an amblyopic eye are:

1. *Visual acuity* is reduced. Recognition acuity is more affected than resolution acuity.
2. *Effect of neutral density filter.* Visual acuity when tested through neutral density filter improves by one or two lines in amblyopia and decreases in patients with organic lesions.
3. *Crowding phenomenon* is present in amblyopics i.e., visual acuity is less when tested with multiple letter charts (e.g., Snellen's chart) than when tested with single charts (optotype).
4. *Fixation pattern* may be central or eccentric. Degree of amblyopia in eccentric fixation is proportionate to the distance of the eccentric point from the fovea.
5. *Colour vision* is usually normal, may be affected in deep amblyopia with vision below 6/36.

Treatment of amblyopia should be started as early as possible (younger the child, better the prognosis). *Occlusion therapy* i.e., occlusion of the sound eye, to force use of amblyopic eye is the main stay in the treatment of amblyopia. However, before the occlusion therapy is started, it should be ensured that:

- Opacity in the media (e.g., cataract), if any, should be removed first, and
- Refractive error, if any, should be fully corrected.

Simplified schedule for occlusion therapy depending on the age is as below:

- Upto 2 years, the occlusion should be done in 2:1, i.e., 2 days in sound eye and one day in amblyopic eye.
- At the age of 3 years, 3:1,
- At the age of 4 years, 4:1,
- At the age of 5 years, 5:1, and
- After the age of 6 years, 6:1

Duration of occlusion should be until the visual acuity develops fully, or there is no further improvement of vision for 3 months.

Abnormal retinal correspondence (ARC)

In a state of normal binocular single vision, there exists a precise physiological relationship between the corresponding points of the two retinae. Thus, the foveae of two eyes act as corresponding points and have the same visual direction. This adjustment is called *normal retinal correspondence* (NRC). When squint develops, patient may experience either diplopia or confusion. To avoid these, sometimes (especially in children with small degree of esotropia), there occurs an active cortical adjustment in the directional values of the two retinae. In this state fovea of the normal eye and an extrafoveal point on the retina of the squinting eye acquire a common visual direction i.e. become corresponding points. This condition is called *abnormal retinal correspondence* (ARC) and the child gets a crude type of binocular single vision.

Tests to detect abnormal retinal correspondence include Worth's four-dot test, titmus stereo test, Bagolini striated glass tests, after image tests and synoptophore tests (see pages 348-350).

Diplopia

Binocular diplopia

Occurs due to formation of image on dissimilar points of the two retinae (see page 351).

Causes of binocular diplopia are:

- *Paralysis or paresis* of the extraocular muscles (commonest cause)
- *Displacement of one eye ball* as occurs in space occupying lesion in the orbit, and fractures of the orbital wall,
- *Mechanical restriction of ocular movements* as caused by thick pterygium, symblepharon and thyroid ophthalmopathy.
- *Deviation of ray of light in one eye* as caused by decentred spectacles.
- *Anisometropia* i.e., disparity of image size between two eyes as occurs in acquired high anisometropia (e.g., uniocular aphakia with spectacle correction).

Types. Binocular diplopia may be crossed or uncrossed.

- ***Uncrossed diplopia.*** In uncrossed (harmonious) diplopia the false image is on the same side as deviation. It occurs in convergent squint.
- ***Crossed diplopia.*** In crossed (unharmonious) diplopia the false image is seen on the opposite side. It occurs in divergent squint.

Uniocular diplopia

Though not an anomaly of binocular vision, but it will not be out of place to describe uniocular diplopia along with binocular diplopia. In uniocular diplopia an object appears double from the affected eye even when the normal eye is closed.

Causes of uniocular diplopia are:

- *Subluxated clear lens* (pupillary area is partially phakic and partially aphakic).
- *Subluxated intraocular lens* (pupillary area is partially aphakic and partially pseudophakic).
- *Double pupil* due to congenital anomaly, or large peripheral iridectomy or iridodialysis.
- *Incipient cataract.* Usually polyopia i.e., multiple images may be seen due to multiple water clefts within the lens.
- *Keratoconus.* Diplopia occurs due to changed refractive power of the cornea in different parts.

Treatment of diplopia

Treat the causative disease. Temporary relief from annoying diplopia can be obtained by occluding the affected eye.

STRABISMUS

DEFINITION AND CLASSIFICATION

Definition

Normally visual axis of the two eyes are parallel to each other in the 'primary position of gaze' and this alignment is maintained in all positions of gaze.

A *misalignment of the visual axes of the two eyes is called squint or strabismus.*

Classification of strabismus

Broadly, strabismus can be classified as below:

I. Apparent squint or pseudostrabismus.
II. Latent squint (Heterophoria)
III. Manifest squint (Heterotropia)
   1. Concomitant squint
   2. Incomitant squint.

PSEUDOSTRABISMUS

In pseudostrabismus (apparent squint), the visual axes are in fact parallel, but the eyes seem to have a squint:

1. ***Pseudoesotropia*** or apparent convergent squint may be associated with:
- *Prominent epicanthal fold* (which covers the normally visible nasal aspect of the globe and gives a false impression of esotropia)
- *Negative angle kappa*, and

2. ***Pseudoexotropia*** or apparent divergent squint may be associated with
- *hypertelorism,* a condition of wide separation of the two eyes (i.e. wide IPD), and
- *Positive angle kappa.*

HETEROPHORIA

Heterophoria also known as '*latent strabismus*', is a condition in which the tendency of the eyes to deviate is kept latent by fusion. Therefore, when the influence of fusion is removed the visual axis of one eye deviates away. O*rthophoria* is a condition of perfect alignment of the two eyes which is maintained even after the removal of influence of fusion. However, orthophoria is a theoretical ideal. Practically a small amount of heterophoria is of universal occurrence and is known as '*physiological heterophoria*'.

Types of heterophoria

1. ***Esophoria***. It is a tendency to converge. It may be:

i. *Convergence excess type* (esophoria greater for near than distance).
ii. *Divergence weakness type* (esophoria greater for distance than near).
iii. *Non-specific type* (esophoria which does not vary significantly in degree for any distance).

2. ***Exophoria***. It is a tendency to diverge. It may be:

i. *Convergence weakness type* (exophoria greater for near than distance).
ii *Divergence excess type* (exophoria greater on distant fixation than the near).
iii *Non-specific type* (exophoria which does not vary significantly in degree for any distance).

3. ***Hyperphoria***. It is a tendency to deviate upwards, while hypophoria is a tendency to deviate downwards. However, in practice it is customary to use the term right or left hyperphoria depending on the eye which remains up as compared to the other.

4. ***Cyclophoria***. It is a tendency to rotate around the anteroposterior axis. When the 12 O'clock meridian of cornea rotates nasally, it is called *incyclophoria* and when it rotates temporally it is called *excyclophoria.*

Etiology

A. *Anatomical factors*

Anatomical factors responsible for development of heterophoria include:

1. Orbital asymmetry.
2. Abnormal interpupillary distance (IPD). A wide IPD is associated with exophoria and small with esophoria.
3. Faulty insertion of extraocular muscle.
4. A mild degree of extraocular muscle weakness.
5. Anomalous central distribution of the tonic innervation of the two eyes.
6. Anatomical variation in the position of the macula in relation to the optical axis of the eye.

B. *Physiological factors*

1. *Age.* Esophoria is more common in younger age group as compared to exophoria which is more often seen in elderly.
2. *Role of accommodation.* Increased accommodation is associated with esophoria (as seen in hypermetropes and individuals doing excessive near work) and decreased accommodation with exophoria (as seen in simple myopes).
3. *Role of convergence.* Excessive use of convergence may cause esophoria (as occurs in bilateral congenital myopes) while decreased use of convergence is often associated with exophoria (as seen in presbyopes).
4. *Dissociation factor* such as prolonged constant use of one eye may result in exophoria (as occurs in individuals using uniocular microscope and watch makers using uniocular magnifying glass).

Factors predisposing to decompensation

- Inadequacy of fusional reserve,
- General debility and lowered vitality,
- Psychosis, neurosis, and mental stress,
- Precision of job, and
- Advancing age.

Symptoms

Depending upon the symptoms heterophoria can be divided into compensated and decompensated.

Compensated heterophoria. It is associated with no subjective symptoms. Compensation of heterophoria depends upon the reserve neuro-muscular power to overcome the muscular imbalance and individual's desire for maintenance of binocular vision.

Decompensated heterophoria. It is associated with multiple symptoms which may be grouped as under:

1. *Symptoms of muscular fatigue.* These result due to continuous use of the reserve neuromuscular power. These include:
   - *Headache and eyeache* after prolonged use of eyes, which is relieved when the eyes are closed.
   - *Difficulty in changing the focus* from near to distant objects of fixation or vice-versa.
   - *Photophobia* due to muscular fatigue is not relieved by using dark glasses, but relieved by closing one eye.
2. *Symptoms of failure to maintain binocular single vision* are:
   - *Blurring* or crowding of words while reading;
   - *Intermittent diplopia* due to temporary manifest deviation under conditions of fatigue; and
   - *Intermittent squint* (without diplopia) which is usually noticed by the patient's close relations or friends.
3. *Symptoms of defective postural sensations* cause problems in judging distances and positions especially of the moving objects. This difficulty may be experienced by cricketers, tennis players and pilots during landing.

Examination of a case of heterophoria

1. *Testing for vision and refractive error.* It is most important, because a refractive error may be responsible for the symptoms of the patient or for the deviation itself. Preferably, refraction should be performed under full cycloplegia, especially in children.

2. *Cover-uncover test.* It tells about the presence and type of heterophoria. To perform it, one eye is covered with an occluder and the other is made to fix an object. In the presence of heterophoria, the eye under cover will deviate. After a few seconds the cover is quickly removed and the movement of the eye (which was under cover) is observed. Direction of movement of the eyeball tells the type of heterophoria (e.g., the eye will move outward in the presence of esophoria) and the speed of movement tells whether recovery is slow or rapid.

3. *Prism cover test.* (see page 347).

4. *Maddox rod test.* Patient is asked to fix on a point light in the centre of Maddox tangent scale (Fig. 13.9) at a distance of 6 metres. A Maddox rod (which consists of many glass rods of red colour set together in a metallic disc) (Fig. 13.10) is placed in front of one eye with axis of the rod parallel to the axis of deviation (Fig. 13.11).

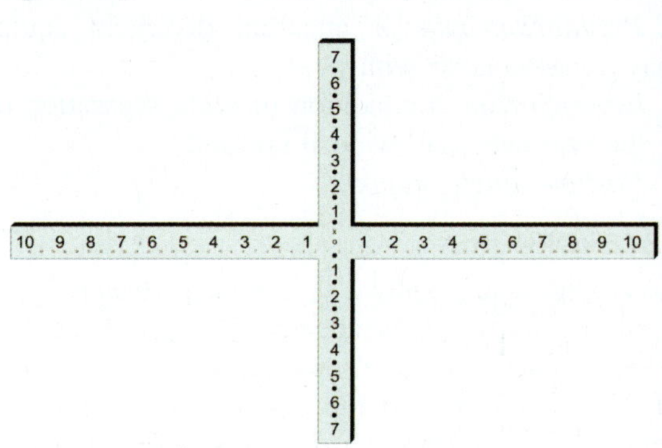

Fig. 13.9. Maddox tangent scale.

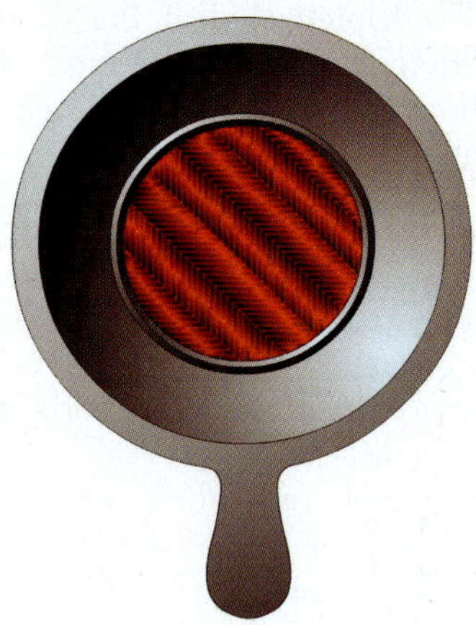

Fig. 13.10. Maddox rod.

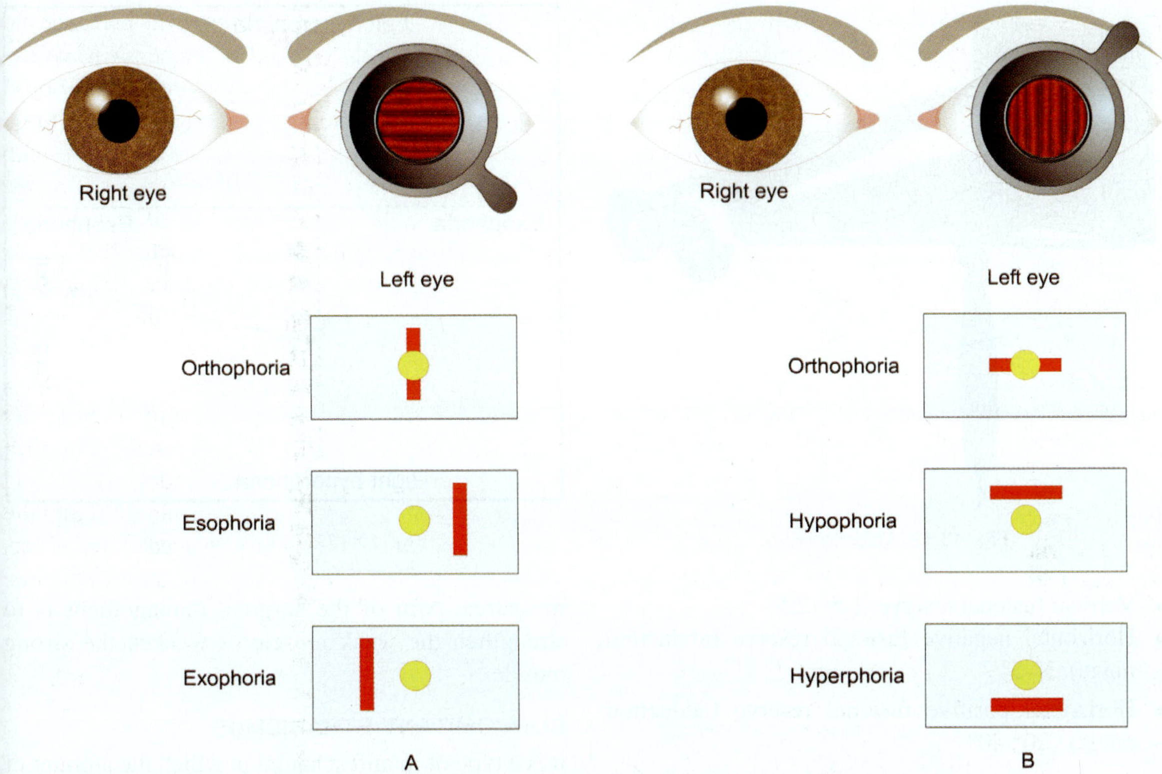

Fig. 13.11. Maddox rod test for horizontal (A) and vertical (B) heterophorias.

The Maddox rod converts the point light image into a line. Thus, the patient will see a point light with one eye and a red line with the other. Due to dissimilar images of the two eyes, fusion is broken and heterophoria becomes manifest. The number on Maddox tangent scale where the red line falls will be the amount of heterophoria in degrees. In the absence of Maddox tangent scale, the dissociation between the point light and red line is measured by the superimposition of the two images by means of prisms placed in front of one eye with apex towards the phoria.

5. *Maddox wing test.* Maddox wing is an instrument (Fig. 13.12) by which the amount of phoria for near (at a distance of 33 cm) can be measured. It is also based on the basic principle of dissociation of fusion by dissimilar objects.

The instrument is designed in such a way that, through its two slits, right eye sees a vertical white arrow and a horizontal red arrow and the left eye sees a vertical and a horizontal line of numbers. The patient is asked to tell the number on the horizontal line which the vertical white arrow is pointing (this will give amount of horizontal phoria) and the number on the vertical line at which the red arrow is pointing (this will measure the vertical phoria). The cyclophoria is measured by asking the patient to align the red arrow with the horizontal line of numbers (Fig. 13.13).

6. *Measurement of convergence and accommodation* is important in planning the management of heterophorias.

- *Near point of convergence* (NPC) can be measured with the help of a RAF rule or the Livingstone binocular gauge. The normal NPC is considered to be around 70 mm.
- *Near point of accommodation* (NPA) should be measured after the NPC. NPA can be measured with the help of a RAF or Prince's rule. Normal NPA varies with the age of patient (see page 42).

7. *Measurement of fusional reserve.* It can be done with the help of a synoptophore or prism bar. The normal values of fusional reserve are as follows:

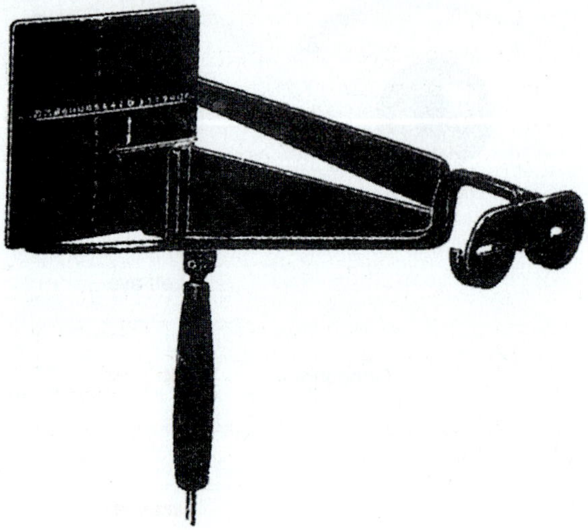

Fig. 13.12. Maddox wing.

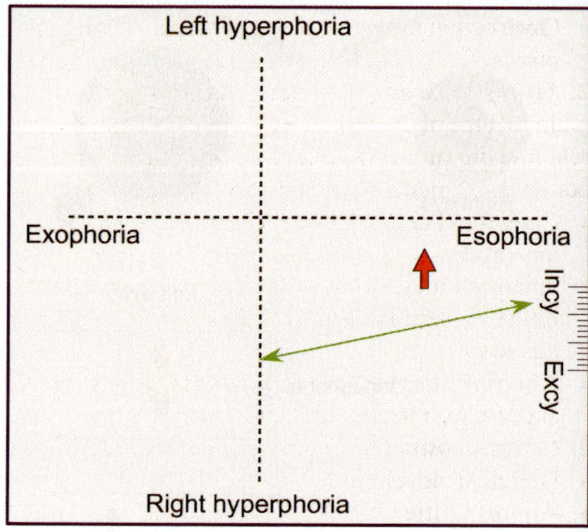

Fig. 13.13. Maddox wing test.

- Vertical fusional reserve: 1.5°-2.5°
- Horizontal negative fusional reserve (abduction range): 3°-5°
- Horizontal positive fusional reserve (adduction range) : 20°-40°

Treatment

Treatment described below, is indicated mainly in patients with decompensated heterophoria (i.e., symptomatic cases).

1. ***Correction of refractive error*** when detected, is most important. It may correct the phoria and/or relieve the symptoms.

2. ***Orthoptic treatment.*** It is indicated in patients with heterophoria without refractive error and in those where heterophoria and/or symptoms are not corrected by glasses. Aim of orthoptic treatment is to improve convergence insufficiency and the fusional reserve. Orthoptic exercises can be done with synoptophore. Simple exercises to be carried out at home should also be taught to the patient.

3. ***Prescription of prism in glasses.*** It may be tried in selected cases of hyperphoria and in troublesome cases of esophoria and exophoria. Prism is prescribed with apex towards the direction of phoria to correct only half or at the most two-thirds of heterophoria.

4. ***Surgical treatment.*** It is undertaken in patients with marked symptoms which are not relieved by other measures. Aim of the surgical management is to strengthen the weak muscle or weaken the strong muscle.

CONCOMITANT STRABISMUS

It is a type of manifest squint in which the amount of deviation in the squinting eye remains constant (unaltered) in all the directions of gaze; and there is no associated limitation of ocular movements.

Etiology

It is not clearly defined. The causative factors differ in individual cases. As we know, the binocular vision and coordination of ocular movements are not present since birth but are acquired in the early childhood. The process starts by the age of 3-6 months and is completed up to 5-6 years. Therefore, any obstacle to the development of these processes may result in concomitant squint. These obstacles can be arranged into three groups, namely: sensory, motor and central.

1. ***Sensory obstacles***. These are the factors which hinder the formation of a clear image in one eye. These include:

- Refractive errors,
- Prolonged use of incorrect spectacles,
- Anisometropia,
- Corneal opacities,
- Lenticular opacities,
- Diseases of macula (e.g., central chorioretinitis),
- Optic atrophy, and

- Obstruction in the pupillary area due to congenital ptosis.

2. *Motor obstacles*. These factors hinder the maintenance of the two eyes in the correct positional relationship in primary gaze and/or during different ocular movements. A few such factors are:

- Congenital abnormalities of the shape and size of the orbit,
- Abnormalities of extraocular muscles such as faulty insertion, faulty innervation and mild paresis,
- Abnormalities of accommodation, convergence and AC/A ratio.

3. *Central obstacles*. These may be in the form of:

- Deficient development of fusion faculty, or
- Abnormalities of cortical control of ocular movements as occurs in mental trauma, and hyperexcitability of the central nervous system during teething.

Clinical features of concomitant strabismus (in general)

The cardinal features of different clinico-etiological types of concomitant strabismus are described separately. However, the clinical features of concomitant strabismus (in general) are as below:

1. *Ocular deviation*. Characteristics of ocular deviation are:

- Unilateral (monocular squint) or alternating (alternate squint).
- Inward deviation (esotropia) or outward deviation (exotropia) or vertical deviation (hypertropia).
- Primary deviation (of squinting eye) is equal to secondary deviation (deviation of normal eye under cover when patient fixes with squinting eye).
- Ocular deviation is equal in all the directions of gaze.

2. *Ocular movements* are not limited in any direction.

3. *Refractive error* may or may not be associated.

4. *Suppression and amblyopia* may develop as sensory adaptation to strabismus. Suppression may be monocular (in monocular squint) and alternating (in alternating strabismus). Amblyopia develops in monocular strabismus only and is responsible for poor visual acuity.

5. *A-V patterns* may be observed in horizontal strabismus. When A-V patterns are associated, the horizontal concomitant strabismus becomes vertically incomitant (see page 354).

Types of concomitant squint

Three common types of concomitant squint are :

1. Convergent squint (esotropia),
2. Divergent squint (exotropia), and
3. Vertical squint (hypertropia).

CONVERGENT SQUINT

Concomitant convergent squint or esotropia denotes inward deviation of one eye (Fig. 13.14). It can be *unilateral* (the same eye always deviates inwards and the second normal eye takes fixation) or *alternating* (either of the eyes deviates inwards and the other eye takes up fixation, alternately).

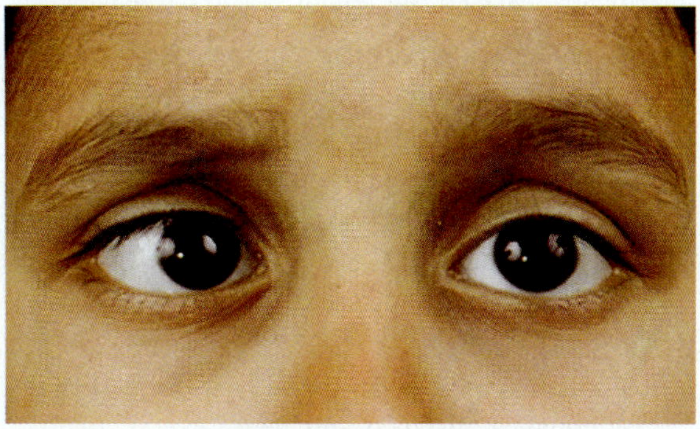

Fig. 13.14. Concomitant squint, (right esotropia).

Clinico-etiological types

Depending upon the clinico-etiological features convergent concomitant squint can be further classified into following types:

1. *Accommodative esotropia*. It occurs due to overaction of convergence associated with accommodation reflex. It is of three types: refractive, non-refractive and mixed.

i. *Refractive accommodative esotropia:* It usually develops at the age of 2 to 3 years and is associated with high hypermetropia (+4 to +7 D). Mostly it is for near and distance (marginally more for near) and fully correctable by use of spectacles.

ii. *Non-refractive accommodative esotropia:* It is caused by abnormal AC/A (accommodative convergence/accommodation) ratio. This may occur even in patients with no refractive error. Esotropia is greater for near than that for distance (minimal or no deviation for distance). It is fully corrected by adding +3 DS for near vision.

iii. *Mixed accommodative esotropia:* It is caused by combination of hypermetropia and high AC/A ratio. Esotropia for distance is corrected by correction of hypermetropia; and the residual esotropia for near is corrected by an addition of +3 DS lens.

2. *Non-accommodative esotropias.* This group includes all those primary esodeviations in which amount of deviation is not affected by the state of accommodation. It includes:

i. *Essential infantile esotropia.* It usually presents at 1-2 months of age. However, it may be detected shortly after birth or any time within the first 6 months of life. Previously, it was known as *congenital esotropia.* It is characterised by fairly large angle of squint (> 30°), alternate fixation in primary gaze and crossed fixation in lateral gaze.

ii. *Essential acquired or late onset esotropia.* It is a common variety of concomitant convergent squint. It typically occurs during first few years of life any time after six months of age. It is of three types:

- *Basic type.* In it the deviation is usually equal at distance and near.
- *Convergence excess type.* In it the deviation is large for near and small or no deviation for distance.
- *Divergence insufficiency type.* It is characterized by a greater deviation for distance than near.

3. *Secondary esotropia* or *sensory deprivation esotropia.* It results from monocular lesions (in childhood) which either prevent the development of normal binocular vision or interfere with its maintenance. Examples of such lesions are: cataract, severe congenital ptosis, aphakia, anisometropia, optic atrophy, retinoblastoma, central chorioretinitis and so on.

4. ***Consecutive esotropia.*** It results from surgical overcorrection of exotropia.

DIVERGENT SQUINT

Concomitant divergent squint (exotropia) is characterised by outward deviation of one eye while the other eye fixates.

Clinico-etiological types

It can be classified into following clinicoetiological types:

1. *Congenital exotropia*

It is rare and almost always present at birth. It is characterised by a fairly large angle of squint, usually alternate with homonymous fixation in lateral gaze, and no amblyopia.

2. *Primary exotropia*

It may be unilateral or alternating and may present as intermittent or constant exotropia.

Intermittent exotropia. It is the most common type of exodeviation with following features:

- Age of onset is usually early between 2 to 5 years.
- Deviation becomes manifest at times and latent at others. Precipitating factors include bright light, fatigue, ill health and day dreaming.
- Sensory testing usually reveals good fusion, stereopsis and no amblyopia.

Constant exotropia. If not treated in time the intermittent exotropia may decompensate to become constant exotropia (Fig. 13.15).

Types. Primary exotropia may be of following three types:

- *Convergence insufficiency* type of exotropia is greater for near than distance,
- *Divergence excess* type of exotropia is greater for distance than near, or
- *Basic non-specific type* exotropia is equal for near and distance.

3. *Secondary (sensory deprivation) exotropia*

It is a constant unilateral deviation which results from long-standing monocular lesions (in adults), associated with low vision in the affected eye. Common causes include: traumatic cataract, corneal

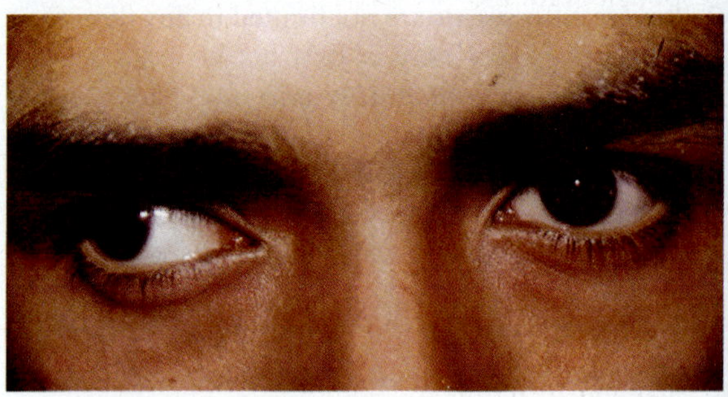

Fig. 13.15. A patient with primary exotropia.

opacity, optic atrophy, anisometropic amblyopia, retinal detachment and organic macular lesions.

4. *Consecutive exotropia*

It is a constant unilateral exotropia which results either due to surgical over-correction of esotropia, or spontaneous conversion of small degree esotropia with amblyopia into exotropia.

EVALUATION OF A CASE OF CONCOMITANT STRABISMUS

I. History

A meticulous history is very important. It should include: age of onset, duration, mode of onset (sudden or gradual), any illness preceding squint (fever, trauma, infections, etc.), intermittent or constant, unilateral or alternating, history of diplopia, family history of squint, history of head tilt or turn and so on.

II. Examination

1. *Inspection*. Large degree squint (convergent or divergent) is obvious on inspection.

2. *Ocular movements*. Both uniocular as well as binocular movements should be tested in all the cardinal positions of gaze.

3. *Pupillary reactions*. These may be abnormal in patients with secondary deviations due to diseases of retina and optic nerve.

4. *Media and fundus examination*. It may reveal associated disease of ocular media, retina or optic nerve.

5. *Testing of vision and refractive error*. It is most important, because a refractive error may be responsible for the symptoms of the patient or for the deviation itself. Preferably, refraction should be performed under full cycloplegia, especially in children.

6. *Cover tests*

i. *Direct cover test* (Fig. 13.16). It confirms the presence of manifest squint. To perform it, the patient is asked to fixate on a point light. Then, the normal looking eye is covered while observing the movement of the uncovered eye. In the presence of squint the uncovered eye will move in opposite direction to take fixation, while in apparent squint there will be no movement. This test should be performed for *near* fixation (i.e., at 33 cm) as well as distance fixation (i.e., at 6 metres).

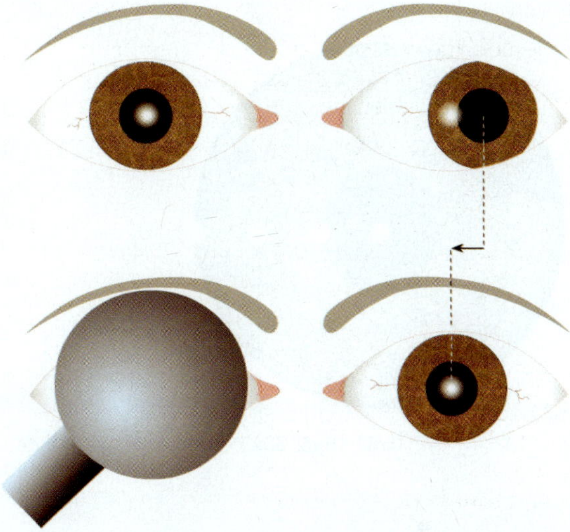

Fig. 13.16. Direct cover test depicting left exotropia.

ii. *Alternate cover test.* It reveals whether the squint is unilateral or alternate and also differentiates concomitant squint from paralytic squint (where secondary deviation is greater than primary).

7. *Estimation of angle of deviation*

i. *Hirschberg corneal reflex test.* It is a rough but handy method to estimate the angle of manifest squint. In it the patient is asked to fixate at point light held at a distance of 33 cm and the deviation of the corneal light reflex from the centre of pupil is noted in the squinting eye. Roughly, the angle of squint is 15° and 45° when the corneal light reflex falls on the border of pupil and limbus, respectively (Fig. 13.17).

ii. *The prism and cover test* (prism bar cover test i.e., PBCT). Prisms of increasing strength with apex towards the deviation are placed in front of one eye and the patient is asked to fixate an object with the other. The cover-uncover test is performed till there is no recovery movement of the eye under cover. This will tell the amount of deviation in prism dioptres. Both heterophoria as well as heterotropia can be measured by this test.

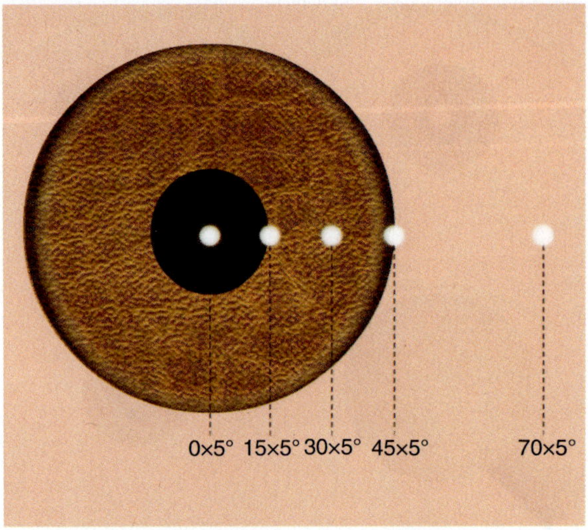

Fig. 13.17. Hirschberg corneal reflex test.

iii. *Krimsky corneal reflex test.* In this test the patient is asked to fixate on a point light and prisms of increasing power (with apex towards the direction of manifest squint) are placed in front of the normal fixating eye till the corneal light reflex is centred in the squinting eye. The power of prism required to centre the light reflex in the squinting eye equals the amount of squint in prism dioptres.

iv. *Measurement of deviation with synoptophore.* All types of heterophorias and heterotropias (both objective and subjective angle of squint) can be measured accurately with it. In addition, many other tests can also be performed with this instrument (for details see page 349).

8. Tests for grade of binocular vision and sensory functions. Normal binocular single vision consists of three grades. Sensory anomalies include disturbances of binocular vision, eccentric fixation, suppression, amblyopia, abnormal retinal correspondence and diplopia. A few common tests for sensory functions are as follows:

i. *Worth's four-dot test.* For this test patient wears goggles with red lens in front of the right and green lens in front of the left eye and views a box with four lights – one red, two green and one white (Fig. 13.18).

Interpretation:

- In *normal binocular single vision*, the patient sees all the four lights in the absence of manifest squint, (Fig. 13.18A).

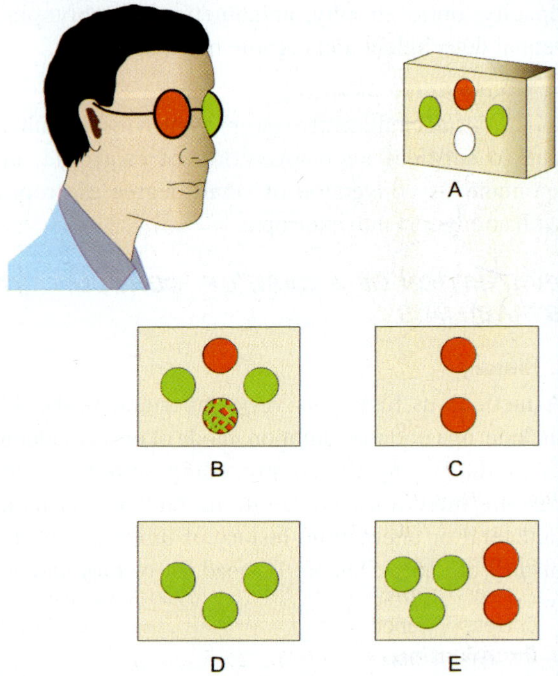

Fig. 13.18. Worth's four-dot test.

- In *abnormal retinal correspondence* (ARC) patient sees four lights even in the presence of a manifest squint.
- In *right suppression* the patient sees only three green lights, (Fig. 13.18D).
- In *left suppression* the patient sees only two red lights, (Fig. 13.18C).
- In *alternating suppression* the patient sees three green lights and two red lights, alternately.
- In *diplopia* the patient sees five lights (2 red and 3 green) (Fig. 13.18E).

ii. *Test for fixation.* It can be tested with the help of a visuoscope or fixation star of the ophthalmoscope. Patient is asked to cover one eye and fix the star with the other eye. Fixation may be centric (normal on the fovea) or eccentric (which may be unsteady, parafoveal, macular, paramacular, or peripheral (Fig. 13.19).

iii. *After-image test.* In this test the right fovea is stimulated with a vertical and left with a horizontal bright light and the patient is asked to draw the position of after-images.

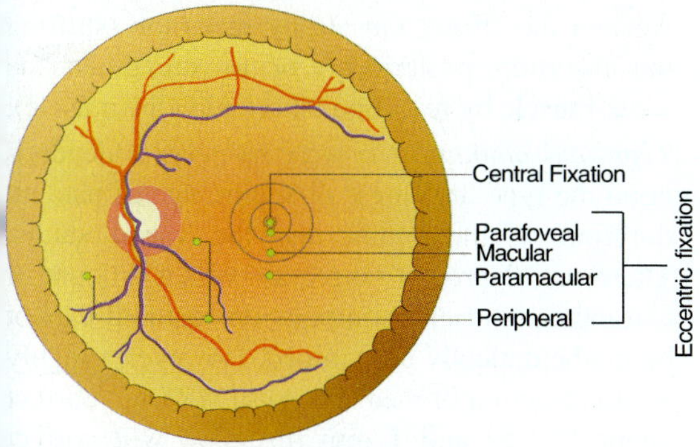

Fig. 13.19. Types of fixation.

Interpretation:

- A patient with normal retinal correspondence will draw a cross (Fig. 13.20A).
- An esotropic patient with abnormal retinal correspondence (ARC) will draw vertical image to the left of horizontal (Fig. 13.20B).
- An exotropic patient with ARC will draw vertical image to the right of horizontal (Fig. 13.20C).

iv. ***Sensory function tests with synoptophore.*** Synoptophore (major amblyoscope) consists of two tubes, having a right-angled bend, mounted on a base (Fig. 13.21). Each tube contains a light source for illumination of slides and a slide carrier at the outer end, a reflecting mirror at the right-angled bend and an eyepiece of +6.5 D at the inner end (Fig. 13.22). The two tubes can be moved separately or together by means of knobs around a semicircular scale. Synoptophore is used for many diagnostic and therapeutic indications in orthoptics.

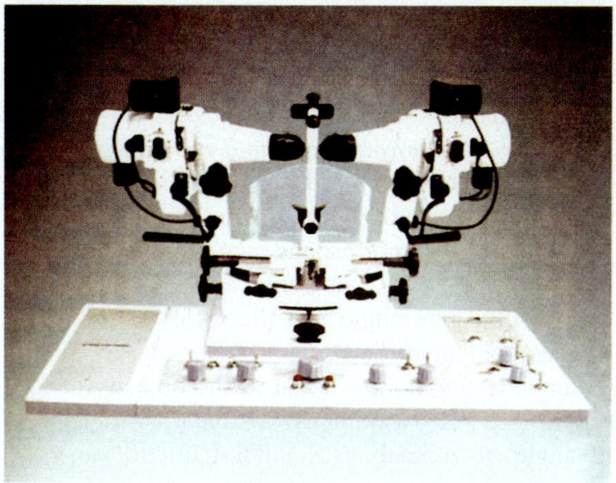

Fig. 13.21. Synoptophore.

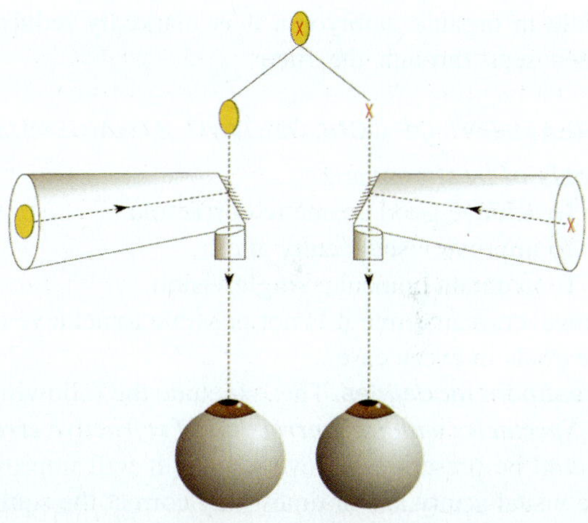

Fig. 13.22. Optical principle of synoptophore.

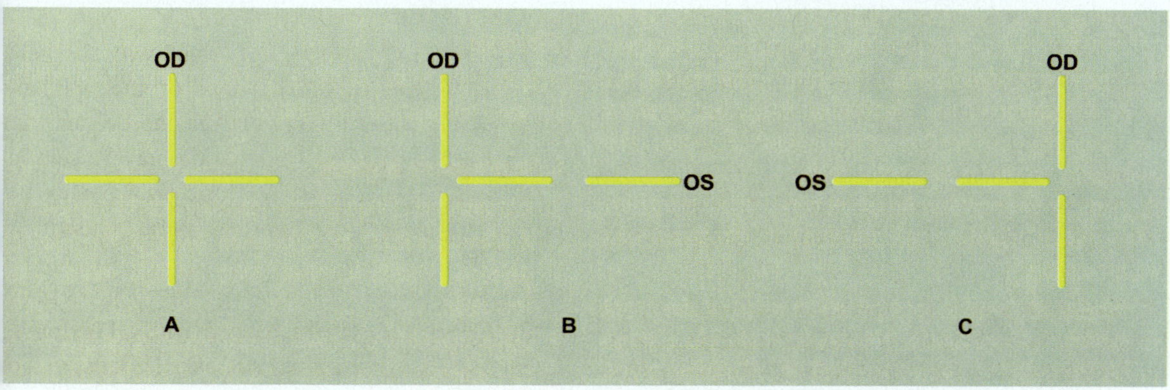

Fig. 13.20. After-image test: A, normal retinal correspondence; B, esotropia with ARC; C, exotropia with ARC.

Synoptophore tests for sensory functions include:

- *Estimation of grades of binocular vision* (page 318).
- *Detection of normal/abnormal retinal correspondence (ARC).* It is done by determining the subjective and objective angles of the squint. In normal retinal correspondence, these two angles are equal. In ARC, objective angle is greater than the subjective angle and the difference between these is called the *angle of anomaly.* When the angle of anomaly is equal to the objective angle, the ARC is harmonious. In unharmonious ARC angle of anomaly is smaller than the objective angle.

v. *Neutral density filter test.* In this test, visual acuity is measured without and with neutral density filter placed in front of the eye. In cases with functional amblyopia visual acuity slightly improves while in organic amblyopia it is markedly reduced when seen through the filter.

TREATMENT OF CONCOMITANT STRABISMUS

Goals of treatment are:

- To achieve good cosmetic correction,
- To improve visual acuity and
- To maintain binocular single vision.

However, many time it is not possible to achieve all the goals in every case.

Treatment modalities. These include the following:

1. *Spectacles with full correction of refractive error* should be prescribed in every case. It will improve the visual acuity and at times may correct the squint partially or completely (as in accommodative squint).

2. *Occlusion therapy.* It is indicated in the presence of amblyopia. After correcting the refractive error, the normal eye is occluded and the patient is advised to use the squinting eye. Regular follow-ups are done in squint clinic. Occlusion helps to improve the vision in children below the age of 10 years. (For occlusion regimen see page 340).

3. *Preoperative orthoptic exercises.* These are given after the correction of amblyopia to overcome suppression.

4. *Squint surgery.* It is required in most of the cases to correct the deviation. However, it should always be instituted after the correction of refractive error, treatment of amblyopia and orthoptic exercises.

- *Basic principles of squint surgery.* These are to weaken the strong muscle by recession (shifting the insertion posteriorly) or to strengthen the weak muscle by resection (shortening the muscle).
- *Type and amount of muscle surgery.* It depends upon the type and angle of squint, age of patient, duration of the squint and the visual status. Therefore, degree of correction versus amount of extraocular muscle manipulation required cannot be mathematically determined. However, roughly 1 mm resection of medial rectus (MR) will correct about 1°-1.5° and 1 mm recession will correct about 2°-2.5°. While 1 mm resection and recession of lateral rectus (LR) muscle will correct 1°-2°. The maximum limit allowed for MR resection is 8 mm and recession is 5.5 mm. The corresponding figures for LR muscle are 10 mm and 8 mm, respectively.

5. *Postoperative orthoptic exercises.* These are required to improve fusional range and maintain binocular single vision.

INCOMITANT SQUINT

It is a type of heterotropia (manifest squint) in which the amount of deviation varies in different directions of gaze. It includes following conditions:

1. Paralytic squint,
2. 'A' and 'V' pattern heterotropias,
3. Restrictive squint.

PARALYTIC STRABISMUS

It refers to ocular deviation resulting from complete or incomplete paralysis of one or more extraocular muscles.

Etiology

The lesions may be neurogenic, myogenic or at the level of neuromuscular junction.

I. *Neurogenic lesions*

1. *Congenital.* Hypoplasia or absence of nucleus is a known cause of third and sixth cranial nerve palsies. Birth injuries may mimic congenital lesions.
2. *Inflammatory lesions.* These may be in the form of encephalitis, meningitis, neurosyphilis or peripheral neuritis (commonly viral). Nerve trunks

may also be involved in the infectious lesions of cavernous sinus and orbit.

3. *Neoplastic lesions.* These include brain tumours involving nuclei, nerve roots or intracranial part of the nerves; and intraorbital tumours involving peripheral parts of the nerves.
4. *Vascular lesions.* These are known in patients with hypertension, diabetes mellitus and atherosclerosis. These may be in the form of haemorrhage, thrombosis, embolism, aneurysms or vascular occlusions. Cerebrovascular accidents are more common in elderly people.
5. *Traumatic lesions.* These include head injury and direct or indirect trauma to the nerve trunks.
6. *Toxic lesions.* These include carbon monoxide poisoning, effects of diphtheria toxins (rarely), alcoholic and lead neuropathy.
7. *Demyelinating lesions.* Ocular palsy may occur in multiple sclerosis and diffuse sclerosis.

II. *Myogenic lesions*

1. *Congenital lesions.* These include absence, hypoplasia, malinsertion, weakness and musculofacial anomalies.
2. *Traumatic lesions.* These may be in the form of laceration, disinsertion, haemorrhage into the muscle substance or sheath and incarceration of muscles in fractures of the orbital walls.
3. *Inflammatory lesions.* Myositis is usually viral in origin and may occur in influenza, measles and other viral fevers.
4. *Myopathies.* These include thyroid myopathy, carcinomatous myopathy and that associated with certain drugs. *Progressive external ophthalmoplegia* is a bilateral myopathy of extraocular muscles; which may be sporadic or inherited as an autosomal dominant disorder.

III. *Neuromuscular junction lesion*

It includes *myasthenia gravis.* The disease is characterised primarily by fatigue of muscle groups, usually starting with the small extraocular muscles, before involving other large muscles.

Clinical features

Symptoms

1. *Diplopia.* It is the main symptom of paralytic squint. It is more marked towards the action of paralysed muscle. It may be crossed (in divergent squint) or uncrossed (in convergent squint). It may be horizontal, vertical or oblique depending on the muscle paralysed. Diplopia occurs due to formation of image on dissimilar points of the two retinae (Fig. 13.23).

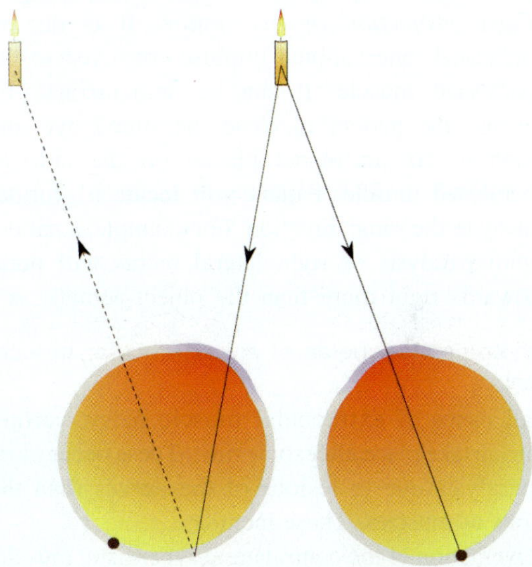

Fig. 13.23. Diplopia.

2. *Confusion.* It occurs due to formation of image of two different objects on the corresponding points of two retinae.
3. *Nausea and vertigo.* These result from diplopia and confusion.
4. *Ocular deviation.* It is of sudden onset.

Signs

1. *Primary deviation.* It is deviation of the affected eye and is away from the action of paralysed muscle, e.g., if lateral rectus is paralysed the eye is converged.
2. *Secondary deviation.* It is deviation of the normal eye seen under cover, when the patient is made to fix with the squinting eye. It is greater than the primary deviation. This is due to the fact that the strong impulse of innervation required to enable the eye with paralysed muscle to fix is also transmitted to the yoke muscle of the sound eye resulting in a greater amount of deviation. This is based on Hering's law of equal innervation of yoke muscles.

3. *Restriction of ocular movement.* It occurs in the direction of the action of paralysed muscles.
4. *Compensatory head posture.* It is adopted to avoid diplopia and confusion. Head is turned towards the direction of action of the paralysed muscle, e.g., if the right lateral rectus is paralysed, patient will keep the head turned towards right.
5. *False projection or orientation.* It is due to increased innervational impulse conveyed to the paralysed muscle. It can be demonstrated by asking the patient to close the sound eye and then to fix an object placed on the side of paralysed muscle. Patient will locate it further away in the same direction. For example, a patient with paralysis of right lateral rectus will point towards right more than the object actually is.

Pathological sequelae of an extraocular muscle palsy

In all cases of extraocular muscle palsy, certain sequelae take place after some time. These occur more in paralysis due to lesions of the nerves than the lesions of muscles. These include:

1. Overaction of the contralateral synergistic muscle.
2. Contracture of the direct antagonist muscle.
3. Secondary inhibitional palsy of the contralateral antagonist muscle.

For example, in paralysis of the right lateral rectus muscle there occurs (Fig 13.24):

- Overaction of the left medial rectus,
- Contracture of the right medial rectus and
- Inhibitional palsy of the left lateral rectus muscle.

Clinical varieties of ocular palsies

1. *Isolated muscle paralysis.* Lateral rectus and superior oblique are the most common muscles to be paralysed singly, as they have separate nerve supply. Isolated paralysis of the remaining four muscles is less common, except in congenital lesions.

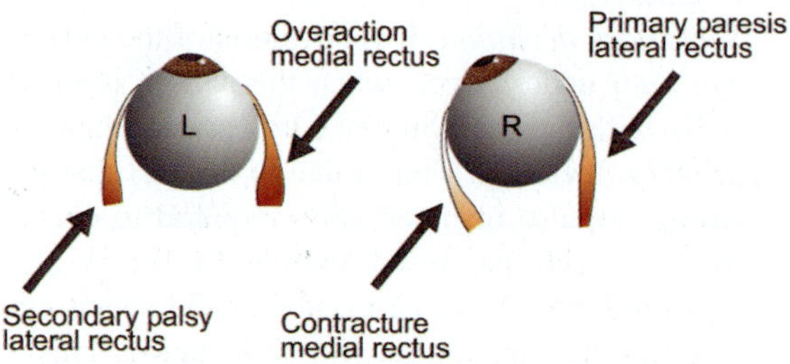

Fig. 13.24. Pathological sequelae of the right lateral rectus muscle paralysis.

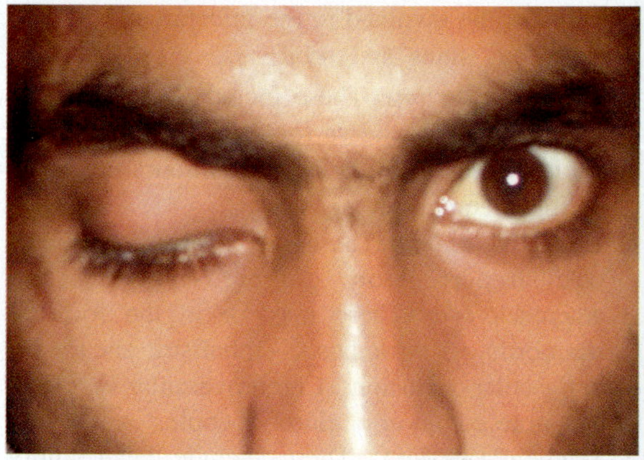

A

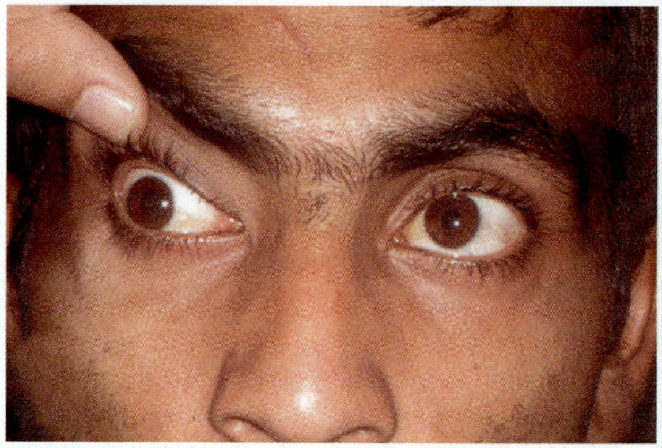

B

Fig. 13.25. A patient with third cranial nerve paralysis showing: A, ptosis; B, divergent squint.

2. *Paralysis of the third cranial nerve.* It is of common occurrence. It may be congenital or acquired. *Clinical features* of third nerve palsy (Fig. 13.25 A and B) include:

- *Ptosis* due to paralysis of the LPS muscle.
- *Deviation.* Eyeball is turned down, out and slightly intorted due to actions of the lateral rectus and superior oblique muscles.
- *Ocular movements* are restricted in all the directions except outward.
- *Pupil* is fixed and dilated due to paralysis of the sphincter pupillae muscle.
- *Accommodation* is completely lost due to paralysis of the ciliary muscle.

- *Crossed diplopia* is elicited on raising the eyelid.
- *Head posture* may be changed if pupillary area remains uncovered.

3. *Double elevator palsy*, also known as monocular elevation deficiency is a congenital condition caused by third nerve nuclear lesion. It is characterised by paresis of the superior rectus and the inferior oblique muscle of the involved eye.

4. *Total ophthalmoplegia*. In this condition all extraocular muscles including LPS and intraocular muscles, viz., sphincter pupillae, and ciliary muscle are paralysed. It results from combined paralysis of third, fourth and sixth cranial nerves. It is a common feature of orbital apex syndrome and cavernous sinus thrombosis.

5. *External ophthalmoplegia*. In this condition, all extraocular muscles are paralysed, sparing the intraocular muscles. It results from lesions at the level of motor nuclei sparing the Edinger-Westphal nucleus.

6. *Internuclear ophthalmoplegia*. In this condition there is lesion of the medial longitudinal bundle. It is the pathway by which various ocular motor nuclei are linked. Internuclear ophthalmoplegia is characterised by: defective action of medial rectus on the side of lesion, horizontal nystagmus of the opposite eye and defective convergence.

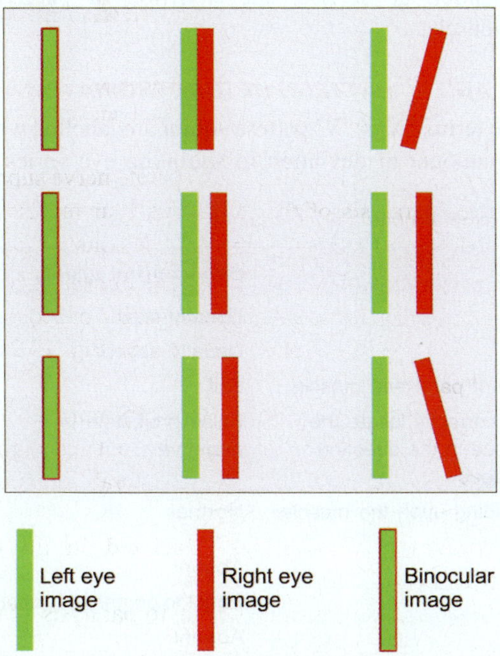

Fig. 13.26. Diplopia chart of a patient with right lateral rectus palsy.

Investigations of a case of paralytic squint

A. *Evaluation for squint*

Every case of squint should be evaluated utilising the tests described on page 327-329. Additional tests required for a case of paralytic squint are:

1. *Diplopia charting.* It is indicated in patients complaining of confusion or double vision. In it patient is asked to wear red and green diplopia charting glasses. Red glass being in front of the right eye and green in front of the left. Then in a semi-dark room, he is shown a fine linear light from a distance of 4 ft. and asked to comment on the images in primary position and in other positions of gaze. Patient tells about the position and the separation of the two images in different fields. Fig. 13.26 shows diplopia charting in a patient with right lateral rectus palsy.
2. *Hess screen test.* Hess screen/Lees screen (Fig. 13.27) test tells about the paralysed muscles and the pathological sequelae of the paralysis, viz., overaction, contracture and secondary inhibitional palsy.

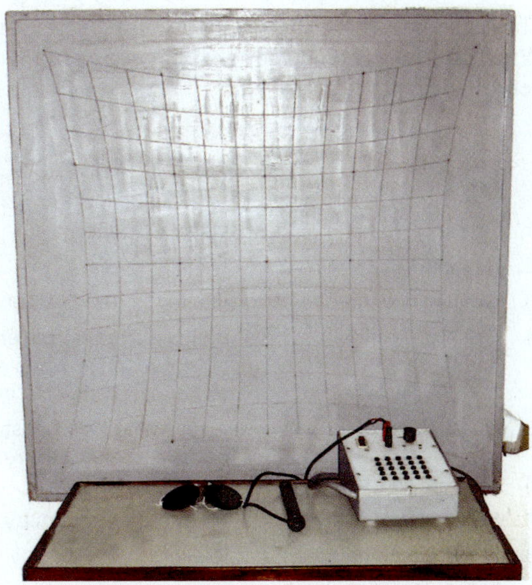

Fig. 13.27. Hess screen.

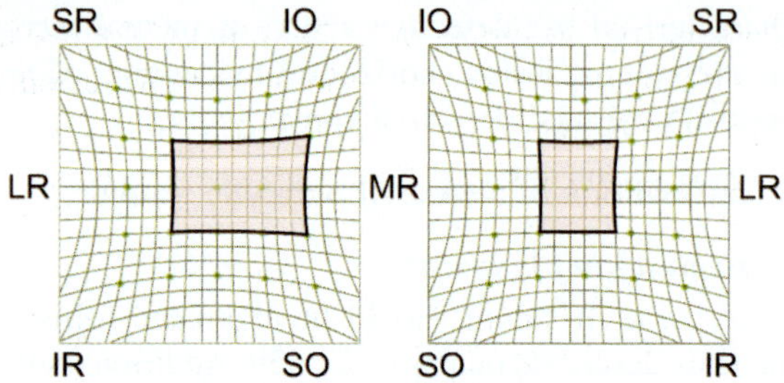

Fig. 13.28. Hess chart in right lateral rectus palsy.

The two charts are compared. The smaller chart belongs to the eye with paretic muscle and the larger to the eye with overacting muscle (Fig. 13.28).

3. *Field of binocular fixation.* It should be tested in patients with paralytic squint where applicable, i.e., if patient has some field of single vision. This test is performed on the perimeter using a central chin rest.
4. *Forced duction test (FDT).* It is performed to differentiate between the incomitant squint due to paralysis of extraocular muscle and that due to mechanical restriction of the ocular movements. FDT is positive (resistance encountered during passive rotation) in cases of incomitant squint due to mechanical restriction and negative in cases of extraocular muscle palsy.

B. *Investigations to find out the cause of paralysis*

These include orbital ultrasonography, orbital and skull computerised tomography scanning and neurological investigations.

Paralytic vs. non-paralytic squint

Differences between paralytic and non-paralytic squint are depicted in Table 13.2.

Management

1. *Treatment of the cause.* An exhaustive investigative work-up should be done to find out the cause and, if possible, treat it.
2. *Conservative measures.* These include: wait and watch for self-improvement to occur for a period of 6 months, vitamin B-complex as neurotonic; and systemic steroids for non-specific inflammations.
3. *Treatment of annoying diplopia.* It includes use of occluder on the affected eye, with intermittent use of both eyes with changed headposture to avoid suppression amblyopia.
4. *Surgical treatment.* It should be carried out in case the recovery does not occur in 6 months. *Aim of treatment* is to provide a comfortable field of binocular fixation, i.e., in central field and lower quadrants. The *principles of surgical treatment* involve strengthening of the paralysed muscle by resection; weakening of the overacting muscle by recession, and transplantation of normal muscle tendon at or near the insertion of paralysed muscle.

'A' AND 'V' PATTERN HETEROTROPIA

The terms 'A' or 'V' pattern squint are labelled when the amount of deviation in squinting eye varies by

Table 13.2. Differences between paralytic and non-paralytic squint

Features	Paralytic squint	Non-paralytic squint
1. Onset	Usually sudden	Usually slow
2. Diplopia	Usually present	Usually absent
3. Ocular movements	Limited in the direction of action of paralysed muscle.	Full
4. False projection	It is positive i.e., patient cannot correctly locate the object in space when asked to see in the direction of paralysed muscle in early stages.	False projection is negative
5. Head posture	A particular head posture depending upon the muscle paralysed may be present.	Normal
6. Nausea and vertigo	Present	Absent
7. Secondary deviation	More than the primary deviation	Equal to primary deviation.
8. In old cases pathological sequelae in the muscles	Present	Absent

more than 10° and 15°, respectively, between upward and downward gaze.

'A' *and* 'V' *esotropia*. In 'A' esotropia the amount of deviation increases in upward gaze and decreases in downward gaze. The reverse occurs in 'V' esotropia.

'A' *and* 'V' *exotropia*. In 'A' exotropia the amount of deviation decreases in upward gaze and increases in downward gaze. The reverse occurs in 'V' exotropia.

Clinical presentations

A and V pattern heterophoria essentially refer to vertically incomitant horizontal strabismus. Thus, the horizontally comitant esotropias and exotropias (described on page 324-326) may be associated with A or V patterns.

RESTRICTIVE SQUINT

In restrictive squint, the extraocular muscle is not paralysed but its movement is mechanically restricted. Restrictive squints are characterized by a smaller ocular deviation in primary position in proportion to the limitation of movement and a positive forced duction test (i.e., a restriction is encountered on passive rotation) (see page 354).

Common causes of restrictive squint are:

- Duane's retraction syndrome,
- Brown's superior oblique tendon sheath syndrome,
- Strabismus fixus,
- Dysthyroid ophthalmopathy (see page 417), and
- Incarceration of extraocular muscle in blow-out fracture of the orbit (see page 425).

1. Duane's retraction syndrome

Duane's retraction syndrome is a congenital ocular motility defect occurring due to fibrous tightening of lateral or medial or both rectus muscles. Its features are:

- Limitation of abduction (type I DRS) or adduction (type II DRS) or both (type III DRS).
- Retraction of the globe and narrowing of the palpebral fissure on attempted adduction.
- Eye in the primary position may be orthotropic, esotropic or exotropic.

2. Brown's superior oblique tendon sheath syndrome

It is congenital ocular motility defect due to fibrous tightening of the superior oblique tendon. It is characterized by limitation of elevation of the eye in adduction (normal elevation in abduction), usually straight eyes in primary position and positive forced duction test on attempts to elevate eye in adduction.

3. Strabismus fixus

It is a rare condition characterised by bilateral fixation of eyes in convergent position due to fibrous tightening of the medial recti.

STRABISMUS SURGERY

Surgical techniques

1. *Muscle weakening procedures* include recession, marginal myotomy and myectomy.
2. *Muscle strengthening procedures* are resection, tucking and advancement.
3. *Procedures that change direction of muscle action.* These include (a) vertical transposition of horizontal recti to correct 'A' and 'V' patterns (b) posterior fixation suture (Faden operation) to correct dissociated vertical deviation; and (c) transplantation of muscles in paralytic squints.

Steps of recession (Fig. 13.29)

1. Muscle is exposed by reflecting a flap of overlying conjunctiva and Tenon's capsule.

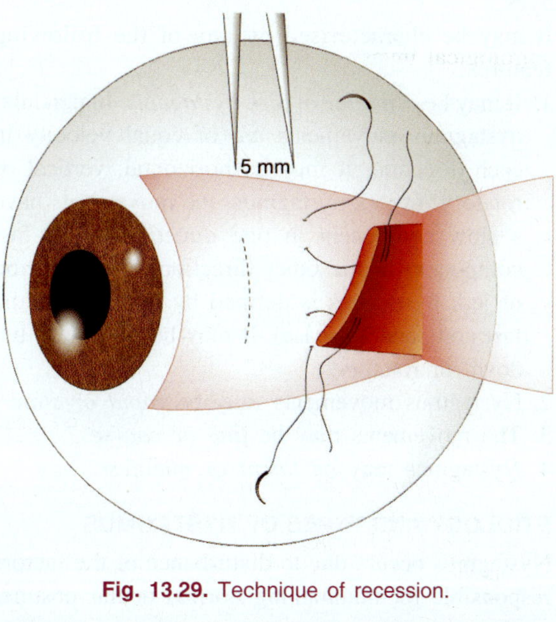

Fig. 13.29. Technique of recession.

2. Two vicryl sutures are passed through the outer quarters of the muscle tendon near the insertion.
3. The muscle tendon is disinserted from the sclera with the help of tenotomy scissors.
4. The amount of recession is measured with the callipers and marked on the sclera.
5. The muscle tendon is sutured with the sclera at the marked site posterior to original insertion.
6. Conjunctival flap is sutured back.

Steps of resection (Fig. 13.30)

1. Muscle is exposed as for recession and the amount to be resected is measured with callipers and marked.
2. Two absorbable sutures are passed through the outer quarters of the muscles at the marked site.
3. The muscle tendon is disinserted from the sclera and the portion of the muscle anterior to sutures is excised.
4. The muscle stump is sutured with the sclera at the original insertion site.
5. Conjunctival flap is sutured back.

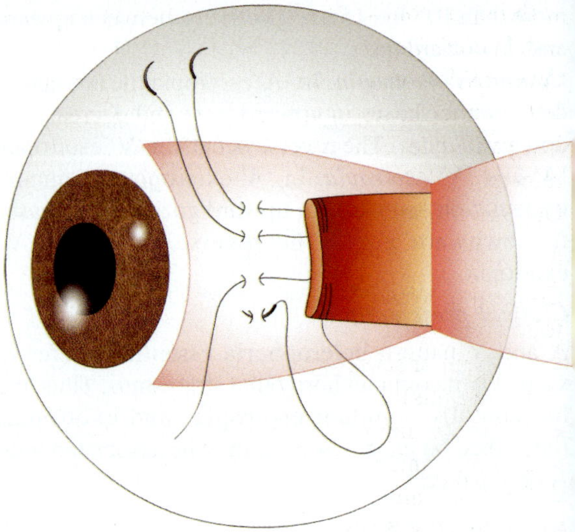

Fig. 13.30. Technique of resection.

NYSTAGMUS

DEFINITION AND FEATURES

Nystagmus is defined as regular and rhythmic to-and-fro involuntary oscillatory movements of the eyes.

It may be characterised by any of the following features:

1. It may be *pendular or jerk nystagmus.* In pendular nystagmus movements are of equal velocity in each direction. It may be horizontal, vertical or rotatory. In jerk nystagmus, the movements have a slow component in one direction and a fast component in the other direction. The direction of jerk nystagmus is defined by direction of the fast component (phase). It may be right, left, up, down or rotatory.
2. Nystagmus movements may be *rapid or slow.*
3. The movements may be *fine or coarse.*
4. Nystagmus may be *latent or manifest.*

ETIOLOGY AND TYPES OF NYSTAGMUS

Nystagmus occurs due to disturbance of the factors responsible for maintaining normal ocular posture. These include disorders of sensory visual pathway, vestibular apparatus, semicircular canals, mid-brain and cerebellum. Nystagmus may be classified into three groups:

- Physiological nystagmus,
- Congenital nystagmus, and
- Acquired nystagmus

I. Physiological nystagmus

Physiological nystagmus occurs normally in a variety of situation including optokinetic nystagmus (OKN), end-gaze nystagmus (EGN) and physiological vestibular nystagmus (vestibulo-ocular reflex i.e., VOR)

1. *Optokinetic nystagmus.* It is a physiological jerk nystagmus induced by presenting to gaze the objects moving serially in one direction, such as strips of a spinning optokinetic drum. The eyes will follow a fixed strip momentarily and then jerk back to reposition centrally to fix up a new strip. Similar condition occurs while looking at outside things from a moving train.

2. *End-gaze nystagmus.* It is a fine jerk horizontal nystagmus seen in normal persons on extreme right or left gaze.

3. *Physiological vestibular nystagmus* (vestibulo-ocular reflex i.e., VOR). It is a jerk nystagmus which can be elicited by stimulating the tympanic membrane with hot or cold water. It forms the basis of caloric test. If cold water is poured into right ear the patient develops left jerk nystagmus (rapid phase towards left), while the reverse happens with warm water, i.e., patient develops right jerk nystagmus. It can be remembered by the mnemonic 'COWS' (Cold–Opposite, Warm–Same).

II. Congenital nystagmus

Congenital nystagmus having onset in infancy is of following types:

- Afferent or sensory nystagmus (congenital ocular nystagmus)
- Idiopathic infantile nystagmus
- Latent/manifest latent nystagmus
- Spasmus nutans
- Nystagmus blockage syndrome

1. *Afferent or sensory nystagmus*

Etiology. Also known as congenital ocular nystagmus, it is usually associated with sensory deprivation due to any of the following causes :

- *Ocular albinism*, chararacterized by iris transillumination defects and foveal hypoplasia.
- *Aniridia* i.e. bilateral near total congenital iris absence.
- *Leber's congenital amaurosis,* characterized by markedly abnormal or flat electroretinogram.
- *Other causes* include, bilateral congenital cataract, achromatopsia, congenital stationary night blindness, bilateral optic nerve hypoplasia, bilateral congenital toxoplasmosis and bilateral macular hypoplasia.

Features. It is characterized by erratic waveform with or without roving eye movements associated with reduced visual acuity due to above mentioned conditions

2. *Idiopathic infantile nystagmus*

Features. Also known as 'idiopathic congenital nystagmus', is characterized by following features:

- *Hereditary* (autosomal dominant, autosomal recessive or X-linked) nystagmus of unknown etiology which persists throughout life.
- *Onset* is early, usually by two months of age.
- *Waveform.* Conjugate horizontal jerk nystagmus, worsens with fixation but improves within 'null zone' and on convergence. The null zone is the direction of gaze in which the nystagmus dampens. Occasionally the nystagmus can be vertical or rotatory.

3. *Latent/manifest latent nystagmus*

- It is not present when both eyes are open. It appears when one eye is covered. It is a jerk nystagmus with rapid phase towards the uncovered eye.
- While testing visual acuity in such patients, one eye should be fogged (by adding plus lenses in front) rather than occluding to minimize induction of latent nystagmus.
- May be associated with congenital esotropia and dissociated vertical deviation (DVD).
- Becomes manifest under monocular viewing conditions i.e., in the presence of decreased vision in one eye as in anisometropic amblyopia, strabismic amblyopia etc.

4. *Spasmus nutans*

It is characterised by fine pendular horizontal nystagmus associated with head nodding and abnormal head posture. It appears in infancy and self-resolves by the age of 3 years.

5. *Nystagmus blockage syndrome*

It is a rare condition in which sudden esotropia develops in infancy to dampen the horizontal nystagmus.

III. Acquired nystagmus

Late onset or acquired nystagmus is usually characterized by oscillopsia, and is often associated with other neurological abnormalities. Acquired nystagmus includes following conditions:

1. *Gaze-evoked nystagmus*

Features. Slow, conjugate horizontal jerk nystagmus in the direction of gaze (no nystagmus in primary gaze). It occurs at smaller angles than physiological end-gaze nystagmus, i.e. around 45° movement.

Causes. It may occur due to :

- *Neurological lesions* of brainstem and posterior fossa, and
- *CNS depression* caused by certain drugs such as alcohol, anticonvulsants, and barbiturates.

2. *Periodic alternating nystagmus*

Features. Conjugate, horizontal jerk nystagmus present in the primary gaze characterized by spontaneous direction changes every 60-90 seconds, with 10-15 second gap or null period, i.e., period of no nystagmus.

Causes. It occurs usually due to vestibulo-cerebellar diseases such as demyelination and Arnold - Chiari malformation. It may also be associated with cervico-medullary junction lesions.

3. *Peripheral vestibular nystagmus*

Features. Conjugate horizontal jerk nystagmus with fast phase away from the side of lesion. Nystagmus improves with fixation and worsens with gaze towards fast phase.

Causes. It is associated with destructive lesions of vestibular system such as labyrinthitis and vestibular neuritis.

4. *Central vestibular nystagmus*

It may be of the following types:

Up beat nystagmus. In primary position of gaze, the fast component is upward. It is usually seen in lesions of central tegmentum of brain stem.

Down beat nystagmus. In primary position of gaze the fast component is downward. It is usually associated with posterior fossa diseases and is typical of compression at the level of foramen magnum. It is a common feature of cerebellar lesions and Arnold Chiari syndrome.

5. *Acquired pendular nystagmus*

Features. Usually disconjugate with horizontal, vertical and torsional components. May be associated with involuntary, repetitive movements of palate, pharynx and face (oculo-palatal myoclonus).

Causes. It is usually associated with brainstem and cerebellar diseases.

6. *See-saw nystagmus*

Features. In it, one eye rises up and intorts, while other shifts down and extorts.

Causes. It is usually associated with upper brain stem lesions.

7. *Convergence retraction syndrome*

Features. It is a jerk nystagmus with bilateral fast component towards the medial side. It is associated with retraction of the globe in convergence.

Causes. Classically associated with pinealoma, but may also occur with other neoplasms, stroke, trauma or multiple sclerosis.

8. *Dissociated or disconjugate nystagmus*

Features. Unilateral or asymmetric nystagmus usually of the abducting and occasionally of the adducting eye.

Causes. It commonly occurs with internuclear ophthalmoplegia (INO)

NYSTAGMOID MOVEMENTS

These are ocular movements which mimic nystagmus. These include:

1. *Ocular flutter* occurs due to interruption of cerebellar connection to brain stem. It is characterized by horizontal oscillation and inability to fixate after change of gaze.

2. *Opsoclonus* refers to combined horizontal, vertical and/or torsional oscillations associated with myoclonic movement of face, arms and legs. It is seen in patients with encephalitis.

3. *Superior oblique myokymia* is characterized by monocular, rapid, intermittent, torsional vertical movements (which are best seen on slit-lamp examination).

4. *Ocular bobbing* refers to rapid downward deviation of the eyes with slow updrift. It occurs due to pontine dysfunctions.

14

CHAPTER

Diseases of the Eyelids

APPLIED ANATOMY

GROSS ANATOMY

The eyelids are mobile tissue curtains placed in front of the eyeballs (Fig. 14.1). These act as shutters protecting the eyes from injuries and excessive light. These also perform an important function of spreading the tear film over the cornea and conjunctiva and also help in drainage of tears by lacrimal pump system.

Parts of eyelid. Each eyelid is divided by a horizontal furrow (sulcus) into an *orbital and tarsal part.*

Position of lids. When the eye is open, the upper lid covers about one-sixth of the cornea and the lower lid just touches the limbus.

Canthi. The two lids meet each other at medial and lateral angles (or outer and inner canthi). In Caucasians with the lids open, the lateral canthus is about 2 mm higher than the medial canthus.

Palpebral aperture. It is the elliptical space between the upper and the lower lid. When the eyes are open it measures about 10-11 mm vertically in the centre and about 28-30 mm horizontally.

The lid margin. It is about 2-mm broad and is divided into two parts by the punctum. The medial, *lacrimal portion* is rounded and devoid of lashes or glands.

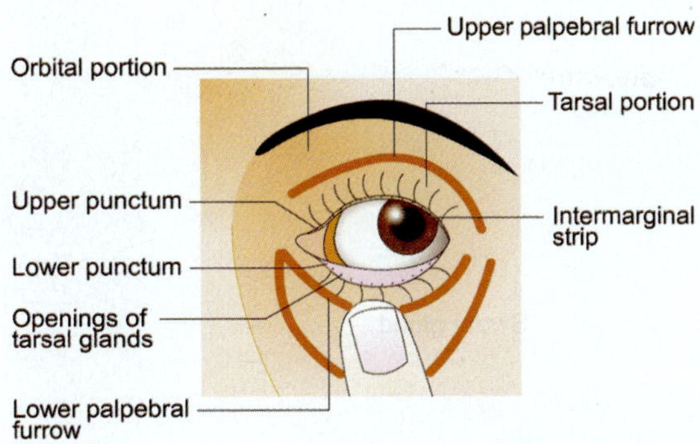

Fig. 14.1. Gross anatomy of the eyelid.

The lateral, *ciliary portion* consists of a rounded anterior border, a sharp posterior border (placed against the globe) and an intermarginal strip (between the two borders). The *grey line* (which marks junction of skin and conjunctiva) divides the intermarginal strip into an anterior strip bearing 2-3 rows of lashes and a posterior strip on which openings of meibomian glands are arranged in a row. The splitting of the eyelids when required in operations is done at the level of grey line.

STRUCTURE

Each eyelid consists (from anterior to posterior) of the following layers (Fig. 14.2):

1. *The skin.* It is elastic having a fine texture and is the thinnest in the body.

2. *The subcutaneous areolar tissue.* It is very loose and contains no fat. It is thus readily distended by oedema or blood.

3. *The layer of striated muscle.* It consists of *orbicularis muscle* which forms an oval sheet across the eyelids. It comprises three portions: the *orbital, palpebral* (pretarsal and preseptal parts) and *lacrimal*. It closes the eyelids and is supplied by zygomatic branch of the facial nerve. Therefore, in paralysis of facial nerve there occurs lagophthalmos which may be complicated by exposure keratitis.

In addition, the upper lid also contains *levator palpebrae superioris* muscle (LPS). It arises from the apex of the orbit and is inserted by three parts on the skin of lid, anterior surface of the tarsal plate and conjunctiva of superior fornix. It raises the upper lid. It is supplied by a branch of oculomotor nerve.

4. *Submuscular areolar tissue.* It is a layer of loose connective tissue. The nerves and vessels lie in this layer. Therefore, to anaesthetise lids, injection is given in this plane.

5. *Fibrous layer.* It is the framework of the lids and consists of two parts: the central tarsal plate and the peripheral septum orbitale (Fig. 14.3).

i. *Tarsal plate.* There are two plates of dense connective tissue, one for each lid, which give shape and firmness to the lids. The upper and lower tarsal plates join with each other at medial and lateral canthi; and are attached to the orbital margins through medial and lateral palpebral ligaments. In the substance of the tarsal plates lie meibomian glands in parallel rows.

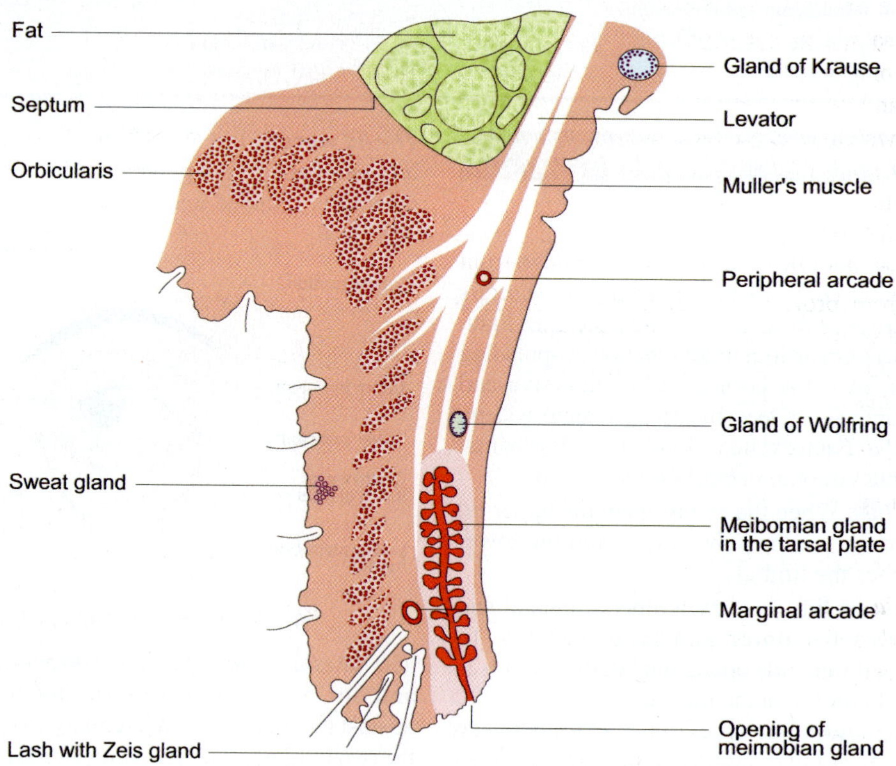

Fig. 14.2. Structure of the upper eyelid.

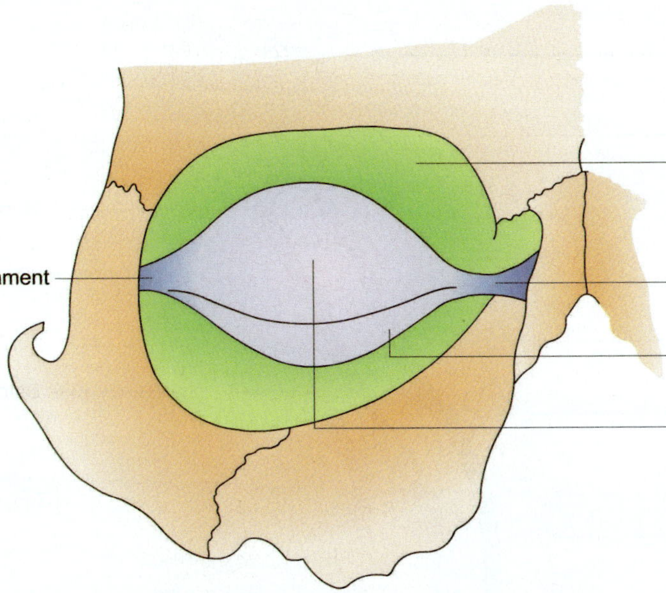

Fig. 14.3. Tarsal plates and septum orbitale.

ii. *Septum orbitale* (palpebral fascia). It is a thin membrane of connective tissue attached centrally to the tarsal plates and peripherally to periosteum of the orbital margin. It is perforated by nerves, vessels and levator palpebrae superioris (LPS) muscle, which enter the lids from the orbit.

6. *Layer of non-striated muscle fibres.* It consists of the palpebral muscle of Muller which lies deep to the septum orbitale in both the lids. In the upper lid it arises from the fibres of LPS muscle and in the lower lid from prolongation of the inferior rectus muscle; and is inserted on the peripheral margins of the tarsal plate. It is supplied by sympathetic fibres.

7. *Conjunctiva.* The part which lines the lids is called *palpebral conjunctiva.* It consists of three parts: marginal, tarsal and orbital. (For structures of conjunctiva see page 52).

GLANDS OF EYELIDS (Fig. 14.4)

1. *Meibomian glands.* These are also known as *tarsal glands* and are present in the stroma of tarsal plate arranged vertically. They are about 30-40 in the upper lid and about 20-30 in the lower lid. They are modified sebaceous glands. Their ducts open at the lid margin. Their secretion constitutes the oily layer of tear film.

2. *Glands of Zeis.* These are also sebaceous glands which open into the follicles of eyelashes.

3. *Glands of Moll.* These are modified sweat glands situated near the hair follicle. They open into the hair follicles or into the ducts of Zeis glands. They do not open directly onto the skin surface as elsewhere.

4. *Accessory lacrimal glands of Wolfring.* These are present near the upper border of the tarsal plate.

BLOOD SUPPLY

The arteries of the lids (medial and lateral palpebral) form *marginal arterial arcades* which lie in the submuscular plane in front of the tarsal plate, 2 mm away from the lid margin, in the upper lid and about 4 mm away in the lower lid. In the upper lid another arcade *(superior arterial arcade)* is formed which lies near the upper border of the tarsal plate. Branches go forward and backward from these arches to supply various structures.

Veins. These are arranged in two plexuses: a post-tarsal which drains into ophthalmic veins and a pre-tarsal opening into subcutaneous veins.

Lymphatics. These are also arranged in two sets: the pre-tarsal and the post-tarsal. Those from lateral half

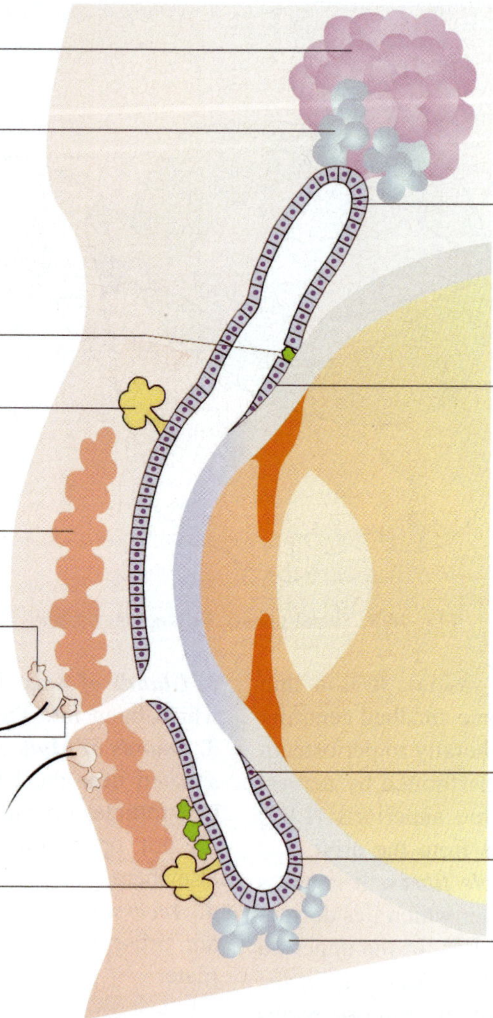

Fig. 14.4. Glands of eyelids.

of the lids drain into preauricular lymph nodes and those from the medial half of the eyelids drain into submandibular lymph nodes.

NERVE SUPPLY

Motor nerves are facial (which supplies orbicularis muscle), oculomotor (which supplies LPS muscle) and sympathetic fibres (which supply the Muller's muscle).

Sensory nerve supply is derived from branches of the trigeminal nerve such as lacrimal, supraorbital and supratrochlear nerves for upper lid; and the infra-orbital nerve with infratrochlear branch for lower lid.

CONGENITAL ANOMALIES

1. *Congenital ptosis.* It is a common congenital anomaly. It is described in detail in the section of ptosis on page 356.

2. *Congenital coloboma.* It is a rare condition characterised by a full thickness triangular gap in the tissues of the lids (Fig. 14.5). The anomaly usually occurs near the nasal side and involves the upper lid more frequently than the lower lid. *Treatment* consists of plastic repair of the defect.

3. *Epicanthus.* It is a semicircular fold of skin which covers the medial canthus. It is a bilateral condition

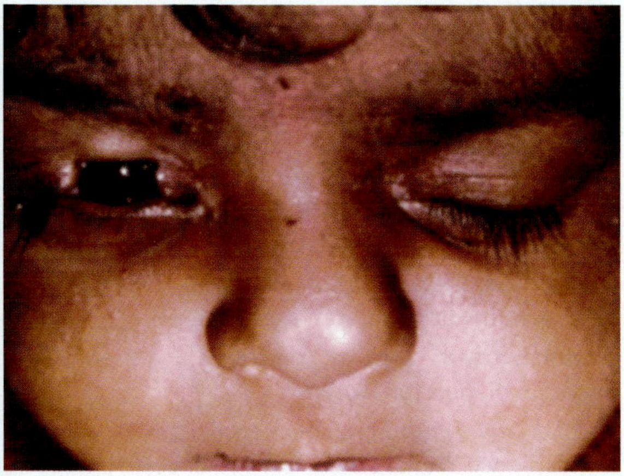

Fig. 14.5. Congenital coloboma upper eyelid.

and may disappear with the development of nose. It is a normal facial feature in Mongolian races. It is the most common congenital anomaly of the lids. *Treatment* consists of plastic repair of the deformity.

4. *Distichiasis.* (see page 370)

5. *Cryptophthalmos.* It is a very rare anomaly in which lids fail to develop and the skin passes continuously from the eyebrow to the cheek hiding the eyeball (Fig. 14.6).

6. *Microblepharon.* In this condition, eyelids are abnormally small. It is usually associated with microphthalmos or anophthalmos. Occasionally the lids may be very small or virtually absent and the condition is called *ablepharon.*

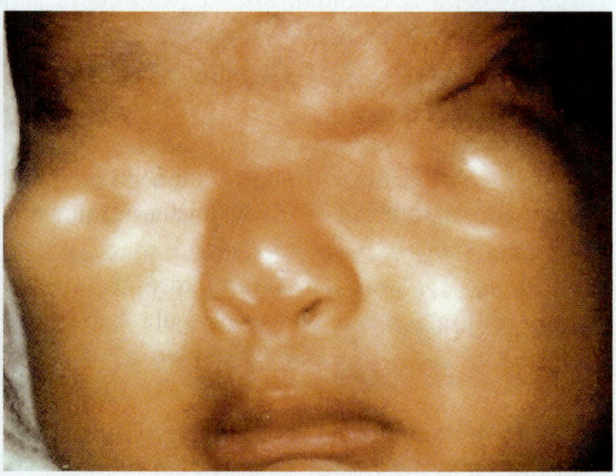

Fig. 14.6. Cryptophthalmos.

7. *Epiblepharon* refers to a congenital anomaly in which a horizontal fold of tissue rides above the lower eyelid margin. It usually disappears with the growth of face and needs no surgical correction.

8. *Euryblepharon* refers to unilateral or bilateral horizontal widening of palpebral fissure. It is usually associated with lateral canthal malposition and lateral ectropion. Congenital euryblepharon usually involves the lateral portion of lower eyelids.

OEDEMA OF THE EYELIDS

Owing to the looseness of the tissues, oedema of the lids is of common occurrence. It may be classified as inflammatory, solid and passive oedema.

I. *Inflammatory oedema.* It is seen in the following conditions.

1. *Inflammations of the lid itself,* which include dermatitis, stye, hordeolum internum, insect bites, cellulitis and lid abscess.
2. *Inflammations of the conjunctiva,* such as acute purulent, membranous and pseudo-membranous conjunctivitis.
3. *Inflammations of the lacrimal sac,* i.e., acute dacryocystitis and lacrimal abscess.
4. *Inflammations of the lacrimal gland,* i.e., acute dacryoadenitis.
5. *Inflammations of the eyeball,* such as acute iridocyclitis, endophthalmitis and panophthalmitis.
6. *Inflammations of the orbit,* which include orbital cellulitis, orbital abscess and pseudo-tumour.
7. *Inflammations of the paranasal sinuses*, e.g., maxillary sinusitis.

II. *Solid oedema of the lids.* It is chronic thickening of the lids, which usually follows recurrent attacks of erysipelas. It resembles oedema of the lids but is harder in consistency.

III. *Passive oedema of the lids.* It may occur due to local or general causes.

1. *Local causes* are: cavernous sinus thrombosis, head injury and angioneurotic oedema.
2. *General causes* are congestive heart failure, renal failure, hypoproteinaemia and severe anaemia.

INFLAMMATORY DISORDERS OF THE EYELIDS

BLEPHARITIS

Blepharitis is a subacute or chronic inflammation of the lid margins. It is an extremely common disease which can be divided into following clinical types:

- Bacterial blepharitis
- Seborrhoeic or squamous blepharitis,
- Mixed staphylococcal with seborrhoeic blepharitis,
- Posterior blepharitis or meibomitis, and
- Parasitic blepharitis.

BACTERIAL BLEPHARITIS

Bacterial blepharitis, also known as chronic anterior blepharitis, or staphylococcal blepharitis or ulcerative blepharitis, is a chronic infection of the anterior part of the lid margin. It is a common cause of ocular discomfort and irritation. The disorder usually starts in childhood and may continue throughout life.

Etiology

Causative organisms, most commonly involved are coagulase positive *Staphylococci*. Rarely, *Streptococci*, *Propionibacterium acnes*, and *Moraxella* may be involved .

Predisposing factors, usually none, may rarely include chronic conjunctivitis and dacryocystitis.

Clinical features

Symptoms include chronic irritation, itching, mild lacrimation, gluing of cilia, and mild photophobia. The symptoms are characteristically worse in the morning. Remissions and exacerbations in symptoms are quite common.

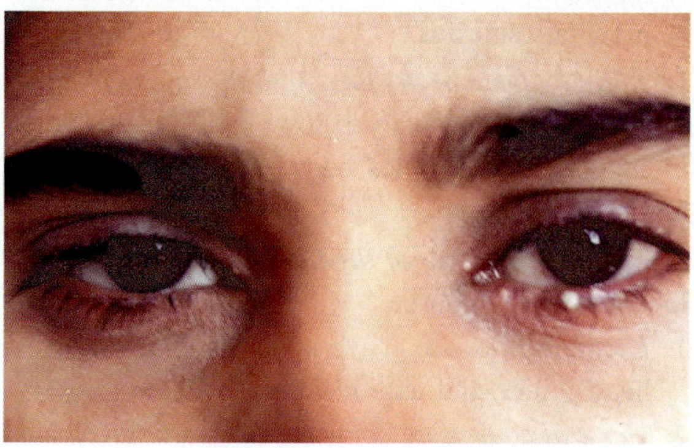

Fig. 14.7. Bacterial blepharitis.

Signs (Fig. 14.7) are as below:

- *Yellow crusts* are seen at the root of cilia which glue them together.
- *Small ulcers*, which bleed easily, are seen on removing the crusts.
- *Red, thickened lid margins* are seen with dilated blood vessels (rosettes).
- *Mild papillary conjunctivitis* and conjunctival hyperemia are common associations .

Complications and sequelae of long standing bacterial blepharitis include:

- *Lash abnormalities* such as madarosis (sparseness or absence of cilia), trichiasis (misdirected cilia), and poliosis (graying of lashes).
- *Tylosis*, i.e. thickening and scarring of lid margin.
- *Eversion of punctum* leading to epiphora.
- *Eczema of skin and ectropion* may develop due to prolonged watering.
- *Recurrent styes* (external hordeola) are a common complication.
- *Marginal Keratitis*, and occasionally phlyctenulosis may develop.
- *Tear film instability*, and dry eye may result.
- *Secondary inflammatory and mechanical changes in the conjunctiva and cornea* are common because of intimate relationship between the lid margins and ocular surface.

Treatment

Bacterial blepharitis should be treated promptly, as below, to avoid complications and sequelae:

1. ***Lid hygiene*** is essential atleast twice daily and should include:
   - *Warm compresses* for 5-10 minutes to soften the crusts,
   - *Crust removal and lid margin cleaning* with the help of cotton buds dipped in the dilute baby shampoo or solution of 3% sodium bicarbonate,
   - *Avoid rubbing of the eyes* or fingering of the lids.
2. ***Antibiotic eye ointment*** should be applied at the lid margin , immediately after removal of the crusts;
   - *Antibiotic eye drops* should be used 3-4 times a day.
   - *Oral antibiotics* such as erythromycin or doxycycline may be useful in unresponsive patients and those complicated by external hordeola and abscess of lash follicle.

3. ***Topial steroids*** (*weak*) such as fluoromethalon may be required in patients with papillary conjunctivitis, marginal keratitis and phlyctenulosis.

4. ***Ocular lubricants***, i.e. artificial tear drops, are required for associated tear film instability and dry eye.

SEBORRHOEIC OR SQUAMOUS BLEPHARITIS

Seborrhoeic blepharitis is primarily anterior blepharitis with some spill over posteriorly. It is of common occurrence.

Etiology. It is usually associated with seborrhoea of scalp (dandruff). Some constitutional and metabolic factors play a part in its etiology. In it, glands of Zeis secrete abnormal excessive neutral lipids which are split by *Corynebacterium acne* into irritating free fatty acids.

Symptoms. Patients usually complain of deposition of whitish material (soft scales) at the lid margin associated with mild discomfort, irritation, occasional watering and a history of falling of eyelashes.

Signs. include:

- *Accumulation of white dandruff-like scales* is seen on the lid margin, among the lashes (Fig. 14.8). On removing these scales underlying surface is found to be hyperaemic and greasy (no ulcers).
- *The lashes fall out easily* but are usually replaced quickly without distortion.
- *Lid margin* is thickened and the sharp posterior border tends to be rounded leading to epiphora, in long standing cases.
- *Signs of bacterial blepharitis*, as described above, may be superadded in patients with mixed seborroeic and bacterial blepheritis.

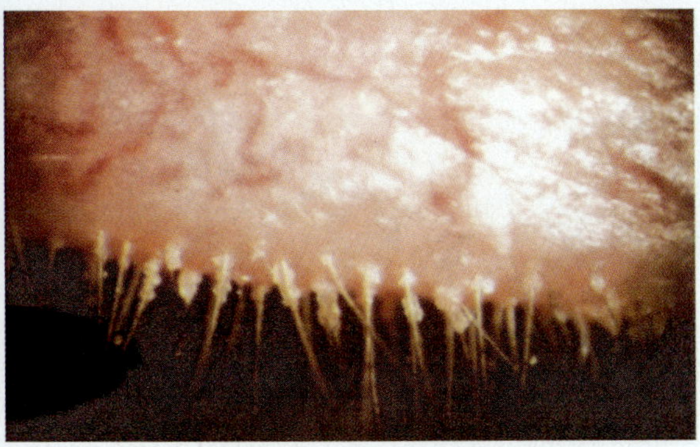

Fig. 14.8. Seborrhoeic blepharitis.

Complications are similar to bacterial blepharitis with comparatively lesser frequency (see page 364).

Treatment.

- *General measures* include improvement of health and balanced diet.
- Associated *seborrhoea of the scalp* should be adequately treated.
- *Local measures* include removal of scales from the lid margin with the help of lukewarm solution of 3 percent soda bicarb or baby shampoo and frequent application of combined antibiotic and steroid eye ointment at the lid margin.
- *Antibiotics,* as described above in bacterial blepharitis, may be required in patients with mixed seborrhoeic and bacterial blepharitis.

POSTERIOR BLEPHARITIS (MEIBOMITIS)

Meibomitis, i.e. inflammation of Meibomian glands occurs in chronic and acute forms.

1. Chronic Meibomitis

Chronic meibomitis is a commonly occurring meibomian gland dysfunction, seen more commonly in middle aged persons, especially those with acne rosacea and/or seborrhoeic dermatitis. Bacterial lipases are being blamed to play main role in the pathogenesis of chronic meibomitis.

Clinical features

Symptoms include chronic irritation, burning, itching, grittiness, mild lacrimation with remissions and exacerbations intermittently. Symptoms are characteristically worse in the morning.

Signs include (Fig 14.9):

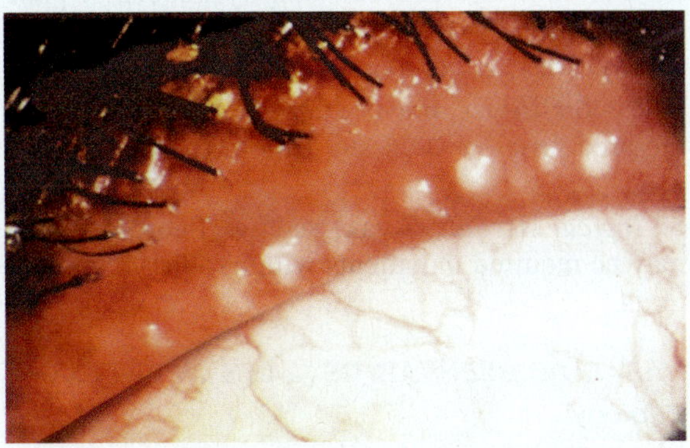

Fig. 14.9. Chronic meibomitis.

- *White frothy (foam like) secretions* are frequently seen on the eyelid margins and canthi (meibomian seborrhoea).
- *Opening of meibomian glands* become prominent with thick secretions which can be expressed out by pressure on the lids giving tooth-paste appearance.
- *Vertical yellowish streaks shinning* through conjunctiva can be seen on eversion of the lids. These represent the meibomian ducts filled with thick secretion.
- *Hyperemia and telangectasia* of posterior lid margin around the orifices of meibomian glands can be seen frequently.

2. Acute meibomitis

Acute meibomitis occurs due to staphylococcal infection. It is characterized by painful swelling around the involved gland. Pressure on it results in expression of pus bead followed by serosanguinous discharge.

Treatment of meibomitis

1. ***Lid hygiene*** is essential at least once a day and should include:

- *Warm compresses* for several minutes.
- *Expression* of accumulated secretions by repeated vertical massage of lids in the form of milking.

2. ***Topical antibiotics*** in the form of eye ointment should be rubbed at the lid margin immediately after massage, and

- Eye drops may be used 3-4 times a day.

3. ***Systemc tetracyclines***, e.g. doxycycline 100 mg b.d. for 1 week and then o.d. for 6-12 weeks, remain the mainstay of treatment of posterior blepharitis because of their ability to block staphylococcal lipase production. Erythromycin may be used where tetracyclines are contraindicated.

4. ***Ocular lubricants*** i.e. artificial tear drops are required for associated tear film instability and dry eye.

5. ***Topical steroids*** (weak) such as fluoromethalon may be required in patients with papillary conjunctivits.

PARASITIC BLEPHARITIS (LASH INFESTATION)

Etiology

Blepharitis associated with infestation of lashes by lice is not uncommon in persons living in poor hygienic conditions. The lice infestations include the following:

- *Phthiriasis palpebrum* refers to the infestation by *phthirus pubis* (crab louse). It is most commonly seen in adults in whom it is usually acquired as a sexually transmitted infection.
- *Pediculosis* refers to the infestation by *pediculus humanus corporis* or *capitis* (head louse). If heavily infested the lice may spread to involve lashes.

Clinical Features

Infestation of lashes with lice causes chronic blepharitis and chronic follicular conjunctivitis.

Symptoms include chronic irritation, itching, burning, and mild lacrimation

Signs are as below (Fig. 14.10).

- *Lid margins* are red and inflamed.
- *Lice* anchoring the lashes with their claws may be seen on slit lamp examination,
- *Nits (eggs)* may be seen as opalescent pearls adherent to the base of cilia.
- *Conjunctival congestion* and follicles may be seen in long standing cases.

Treatment

- *Mechanical removal* of the lices and nits with forceps.
- *Application of antibiotic ointment* and yellow mercuric oxide 1% to the lid margins and lashes.
- *Delousing* of the patient, family members, clothing and bedding is important to prevent recurrences.

EXTERNAL HORDEOLUM (STYE)

It is an acute suppurative inflammation of lash follicle and its associated glands of Zeis or Moll.

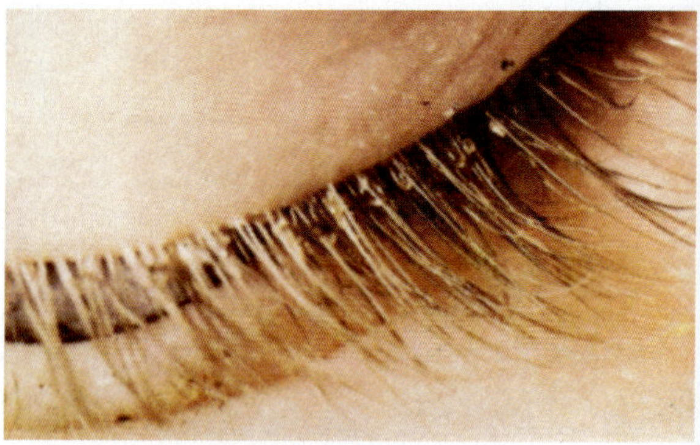

Fig. 14.10. Phthiriasis palpebrum.

Etiology

1. ***Predisposing factors***. It is more common in children and young adults (though no age is bar) and in patients with eye strain due to muscle imbalance or refractive errors. Habitual rubbing of the eyes or fingering of the lids and nose, chronic blepharitis and diabetes mellitus are usually associated with recurrent styes. Metabolic factors, chronic debility, excessive intake of carbohydrates and alcohol also act as predisposing factors.
2. ***Causative organism*** commonly involved is *Staphylococcus aureus*.

Clinical features

Symptoms include acute pain associated with swelling of lid, mild watering and photophobia.

Signs are as follows:

- *Stage of cellulitis* is characterised by localised, firm, red, tender swelling at the lid margin associated with marked oedema (Fig. 14.11). Usually there is one stye, but occasionally, these may be multiple.

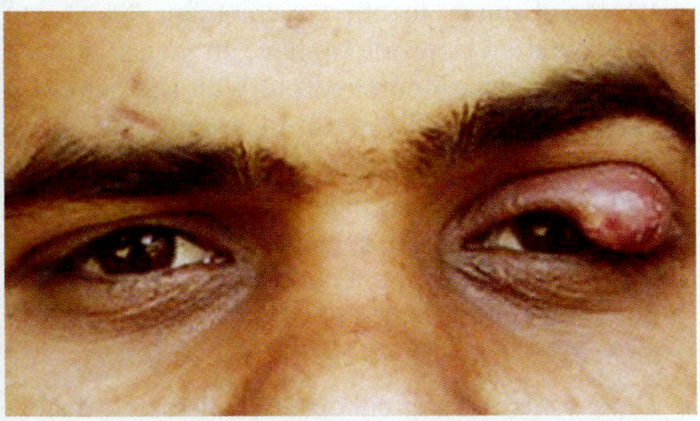

Fig. 14.11. Hordeolum externum (stye) upper eyelid.

- *Stage of abscess* formation is characterised by a visible pus point on the lid margin in relation to the affected cilia.

Treatment

- *Hot compresses* 2-3 times a day are very useful in cellulitis stage.
- *Evacuation* of the pus should be done by epilating the involved cilia, when the pus point is formed. *Surgical incision* is required rarely for a large abscess.
- *Antibiotic* eye drops (3-4 times a day) and eye ointment (at bed time) should be applied to control the infection.
- *Systemic anti-inflammatory and analgesics* relieve pain and reduce oedema.
- *Systemic antibiotics* should be used for early control of infection.
- *In recurrent styes,* try to find out and treat the associated predisposing condition.

CHALAZION

Chalazion, also called a *tarsal* or *meibomian cyst*, is a chronic non-infective granulomatous inflammation of the meibomian gland. This is the commonest of all lid lumps.

Etiology

1. *Predisposing factors* are similar to hordeolum externum.
2. *Pathogenesis.* Usually, first there occurs mild grade infection of the meibomian gland by organisms of very low virulence. As a result, there occurs proliferation of the epithelium and infiltration of the walls of the ducts, which are blocked. Consequently, there occurs retention of secretions (sebum) in the gland, causing its enlargement. The pent-up secretions (fatty in nature) act like an irritant and excite non-infective lipogranulomatous inflammation of the blocked meibomian glands.

Clinical picture

Symptoms include:

- *Painless swelling* in the eyelid, gradually increasing in size is the main presenting symptom.
- *Mild heaviness* in the lid may be felt with moderately large chalazion.
- *Blurred vision* may occur occasionally due to induced astigmatism by a very large chalazion pressing on the cornea.
- *Watering* (*epiphora*) may occur sometimes due to eversion of lower punctum caused by a large chalazion of the lower eyelid .

Signs include:

- *Nodule* is noted slightly away from the lid margin (Fig. 14.12) which is firm to hard and non tender on palpation. Upper lid is involved more commonly than the lower lid probably because of the fact that upper lid contains more meibomian glands than the lower lid. Frequently multiple chalazia may be seen.
- *Reddish purple area*, where the chalazion usually points, is seen on the palpebral conjunctiva after eversion of the lid.

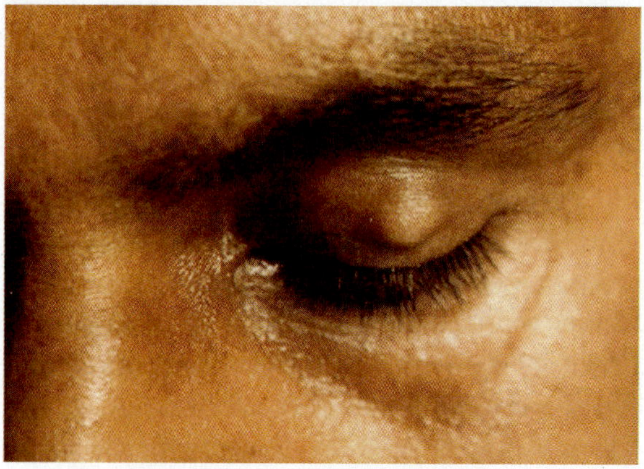

Fig. 14.12. Chalazion upper eye lid.

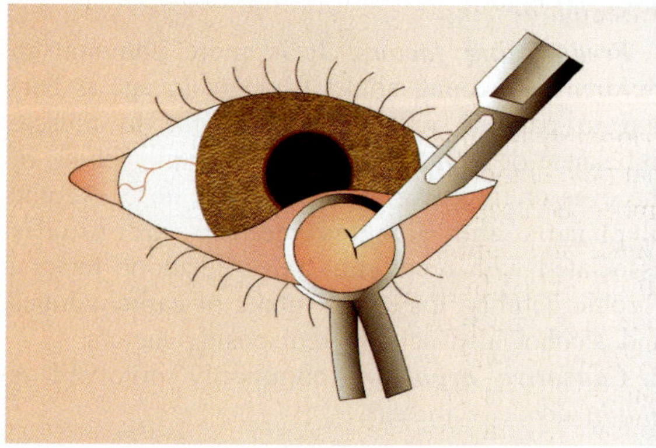

Fig. 14.13. Incision and curettage of chalazion from the conjunctival side.

- *Projection* of the main bulk of the swelling on the skin side may be seen rarely instead of conjunctival side.
- *Marginal chalazion*, occurring occasionally, may present as small reddish grey nodule on the lid margin.

Clinical course and complications

- *Complete spontaneous resolution* may occur rarely.
- *Slow increase in size* is often seen and eventually it may becomes very large.
- *Fungating mass of granulation tissue* may be formed occasionally when the lesion bursts on the conjunctival side.
- *Secondary infection* may lead to formation of hordeolum internum.
- *Calcification* may occur, though very rarely.
- *Malignant change* into meibomian gland carcinoma may be seen occasionally in elderly people.

Treatment

1. *Conservative treatment.* In a small, soft and recent chalazion, self-resolution may be helped by conservative treatment in the form of hot fomentation, topical antibiotic eyedrops and oral anti-inflammatory drugs.
2. *Intralesional injection of long-acting steroid* (triamcinolone) is reported to cause resolution in about 50 percent cases, especially in small and soft chalazia of recent onset, located near the puncta, where incision and curretage may cause damage.
3. *Incision and curettage* (Fig. 14.13) is the conventional and effective treatment for chalazion. Surface anaesthesia is obtained by instillation of xylocaine drops in the eye and the lid in the region of the chalazion is infiltrated with 2 percent xylocaine solution. An incision is made with a sharp blade, which should be vertical on the conjunctival side (to avoid injury to other meibomian ducts) and horizontal on skin side (to have an invisible scar). The contents are curetted out with the help of a chalazion scoop. To avoid recurrence, its cavity should be cauterised with carbolic acid. An antibiotic ointment is instilled and eye padded for about 12 hours. To decrease postoperative discomfort and prevent infection, antibiotic eyedrops, hot fomentation and oral anti-inflammatory and analgesics may be given for 3-4 days.
4. *Diathermy.* A marginal chalazion is better treated by diathermy.
5. *Oral tetracycline* should be given as prophylaxis in recurrent chalazia, especially if associated with acne rosacea.

INTERNAL HORDEOLUM

It is a suppurative inflammation of the meibomian gland associated with blockage of the duct.

Etiology.

Predisposing factors are similar to hordeolum externum (see page 367).

Causative mechanism. Hordeolum internum may occur as:

- *Primary Staphylococcal infection* of the meibomian gland or due to

- *Secondary infection in a chalazion* (infected chalazion).

Clinical picture

Symptoms are similar to hordeolum externum, except that pain is more intense, due to the swelling being embedded deeply in the dense fibrous tissue.

Signs. On examination, hordeolum internum can be differentiated from hordeolum externum by the fact that in it, the point of maximum tenderness and swelling is away from the lid margin and that pus usually points on the tarsal conjunctiva (seen as yellowish area on everting the lid) and not on the root of cilia (Fig. 14.14). Sometimes, pus point may be seen at the opening of involved meibomian gland or rarely on the skin.

Treatment

It is similar to hordeolum externum (see page 367), except that, when pus is formed, it should be drained by a vertical incision from the tarsal conjunctiva.

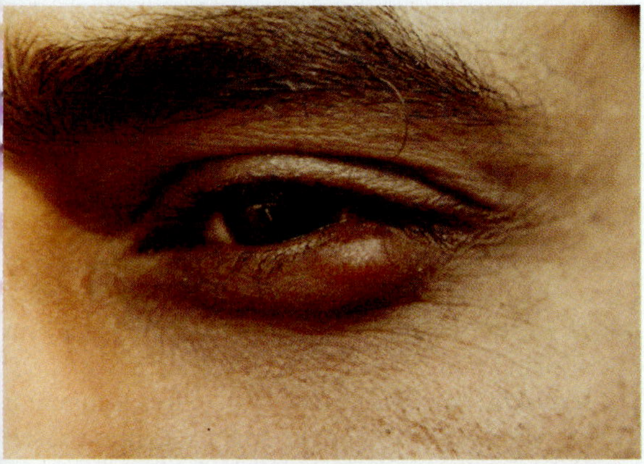

Fig. 14.14. Hordeolum internum lower eyelid.

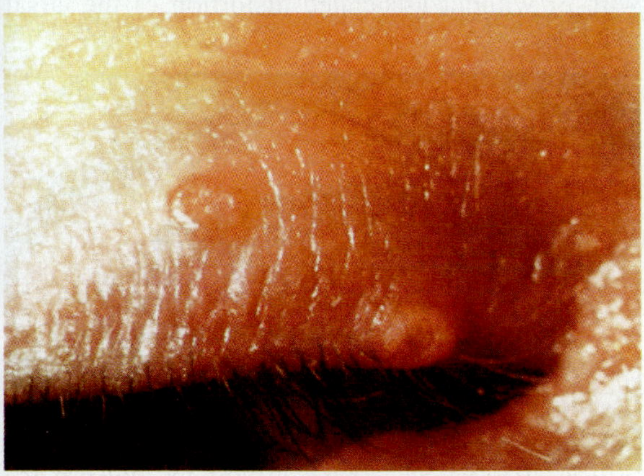

Fig. 14.15. Molluscum contagiosum of the lids.

MOLLUSCUM CONTAGIOSUM

Etiology. It is a viral infection of the lids, commonly affecting children. It is caused by a large poxvirus.

Clinical features. Its typical lesions are multiple, pale, waxy, umbilicated swellings scattered over the skin near the lid margin (Fig. 14.15).

Complications include chronic follicular conjunctivitis and superficial keratitis.

Treatment. The skin lesions should be incised and the interior cauterised with tincture of iodine or pure carbolic acid.

EYELASH DISORDERS

TRICHIASIS

It refers to inward misdirection of cilia (which rub against the eyeball) with normal position of the lid margin (Fig. 14.16).

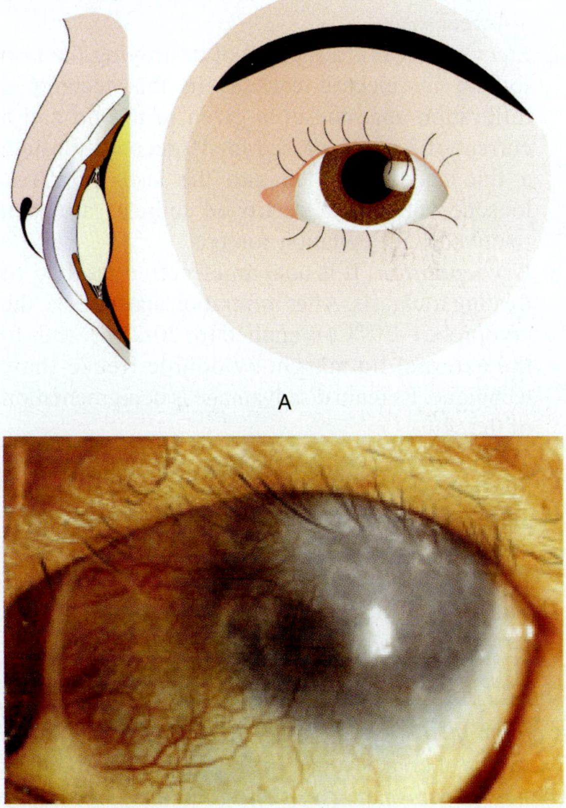

A

B

Fig. 14.16. Trichiasis; A, diagramatic depiction; B, clinical photograph.

Etiology. Common causes of trichiasis are: cicatrising trachoma, ulcerative blepharitis, healed membranous conjunctivitis, hordeolum externum, mechanical injuries, burns, and operative scar on the lid margin.

Symptoms. These include foreign body sensation and photophobia. Patient may feel troublesome irritation, pain and lacrimation.

Signs. Examination reveals one or more misdirected cilia touching the cornea. Reflex blepharospasm and photophobia occur when cornea is abraded. Conjunctiva may be congested. Signs of causative disease viz. trachoma, blepharitis etc. may be present.

Complications. These include recurrent corneal abrasions, superficial corneal opacities, corneal vascularisation (Fig. 14.16B) and non-healing corneal ulcer.

Treatment. A few misdirected cilia may be treated by any of the following methods:

1. *Epilation* (mechanical removal with forceps). It is a temporary measure, as recurrence occurs within 3-4 weeks.
2. *Electrolysis.* It is a method of destroying the lash follicle by electric current. In this technique, infiltration anaesthesia is given to the lid and a current of 2 mA is passed for 10 seconds through a fine needle inserted into the lash root. The loosened cilia with destroyed follicles are then removed with epilation forceps.
3. *Cryoepilation.* It is also an effective method of treating trichiasis. After infiltration anaesthesia, the cryoprobe (–20 °C) is applied for 20-25 seconds to the external lid margin by double freeze-thaw technique. Its main disadvantage is depigmentation of the skin.
4. *Surgical correction.* When many cilia are misdirected operative treatment similar to cicatricial entropion should be employed.

PSEUDOTRICHIASIS

The inward turning of lashes along with the lid margin (seen in entropion) is called *pseudotrichiasis.*

DISTICHIASIS

Congenital distichiasis is a rare anomaly in which an extra row of cilia occupies the position of Meibomian glands which open into their follicles as ordinary sebaceous glands. These cilia are usually directed backwards and when rubbing the cornea, should be electroepilated or cryoepilated.

Acquired distichiasis (metaplastic lashes) occurs when due to metaplasia and differentiation, the meibomian glands are transformed into hair follicles. The most important cause is late stage of cicatrizing conjunctivitis associated with chemical injury, Stevens-Johnson syndrome and ocular cicatricial pemphigoid.

MADAROSIS

Madarosis refers to partial or complete loss of eyelashes.

Causes can be local or systemic.

- *Local causes* of madarosis include cicatrizing conjunctivitis, and complication of cryotherapy, radiotherapy or surgery done for any eyelid lesion.
- *Systemic causes* of madarosis are alopecia (patchy, totalis/universalis), psoriasis, hypothyroidism and leprosy.

ANOMALIES IN THE POSTION OF LID MARGINS

ENTROPION

Entropion refers to inturning of the lid margin.

Etiological types

1. *Congenital entropion.* It is a rare condition seen since birth. In it, pretarsal orbicularis is hypertrophied, forming a marked rigid. It may be associated with micro-phthalmos.

2. *Cicatricial entropion* (Fig. 14.17). It is a common variety usually involving the upper lid. It is caused by cicatricial contraction of the palpebral conjunctiva, with or without associated distortion of the tarsal plate.

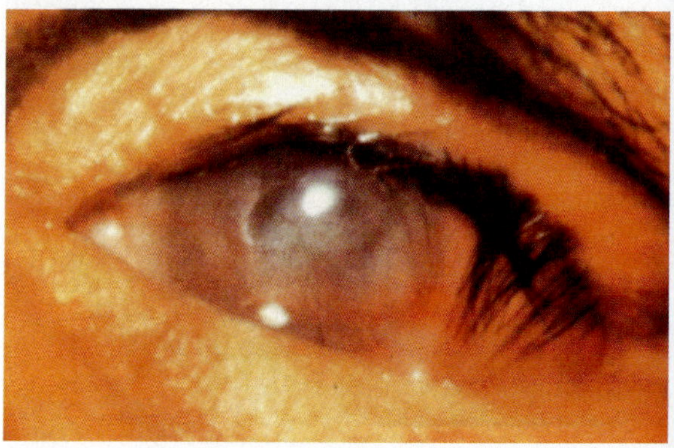

Fig. 14.17. Cicatricial entropion.

Common causes are trachoma, membranous conjunctivitis, chemical burns, pemphigus and Stevens-Johnson syndrome.

3. *Senile (involutional) entropion.* It is common occurence and affects only the lower lid in elder people (Fig. 14.18).

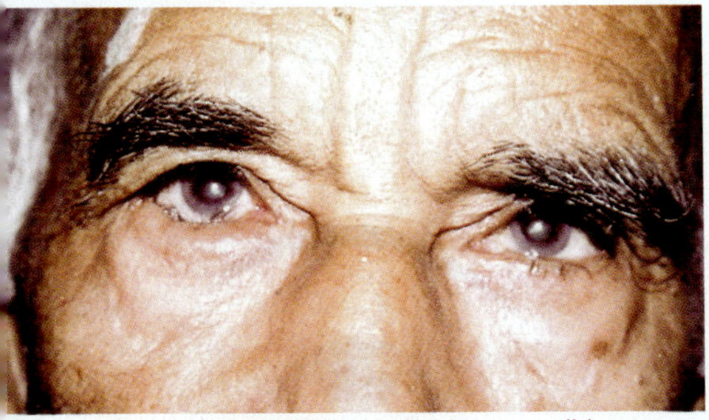

Fig. 14.18. Senile entropion lower eyelid.

Etiological factors which contribute for its development are:

- *Horizontal laxity* of the lid due to weakening of orbicularis muscle.
- *Vertical lid instability* due to weakening or dehiscence of capsulopalpebral fascia (lower lid retractor);
- *Over-riding of pretarsal orbicularis.* Degeneration of palpebral connective tissue separates the orbicularis muscle fibres and thus allowes pre-septal fibres to over-ride the pretarsal fibres; and

4. *Mechanical entropion.* It occurs due to lack of support provided by the globe to the lids. Therefore, it may occur in patients with phthisis bulbi, enophthalmos and after enucleation or evisceration operation.

Clinical picture

Symptoms occur due to rubbing of cilia against the cornea and conjunctiva and are thus similar to trichiasis. These include foreign body sensation, irritation, lacrimation and photophobia.

Signs. are as follows:

1. *Inturning of lid margins.* On examination, lid margin is found inturned. Depending upon the degree of inturning it can be divided into three grades:
   - *Grade I entropion*, only the posterior lid border is inrolled.
   - *Grade II entropion*, includes inturning up to the inter-marginal strip and
   - *Grade III entropion*, in which the whole lid margin including the anterior border is inturned.
2. *Signs of causative disease* e.g. scarring of palpebral conjunctiva in cicatricial entropion, and horizontal lid laxity in involutional entropion may be seen.
3. *Signs of complications* include recurrent corneal abrasions, superficial corneal opacities, corneal vascularization and even corneal ulceration.

Treatment

1. *Congenital entropion* may resolve with time without need of any intervention or may require plastic reconstruction of the lid crease and correction of the underlying defect.

2. *Cicatricial entropion.* It is treated by a plastic operation, which is based on any of the following basic principles:

- Altering the direction of lashes, or
- Transplanting the lashes, or
- Straightening the distorted tarsus.

Surgical techniques employed for correcting cicatricial entropion are as follows:

i. *Anterior lamellar resection.* It is the simplest operation employed to correct mild degree of entropion. In this operation, an elliptical strip of skin and orbicularis muscle is resected 3 mm away from the lid margin.

ii. *Tarsal wedge resection.* It corrects moderate degree of entropion associated with atrophic tarsus. In this operation, in addition to the elliptical resection of skin and muscle, a wedge of tarsal plate is also removed (Fig. 14.19).

iii. *Transposition of tarsoconjunctival wedge.* (Modified Ketssey's operation) (Fig. 14.20): This is indicated to treat mild to moderate amount of cicatricial entropion. It basically involves tarsal fracture and eversion of distal tarsus. A horizontal incision is made along the whole length of sulcus subtarsalis (2-3 mm above the lid margin) involving conjunctiva and tarsal plate (Fig. 14.20A). The lower piece of tarsal plate is undermined up to lid margin. Mattress sutures are then passed from the upper cut end of the tarsal plate to emerge on the skin 1 mm above the lid margin (Fig. 14.20B). When sutures are tied the entropion is corrected by transposition of tarsoconjunctival wedge (Fig. 14.20C).

iv. *Posterior lamellar graft.* Indications of this operation includes severe entropion with upper eyelid retraction. In this operation the deficient or keratinized conjunctiva and the scarred and contracted tarsus are replaced by a composite

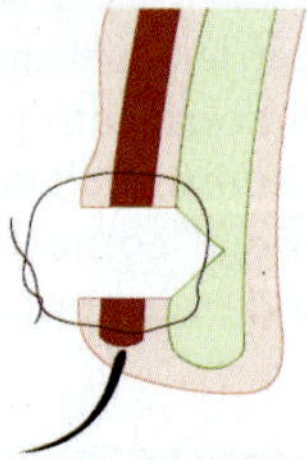

Fig. 14.19. Tarsal wedge resection

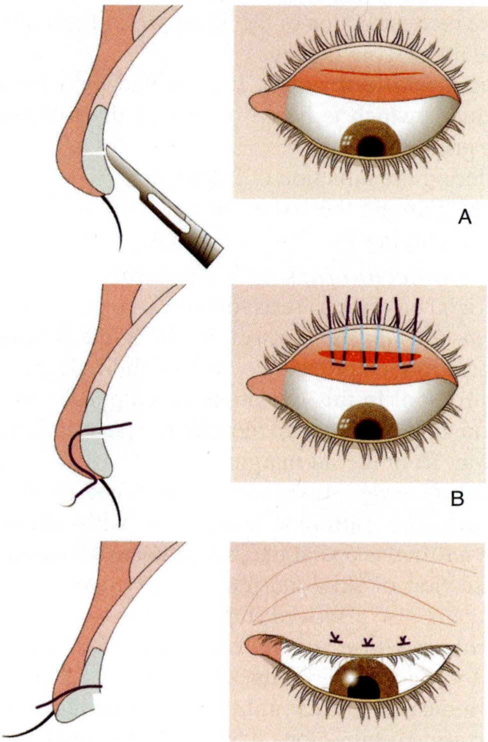

Fig. 14.20. Transposition of tarsoconjunctival wedge

posterior lamellar graft. Tarsus may be replaced by preserved sclera or ear cartilage or hard palate alongwith conjunctival or mucous membrane graph.

3. *Senile entropion.* Surgical techniques are as below:

i. *Transverse everting suture.* These offer temporary cure (upto 18 months) and are thus indicated in very old patients. The transverse sutures are applied through full thicknes of the lids (Fig 14.21) to prevent overriding of the preseptal muscles.

ii. *Wies operation* (Transverse lid split and everting sutures). This operation is indicated for long term

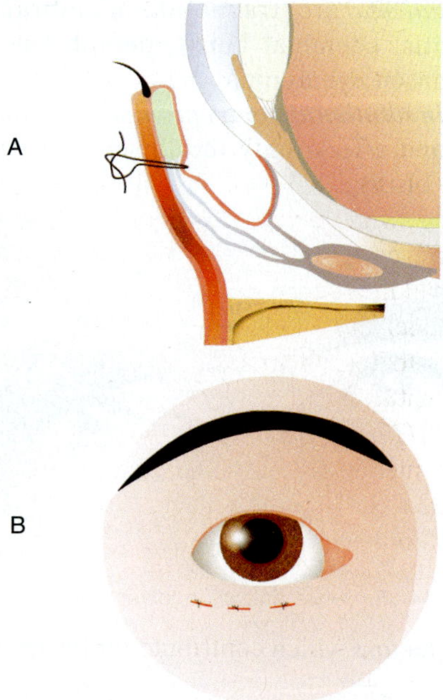

Fig. 14.21. Transverse lid everting sutures. A, diagrammatic section; and B, frontal view to show the position of sutures.

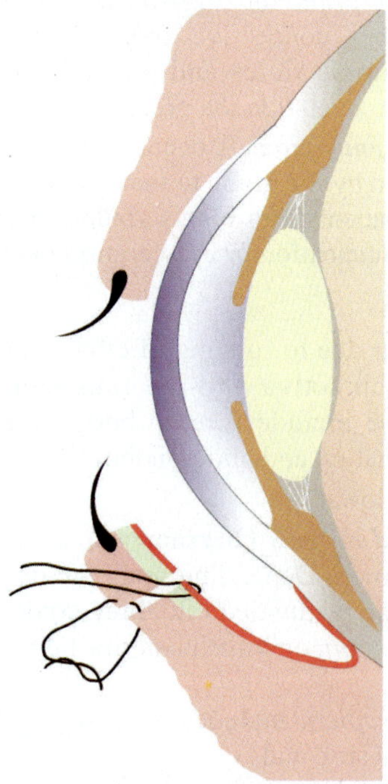

Fig. 14.22. Wies operation.

cure in patients with little horizontal laxity. In this operation, an incision involving skin, orbicularis and tarsal plate is given 3 mm below the lid margin, along the whole length of the eyelid. Mattress sutures are then passed through the lower cut end of the tarsus to emerge on the skin, 1 mm below the lid margin and are tied firmly (Fig. 14.22). The entropion is corrected by prevention of over-riding of preseptal muscle by the horizontal fibrous scar tissue barrier and transferring of the pull of lid retractors to the upper border of tarsus by the everting sutures.

iii. *Plication of lower lid retractors* (Jones, operation). It is performed in severe cases or when recurrence occurs after the above described operations. In this operation, the lower lid retractors are exposed

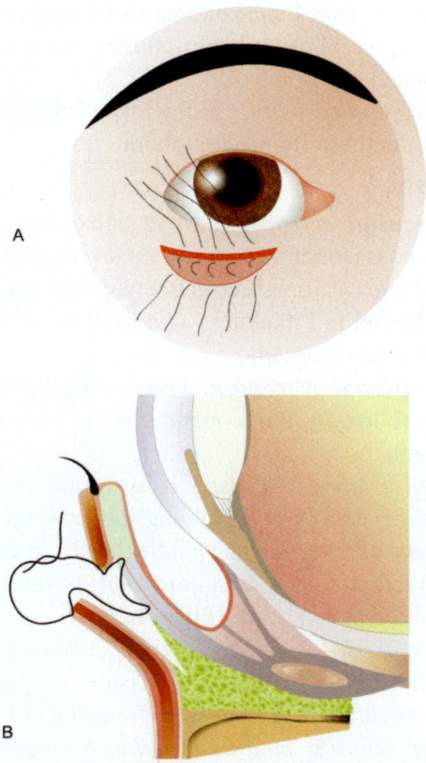

Fig. 14.23. Plication of lower lid retractors: A, front view; B, cut section.

via horizontal skin incision at the lower border of the tarsal plate, shortened and the sutures are used to create a barrier to prevent over-riding of the pre-septal muscle. (Fig. 14.23)

iv. *Quickert procedure*. This is indicated in patients having associated marked horizontal lid laxity. This operation consists of transverse lid split to create barrier for over-riding of pre-septal muscle, everting sutures to transfer pull of lower lid retractors to upper border of tarsus and horizontal lid shortening to correct the laxity (Fig 14.24). Thus quickert procedure basically combines horizontal lid shortening with Weiss procedure.

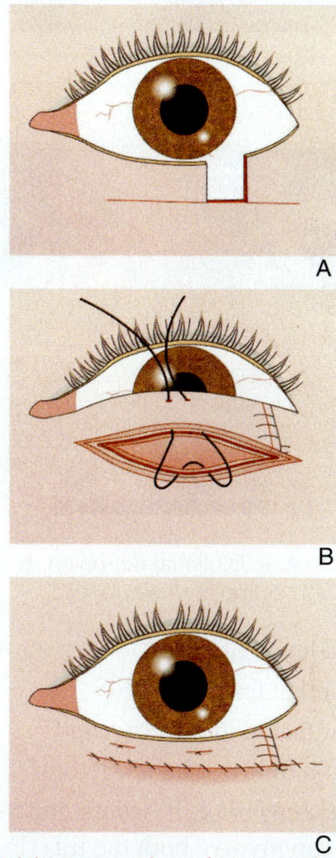

Fig. 14.24. Quickert procedure: A, two vertical incisions for horizontal lid shortening and horizontal slit incision; B, passage of lid everting suture after completion of horizontal lid resection and C, final position of the sutures.

ECTROPION

Out rolling or outward turning of the lid margin is called ectropion.

Etiological types

1. ***Congenital ectropion***. This is very rare, but may be seen in Down syndrome and blepharophimosis syndrome. It may occur in both the upper and lower lids and is due to a congenital shortage of the skin.

2. ***Involutional ectropion.*** It is the commonest variety and involves only the lower lids (Fig. 14.25 A). It occurs due to following age-related changes:

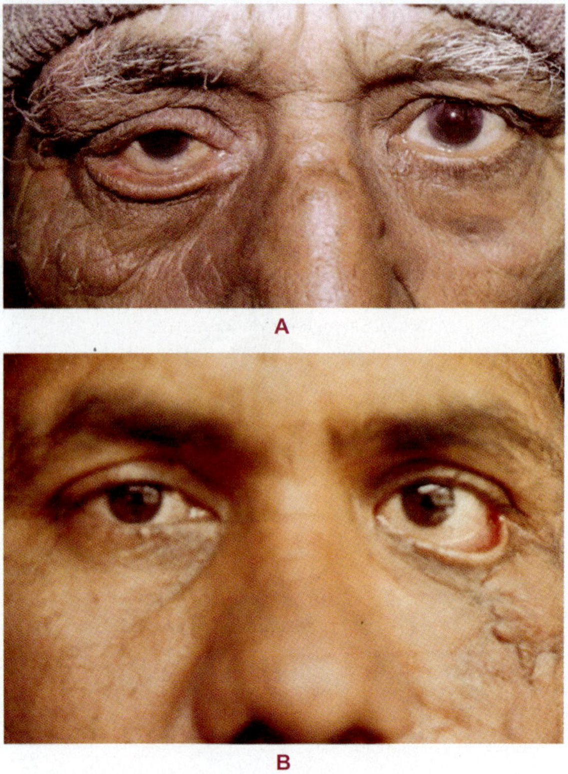

Fig. 14.25. A. involutional ectropion, B. cicatricial ectropion lower eyelid.

- Horizontal laxity of eyelid,
- Medial canthal tendon laxity,
- Lateral canthal tendon laxity, and
- Disinsertion of lower lid retractors.

3. ***Cicatricial ectropion.*** It occurs due to scarring of the skin and can involve both the lids (Fig. 14.25 B). *Common causes* of skin scarring are: thermal burns, chemical burns, lacerating injuries and skin ulcers.

4. ***Paralytic ectropion.*** It results due to paralysis of the seventh nerve. It mainly occurs in the lower lids. *Common causes* of facial nerve palsy are: Bell's palsy, head injury and infections of the middle ear.

5. ***Mechanical ectropion.*** It occurs in conditions where either the lower lid is pulled down (as in tumours) or pushed out and down (as in proptosis and marked chemosis of the conjunctiva).

Clinical picture

Symptoms.

- *Epiphora* is the main symptom in ectropion of the lower lid.
- *Symptoms due to associated chronic conjunctivitis* include: irritation, discomfort and mild photophobia.

Signs.

1. *Lid margin is outrolled*. Depending upon the degree of outrolling, ectropion can be divided into three grades:
   - *Grade-I*: In it only punctum is everted.
   - *Grade-II*: Lid margin is everted and palpebral conjunctiva is visible.
   - *Grade-III*: The fornix is also visible.
2. *Signs of the etiological condition* such as:
   - *Skin scars* in cicatricial ectropion and
   - *Seventh nerve palsy* in paralytic ectropion may also be seen.

Complications

- *Dryness and thickening* of conjunctiva and corneal ulceration (exposure keratitis) may occur due to prolonged exposure.
- *Eczema and dermatitis* of the lower lid skin may occur due to prolonged epiphora.

Treatment

1. Congenital ectropion. Mild ectropion often requires no treatment. Moderate or severe ectropion is treated like cicatricial ectropion with horizontal lid tightening and full thickness skin graft to vertically lengthen anterior lamella.

2. ***Involutional ectropion.*** Depending upon the severity, following three operations are commonly performed:

i. *Medial conjunctivoplasty*. It is useful in mild cases of ectropion involving punctal area. It consists of excising a spindle-shaped piece of conjunctiva and subconjunctival tissue from below the punctal area (Fig. 14.26).

ii. *Horizontal lid shortening.* It is performed by a full thickness pentagonal excision in patients with moderate degree of ectropion (Fig. 14.27).

iii. *Byron Smith's modified Kuhnt-Szymanowski operation.* It is performed for severe degree of ectropion which is more marked over the lateral half of the lid. In it, a base up pentagonal full thickness excision from the lateral third of the eyelid is combined with triangular excision of the skin from the area just lateral to lateral canthus to elevate the lid (Fig. 14.28).

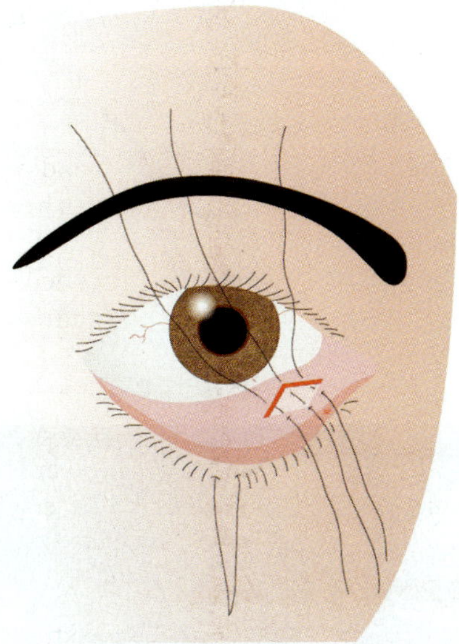

Fig. 14.26. Medial conjunctivoplasty.

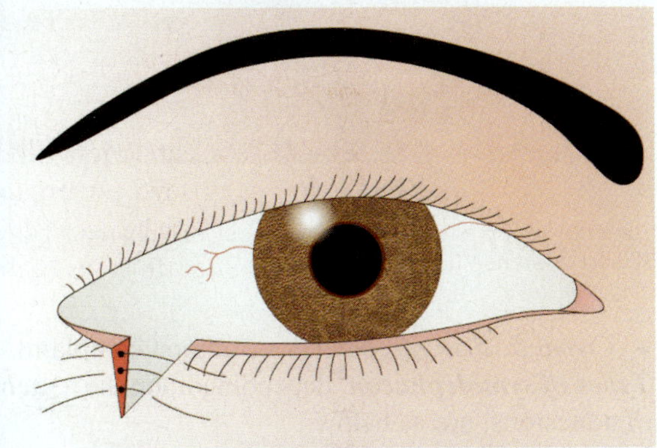

Fig. 14.27. Horizontal lid shortening.

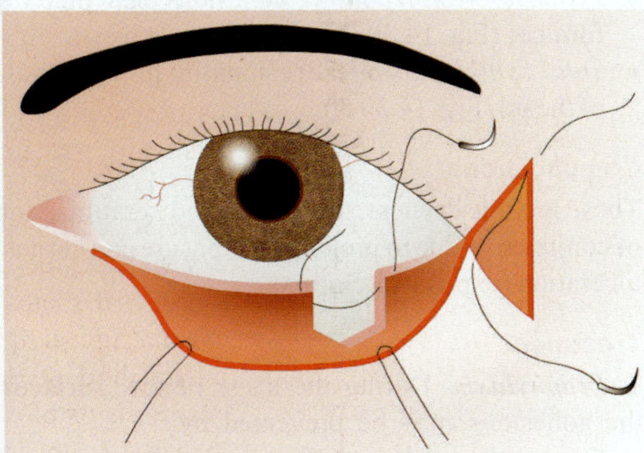

Fig. 14.28. Modified Kuhnt-Szymanowski operation.

3. *Paralytic ectropion*. Paralytic ectropion often resolves spontaneously within 6 months especially when due to Bells palsy. Therefore, temporary measures are taken initially. Permanent surgical treatment is required only in non-resolving cases.

Temporary measures include:

- Topical lubricants,
- Taping temporal side of eyelid, and
- Suture tarsorraphy.

Permanent measures include: lateral tarsorrhaphy, canthoplasty, horizontal lid tightening with or without middle lamellar buttress such as ear cartilage or palpebral sling operation, in which a fascia lata sling is passed in the subcutaneous layer all around the lid margins.

4. *Cicatricial ectropion*. Depending upon the degree it can be corrected by any of the following operations:

i. *V-Y operation.* It is indicated in mild degree ectropion. In it a V-shaped incision is given, skin is undermined and sutured in a Y-shaped pattern (Fig. 14.29).

ii. *Z-plasty (Elschnig's operation).* It is useful in mild to moderate degree of ectropion.

iii. *Excision of scar tissue and full thickness skin grafting.* It is performed in severe cases. Skin graft may be taken from the upper lid, behind the ear, or inner side of upper arm.

5. *Mechanical ectropion*. It is corrected by treating the underlying mechanical force causing ectropion.

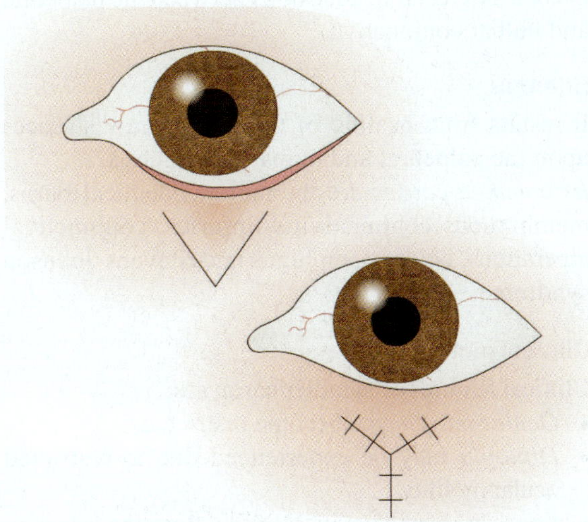

Fig. 14.29. V-Y operation.

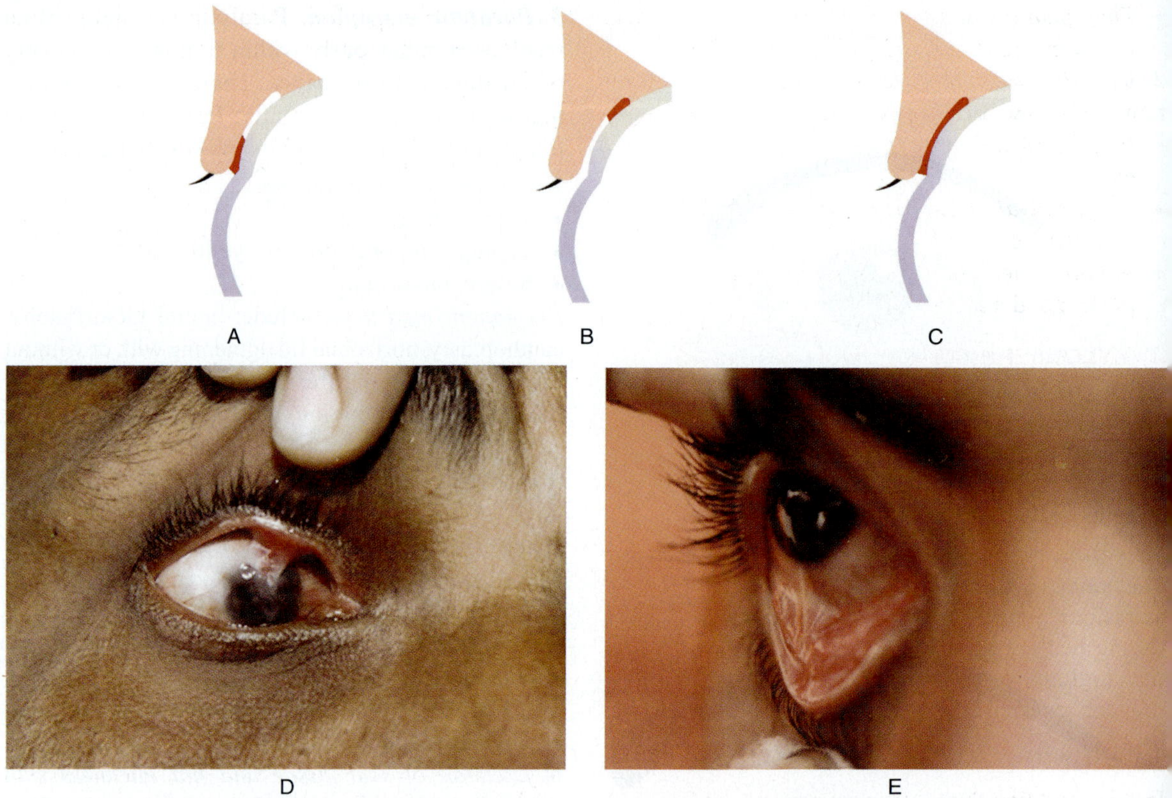

Fig. 14.30. Symblepharon: Diagrammatic depiction of anterior (A), posterior (B) and total symblepharon (C); clinical photographs of anterior (D) and posterior (E) symblepharon.

SYMBLEPHARON

In this condition, lids become adherent with the eyeball as a result of adhesions between the palpebral and bulbar conjunctiva.

Etiology

It results from healing of the kissing raw surfaces upon the palpebral and bulbar conjunctiva.

Its common causes are thermal or chemical burns, membranous conjunctivitis, injuries, conjunctival ulcerations, ocular pemphigus and Stevens-Johnson syndrome.

Clinical picture

Clinical features of symblepharon are:

- *Ocular movements* become restricted,
- *Diplopia* may be experienced due to restricted ocular motility,
- *Lagophthalmos* i.e. inability to close the lids may occur due to adhesions.
- *Cosmetic disfigurement* is a common complaint.

Types of symblepharon, depending upon the extent of adhesions, are as below:

- *Anterior symblepharon*–adhesions present only in the anterior part (Fig. 14.30 A and D).
- *Posterior symblepharon*–adhesions present in the fornices (Fig. 14.30 B and E).
- *Total symblepharon*–adhesions involving whole of the lid (Fig. 14.30 C).

Complications

These include dryness, thickening and keratinisation of conjunctiva due to prolonged exposure and corneal ulceration (exposure keratitis).

Treatment

1. *Prophylaxis*. During the stage of raw surfaces, the adhesions may be prevented by:

- *Sweeping a glass rod* coated with lubricant around the fornices several times a day.

- *Therapeutic soft contact lens* of large size, also helps in preventing the adhesions.

2. *Curative treatment* consists of symblepharectomy. The raw area created may be covered by:

- *Mobilising the surrounding conjunctiva* in mild cases.
- *Conjunctival or buccal mucosal graft* is required in severe cases.
- *Amniotic membrane transplantation* (AMT), also gives good results.

ANKYLOBLEPHARON

It refers to the adhesions between margins of the upper and lower lids. It may occur as a congenital anomaly or may result after healing of chemical burns, thermal burns, ulcers and traumatic wounds of the lid margins. Ankyloblepharon may be complete or incomplete. It is usually associated with symblepharon.

Treatment. Lids should be separated by excision of adhesions between the lid margins and kept apart during healing process. When adhesions extend to the angles, epithelial grafts should be given to prevent recurrences.

BLEPHAROPHIMOSIS

In this condition the extent of the palpebral fissure is decreased. It appears contracted at the outer canthus.

Etiology. It may be congenital (see page 378) or acquired, due to formation of a vertical skin fold at the lateral canthus (epicanthus lateralis) following eczematous contractions.

Treatment. Usually no treatment is required. In marked cases, canthoplasty operation is performed.

LAGOPHTHALMOS

This condition is characterised by inability to close the eyelids voluntarily.

Etiology. It occurs in patients with paralysis of orbicularis oculi muscle, cicatricial contraction of the lids, symblepharon, severe ectropion, proptosis, following over-resection of the levator muscle for ptosis, and in comatosed patients. Physiologically some people sleep with their eyes open (nocturnal lagophthalmos).

Clinical picture. It is characterised by incomplete closure of the palpebral aperture associated with features of the causative disease.

Complications include conjunctival and corneal xerosis and exposure keratitis.

Treatment is as below:

1. *Measures to prevent exposure keratitis*

- *Atificial tear drops* should be instilled frequently and the open palpebral fissure should be filled with an antibiotic eye ointment during sleep and in comatosed patients.
- *Soft bandage contact lens* may be used to prevent exposure keratitis.
- *Tarsorrhaphy* may be performed to cover the exposed cornea when indicated.

2. *Measures to treat the cause* of lagophthalmos, wherever possible should be taken.

TARSORRHAPHY

In this operation adhesions are created between a part of the lid margins with the aim to narrow down or almost close the palpebral aperture. It is of two types: temporary and permanent.

1. Temporary tarsorrhaphy

Indications. (i) To protect the cornea when seventh nerve palsy is expected to recover. (ii) To assist healing of an indolent corneal ulcer. (iii) To assist in healing of skin-grafts of the lids in the correct position.

Surgical techniques. This can be carried out as median or paramedian tarsorrhaphy (Fig. 14.31).

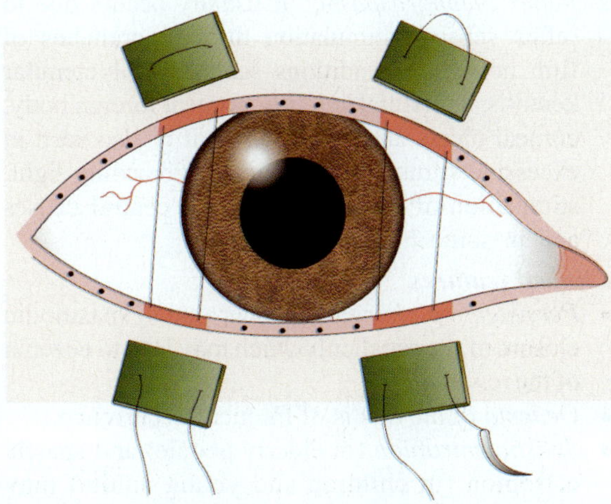

Fig. 14.31. Surgical technique of paramedian tarsorrhaphy.

1. *Incision.* For paramedian tarsorrhaphy, about 5 mm long incision site is marked on the corresponding parts of the upper and lower lid margins, 3-mm on either side of the midline. An incision 2-mm deep is made in the grey line on the marked site and the marginal epithelium is then excised taking care not to damage the ciliary line anteriorly and the sharp lid border posteriorly.
2. *Suturing.* The raw surfaces thus created on the opposing parts of the lid margins are then sutured with double-armed 6-0 silk sutures passed through a rubber bolster.

2. Permanent tarsorrhaphy

Indications. (i) Established cases of VII nerve palsy where there is no chance of recovery; and (ii) established cases of neuroparalytic keratitis with severe loss of corneal sensations.

Technique. It is performed at the lateral canthus to create permanent adhesions. The eyelids are overlapped after excising a triangular flap of skin and orbicularis from the lower lid and corresponding triangular tarso-conjunctival flap from the upper lid.

BLEPHAROSPASM

It refers to the involuntary, sustained and forceful closure of the eyelids.

***Etiology*.** Blepharospasm occurs in two forms:

1. *Essential (spontaneous) blepharospasm.* It is a rare idiopathic condition involving patients between 45 and 65 years of age.
2. *Reflex blepharospasm.* It usually occurs due to reflex sensory stimulation through branches of fifth nerve, in conditions such as: phlyctenular keratitis, interstitial keratitis, corneal foreign body, corneal ulcers and iridocyclitis. It is also seen in excessive stimulation of retina by dazzling light, stimulation of facial nerve due to central causes and in some hysterical patients.

Clinical features.

- *Persistent epiphora* may occur due to spasmodic closure of the canaliculi which may lead to eczema of the lower lid.
- *Oedema of the lids* is of frequent occurrence.
- *Spastic entropion* (in elderly people) and spastic ectropion (in children and young adults) may develop in long-standing cases.
- *Blepharophimosis* may result due to contraction of the skin folds following eczema.

Treatment

Treatment of essential blepharospasm:

- *Botulinum toxin,* injected subcutaneously over the orbicularis muscle, blocks the neuromuscular junction and relieves the spasm.
- *Facial denervation* may be required in severe cases.

Treatment of reflex blepharospasm:

- *Causative disease* should be treated to prevent recurrences.
- *Associated complications* should also be treated.

PTOSIS

Abnormal drooping of the upper eyelid is called ptosis. Normally, upper lid covers about upper one-sixth of the cornea, i.e., about 2 mm. Therefore, in ptosis it covers more than 2 mm.

Types and etiology

I. *Congenital ptosis*

It is associated with congenital weakness (mal development) of the levator palpebrae superioris (LPS). It may occur in the following forms:

1. *Simple congenital ptosis* (not associated with any other anomaly) (Fig. 14.32A).
2. Congenital ptosis with associated weakness of superior rectus muscle.
3. As a part of *blepharophimosis syndrome*, which comprises congenital ptosis, blepharophimosis, telecanthus and epicanthus inversus (Fig. 14.32B).
4. *Congenital synkinetic ptosis* (Marcus Gunn jaw-winking ptosis). In this condition there occurs retraction of the ptotic lid with jaw movements i.e., with stimulation of ipsilateral pterygoid muscle.

II. *Acquired ptosis*

Depending upon the cause it can be neurogenic, myogenic, aponeurotic or mechanical.

1. *Neurogenic ptosis*. It is caused by innervational defects such as third nerve palsy, Horner's syndrome, ophthalmoplegic migraine and multiple sclerosis.

Horner's syndrome, occuring due to oculo-sympathetic paresis, is characterised by mild ptosis (due to paralysis of Muller's muscles), miosis (due to paralysis of dilator pupillae), and reduced ipsilateral sweating (anhydrosis), mild enophthalmos and loss of ciliospinal reflex.

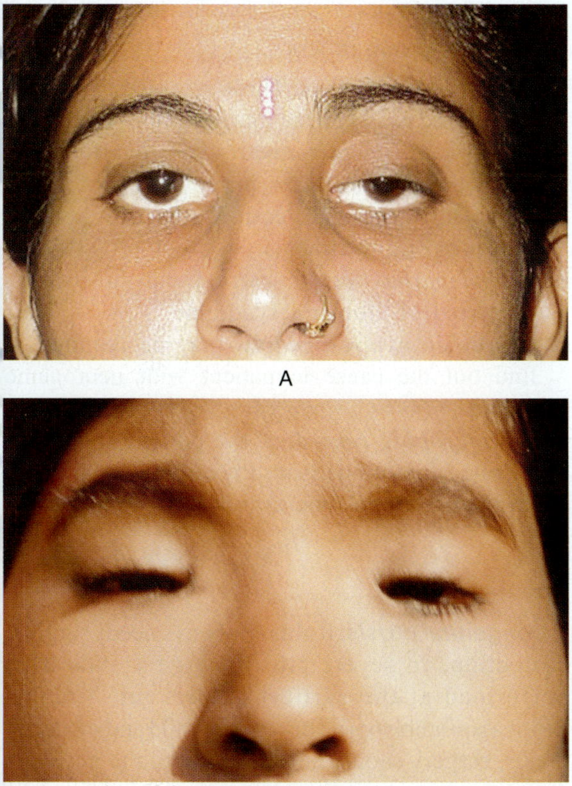

A

B

Fig. 14.32. Congenital ptosis: A, simple; B, blepharophimosis syndrome.

2. *Myogenic ptosis.* It occurs due to acquired disorders of the LPS muscle or of the myoneural junction. It may be seen in patients with myasthenia gravis, dystrophia myotonica, ocular myopathy, oculo-pharyngeal muscular dystrophy and following trauma to the LPS muscle.

3. *Aponeurotic ptosis.* It develops due to defects of the levator aponeurosis in the presence of a normal functioning muscle. It includes:

- *Involutional (senile) ptosis,*
- *Postoperative ptosis* (which is rarely observed after cataract and retinal detachment surgery),
- *Ptosis* due to aponeurotic weakness associated with blepharochalasis, and
- *Traumatic dehiscence* or disinsertion of the aponeurosis.

4. *Mechanical ptosis.* It may result due to excessive weight on the upper lid as seen in patients with lid tumours, multiple chalazia and lid oedema. It may also occur due to scarring (cicatricial ptosis) as seen in patients with ocular pemphigoid and trachoma.

Clinical evaluation

Following scheme may be adopted for work up of a ptosis patient:

I. *History*. It should include age of onset, family history, history of trauma, eye surgery and variability in degree of the ptosis.

II. *Examination*

1. *Exclude pseudoptosis* (simulated ptosis) on inspection. Its common causes are:

- *Ipsilateral conditions* such a microphthalmos, phthisis bulbi, enophthalmos, prosthesis, brow ptosis, dermatochalasis, and hypotropia.
- *Contralateral conditions* include: eyelid retraction, high myopia, and proptosis.

2. *Observe the following points* in each case:

- Whether ptosis is unilateral or bilateral.
- Function of orbicularis oculi muscle.
- Eyelid crease is present or absent.
- Jaw-winking phenomenon is present or not.
- Associated weakness of any extraocular muscle.
- Bell's phenomenon (up and outrolling of the eyeball during forceful closure) is present or absent.

3. *Measurement of amount (degree) of ptosis.* In unilateral cases, difference between the vertical height of the palpebral fissures of the two sides indicates the degree of ptosis (Fig. 14.33). In bilateral cases it can be determined by measuring the amount of cornea

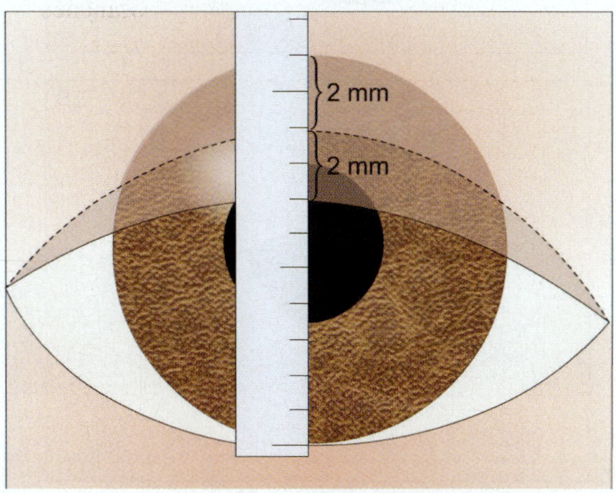

Fig. 14.33. Measurement of degree of ptosis in millimetres.

covered by the upper lid and then subtracting 2 mm. *Ptosis is graded* depending upon its amount as:

- Mild ptosis : 2 mm
- Moderate ptosis : 3 mm
- Severe ptosis : 4 mm

4. *Margin reflex distance* (MRD) refers to the distance between the upper lid margins and corneal light reflex (of a pen torch held in front, on which patient is looking). Normal value of MRD is 4-5 mm.

5. *Assessment of levator function.* It is determined by the lid excursion caused by LPS muscle (Burke's method). Patient is asked to look down, and thumb of one hand is placed firmly against the eyebrow of the patient (to block the action of frontalis muscle) by the examiner. Then the patient is asked to look up and the amount of upper lid excursion is measured with a ruler (Fig. 14.34) held in the other hand by the examiner. *Levator function is graded* as follows:

- Normal : 15 mm
- Good : 8 mm or more
- Fair : 5-7 mm
- Poor : 4 mm or less

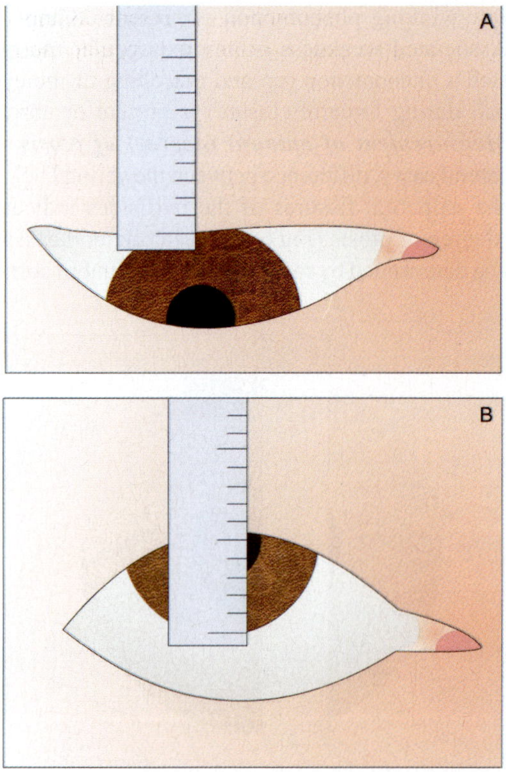

Fig. 14.34. Assessment of levator function: A, looking down; B, looking up.

6. *Special investigations.* Those required in patients with acquired ptosis are as follows:

i. *Tensilon test* is performed when myasthenia is suspected. There occurs improvement of ptosis with intravenous injection of edrophonium (Tensilon) in myasthenia.

ii. *Phenylephrine test* is carried out in patients suspected of Horner's syndrome.

iii. *Neurological investigations* may be required to find out the cause in patient with neurogenic ptosis.

7. *Photographic record* of the patient should be maintained for comparison. Photographs should be taken in primary position as well as in up and down gazes.

Treatment

I. *Congenital ptosis.* It almost always needs surgical correction. In severe ptosis, surgery should be performed at the earliest to prevent stimulus deprivation amblyopia. However, in mild and moderate ptosis, surgery should be delayed until the age of 3-4 years, when accurate measurements are possible. Congenital ptosis can be treated by any of the following operations:

1. *Tarso-conjunctivo-Mullerctomy (Fasanella-Servat operation)* It is performed in cases having mild ptosis (1.5-2mm) and good levator function. In it, upper lid is everted and the upper tarsal border along with its attached Muller's muscle and conjunctiva are resected (Fig. 14.35).

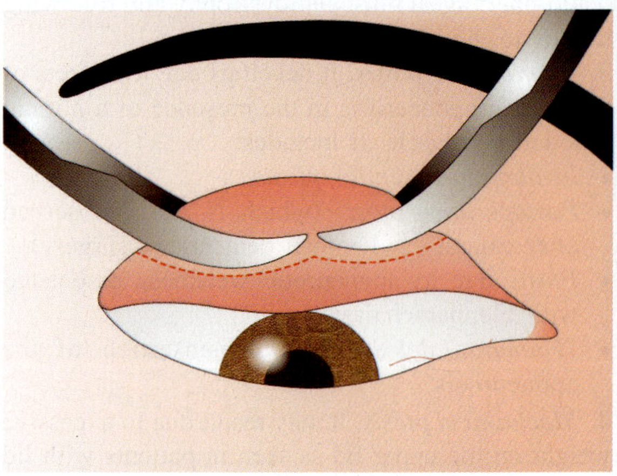

Fig. 14.35. Fasanella-Servat operation.

2. *Levator resection.* It is a very commonly performed operation for moderate and severe grades of ptosis. It is contraindicated in patients having severe ptosis with poor levator function.

Amount of levator resection required: Most of the surgeons find it out by adjusting the lid margin in relation to cornea during operation on the table in individual case. However, a rough estimate in different grades of ptosis can be made:

- *Moderate ptosis.* Depending on the level of LPS function the amount of LPS to be resected is as below:
  - Good function : 16-17 mm (minimal)
  - Fair function : 18-22 mm (moderate)
  - Poor function : 23-24 mm (maximum)
- *Severe ptosis.* Fair levator function: 23-24 mm (maximum LPS resected).

Techniques. Levator muscle may be resected by either conjunctival or skin approach.

i. *Conjunctival approach* (Blaskowics' operation): This technique is comparatively easy but not suitable for large amount of resection. In it LPS muscle is exposed by an incision made through the conjunctiva near the upper tarsal border, after the upper lid is doubly everted over a Desmarre's lid retractor (Fig. 14.36).
ii. *Skin approach (Everbusch's operation)*: It is a more frequently employed technique. It allows comparatively better exposure of the LPS muscle through a skin incision along the line of future lid crease (Fig. 14.37).

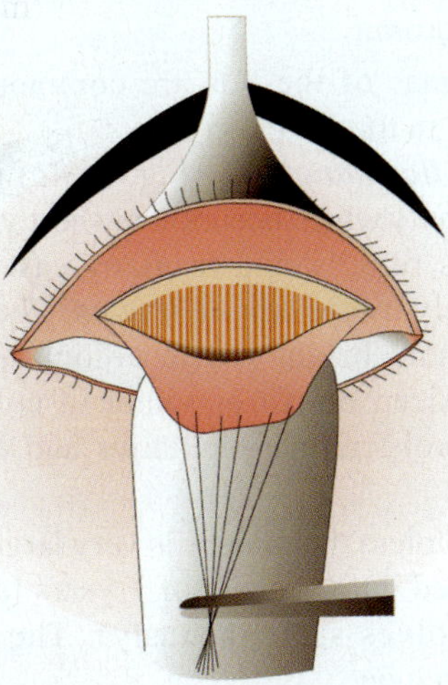

Fig. 14.36. Conjunctival approach for levator resection.

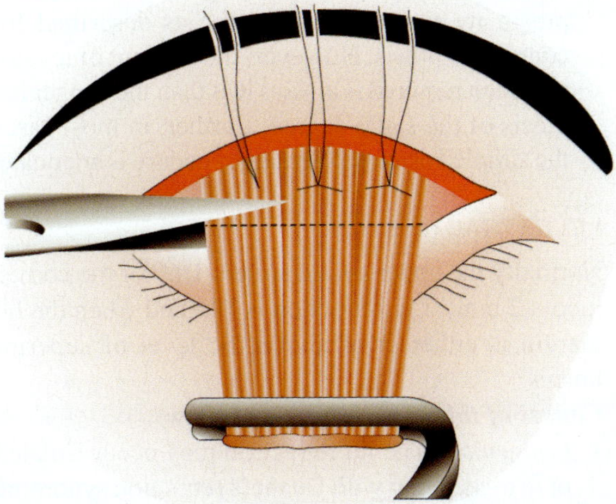

Fig. 14.37. Skin approach for levator resection.

3. *Frontalis sling operation* (Brow suspension): This is performed in patients having severe ptosis with no levator function. In this operation, lid is anchored to the frontalis muscle via a sling (Fig. 14.38). Fascia lata or some non-absorbable material (e.g., supramide suture, silicon rod) may be used as sling.

II. *Acquired ptosis*

- *Treat the underlying cause* where ever possible.
- *Conservative treatment* should be carried out and surgery deferred at least for 6 months in neurogenic ptosis.

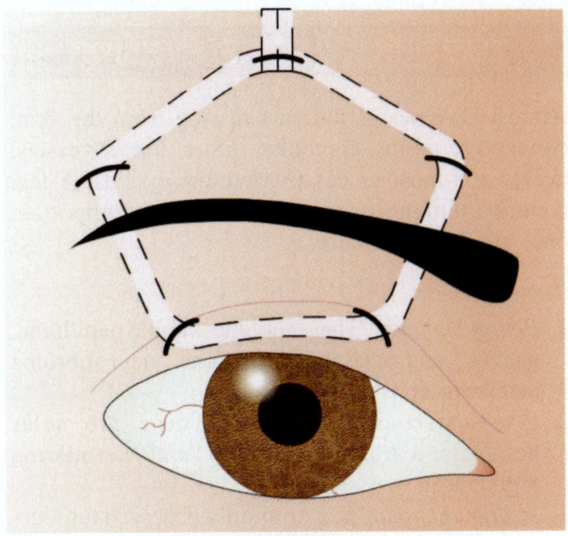

Fig. 14.38. Frontalis sling operation.

- *Surgical procedures* (when required) for acquired ptosis are essentially the same as described for congenital ptosis. However, the amount of levator resection required is always less than the congenital ptosis of the same degree. Further, in most cases the simple Fasanella-Servat procedure is adequate.

LID RETRACTION

Normally the upper eyelid covers 1/6th of the cornea (about 2 mm). Lid retraction is labelled when the lid margin is either at or above the level of superior limbus.

Causes of lid retraction are as below:

1. *Congenital.* The lid retraction may occur isolated or in association with Duane's retraction syndrome and Down's syndrome.
2. *Thyroid eye disease* is the more common cause.
3. *Mechanical causes* of lid retraction are:
   - Surgical overcorrection of ptosis, and
   - Scarring of the upper eyelid skin after burns, trauma or infection.
4. *Neurogenic causes* include:
   - Facial palsy (due to unopposed levator action),
   - Third nerve misdirection,
   - Marcus-Gunn jaw winking syndrome,
   - Parinaud syndrome, and
   - Effect of sympathomimetic eye drops
5. *Systemic causes:*
   - Uraemia

TUMOURS OF THE EYELIDS

Almost all types of tumours arising from the skin, connective tissue, glandular tissue, blood vessels, nerves and muscles can involve the eyelids. A few common tumours are listed and only the important ones are described here.

Classification

1. *Benign tumours.* These include; simple papilloma, naevus, angioma, haemangioma, neurofibroma and sebaceous adenoma.
2. *Pre-cancerous conditions.* These are solar keratosis, carcinoma *in-situ* and xeroderma pigmentosa.
3. *Malignant tumours.* Commonly observed tumours include squamous cell carcinoma, basal cell carcinoma, malignant melanoma and sebaceous gland adenocarcinoma.

BENIGN TUMOURS

1. Papillomas

Papillomas are the most common benign tumours arising from the surface epithelium. These occur in two forms: squamous papillomas and seborrhoeic keratosis.

i. *Squamous papillomas* derived from squamous cells occur in adults, as very slow growing or stationary, raspberry-like growths or as a pedunculated lesion, usually involving the lid margin. These may be non-specific or related to human papilloma virus (viral wart or verruca vulgaris). Its treatment consists of simple excision.
ii. *Seborrhoeic keratosis* (basal cell papilloma), derived from basal cells occurs in middle-aged and older persons. Their surface is friable, verrucous and slightly pigmented.

2. Xanthelasma

These are creamy-yellow plaque-like lesions which frequently involve the skin of upper and lower lids near the inner canthus (Fig. 14.39). Xanthelasma occurs more commonly in middle-aged women. Xanthelasma represents lipid deposits in histiocytes in the dermis of the lid. These may be associated with diabetes mellitus or high cholesterol levels.

Treatment: Excision may be advised for cosmetic reasons; but recurrences are common.

3. Haemangioma

Haemangiomas of the lids are common tumours. These occur in three forms:

i. *Capillary haemangioma* (Fig. 14.40) is the most common variety which occurs at or shortly after birth, often grows rapidly and in many cases resolves spontaneously by the age of 7 years. These may be superficial and bright red in colour (strawberry naevus) or deep bluish or violet in colour. They consist of proliferating capillaries and endothelial cells.

Treatment. Unless the tumour is very large it may be left untouched until the age of 7 years (as in many cases it resolves spontaneously). The treatment modalities include:

- *Excision*: It is performed in small tumours.

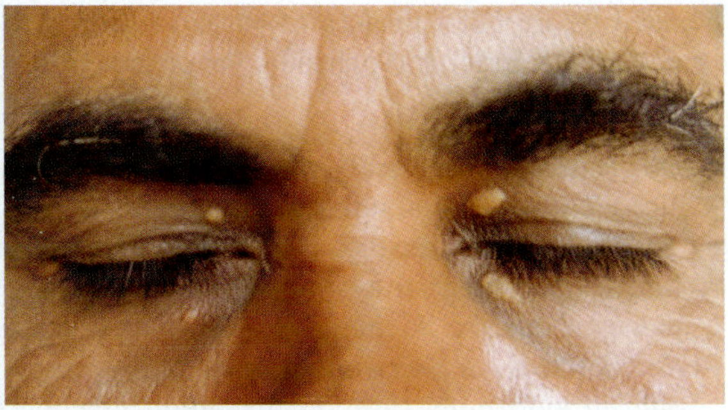

Fig. 14.39. Xanthelasma

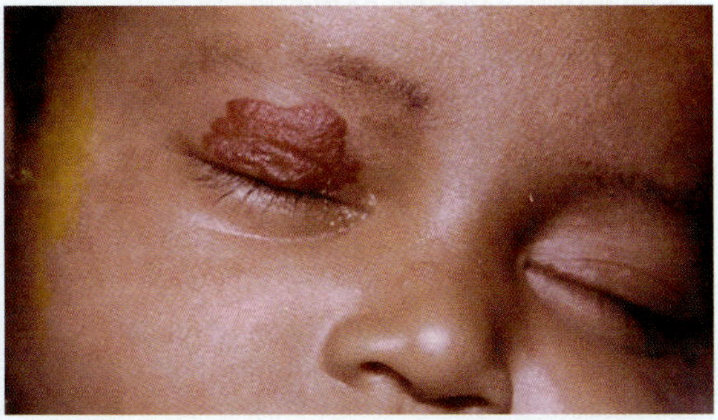

Fig. 14.40. Capillary haemangioma.

- *Intralesional steroid* (triamcinolone) injection is effective in small to medium size tumours.
- Alternate day high dose *steroid therapy* regimen is recommended for large diffuse tumours.
- *Superficial radiotherapy* may also be given for large tumours.

ii. ***Naevus flammeus*** (port wine stain). It may occur pari passu or more commonly as a part of Sturge-Weber syndrome. It consists of dilated vascular channels and does not grow or regress like the capillary haemangioma.

iii. ***Cavernous haemangiomas*** are developmental and usually occur after first decade of life. It consists of large endothelium-lined vascular channels and usually does not show any regression. Treatment is similar to capillary haemangiomas.

4. Neurofibroma

Lids and orbits are commonly affected in neurofibromatosis (von Recklinghausen's disease). The tumour is usually of plexiform type (Fig. 14.41).

5. Keratoacanthomas

Keratoacanthomas occur as non-pigmented protrusions with a keratin filled central crater . These are comparatively uncommon tumors that grow rapidly for 2 to 6 weeks and then spontaneously involute over a few months.

Differential diagnosis need to be made sometimes from the squamous cell carcinoma.

Treatment consists of complete excision and biopsy. Incomplete specimen may be indistinguishable from a squamous cell carcinoma on histopathological examination.

6. Naevi

Naevi are common cutaneous lesions that arise from the arrested epidermal melanocytes .

Types. Depending upon the depth of involvement, naevi are of three types:

- *Junctional naevi*, located at the epidermis/dermis junction, are flat, brown in appearance.
- *Dermal naevi*, located within the dermis, are elevated lesions which may not be visibly pigmented.
- *Compound naevi*, are slightly elevated and share features of junctional and dermal naevi.

PREMALIGNANT TUMOURS

Actinic (solar) keratosis

Actinic Keratosis, though a common lesion of sun exposed skin is relatively uncommon on the eyelids.

Clinical features include a flat, scaly lesion with hyperkeratosis with or without keratin horn.

Histologically, it is characterized by parakeratosis and cellular atypia but no invasion.

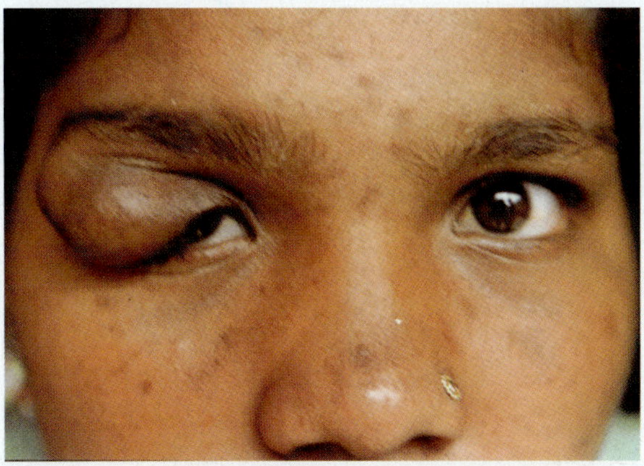

Fig. 14.41. Neurofibroma upper eyelid.

Xeroderma pigmentosa

Characteristic features of this autosomal recessive (AR) disease are:

- *Progressive cutaneous pigmentation* resulting from damage on exposure to natural sunlight.
- *Bird like facies* is typical of this condition.
- *Predisposition* to develop lid tumors (basal cell carcinoma, squamous cell carcinoma and melanoma) and conjunctival malignancies.

MALIGNANT TUMOURS

1. Basal-cell carcinoma

It is the commonest malignant tumour of the lids (90%) usually seen in elderly people. It is locally malignant and involves most commonly lower lid (50%) followed by medial canthus (25%), upper lid (10-15%) and outer canthus (5-10%).

Predisposing factors include increasing age, white skin, sun exposure, xeroderma pigmentosa and basal cell naevus syndrome.

Clinical features. It may present in four forms:

- *Non-ulcerated nodular form,*
- *Sclerosing or morphea type*
- *Pigmented basal cell carcinoma.*

(rare presentation,)

- *Noduloulcerative basal cell carcinoma* is the most common presentation. It starts as a small nodule which undergoes central ulceration with pearly rolled margins. The tumour grows by burrowing and destroying the tissues locally like a rodent and hence the name rodent ulcer (Fig. 14.42).

Histological features. The most common pattern is solid basal cell carcinoma in which the dermis is invaded by irregular masses of basaloid cells with characteristic peripheral palisading appearance.

Treatment

- *Surgery.* Local surgical excision of the tumour along with a 3 mm surrounding area of normal skin with primary repair is the treatment of choice. Mohs' microsurgical technique or frozen section biopsy should be adopted for complete removal.
- *Radiotherapy and cryotherapy* should be given only in inoperable cases for palliation.

2. Squamous cell carcinoma

It forms the second commonest malignant tumour of the lid. Its incidence (5%) is much less than the basal cell carcinoma. It commonly arises from the lid margin (mucocutaneous junction) in elderly patients *de novo* or from pre-existing lesion such as actinic keratosis, Bowen's disease and radiation dermatosis. It affects lower lids more frequently.

Risks Factors include sun exposure, radiation, fair skin, injury or other irritative insults. There is a male predilection.

Clinial features. It may present in two forms:

- *Ulcerated, scaly, erythematous plaque like growth* with elevated and indurated margins is the common presentation (Fig. 14.43).
- *Fungating or polypoid* verrucous lesion without ulceration, is a rare presentation.

Metastasis. It is metastasized in preauricular and sub-mandibular lymph nodes.

Histological features. It is characterised by an irregular downward proliferation of epidermal cells into the dermis. In well-differentiated form, the

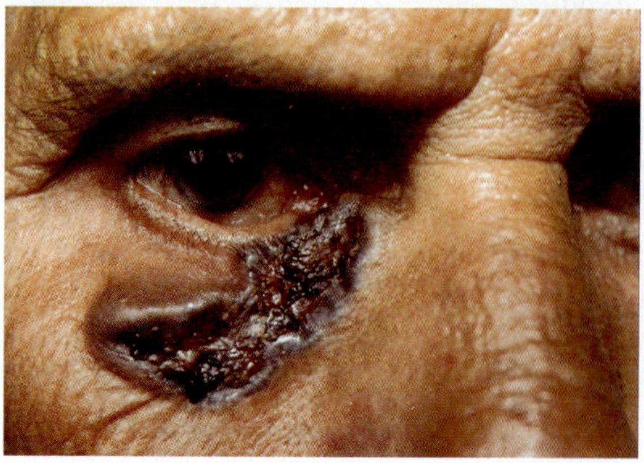

Fig. 14.42. Basal cell carcinoma lower eyelid.

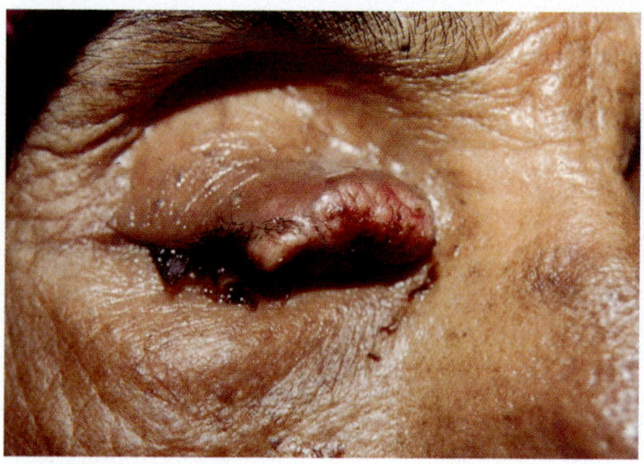

Fig. 14.43. Squamous cell carcinoma of upper lid.

malignant cells have a whorled arrangement forming epithelial pearls which may contain laminated keratin material in the centre.

Treatment is on the lines of basal cell carcinoma.

3. Sebaceous gland carcinoma

It is a rare tumour arising from the meibomian glands (western literature). However, *Indian literature reports* the sebaceous gland carcinoma being the commonest malignancy of eyelid followed by basal cell and squamous cell carcinoma.

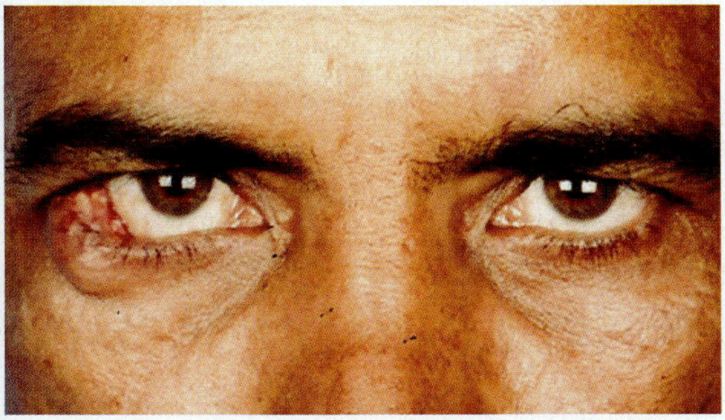

Fig. 14.44. Meibomian gland carcinoma lower eyelid.

Clinical features. It usually presents initially as a nodule (which may be mistaken for a chalazion), more frequently on the upper eye lid. Which then grows to form a big growth (Fig. 14.44). Rarely, a diffuse tumour along the lid margin may be mistaken as chronic blepharitis.

Treatment. Surgical excision with reconstruction of the lids is the treatment of choice. Recurrences are common.

4. Malignant melanoma (melanocarcinoma)

It is a rare tumour of the lid (less than 1% of all eyelid lesions). It may arise from a pre-existing naevus, but usually arises *de novo* from the melanocytes present in the skin.

Clinical features. It may present in three forms:

- *Lentigo maligna type* is characterized initially by a flat, pigmented , well defined lesion which later on becomes elevated as it invades the dermis.
- *Superficial spreading type* is characterized by mildly elevated, pigmented lesion with irregular margins.
- *Nodular type* is characterized by a rapidly growing lesion (may not be visibly pigmented), which ulcerates and bleeds frequently.

Metastasis. The tumour spreads locally as well as to distant sites by lymphatics and blood stream.

Treatment. It is a radio-resistant tumour. Therefore, surgical excision with 10 mm margins (confirmed on frozen section) with reconstruction of the lid is the treatment of choice.

15

CHAPTER

Diseases of the Lacrimal Apparatus

APPLIED ANATOMY

The lacrimal apparatus comprises
- Main lacrimal gland,
- Accessory lacrimal glands, and
- Lacrimal passages, which include: puncta, canaliculi, lacrimal sac and nasolacrimal duct (NLD) (Fig. 15.1).

Main lacrimal gland

It consists of an upper orbital and a lower palpebral part.

1. *Orbital part* is larger, about the size and shape of a small almond, and is situated in the fossa for lacrimal gland at the outer part of the orbital plate of frontal bone. It has got two surfaces — superior and inferior. The superior surface is convex and lies in contact with the bone. The inferior surface is concave and lies on the levator palpebrae superioris muscle.

2. *Palpebral part* is small and consists of only one or two lobules. It is situated upon the course of the ducts of orbital part from which it is separated by LPS muscle. Posteriorly, it is continuous with the orbital part.

Ducts of lacrimal gland. Approximately 10-12 ducts pass downward from the main gland to open in the lateral part of superior fornix. One or two ducts also open in the lateral part of inferior fornix.

Accessory lacrimal glands (Fig. 14.4)

1. *Glands of Krause.* These are microscopic glands lying beneath the palpebral conjunctiva between fornix and the edge of tarsus. These are about 42 in the upper fornix and 6-8 in the lower fornix.
2. *Glands of Wolfring.* These are present near the upper border of the superior tarsal plate and along the lower border of inferior tarsus.

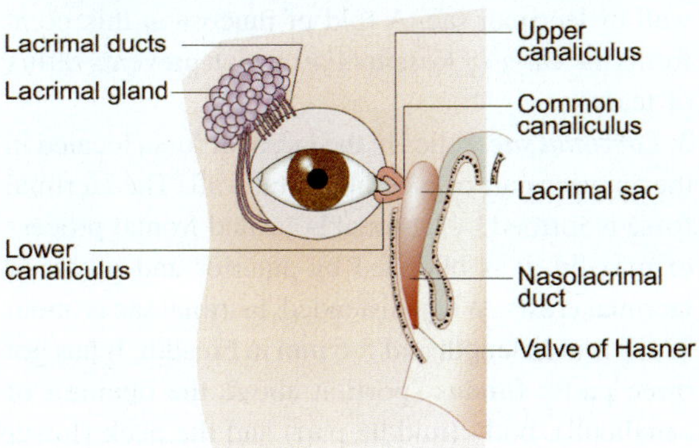

Fig. 15.1. The lacrimal apparatus.

Structure, blood supply and nerve supply

Structure. All lacrimal glands are serous acini, similar in structure to the salivary glands. Microscopically these consist of glandular tissue (acini and ducts), connective tissue and puncta.

Blood supply. Main lacrimal gland is supplied by lacrimal artery which is a branch of ophthalmic artery.

Nerve supply.

1. *Sensory supply* comes from lacrimal nerve, a branch of the ophthalmic division of the fifth nerve.
2. *Sympathetic supply* comes from the carotid plexus of the cervical sympathetic chain.
3. *Secretomotor fibres* are derived from the superior salivary nucleus (pons) → greater petrosal nerve → synapse at pterygopalatine ganglion → Zygomatic nerve → Lacrimal nerve → lacrimal gland.

Lacrimal passages

1. *Lacrimal puncta.* These are two small, rounded or oval openings on upper and lower lids, about 6 and 6.5 mm, respectively, temporal to the inner canthus. Each punctum is situated upon a slight elevation called lacrimal papilla which becomes prominent in old age. Normally the puncta dip into the lacus lacrimalis (collection of tear fluid in the inner canthus).

2. *Lacrimal canaliculi.* Superior and inferior canaliculi join the puncta to the lacrimal sac. Each canaliculus has two parts: vertical (1-2 mm) and horizontal (6-8 mm) which lie at right angle to each other. The horizontal part converges towards inner canthus to open in the sac. The two canaliculi may open separately or may join to form common canaliculus which opens immediately into the outer wall of lacrimal sac. A fold of mucosa at this point forms the *valve of Rosenmuller* which prevents reflux of tears.

3. *Lacrimal sac.* It lies in the lacrimal fossa located in the anterior part of medial orbital wall. The lacrimal fossa is formed by lacrimal bone and frontal process of maxilla. It is bounded by anterior and posterior lacrimal crests. When distended, lacrimal sac is about 12-15 mm in length and 5-6 mm in breadth. It has got three parts: fundus (portion above the opening of canaliculi), body (middle part) and the neck (lower small part which is narrow and continuous with the nasolacrimal duct).

4. *Nasolacrimal duct (NLD)*. It extends from neck of the lacrimal sac to inferior meatus of the nose. It is about 15-18 mm long and lies in a bony canal formed by the maxilla and the inferior turbinate. Direction of the NLD is downwards, backwards and laterally. Externally its location is represented by a line joining inner canthus to the ala of nose. The upper end of the NLD is the narrowest part.

There are numerous membranous valves in the NLD, the most important is the *valve of Hasner*, which is present at the lower end of the duct and prevents reflux from the nose.

TEAR FILM

Structure of tear film

Wolff was the first to describe the detailed structure of the fluid covering the cornea and called it precorneal film. He described this film to consist of three layers, which from posterior to anterior are mucus layer, aqueous layer and lipid or oily layer (Fig. 15.2).

1. *Mucus layer.* It is the innermost and thinnest stratum of the tear film. It consists of mucin secreted by conjunctival goblet cells and glands of Manz. It converts the hydrophobic corneal surface into hydrophilic one.

2. *Aqueous layer.* The bulk of tear film is formed by this intermediate layer which consists of tears secreted by the main and accessory lacrimal glands. *The tears* mainly comprise of water and small quantities of solutes such as sodium chloride, sugar, urea and proteins. Therefore, it is alkaline and salty

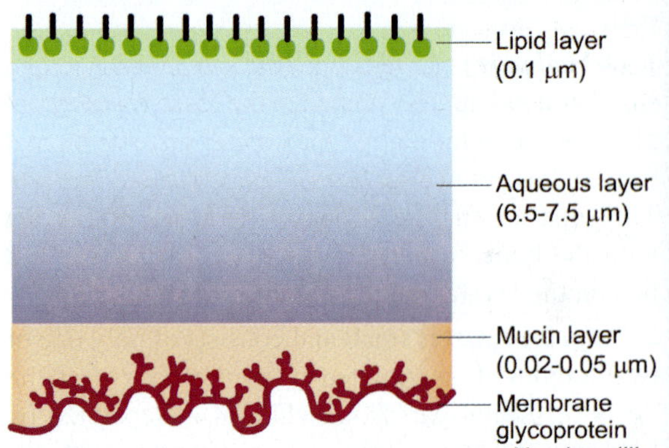

Fig. 15.2. Structure of the tear film.

in taste. It also contains antibacterial substances like lysozyme, betalysin and lactoferrin.

3. ***Lipid or oily layer.*** This is the outermost layer of tear film formed at air-tear interface from the secretions of Meibomian, Zeis, and Moll glands. This layer prevents the overflow of tears, retards their evaporation and lubricates the eyelids as they slide over the surface of the globe.

Functions of tear film

1. Keeps the cornea and conjunctiva moist.
2. Provides oxygen to the corneal epithelium.
3. Washes away debris and noxious irritants.
4. Prevents infection due to presence of antibacterial substances.
5. Facilitates movements of the lids over the globe.

Secretion of tears

Tears are continuously secreted throughtout the day by accessory (*basal secretion*) and main (*reflex secretion*) lacrimal glands. Reflex secretion is in response to sensations from the cornea and conjunctiva, probably produced by evaporation and break-up of tear film. *Hyperlacrimation* occurs due to irritative sensations from the cornea and conjunctiva. *Afferent pathway* of this secretion is formed by fifth nerve and efferent by parasympathetic (secreto-motor) supply of lacrimal gland.

Elimination of tears

Tears flow downwards and laterally across the ocular surface. A variable amount of tears is lost by evaporation from the ocular surface. The remainder of tears flow along the superior and inferior marginal strips and collects as lacus lacrimalis in the inner canthus (Fig 15.3A), from where it is drained by the lacrimal passage into the nasal cavity. About 70% tears is drained via inferior canaliculus and 30% via the superior canaliculus by an active lacrimal pump mechanism constituted by the fibers of orbicularis as below:

When the eyelids close with each blink there occurs:

- *Contraction of pretarsal orbicularis oculi* which compresses the ampulla and shortens the canaliculi. This movement propels the tear fluid present in the ampulla and horizontal part of canaliculi towards the lacrimal sac .
- *Contraction of preseptal fibers of orbicularis* distends the lacrimal sac and creates therein a negative pressure which draws the tear fluid from canaliculi into the lacrimal sac (Fig15.3B).

When the eyelids open following events occur:

- *Relaxation of pretarsal orbicularis* allows the canaliculi and ampulla to expand and reopen, and to draw the tear fluid from the lacus lacrimalis and marginal tear strips.
- *Relaxation of preseptal fibers (Horner's muscle)* results in collapse of sac, as a consequence a positive pressure is created which forces the tears down the nasolacrimal duct (NLD) into the nose (Fig15.3C). Gravity also helps in downward flow of tears along the NLD.

  Note: In atonia of sac, tears are not drained through the lacrimal passages, in spite of anatomical patency; resulting in epiphora.

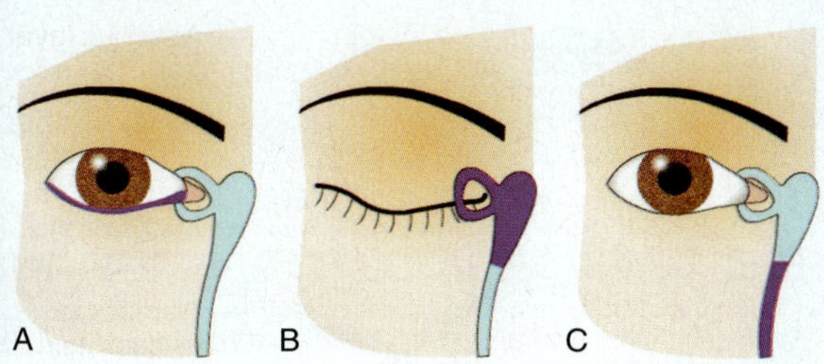

Fig. 15.3. Elimination of tears by lacrimal pump mechanism.

THE DRY EYE

The dry eye per se is not a disease entity, but a symptom complex occurring as a sequelae to deficiency or abnormalities of the tear film.

Etiology

According to International Dry Eye Workshop report (DEWS report 2007), the causes of dry eye can be classified as below:

I. ***Aqueous deficiency dry eye*** also known as keratoconjunctivitis sicca (KCS). Its causes include

1. ***Sjogren's syndrome*** (Primary keratoconjunctivitis sicca)

2. ***Non Sjogren's keratoconjunctivitis sicca***. Causes can be grouped as below:

i. *Lacrimal gland deficiencies* as seen in congenital alacrimia, familial dysautonomia (Riley-Day syndrome), age related dry eye and infiltrations of lacrimal gland e.g. in sarcoidosis, tumours and post radiation fibrosis of lacrimal gland.

ii. *Lacrimal gland duct obstruction* as seen in old trachoma, chemical burns, cicatricial pemphigoid and Stevens-Johnson syndrome.

iii. *Reflex hyposecretion* (neurogenic causes) as seen in reflex sensory block, reflex motor blade, 7th cranial nerve damage, reduced corneal sensations after refractive surgery and corneal lens wear.

II. *Evaporative dry eye*

It is caused by the conditions which decrease tear film stability and thus increase evaporation.

Causes can be grouped as:

1. *Meibomian gland dysfunction* as seen in chronic posterior blepharitis, rosacea, and congenital absence of meibomian glands.
2. *Lagophthalmos* as seen in facial nerve palsy, severe proptosis, symblepharon and eyelid scarring.
3. *Defective blinking* such as low blink rate as seen in prolonged computer users and other causes.
4. *Vitamin A deficiency and other factors* affecting ocular surface e.g. topical drugs, preservatives, contact lens wear, ocular surface allergic disease and scarring disorders.

Clinical features

Symptoms suggestive of dry eye include irritation, foreign body (sandy) sensation, feeling of dryness, itching, non-specific ocular discomfort and chronically sore eyes not responding to a variety of drops instilled earlier.

Signs of dry eye are as below:

- *Tear film signs.* It may show presence of stingy mucous and particulate matter. Marginal tear strip is reduced or absent (normal height is 1mm). Froth in the tears along the lid margin is a sign of meibomian gland dysfunction.
- *Conjunctival signs.* It becomes lustureless, mildly congested, conjunctival xerosis and keratinization may occur. Rose Bengal or lisamin green staining may be positive (details given in tear film tests).
- *Corneal signs.* It may show punctuate epithelial erosions, filaments and mucus plaques. Cornea may loose lusture. Vital stains, fluorescein, Rose Bengal or Lisamin green may delineate the above lesions.
- *Signs of causative disease* such as posterior blepharitis, conjunctival scarring diseases (trachoma, Stevens Johnson syndrome, chemical burns, ocular pemphigoid) and lagophthalmos may be depicted.

Tear film tests

These include tear film break-up time (BUT), Schirmer-I test, vital staining with Rose Bengal, tear levels of lysozyme and lactoferrin, tear osmolarity and conjunctival impression cytology. Out of these BUT, Schirmer-I test and Rose Bengal staining are most important and when any two of these are positive, diagnosis of dry eye syndrome is confirmed.

1. *Tear film break-up (BUT).* It is the interval between a complete blink and appearance of first randomly distributed dry spot on the cornea. It is noted after instilling a drop of fluorescein and examining in a cobalt-blue light of a slit-lamp. BUT is an indicator of adequacy of mucin component of tears. Its normal values range from 15 to 35 seconds. Values less than 10 seconds imply an unstable tear film.

2. *Schirmer-I test*. It measures total tear secretions. It is performed with the help of a 5 × 35 mm strip of Whatman-41 filter paper which is folded 5 mm from one end and kept in the lower fornix at the junction of lateral one-third and medial two-thirds. The patient is asked to look up and not to blink or close the eyes (Fig. 15.4). After 5 minutes wetting of the filter paper strip from the bent end is measured. Normal values of Schirmer-I test are more than 15 mm. Values of 5-10 mm are suggestive of moderate to mild kerato-conjunctivitis sicca (KCS) and less than 5 mm of severe KCS.

3. *Rose Bengal staining.* It is a very useful test for detecting even mild cases of KCS. Depending upon the severity of KCS three staining patterns A, B and C have been described: 'C' pattern represents mild or

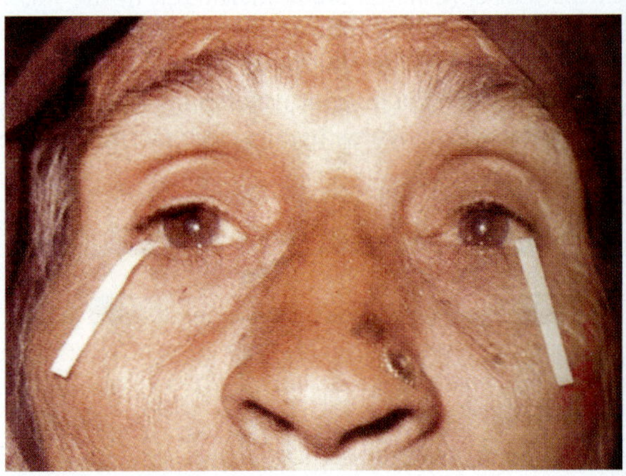

Fig. 15.4. Schirmer test.

early cases with fine punctate stains in the interpalpebral area; 'B' the moderate cases with extensive staining; and 'A' the severe cases with confluent staining of conjunctiva and cornea.

Grading of dry eye severity

Various criteria have been proposed to grade severity of dry eye. Recently accepted system based on severity of signs and tear film tests recommended by Dry Eye Workshop (DREWS) Report (2007) grades the severity of dry eye into 4 levels:

- Level 1 (mild dry eye)
- Level 2 (moderate dry eye)
- Level 3 (severe dry eye), and
- Level 4 (very severe dry eye)

Treatment

At present, there is no cure for dry eye. The following treatment modalities have been tried with variable results:

1. *Supplementation with tear substitutes.* Artificial tears remains the mainstay in the treatment of dry eye. These are available as drops, ointments and slow-release inserts. Mostly available artificial tear drops contain either cellulose derivatives (e.g., 0.25 to 0.7% methyl cellulose and 0.3% hypromellose) or polyvinyl alcohol (1.4%).

2. *Topical cyclosporine* (0.05%, 0.1%) is reported to be very effective drug for dry eye in many recent studies. It helps by reducing the cell-mediated inflammation of the lacrimal tissue.

3. *Mucolytics,* such as 5 percent acetylcystine used 4 times a day helps by dispersing the mucus threads and decreasing tear viscosity.

4. *Preservation of existing tears by reducing evaporation and decreasing drainage.*

- *Evaporation can be reduced* by decreasing room temperature, use of moist chambers and protective glasses.
- *Punctal occlusion* to decrease drainage can be carried out by collagen implants, cynoacrylate tissue adhesives, electrocauterisation, argon laser occlusion and surgical occlusion to decrease the drainage of tears in patients with very severe dry eye.
- *Permanent lateral tarsorrhaphy* may be required in very severe cases.

5. *Treatment of the causative disease* of dry eye when discovered is very useful. e.g.:

- *Systemic tetracyclines* and *lid hygiene* in patients with chronic posterior blepharitis
- *Vitamin A supplement* for the deficiency
- *Treat the cause* of lagophthalmos.

SJOGREN'S SYNDROME

It is an autoimmune chronic inflammatory disease with multi-system involvement. It typically occurs in women between 40 and 50 years of age. Its main feature is an aqueous deficiency dry eye — the keratoconjunctivitis sicca (KCS). In *primary Sjogren's syndrome* patients present with sicca complex– a combination of KCS and xerostomia (dryness of mouth). In *secondary Sjogren's syndrome* dry eye and/or dry mouth are associated with an autoimmune disease, commonly rheumatoid arthritis. Its *pathological features* include focal accumulation and infiltration by lymphocytes and plasma cells with destruction of lacrimal and salivary glandular tissue.

THE WATERING EYE

It is characterised by overflow of tears from the conjunctival sac. The condition may occur either due to excessive secretion of tears (hyperlacrimation) or may result from obstruction to the outflow of normally secreted tears (epiphora).

Etiology

(A) *Causes of hyperlacrimation*

1. *Primary hyperlacrimation.* It is a rare condition which occurs due to direct stimulation of the lacrimal gland. It may occur in early stages of lacrimal gland tumours and cysts and due to the effect of strong parasympathomimetic drugs.

2. *Reflex hyperlacrimation.* It results from stimulation of sensory branches of fifth nerve due to irritation of cornea or conjunctiva. It may occur in multitude of conditions which include:

- *Affections of the lids:* Stye, hordeolum internum, acute meibomitis, trichiasis, concretions and entropion.
- *Affections of the conjunctiva:* Conjunctivitis which may be infective, allergic, toxic, irritative or traumatic.

- *Affections of the cornea:* These include, corneal abrasions, corneal ulcers and non-ulcerative keratitis.
- *Affections of the sclera:* Episcleritis and scleritis.
- *Affections of uveal tissue:* Iritis, cyclitis, iridocyclitis.
- *Acute glaucomas.*
- *Endophthalmitis and panophthalmitis.*
- *Orbital cellulitis.*

3. *Central lacrimation* (psychical lacrimation). The exact area concerned with central lacrimation is still not known. It is seen in emotional states, voluntary lacrimation and hysterical lacrimation.

(B) *Causes of epiphora*

Inadequate drainage of tears may occur due to physiological or anatomical (mechanical) causes.

I *Physiological cause* is 'lacrimal pump' failure due to lower lid laxity or weakness of orbicularis muscle.

II *Mechanical obstruction* in lacrimal passages may lie at the level of punctum, canaliculus, lacrimal sac or nasolacrimal duct.

1. *Punctal causes* include:
   - *Eversion of lower punctum:* It is commonly seen in old age due to laxity of the lids. It may also occur following chronic conjunctivitis, chronic blepharitis and due to any cause of ectropion.
   - *Punctal obstruction:* There may be congenital absence of puncta or cicatricial closure following injuries, burns or infections. Rarely a small foreign body, concretion or cilia may also block the punctum. Prolonged use of drugs like idoxuridine and pilocarpine is also associated with punctal stenosis.
2. *Causes in the canaliculi.* Canalicular obstruction may be congenital or acquired due to foreign body, trauma, idiopathic fibrosis and canaliculitis. Commonest cause of canaliculitis is actinomyces.
3. *Causes in the lacrimal sac.* These include congenital mucous membrane folds, traumatic strictures, dacryocystitis, specific infections like tuberculosis and syphilis, dacryolithiasis and tumours (Atonia of the sac is a physiological cause).
4. *Causes in the nasolacrimal duct.* Congenital lesions include non-canalization, partial canalization or imperforated membranous valves. Acquired causes of obstruction are traumatic strictures, inflammatory strictures, idiopathic stenosis, tumours and diseases of the surrounding bones.

Clinical evaluation of a case of 'Watering eye'

1. *Ocular examination with diffuse illumination using magnification* should be carried to rule out any cause of reflex hypersecretion located in lids, conjunctiva, cornea, sclera, anterior chamber, uveal tract and so on. This examination should also exclude punctal causes of epiphora and any swelling in the sac area.

2. *Regurgitation test.* A steady pressure with index finger is applied over the lacrimal sac area above the medial palpebral ligament. Reflux of mucopurulent discharge indicates chronic dacryocystitis with obstruction at lower end of the sac or the nasolacrimal duct.

3. *Fluorescein dye disappearance test (FDDT).* In this test 2 drops of fluorescein dye are instilled in both the conjunctival sacs and observations are made after 2 minutes. Normally, no dye is seen in the conjunctival sac. A prolonged retention of dye in conjunctival sac indicates inadequate drainage which may be due to atonia of sac or mechanical obstruction.

4. *Lacrimal syringing test.* It is performed after topical anaesthesia with 4 percent xylocaine (Fig. 15.5). Normal saline is pushed into the lacrimal sac from lower punctum with the help of a syringe and lacrimal cannula.

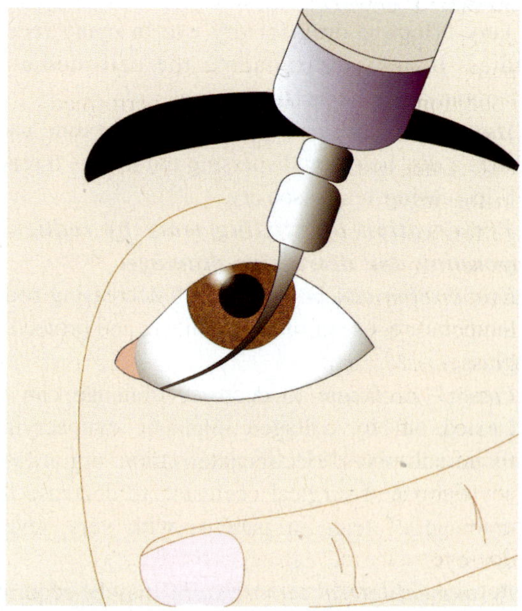

Fig. 15.5. Technique of lacrimal syringing.

- A free passage of saline through lacrimal passages into the nose rules out any mechanical obstruction.
- In the presence of partial obstruction, saline passes with considerable pressure on the syringe.
- In the presence of obstruction no fluid passes into nose and it may reflux through same punctum (indicating obstruction in the same or common canaliculus) or through opposite punctum (indicating obstruction in the lower sac or nasolacrimal duct).

5. *Jones dye tests.* These are performed when partial obstruction is suspected. Jones dye tests are of no value in the presence of total obstruction.

i. *Jones primary test (Jones test I).* It is performed to differentiate between watering due to partial obstruction of the lacrimal passages from that due to primary hypersecretion of tears. Two drops of 2 percent fluorescein dye are instilled in the conjunctival sac and a cotton bud dipped in 1 percent xylocaine is placed in the inferior meatus at the opening of nasolacrimal duct. After 5 minutes the cotton bud is removed and inspected. A dye-stained cotton bud indicates adequate drainage through the lacrimal passages and the cause of watering is primary hypersecretion (further investigations should aim at finding the cause of primary hypersecretion). While the unstained cotton bud (negative test) indicates either a partial obstruction or failure of lacrimal pump mechanism. To differentiate between these conditions, Jones dye test-II is performed.

ii. *Jones secondary test (Jones test II).* When primary test is negative, the cotton bud is again placed in the inferior meatus and lacrimal syringing is performed. A positive test suggests that dye was present in the sac but could not reach the nose due to partial obstruction. A negative test indicates presence of lacrimal pump failure.

6. *Dacryocystography.* It is valuable in patients with mechanical obstruction. It tells the exact site, nature and extent of block (Fig. 15.6). In addition, it also gives information about mucosa of the sac, presence of any fistulae, diverticulae, stone, or tumour in the sac.

To perform it a radiopaque material such as lipiodol, pentopaque, dianosil or condray-280 is pushed in the sac with the help of a lacrimal cannula and X-rays are taken after 5 minutes and 30 minutes to visualize the entire passage. For better anatomical visualization the modified technique known as *substraction macrodacryocystography* with canalicular catheterisation should be preferred.

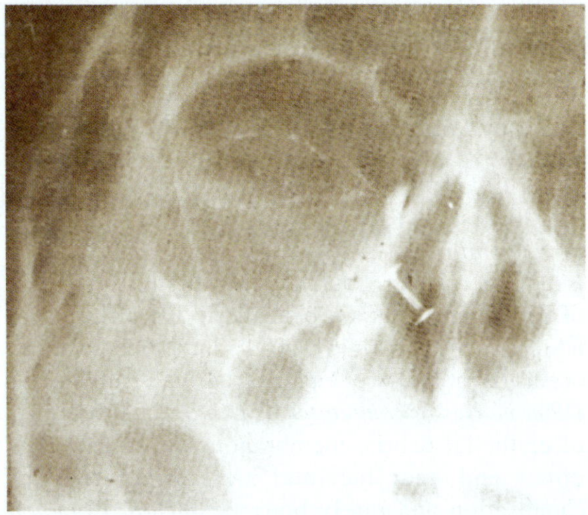

Fig. 15.6. Normal dacryocystogram.

7. *Radionucleotide dacryocystography* (lacrimal scintillography). It is a non-invasive technique to assess the functional efficiency of lacrimal drainage apparatus. A radioactive tracer (sulphur colloid or technitium) is instilled into the conjunctival sac and its passage through the lacrimal drainage system is visualised with an Anger gamma camera (Fig. 15.7).

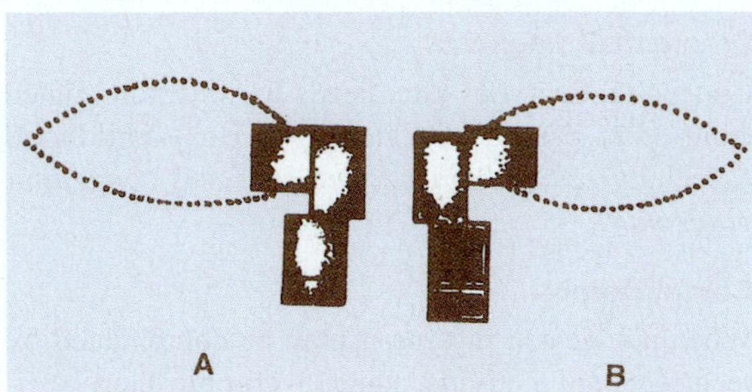

Fig. 15.7. Lacrimal scintillography showing: A, normal lacrimal excretory system on right side; B, obstruction at the junction of lacrimal sac and nasolacrimal on left side.

DACRYOCYSTITIS

Inflammation of the lacrimal sac is not an uncommon condition. It may occur in two forms: congenital and adult dacryocystitis.

CONGENITAL DACRYOCYSTITIS

It is an inflammation of the lacrimal sac occuring in newborn infants; and thus also known as *dacryocystitis neonatorum.*

Etiology

It follows stasis of secretions in the lacrimal sac due to *congenital blockage in the nasolacrimal duct*. It is of very common occurrence. As many as 30 percent of newborn infants are believed to have closure of nasolacrimal duct at birth; mostly due to 'membranous occlusion' at its lower end, near the valve of Hasner. *Other causes of congenital NLD block* are: presence of epithelial debris, membranous occlusion at its upper end near lacrimal sac, complete non-canalisation and rarely bony occlusion. *Common bacteria* associated with congenital dacryocystitis are *Staphylococci*, *Pneumococci* and *Streptococci*.

Clinical picture

Congenital dacryocystitis usually presents as a mild grade chronic inflammation. It is characterised by:

1. *Epiphora,* usually developing after seven days of birth. It is followed by copious *mucopurulent discharge* from the eyes.
2. *Regurgitation test* is usually positive, i.e., when pressure is applied over the lacrimal sac area, purulent discharge regurgitates from the lower punctum.
3. *Swelling* on the sac area may appear eventually.

Differential diagnosis

Congenital dacryocystitis needs to be differentiated from other causes of watering in early childhood especially *ophthalmia neonatorum* and *congenital glaucoma.*

Complications

When not treated in time it may be complicated by recurrent conjunctivitis, acute on chronic dacryocystitis, lacrimal abscess and fistulae formation.

Treatment

It depends upon the age at which the child is brought. The treatment modalities employed are as follows:

1. *Massage over the lacrimal sac area and topical antibiotics* constitute the treatment of congenital NLD block, up to 3-4 weeks of age. Massage increases the hydrostatic pressure in the sac and helps to open up the membranous occlusions. It should be carried out at least 4 times a day to be followed by instillation of antibiotic drops. This conservative treatment cures obstruction in about 90 percent of the infants.

2. *Lacrimal syringing (irrigation) with normal saline and antibiotic solution.* It should be added to the conservative treatment if the condition is not cured up to the age of 2 months. Lacrimal irrigation helps to open the membranous occlusion by exerting hydraulic pressure. Syringing may be carried out once a week or in two weeks.

3. *Probing of NLD with Bowman's probe.* It should be performed, in case the condition is not cured by the age of 3-4 months. Some surgeons prefer to wait till the age of 6 months. It is usually performed under general anaesthesia. While performing probing, care must be taken not to injure the canaliculus. In most instances a single probing will relieve the obstruction. In case of failure, it may be repeated after an interval of 3-4 weeks.

4. *Balloon catheter dilation,* with the help of a probe carrying inflatable balloon, may be carried out in children where repeated probing is failure or directly in cases where the obstruction seems to be due to scarring or constriction rather than merely by a distal membrane.

5. *Intubation with silicone tube* may be performed if repeated probings and balloon catheter dilation are failure. The silicone tube should be kept in the NLD for about six months.

6. *Dacryocystorhinostomy (DCR) operation:* When the child is brought very late or repeated probing, balloon catheter dilation and intubation are a failure, then conservative treatment by massaging, topical antibiotics and intermittent lacrimal syringing should be continued till the age of 4 years. After this, DCR operation should be performed.

ADULT DACRYOCYSTITIS

Adult dacryocystitis may occur in an acute or a chronic form.

CHRONIC DACRYOCYSTITIS

Chronic dacryocystitis is more common than the acute dacryocystitis.

Etiology

The etiology of chronic dacryocystitis is multi-factorial. The well-established fact is a vicious cycle of *stasis and mild infection* of long duration. The etiological factors can be grouped as under:

A. ***Predisposing factors***

1. *Age*. It is more common between 40 and 60 years of age.
2. *Sex*. The disease is predominantly seen in females (80%) probably due to comparatively narrow lumen of the bony canal.
3. *Race*. It is rarer among Negroes than in Whites; as in the former NLD is shorter, wider and less sinuous.
4. *Heredity*. It plays an indirect role. It affects the facial configuration and so also the length and width of the bony canal.
5. *Socio-economic status*. It is more common in low socio-economic group.
6. *Poor personal hygiene*. It is also an important predisposing factor.

B. ***Factors responsible for stasis of tears in lacrimal sac***

1. *Anatomical factors,* which retard drainage of tears include: comparatively narrow bony canal, partial canalization of membranous NLD and excessive membranous folds in NLD.
2. *Foreign bodies* in the sac may block opening of NLD.
3. *Excessive lacrimation,* primary or reflex, causes stagnation of tears in the sac.
4. *Mild grade inflammation* of lacrimal sac due to associated recurrent conjunctivitis may block the NLD by epithelial debris and mucus plugs.
5. *Obstruction of lower end of the NLD* by nasal diseases such as polyps, hypertrophied inferior concha, marked degree of deviated nasal septum, tumours and atrophic rhinitis causing stenosis may also cause stagnation of tears in the lacrimal sac.

C. ***Source of infection.*** Lacrimal sac may get infected from the conjunctiva, nasal cavity (retrograde spread), or paranasal sinuses.

D. ***Causative organisms***. These include: *Staphylococci*, *Pneumococci*, *Streptococci* and *Pseudomonas pyocyanea*. Rarely chronic granulomatous infections like tuberculosis, syphilis, leprosy and occasionally rhinosporiodosis may also cause dacryocystitis.

Clinical picture

Clinical picture of chronic dacryocystitis may be divided into four stages:

1. *Stage of chronic catarrhal dacryocystitis.* It is characterised by mild inflammation of the lacrimal sac associated with blockage of NLD. In this stage the only symptom is *watering eye* and sometimes mild redness in the inner canthus. On *syringing* the lacrimal sac, either clear fluid or few fibrinous mucoid flakes regurgitate. *Dacryocystography* reveals block in NLD, a normal-sized lacrimal sac with healthy mucosa.

2. *Stage of lacrimal mucocoele.* It follows chronic stagnation causing distension of lacrimal sac. It is characterised by constant *epiphora* associated with a *swelling* just below the inner canthus (Fig. 15.8). Milky or gelatinous mucoid fluid regurgitates from the lower punctum on pressing the swelling. *Dacryocystography* at this stage reveals a distended sac with blockage somewhere in the NLD.

Sometimes due to continued chronic infection, opening of both the canaliculi into the sac are blocked and a large fluctuant swelling is seen at the inner canthus with a negative regurgitation test. This is called *encysted mucocele.*

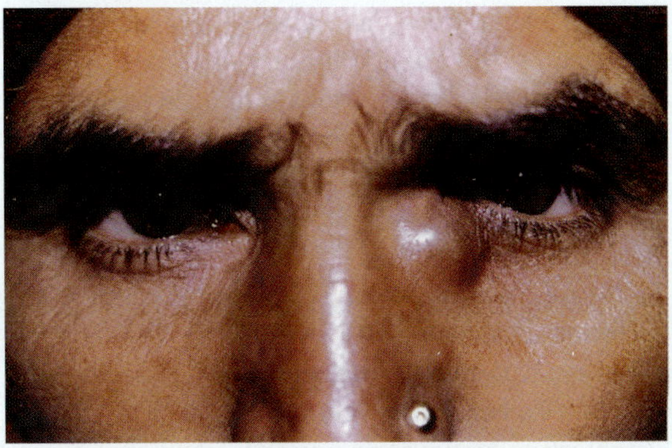

Fig. 15.8. Lacrimal mucocele.

3. *Stage of chronic suppurative dacryocystitis.* Due to pyogenic infection, the mucoid discharge becomes purulent, converting the mucocele into 'pyocoele'. The condition is characterised by epiphora, associated recurrent conjunctivitis and swelling at the inner canthus with mild erythema of the overlying skin. On regurgitation a frank purulent discharge flows from the lower punctum. If openings of canaliculi are blocked at this stage the so called *encysted pyocoele* results.

4. ***Stage of chronic fibrotic sac.*** Low grade repeated infections for a prolonged period ultimately result in a small fibrotic sac due to thickening of mucosa, which is often associated with persistent epiphora and discharge. Dacryocystography at this stage reveals a very small sac with irregular folds in the mucosa.

Complications

- Chronic intractable conjunctivitis, acute on chronic dacryocystitis.
- Ectropion of lower lid, maceration and eczema of lower lid skin due to prolonged watering.
- Simple corneal abrasions may become infected leading to hypopyon ulcer.
- If an intraocular surgery is performed in the presence of dacryocystitis, there is high risk of developing endophthalmitis. Because of this, syringing of lacrimal sac is always done in suspected cases before attempting any intraocular surgery.

Treatment

1. ***Conservative treatment*** by repeated lacrimal syringing. It may be useful in recent cases only. Long-standing cases are almost always associated with blockage of NLD which usually does not open up with repeated lacrimal syringing or even probing.

2. ***Balloon catheter dilation*** also known as balloon dacryocystoplasty can be tried in patient with partial nasolacrimal duct obstruction. Success rate reported in adults is about 50%.

3. ***Dacryocystorhinostomy (DCR).*** It should be the operation of choice as it re-establishes the lacrimal drainage. However, before performing surgery, the infection especially in pyocoele should be controlled by topical antibiotics and repeated lacrimal syringings.

4. ***Dacryocystectomy (DCT).*** It should be performed only when DCR is contraindicated. *Indications of DCT* include: (i) Too young (less than 4 years) or too old (more than 60 years) patient. (ii) Markedly shrunken and fibrosed sac. (iii) Tuberculosis, syphilis, leprosy or mycotic infections of sac. (iv) Tumours of sac. (v) Gross nasal diseases like atrophic rhinitis (vi) An unskilled surgeon, because it is said that, a good 'DCT' is always better than a badly done 'DCR'.

5. ***Conjunctivodacryocystorhinostomy (CDCR).*** It is performed in the presence of blocked canaliculi.

ACUTE DACRYOCYSTITIS

Acute dacryocystitis is an acute suppurative inflammation of the lacrimal sac, characterised by presence of a painful swelling in the region of sac.

Etiology

It may develop in two ways:

1. *As an acute exacerbation of chronic dacryocystitis.*
2. *As an acute peridacryocystitis due to direct involvement from the neighbouring infected structures* such as: paranasal sinuses, surrounding bones and dental abscess or caries teeth in the upper jaw.

Causative organisms. Commonly involved are *Streptococcus haemolyticus*, *Pneumococcus* and *Staphylococcus*.

Clinical picture

Clinical picture of acute dacryocystitis can be divided into 3 stages:

1. ***Stage of cellulitis.*** It is characterised by a *painful swelling* in the region of lacrimal sac associated with *epiphora* and constitutional symptoms such as *fever and malaise.* The swelling is red, hot, firm and tender. Redness and oedema also spread to the lids and cheek. When treated resolution may occur at this stage. However, if untreated, self-resolution is rare.

2. ***Stage of lacrimal abscess.*** Continued inflammation causes occlusion of the canaliculi due to oedema. The sac is filled with pus, distends and its anterior wall ruptures forming a pericystic swelling. In this way, a large fluctuant swelling the lacrimal abscess is formed. It usually points below and to the outer side of the sac, owing to gravitation of pus and presence of medial palpebral ligament in the upper part (Fig. 15.9).

3. ***Stage of fistula formation.*** When the lacrimal abscess is left unattended, it discharges spontaneously, leaving an *external fistula* below the medial palpebral ligament (Fig. 15.10). Rarely, the abscess may open up into the nasal cavity forming an *internal fistula.*

Complications

These include:

- Acute conjunctivitis,

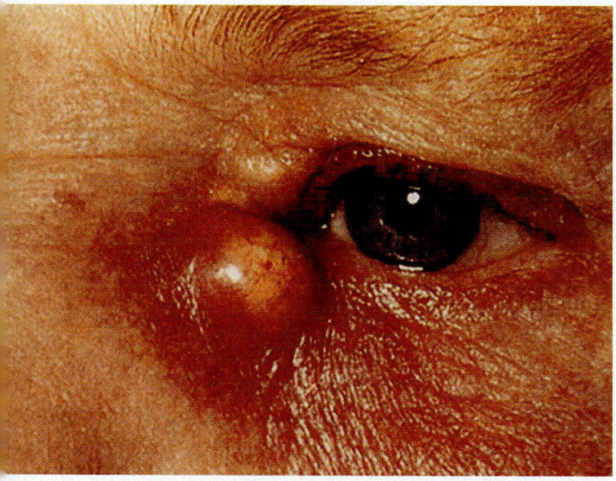

Fig. 15.9. Acute dacryocystitis: Stage of lacrimal abscess.

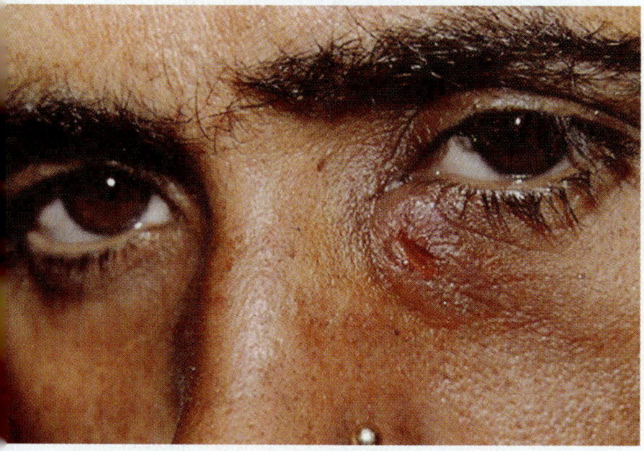

Fig. 15.10. Acute dacryocystitis: Stage of external lacrimal fistula.

- Corneal abrasion which may be converted to corneal ulceration,
- Lid abscess,
- Osteomyelitis of lacrimal bone,
- Orbital cellulitis,
- Facial cellulitis and acute ethmoiditis.
- Rarely cavernous sinus thrombosis and very rarely generalized septicaemia may also develop.

Treatment

1. *During cellulitis stage.* It consists of systemic and topical antibiotics to control infection; and systemic anti-inflammatory analgesic drugs and hot fomentation to relieve pain and swelling.
2. *During stage of lacrimal abscess.* In addition to the above treatment when pus starts pointing on the skin, it should be drained with a small incision. The pus should be gently squeezed out, the dressing done with *betadine* soaked roll gauze.

   Later on depending upon condition of the lacrimal sac either DCT or DCR operation should be carried out, otherwise recurrence will occur.
3. *Treatment of external lacrimal fistula.* After controlling the acute infection with systemic antibiotics, fistulectomy along with DCT or DCR operation should be performed.

SURGICAL TECHNIQUE OF DACRYOCYSTORHINOSTOMY

Dacryocystorhinostomy (DCR) operation can be performed by two techniques:

- Conventional external approach DCR, and
- Endonasal DCR
- Endocanalicular laser DCR.

Conventional external approach DCR (Fig. 15.11)

1. *Anaesthesia.* General anaesthesia is preferred, however, it may be performed with local infiltration anaesthesia in adults.
2. *Skin incision.* Either a curved incision along the anterior lacrimal crest or a straight incision 8 mm medial to the medial canthus is made.
3. *Exposure of medial palpebral ligament (MPL) and anterior lacrimal crest.* MPL is exposed by blunt dissection and cut with scissors to expose the anterior lacrimal crest.
4. *Dissection of lacrimal sac.* Periosteum is separated from the anterior lacrimal crest and along with the lacrimal sac is reflected laterally with blunt dissection exposing the lacrimal fossa.
5. *Exposure of nasal mucosa.* A 15 mm × 10 mm bony osteum is made by removing the anterior lacrimal crest and the bones forming lacrimal fossa, exposing the thick pinkish white nasal mucosa.
6. *Preparation of flaps of sac.* A probe is introduced into the sac through lower canaliculus and the sac is incised vertically. To prepare anterior and posterior flaps, this incision is converted into H shape.
7. *Fashioning of nasal mucosal flaps* is also done by vertical incision converted into H shape.
8. *Suturing of flaps.* Posterior flap of the nasal mucosa is sutured with posterior flap of the sac

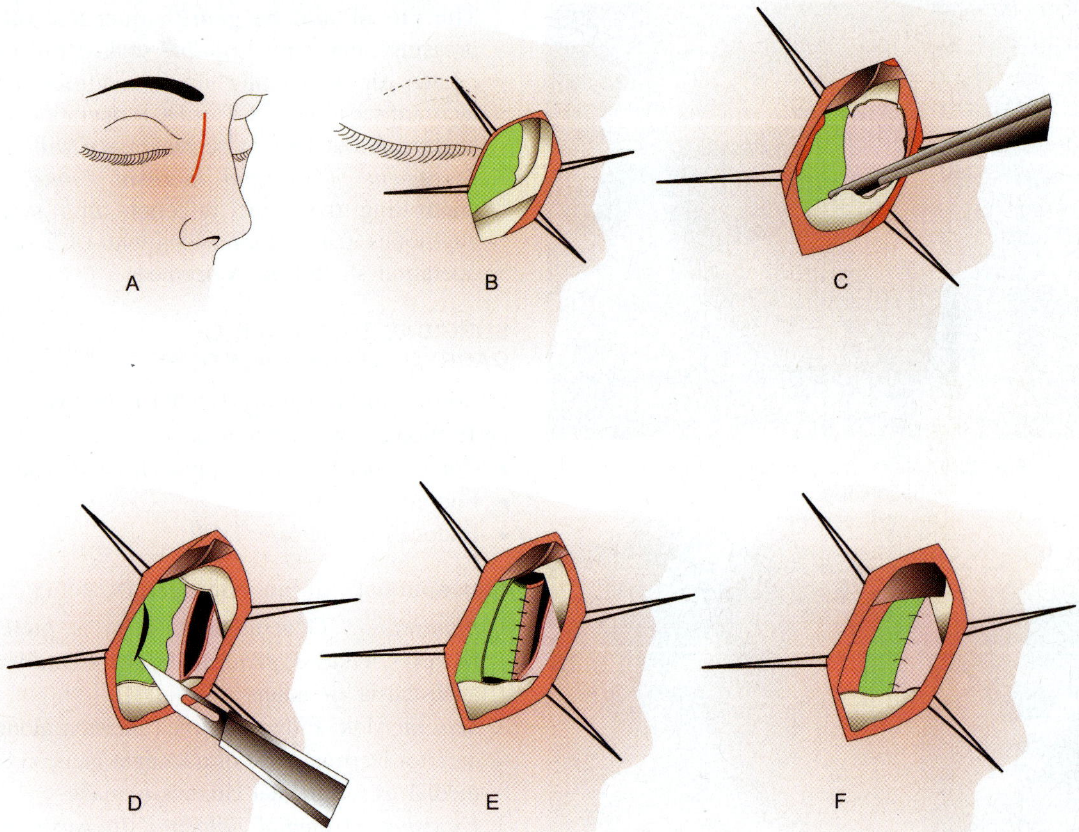

Fig. 15.11. Surgical steps of external dacryocystorhinostomy: A, skin incision; B, exposure of bony lacrimal fossa; C, preparation of bony osteum and exposure of nasal mucosa; D, preparation of flaps of the nasal mucosa and lacrimal sac; E, suturing of posterior flaps; F, suturing of anterior flaps.

using 6-0 vicryl or chromic cat gut sutures. It is followed by suturing of the anterior flaps.

9. *Closure.* MPL is sutured to periosteum, orbicularis muscle is sutured with 6-0 vicryl and skin is closed with 6-0 silk sutures.

Endonasal DCR

Presently many eye surgeons, alone or in collaboration with the ENT surgeons, are preferring endonasal DCR over conventional external approach DCR because of its advantages (described below).

Surgical steps of endonasal DCR are (Fig. 15.12):

1. ***Preparation and anaesthesia.*** Nasal mucosa is prepared for 15-30 minutes before operation with nasal decongestant drops and local anaesthetic agent. Conjunctival sac is anaesthetised with topically instilled 2% lignocaine. Then 3 ml of lignocaine 2% with 1 in 2 lac adrenaline is injected into the medial parts of upper and lower eyelids and via sub-caruncular injection to the lacrimal fossa region.

2. ***Identification of sac area.*** A 20-gauge light pipe is inserted via the upper canaliculi into the sac. With the help of endoscope, the sac area which is transilluminated by the light pipe is identified (Fig. 15.12A) and a further injection of lignocaine with adrenaline is made below the nasal mucosa in this area.

3. ***Creation of opening in the nasal mucosa, bones forming the lacrimal fossa and posteromedial wall of sac*** can be accomplished by two techniques:

i *By cutting* the tissues with appropriate instruments or

ii *By ablating* with Holmium YAG laser (endoscopic laser assisted DCR).

Note: The size of opening is about 12 mm × 10 mm (Fig. 15.12B).

4. *Stenting of rhinostomy opening.* The outflow system is then stinted using fine silicone tubes passed via the superior and inferior canaliculi into the rhinostomy and secured with a process of knotting (Fig. 15.12C). Nasal packing and dressing is done.

5. *Postoperative care and removal of sialistic lacrimal stents.* After 24 hours of operation nasal packs are removed and patient is advised to use decongestent, antibiotic and steroid nasal drops for 3-4 weeks. The sialistic lacrimal stents are removed 8-12 weeks after surgery and the nasal drops are continued further for 2-3 weeks.

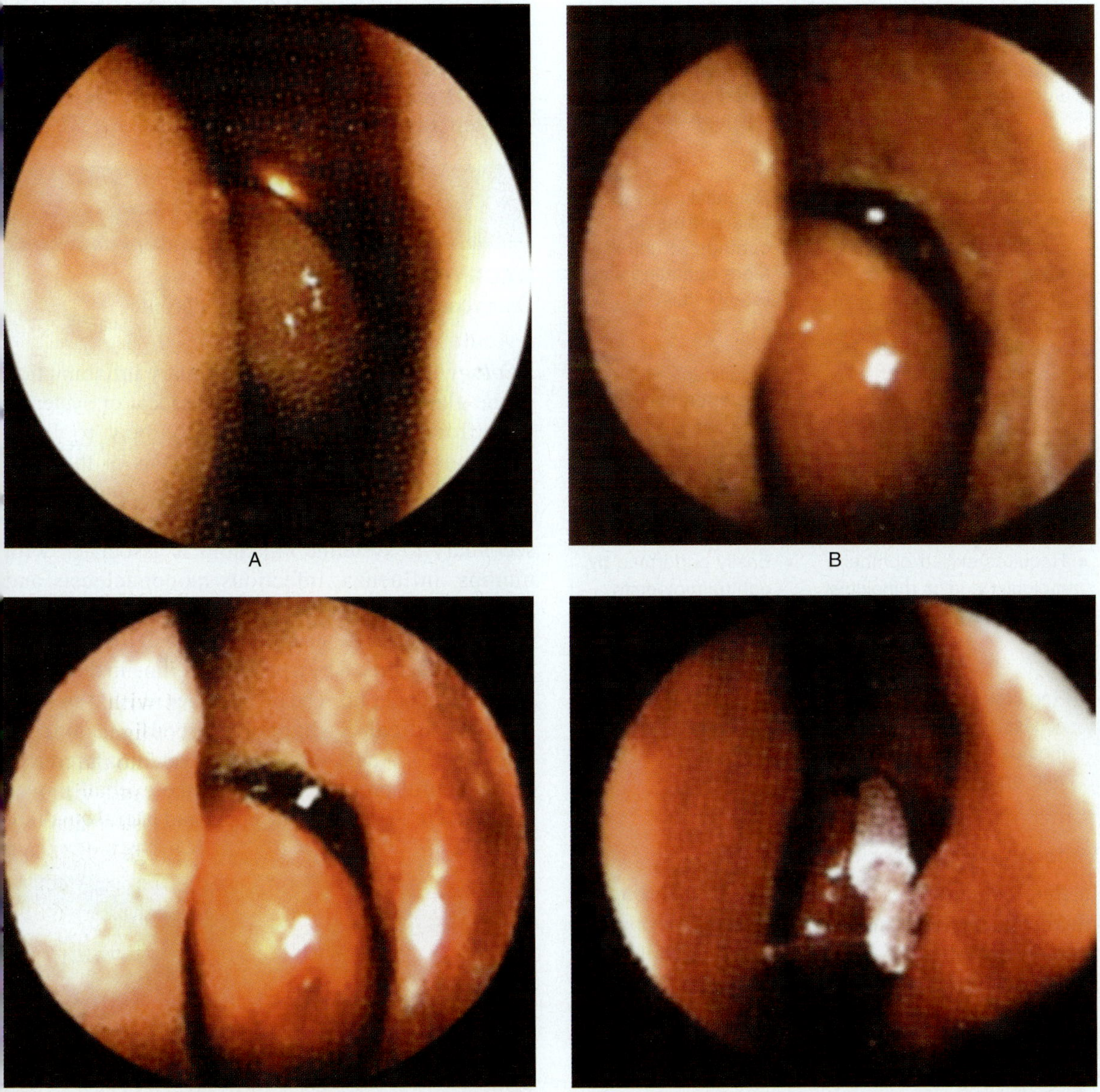

A B C D

Fig. 15.12. Surgical steps of endonasal DCR: A, endoscopic identification of sac area in the middle meatus; B, opening created in the middle meatus; C, stenting of rhinostomy opening with fine silicone tubes.

Advantages and disadvantages of endoscopic DCR vis-a-vis external DCR

Advantages and disadvantages of endoscopic DCR vis-a-vis external DCR are summerized in Table 15.1.

Table 15.1. Advantages and disadvantages of endonasal DCR vis-a-vis external DCR

Endoscopic DCR	*External DCR*
Advantages	*Disadvantages*
• No external scar	• Cutaneous scar
• Relatively blood less surgery	• Relatively more bleeding during surgery
• Better visualisation of nasal pathology	
• Less chances of injury to ethmoidal vessels and cribri form plate.	• Potential injury to adjacent medial canthus structures
• Less time consuming (15-30 mins) since nasal mucosal flaps and sac wall flaps are not made.	• More operating time (45-60 minutes)
• No post operative morbidity	• Significant postoperative morbidity
Disadvantages	*Advantages*
• Less success rate (70-90%)	• More success rate (95%)
• Requires skilled ophthalmologist and/or rhinologist.	• Easily performed by ophthalmologists
• Expensive equipment	• Cheap (expensive equipment not required)
• Requires reasonable access to middle meatus and familiarity with endoscopic anatomy.	• Does not require familiarity with endoscopic anatomy

Endocanlicular Laser DCR

In this technique laser probe is passed through a canaliculus upto the medial wall of sac. An opening is created by ablating the posteriomedial wall of the sac, bone forming the lacrimal fossa and adjacent nasal mucosa. It is performed with a Holmium YAG or KTP laser. This is a quick procedure and can be carried out under local anaesthesia. It is particularly useful for the elderly patients. Success rate is only 70%. Failure can be tackled by endonasal DCR or conventional external DCR.

SURGICAL TECHNIQUE OF DACRYOCYSTECTOMY (DCT)

1 *to* 4 *steps* are same as for external DCR operation.

5. *Removal of lacrimal sac.* After exposing the sac, it is separated from the surrounding structures by blunt dissection followed by cutting its connections with the lacrimal canaliculi. It is then held with artery forceps and twisted 3-4 times to tear it away from the nasolacrimal duct (NLD).
6. *Curettage of bony NLD.* It is done with the help of a lacrimal curette to remove the infected parts of membranous NLD.
7. *Closure.* It is done as for external DCR (Step 9).

SWELLINGS OF THE LACRIMAL GLAND

DACRYOADENITIS

Dacryoadenitis may be acute or chronic.

I. Acute dacryoadenitis

Etiology. It may develop as a primary inflammation of the gland or secondary to some local or systemic infection. Dacryoadenitis secondary to local infections occurs in trauma, erysipelas of the face, conjunctivitis (especially gonococcal and staphylococcal) and orbital cellulitis. Dacryoadenitis secondary to systemic infections is associated with mumps, influenza, infectious mononucleosis and measles.

Clinical picture. Acute inflammation of the palpebral part is characterised by a painful swelling in the lateral part of the upper lid. The lid becomes red and swollen with a typical S-shaped curve of its margin (Fig. 15.13). Acute orbital dacryoadenitis produces some painful proptosis in which the eyeball moves down and in. A fistula in the upper and lateral quadrant

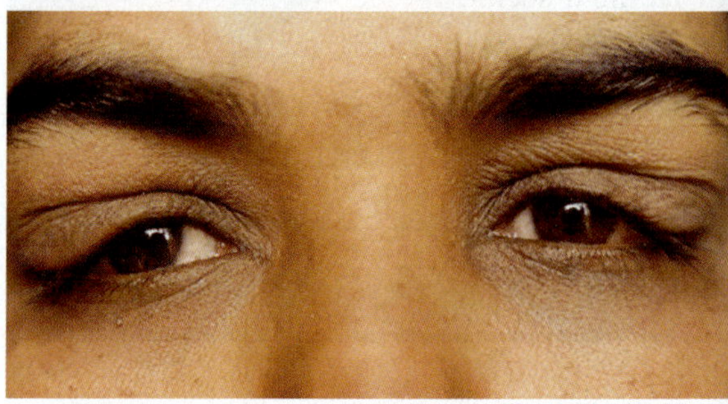

Fig. 15.13. A patient with bilateral dacryoadenitis: note, s-shaped curve of upper eyelid.

of the upper lid may develop as a complication of suppurative dacryoadenitis.

Treatment. It consists of a course of appropriate systemic antibiotic, analgesic and anti-inflammatory drugs along with hot fomentation. When pus is formed, incision and drainage should be carried out.

II. Chronic dacryoadenitis

It is characterised by engorgement and simple hypertrophy of the gland.

Etiology. Chronic dacryoadenitis may occur: (i) as sequelae to acute inflammation; (ii) in association with chronic inflammations of conjunctiva and; (iii) due to systemic diseases such as tuberculosis, syphilis and sarcoidosis.

Clinical features. These include (i) a painless swelling in upper and outer part of lid associated with ptosis; (ii) eyeball may be displaced down and in; and (iii) diplopia may occur in up and out gaze.
On palpation, a firm lobulated mobile mass may be felt under the upper and outer rim of the orbit.

Differential diagnosis from other causes of lacrimal gland swellings is best made after fine needle aspiration biopsy or incisional biopsy.

Treatment consists of treating the cause.

MIKULICZ'S SYNDROME

It is characterised by bilaterally symmetrical enlargement of the lacrimal and salivary glands associated with a variety of systemic diseases. These include: leukaemias, lymphosarcomas, benign lymphoid hyperplasia, Hodgkin's disease, sarcoidosis and tuberculosis.

DACRYOPES

It is a cystic swelling, which occurs due to retention of lacrimal secretions following blockage of the lacrimal ducts.

TUMOURS OF THE LACRIMAL GLAND

These are not so common and in a simplified way can be classified as below:

I. *Epithelial tumours of lacrimal gland*. These account for 50% tumourous swellings of lacrimal gland and include:

1. *Benign epithelial tumours.* These include 'benign mixed tumour' which accounts for 50% of epithelial tumours and 25% of all tumours of lacrimal gland.
2. *Malignant epithelial tumours*. These also constitute 25% of all cases and 50% of epithelial tumours and include: malignant mixed tumour, adenoid cystic carcinoma, mucoepidermoid carcinoma and adenocarcinoma.

II. *Non epithelial tumours of lacrimal gland.* Constitute approximately 50% of all cases. These include:

1. *Lymphoproliferative tumours* (see page 424) and
2. *Inflammatory conditions* such as idiopathic orbital inflammatory disease (see page 416), sarcoidosis, and Mikulicz's syndrome.

Epithelial Tumours of Lacrimal Gland

Benign mixed tumour

It is also known as *pleomorphic adenoma* and occurs predominantly in young adult males.

Clinically it presents as a slowly progressive painless swelling in the upper-outer quadrant of the orbit displacing the eyeball downwards and inwards (Fig. 15.14). It is locally invasive and may infiltrate its own pseudocapsule to involve the adjacent periosteum. *Histologically,* it is characterised by presence of pleomorphic myxomatous tissue, just like benign mixed tumour of salivary gland.

Treatment consists of complete surgical removal with the capsule. Recurrences are very common following incomplete removal.

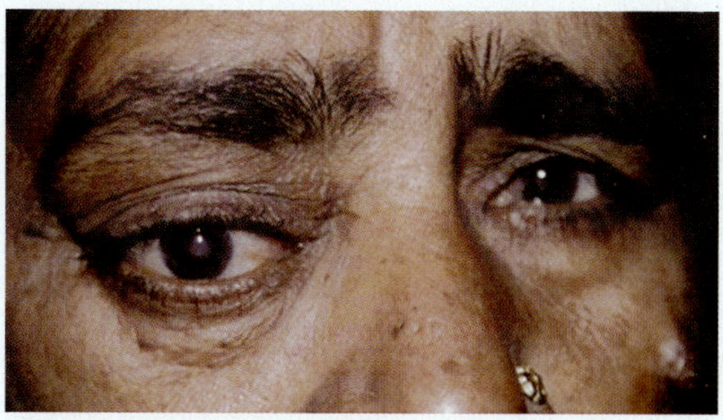

Fig. 15.14. Down and in displacement of right eyeball in a patient with benign mixed tumour.

Malignant mixed tumour

It occurs in the older age group as compared to the benign mixed tumour. It presents as a painful swelling of short duration. Histologically, areas resembling benign mixed tumour are seen along with the adenocarcinomatous areas.

16

CHAPTER

Diseases of the Orbit

APPLIED ANATOMY

BONY ORBIT

The bony orbits are quadrangular truncated pyramids situated between the anterior cranial fossa above and the maxillary sinuses below (Fig. 16.1). Each orbit is about 40 mm in height, width and depth and is formed by portions of seven bones: (1) frontal, (2) maxilla, (3) zygomatic, (4) sphenoid, (5) palatine, (6) ethmoid and (7) lacrimal. It has four walls (medial, lateral, superior and inferior), base and an apex.

Medial walls of the two orbits are parallel to each other and, being thinnest, are frequently fractured during injuries as well as during orbitotomy operations and, it also accounts for ethmoiditis being the commonest cause of orbital cellulitis.

Inferior orbital wall (floor) is triangular in shape and being quite thin is commonly involved in blow-out fractures and is easily invaded by tumours from the maxillary antrum.

Lateral wall of the orbit is triangular in shape. It covers only posterior half of the eyeball. Therefore, palpation of the retrobulbar tumours is easier from this side. Because of its advantageous anatomical position, a surgical approach to the orbit by lateral orbitotomy is popular.

Roof of the orbit is triangular in shape and is formed mainly by the orbital plate of frontal bone.

Base of the orbit is the anterior open end of the orbit. It is bounded by thick orbital margins.

Orbital apex (Fig. 16.2). It is the posterior end of orbit where the four orbital walls converge. It has two orifices, the *optic canal* which transmits optic nerve and ophthalmic artery and the *superior orbital fissure* which transmits a number of nerves, arteries and veins (Fig. 13.2).

ORBITAL FASCIA

It is a thin connective tissue membrane lining various intraorbital structures. Though, it is one continuous tissue, but for the descriptive convenience it has been

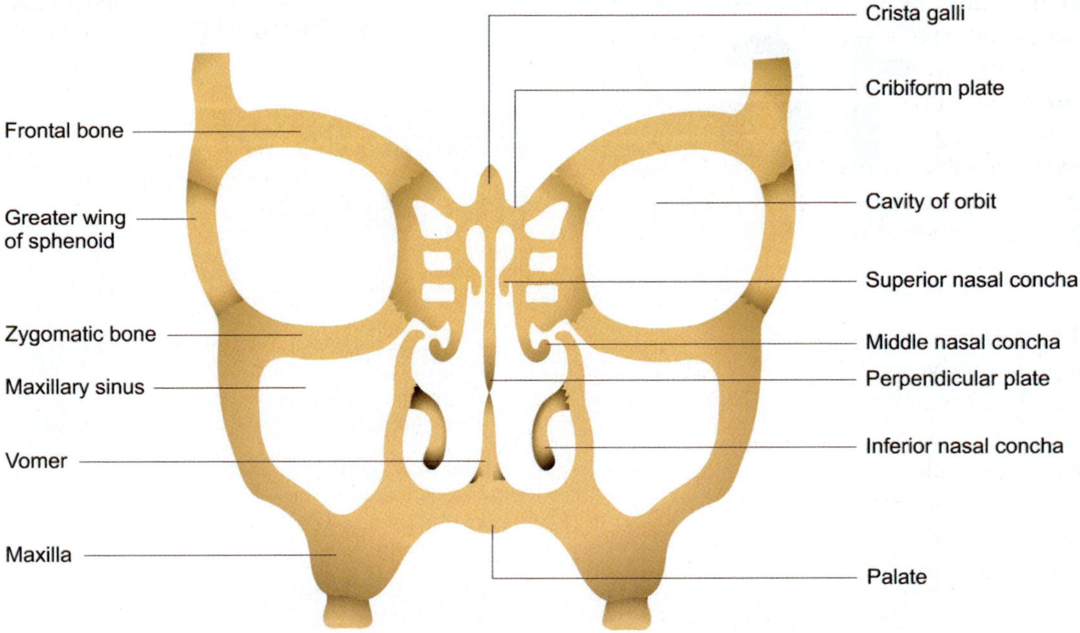

Fig. 16.1. Schematic coronal section through the orbits and nasal cavity.

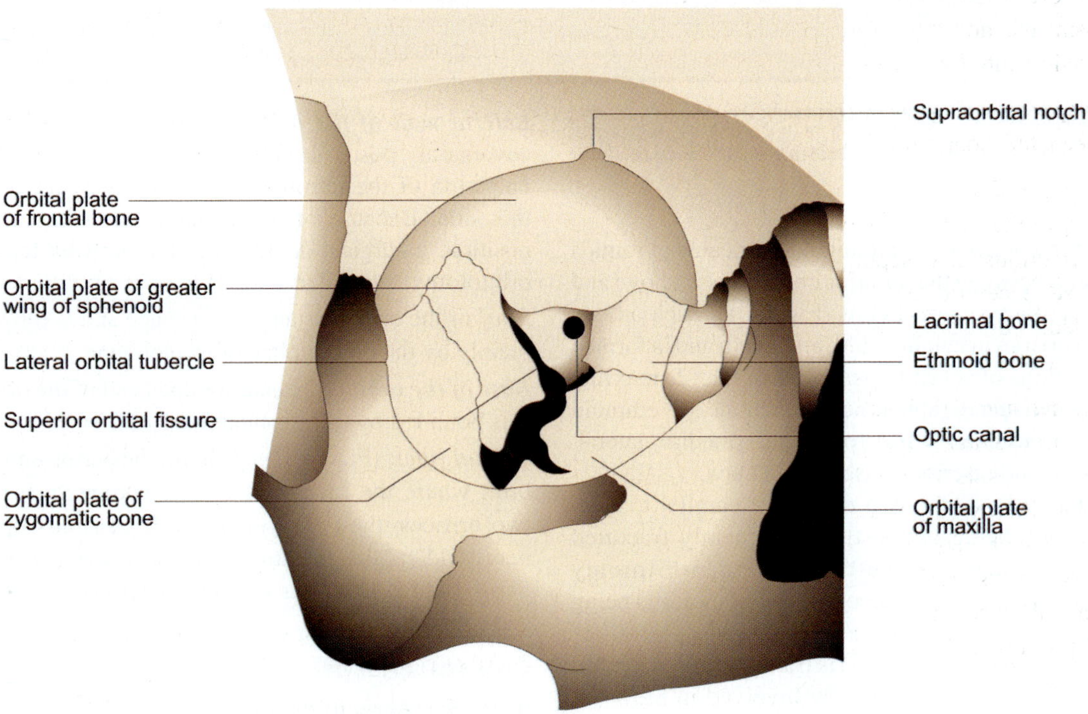

Fig. 16.2. A schematic view of the orbital cavity and orbital rim.

divided into fascia bulbi, muscular sheaths, intermuscular septa, membranous expansions of the extraocular muscles and ligament of Lockwood. ***Fascia bulbi*** (Tenon's capsule) envelops the globe from the margins of cornea to the optic nerve. Its lower part is thickened to form a sling or hammock on which the globe rests; this is called '*suspensory ligament of Lockwood*'.

CONTENTS OF THE ORBIT

The *volume* of each orbit is about 30 cc. Approximately one-fifth of it is occupied by the eyeball. Other contents of the orbit include: part of optic nerve, extraocular muscles, lacrimal gland, lacrimal sac, ophthalmic artery and its branches, third, fourth and sixth cranial nerves and ophthalmic and maxillary divisions of the fifth cranial nerve, sympathetic nerve, orbital fat and fascia.

SURGICAL SPACES IN THE ORBIT

These are of importance as most orbital pathologies tend to remain in the space in which they are formed. Therefore, their knowledge helps the surgeon in choosing the most direct surgical approach. Each orbit is divisible into four surgical spaces (Fig. 16.3).

1. *Subperiosteal space.* This is a potential space between the bone and the periorbita (periosteum).

2. *Peripheral space.* It is bounded peripherally by the periorbita and internally by the four recti with thin intermuscular septa. Tumours present here produce eccentric proptosis and can usually be palpated. For peribulbar anaesthesia, injection is made in this space.

3. *Central space.* It is also called *muscular cone* or *retrobulbar space*. It is bounded anteriorly by the Tenon's capsule lining back of the eyeball and peripherally by the four recti muscles and their intermuscular septa in the anterior part. In the posterior part, it becomes continuous with the peripheral space. Tumours lying here usually produce axial proptosis. Retrobulbar injections are made in this space.

4. *Tenon's space.* It is a potential space around the eyeball between the sclera and Tenon's capsule.

PROPTOSIS

Proptosis is defined as forward displacement of the eyeball beyond the orbital margins. Though the word exophthalmos (out eye) is synonymous with it; but somehow it has become customary to use the term exophthalmos for the displacement associated with thyroid eye disease.

CLASSIFICATION

Proptosis can be divided into following clinical groups:

- Unilateral proptosis
- Bilateral proptosis
- Acute proptosis
- Intermittent proptosis
- Pulsating proptosis

ETIOLOGY

Important causes of proptosis in each clinical group are listed here:

A. *Causes of unilateral proptosis*

1. *Congenital conditions.* These include: dermoid cyst, congenital cystic eyeball, and orbital teratoma.
2. *Traumatic lesions.* These are: orbital haemorrhage, retained intraorbital foreign body, traumatic aneurysm and emphysema of the orbit.
3. *Inflammatory lesions.* Acute inflammations are orbital cellulitis, abscess, thrombophlebitis, panophthalmitis, and cavernous sinus thrombosis (proptosis is initially unilateral but ultimately becomes bilateral). Chronic inflammatory lesions include: pseudotumours, tuberculoma, gumma and sarcoidosis.
4. *Circulatory disturbances and vascular lesions.* These are: angioneurotic oedema, orbital varix and aneurysms.
5. *Cysts of orbit.* These include: haematic cyst, implantation cyst and parasitic cyst (hydatid cyst and cysticercus cellulosae).
6. *Tumours of the orbit.* These can be primary, secondary or metastatic (see page 419).
7. *Mucoceles of paranasal sinuses,* especially frontal (most common), ethmoidal and maxillary sinus are common causes of unilateral proptosis.

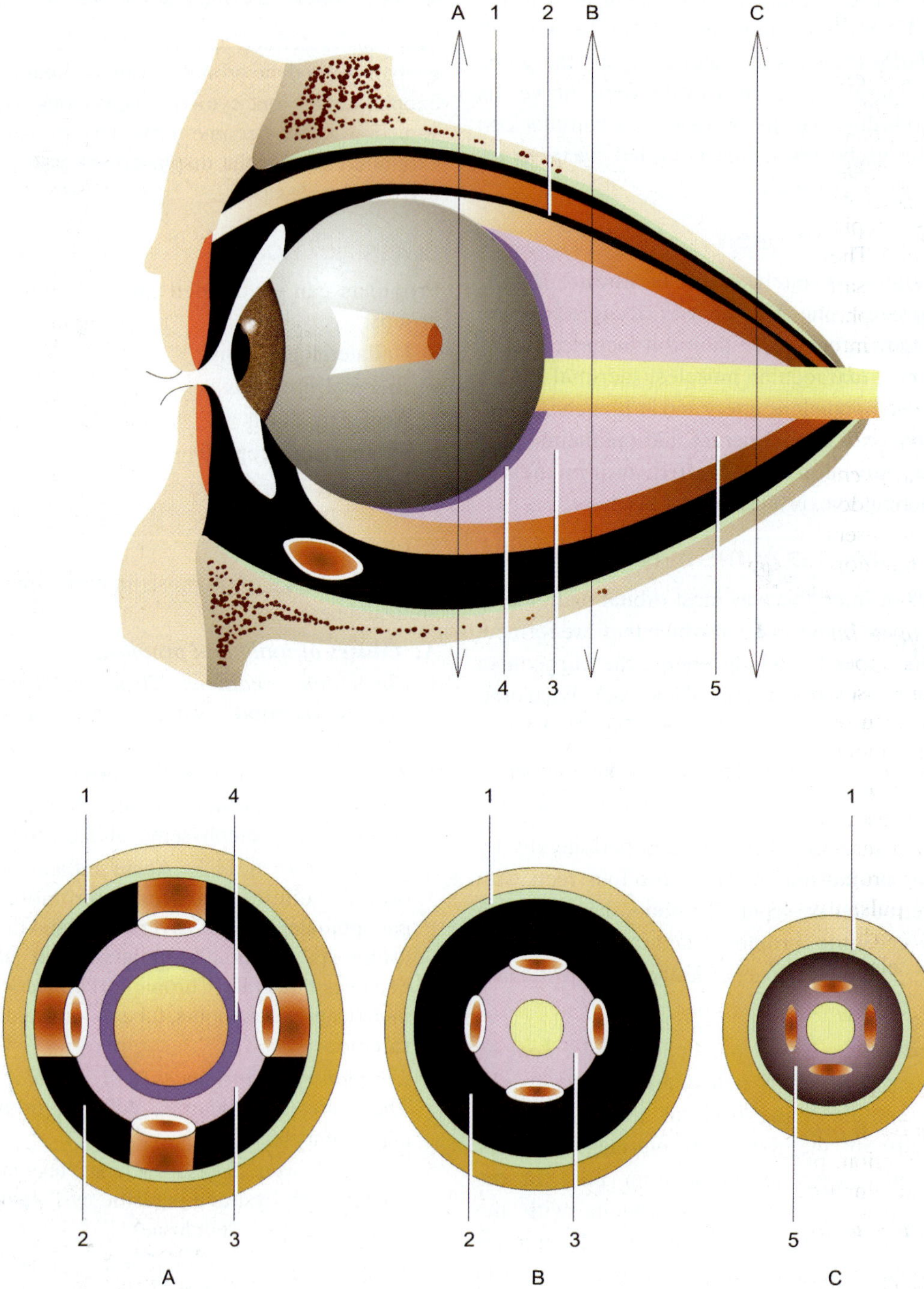

Fig. 16.3. Schematic sections of the orbital cavity to demonstrate surgical spaces of the orbit. Above sagittal section; below coronal sections at levels A, B, C (1. subperiosteal space; 2. peripheral space; 3. central space; 4. Tenon's space; 5. peripheral and central spaces merged with each other at the orbital apex).

B. *Causes of bilateral proptosis*

1. *Developmental anomalies of the skull*: craniofacial dysostosis e.g., oxycephaly (tower skull).
2. *Osteopathies*: Osteitis deformans, rickets and acromegaly.
3. *Inflammatory conditions*: Mikulicz's syndrome and late stage of cavernous sinus thrombosis.
4. *Endocrinal exophthalmos*: It may be thyrotoxic or thyrotropic.
5. *Tumours*: These include symmetrical lymphoma or lymphosarcoma, secondaries from neuroblastoma, nephroblastoma, Ewing's sarcoma and leukaemic infiltration.
6. *Systemic diseases*: Histiocytosis, systemic amyloidosis, xanthomatosis and Wegener's granulomatosis.

C. *Causes of acute proptosis.* It develops with extreme rapidity (sudden onset). Its common causes are: orbital emphysema, fracture of the medial orbital wall, orbital haemorrhage and rupture of ethmoidal mucocele.

D. *Cause of intermittent proptosis.* This type of proptosis appears and disappears of its own. Its common causes are: orbital varix, periodic orbital oedema, recurrent orbital haemorrhage and highly vascular tumours.

E. *Causes of pulsating proptosis.* It is caused by pulsating vascular lesions such as caroticocavernous fistula and saccular aneurysm of ophthalmic artery. Pulsating proptosis also occurs due to transmitted cerebral pulsations in conditions associated with deficient orbital roof. These include congenital meningocele or meningoencephalocele, neurofibromatosis and traumatic or operative hiatus.

INVESTIGATIONS

I. *Clinical evaluation*

(A) *History*. It should include: age of onset, nature of onset, duration, progression, chronology of orbital signs and symptoms, and associated symptoms.

(B) *Local examination*. It should be carried out as follows:

1. *Inspection.* (i) To differentiate proptosis from pseudoproptosis which is seen in patients with buphthalmos, axial high myopia, retraction of upper lid and enophthalmos of the opposite eye; (ii) to ascertain whether the proptosis is unilateral or bilateral; (iii) to note the shape of the skull; and (iv) to observe whether proptosis is axial or eccentric.
2. *Palpation.* It should be carried out for retrodisplacement of globe to know compressibility of the tumour, for orbital thrill, for any swelling around the eyeball, regional lymph nodes and orbital rim.
3. *Auscultation.* It is primarily of value in searching for abnormal vascular communications that generate a bruit, such as caroticocavernous fistula.
4. *Transillumination.* It is helpful in evaluating anterior orbital lesions.
5. *Visual acuity.* Orbital lesions may reduce visual acuity by three mechanisms: refractive changes due to pressure on back of the eyeball, optic nerve compression and exposure keratopathy.
6. *Pupil reactions.* The presence of Marcus Gunn pupil is suggestive of optic nerve compression.
7. *Fundoscopy.* It may reveal venous engorgement, haemorrhage, disc oedema and optic atrophy. Choroidal folds and opticociliary shunts may be seen in patients with meningiomas.
8. *Ocular motility.* It is restricted in thyroid ophthalmopathy, extensive tumour growths and neurological deficit.
9. *Exophthalmometry.* It measures protrusion of the apex of cornea from the outer orbital margin (with the eyes looking straight ahead). Normal values vary between 10 and 21 mm and are symmetrical in both eyes. A difference of more than 2 mm between the two eyes is considered significant. The simplest instrument to measure proptosis is *Luedde's exophthalmometer* (Fig. 16.4). However, the *Hertel's exophthalmometer* (Fig. 16.5) is the most commonly used instrument. Its advantage is that it measures the two eyes simultaneously.

(C) *Systemic examination*. A thorough examination should be conducted to rule out systemic causes of proptosis such as thyrotoxicosis, histiocytosis, and primary tumours elsewhere in the body (secondaries in orbits). Otorhinolaryngological examination is necessary when the paranasal sinus or a nasopharyngeal mass apears to be a possible etiological factor.

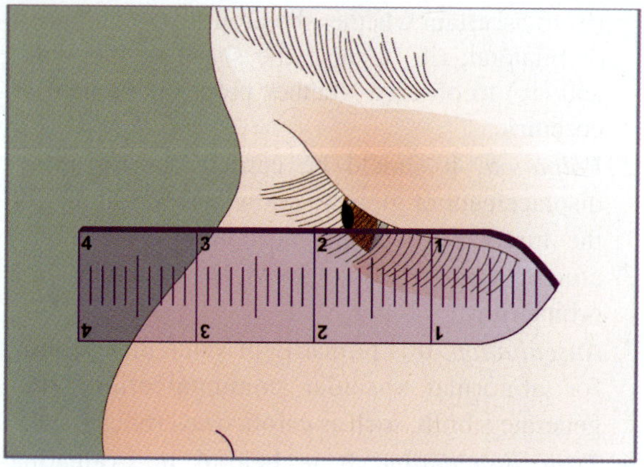

Fig. 16.4. Luedde's exophthalmometer.

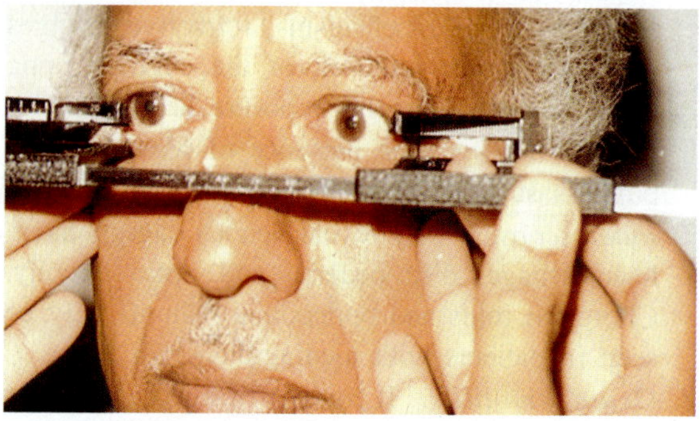

Fig. 16.5. Hertel's exophthalmometer.

II. *Laboratory investigations*

These should include:

- Thyroid function tests,
- Haematological studies (TLC, DLC, ESR, VDRL test),
- Casoni's test (to rule out hydatid cyst),
- Stool examination for cysts and ova, and
- Urine analysis for Bence Jones proteins for multiple myeloma.

III. *Imaging Techniques*

(A) *Non-invasive techniques*

1. *Plain X-rays.* It is still the most frequently used initial radiological examination. Commonly required exposures are in the *Caldwell view,* the *Water's view,* a lateral view and the Rhese view (for optic foramina). X-ray signs of orbital diseases include enlargement of orbital cavity, enlargement of optic foramina, calcification and hyperostosis.
2. *Computed tomography scanning.* It is very useful for determining the location and size of an orbital mass. A combination of axial (CAT) and coronal (CCT) cut enables a three-dimensional visualisation. CT scan is capable of visualising various structures like globe, extraocular muscles and optic nerves. Further, this technique is also useful in examining areas adjacent to the orbits such as orbital walls, cranial cavity, paranasal sinuses and nasal cavity. Its main disadvantage is the inability to distinguish between pathologically soft tissue masses which are radiologically isodense.
3. *Ultrasonography.* It is a non-radiational non-invasive, completely safe and extremely valuable initial scanning procedure for orbital lesions. In the diagnosis of orbital lesions, it is superior to CT scanning in actual tissue diagnosis and can usually differentiate between solid, cystic, infiltrative and spongy masses.
4. *Magnetic resonance imaging (MRI).* It is a major advance in the imaging techniques. It is very sensitive for detecting differences between normal and abnormal tissues and has excellent image resolution. The technique produces tomographic images which are superficially very similar to CT scan but rely on entirely different physical principles for their production.

   MR angiography is useful in vascular lesions of the orbit.

(B) *Invasive procedures*

Before the advent of CT and MR angiography , the invasive investigations were needed for vascular lesions as below:

- *Orbital venography* for the suspected orbital varix,
- *Carotid angiography* for suspected arteriovenous malformations, aneurysm and arteriovenous fistulas.
- *Radioisotope arteriography* in proptosis of vascular lesions.

However, because of the availability of non-invasive techniques of *CT* and *MR angiography*, most of the vascular lesions can now be easily evaluated without the need of potentially dangerous above mentioned invasive procedures.

IV. *Histopathological studies*

The exact diagnosis of many orbital lesions cannot be made without the help of histopathological studies which can be accomplished by following techniques:

1. *Fine-needle aspiration biopsy* (FNAB). It is a reliable, accurate (95%), quick and easy technique for cytodiagnosis in orbital tumours. The biopsy aspirate is obtained under direct vision in an obvious mass and under CT scan or ultrasonographic guidance in retrobulbar mass using a 23-gauge needle.
2. *Incisional biopsy*. Undoubtedly, for accurate tissue diagnosis a proper biopsy specimen at least 5 to 10 mm in length is required. However, the scope of incisional biopsy in the diagnosis of orbital tumours is not clearly defined. It may be undertaken along with frozen tissue study in infiltrative lesions which remain undiagnosed.
3. *Excisional biopsy*. It should always be preferred over incisional biopsy in orbital masses which are well encapsulated or circumscribed. It is performed by anterior orbitotomy for a mass in the anterior part of orbit and by lateral orbitotomy for a retrobulbar mass.

ENOPHTHALMOS

It is the inward displacement of the eyeball. About 50 percent cases of mild enophthalmos are misdiagnosed as having ipsilateral ptosis or contralateral proptosis. ***Common causes*** are:

1. *Congenital*. Microphthalmos and maxillary hypoplasia.
2. *Traumatic*. Blow out fractures of floor of the orbit.
3. *Post-inflammatory*. Cicatrization of extraocular muscles as in the pseudotumour syndromes.
4. *Paralytic enophthalmos*. It is seen in Horner's syndrome (due to paralysis of cervical sympathetics).
5. *Atrophy of orbital contents*. Senile atrophy of orbital fat, atrophy due to irradiation of malignant tumours, following cicatrizing metastatic carcinoma and due to scleroderma.

DEVELOPMENTAL ANOMALIES OF THE ORBIT

Developmental anomalies of the orbit are commonly associated with abnormalities of skull and facial bones. They are frequently hereditary (autosomal dominant) in origin.

Details of such anomalies are beyond the scope of the book. However, a few salient features of some anomalies are mentioned below:

Craniosynostosis

Craniosynostosis results from premature closure of one or more cranial sutures. Depending upon the suture involved craniosynostosis may be of following types:

Anomaly	*Suture closed prematurely*
• Brachycephaly (clover-leaf skull)	Coronal sutures
• Oxycephaly (tower-shaped skull)	Coronal suture
• Scophocephaly (boat-shaped skull)	Sagittal suture
• Trigonocephaly (egg-shaped skull)	Frontal suture
• Acrocephaly	Multiple cranial sutures

Craniofacial dysostosis

Craniofacial dysostosis (Crouzon syndrome) refers to premature closure of coronal and saggital sutures (brachycephaly) associated with maxillary hypoplasia. Inheritance is autosomal dominant, but 25% of cases occurs as fresh mutation.

Ocular features include:

- Proptosis due to shallow orbits,
- V-pattern exotropia and hypertropia,
- Hypertelorism i.e., widely separated eyeballs (increased interpupillary distance), and
- Optic atrophy may occur due to compression at optic foraman.

Ocular associations include blue sclera, megalocornea, aniridia, glaucoma, cataract, ectopia lentis and optic nerve hypoplasia.

Systemic features are:

- Mental retardation,

- High-arched palate,
- Irregular dentition, and
- Hooked (parrot beak) nose.

Mandibulofacial dysostosis

Mandibulofacial dysostosis (Treacher-Collin syndrome) refers to a condition resulting from hypoplasia of zygoma and mandible.

Ocular features include:
- Indistinct inferior orbital margin,
- Coloboma of the lower eyelid, and
- Anti-mongoloid slant.

Systemic features are:
- Macrostomia with high-arched palate,
- External ear deformity, and
- Bird-like face.

Median facial cleft syndrome

Main ocular features of this anomaly are:
- Hypertelorism,
- Telecanthus, and
- Divergent squint.

Main systemic features include:
- Cleft-nose, lip and palate; and
- V-shaped frontal hair line (widow's peak).

Acrocephaly-syndactyle (Apert syndrome)

It is the most severe of craniosynostosis in which all the cranial sutures may be involved.

Systemic features include:
- Tower skull with flat occiput,
- Mental retardation,
- Ventricular septal defect,
- High arched palate, and
- Syndactyly of the fingers and toes.

Ocular features are:
- Hypertelorism—increased IPD,
- Bilateral proptosis due to shallow orbits,
- Congenital ptosis,
- Antimongoloid slant, and
- Divergent squint.

Ocular associations include keratoconus, congenital glaucoma and ectopia lentis.

Hypertelorism

It is a condition of widely separated eyeballs resulting from widely separated orbits and broad nasal bridge. Hypertelorism may occur de novo or as a part of various syndromes such as Apert syndrome, Crouzons syndrome and median facial cleft syndrome.

Ocular features of hypertelorism are:
- Increased interpupillary distance (IPD)—may be 85 mm (normally, average IPD in an adult is 60 mm),
- Telecanthus,
- Divergent squint,
- Anti-mongoloid slant, and
- Optic atrophy may be associated in some cases due to narrow optic canal.

ORBITAL INFECTIONS AND INFLAMMATIONS

CLASSIFICATION

A. *Orbital Infections*

I. *Acute orbital and related infections*
1. Pre-septal cellulitis
2. Orbital cellulitis and intraorbital abscess
3. Orbital osteoperiostitis
4. Orbital thrombophlebitis
5. Tenonitis
6. Cavernous sinus thrombosis

II. *Chronic orbital infections*
1. Tuberculosis
2. Syphilis
3. Actinomycosis
4. Mycotic infections e.g., mucormycosis
5. Parasitic infestations

B. *Orbital inflammations (non-infective)*

I. *Isolated orbital inflammations*

a. Diffuse
- Idiopathic orbital inflammatory disease (IOID)
- Idiopathic sclerosing inflammation of the orbit

b. Focal
- Myositis
- Dacryoadenitis
- Tolosa- Hunt Syndrome

II. *Systemic inflammations*
- Thyroid eye disease,
- Wegner's granulomatosis, and
- Sarcoidosis.

Salient features of some infections and inflammations of the orbit are described here.

PRESEPTAL CELLULITIS

Preseptal (or periorbital) cellulitis refers to infection of the subcutaneous tissues anterior to the orbital septum. Strictly speaking it is not an orbital disease but is included here under because the facial veins are valveless and preseptal cellulitis may spread posteriorly to produce orbital cellulitis.

Etiology

Causative organisms are usually *Staphylococcus aureus* or *Sreptococcus pyogenes* and occasionally *Haemophilus influenzae*.

Modes of infection. The organisms may invade the preseptal tissue by any of the following modes.

1. *Exogenous infection* may result following skin lacerations, insect bites and eyelid operations.
2. *Extension from local infections* such as from an acute hordeolum or acute dacryocystitis.
3. *Endogenous infection* may occur by haematogenous spread from remote infection of the middle ear or upper respiratory tract.

Clinical features

Preseptal cellulitis presents as inflammatory oedema of the eyelids and periorbital skin with no involvement of the orbit.

Characteristic features are (Fig. 16.6):

- Painful acute periorbital swelling,
- Erythema and hyperaemia of the lids,
- Fever and leukocytosis may be associated,
- Proptosis is absent,
- Ocular moments are normal,
- Conjunctiva is usually not congested, and
- Visual acuity is normal.

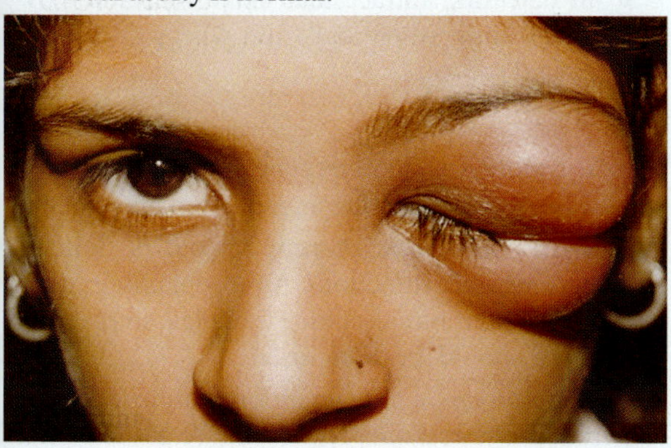

Fig. 16.6. Preseptal cellulitis.

Treatment

- *Systemic antibiotics*, oral—for mild to moderate cases, and injectable—for severe cases, form the mainstay of treatment.
- *Systemic analgesics* and anti-inflammatory drugs help in reducing pain and swelling.
- *Topical antibiotics* may be used for associated conjunctivitis.
- *Warm compresses*, 2-3 times a day, have a soothing effect.
- *Surgical exploration* and debridement is required in the presence of a fluctulant mass or abscess, or when retained foreign body is suspected.

ORBITAL CELLULITIS AND INTRAORBITAL ABSCESS

Orbital cellulitis refers to an acute infection of the soft tissues of the orbit behind the orbital septum. Orbital cellulitis may or may not progress to a subperiosteal abscess or orbital abscess.

Etiology

Modes of infection

1. *Exogenous infection.* It may result from penetrating injury especially when associated with retention of intraorbital foreign body, and following operations like evisceration, enucleation, dacryocystectomy and orbitotomy.
2. *Extension of infection from neighbouring structures.* These include paranasal sinuses, teeth, face, lids, intracranial cavity and intraorbital structures. It is the commonest mode of orbital infections.
3. *Endogenous infection.* It may rarely develop as metastatic infection from breast abscess, puerperal sepsis, thrombophlebitis of legs and septicaemia.

Causative organisms. Those commonly involved are: *Streptococcus pneumoniae*, *Staphylococcus aureus*, *Streptococcus pyogenes* and *Haemophilus influenzae*.

Pathology

Pathological features of orbital cellulitis are similar to suppurative inflammations of the body in general, except that:

- Due to the absence of a lymphatic system the protective agents are limited to local phagocytic elements provided by the orbital reticular tissue;

- Due to tight compartments, the intraorbital pressure is raised which augments the virulence of infection causing early and extensive necrotic sloughing of the tissues; and
- In most cases the infection spreads as thrombophlebitis from the surrounding structures, therefore, a rapid spread with extensive necrosis is the rule.

Clinical features

Symptoms include:

- *Swelling and severe pain* (which is increased by movements of the eyeball or pressure) are main symptoms.
- *Other associated symptoms* include fever, nausea, vomiting, prostrations and sometimes loss of vision.

Signs of orbital cellulitis (Fig. 16.7) are:

- *Swelling of lids*, characterised by woody hardness and redness, is usually marked.
- *Chemosis of conjunctiva,* which may protrude and become desiccated or necrotic.
- *Axial proptosis* of varying degree is present.
- *Restriction of ocular movements*, mild to severe, is frequently present.
- *Fundus examination* may show congestion of retinal veins and signs of papillitis or papilloedema.

Complications

These are quite common if not treated promptly.

1. *Ocular complications* are usually blinding and include exposure keratopathy, optic neuritis and central retinal artery occlusion.

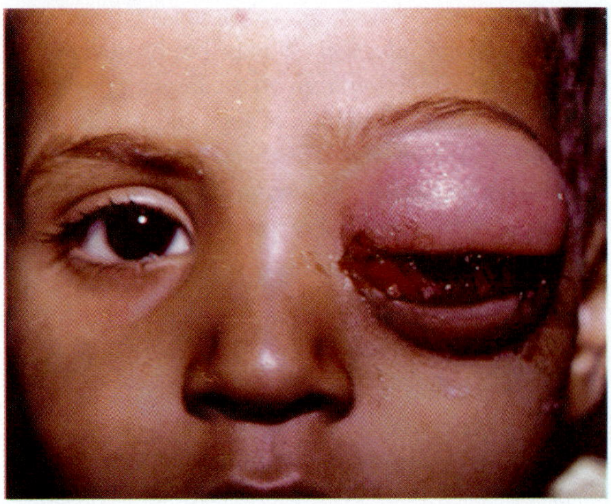

Fig. 16.7. Orbital cellulitis in a three-year-old female child.

2. *Orbital complications* are progression of orbital cellulitis into subperiosteal abscess and/or orbital abscess:

i. *Subperiosteal abscess* is collection of purulent material between the orbital bony wall and periosteum, most frequently located along the medial orbital wall. Clinically, subperiosteal abscess is suspected when clinical features of orbital cellulitis are associated with eccentric proptosis; but the diagnosis is confirmed by CT scan.

ii. *Orbital abscess* is collection of pus within the orbital soft tissue. Clinically it is suspected by signs of severe proptosis, marked chemosis, complete ophthalmoplegia, and pus points below the conjunctiva, but is confirmed by CT scan.

3. *Temporal or parotid abscesses* may occur due to spread of infection around the orbit.

4. *Intracranial complications* include cavernous sinus thrombosis, meningitis and brain abscesses.

5. *General septicemia or pyaemia* may occur eventually in few cases.

Investigations

1. *Bacterial cultures* should be performed from nasal and conjunctival swabs and blood samples.
2. *Complete haemogram* may reveal leukocytosis.
3. *X-ray PNS* to identify associated sinusitis.
4. *Orbital ultrasonography* to detect intra-orbital abscess.
5. *CT scan and MRI* are useful:
   - in differentiating preseptal and postseptal cellulitis;
   - in detecting subperiosteal abscesses and orbital abscesses.
   - in detecting intracranial extension; and
   - in deciding when and from where to drain an orbital abscess.

Treatment

Orbital cellulitis is an emergency and so the patient should be hospitalised for aggresive management.

1. *Intensive antibiotic therapy* should be initiated to overcome the infection. After obtaining nasal, conjunctival and blood culture samples, intravenous antibiotics should be administered:

- *For Staphylococcal infections* high doses of penicillinase-resistant antibiotic (e.g., oxacillin) combined with ampicillin should be given.

- Cefotaxime, ciprofloxacin or vancomycin may be used alternative to oxacillin and penicillin combination.
- *To cover H. influenzae* especially in children, chloramphenicol or clavulanic acid should also be added.
- *To cover anaerobes* oral metronidazole 500 mg every 8 hrs. should be added.

2. ***Analgesic and anti-inflammatory drugs*** are helpful in controlling pain and fever.

3. ***Topical antibiotic eye ointment,*** QID, for corneal exposure and chemosis when there is severe proptosis.

4. ***Nasal decongestant drops*** should be started.

5. ***Revaluation***, atleast twice to thrice daily in the hospital, is required to monitor the response and modify the treatment accordingly.

6. ***Surgical intervention***. Its indications include unresponsiveness to antibiotics, decreasing vision and presence of an orbital or subperiosteal abscess. Surgical intervention may be required as below:

- *Immediate canthotomy/cantholysis* may be needed, if the orbit is tight, an optic neuropathy is present, or the IOP is severely elevated.
- *A free incision into the abscess* should be made when it points under the skin or conjunctiva.
- *Subperiosteal abscess is drained* by a 2-3 cm curved incision in the upper medial aspect.
- In most cases it is necessary to drain both the orbit as well as the infected paranasal sinuses.

ORBITAL MUCORMYCOSIS

Etiology. Mucormycosis, also known as phacomycosis is a severe fungal infection of the orbit. The most common fungal genera causing are *Mucor* (mucormycosis) and *Rhizopus*. Infection usually begins in the sinuses and erodes into the orbital cavity. The organisms have a tendency to invade vessels and cause ischemic necrosis. A necrotizing reaction destroys muscles, bone and soft tissue, frequently without causing signs of orbital cellulitis.

Clinical features. The patients prone to such infections are diabetics and immuno-compromised such as those with renal failure, malignant tumours and those on antimetabolite or steroid therapy; so most of the patients are seriously ill and present with:

- *Pain and proptosis*, and

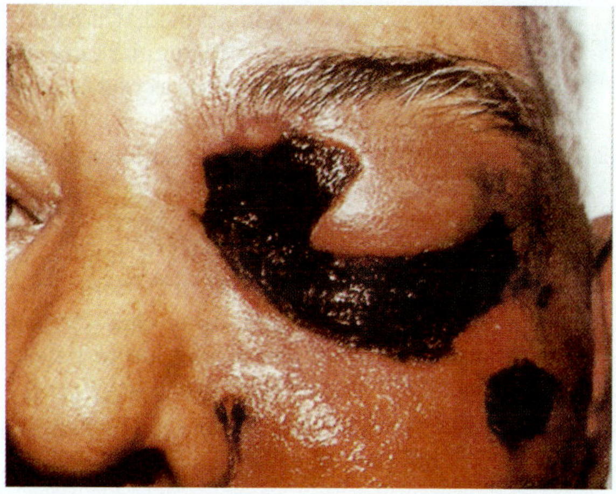

Fig. 16.8. Areas of black ischar and necrosis on the eyelids in a patient with rhino-orbital mucormycosis.

- *Necrotic areas with black eschar* formation may be seen on the mucosa of palate, turbinates and nasal septum and skin of eyelids (Fig. 16.8).

Complications. If not treated energetically, patient develops meningitis, brain abscess and dies within days to weeks.

Diagnosis is made clinically and confirmed by biopsy of the involved area and finding of nonseptate broad branching hyphae.

Treatment is often difficult and inadequate. Therefore, recurrences are common. Treatment includes:

- *Correction of underlying disease* (e.g. diabetic ketoacidosis) if possible;
- *Surgical excision* of the involved tissue; and
- *Intravenous amphotericin B* or other appropriate antifungal drug.
- *Exentration* may be required in severe unresponsive cases.

ORBITAL PERIOSTITIS

Orbital periostitis, i.e., inflammation of the periorbita, is not very common. It may rarely involve the surrounding bones producing orbital osteoperiostitis.

Etiology. It may result from injuries or as an extension of infection from the surrounding structures (similar to orbital cellulitis). Tubercular periostitis is known in children and syphilitic in adults.

Clinical picture. It may present in two forms:

1. *Anterior orbital periostitis*. It involves the orbital margin and is characterised by severe pain, tenderness and swelling of the inflamed area.

Subperiosteal abscess, when formed, frequently bursts on the skin surface. Tubercular anterior orbital periostitis usually manifests as non-healing fistula.

2. *Posterior (deep) periostitis.* It is characterised by deep-seated orbital pain, mild to moderate proptosis and slight limitation of ocular movements. When the orbital apex is implicated in addition, the typical picture of '*orbital apex syndrome*' is also produced. It is characterised by a triad of: (i) ophthalmoplegia due to paresis of third, fourth and sixth cranial nerves; (ii) anaesthesia in the region of supply of ophthalmic division of fifth nerve; and (iii) amaurosis due to involvement of optic nerve.

Treatment. It is on the lines of orbital cellulitis.

CAVERNOUS SINUS THROMBOSIS

Septic thrombosis of the cavernous sinus is a disastrous sequela, resulting from spread of sepsis travelling along its tributaries.

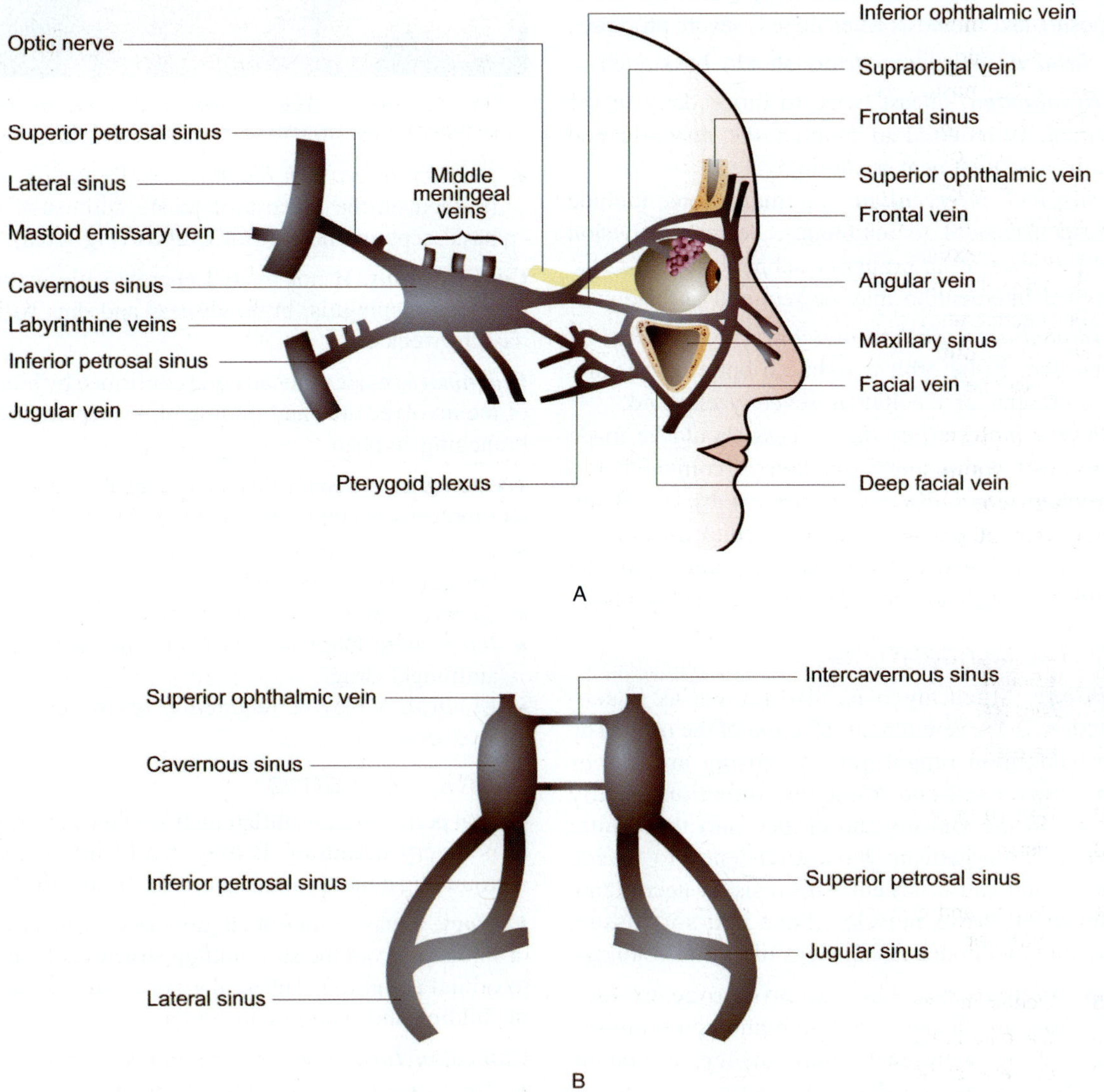

Fig. 16.9. Tributaries of the cavernous sinus: (A) lateral view; (B) superior view.

Communications of cavernous sinus and sources of infection (Fig. 16.9 A and B)

1. *Anteriorly,* the superior and inferior ophthalmic veins drain in the sinus. These veins receive blood from face, nose, paranasal sinuses and orbits. Therefore, infection to cavernous sinus may spread from infected facial wounds, erysipelas, squeezing of stye, furuncles, orbital cellulitis and sinusitis.
2. *Posteriorly,* the superior and inferior petrosal sinuses leave it to join the lateral sinus. Labyrinthine veins opening into the inferior petrosal sinuses bring infections from the middle ear. Mastoid emissary veins may spread infection from the mastoid air cells.
3. *Superiorly,* the cavernous sinus communicates with veins of the cerebrum and may be infected from meningitis and cerebral abscesses.
4. *Inferiorly,* the sinus communicates with pterygoid venous plexus.
5. *Medially,* the two cavernous sinuses are connected with each other by transverse sinuses which account for transfer of infection from one side to the other.

Clinical picture

Cavernous sinus thrombosis starts initially as a unilateral condition, which soon becomes bilateral in more than 50 percent of cases due to intercavernous communication. The condition is characterised by general and ocular features.

General features. Patient is seriously ill having high grade fever with rigors, vomiting and headache.

Ocular features. Patient develops:

- *Severe pain* in the eye and forehead on the affected side.
- *Conjunctiva* is swollen and congested.
- *Proptosis* develops rapidly.
- *Palsy* of third, fourth and sixth cranial nerves occurs frequently.
- *Oedema in mastoid region* is a pathognomic sign. It is due to back pressure in the mastoid emissary vein.
- *Fundus* may be normal with unimpaired vision in early cases. In advanced cases, retinal veins show congestion and there may appear papilloedema.

Complications

At any stage, the hyperpyrexia and signs of meningitis or pulmonary infarction may precede death.

Differential diagnosis

The rapidly developing, acute inflammatory type of proptosis seen in cavernous sinus thrombosis needs to be differentiated from orbital cellulitis and panophthalmitis as summarised in Table 16.1.

Table 16.1. Differential diagnosis of acute inflammatory proptosis

	Clinical features	*Cavernous sinus thrombosis*	*Orbital cellulitis*	*Panophthalmitis*
1.	Laterality	Initially unilateral, but soon becomes bilateral	Unilateral	Unilateral
2.	Degree of proptosis	Moderate	Marked	Moderate
3.	Vision	Not affected in early stage	Not affected in early stage	Complete loss of vision from the beginning
4.	Cornea and anterior chamber	Clear in early stages	Clear in early stages	Hazy due to corneal oedema. Pus in the anterior chamber
5.	Ocular movements	Complete limitation to palsy	Marked limitation	Painful and limited
6.	Oedema in mastoid region	Present	Absent	Absent
7.	General symptoms with fever, and prostrations	Marked	Mild	Mild

Treatment

1. *Antibiotics* are the sheet anchor of treatment. Massive doses of modern potent broad spectrum antibiotics should be injected intravenously.
2. *Analgesics* and anti-inflammatory drugs control pain and fever.
3. *Anticoagulants' role* is controversial.

SPECIFIC CHRONIC ORBITAL INFLAMMATIONS

These include: foreign body granuloma, orbital sarcoidosis, orbital vasculitis, Wegener's granulomatosis, specific granulomatous inflammation caused by tuberculosis, syphilis, fungi, viruses, parasites, leaking dermoid cyst, polyarteritis nodosa and so on. At one time or another all these conditions were diagnosed as pseudotumours.

IDIOPATHIC ORBITAL INFLAMMATORY DISEASE (PSEUDOTUMOUR)

The term '*pseudotumour*' was coined for those conditions of the orbit which clinically presented as tumours but histopathologically proved to be chronic inflammations. However, recently, the use of this term has been restricted for an idiopathic localized inflammatory disease consisting principally of a lymphocytic infiltration associated with a polymorphonuclear cellular response and a fibrovascular tissue reaction that has a variable but self-limiting course. Presently, *idiopathic orbital inflammatory disease (IOID)* is a term being preferred to denote this condition.

Clinical features (Fig. 16.10): Pseudotumour can occur throughout the orbit from the region of lacrimal gland to the orbital apex and thus produce varied clinical presentations. The most commonly noted features are:

- *Age*. The condition typically affects individuals between 40 and 50 years; however, age is no bar.
- *Laterality*. Most cases are unilateral, although both sides may be involved occasionally.
- *Presenting features* are swelling or puffiness of the eyelids, proptosis, orbital pain, restricted ocular movements, diplopia, chemosis and redness.
- *Spontaneous remissions*. After few weeks, are known in pseudotumour.

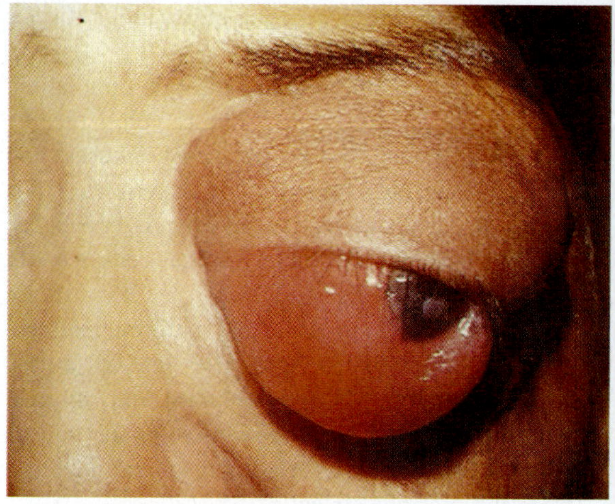

Fig. 16.10. Pseudotumour involving the right orbit.

- *Recurrences* are also common.
- *Severe prolonged inflammation* in some patients may cause progressive fibrosis of the orbital tissues leading to a frozen orbit with visual impairment.

Diagnosis

- *Clinically* pseudotumour is suspected only by exclusion of the known conditions.
- *Ultrasonic and CT-scanning* show a diffuse infiltrative lesion with irregular ill-defined margins and variable density.
- *MRI* shows hypointense lesion c.f. muscle on T1 and hyperintense lesion c.f. muscle on T2. There occurs moderate enhancement with gadolinium.
- *Fine-needle aspiration biopsy* may give histological clue.
- *Incisional biopsy* may be needed to confirm the diagnosis.

Treatment

- *Systemic corticosteroids*, 60-80 mg of prednisolone per day for 2 weeks, initially and then to be tapered gradually forms the mainstay of treatment. Usually, more than half of the patients show a positive response.
- *Radiotherapy* is usually effective in patients non-responsive to steroids.
- *Cytotoxic agents* may be required in a few recalcitrant cases.

GRAVES' OPHTHALMOPATHY

This term is coined to denote typical ocular changes which include lid retraction, lid lag, and proptosis. These changes have also been labelled as: endocrine exophthalmos, malignant exophthalmos, dysthyroid ophthalmopathy, ocular Graves' disease (OGD), and thyroid eye disease (TED), and thyroid-associated ophthalmopathy (TAO).

ETIOPATHOGENESIS

Thyroid eye disease may be associated with hyperthyroidism (in 90% cases), hypothyroidism (4%) or even euthyroidism (6%).

Risk factors

- *Female sex* (4-6 times more common than males)
- *Smoking* (risk is directly related to the number of cigarettes smoked per day)
- *Middle age* (most cases occur in middle age)
- *Autoimmune thyroid disease*
- *HLA- DR3 and HLA-B8*

Pathogenesis

Thyroid eye disease is being considered an autoimmune disease with orbital fibroblasts as the primary target of inflammatory attack and extraocular muscles being secondarily involved. It is probable that the target antigen is shared between the thyroid follicular cells and orbital fibroblasts. The activated T-cells probably act on the fibroblast-adipocyte lineage within the orbit and stimulate adipogenesis, fibroblast proliferation, and glycosaminoglycan synthesis. As a consequence, the extraocular muscles are enlarged due to edema and infiltration with round cells. The orbital soft tissue shows increased amounts of acid mucopolysaccharide and infiltration with lymphocytes , plasma cells , macrophages and mast cells.

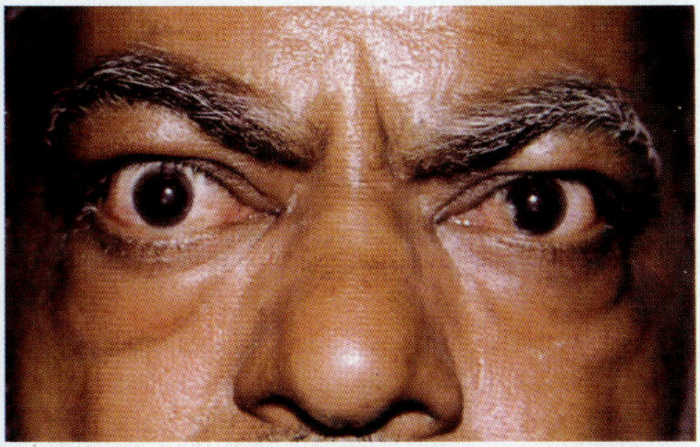

Fig. 16.11. A patient with Graves' ophthalmopathy having bilateral exophthalmos and lid retraction.

CLINICAL PROFILE

Clinical features (Fig. 16.11)

1. *Lid signs.* These are:
   - *Retraction of the upper lids* producing the characteristic staring and frightened appearance (Dalrymple's sign); is the most common clinical features (90% of cases).
   - *Lid lag* (von Graefe's sign) i.e., when globe is moved downward, the upper lid lags behind (50% cases).
   - *Fullness of eyelids* due to puffy oedematous swelling (Enroth's sign);
   - *Difficulty in eversion* of upper lid (Gifford's sign);
   - *Infrequent blinking* (Stellwag's sign).
2. *Conjunctival signs.* These include 'deep injection' and 'chemosis'.
3. *Pupillary signs.* These are of less importance and may be evident as inequality of dilatation of pupils.
4. *Ocular motility defects.* These range from convergence weakness (Mobius's sign) to partial or complete immobility of one or all of the extrinsic ocular muscles (40% of cases). The most common ocular motility defect is a unilateral elevator palsy caused by an involvement of the inferior rectus muscle followed by failure of abduction due to involvement of medial rectus muscle.
5. *Exophthalmos.* It is a common (60%) and classical sign of the disease. As a rule both eyes are symmetrically affected; but it is frequent to find one eye being more porminent than the other. Even unilateral proptosis is not uncommon. In majority of cases it is self-limiting.
6. *Exposure keratitis and symptoms of ocular surface discomfort.* These include sandy or gritty sensation, lacrimation and photophobia. Corneal exposure has been attributed to upper lid retraction, exophthalmos, lagophthalmos, inability to elevate the eyes and a decreased blink rate.
7. *Optic neuropathy.* It occurs in about 60% of cases due to direct compression of the nerve or its blood supply by the enlarged rectus muscles at the orbital apex. It may manifest as papilloedema or optic atrophy with associated slowly progressive impairment of vision.

Classification

American Thyroid Association (ATA) has classified Graves' ophthalmopathy, irrespective of the hormonal status into following classes, characterised by the acronym 'NOSPECS'.

Class 0 : N : No signs and symptoms.
Class 1 : O : Only signs, no symptoms (signs are limited to lid retraction, with or without lid lag and mild proptosis).
Class 2 : S : Soft tissue involvement with signs (as described in Class-1) and symptoms including lacrimation, photophobia, lid or conjunctival swelling.
Class 3 : P : Proptosis is well established.
Class 4 : E : Extraocular muscle involvement (limitation of movement and diplopia).
Class 5 : C : Corneal involvement (exposure keratitis).
Class 6 : S : Sight loss due to optic nerve involvement with disc pallor or papilloedema and visual field defects.

For practical purposes it has been described as '*early*' (which include ATA Class 1 and 2) and '*Late Graves' ophthalmopathy*' (Class 3 to 6).

Clinical course

Thyroid eye disease (TED) is a self limiting disease that lasts from 1-5 years (longer in smokers as compared to non-smokers). Its clinical course is divided into three phases:

1. *Active phase* of increasing severity is characterized by active inflammation with marked lid edema, conjunctival chemosis and congestion and increasing exophthalmos .

2. *Regression phase* is of declining severity in which all of the above signs slowly settles down.

3. *Inactive plateau phase*, also known as quiescent burnt-out phase, ensues after regression phase.

Reactivation of inflammation occurs in approximately 5 to 10% of patients over their lifetime.

Rundle's curve refers to the time course of the above phases can be plotted graphically for each patient. Based on this the patients can be broadly categorized in mild, moderate, marked or severe disease (Rundle a-d).

MANAGEMENT

Diagnosis

Clinical diagnosis is not difficult in advanced cases of Graves' ophthalmopathy with bilateral proptosis. However, early cases having unilateral proptosis need to be differentiated from other causes of unilateral proptosis of adulthood onset (see page 405).

Investigations

1. *Thyroid function tests.* These should include: serum T3, T4, TSH and estimation of radioactive iodine uptake.
2. *Positional tonometry.* An increase in intra-ocular pressure in upgaze helps in diagnosis of subclinical cases.
3. *Ultrasonography.* It can detect changes in extraocular muscles even in class 0 and class 1 cases and thus helps in early diagnosis. In addition to the increase in muscle thickness, erosion of temporal wall of orbit, accentuation of retrobulbar fat and perineural inflammation of optic nerve can also be demonstrated in some early cases.
4. *Computerised tomographic scanning.* It may show proptosis, muscle thickness, thickening of optic nerve and anterior prolapse of the orbital septum (due to excessive orbital fat and/or muscle swelling).
5. *MRI* (T2-weighted and STIR) gives better soft tissue resolution and identifies active disease.
6. *Orthoptic work-up* may include field of binocular single vision, field of uniocular fixation, and Hess/ Lee charting.

Treatment

It is in addition to and independent of the therapy for the associated thyroid dysfunction; as the latter usually does not alter the course of ophthalmic features. The treatment modalities employed are as follows:

(A) *Non-surgical management*

1. *Smoking cessation* should be insisted with the patients as it may markedly influence the course of disease.
2. *Head elevation* at night and *cold compresses* in the morning help in reducing periorbital edema.
3. *Lubricating artificial tear drops* instilled frequently in the day time and ointment at bed time are useful for relief of foreign body sensation and other symptoms of dry ocular surface.
4. *Eyelid taping* at night prevents complication of exposure.

5. *Guanethidine 5% eyedrops* may decrease the lid retraction caused by overaction of Muller's muscle.
6. *Prisms* may be prescribed to alleviate annoying diplopia till the quiscent phase is reached.
7. *Systemic steroids* may be indicated in acutely inflamed orbit with rapidly progressive chemosis and proptosis with or without optic neuropathy.
8. *Radiotherapy.* 2000 rads given over 10 days period may help in reducing orbital oedema in patients where steroids are contraindicated. However, radiotherapy may transiently worsen the disease.
9. *Combined threapy* with low dose steroids, azathioprine and irradiation is reported to be more effective than steroids or radiotherapy alone.

(B) *Surgical management*

- *During active phase*, orbital decompression may be required for an acutely progressive optic neuropathy and/or exposure keratitis, in patients who do not respond to energetic steroid therapy.
- *During quiescent burnt-out phase* the surgical management is required to improve function and cosmesis.
- *A stepwise surgical approach*, starting with orbital decompression (if required to restore normal globe position) followed by extraocular muscle surgery (for diplopia if still persisting) followed by eyelid surgery is recommended. Alteration of this sequence may lead to unpredictable results.

1. *Orbital decompression* may be carried out by an external or endoscopic approach and may involve 2, 3 or 4 walls:

- *Two-wall decompression*, in which part of the orbital floor and medial wall are removed, allows 3-6 mm of replacement of the globe.
- *Three-wall decompression* involves removal of parts of the floor , medial wall and lateral wall, and allows about 6-10 mm of retroplacement of the globe.
- *Four-wall decompression* involves removal of lateral half of roof and large portion of sphenoid at the apex, in addition to three-wall removal as above. This allows 10-16 mm of retroplacement of the globe and is indicated very rarely in patients with severe proptosis.

2. *Extraocular muscle surgery* should always be carried out after the orbital decompression, since the latter may alter extraocular motility. Extraocular muscle surgery is required to achieve binocular single vision in the primary gaze and reading position.

3. *Eyelid surgery*, when required, should be undertaken last, as the extraocular muscle surgery may affect eyelid retraction. As temporary measures, before the definitive surgical correction, *the botulinum toxin* injection aimed at Muller's muscle and LPS muscle may be used, if so desired by the patient. Eyelid surgery for definitive correction may include:

- *Mullerotomy* i.e. disinsertion of Muller's muscle is required for mild lid retraction.
- *Levator recession/disinsertion* may be required for moderate to severe upper eye lid retraction.
- *Scleral grafts* with LPS recession may be required in very severe cases.
- *Recession of lower eyelid retractors* may be required to correct more than 2 mm retraction of lower eyelid.
- *Blepharoplasty.* It may be performed by removal of excess fatty tissue and redundant skin from around the eyelids.

ORBITAL TUMOURS

Orbital tumours are not very common. These include primary, secondary and metastatic tumours.

(A) *Primary tumours.* Those arising from the various orbital structures are as follows:

1. *Developmental tumours*: Dermoid, epidermoid, lipodermoid and teratoma.
2. *Vascular tumours*: Capillary and cavernous haemangioma, haemangiopericytoma and lymphangioma.
3. *Adipose tissue tumours*: Liposarcoma
4. *Fibrous tissue tumours*: Fibroma, fibrosarcoma and fibromatosis.
5. *Osseous and cartilaginous tumours*: Osteoma, chondroma, osteoblastoma, osteogenic sarcoma after irradiation, fibrous dysplasia of bone, and Ewing's sarcoma.
6. *Mesenchymal tumours*: Rhabdomyoma and fibrous histiocytoma.
7. *Neural tumours*: Optic nerve glioma, meningioma, neurofibroma, neurofibromatosis and schwannoma.

8. *Tumours of lacrimal gland include*: Epithelial tumours (benign and malignant mixed tumours and adenocarcinoma) and non epithelial tumours.
9. *Lymphoproliferative disorders include:* Benign reactive lymphoid hyperplasia, Malignant orbital lymphomas, Langerhan cell histiocytosis, Plasma cell tumours and, Xanthogranuloma.

(B) ***Secondary tumours,*** spreading from surrounding structures.

(C) ***Metastatic tumours,*** from distant primary tumours.

(A) PRIMARY ORBITAL TUMOURS

I. Developmental tumours

1. *Dermoids.* These are common developmental tumours which arise from an embryonic displacement of the epidermis to a subcutaneous location. The cystic component is lined with keratinizing epithelium and may contain one or more dermal adnexal structures such as hair follicles and sebaceous glands. Dermoids are of two types:

(a) ***Superficial dermoid.*** It is seen in infancy. Appears as a firm, round, localised lesion in the upper temporal or upper nasal aspect of the orbit. These do not extend deep into the orbit and are not associated with bony defects. Displacement of globe is also not seen as these are located anterior to the orbital septum (Fig. 16.12).

(b) ***Deep dermoids.*** These are present in adolescence with proptosis or a mass lesion having indistinct posterior margins (as they arise from deeper sites). They may be associated with bony defects. *Treatment of dermoids* is surgical excision. Care should be taken not to leave behind the contents of cyst which are potentially irritating.

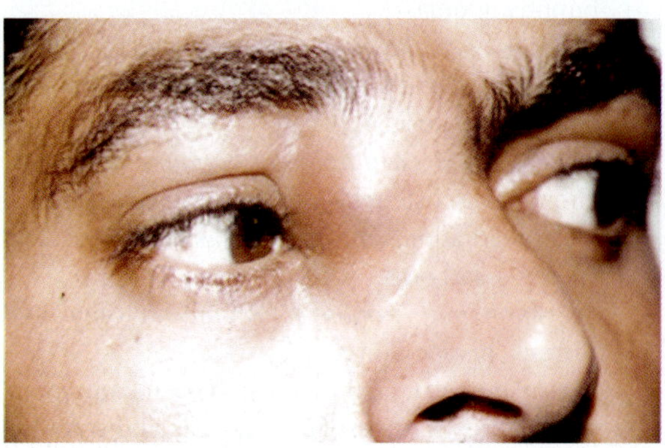

Fig. 16.12. Dermoid right orbit.

2. *Epidermoid.* It is composed of epidermis without any epidermal appendages in the wall of the cyst. These are almost always cystic. The cyst wall contains keratin debris. *Treatment* is surgical excision.

3. *Lipodermoids.* These are solid tumours usually seen beneath the conjunctiva. These are mostly located adjacent to the superior temporal quadrant of the globe (Fig. 16.13). These do not require any surgical intervention unless they enlarge significantly. (Also see page 85).

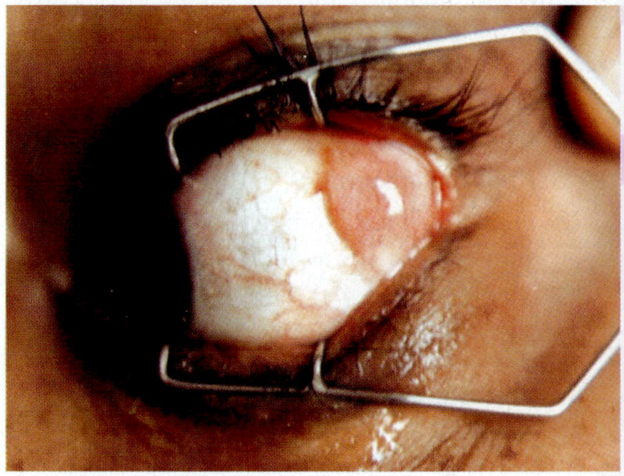

Fig. 16.13. Lipodermoid.

4. *Teratomas* (Fig. 16.14). These are composed of ectoderm, mesoderm and endoderm. These may be solid, cystic or a mixture of both. The cystic form is more prevalent. Most of these are benign but some solid tumours in newborns are malignant. Exenteration is usually performed for solid tumours to effect a permanent cure. Cystic tumours may be excised without removing the eyeball.

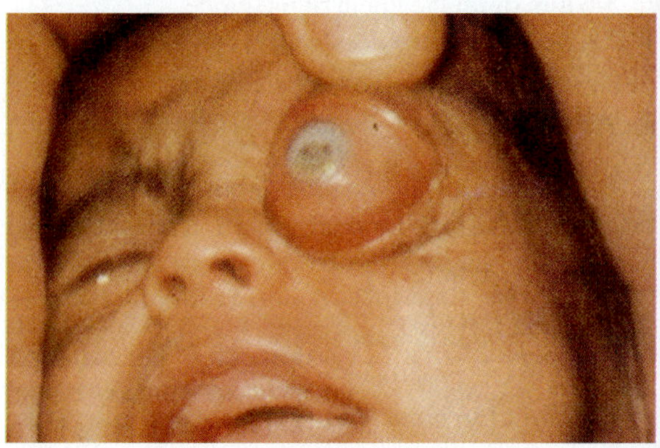

Fig. 16.14. Congenital teratoma.

II. Vascular tumours

These are the most common primary benign tumours of the orbit. These can be either haemangiomas or lymphangiomas. *Haemangiomas* are further divided into two types — capillary and cavernous.

1. *Capillary haemangioma.* It is commonly seen at birth or during the first month. It appears as periocular swelling in the anterior part of the orbit. It tends to increase in size on straining or crying. This tumour may initially grow in size followed by stabilization and then regression and disappearance.

Treatment. These tumours usually do not require any treatment. *Indications for treatment* are: optic nerve compression, exposure keratitis, ocular dysfunction or cosmetic blemish. *Mode of therapy* are: systemic and/or intralesional steroids, low-dose superficial radiations, surgery and cryotherapy.

2. *Cavernous haemangioma.* It is the commonest benign orbital tumour among adults with female preponderance (70%). The tumour is usually located in the retrobulbar muscle cone. So, it presents as a slowly progressing unilateral axial proptosis in the second to fourth decade. It may occasionally compress the optic nerve without causing proptosis.

Treatment. Surgical excision of the tumour is undertaken via lateral orbitotomy approach. Since the tumour is well encapsulated, complete removal is generally possible.

3. *Lymphangioma.* It is an uncommon tumour presenting with slowly progressive proptosis in a young person. It often enlarges because of spontaneous bleed within the vascular spaces, leading to formation of 'chocolate cysts' which may regress spontaneously.

III. Mesenchymal tumours

Rhabdomyosarcoma. It is a highly malignant tumour of the orbit arising from the pluripotent mesenchymal cells which have the potential to differentiate into striated muscles. It is the most common primary orbital tumour among children, usually occurring below the age of 15 years (90%), slightly more common in males.

Histopathologically rhabdomyosarcoma may be of three types:

- *Embryonal sarcoma*, (commonest), followed by,
- *Alveolar sarcoma*, and
- *Pleomorphic sarcoma* (least common)

Clinical features. It classically presents as rapidly progressive proptosis of sudden onset in a child of 7-8 years (Fig. 16.15). The clinical presentation mimics an acute inflammatory process. The tumour commonly involves the superionasal quadrant; but may invade any part of the orbit.

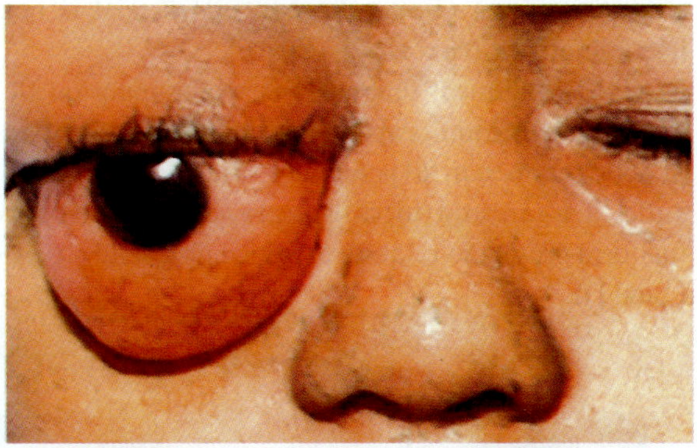

Fig. 16.15. Massive proptosis due to rhabdomyosarcoma located in the superonasal quadrant (mimmicking acute inflammatory process).

Diagnosis. The clinical suspicion is supported by X-rays showing bone destruction and CT/MRI scan demonstrating irregular but well defined tumour with adjacent bone destruction. Diagnosis is confirmed by biopsy.

Treatment.

- *Surgical excision* is possible only for a well circumscribed localised tumour.
- *Radiation therapy* in high dose (5000 rads in 5 weeks) combined with systemic chemotherapy is very effective.
- *Chemotherapy* regime consists of Vincristine 2 mg/m^2 on day 1 and 5, actinomycin-D 0.015 mg/kg IV once a day for 5 days and cyclophosphamide 10 mg/kg once a day for 3 days; to be repeated every 4 weeks for a period of 2 years.
- *Exenteration* is required in a few unresponsive patients.

IV. Neural Tumours

1. *Optic nerve glioma.* It is a slow growing tumour arising from the astrocytes. It usually occurs in first decade of life. It may present either as a solitary tumour or as a part of von Recklinghausen's neurofibromatosis (30%). Optic nerve alone is affected in 28% of cases, 72% involve the optic chiasma, often with mid-brain and hypothalamic involvement.

Clinical features. It is characterised by gradual visual loss associated with a gradual, painless, unilateral axial proptosis occurring in a child usually between 4 and 8 years of age (Fig. 16.16A). Fundus examination may show optic atrophy (more common) or papilloedema and venous engorgement. Intracranial extension of the glioma through optic canal is not uncommon.

Diagnosis. Clinical diagnosis is well supported by X-rays showing uniform regular rounded enlargement of optic foramen in 90 percent of cases (Fig. 16.16 B) and CT scan and ultrasonography depicting a fusiform growth in relation to optic nerve (Fig. 16.16 C and D).

Treatment.

- *Observation*, without any treatment, is recommended for patients having stationary tumour, with good vision, and non-disfiguring proptosis.
- *Surgical excision* of the tumour mass with preservation of the eyeball, by lateral orbitotomy when the cosmetically unacceptable proptosis is present in a blind eye (due to optic atrophy). Tumours with intracranial extensions are dealt with the neurosurgeons.
- *Radiotherapy* should be given in unoperable cases.

2. *Meningiomas*. These are invasive tumours arising from the arachnoidal villi. Meningiomas invading the orbit are of two types: primary and secondary.

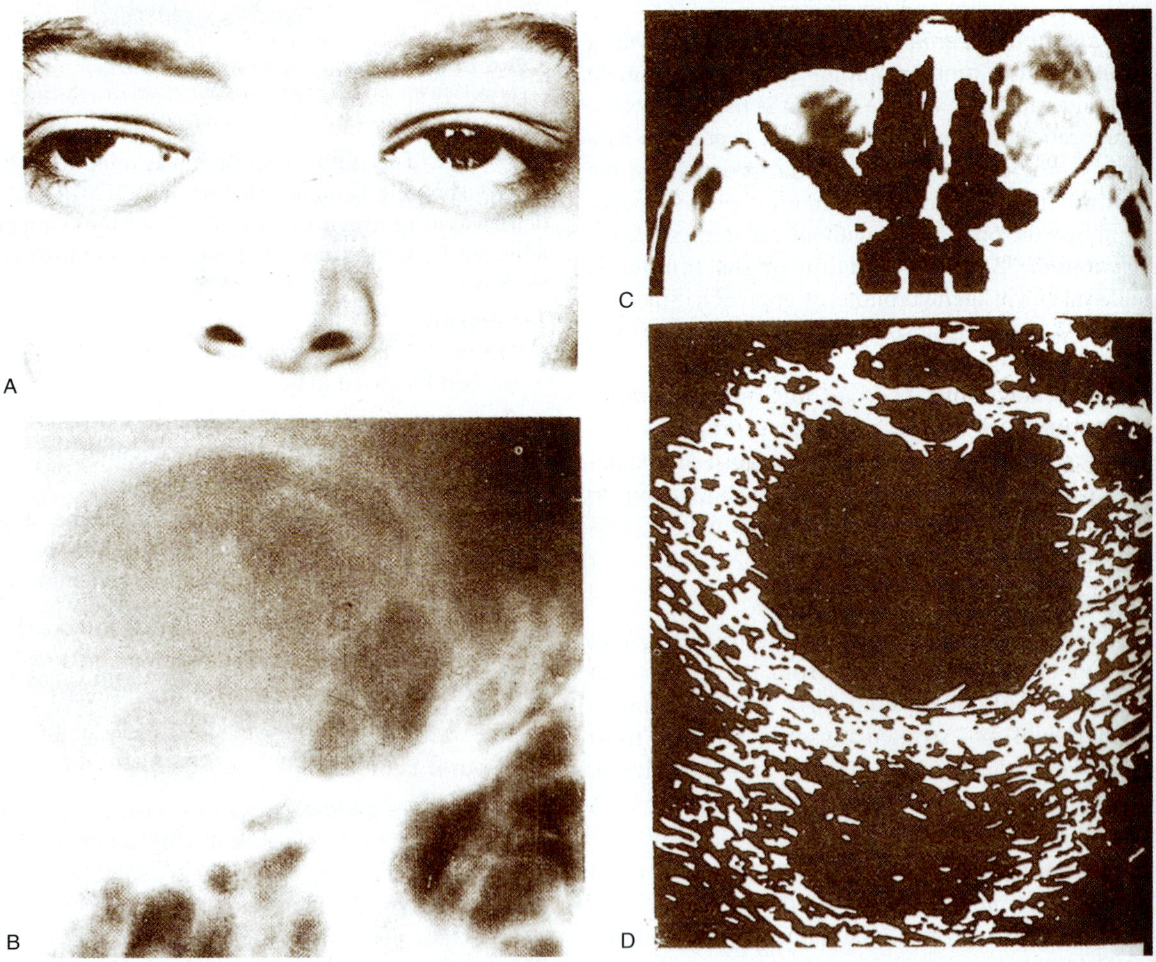

Fig. 16.16. Optic nerve glioma : A, clinical photograph; B, X-rays optic foramina; C. CT scan; D, ultrasonography B scan.

(a) *Primary intraorbital meningiomas*, also known as '*optic nerve sheath meningiomas*' is a rare benign tumour of meningothelial cells of the meninges that usually occur in mid age and has slight female preponderance. There is an assocation with neurofibrometasis-2. This tumour usually presents with early visual loss associated with limitation of ocular movements, optic disc oedema or atrophy, and a slowly progressive unilateral proptosis. During the intradural stage, it is clinically indistinguishable from optic nerve glioma. However, the presence of opticociliary shunt is pathognomic of an optic nerve sheath meningioma.

Treatment is as below:

- *Observation* is recommended if visual acuity is good.
- *Surgical excision* is recommended for severe proptosis with blind eye, or threat to the chiasma

Prognosis for life is good.

(b) *Secondary orbital meningiomas.* Those intracranial meningiomas which secondarily invade the orbit either arise from the sphenoid bone or involve it enroute to the orbit. Orbital invasion may occur through: floor of anterior cranial fossa, superior orbital fissure and optic canal. Meningioma enplaque, affecting the greater and lesser wings of sphenoid and taking origin in the region of pterion, is the most common variety affecting the orbit secondarily. These tumours typically occur in middle-aged women.

Clinical features. These are characterised by greater proptosis and lesser visual impairment than the primary intraorbital meningiomas. Other characteristic features of these tumours are boggy eyelid swelling and an ipsilateral swelling in the temporal region of the face, especially when the intracranial tumour arises from the lateral part of sphenoid ridge (Fig. 16.17A). In such cases proptosis is due to hyperostosis on the lateral wall and roof of the orbit. CT scan is very useful in assessing the extent of tumour (Figs. 16.17 B and C).

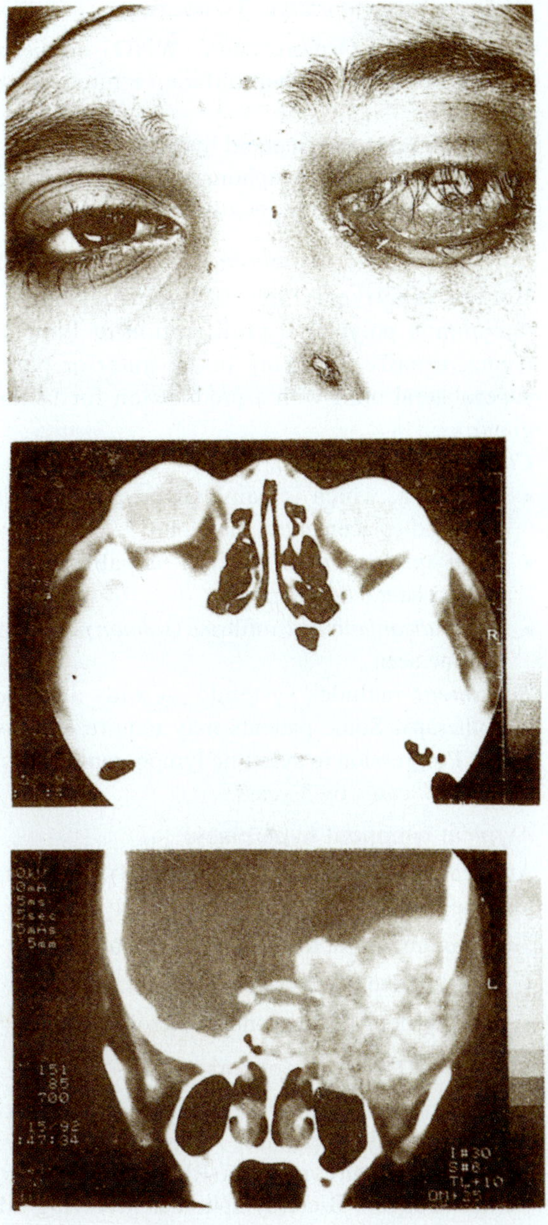

A B C

Fig. 16.17. Secondary orbital involvement in a patient with sphenoidal ridge meningioma, clinical photograph: (A) CT scan, coronal (B) and axial (C) sections.

Management of secondary orbital (sphenoid wing) meningiomas is as below:

- *Observation* is recommended till they produce functional consequences.
- *Subtotal resection* through a combined approach to the intracranial and orbital component, in collaboration with neurosurgeon, is recommended when they produce profound proptosis, compressive optic neuropathy, motility impairment or cerebral edema .
- *Postoperative radiotherapy* is advocated to reduce the risk of recurrences of the residual tumour.

V. Lymphoproliferative Tumours

World Health Organization (WHO) consensus classification of lymphoproliferative tumours is as below:

- Benign reactive lymphoid hyperplasia
- Malignant orbital lymphomas, and
- Langerhan's cell histiocytosis

Benign Reactive Lymphoid Hyperplasia (BRLH)

Benign reactive lymphoid hyperplasia, is an uncommon polyclonal proliferation of lymphoid tissue, usually occurring in the anterior part of superolateral orbit with a predilection for lacrimal gland.

Clinical features include:

- *Proptosis*, which is painless, progressive with medial displacement of the globe.
- *Firm rubbery mass* is often palpable beneath supero-lateral orbital rim.
- *Pink subconjunctival* infiltrate (*salmon patch*) may also be seen .

Treatment includes systemic steroids and local radiotherapy. Some patients may require cytotoxic drugs. Progression to systemic lymphomas occurs in about 25% cases by 5 years.

Atypical lymphoid hyperplasia

Atypical lymphoid hyperplasia (ALH) is an intermediate between BRLH and malignant lymphoma.

Features are similar to BRLH except that:

- May involve other systemic organs, and
- Usually does not respond to steroids.

Malignant Orbital Lymphomas

Orbit is mainly (90%) involved by malignant non-Hodgkin B-cell lymphomas. According to 'Revised European American Lymphoma (REAL)' classification, the non-Hodgkin B-cell lymphomas involving orbit are as follows:

1. *Mucosa Associated Lymphoid Tissue* (MALT) *lymphoma*

- *Accounts* for 40-70% of all orbital lymphomas.
- *Usually unilateral*, but bilateral involvement may occur in 25% cases.
- *Present* with gradual proptosis and/or palpable firm rubbery masses.
- *Systemic involvement* occurs in 50% of cases.
- *Treatment* includes radiotherapy or chemotherapy depending upon the grade and spread of tumour.

2. *Chronic lymphocytic lymphoma* (CLL). It also represents a low-grade lesion of small mature appearing lymphocytes.

3. *Follicular center lymphoma*. It represents a low-grade lesion with follicular centers.

4. *High grade lymphomas* involving orbit include large cell lymphoma, lymphoblastic lymphoma and Burkitt's lymphoma.

Langerhan's Cell Histiocytosis

Langerhan's cell histiocytosis, formerly known as *histiocytosis* X, is a group of diseases characterised by an idiopathic abnormal proliferation of histiocytes with granuloma formation. These diseases primarily affect children with an orbital involvement in 20 per cent of cases. This group includes following three diseases:

1. *Hand-Schuller-Christian disease*. It is a chronic disseminated form of histiocytosis involving both soft tissues and bones in older children of either sex. It is characterised by a triad of proptosis, diabetes insipidus and bony defects in the skull.

2. *Letterer-Siwe disease*. Now termed as '*diffuse soft tissue histiocytosis*' is a systemic form of histiocytosis characterised by widespread soft tissue and visceral involvement with or without bony changes. The disease has a slight male preponderance and often occurs in the first three years of life. Orbital involvement is comparatively rare.

3. *Unifocal or multifocal eosinophilic granuloma* is characterised by a solitary or multiple granulomas involving the bones. The disease occurs in elder children and frequently involves the orbital bones.

(B) SECONDARY ORBITAL TUMOURS

These may arise from the following structures:

1. *Tumours of eyeball:* Retinoblastoma (Fig. 11.36) and malignant melanoma (Fig. 7.24).
2. *Tumours of the eyelids:* Squamous cell carcinoma and basal cell carcinoma.
3. *Tumours of nose and paranasal sinuses:* These tumours very commonly involve the orbit (50%). These include: carcinomas, sarcomas and osteomas.

4. *Tumours of nasopharynx.* Carcinoma of nasopharynx is the commonest tumour involving the orbit. Thirty-eight percent cases with this tumour show ophthalmoneurological symptoms which include proptosis and involvement of fifth and sixth cranial nerves. Rarely, third, fourth and second cranial nerves are also involved.
5. *Tumours of cranial cavity* invading orbit are glioma and meningioma.

(C) METASTATIC ORBITAL TUMOURS

These involve the orbit by haematogenous spread from a distant primary focus and include the following:

I. *Metastatic tumours in children*

1. *Neuroblastoma*— from adrenals and sympathetic chain.
2. *Nephroblastoma*—from kidneys.
3. *Ewing's sarcoma*—from the bones.
4. *Leukaemic infiltration.*

II. *Metastatic tumours in adults*

1. *Carcinoma* — from lungs, breast, prostate, thyroid and rectum.
2. *Malignant melanoma*—from skin.

ORBITAL BLOW-OUT FRACTURES

Blow-out fractures are isolated comminuted fractures which occur when the orbital walls are pressed indirectly. These mainly involve orbital floor and medial wall.

Etiology

Blow-out orbital fractures generally result from trauma to the orbit by a relatively large, often rounded object, such as tennis ball, cricket ball, human fist (Fig. 16.18) or part of an automobile. The force of the blow causes a backward displacement of the eyeball and an increase in the intraorbital pressure; with a resultant fracture at the weakest point of the orbital wall. Usually this point is the orbital floor, but this may be the medial wall also.

Classification

1. *Pure blow-out fractures*: These are not associated with involvement of the orbital rim.
2. *Impure blow-out fractures*: These are associated with other fractures about the middle third of the facial skeleton.

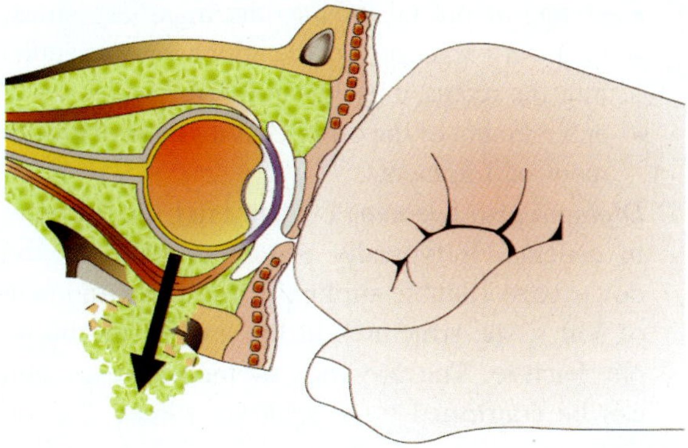

Fig. 16.18. Mechanism of blow-out-fracture of the orbital floor.

Clinical features

1. *Periorbital oedema and blood extravasation* in and around the orbit (such as subconjunctival ecchymosis) occur immediately. This may mask certain signs and symptoms seen later.
2. *Emphysema* of the eyelids occurs more frequently with medial wall than floor fractures. It may be made worse by blowing of the nose.
3. *Paraesthesia and anaesthesia* in the distribution of infraorbital nerve (lower lid, cheek, side of nose, upper lip and upper teeth) are very common.
4. *Ipsilateral epistaxis* as a result of bleeding from maxillary sinus into the nose is frequently noted in early stages.
5. *Proptosis* of variable degree may also be present initially because of the associated orbital oedema and haemorrhage.
6. *Enophthalmos and mechanical ptosis.* After about 10 days, as the oedema decreases, the eyeball sinks backward and somewhat inferiorly resulting in enophthalmos and mechanical ptosis (Fig. 16.19). Three factors responsible for producing enophthalmos are:

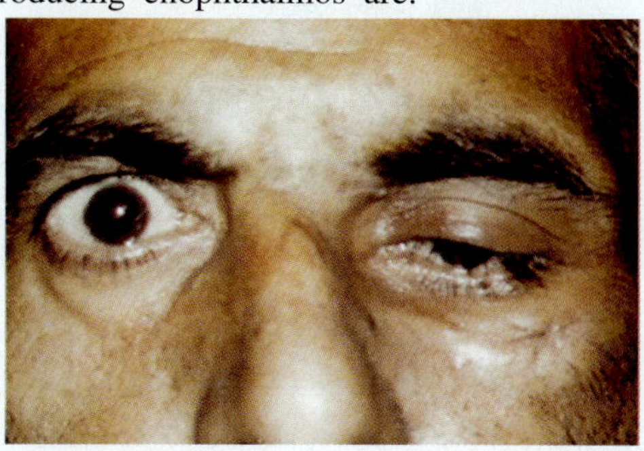

Fig. 16.19. Enophthalmos and mechanical ptosis in a patient with blow-out-fracture of orbit.

- escape of orbital fat into the maxillary sinus;
- backward traction on the globe by entrapped inferior rectus muscle; and
- enlargement of the orbital cavity from displacement of fragments.

7. *Diplopia* also becomes evident after the decrease in oedema. It typically occurs in both up and down gaze (double diplopia) due to entrapment of soft tissue structures in the area of the blow-out fracture. The presence of muscle restriction can be confirmed by a positive *'forced duction test'*.
8. *Severe ocular damage* associated with blowout fracture is rare. This is because a 'blow-out fracture' is nature's way of protecting the globe from injury. Nevertheless, the eye should be carefully examined to exclude the possibility of intraocular damage.

Orbital Imaging

1. *Plain X-rays.* The most useful projection for detecting an orbital floor fracture is a nose-chin (Water's) view. The common Roentgen findings are: fragmentation and irregularity of the orbital floor; depression of bony fragments and 'hanging drop' opacity of the superior maxillary antrum from orbital contents herniating through the floor (Fig. 16.20).

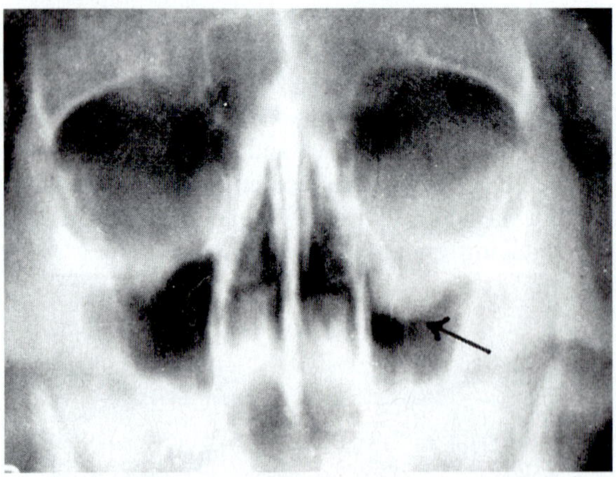

Fig. 16.20. Plain X-ray orbit (AP view) showing herniated orbital contents (arrow) with blow-out fracture of the orbital floor.

2. *Computerised tomography scanning and magnetic resonance imaging (MRI).* These are of greater value for detailed visualisation of soft tissues. Coronal sections are particularly useful in evaluating the extent of the fracture.

Management

I. *General measures and medical treatment*

1. *Avoid nose blowing* should be advised to each patient, as the nose blowing may contribute to surgical emphysema and herniation of soft tissue.
2. *Systemic antibiotics* should be given to prevent secondary infection from the maxillary sinus.
3. *Analgesics and anti-inflammatory drugs* to decrease pain and swelling.
4. *Cold compresses*, immediately following trauma may decrease swelling by causing vasoconstriction.

II. *Surgical management*

Surgical repair to restore continuity of the orbital floor may be made with or without implants. It may not be required in many cases. The optimal time for surgery, when indicated, is after 10-14 days of injury.

Indications of surgical intervention include:

1. Diplopia not resolving significantly in the early days after trauma.
2. A fracture with a large herniation of tissues into the antrum.
3. Incarceration of tissues in the fracture resulting in globe retraction and increased appla- nation tension on attempted upward gaze.
4. Enophthalmos greater than 3 mm.

Any of these factors, alone or combinedly could indicate that early orbital repair is necessary.

ORBITAL SURGERY

ORBITOTOMY

Orbitotomy operation refers to surgical approach for an orbital mass lesion. There are four surgical approaches to the orbit:

1. *Anterior orbitotomy.* It is indicated only when the lesion is readily palpable through the eyelids and is judged to be mainly in front of the equator of eyeball. Depending upon the location of the lesion the anterior orbitotomy can be performed by any of the following approaches:

(i) *Superior approach* is used for the lesions located in the superoanterior part of the orbit. It can be performed through:
- Transcutaneous route, (Fig. 16.21 A) or
- Trans conjunctival route.

(ii) *Inferior approach* is suitable for the lesions located in the inferoanterior part of the orbit. It can be performed through:
- Transcutaneous route, (Fig. 16.21 B) or
- Trans conjunctival route

(iii) *Medial approach* can be performed through:
- Transcutaneous route, (Fig. 16.21 C)
- Trans conjunctival route, or
- Trans caruncular route

(iv) *Lateral approach* is performed through a lateral canthotomy incision (Fig. 16.21 D).

2. *Lateral orbitotomy.* In this approach lateral half of the supraorbital margin with the quadrilateral piece of bone forming the lateral orbital wall is temporarily removed. This approach provides an adequate exposure to the orbital contents and is particularly valuable for the retrobulbar lesions. The classical technique of lateral orbitotomy using S-shaped brow skin incision (Fig. 16.21E) is called *Kronlein's operation.* This incision allows good exposure but leaves noticeable scar. Therefore, presently the preferred incisions are:

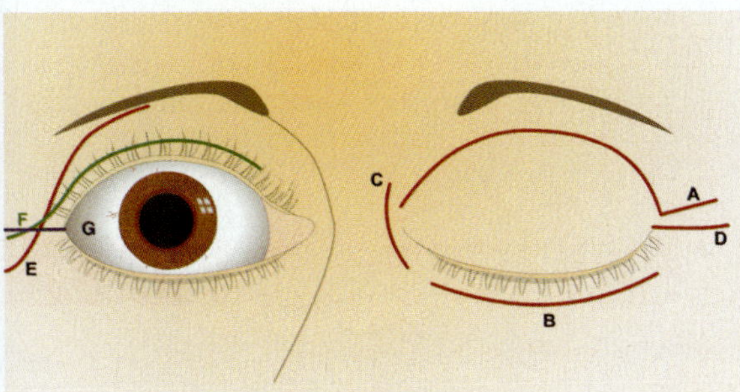

Fig. 16.21. Incision site for: *Anterior orbitotomy* (A. superior approach, upper eyelid crease incision; B, inferior approach, subciliary incision; C. medial i.e. frontoethmoidal approach; D. lateral approach by lateral canthotomy) and *Lateral orbitotomy*: (E. S-shaped brow skin incision; F. upper eyelid crease incision, and G. lateral canthotomy incision)

- Upper eyelid crease incision (Fig. 16.21F), or
- Lateral canthotomy incision (Fig. 16.21G)

3. *Transfrontal orbitotomy.* In this technique orbit is opened through its roof and thus mainly the domain of neurosurgeons. Transfrontal orbitotomy is used to decompress the roof of the optic canal and to explore and remove when possible tumours of the sphenoidal ridge involving the superior orbital fissure.

4. *Temporofrontal orbitotomy*. This approach provides an access to the orbit (through its roof) and anterior and middle cranial fossa simultaneously.

EXENTERATION

It is a mutilating surgery in which all the contents of the orbits along with the periorbita are removed through an incision made along the orbital margins (Fig. 16.22). Exenteration is indicated for malignant tumours arising from the orbital structures or spreading from the eyeball. Now-a-days, debulking of the orbit is preferred over exenteration.

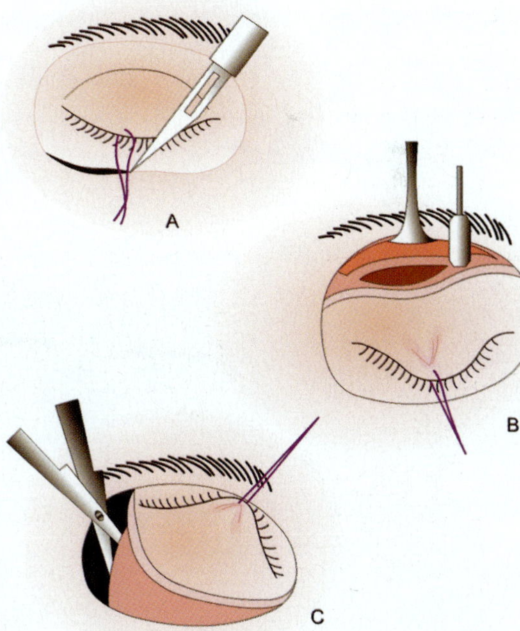

Fig. 16.22. Exenteration of the orbit : A, skin incision; B, periosteal reflection and C, amputation of the orbital contents.

17 CHAPTER

Ocular Injuries

MECHANICAL INJURIES
- Extraocular foreign bodies
- Blunt trauma
- Open globe injuries
- Sympathetic ophthalmitis

CHEMICAL INJURIES
- Alkali burns
- Acid burns

THERMAL INJURIES

ELECTRICAL INJURIES

RADIATIONAL INJURIES
- Ultraviolet radiations
- Infrared radiations
- Ionizing radiational injuries

MECHANICAL INJURIES

In this era of high speed traffic and industrialization, the incidence of injuries is increasing in general. Like any other part of the body, eyes are also not exempted from these injuries; in spite of the fact that they are well protected by the lids, projected margins of the orbit, the nose and a cushion of fat from behind.

The mechanical ocular injuries can be discussed under following headings:

- Extraocular foreign bodies
- Blunt trauma
- Open globe injuries
- Sympathetic ophthalmitis

Ocular Trauma Terminologies

Before going into details of the mechanical injuries, it will be worthwhile to become familiar with the new ocular trauma terminology system proposed by the 'Birmingham Eye Trauma Terminology' (BETT). The term ***eyewall*** has been restricted for the outer fibrous coat (cornea and sclera) of the eyeball. The definitions proposed by the BETT and as such adopted by 'American Ocular Trauma Society' for mechanical ocular injuries are as follows:

1. *Closed-globe injury* is the one in which eyewall (sclera and cornea) does not have a full thickness wound but there is intraocular damage. It includes contusion and lamellar laceration.

- *Contusion* refers to the closed-globe injury resulting from blunt trauma. Damage may occur at the site of impact or at a distant site.
- *Lamellar laceration* is a closed globe injury characterized by a partial thickness wound of the eyewall caused by a sharp object or blunt trauma.

2. *Open-globe injury* is associated with a full thickness wound of the sclera or cornea or both. It includes rupture and laceration of eye wall.

i. *Rupture* refers to a full-thickness wound of eyewall caused by the impact of blunt trauma. The wound occurs due to markedly raised intraocular pressure by an inside-out injury mechanism.

ii. *Laceration* refers to a full-thickness wound of eyewall caused by a sharp object. The wound occurs at the impact site by an outside-in mechanism. It includes penetrating and perforating injuries.

- *Penetrating injury* refers to a single laceration of eyewall caused by a sharp object.
- *Perforating injury* refers to two full thickness lacerations (one entry and one exit) of the eyewall caused by a sharp object or missile. The two

wounds must have been caused by the same agent.

- *Intraocular foreign body injury* is technically a penetrating injury associated with retained intraocular foreign body. However, it is grouped separately because of different clinical implications.

EXTRAOCULAR FOREIGN BODIES

Extraocular foreign bodies are quite common in industrial and agricultural workers. Even in day-to-day life, these are not uncommon.

Common sites. A foreign body may be impacted in the conjunctiva or cornea (Fig. 17.1).

- *On the conjunctiva,* it may be lodged in the sulcus subtarsalis, fornices or bulbar conjunctiva.
- *In the cornea,* it is usually embedded in the epithelium, or superficial stroma and rarely into the deep stroma.

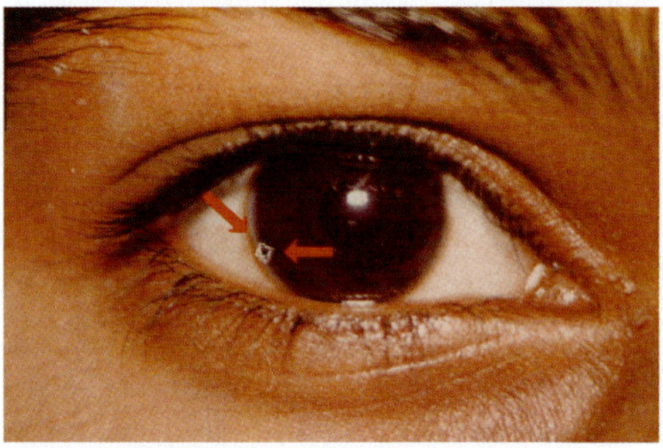

Fig. 17.1. Foreign body on the cornea.

Common types. The usual foreign bodies:

- *In industrial workers* are particles of iron (especially in lathe and hammer-chisel workers), emery and coal.
- *In agriculture workers,* these are husk of paddy and wings of insects.
- *Other common foreign bodies* are particles of dust, sand, steel, glass, wood and small insects (mosquitoes).

Symptoms. A foreign body produces immediate:

- *Discomfort,* profuse *watering and redness* in the eye.
- *Pain and photophobia* are more marked in corneal foreign body than the conjunctival.
- *Defective* vision occurs when it is lodged in the centre of cornea.

Signs. Examination reveals marked blepharospasm and conjunctival congestion. A foreign body can be localized on the conjunctiva or cornea by oblique illumination. Slit-lamp examination after fluorescein staining is the best method to discover corneal foreign body. Double eversion of the upper lid is required to discover a foreign body in the superior fornix.

Complications include:

- *Acute bacterial conjunctivitis* may occur from infected foreign bodies or due to rubbing with infected hands.
- *Corneal ulceration* may occur as a complication of corneal foreign body.
- *Pigmentation and/or opacity* may be left behind by an iron or emery particles embedded in the cornea.

Treatment. Extraocular foreign bodies should be removed as early as possible.

1. ***Removal of conjunctival foreign body.*** A foreign body lying loose in the lower fornix, sulcus subtarsalis or in the canthi may be removed with a swab stick or clean handkerchief even without anaesthesia. Foreign bodies impacted in the bulbar conjunctiva need to be removed with the help of a hypodermic needle after topical anaesthesia.

2. ***Removal of corneal foreign body.*** Eye is anaesthetised with topical instillation of 2 to 4 percent xylocaine and the patient is made to lie supine on an examination table. Lids are separated with universal eye speculum, the patient is asked to look straight upward and light is focused on the cornea. First of all, an attempt is made to remove the foreign body with the help of a wet cotton swab stick. If it fails then foreign body spud or hypodermic needle is used. Extra care is taken while removing a deep corneal foreign body, as it may enter the anterior chamber during manoeuvring. If such a foreign body happens to be magnetic, it is removed with a hand-held magnet. After removal of foreign body, pad and bandage with antibiotic eye ointment is applied for 24 to 48 hours. Antibiotic eyedrops are instilled 3-4 times a day for about a week.

Prophylaxis. Industrial and agricultural workers should be advised to use special protective glasses. Cyclists and scooterists should be advised to use protective plain glasses or tinted goggles. Special guards should be put on grinding machines and use of tools with overhanging margins should be banned. Eye healthcare education should be imparted, especially to the industrial and agricultural workers.

BLUNT TRAUMA

Modes of injury

Blunt trauma may occur following:

- *Direct blow* to the eye ball by fist, ball or blunt instruments like sticks, and big stones.
- *Accidental blunt trauma* to eyeball may also occur in roadside accidents, automobile accidents, injuries by agricultural and industrial instruments/ machines and fall upon the projecting blunt objects.

Mechanics of blunt trauma to eyeball

Blunt trauma of eyeball produces damage by different forces as described below:

1. *Direct impact on the globe.* It produces maximum damage at the point where the blow is received (Fig. 17.2A).

2. *Compression wave force.* It is transmitted through the fluid contents in all the directions and strikes the angle of anterior chamber, pushes the iris-lens diaphragm posteriorly, and also strikes the retina and choroid (Fig. 17.2B). This may cause considerable damage. Sometimes the compression wave may be so explosive, that maximum damage may be produced at a point distant from the actual place of impact. This is called *contre-coup damage*.

3. *Reflected compression wave force.* After striking the outer coats the compression waves are reflected towards the posterior pole and may cause foveal damage (Fig. 17.2C).

4. *Rebound compression wave force.* After striking the posterior wall of the globe, the compression waves rebound back anteriorly. This force damages the retina and choroid by forward pull and lens-iris diaphragm by forward thrust from the back (Fig. 17.2D).

5. *Indirect force.* Ocular damage may also be caused by the indirect forces from the bony walls and elastic contents of the orbit, when globe suddenly strikes against these structures.

Modes of damage

The different forces of the blunt trauma described above may cause damage to the structures of the globe by one or more of the following modes:

1. *Mechanical tearing of the tissues* of eyeball.
2. *Damage to the tissue cells* sufficient to cause disruption of their physiological activity.
3. *Vascular damage* leading to ischaemia, oedema and haemorrhages.
4. *Trophic changes* due to disturbances of the nerve supply.
5. *Delayed complications* of blunt trauma such as secondary glaucoma, haemophthalmitis, late rosette cataract and retinal detachment.

Traumatic lesions of blunt trauma

Traumatic lesions produced by blunt trauma can be grouped as follows:

- Closed globe injury
- Globe rupture
- Extraocular lesions

A. Closed-globe injury

Either there is no corneal or scleral wound at all (contusion) or it is only of partial thickness (lamellar

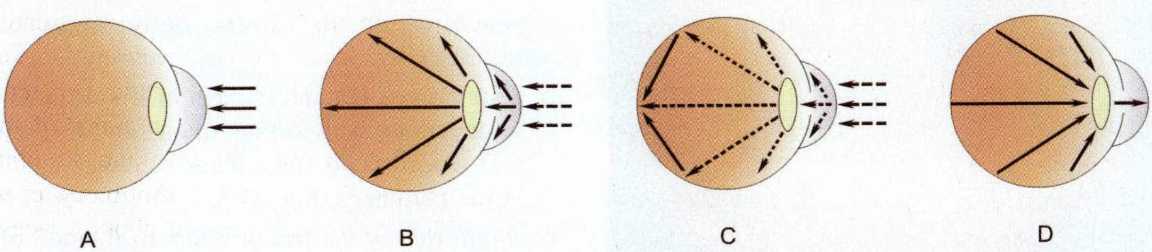

Fig. 17.2. Mechanics of blunt trauma to eyeball: A, direct impact; B, compression wave force; C, reflected compression wave; D, rebound compression wave.

laceration). Contusional injuries may vary in severity from a simple corneal abrasion to an extensive intraocular damage. Lesions seen in closed-globe injury are briefly enumerated here structurewise.

I. *Cornea*

1. *Simple abrasions.* These are very painful and diagnosed by fluorescein staining. These usually heal up within 24 hours with 'pad and bandage' applied after instilling antibiotic ointment.
2. *Recurrent corneal erosions* (recurrent keractalgia). These may sometimes follow simple abrasions, especially those caused by fingernail trauma. Patient usually gets recurrent attacks of acute pain and lacrimation on opening the eye in the morning. This occurs due to abnormally loose attachment of epithelium to the underlying Bowman's membrane.
   Treatment. Loosely attached epithelium should be removed by debridement and 'pad and bandage' applied for 48 hours, so that firm healing is established.
3. *Partial corneal tears* (lamellar corneal laceration). These may also follow a blunt trauma.
4. *Blood staining of cornea.* It may occur occasionally from the associated hyphaema and raised intraocular pressure. Cornea becomes reddish brown (Fig. 17.3) or greenish in colour and in later stages simulates dislocation of the clear lens into the anterior chamber. It clears very slowly from the periphery towards the centre, the whole process may take even more than two years.

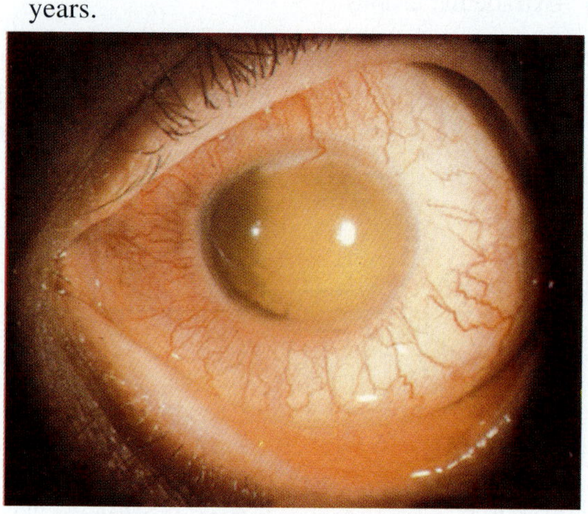

Fig. 17.3. Blood staining of cornea.

5. *Deep corneal opacity.* It may result from oedema of corneal stroma or occasionally from folds in the Descemet's membrane.

II. *Sclera*

Partial thickness scleral wounds (lamellar scleral lacerations) may occur alone or in association with other lesions of closed-globe injury.

III. *Anterior chamber*

1. *Traumatic hyphaema* (blood in the anterior chamber). It occurs due to injury to the iris or ciliary body vessels (Fig. 17.4).
2. *Exudates.* These may collect in the anterior chamber following traumatic uveitis.

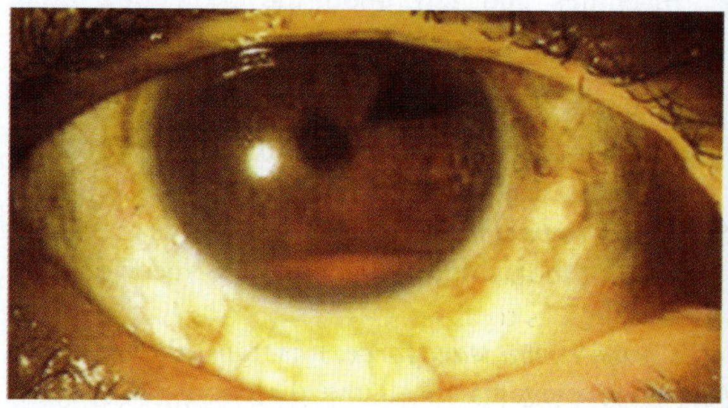

Fig. 17.4. Photograph of a patient with hyphaema.

IV. *Iris, pupil and ciliary body*

1. *Traumatic miosis.* It occurs initially due to irritation of ciliary nerves. It may be associated with spasm of accommodation.
2. *Traumatic mydriasis* (Iridoplegia). It is usually permanent and may be associated with traumatic cycloplegia.
3. *Rupture of the pupillary margin* is a common occurrence in closed-globe injury.
4. *Radiating tears in the iris stroma,* sometimes reaching up to ciliary body, may occur occasionally.
5. *Iridodialysis* i.e., detachment of iris from its root at the ciliary body occurs frequently. It results in a D-shaped pupil and a black biconvex area seen at the periphery (Fig. 17.5).
6. *Antiflexion of the iris.* It refers to rotation of the detached portion of iris, in which its posterior surface faces anteriorly. It occurs following extensive iridodialysis.

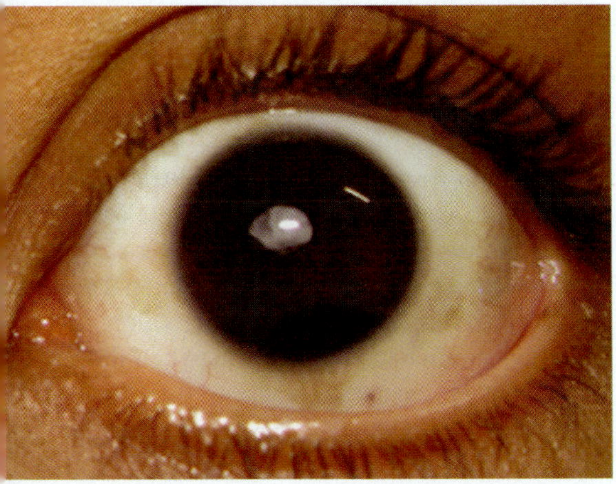

Fig. 17.5. Traumatic cataract and iridodialysis following contusional injury.

7. *Retroflexion of the iris.* This term is used when whole of the iris is doubled back into the ciliary region and becomes invisible.
8. *Traumatic aniridia or iridremia.* In this condition, the completely torn iris (from ciliary body) sinks to the bottom of anterior chamber in the form of a minute ball.
9. *Angle recession* refers to the tear between longitudinal and circular muscle fibres of the ciliary body. It is characterized by deepening of the anterior chamber and widening of the ciliary body band on gonioscopy. Later on it is complicated by glaucoma.
10. *Inflammatory changes.* These include traumatic iridocyclitis, haemophthalmitis, post-traumatic iris atrophy and pigmentary changes.

Treatment. It consists of atropine, antibiotics and steroids. In the presence of ruptures of pupillary margins and subluxation of lens, atropine is contraindicated.

V. *Lens*

It may show following changes:

1. *Vossius ring.* It is a circular ring of brown pigment seen on the anterior capsule. It occurs due to striking of the contracted pupillary margin against the crystalline lens. It is always smaller than the size of the pupil.
2. *Concussion cataract.* It occurs mainly due to imbibition of aqueous and partly due to direct mechanical effects of the injury on lens fibres. It may assume any of the following shapes:
   - *Discrete subepithelial opacities* are of most common occurrence.
   - *Early rosette cataract* (punctate). It is the most typical form of concussion cataract. It appears as feathery lines of opacities along the star-shaped suture lines; usually in the posterior cortex (Fig. 17.6).
   - *Late rosette cataract.* It develops in the posterior cortex 1 to 2 years after the injury. Its sutural extensions are shorter and more compact than the early rosette cataract.
   - *Traumatic zonular cataract.* It may also occur in some cases, though rarely.
   - *Diffuse (total) concussion cataract.* It is of frequent occurrence.
   - *Early maturation of senile cataract* may follow blunt truma.

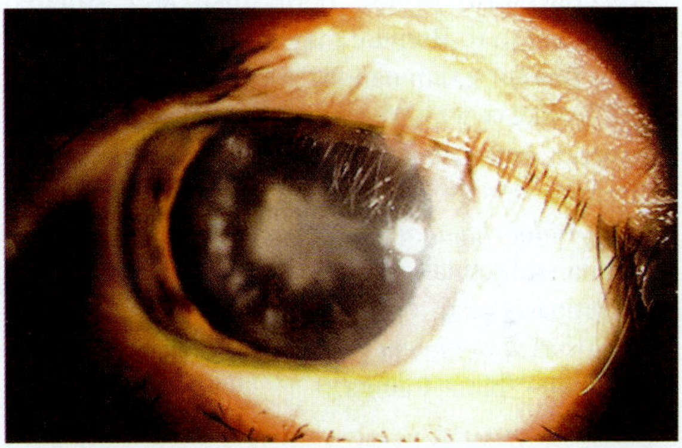

Fig. 17.6. Rosette-shaped cataract following blunt trauma.

Treatment of traumatic cataract is on general lines (see pages 193-214).

3. *Traumatic absorption of the lens.* It may occur sometimes in young children resulting in aphakia.
4. *Subluxation of the lens* (Fig. 8.31A). It may occur due to partial tear of zonules. The subluxated lens is slightly displaced but still present in the pupillary area. On dilatation of the pupil its edge may be seen. Depending upon the site of zonular tear subluxation may be vertical (upward or downward), or lateral (nasal or temporal).
5. *Dislocation of the lens.* It occurs when rupture of the zonules is complete. It may be intraocular (commonly) or extraocular (sometimes). Intraocular dislocation may be anterior (into the anterior

chamber, Fig. 8.31B) or posterior (into the vitreous, Fig. 8.31C). Extraocular dislocation may be in the subconjunctival space (phakocele) or it may fall outside the eye.

For treatment of the subluxated or dislocated lens see page 216.

VI. *Vitreous*

1. *Liquefaction and appearance of clouds* of fine pigmentary opacities (a most common change).
2. *Detachment* of the vitreous either anterior or posterior.
3. *Vitreous haemorrhage.* It is of common occurrence (see page 260).
4. *Vitreous herniation* in the anterior chamber may occur with subluxation or dislocation of the lens.

VII. *Choroid*

1. *Rupture of the choroid.* The rupture of choroid is concentric to the optic disc and situated temporal to it. Rupture may be single or multiple. On fundus examination, the choroidal rupture looks like a whitish crescent (due to underlying sclera) with fine pigmentation at its margins. Retinal vessels pass over it (Fig. 17.7).
2. *Choroidal haemorrhage* may occur under the retina (subretinal) or may even enter the vitreous if retina is also torn.
3. *Choroidal detachment* is also known to occur following blunt trauma.

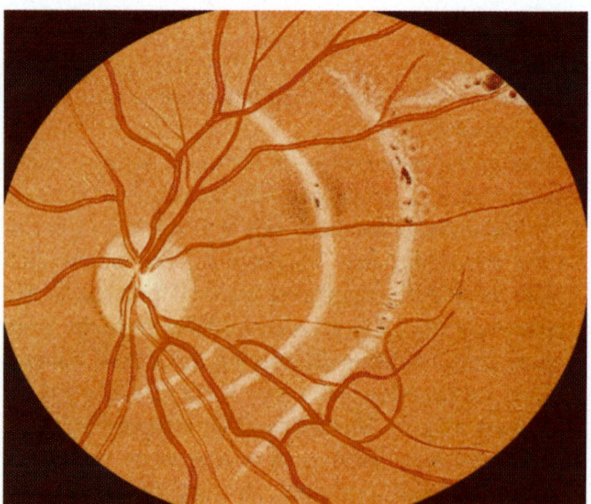

Fig. 17.7. Choroidal rupture following blunt trauma.

4. *Traumatic choroiditis* may be seen on fundus examination as patches of pigmentation and discoloration after the eye becomes silent.

VIII. *Retina*

1. *Commotio retinae* (Berlin's oedema). It is of common occurrence following a blow on the eye. It manifests as milky white cloudiness involving a considerable area of the posterior pole with a '*cherry-red spot*' in the foveal region. It may disappear after some days or may be followed by pigmentary changes.
2. *Retinal haemorrhages.* These are quite common following concussion trauma. Multiple haemorrhages including flame-shaped and pre-retinal (subhyaloid) D-shaped haemorrhage may be associated with traumatic retinopathy.
3. *Retinal tears.* These may follow a contusion, particularly in the peripheral region, especially in eyes already suffering from myopia or senile degenerations.
4. *Traumatic proliferative retinopathy* (Retinitis proliferans). It may occur secondary to vitreous haemorrhage, forming tractional bands.
5. *Retinal detachment.* It may follow retinal tears or vitreo-retinal tractional bands.
6. *Concussion changes at macula.* Traumatic macular oedema is usually followed by *pigmentary degeneration.* Sometimes, a *macular cyst* is formed, which on rupture may be converted into a lamellar or full thickness *macular hole.*

IX. *Intraocular pressure changes in closed-globe injury*

1. *Traumatic glaucoma.* It may occur due to multiple factors, which are described in detail on page 235.
2. *Traumatic hypotony.* It may follow damage to the ciliary body and may even result in phthisis bulbi.

X. *Traumatic changes in the refraction*

1. *Myopia* may follow ciliary spasm or rupture of zonules or anterior shift of the lens.
2. *Hypermetropia* and loss of accommodation may result from damage to the ciliary body (cycloplegia).

B. Globe rupture

Globe rupture is a full-thickness wound of the eye-wall (sclera, cornea or both) caused by a blunt object. Globe rupture may occur in two ways:

1. *Direct rupture* may occur, though rarely, at the site of injury.

2. *Indirect rupture* is more common and occurs because of the compression force. The impact results in momentary increase in the intraocular pressure and an inside-out injury at the weakest part of eyewall, i.e., in the vicinity of canal of Schlemm concentric to the limbus. The superonasal limbus is the most common site of globe rupture (contrecoup effect—the lower temporal quadrant being most exposed to trauma). Rupture of the globe may be associated with prolapse of uveal tissue, vitreous loss, intraocular haemorrhage and dislocation of the lens.

***Treatment*.** A badly damaged globe should be enucleated. In less severe cases, repair should be done under general anaesthesia. Postoperatively atropine, antibiotics and steroids should be used.

C. Extraocular lesions

Extraocular lesions caused by blunt trauma are as follows:

1. *Conjunctival lesions.* *Subconjunctival haemorrhage* occurs very commonly. It appears as a bright red spot. *Chemosis and lacerating wounds* of conjunctiva (tears) are also not uncommon.

2. *Eyelid lesion.* *Ecchymosis* of eyelids is of frequent occurrence. Because of loose subcutaneous tissue, blood collects easily into the lids and produces 'black-eye'. There may occur *laceration and avulsion* of the lids. *Traumatic ptosis* may follow damage to the levator muscle.

3. *Lacrimal apparatus lesions.* These include dislocation of lacrimal gland and lacerations of lacrimal passages especially the canaliculi.

4. *Optic nerve injuries.* These are commonly associated with fractures of the base of skull. These may be in the form of traumatic papillitis, lacerations of optic nerve, optic nerve sheath haemorrhage and avulsion of the optic nerve from back of the eye.

5. *Orbital injury.* There may occur fractures of the orbital walls; commonest being the '*blow-out fracture*' of the orbital floor (see page 425). Orbital *haemorrhage* may produce sudden proptosis. *Orbital emphysema* may occur following ethmoidal sinus rupture.

OPEN-GLOBE INJURIES

Open-globe injury is defined as a full thickness wound of the eye-wall (sclera or/and cornea). It includes:

1. ***Globe rupture***, i.e. full thickness wound of the eye wall caused by blunt trauma. It is covered with blunt trauma, see page 435.
2. ***Globe laceration*** refers to full-thickness wound of eyewall caused by sharp objects. It includes:
   i. Penetrating injury
   ii. Perforating injury, and
   iii. Intraocular foreign bodies.

PENETRATING AND PERFORATING INJURIES

As mentioned earlier, penetrating injury is defined as a single full-thickness wound of the eyewall caused by a sharp object. While perforating injury refers to two full-thickness wounds (one entry and one exit) of the eyewall caused by a sharp object or missile.

These can cause severe damage to the eye and so should be treated as *serious emergencies*.

Modes of injury

1. *Trauma by sharp and pointed instruments* like needles, knives, nails, arrows, screw-drivers, pens, pencils, compasses, glass pieces and so on.
2. *Trauma by foreign bodies travelling at very high speed* such as bullet injuries and iron foreign bodies in lathe workers.

Effects of penetrating/perforating injury

Damage to the ocular structures may occur by following effects:

1. *Mechanical effects of the trauma* or physical changes. These are discussed later in detail.
2. *Introduction of infection.* Sometimes, pyogenic organisms enter the eye during perforating injuries, multiply there and can cause varying degree of infection depending upon the virulence and host defence mechanism. These include: ring abscess of the cornea, sloughing of the cornea, purulent iridocyclitis, endophthalmitis or panophthalmitis (see pages 168-171).

   Rarely tetanus and infection by gas-forming organisms (*Clostridium welchii*) may also occur.
3. *Post-traumatic iridocyclitis.* It is of frequent occurrence and if not treated properly can cause devastating damage.

4. *Sympathetic ophthalmitis.* It is a rare but most dangerous complication of a perforating injury. It is described separately (see page 441).

Mechanical effects

Mechanical effects of penetrating/perforating trauma on the different ocular structures with their management are enumerated here briefly.

1. *Wounds of the conjunctiva.* These are common and usually associated with subconjunctival haemorrhage. A wound of more than 3 mm should be sutured.

2. *Wounds of the cornea.* These can be divided into uncomplicated and complicated wounds.

i. *Uncomplicated corneal wounds.* These are not associated with prolapse of intraocular contents. Margins of such wounds swell up and lead to automatic sealing and restoration of the anterior chamber.

   Treatment. A small central wound does not need stitching. The only treatment required is pad and bandage with atropine and antibiotic ointments.

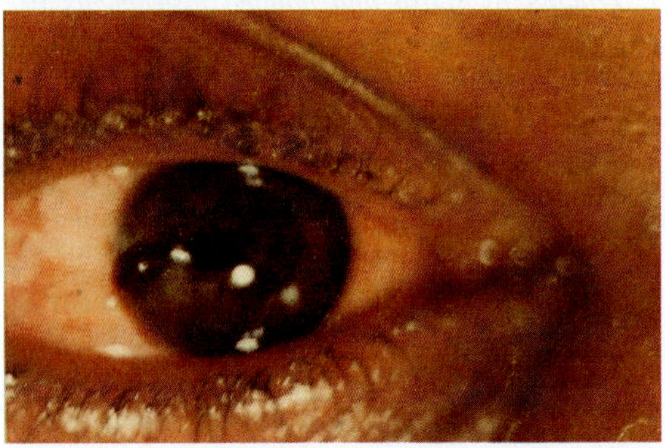

Fig. 17.8. Corneal tear with iris prolapse.

   A large corneal wound (more than 2 mm) should always be sutured.

ii. *Complicated corneal wounds.* These are associated with prolapse of iris (Fig. 17.8), sometimes lens matter and even vitreous.

   Treatment. Corneal wounds with iris prolapse should be sutured meticulously after abscising the iris. The prolapsed iris should never be reposited; since it may cause infection. When associated with lens injury and vitreous loss, lensectomy and anterior vitrectomy may be performed along with repair of the corneal wound.

3. *Wounds of the sclera.* These are usually associated with corneal wounds and should be managed as above. In corneo-scleral tear, first suture should be applied at the limbus.

4. *Wounds of the lens.* Extensive lens ruptures with vitreous loss should be managed as above. Small wounds in the anterior capsule may seal and lead on to traumatic cataract; which may be in the form of a localised stationary cataract, early or late rosette cataract, or complete (total) cataract. These should be treated on general lines (pages 183-202).

5. *A badly (severely) wounded eye.* It refers to extensive corneo-scleral tears associated with prolapse of the uveal tissue, lens rupture, vitreous loss and injury to the retina and choroid. Usually there seems to be no chance of getting useful vision in such cases. So, preferably such eyes should be excised.

INTRAOCULAR FOREIGN BODIES

Penetrating injuries with foreign bodies are not infrequent. Seriousness of such injuries is compounded by the retention of intraocular foreign bodies (IOFB).

Common foreign bodies responsible for such injuries include: chips of iron and steel (90%) particles of glass stone, lead pellets, copper percussion caps aluminium, plastic and wood.

Modes of damage

A penetrating/perforating injury with retained foreign body may damage the ocular structures by the following modes:

A. Mechanical effects.
B. Introduction of infection.
C. Reaction of foreign bodies.
D. Post-traumatic iridocyclitis.
E. Sympathetic ophthalmitis (see page 441).

A. *Mechanical effects*

Mechanical effects depend upon the size, velocity and type of the foreign body. Foreign bodies greater than 2 mm in size cause extensive damage. The lesions caused also depend upon the route of entry and the site up to which a foreign body has travelled. In general these include:

- Corneal or/and scleral perforation, hyphaema, iris hole;

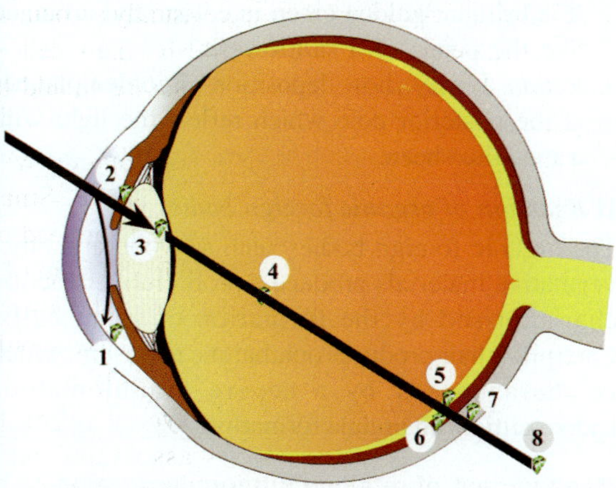

Fig. 17.9. Common sites for retention of an intraocular foreign body: 1, anterior chamber; 2, iris; 3, lens; 4, vitreous; 5, retina; 6, choroid; 7, sclera; 8, orbital cavity.

- Rupture of the lens and traumatic cataract;
- Vitreous haemorrhage and/or degeneration;
- Choroidal perforation, haemorrhage and inflammation;
- Retinal hole, haemorrhages, oedema and detachment.

Locations of IOFB. Having entered the eye through the cornea or sclera a foreign body may be retained at any of the following sites (Fig. 17.9):

1. *Anterior chamber.* In the anterior chamber, the IOFB usually sinks at the bottom. A tiny foreign body may be concealed in the angle of anterior chamber, and visualised only on gonioscopy.
2. *Iris.* Here the foreign body is usually entangled in the stroma.
3. *Posterior chamber.* Rarely a foreign body may sink behind the iris after entering through pupil or after making a hole in the iris.
4. *Lens.* Foreign body may be present on the anterior surface or inside the lens. Either an opaque track may be seen in the lens or the lens may become completely cataractous.
5. *Vitreous cavity.* A foreign body may reach here through various routes, which are depicted below (Fig. 17.10):
6. *Retina, choroid and sclera.* A foreign body may obtain access to these structures through corneal route or directly from scleral perforation.

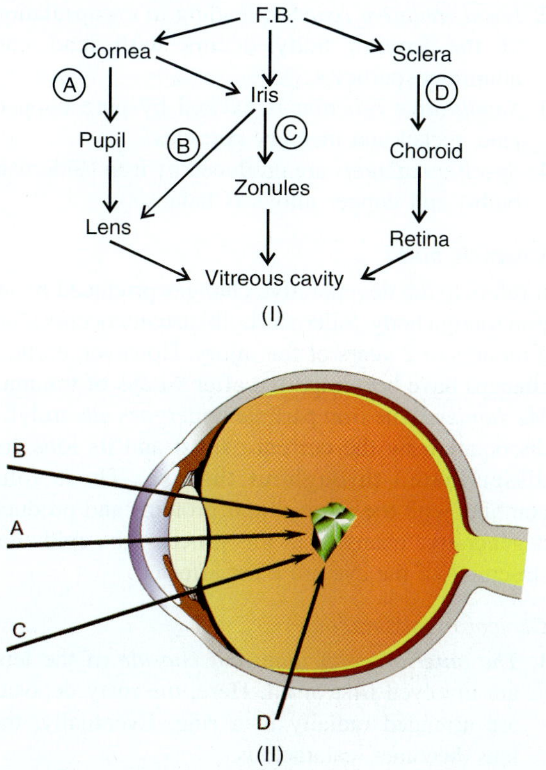

Fig. 17.10. Logarthmic (I) and diagrammatic (II) depiction of routes of access of a foreign body in the vitreous, through: A, cornea, pupil, lens; B, cornea, iris, lens; C, cornea, iris, zonules; D, sclera, choroid, retina.

7. *Orbital cavity.* A foreign body piercing the eyeball may occasionally cause double perforation and come to rest in the orbital tissues.

B. Introduction of Infection

Intraocular infection is the real danger to the eyeball. Fortunately, small flying metallic foreign bodies are usually sterile due to the heat generated on their commission. However, pieces of the wood and stones carry a great chance of infection. Unfortunately, once intraocular infection is established it usually ends in endophthalmitis or even panophthalmitis.

C. Reactions of the foreign body

I. *Inorganic foreign body*

Depending upon its chemical nature following 4 types of reactions are noted in the ocular tissues:

1. *No reaction* is produced by the inert substances which include glass, plastic, porcelain, gold silver and platinum.

2. *Local irritative reaction* leading to encapsulation of the foreign body occurs with lead and aluminium particles.
3. *Suppurative reaction* is excited by pure copper, zinc, nickel and mercury particles.
4. *Specific reactions* are produced by iron (Siderosis bulbi) and copper alloys (Chalcosis).

Siderosis bulbi

It refers to the degenerative changes produced by an iron foreign body. Siderosis bulbi usually occurs after 2 months to 2 years of the injury. However, earliest changes have been reported after 9 days of trauma.
Mechanism. The iron particle undergoes electrolytic dissociation by the current of rest and its ions are disseminated throughout the eye. These ions combine with the intracellular proteins and produce degenerative changes. In this process, the epithelial structures of the eye are most affected.

Clinical manifestations

1. *The anterior epithelium and capsule* of the lens are involved first of all. Here, the rusty deposits are arranged radially in a ring. Eventually, the lens becomes cataractous.
2. *Iris.* It is first stained greenish and later on turns reddish brown.
3. *Retina develops pigmentary degeneration* which resembles retinitis pigmentosa.
4. *Secondary open angle type of glaucoma* occurs due to degenerative changes in the trabecular meshwork.

Chalcosis

It refers to the specific changes produced by the alloy of copper in the eye.
Mechanism. Copper ions from the alloy are dissociated electrolytically and deposited under the membranous structures of the eye. Unlike iron ions these do not enter into a chemical combination with the proteins of the cells and thus produce no degenerative changes.

Clinical manifestations

1. *Kayser-Fleischer ring.* It is a golden brown ring which occurs due to deposition of copper under peripheral parts of the Descemet's membrane of the cornea.
2. *Sunflower cataract.* It is produced by deposition of copper under the posterior capsule of the lens. It is brilliant golden green in colour and arranged like the petals of a sunflower.
3. *Retina.* It may show deposition of golden plaques at the posterior pole which reflect the light with a metallic sheen.

II *Reaction of organic foreign bodies*

The organic foreign bodies such as wood and other vegetative materials produce a proliferative reaction characterised by the formation of giant cells. Caterpillar hair produces ophthalmia nodosum, which is characterised by a severe granulomatous iridocyclitis with nodule formation.

Management of retained intraocular foreign bodies (IOFB)

Diagnosis

It is a matter of extreme importance particularly as the patient is often unaware that a particle has entered the eye. To come to a correct diagnosis following steps should be taken:

1. *History.* A careful history about the mode of injury may give a clue about the type of IOFB.

2. *Ocular examination.* A thorough ocular examination with slit-lamp including gonioscopy should be carried out. The signs which may give some indication about IOFB are: subconjunctival haemorrhage, corneal scar, holes in the iris, and opaque track through the lens. With clear media, sometimes IOFB may be seen on ophthalmoscopy in the vitreous or on the retina. IOFB lodged in the angle of anterior chamber may be visualised by gonioscopy.

3. *Plain X-rays orbit.* Antero-posterior and lateral views are still being recommended for the location of IOFB, as most foreign bodies are radio opaque. However, many workers feel there is no use of plain film radiology (PFR), as CT images are required for suspected IOFB, even if PFR is negative

4. *Localization of IOFB*. Once IOFB is suspected clinically and later confirmed, on fundus examination and/or X-rays, its exact localization is mandatory to plan the proper removal. Following techniques may be used:

- *Radiographic localization.* Before the advent of ultrasonography and CT scan, different specialized radiographic techniques were used to localize IOFBs; which are now obsolete. However, a simple limbal ring method which is still used (most centers

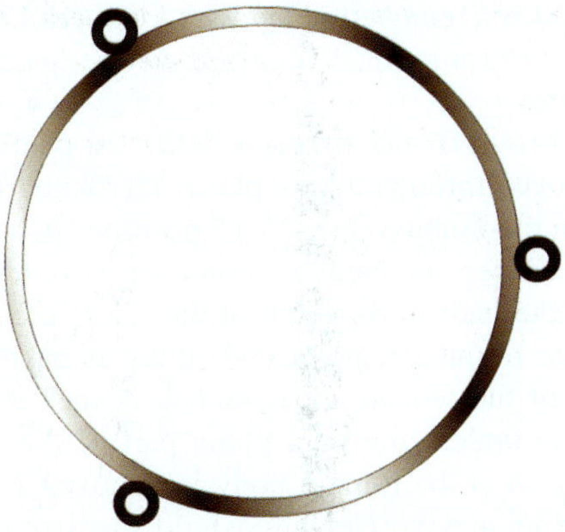

Fig. 17.11. Limbal ring used for localization of an intraocular foreign body.

have discarded it) is described below:

Limbal ring method. It is the most simple but now-a-days, sparingly employed technique. A metallic ring of the corneal diameter (Fig. 17.11) is stitched at the limbus and X-rays are taken. One exposure is taken in the anteroposterior view. In the lateral view three exposures are made one each while the patient is looking straight, upwards and downwards, respectively. The position of the foreign body is estimated from its relationship with the metallic ring in different positions (Fig. 17.12).

- *Ultrasonographic localization.* It is being used increasingly these days. It can tell the position of even non-radioopaque foreign bodies.
- *CT scan.* With axial and coronal cuts, CT scan is presently the best method of IOFB localization. It provides cross-sectional images with a sensitivity and specificity that are superior to plain radiography and ultrasonography.
- *Magnetic resonance imaging* (MRI) is not recommended as a general screening tool, since it can cause further damage by producing movement of a magnetic IO foreign body. However, after the CT has excluded the presence of a metallic IO foreign body; MRI has a special role in localizing small plastic or wooden IO foreign bodies.

Treatment

IOFB should always be removed, except when it is inert and probably sterile or when little damage has

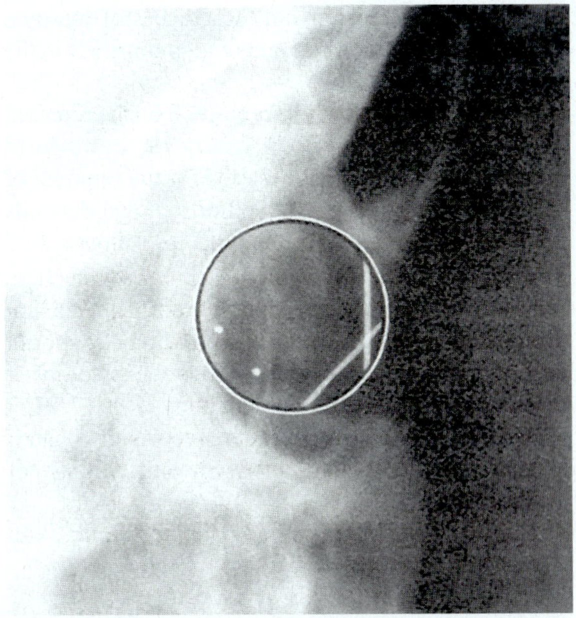

Fig. 17.12. Limbal ring method of radiographic localization of IOFB: Lateral view with eyeball in straight position; superimposed over lateral view with eyeball in down gaze.

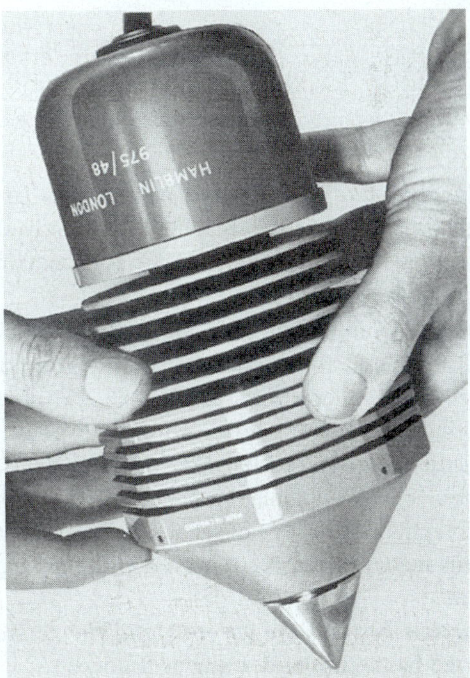

Fig. 17.13. Hand-held magnet.

been done to the vision and the process of removal may be risky and destroy sight (e.g., minute FB in the retina).

Removal of magnetic IOFB is easier than the removal of non-magnetic FB. Usually a hand-held electromagnet (Fig. 17.13) is used for the removal of magnetic foreign body. Method of removal depends upon the site (location) of the IOFB as follows:

1. *Foreign body in the anterior chamber.* It is removed through a corresponding corneal incision directed straight towards the foreign body. It should be 3 mm internal to the limbus and in the quadrant of the cornea lying over the foreign body (Fig. 17.14).

- *Magnetic* foreign body is removed with a hand-held magnet. It may come out with a gush of aqueous.
- *Non-magnetic* foreign body is picked up with toothless forceps.

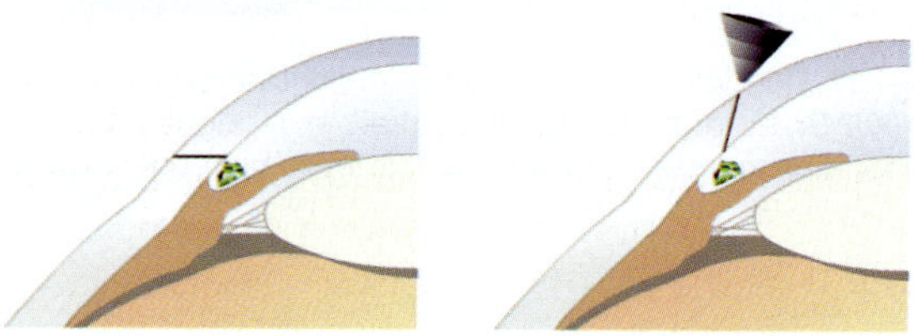

A B

Fig. 17.14. Removal of a magnetic intraocular foreign body from the anterior chamber: A, the wrong incision; B, correct incision.

2. *Foreign body entangled in the iris tissue* (magnetic as well as non-magnetic) is removed by performing sector iridectomy of the part containing foreign body.

3. *Foreign body in the lens.* Magnet extraction is usually difficult for intralenticular foreign bodies. Therefore, magnetic foreign body should also be treated as non-magnetic foreign body. An extracapsular cataract extraction (ECCE) with intraocular lens implantation should be performed. The foreign body may be evacuated itself along with the lens matter or may be removed with the help of forceps.

4. *Foreign body in the vitreous and the retina* is removed by the posterior route as follows:

i. *Magnetic removal.* This technique is used to remove a magnetic foreign body that can be well localized and removed safely with a powerful magnet without causing much damage to the intraocular structures.

- *An intravitreal foreign body* is preferably removed through a pars plana sclerotomy (5 mm from the limbus) (Fig. 17.15 position 'A'). At the site chosen for incision, conjunctiva is reflected and the incision is given in the sclera concentric to the limbus. A preplaced suture is passed and lips of the wound are retracted. A nick is given in the underlying pars plana part of the ciliary body. And the foreign body is removed with the help of a powerful hand-held electromagnet. Preplaced suture is tied to close the scleral wound. Conjunctiva is stitched with one or two interrupted sutures.
- *For an intraretinal foreign body*, the site of incision should be as close to the foreign body as possible (Fig. 17.15 position 'B'). A trapdoor scleral flap is created, the choroidal bed is treated with diathermy, choroid is incised and foreign body is removed with either forceps or external magnet.

ii. *Forceps removal with pars plana vitrectomy*. This technique is used to remove all non-magnetic foreign bodies and those magnetic foreign bodies that can not be safely removed with a magnet. In this technique, the foreign body is removed with vitreous

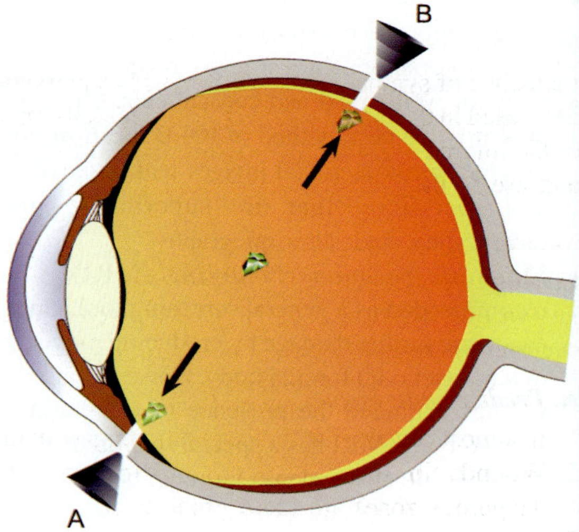

Fig. 17.15. Removal of a magnetic intraocular foreign body from posterior segment.

forceps after performing three-pore pars plana vitrectomy under direct visualization using an operating microscope (Fig. 17.16).

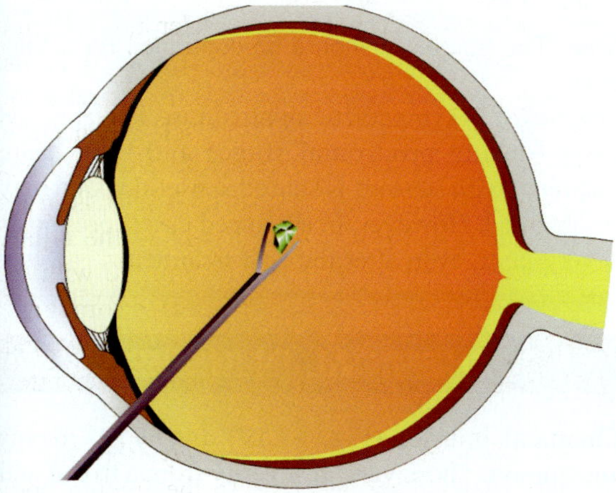

Fig. 17.16. Removal of a non-magnetic foreign body through pars plana.

SYMPATHETIC OPHTHALMITIS

Sympathetic ophthalmitis is a serious bilateral granulomatous panuveitis which follows a penetrating ocular trauma. The injured eye is called *exciting eye* and the fellow eye which also develops uveitis is called *sympathizing eye.* Very rarely, sympathetic ophthalmitis can also occur following an intraocular surgery.

Incidence

Incidence of sympathetic ophthalmitis has markedly decreased in the recent years due to meticulous repair of the injured eye utilizing microsurgical techniques and use of the potent steroids.

Etiology

Etiology of sympathetic ophthalmitis is still not known exactly. However, the facts related with its occurrence are as follows:

A. ***Predisposing factors***

1. It almost always follows a penetrating wound.
2. Wounds in the ciliary region (the so-called dangerous zone) are more prone to it.
3. Wounds with incarceration of the iris, ciliary body or lens capsule are more vulnerable.
4. It is more common in children than in adults.
5. It does not occur when actual suppuration develops in the injured eye.

B. ***Pathogenesis.*** Various theories have been put forward. Most accepted one is *allergic theory,* which postulates that the uveal pigment acts as allergen and excites plastic uveitis in the sound eye.

Pathology

It is characteristic of granulomatous uveitis, i.e., there is nodular aggregation of lymphocytes, plasma cells, epitheloid cells and giant cells scattered throughout the uveal tract.

Dalen-Fuchs' nodules are formed due to proliferation of the pigment epithelium (of the iris, ciliary body and choroid) associated with invasion by the lymphocytes and epitheloid cells. Retina shows perivascular cellular infiltration (sympathetic perivasculitis).

Clinical picture

I. *Exciting (injured) eye.* It shows clinical features of persistent low grade plastic uveitis, which include ciliary congestion, lacrimation and tenderness. Keratic precipitates may be present at the back of cornea (dangerous sign).

II. Sympathizing (sound) eye. It is usually involved after 4-8 weeks of injury in the other eye. Earliest reported case is after 9 days of injury. Most of the cases occur within the first year. However, delayed and very late cases are also reported. Sympathetic ophthalmitis, almost always, manifests as acute plastic iridocyclitis. Rarely it may manifest as neuroretinitis or choroiditis. Clinical picture of the iridocyclitis in sympathizing eye can be divided into two stages:

1. *Prodromal stage.* *Symptoms.* Sensitivity to light (photophobia) and transient indistinctness of near objects (due to weakening of accommodation) are the earliest symptoms.

Signs. In this stage the first sign may be presence of retrolental flare and cells or the presence of a few keratic precipitates (KPs) on back of cornea. Other signs includes mild ciliary congestion, slight tenderness of the globe, fine vitreous haze and disc oedema which is seen occasionally.

2. *Fully-developed stage.* It is clinically characterised by typical signs and symptoms consistent with acute plastic iridocyclitis (see page 149).

Treatment

A. *Prophylaxis*

I. *Early excision of the injured eye*. It is the best prophylaxis when there is no chance of saving useful vision.

II. *When there is hope of saving useful vision*, following steps should be taken:

1. A *meticulous repair* of the wound using microsurgical technique should be carried out, taking great care that uveal tissue is not incarcerated in the wound.
2. *Immediate expectant treatment* with topical as well as systemic steroids and antibiotics along with topical atropine should be started.
3. *When the uveitis is not controlled* after 2 weeks of expectant treatment, i.e., lacrimation, photophobia and ciliary congestion persist and if KPs appear, this injured eye should be excised immediately.

B. *Treatment when sympathetic ophthalmitis has already supervened*

I. *If the case is seen shortly after the onset of inflammation* (i.e., during prodromal stage) in the sympathizing eye, and the injured eye has no useful vision, this useless eye should be excised at once.

II. *Conservative treatment of sympathetic ophthalmitis* on the lines of iridocyclitis should be started immediately, as follows:

1. *Corticosteroids* should be administered by all routes, i.e., systemic, periocular injections and frequent instillation of topical drops.

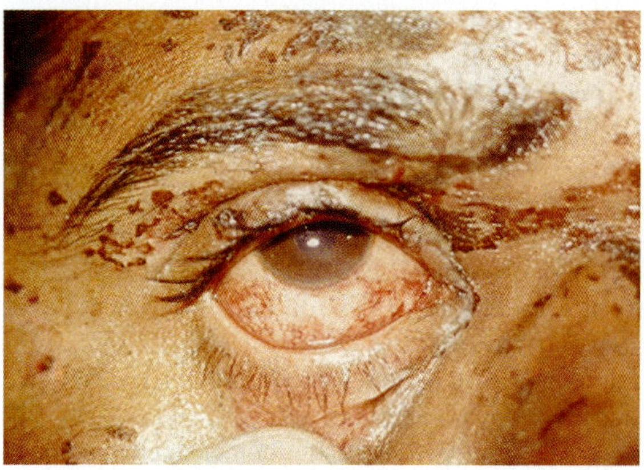

Fig. 17.17. A patient with chemical injury face including eyes.

2. *Immunosuppressant* drugs should be started in severe cases, without delay.
3. *Atropine* should be instilled three times a day in all cases.

Note. The treatment should be continued for a long time.

Prognosis. If sympathetic ophthalmitis is diagnosed early (during prodromal stage) and immediate treatment with steroids is started, a useful vision may be obtained. However, in advanced cases, prognosis is very poor, even after the best treatment.

CHEMICAL INJURIES

Chemical injuries (Fig. 17.17) are by no means uncommon. These vary in severity from a trivial and transient irritation of little significance to complete and sudden loss of vision.

Modes of injury

These usually occur due to external contact with chemicals under following circumstances:

1. *Domestic accidents,* e.g., with ammonia, solvents, detergents and cosmetics.
2. *Agricultural accidents,* e.g., due to fertilizers, insecticides, toxins of vegetable and animal origin.
3. *Chemical laboratory accidents,* with acids and alkalies.
4. *Deliberate chemical attacks,* especially with acids to disfigure the face.
5. *Chemical warfare* injuries.
6. *Self-inflicted chemical* injuries are seen in malingerers and psychopaths.

Types

In general, the serious chemical burns mainly comprise alkali and acid burns.

A. *Alkali burns*

Alkali burns are among the most severe chemical injuries known to the ophthalmologists. Common alkalies responsible for burns are: lime, caustic potash or caustic soda and liquid ammonia (most harmful).

Mechanisms of damage produced by alkalies includes:

1. Alkalies dissociate and saponify fatty acids of the cell membrane and, therefore, destroy the structure of cell membrane of the tissues.

2. Being hygroscopic, they extract water from the cells, a factor which contributes to the total necrosis.
3. They combine with lipids of cells to form soluble compounds, which produce a condition of softening and gelatinisation.

The above effects result in an increased deep penetration of the alkalies into the tissues. Alkali burns, therefore, spread widely, their action continues for some days and their effects are difficult to circumscribe. Hence, prognosis in such cases must always be guarded.

Clinical picture. It can be divided into three stages:

1. *Stage of acute ischaemic necrosis.* In this stage;
   i. *Conjunctiva* shows marked oedema, congestion, widespread necrosis and a copious purulent discharge.
   ii. *Cornea* develops widespread sloughing of the epithelium, oedema and opalescence of the stroma.
   iii. *Iris* becomes violently inflamed and in severe cases both iris and ciliary body are replaced by granulation tissue.
2. *Stage of reparation.* In this stage conjunctival and corneal epithelium regenerate, there occurs corneal vascularization and inflammation of the iris subsides.
3. *Stage of complications.* This is characterised by development of symblepharon, recurrent corneal ulceration and development of complicated cataract and secondary glaucoma.

B. *Acid burns*

Acid burns are less serious than alkali burns. Common acids responsible for burns are: sulphuric acid, hydrochloric acid and nitric acid.

Chemical effects. The strong acids cause instant coagulation of all the proteins which then act as a barrier and prevent deeper penetration of the acids into the tissues. Thus, the lesions become sharply demarcated.

Ocular lesions

1. *Conjunctiva.* There occurs immediate necrosis followed by sloughing. Later on symblepharon is formed due to fibrosis.
2. *Cornea.* It is also necrosed and sloughed out. The extent of damage depends upon the concentration of acid and the duration of contact.

Table 17.1. Grades of chemical burns (Roper-Hall classification)

Grade	*Corneal appearance*	*Limbal ischaemia*	*Visual prognosis*
I.	Clear corneal	Nil	Good
II.	Hazy but iris details visible	< 1/3	Good
III.	Opaque cornea. Iris details obscured	1/3 to 1/2	Doubtful
IV.	Opaque, no view of the iris and pupil	>1/2	Poor

In severe cases, the whole cornea may slough out followed by staphyloma formation.

Grading of chemical burns

Depending upon the severity of damage caused to the limbus and cornea, the extent of chemical burns may be graded in Roper-Hall classification as follows (Table 17.1):

Treatment of chemical burns

1. *Immediate and thorough irrigation* with the available clean water or saline delivered through an I.V. tubing. Deliver minimum of $2\,L$ of water or until pH is restored.
   Note: Do not waste time on history and examination of the patient; it should be done after the irrigation.
2. *Mechanical removal of contaminant.* If any particles are left behind, particularly in the case of lime, these should be removed carefully with a swab stick.
3. *Removal of contaminated and necrotic tissue.* Necrosed conjunctiva should be excised. Contaminated and necrosed corneal epithelium should be removed with a cotton swab stick.
4. *Maintenance of favourable conditions* for rapid and uncomplicated healing by frequent application of topical atropine, corticosteroids, antibiotics and lubricants.
5. *Prevention of symblepharon* can be done by using a glass shell or sweeping a glass rod in the fornices twice daily.
6. *Treatment of complications*
   i. *Secondary glaucoma* should be treated by topical 0.5 percent timolol, instilled twice a day

along with oral acetazolamide 250 mg 3-4 times a day.

ii. *Poor corneal healing* with limbal stem cell deficiency may be treated by amniotic membrane transplantation with or without limbal stem cell transplantation.

iii. *Pseudopterygium*, when formed, should be excised together with conjuctival autograft (if adequate host conjuctiva) or amniotic membrane facilitated by antimitotic drugs (e.g. mitomycin-C).

iv. *Treatment* of *symblepharon* (see page 376).

v. *Corneal opacity* may be treated by keratoplasty if adequate tear film and stem cell population available.

vi. *Keratoprosthesis* remains a surgical option in severely damaged eyes.

THERMAL INJURIES

Thermal injuries are usually caused by fire, or hot fluids. The main brunt of such injuries lies on the lids. Conjunctiva and cornea may be affected in severe cases.

Treatment for burns of lids is on general lines. When cornea is affected, it should be treated with atropine, steroids, antibiotics and lubricants.

ELECTRICAL INJURIES

The passage of strong electric current from the area of eyes may cause following lesions:

1. *Conjunctiva* becomes congested.
2. *Cornea* develops punctate or diffuse interstitial opacities.
3. *Iris and ciliary body* are inflamed.
4. *Lens* may develop 'electric cataract' after 2-4 months of accident.
5. *Retina* may show multiple haemorrhages.
6. *Optic nerve* may develop neuritis.

RADIATIONAL INJURIES

1. *Ultraviolet radiations.* These may cause (i) photo-ophthalmia (see page 113) and (ii) may be responsible for senile cataract.
2. *Infrared radiations.* These may cause solar macular burns (see page 287).
3. *Ionizing radiational injuries.* These are caused following radiotherapy to the tumours in the vicinity of the eyes. The common ocular lesions include:
   - Radiation keratoconjunctivitis;
   - Radiation dermatitis of lids; and
   - Radiation cataract.

18 CHAPTER

Ocular Therapeutics, Lasers and Cryotherapy in Ophthalmology

OCULAR THERAPEUTICS

- Modes of administration
- Antibacterial agents
- Antiviral drugs
- Ocular antifungal agents
- Mydriatics and cycloplegics
- Anti-glaucoma drugs
- Corticosteroids
- Nonsteroidal anti-inflammatory drugs
- Intraocular irrigating solutions
- Viscoelastic substances
- Anti-VEGF

LASERS IN OPTHALMOLOGY

- Production of laser beam
- Types of lasers
- Mechanisms of laser effects and their therapeutic applications

CRYOTHERAPY IN OPHTHALMOLOGY

- Principle
- Cryounit
- Mode of action
- Uses

OCULAR THERAPEUTICS

MODES OF ADMINISTRATION

Ocular pharmacotherapeutics can be delivered by four methods: topical instillation into the conjunctival sac, periocular injections, intraocular injections and systemic administration.

1. Topical instillation into the conjunctival sac

This is the most commonly employed mode of administration for ocular therapeutics. The drugs can be administered topically in the form of eyedrops, ointments, gels, ocuserts and with the help of soft contact lenses.

(a) ***Eyedrops (gutta).*** This is the simplest and most convenient method of topical application, especially for daytime use. Eyedrops may be in the form of aqueous solutions (drug totally dissolved) or aqueous suspensions (drug is present as small particles kept suspended in the aqueous medium) or oily solutions. Application in the form of eyedrops makes the drug available for immediate action but it is quickly diluted by tears within about a minute.

(b) ***Eye ointment (oculenta or ung).*** Topical application in the form of an eye ointment increases the bioavailability of the drug by increasing tissue contact time and by preventing dilution and quick absorption. However, the drug is not available for immediate use and ointments blur the vision. These are best for bedtime application or when ocular bandage is to be applied.

(c) ***Gels.*** These have prolonged contact time like ointments and do not cause much blurring of vision. However, they are costly and difficult to prepare.

(d) ***Ocuserts.*** These form a system of drug delivery through a membrane. These can be placed in the upper or lower fornix up to a week and allow a drug to be released at a relatively constant rate. Pilocarpine ocuserts have been found very useful in patients with primary open-angle glaucoma; by efficiently controlling intraocular pressure with comparatively fewer side-effects.

(e) ***Soft contact lenses.*** These are very good for delivering higher concentrations of drugs in emergency treatment. A pre-soaked soft contact lens in 1 percent pilocarpine has been found as effective as 4 percent pilocarpine eyedrops in patients with acute angle closure glaucoma. Soft contact lenses are also used to deliver antibiotics and antiviral drugs in patients with corneal ulcers.

Intraocular penetration of topically instilled drugs

Topically instilled medications largely penetrate intraocularly through the cornea. The main barrier through cornea is its epithelium, which is lipophilic, and crossed readily by non-polar drugs. Stroma being hydrophilic allows rapid passage of the drug through endothelium into the anterior chamber. So following features will allow better penetration of drugs through the cornea:

- Drugs which are soluble both in water and fats.
- Pro-drug forms are lipophilic and after absorption through epithelium are converted into proper drugs which can easily pass through stroma.
- Agents that reduce surface tension increase corneal wetting and therefore present more drug for absorption. Benzalkonium chloride used as preservative also acts as a wetting agent and thus increases the drug absorption.

2. Periocular injections

These are not infrequently employed to deliver drugs. These include subconjunctival, sub-Tenon, retrobulbar and peribulbar injections.

(a) *Subconjunctival injections.* These are commonly used to achieve higher concentration of drugs. Further, the drugs which cannot penetrate the cornea owing to large-sized molecules can easily pass through the sclera.

(b) *Sub-Tenon injections.* These are preferred over subconjunctival injection. Anterior sub-Tenon injections are used mainly to administer steroids in the treatment of severe or resistant anterior uveitis. Posterior sub-Tenon injections are indicated in patients with intermediate and posterior uveitis.

(c) *Retrobulbar injections.* Now-a-days, these are sparingly used to deliver drugs for optic neuritis, papillitis, posterior uveitis and also for administering retrobulbar block anaesthesia.

(d) *Peribulbar injections.* These are now frequently used for injecting anaesthetic agents. Peribulbar anaesthesia has almost replaced the retrobulbar and facial block anaesthesia.

3. Intraocular injections

Such injections are made in desperate cases (e.g., endophthalmitis) to deliver the drugs in maximum concentration at the target tissue. These include: *intracameral injection* (into the anterior chamber), and *intravitreal injection* (into the vitreous cavity).

4. Systemic administration

The systemic routes include oral intake and intramuscular and intravenous injections. The intraocular penetration of systemically administered drugs mainly depends upon the blood-aqueous barrier. The passage through blood-aqueous barrier in turn is influenced by the molecular weight and the lipid solubility of the drug.

Only low molecular weight drugs can cross this blood-aqueous barrier. No passage is allowed to large-sized molecules, such as penicillin. Out of the borderline molecular weight drugs, those with high lipid solubility can pass easily e.g., sulphonamides have the same molecular weight as sucrose but are 16 times more permeable due to their lipid solubility. Similarly, chloramphenicol being lipid soluble also enters the eye easily.

COMMON OCULAR THERAPEUTICS

The agents commonly used in ophthalmic practice include: antibacterial, antiviral, antifungal, antiglaucoma, corticosteroids, nonsteroidal anti-inflammatory drugs (NSAIDs) and viscoelastic substances.

ANTIBACTERIAL AGENTS

Antimicrobial drugs are the greatest contribution of the present century to therapeutics. As there are a wide range of microorganisms, there are also specific antibiotics for almost each organism. Depending on the type of action, these can be either *bacteriostatic* or *bactericidal.* A few common antimicrobials described here are grouped on the basis of their chemical structure.

Sulphonamides

These are *bacteriostatic* agents that act by competing with PABA (para-aminobenzoic acid) which is essential for the bacterial cell nutrition. Thus, they prevent susceptible microorganisms from synthesizing folic acid.

In ophthalmic practice, these are used topically and systemically in the treatment of chlamydial infections, viz., trachoma and inclusion conjunctivitis. They are also helpful as an adjunct to pyrimethamine in the treatment of toxoplasmosis.

Beta-lactam antibiotics

These antibiotics have a beta-lactam ring. The two important groups are penicillins, and cephalosporins.

All beta-lactam antibiotics act by interfering with the synthesis of bacterial cell wall.

A. *Penicillins*. These are produced by growing one of the penicillium moulds in deep tanks. These may be categorised as: natural penicillins and semisynthetic penicillins.

In deep-seated inflammations of the orbit or lids, penicillin is given parenterally. In superficial inflammations of the conjunctiva and cornea it is administered locally as *drops* or *ointments*. In intraocular infections it is given as subconjunctival injections. Commonly used preparations are as follows:

1. *Benzyl penicillin.* A dose of 500,000 units twice daily is sufficient for sensitive infections and produces high levels in all tissues except CNS and eye.
2. *Procaine penicillin.* This is an intramuscular depot preparation which provides tissue levels up to 24 hours.
3. *Methicillin, cloxacillin and flucloxacillin.* These penicillins are not affected by penicillinase and are, therefore, used for staphylococcal infections which are resistant to other penicillins.
4. *Carbenicillin.* It is resistant to the penicillinase produced by some strains of *Proteus, Pseudomonas* and coliform organisms. It is ineffective by mouth.
5. *Ampicillin.* It is a broad-spectrum penicillinase-sensitive penicillin. It is acid resistant and usually administered orally.

   Its dosage is 0.25-2 g oral/I.M./I.V. depending upon the severity of infection every 6 hours. Paediatric dose is 25-50 mg/kg/day.
6. *Amoxicillin.* Its spectrum is similar to ampicillin except that it is less effective against *Shigella* and *H. influenzae*. Its oral absorption is better than ampicillin and thus higher and more sustained blood levels are produced. Incidence of diarrhoea is less with it than with ampicillin and is thus better tolerated orally.

B. *Cephalosporins*. These drugs have a similar structure and mode of action as penicillin. All the cephalosporins have a bactericidal action against a wide range of organisms. By convention these have been categorised into three generations of broadly similar antibacterial and pharmacokinetic properties:

1. *First-generation (narrow spectrum) cephalosporins.* These are very active against Gram-positive cocci and thus have useful antistaphylococcal activity. These include cefazolin, cephradine, cephalexin and cephadroxyl.
2. *Second-generation (intermediate spectrum) cephalosporins.* These have antistaphylococcal activity and are also effective against certain Gram-negative organisms. They comprise cefuroxime, cefamandole and cefoxitin.
3. *Third-generation (wide spectrum) cephalosporins.* These are mainly effective against Gram-negative organisms but not against *Staphylococci*. These include: cefotaxime, cefixime and cefotetan.

Side-effects. Cephalosporins have a low frequency of adverse effects in comparison to antimicrobials in general. The most usual are allergic reactions of the penicillin type. If these are continued for more than 2 weeks, thrombocytopenia, neutropenia, interstitial nephritis or abnormal liver function tests may occur. These resolve on stopping the drug.

Aminoglycosides

These are bactericidal and act primarily against Gram-negative bacilli. These are not absorbed orally, distributed mainly extracellularly and are excreted unchanged in the urine. These are ototoxic and nephrotoxic. Certain aminoglycosides are too toxic for systemic use and hence used only topically. Commonly used preparations are as follows:

1. *Streptomycin.* It is used mainly in tuberculosis.
2. *Gentamicin.* It has become the most commonly used aminoglycoside for acute infections. It has a broader spectrum of action and is effective against *Pseudomonas aeruginosa*. It is nephrotoxic, therefore, its dose must be precisely calculated according to body weight and renal function. For an average adult with normal renal function, the dose is 1-1.5 mg/kg intramuscularly, 8 hourly. Topically, it is used as 0.3% eyedrops.
3. *Tobramycin.* It is 2-4 times more active against *Pseudomonas aeruginosa* and *Proteus* as compared to gentamicin. Topically, it is used as 1% eyedrops.
4. *Amikacin.* It is recommended as a reserve drug for hospital acquired infections with gram-negative bacilli, where gentamicin resistance is increasing.

5. *Neomycin.* It is a widespectrum aminoglycoside, active against most Gram-negative bacilli and some Gram-positive cocci. However, *Pseudomonas* and *Streptococcus pyogenes* are not sensitive to it. It is highly toxic to internal ear and kidney and hence used only topically (0.3-0.5%).
6. *Framycetin.* It is very similar to neomycin. It is also too toxic for systemic use and hence used only topically. It is available as 1 percent skin cream; 0.5 percent eye ointment and eyedrops.

Tetracyclines

These are broad-spectrum bacteriostatic agents with a considerable action against both Gram-positive and Gram-negative organisms as well as some fungi, *Rickettsiae* and *Chlamydiae*. This group includes tetracycline, chlortetracycline and oxytetracycline.

Chloramphenicol

It is also a broad-spectrum antibiotic, primarily bacteriostatic, effective against Gram-positive as well as Gram-negative bacteria, *Rickettsiae*, *Chlamydiae* and *Mycoplasma*.

Its molecule is relatively small and lipid soluble. Therefore, on systemic administration, it enters the eye in therapeutic concentration. Topically it is used as 0.5% eyedrops.

Polypeptides

These are powerful bactericidal agents, but rarely used systemically due to toxicity. Clinically used polypeptides are polymyxin B, bacitracin, colistin and tyrothricin.

1. *Polymyxin B and colistin.* These are active against most Gram-negative bacteria, notably *Pseudomonas*.
2. *Neosporin* (neomycin-polymyxin-bacitracin). It is an effective broad-spectrum antimicrobial but suffers the disadvantage of a high incidence (6-8%) of sensitivity due to neomycin.

Fluoroquinolones

Fluoroquinolones are potent synthetic agents having broad spectrum of activity against Gram-positive and Gram-negative organisms.

Mechanism of action. Fluoroquinolones are bactericidal drugs. They inhibit the bacterial DNA synthesis.

Preparations. Fluroquinolones by convention have been grouped into four generations (Table 18.1).

Table 18.1. Commonly used fluoroquinolones

Generation and drug	*Preparation and doses*	
	Topical	*Systemic*
First generation		
• Ciprofloxacin	0.3%, 1 to 4 hrly.	500 mg orally 12 hrly. 200 mg I/V 12 hrly.
• Norfloxacin	0.3%, 1 to 4 hrly.	400 mg orally 12 hrly.
Second generation		
• Ofloxacin	0.3%, 1 to 4 hrly.	200-400 mg orally 12 hrly. 200 mg I/V 12 hrly.
• Lomefloxacin	0.3%, 1 to 4 hrly.	400 mg orally OD
• Pefloxacin	0.3%, 1 to 4 hrly.	400 mg orally or I/V 12 hrly.
Third generation		
• Sparfloxacin	0.3% 1 to 4 hrly.	400 mg orally on day 1 followed by 200 mg OD
Fourth generation		
• Gatifloxacin	0.3% 1 to 4 hrly.	400 mg OD
• Moxifloxacin	0.5% 1 to 4 hrly.	400 mg OD

ANTIVIRAL DRUGS

These are more often used locally in the eye. Currently available antiviral agents are virostatic. They are active against DNA viruses; especially herpes simplex virus. Antiviral drugs used in ophthalmology can be grouped as below:

For herpes simplex virus infection

- Idoxuridine
- Vidarabine
- Trifluridine
- Acyclovir
- Famiciclovir

For herpes zoster virus infection

- Acyclovir
- Famiciclovir
- Valaciclovir
- Vidarabine
- Sorvudine

For CMV retinitis

- Ganciclovir
- Foscarnet
- Zidovudin

Non selective

- Interferons
- Immunoglobulins

Some of the antiviral drugs are described in brief.

1. *Idoxuridine (IDU, 5-iodo-2 deoxyuridine).* It is a halogenated pyrimidine resembling thymidine. *Mechanism of action.* It inhibits viral metabolism by substituting for thymidine in DNA synthesis and thus prevents replication of virus.

Topically it is used as 10% eye drops.

Preparations. It is available as 0.1 percent eye drops and 0.5 percent eye ointment.

Indications and doses: Since the intraocular penetration of topically applied IDU is very poor, it is not of much value in the treatment of chronic stromal herpetic keratitis. It is mainly used in acute epithelial herpetic keratitis. IDU drops are used one hourly during day and two hourly during night and has to be continued till microscopic staining disappears.

Side-effects include follicular conjunctivitis, lacrimal punctal stenosis and irritation with photophobia.

Contraindications. It is known to inhibit corneal stromal healing, hence its use is not advisable during first few weeks after keratoplasty.

2. *Adenine arabinoside (Ara-A, Vidarabine).* It is a purine nucleoside. It has antiviral activity against herpes simplex, cytomegalo, vaccinia and zoster viruses. It is more potent and less toxic than IDU and is also effective in IDU resistant cases. It has no cross allergenicity with IDU or TF_3 and thus can be used with IDU.

Mechanism of action: It is metabolized to triphosphate form which inhibits DNA polymerase and thus the growth of viral DNA is arrested. *Preparations:* It is available as 3% ophthalmic ointment.

Dose: It is used 5 times a day till epithelization occurs and then reduced to once or twice daily for 4-5 days to prevent recurrences. *Side-effects* are superificial punctate keratitis and irritation on prolonged application.

3. *Cytosine-Arabinoside (Cytarabine).* It is a purine nucleoside.

Mechanism of action: It blocks nucleic acid synthesis by preventing conversion of cytosine ribose to cytosine deoxyribose.

Preparation: It is not commercially available at present. 5 percent solution used as drops has been found experimentally effective for treatment of herpes simplex keratitis.

Side-effects. It causes profound corneal epithelial toxicity with superficial punctate keratitis and iritis. So it is not recommended for clinical use.

4. *Trifluorothymidine (TF_3).* It is a pyrimidine nucleoside. It has the advantage over IDU of higher solubility, greater potency, lack of toxicity and allergic reactions. It is also effective in IDU-resistant cases.

Mechanism of action: It is a DNA inhibitor with same mechanism as IDU.

Preparation: It is available as 1 per cent eyedrops.

Dose: One drop is instilled 4 hourly. If no improvement occurs in 14 days, it is better to change to some other antiviral drug.

Toxicity: It is least toxic. It may cause mild superficial punctate keratitis on prolonged use.

5. *Acyclovir (Acycloguanosine).* It has proved to be an extremely safe and effective agent and is effective in most forms of herpes simplex and herpes zoster infections.

Mechanism of action: It inhibits viral DNA, preferentially entering the infected cells, with little effect on normal cells. It penetrates into deeper layers and thus is very effective in stromal keratitis.

Preparation. It is available as 3 percent ophthalmic ointment and also as tablet for oral use and injection for intravenous use.

Indications and doses: (a) Topical 3 percent ointment is used 5 times a day for epithelial as well as stromal herpes simplex keratitis (b) Oral acyclovir four tablets of 200 mg each, 5 times a day for 5-7 days, may be considered in following situations: (i) After penetrating keratoplasty in patients suffering from herpes simplex keratitis. (ii) Recalcitrant stromal or uveal disease caused by HSV. (iii) To reduce ocular complications of keratitis and uveitis in herpes zoster ophthalmicus.

Side-effects: A few cases show slight punctate epithelial keratopathy which ceases once the drug is stopped.

6. *Valaciclovir.* It is used for treatment of herpes zoster ophthalmicus in a dose of 500-700 mg TDS for 7 days. It is as effective as acyclovir in acute disease and is more effective in reducing late neuralgia.

7. *Famiciclovir.* Its use, dose and effectivity is similar to valaciclovir.

8. *Interferons.* These are non-toxic, species-specific proteins possessing broad-spectrum antiviral activity. However, it is still not available for commercial use.

9. *Immunoglobulins.* These preparations may be useful in the treatment or prophylaxis of certain viral diseases especially in patients with immune deficiencies.

10. *Ganciclovir.* It is used for the treatment of CMV retinitis in immunocompromised individuals. *Dose:* 5 mg/kg body weight every 12 hours for 2-3 weeks, followed by a permanent maintenance dose of 5 mg/kg once daily for 5 out of 7 days.

11. *Foscarnet (Phosphonoformic acid; PFA).* It is as effective as ganciclovir in the treatment of CMV retinitis in AIDS patients.

12. *Zidovudin (azidothymidine; AZT).* It has been recently recommended for selected AIDS patients with non-vision threatening retinitis who have no evidence of systemic CMV infection.

OCULAR ANTIFUNGAL AGENTS

A number of antifungal agents have become available in the recent years. These can be broadly classified on the basis of their chemical structure into polyene antibiotics, imidazole derivatives, pyrimidines and silver compounds.

I. Polyene antifungals

These have been the mainstay of antifungal therapy. These are isolated from various species of *Streptomyces* and consist of a large, conjugated, double-bond system in a lactose ring linked to an amino acid sugar.

Mechanism of action. They work by binding to the sterol groups in fungal cell membranes, rendering them permeable. This occurrence leads to lethal imbalances in cell contents. Polyenes do not penetrate well into the cornea and are not beneficial in deep stromal keratitis.

Preparations. This group includes following drugs:

1. *Nystatin.* It is fungistatic and is well tolerated in the eye as 3.5 percent ointment. It has a medium level of activity in ocular infections caused by *Candida* or *Aspergillus* isolates. Because of its narrow spectrum and poor intraocular penetration its use is restricted.
2. *Amphotericin B (Fungizone).* This antibiotic may act as fungistatic or fungicidal depending upon the concentration of the drug and sensitivity of the fungus. Topically, it is effective in superficial infections of the eye in the concentration of 0.075 to 0.3 percent drops. Subconjunctival injections are quite painful and more than 300 mg is poorly tolerated.

   Amphotericin B may be given intravitreally or/and intravenously for treatment of intraocular infections caused by *Candida*, *Histoplasma*, *Cryptococcus* and some strains of *Aspergillus* and others. For intravenous administration a solution of 0.1 mg/ml in 5 percent dextrose with heparin is used.
3. *Natamycin (Pimaricin).* It is a broad-spectrum antifungal drug having activity against *Candida*, *Aspergillus, Fusarium* and *Cephalosporium*. Topical application of 5 percent pimaricin suspension produces effective concentrations within the corneal stroma but not in intraocular fluid. It is the drug of choice for *Fusarium solani* keratitis. It adheres well to the surface of the ulcer, making the contact time of the antifungal agent with the eye greater. It is not recommended for injection.

II. Imidazole antifungal drugs

Various imidazole derivatives available for use in ocular fungal infections include: miconazole, clotrimazole, ketoconazole, econazole and itraconazole.

1. *Miconazole.* It possesses a broad antifungal spectrum and is fungicidal to various species of *Candida, Aspergillus, Fusarium, Cryptococcus, Cladosporium, Trichophyton* and many others. Topical (1%) and subconjunctival (10 mg) application of miconazole produces high levels of drug in the cornea which is more dramatic in the presence of epithelial defect.
2. *Clotrimazole.* It is fungistatic and is effective against *Candida, Aspergillus* and many others. Its 1 percent suspension is effective topically and is the treatment of choice in *Aspergillus* infections of the eye.
3. *Econazole.* It also has broad-spectrum antifungal activity and is used topically as 1 percent econazole nitrate ointment. Because of its poor intraocular penetration, it is effective only in superficial infections of the eye.

4. *Ketoconazole.* It is effective after oral administration and possesses activity against common fungi. It is given as single oral dose of 200-400 mg daily up to at least one week after the symptoms have disappeared. It is an adjunctive systemic antifungal agent in fungal keratitis complicated by endophthalmitis.
5. *Fluconazole.* It is fungistatic drug active against *Candida, Aspergillus* and *Cryptococcus*. It is available for oral use (50-100 mg tablets) and also for topical use (0.2% eyedrops).
6. *Itraconazole.* It is prescribed for treatment of fungal infections caused primarily by *Aspergillus*, *Histoplasmosis*, *Blastomycosis*. It has moderate effect against *Candida* and *Fusarium* infections. It is available for oral and topical use. Oral dose is 200 mg twice daily for a week. Topically it is used as 1% eye drops.

III. Pyridine

This group includes ***flucystosine***, which is a fluorinated salt of pyrimidine. Its mechanism of action is not clear. The drug is very effective against *Candida* species and yeasts. It is used as 1.5 percent aqueous drops hourly. It can also be given orally or intravenously in doses of 200 mg/kg/day.

IV. Silver compounds

Combination of silver with sulfonamides and with other anti-microbial compounds significantly increases the activity against bacterial and fungal infections. In this context several silver compounds have been synthesized. Most frequently used is *silver sulphadiazine* which is reported to be highly effective against *Aspergillus* and *Fusarium* species.

MYDRIATICS AND CYCLOPLEGICS

(See pages 99, 155 and 582)

ANTI-GLAUCOMA DRUGS

Classification

A. Parasympathomimetic drugs (Miotics)
B. Sympathomimetic drugs (Adrenergic agonists)
C. β-blockers
D. Carbonic anhydrase inhibitors
E. Hyperosmotic agents
F. Prostaglandins
G. Calcium channel blockers

A. Parasympathomimetic drugs (Miotics)

Parasympathomimetics, also called as *cholinergic drugs*, either imitate or potentiate the effects of acetylcholine.

Classification

Depending upon the mode of action, these can be classified as follows:

1. *Direct-acting* or agonists e.g., pilocarpine.
2. *Indirect-acting parasympathomimetics or cholinesterase inhibitors:* As the name indicates these drugs act indirectly by destroying the enzyme cholinesterase; thereby sparing the naturally acting acetylcholine for its actions. These drugs have been divided into two subgroups, designated as *reversible* (e.g., physostigmine) and *irreversible* (e.g., echothiophate iodide, demecarium and diisopropyl-fluorophosphate, DFP_3) anti-cholinesterases.
3. *Dual-action parasympathomimetics, i.e.,* which act as both a muscarinic agonist as well as a weak cholinesterase inhibitor e.g., carbachol.

Mechanism of action

1. *In primary open-angle glaucoma* the miotics reduce the intraocular pressure (IOP) by enhancing the aqueous outflow facility. This is achieved by changes in the trabecular meshwork produced by a pull exerted on the scleral spur by contraction of the longitudinal fibres of ciliary muscle.
2. *In primary angle-closure glaucoma* these reduce the IOP due to their miotic effect by opening the angle. The mechanical contraction of the pupil moves the iris away from the trabecular meshwork.

Side-effects

1. *Systemic side-effects* noted are: bradycardia, increased sweating, diarrhoea, excessive salivation and anxiety. The only serious complication noted with irreversible cholinesterase inhibitors is 'scoline apnoea', i.e., inability of the patient to resume normal respiration after termination of general anaesthesia.
2. *Local side-effects* are encountered more frequently with long-acting miotics (i.e. irreversible cholinesterase inhibitors). These include problems due to miosis itself (e.g. reduced visual acuity in the presence of polar cataracts, impairment of night vision and generalized contraction of visual

fields), spasm of accommodation which may cause myopia and frontal headache, retinal detachment, lenticular opacities, iris cyst formation, mild iritis, lacrimation and follicular conjunctivitis.

Preparations

1. *Pilocarpine*. It is a direct-acting parasympathomimetic drug. Earlier it was the most commonly used and the most extensively studied miotic. However, presently, due to availability of many better drugs, it is not being preferred as the option for treatment in POAG. Even in PNAG, many glaucoma experts are discouraging its use. *Indications:* (i) Primary open-angle glaucoma; (ii) Acute angle-closure glaucoma; (iii) Chronic synechial angle-closure glaucoma. *Contraindications:* inflammatory glaucoma, malignant glaucoma and known allergy. *Available preparations* and dosage are: (a) *Eyedrops* are available in 1%, 2% and 4% strengths. Except in very darkly pigmented irides maximum effect is obtained with a 4 percent solution. In POAG, therapy is usually initiated with 1 percent concentration. The onset of action occurs in 20 minutes, peak in 2 hours and duration of effect is 4-6 hours. Therefore, the eyedrops are usually prescribed every 6 or 8 hourly. (b) *Ocuserts* are available as pilo-20 and pilo-40. These are changed once in a week. Pilo-20 is generally used in patients controlled with 2 percent or less concentration of eyedrops; and pilo-40 in those requiring higher concentration of eyedrops. (c) *Pilocarpine gel* (4%) is a bedtime adjunct to the daytime medication.

2. *Carbachol*. It is a dual-action (agonist as well as weak cholinesterase inhibitor) miotic. *Indications.* It is a very good alternative to pilocarpine in resistant or intolerant cases. *Preparations.* It is available as 0.75 percent and 3 percent eyedrops. *Dosage:* The action ensues in 40 minutes and lasts for about 12 hours. Therefore, the drops are instilled 2 or 3 times a day.

3. *Echothiophate iodide (Phospholine iodide)*. It is a long acting cholinesterase inhibitor. *Indications:* It is very effective in POAG. *Preparations:* Available as 0.03, 0.06 and 0.125 percent eyedrops. *Dosage:* The onset of action occurs within 2 hours and lasts up to 24 hours. Therefore, it is instilled once or twice daily.

4. *Demecarium bromide*. It is similar to ecothiopate iodide and is used as 0.125 percent or 0.25 percent eyedrops.

5. *Physostigmine* (eserine). It is a reversible (weak) cholinesterase inhibitor. It is used as 0.5 percent ointment twice a day.

B. Sympathomimetic drugs

Sympathomimetics, also known as *adrenergic agonists,* act by stimulation of alpha, beta or both the receptors.

Classification

Depending upon the mode of action, these can be classified as follows:

1. Both alpha and beta-receptor stimulators e.g., epinephrine.
2. Direct alpha-adrenergic stimulators e.g., norepinephrine and clonidine hydrochloride.
3. Indirect alpha-adrenergic stimulators e.g., pargyline.
4. Beta-adrenergic stimulator e.g., isoproterenol.

Mechanisms of action

1. Increased aqueous outflow results by virtue of both alpha and beta-receptor stimulation.
2. Decreased aqueous humour production occurs due to stimulation of alpha-receptors in the ciliary body.

Side-effects

1. *Systemic side-effects* include hypertension, tachycardia, headache, palpitation, tremors, nervousness and anxiety.
2. *Local side-effects* are burning sensation, reactive hyperaemia of conjunctiva, conjunctival pigmentation, allergic blepharo conjunctivitis, mydriasis and cystoid macular oedema (in aphakics).

Preparations

1. *Epinephrine*. This direct-acting sympathomimetic drug stimulates both alpha and beta- adrenergic receptors. *Indications:* (i) It is one of the standard drugs used for the management of POAG. (ii) It is also useful in most of the secondary glaucomas. *Preparations:* It is available as 0.5 percent, 1 percent and 2 percent eyedrops. *Dosage:* The action starts within 1 hour and lasts up to 12-24 hours. Therefore, it is instilled twice daily.

2. *Dipivefrine* (Propine or dipivalylepinephrine). It is a prodrug which is converted into epinephrine after its absorption into the eye. It is more lipophilic than epinephrine and thus its corneal penetration is increased by 17 times. *Preparations:* It is available as 0.1 percent eyedrops. *Dosage:* Action and efficacy is similar to 1 percent epinephrine. It is instilled twice daily.

3. *Clonidine hydrochloride.* It is a centrally-acting systemic antihypertensive agent, which has been shown to lower the IOP by decreasing aqueous humour production by stimulation of alpha-receptors in the ciliary body. *Preparations and dosage:* It is used as 0.125 percent and 0.25 percent eye drops, twice daily.

4. *Brimonidine* (0.2%). *Mechanism of action*. It is a selective alpha-2 adrenergic agonist and lowers IOP by decreasing aqueous production and enhancing uveoscleral outflow. It has an additive effect to beta-blockers. *Dosage:* It has a peak effect of 2 hours and action lasts for 12 hours; so it is administered twice daily.

5. *Apraclonidine* (0.5%, 1%). It is also alpha-2 adrenergic agonist like brimonidine. It is an extremely potent ocular hypotensive drug and is commonly used prophylactically for prevention of IOP elevation following laser trabeculoplasty, YAG laser iridotomy and posterior capsulotomy. It is of limited use for long-term administration because of the high rate of ocular side-effects.

C. Beta-adrenergic blockers

These are, presently, the most frequently used antiglaucoma drugs. The commonly used preparations are timolol and betaxolol. Other available preparations include levobunolol, carteolol and metipranolol.

Mechanism of action. Timolol and levobunolol are non-selective beta-1 (Cardiac) and beta-2 (smooth muscle, pulmonary) receptor blocking agents. Betaxolol has 10 times more affinity for beta-1 than beta-2 receptors.

The drugs timolol and levobunolol lower IOP by blockade of beta-2 receptors in the ciliary processes, resulting in decreased aqueous production. The exact mechanism of action of betaxolol (cardioselective beta-blocker) is unknown.

Indications. Beta adrenergic blockers are useful in all types of glaucomas, viz., developmental, primary and secondary; narrow as well as open angle. Unless contraindicated due to systemic diseases, beta-blockers are frequently used as the first choice drug in POAG and all secondary glaucomas.

Contraindications. These drugs should be used with caution or not at all, depending on the severity of the systemic disease in patients with bronchial asthma, emphysema, COPD, heart blocks, congestive heart failure or cardiomyopathy. Betaxolol is the beta blocker, of choice in patients at risk for pulmonary diseases. The other contraindication includes known drug allergies.

Additive effects. Beta-blockers have very good synergistic effect when combined with miotics; and are thus often used in combination in patients with POAG, unresponsive to the single drug.

Side-effects

1. *Ocular side-effects* are not frequent. These include burning and conjunctival hyperaemia, superficial punctate keratopathy and corneal anaesthesia.

2. *Systemic side-effects* are also unusually low. However, these are reported more often than ocular side-effects. These include (i) *Cardiovascular effects* which result from blockade of beta-1 receptors. These are bradycardia, arrhythmias, heart failure and syncope. (ii) *Respiratory reactions:* These include bronchospasm and airway obstruction, especially in asthmatics. These occur due to blockade of beta-2 receptors; and thus are not known with betaxolol. (iii) *Central nervous system effects.* These include depression, anxiety, confusion, drowsiness, disorientation, hallucinations, emotional lability, dysarthria and so on. (iv) *Miscellaneous effects* are nausea, diarrhoea, decreased libido, skin rashes, alopecia and exacerbation of myasthenia gravis.

Preparations

1. *Timolol.* It is a non-selective beta-1 and beta-2 blocker. It is available as 0.25 per cent and 0.5 percent eye drops. The salt used is timolol maleate. Its action starts within 30 minutes, peak reaches in 2 hours and effects last up to 24 hours. Therefore, it is used once or twice daily. The drug is very effective, however, the phenomenon of 'short-term escape' and 'long-term drift' are well known. '*Short-term escape*' implies marked initial fall in IOP, followed by a transient rise with continued moderate fall in IOP. The '*long-term drift*' implies a slow rise in IOP in patients who were well controlled with many months of therapy.

2. *Betaxolol.* It is a cardioselective beta-blocker and thus can be used safely in patients prone to attack of bronchial asthma; an advantage over timolol. It is available as 0.5 percent suspension, and 0.25 percent suspension, and is used twice daily. Its action starts within 30 minutes, reaches peak in 2 hours and lasts for 12 hours. It is slightly less effective than timolol in lowering the IOP.

3. *Levobunolol.* It is available as 0.5 percent solution and its salient features are almost similar to timolol.

4. *Carteolol.* It is available as 1 percent and 2 per cent solution and is almost similar to timolol except that it induces comparatively less bradycardia.

5. *Metipranolol.* It is available as 0.1 percent, 0.3 percent and 0.6 percent solution and is almost similar to timolol in all aspects.

D. Carbonic anhydrase inhibitors (CAIs)

These are potent and most commonly used systemic antiglaucoma drugs. These include acetazolamide (most frequently used), methazolamide, dichlorphenamide and ethoxzolamide.

Mechanism of action. As the name indicates CAIs inhibit the enzyme carbonic anhydrase which is related to the process of aqueous humour production. Thus, CAIs lower the IOP by reducing the aqueous humour formation.

Indications. These are used as additive therapy for short term in the management of all types of acute and chronic glaucomas. Their long-term use is reserved for patients with high risk of visual loss, where all other treatments fail.

Side-effects. Unfortunately, 40-50 percent of patients are unable to tolerate CAIs for long term because of various disabling side-effects. These include:

1. *Paresthesias* of the fingers, toes, hands, feet and around the mouth are experienced by most of the patients. However, these are transient and of no consequence.

2. *Urinary frequency* may also be complained by most of patients due to the diuretic effect.

3. *Serum electrolyte imbalances* may occur with higher doses of CAIs. These may be in the form of (i) *Bicarbonate depletion* leading to metabolic acidosis. This is associated with '*malaise symptom complex*', which includes: malaise, fatigue, depression, loss of libido, anorexia and weight loss. Treatment with sodium bicarbonate or sodium acetate may help to minimize this situation in many patients. (ii) *Potassium depletion.* It may occur in some patients, especially those simultaneously getting corticosteroids, aspirin or thiazide diuretics. Potassium supplement is indicated only when significant hypokalemia is documented. (iii) *Serum sodium and chloride* may be transiently reduced; more commonly with dichlorphenamide.

4. *Gastrointestinal symptom complex.* It is also very common. It is not related to the malaise symptom complex caused by biochemical changes in the serum. Its features include—vague abdominal discomfort, gastric irritation, nausea, peculiar metallic taste and diarrhoea.

5. *Sulfonamide related side-effects of CAIs,* seen rarely, include renal calculi, blood dyscrasias, Stevens-Johnson syndrome, transient myopia, hypertensive nephropathy and teratogenic effects.

Preparations and doses

1. *Acetazolamide* (diamox). It is available as tablets, capsules and injection for intravenous use. The acetazolamide 250 mg tablet is used 6 hourly. Its action starts within 1 hour, peak is reached in 4 hours and the effect lasts for 6-8 hours.

2. *Dichlorphenamide.* It is available as 50 mg tablets. Its recommended dose is 25 to 100 mg three times a day. It causes less metabolic acidosis but has a sustained diuretic effect.

3. *Methazolamide.* It is also available as 50 mg tablets. It has a longer duration of action than acetazolamide. Its dose is 50-100 mg, 2 or 3 times a day.

4. *Ethoxzolamide.* It is given in a dosage of 125 mg every 6 hours and is similar to acetazolamide in all aspects.

5. *Dorzolamide* (2%). It is a topical carbonic anhydrase inhibitor. It is water soluble, stable in solution and has excellent corneal penetration. It decreases IOP by 22% and has got additive effect with timolol. It is administered thrice daily. Its *side effects* include burning sensation and local allergic reaction.

6. *Brinzolamide* (1%). It is also a topical CAI which decreases IOP by decreasing aqueous production. It is administered twice daily (BD).

E. Hyperosmotic agents

These are the second class of compounds, which are administered systemically to lower the IOP. These include: glycerol, mannitol, isosorbide and urea.

Mechanism of action. Hyperosmotic agents increase the plasma tonicity. Thus, the osmotic pressure gradient created between the blood and vitreous draws sufficient water out of the eyeball, thereby significantly lowering the IOP.

Indications. These are used as additive therapy for rapidly lowering the IOP in emergency situations, such as acute angle-closure glaucoma or secondary glaucomas with very high IOP. They are also used as a prophylactic measure prior to intraocular surgery.

Preparations and doses

1. ***Glycerol.*** It is a frequently used oral hyperosmotic agent. Its recommended dose is 1-1.5 gm/kg body weight. It is used as a 50 percent solution. So, glycerol (50 to 80 ml in adults) is mixed with equal amount of lemon juice (preferably) or water before administering orally. Its action starts in 10 minutes, peaks in 30 minutes and lasts for about 5-6 hours. It can be given repeatedly. It is metabolised to glucose in the body. Thus, its repeated use in diabetics is not recommended.

2. ***Mannitol.*** It is the most widely used intravenous hyperosmotic agent. It is indicated when the oral agents are felt to be insufficient or when they cannot be taken for reasons such as nausea. Its recommended dose is 1-2 gm/kg body weight. It is used as a 20 percent solution. It should be administered very rapidly over 20-30 minutes. Its action peaks in 30 minutes and lasts for about 6 hours. It does not enter the glucose metabolism and thus is safe in diabetics. However, it should be used cautiously in hypertensive patients.

3. ***Urea.*** When administered intravenously it also lowers the IOP. However, because of lower efficacy and more side-effects than mannitol, it is not recommended for routine use.

4. ***Isosorbide.*** It is an oral hyperosmotic agent, similar to glycerol in action and doses. However, metabolically it is inert and thus can be used repeatedly in diabetics.

F. Prostaglandin derivatives

1. ***Latanoprost*** (0.005%). It is a synthetic drug which is an ester analogue of prostaglandin F_2-α. It acts by increasing uveoscleral outflow and by causing reduction in episcleral venous pressure. It is as effective as timolol. It has additive effect with pilocarpine and timolol. Its duration of action is 24 hours and is, thus, administered once daily. Its side-effects include conjunctival hyperaemia, foreign body sensation and increased pigmentation of the iris.

2. ***Bimatoprost*** (0.03%). It is a prostamide which decreases IOP by decreasing ocular outflow resistance. It is used once a day (OD).

3. ***Travoprost*** (0.004%). It is a synthetic prostaglandin F_2 analogue and decreases IOP by increasing uveoscleral outflow of aqueous.

4. ***Unoprostive isopropyl*** (0.12%). It is a dolosanoid related in structure to prostaglandin F_2-α. It lowers IOP by increasing uveoscleral outflow of aqueous. It also increases retinal blood flow.

G. Calcium channel blockers

Calcium channel blockers such as nifedipine, diltiazem and verapamil are commonly used antihypertensive drugs. Recently, some of these have been used as anti-glaucoma drugs.

Mechanism of action. The exact mechanism of lowering IOP of topically used calcium channel blockers remains to be elucidated. It might be due to its effects on secretory ciliary epithelium.

Preparations. Verapamil has been tried as 0.125 percent and 0.25 percent eyedrops twice a day.

Indications. Though the IOP lowering effect of verapamil is not superior than the standard topical antiglaucoma drugs, it has a place in the mangement of patients with POAG, where miotics, beta-blockers and sympathomimetics are all contraindicated e.g., in patients suffering simultaneously from axial cataract, bronchial asthma and raised blood pressure. It can also be used for additive effect with pilocarpine and timolol.

Antiglaucoma drugs: Mechanism of lowering IOP at a glance

Drugs which increase trabecular outflow

- Miotics (e.g., pilocarpine)
- Epinephrine, Dipivefrine
- Bimatoprost

Drugs which increase uveoscleral outflow

- Prostaglandins (latanoprost)
- Epinephrine, Dipivefrine
- Brimonidine
- Apraclonidine

Drugs which decrease aqueous production

- *Carbonic anhydrase inhibitors* (e.g., acetazolamide, dorzolamide).
- *Alpha receptor stimulators* in ciliary process (e.g., epinephrine, dipivefrine, clonidine, brimonidine, apraclonidine.
- *Beta blockers* (e.g., timolol, betaxolol, levobunolol).

Hyperosmotic agents (e.g., glycerol, mannitol, urea).

CORTICOSTEROIDS

These are 21-C compounds secreted by the adrenal cortex. They have potent anti-inflammatory, anti-allergic and anti-fibrotic actions. Corticosteroids reduce inflammation by reduction of leukocytic and plasma exudation, maintenance of cellular membrane integrity with inhibition of tissue swelling, inhibition of lysosome release from granulocytes, increased stabilisation of intracellular lysosomal membranes and suppression of circulating lymphocytes.

Classification and relative anti-inflammatory drug potency (Table 18.2)

Table 18.2. Corticosteroids: equivalent anti-inflammatory oral dose (mg) and relative anti-inflammatory potency

Drug	*Equivalent anti-inflammatory oral dose (mg)*	*Relative anti-inflammatory potency*
I. *Glucocorticoids*		
1. *Short acting*		
Hydrocortisone (Cortisol)	20	1
Cortisone	25	0.8
Prednisolone	5	4
Prednisone	5	4
Methylprednisolone	4	5
2. *Intermediate-acting*		
Triamcinolone	4	5
Fluprednisolone	1.5	15
3. *Long-acting*		
Dexamethasone	0.75	26
Betamethasone	0.60	33
II. *Mineralocorticoids*		
Fludrocortisone	2	10

Preparations and modes of administration

Corticosteroids may be administered locally in the form of drops, ointments or injections and systemically in the form of tablets or injections.

(A) *Topical ophthalmic preparations used commonly are as follows:*

Cortisone acetate	As 0.5% suspension and 1.5% ointment
Hydrocortisone	As 0.5% suspension acetate and 0.2% solution
Dexamethasone	As 0.1% solution and sodium phosphate 0.5% ointment
Betamethasone	As 0.1% solution and sodium phosphate 0.1% ointment
Medryson	1% suspension
Flurometholone	0.1% suspension
Loteprednol	0.5% suspension

(B) *Systemic corticosteroid preparations used commonly are:*

Prednisolone	As 5 mg, 10 mg tab and solution for injection in the strength of 20 mg/ml
Dexamethasone	As 0.5 mg tab and solution for injection in the strength of 4 mg/ml
Betamethasone	0.5 mg and 1 mg tab

Ocular indications

1. *Topical preparations* are used in uveitis, scleritis, allergic conjunctivitis (vernal catarrh and phlyctenular conjunctivitis), allergic keratitis, cystoid macular oedema and after intraocular surgery.
2. *Systemic preparations* are indicated in posterior uveitis, sympathetic ophthalmia, Vogt-Koyanagi-Harada syndrome (VKH), papillitis, retrobulbar neuritis, anterior ischaemic optic neuropathy, scleritis, malignant exophthalmos, orbital pseudotumours, orbital lymphangioma and corneal graft rejections.

Side-effects

Injudicious use of *topical steroids* may cause glaucoma, cataract, activation of infection (if given in herpetic, fungal and bacterial keratitis), dry eye and ptosis.

Misuse of *systemic corticosteroids* may cause ocular and systemic side-effects. Ocular complications include cataract, glaucoma, activation of infection, delayed wound healing, papilloedema, and central retinal vein occlusion.

Systemic complications include peptic ulcer, hypertension, osteoporosis, aggravation of diabetes mellitus, mental changes, cushingoid state and reactivation of tuberculosis and other infections.

NONSTEROIDAL ANTI-INFLAMMATORY DRUGS

Nonsteroidal anti-inflammatory drugs (NSAIDs), often referred to as 'aspirin-like drugs', are a heterogeneous group of anti-inflammatory, analgesic and antipyretic compounds. These are often chemically unrelated (although most of them are organic acids), but share certain therapeutic actions and side-effects.

Mechanisms of action

The NSAIDs largely act by irreversibly blocking the enzyme cyclo-oxygenase, thus inhibiting the prostaglandin biosynthesis. They also appear to block other local mediators of the inflammatory response such as polypeptides of the kinin system, lysosomal enzymes, lymphokinase and thromboxane A2; but not the leukotrienes.

Preparations

A. *NSAIDs available for systemic use* can be grouped as follows:

1. *Salicylates* e.g., aspirin.
2. *Pyrazolone derivatives* e.g., phenylbutazone, oxyphenbutazone, aminopyrine and apazone.
3. *Para-aminophenol derivatives* e.g., phenacetin and acetaminophen.
4. *Indole derivatives* e.g., indomethacin and sulindac.
5. *Propionic acid derivatives* e.g., ibuprofen, naproxen and flurbiprofen.
6. *Anthranilic acid derivatives* e.g., mefenamic acid and flufenamic acid.
7. *Other newer NSAIDs* e.g., ketorolac tromethamine, carprofen and diclofenac.

B. *Topical ophthalmic NSAIDs preparations* available include:

1. *Indomethacin* suspension (0.1%)
2. *Flurbiprofen,* 0.3% eyedrops
3. *Ketorolac tromethamine,* 0.5% eyedrops
4. *Diclofenac sodium,* 0.1% eyedrops
5. *Bromefenac*, 0.09% eyedrops
6. *Nepafenac*, 0.1% eyedrops

Ophthalmic indications of NSAIDs

1. *Episcleritis and scleritis.* Recalcitrant cases of episcleritis may be treated with systemic NSAIDs such as oxyphenbutazone 100 mg TDS or indomethacin 25 mg BD.

   NSAIDs may also suppress the inflammation in diffuse and nodular varieties of scleritis, but are not likely to control the necrotizing form.
2. *Uveitis.* NSAIDs are usually not used as the primary agents in therapy of uveitis. They are, however, useful in the long-term therapy of recurrent anterior uveitis, initially controlled by steroid therapy. Phenylbutazone is of use in uveitis associated with ankylosing spondylitis.
3. *Cystoid macular oedema (CME).* Topical and/or systemic antiprostaglandin drugs are effective in preventing the postoperative CME occurring after cataract operation. The drug (e.g., 0.03% flurbiprofen eyedrops) is started 2 days preoperatively and continued for 6-8 weeks post-operatively.
4. *Pre-operatively to maintain dilatation of the pupil.* Flurbiprofen drops used every 5 minutes for 2 hours preoperatively are very effective in maintaining the pupillary dilatation during the operation of extracapsular cataract extraction with or without intraocular lens implantation.
5. *Spring catarrh.* Sodium cromoglycate 2 percent inhibits degranulation of the mast cells and thus is more useful when used prophylactically in patients with spring catarrh. Topical antiprostaglandins are effective in the treatment of spring catarrh.
6. *Topical antihistaminics* are helpful in cases of mild allergic conjunctivitis.

INTRAOCULAR IRRIGATING SOLUTIONS

Functions

Intraocular irrigating solutions are the most essential tools for the modern cataract surgery and other intraocular surgeries. These are aqueous solutions which sub-serve the following functions:

- *Clear and maintain moisture* of the ocular tissues.
- *Maintain physiological and anatomical integrity* of the intraocular tissues and chamber.
- *Provide cellular nutrients* required for intercellular and intracellular functions during prolonged intraocular surgery.
- *Maintain corneal transparency* during intraocular surgery by maintaining endothelial cell metabolism and then avoiding corneal clouding .
- Maintain intraocular pressure during the surgery.

Indications/Uses

- *Cataract surgery.* Irrigating solutions are essential for each and every step of modern cataract surgery with IOL implantation.

- *Glaucoma surgery*. In trabeculectomy and other invasive filteration surgery, irrigation solution helps to maintain the chamber, wash detirious substances and maintain tissues moisture
- *Corneal surgery* and anterior segment reconstruction.
- *Vitrectomy and posterior segment surgery.*

Commercially available intraocular irrigating solutions

Commercially available irrigating solutions suitable for intraocular use include:

- Lactated Ringers solution
- Balanced salt solution (BSS)
- Balanced salt solution plus(BSS-Plus)

Salient features of commercially available irrigating solutions:

1. *Lactated Ringers solution*

Composition in mMoles/liter is: NaCl (102), KCl(4), $CaCl_2$ (3), and sodium lactate (28).

pH of lactate Ringers solution is 7.2

Osmolality is 279

Advantages: Maintains the integrity of intraocular tissues.

Disadvantages: Since it contains sodium lactate in much higher concentration than aqueous humour , so prolonged perfusion causes endothelial cell break down and corneal swelling.

2. *Balanced salt solution(BSS)*

Composition in mmol/liter is: NaCl(110), KCl(10), $CaCl_3$(3), $MgCl_2$(1.5), Sodium citrate (8) and sodium acetate (29),

pH of BSS is 7.4,

Osmolality is 305.

Advantages: It is better tolerated irrigant which helps to maintain the integrity of intraocular tissues.

Disadvantages: BSS is less protective to corneal endothelial cells as compared to BSS plus as it lacks the bicarbonate, glucose and glutathione. After prolonged exposure it may result in:

- *Polymegathism*, i.e., a significant increase in the co-efficient of variation of cell area;
- *Pleomorphism*, i.e., a significant decrease in the percentage of hexagonal cells; and
- *Stressed endothelial monolayer*, which may be more susceptible to additional surgical trauma

3. *Balanced salt solution (BSS) plus*

Composition: The concentration of constituents of BSS Plus, also known as GBR (glutathione, bicarbonate, Ringers) in mMole/L is NaCl(122.2.2), KCl(5.08), $MgCl_2$ (0.98), disodium phosphate (2.5), dextrose (5.11), oxidized glutathione (0.30), and sodium bicarbonate (25)

pH of BSS plus is 7.4,

Osmolality (mosm) is 305

Advantages of BSS plus are as below:

- *Iso-osmotic* with intraocular tissues.
- *Corneal endothelium functioning is maintained* even on prolonged irrigation and thus minimal changes occur in endothelial morphologic characteristics.
- *Lens clarity is maintained* in posterior segment surgery.
- *Blood aqueous barrier is maintained* by glutathione which protects the cells against oxidative stress and thus inflammation is minimized.

VISCOELASTIC SUBSTANCES

Use of viscous or viscoelastic substances has become almost mandatory in the modern microphthalmic surgery, especially intraocular lens implantation, which involves a risk of involuntary tissue damage due to intraocular manipulations.

Properties of viscoelastic substances

An ideal viscoelastic substance should have the following properties:

1. *Chemically* the material should be inert, iso-osmotic, free from particulate matter, non-pyrogenic, non-antigenic, non-toxic and sterile.
2. *Optically* clear.
3. *Viscosity* of the substances should be enough to provide sufficient space for manipulation within the eye.
4. *Hydrophilic* and dilutable properties are necessary to irrigate the material out of the eye after the operation.
5. *Protectability and maintenance of space.* It should protect the endothelium, separate the tissues, maintain the space and act as a lubricant.

Preparations

1. *Methylcellulose.* It is the most commonly used substance. It is only a viscous and not a

viscoelastic substance. Its active ingredient is highly purified 2% hydroxypropyl methylcellulose.

2. *Sodium hyaluronate (1%) (Healon).* Being extremely viscoelastic and non-inflammatory, it is the best available viscoelastic substance. However, being expensive, it is less popular than methylcellulose.
3. *Hypromellose (2%).* It is a viscous substance similar to methylcellulose.
4. *Chondroitin sulfate (20% and 50%).* It is a viscoelastic substance similar to sodium hyaluronate. It is also available as 1:3 mixture of 4% chondroitin sulfate and 3% sodium hyaluronate (Viscoat) and in combination with methylcellulose (Ocugel).

Alternatives to viscoelastic substances

Substances used as alternative to viscoelastics for maintenance of anterior chamber are air, serum and other blood products and balanced salt solution. However, none of these match the properties of viscoelastic substances.

Clinical uses

1. *Cataract surgery with or without IOL implantation.* It is the most important indication. Here the viscoelastic substance is used for:
   - i. Maintenance of anterior chamber;
   - ii. Protection of corneal endothelium;
   - iii. Coating the IOL
   - iv. Preventing the entry of blood and fluid in the anterior chamber.
2. *Other uses.* Viscoelastic substances are also useful in glaucoma surgery, keratoplasty, retinal detachment surgery and repair of the globe in perforating injuries.

Side-effects

Post-operative rise in intraocular pressure may occur if a considerable amount of viscoelastic substance is left inside the anterior chamber; so it must be washed off after surgery.

VITREOUS SUBSTITUTES

(See page 262).

ANTI-VASCULAR ENDOTHELIAL GROWTH FACTOR AGENTS (Anti-VEGF)

The vascular endothelial growth factors (VEGF-A) are the key factors blamed for producing neovascularization disorders e.g. choroidal neovascularization (wet ARMD), retinal neovascularization (diabetic retinopathy, sickle cell retinopathy, neovascular glaucoma in CRVO etc.). There are 9 isoforms of VEGF-A of which VEGF-165 is the most abundantly expressed but all isoforms are thought to contribute to ocular angiogenesis.

Anti-vascular endothelial growth factor (anti-VEGF) agents, which have revolutionized the treatment of ocular diseases associated with neovascularization include:

- Ranibizumab (Lucentis),
- Pegaptanib (Macugen), and
- Bevacizumab (Avastin).

Ranibizumab

Ranibizumab (marketed as Lucentis by Genentech, USA) is a humanized monoclonal antibody fragment (fab). Its production is by an *E.Coli* expression system in a nutrient medium. Its molecular weight is 48KD and it has a short half-life of 2 hours.

Mechanism of action. Ranibizumab binds to all isoforms of VEGF-A and inhibits their biological activity.

Dose. It is the only FDA approved non-selective anti-VEGF agent for the treatment of choroidal neovascularization or as multiple intra-vitreal injection (every 8 weeks) in the dose of 0.5 mg/0.05 ml. Available as 0.23 ml vial containing 10 mg/ml of the drug.

Pegaptanib

Pegaptanib (marketed as Macugen by Eyetech pharmaceuticals, USA) is a pegylatedaptamer (i.e. an oligonucleotide with polyethylene glycol covalently attached). Its molecular weight is 50 KD.

Mechanism of action. It binds with high affinity to VEGF-165 isoform of VEGF-A and inhibits its activity thereby inhibiting angiogenesis.

Intravitreal dose is 0.3 mg in 90 µl (multiple injections every 6 weeks).

Bevacizumab

Bevacizumab (marketed as Avastin by Gentech,USA) is a full length recombinant humanized monoclonal antibody (IgG1) against VEGF-A. Its molecular weight is 149KD. It is currently approved for colorectal cancers as an intravitreous injection. Its off-label use in ocular neovascular disorders, e.g. wet ARMD have shown its effectivity.

Mechanism of action. It binds to all isoforms of VEGF-A and inhibits their activity.

Intravitreal dose. Available as 4 ml vial containing 100 mg of the drug. Its intravitreal dose is 1.25 mg (0.05 ml).

Indications for anti-VEGF agents include Neovascular Age Related Macular Degeneration (common indication), diabetic retinopathy, retinal vein occlusion, neovascular glaucoma, myopic CNV, inflammatory CNV, choroidalosteoma, juxtafoveal telangiectasia, ROP, idiopathic polypoidalchoroidopathy, pseudophakic cystoid edema and central serous retinopathy.

Complications of intravitreal injection of anti-VEGF agents include cataract, glaucoma, vitreous haemorrhage, endophthalmitis, retinal detachment etc.

LASERS IN OPHTHALMOLOGY

The word LASER is an acronym for 'Light Amplification by Stimulated Emission of Radiation'. Laser light is characterised by monochromaticity, coherence and collimation. These properties make it the brightest existing light.

PRODUCTION OF LASER BEAM

In the laser system atomic environments of various types are stimulated to produce laser light. A laser system consists of a transparent crystal rod or a gas or liquid filled cavity constructed with a fully reflective mirror at one end and a partially reflective mirror at the other. Surrounding the rod or cavity is an optical or electrical source of energy that will raise the energy level of the atoms within the cavity or rod to a high and unstable level. This phenomenon is called *population inversion.* From this level, the atoms spontaneously decay back to a lower energy level, releasing the excess energy in the form of light which is amplified to an appropriate wavelength. Thus, laser is created mainly by two means: population inversion in active medium and amplification of appropriate wavelength of light.

TYPES OF LASERS

There are various types of lasers depending upon the type of atomic environment stimulated to produce the laser beam. Common types of lasers are depicted in Table 18.3.

Table 18.3. Lasers used in ophthalmology

Type of laser	*Atomic environment used*	*Effects produced*
1. Argon	Argon gas	Photocoagulation
2. Krypton	Krypton gas	Photocoagulation
3. Diode	Diode crystal	Photocoagulation
4. Diode-pumped frequency doubled Nd:YAG	Diode and Nd:YAG crystals	Photocoagulation
5. Nd:YAG	A liquid dry or a solid compound of yttrium-aluminium garnet and neodymium	Photodisruption
6. Excimer	Helium and flourine gas	Photoablation

MECHANISMS OF LASER EFFECTS AND THEIR THERAPEUTIC APPLICATIONS

1. *Photocoagulation*. The principal lasers used in ophthalmic therapy are the thermal lasers, which depend upon absorption of the laser light by tissue pigments. The absorbed light is converted into heat, thus raising the temperature of the target tissue high enough to coagulate and denature cellular elements. Argon, diode, krypton and diode pump frequency doubled Nd-YAG lasers are based on this mechanism.

Modes of action. Photocoagulation is effective in treating ocular diseases by production of a scar, occlusion of vessels, tissue atrophy, and tissue contraction.

Therapeutic applications based on photocoagulation are as follows:

1. *Eyelid lesions* such as haemangioma.
2. *Corneal conditions e.g.,* reduction of postoperative astigmatism from cataract sutures—by Argon laser suturotomy and treatment of corneal neovascularisation.
3. *Laser for glaucoma.* Procedures employed include laser iridotomy for narrow-angle glaucoma, argon

laser trabeculoplasty (ALT) for open-angle glaucoma, laser goniopunctures for developmental glaucoma, prophylactic pan-retinal photocoagulation to prevent neovascular glaucoma in patients with retinal hypoxic states (e.g., central retinal vein occlusion) and cyclophotocoagulation for absolute or near absolute glaucoma.

4. *Lesions of iris.* These include laser coreoplasty for updrawn pupil, photomydriasis for pathologic miotic pupil, laser sphincterotomy and laser shrinkage of iris cyst.
5. *Lesions of retina and choroid.* These form the most important indications. Common conditions are:
   - Diabetic retinopathy in which pan-retinal photocoagulation (PRP) is carried out for proliferative retinopathy and focal or grid-photocoagulation for exudative maculopathy.
   - Peripheral retinal vascular abnormalities such as Eales' disease, proliferative sickle cell disease, Coats' disease and retinopathy of prematurity.
   - Intraocular tumours such as retinoblastoma, malignant melanoma and choroidal haemangioma.
   - Macular diseases, such as central serous retinopathy, and age-related macular degeneration (ARMD).
   - For sealing of holes in retinal detachment.

***Complications of laser photocoagulation*.** These include: accidental foveal burns, macular oedema and macular pucker, pre-retinal fibrosis, haemorrhage from retina and choroid, retinal hole formation, ischaemic papillitis, localised opacification of lens and accidental corneal burns.

2. *Photodisruption*. Laser based on this mechanism ionize the electrons of the target tissue producing a physical state called *plasma*. This plasma expands with momentary pressures as high as 10 kilobars, exerting a cutting/incising effect upon the tissues. Nd:YAG laser is based on this mechanism.

Therapeutic applications of Nd:YAG laser include capsulotomy for thickened posterior capsule and membranectomy for pupillary membranes. Recently it has also been tried for phacolysis (laser phaco surgery) in phacoemulsification technique of cataract extraction.

3. *Photoablation*. Lasers based on this mechanism produce UV light of very short wavelength which breaks chemical bonds of biologic materials, converting them into small molecules that diffuse away. These lasers are collectively called *excimer* (excited dimer) *lasers*. These act by tissue modelling. ***Therapeutic applications of excimer lasers*** are: photorefractive keratectomy (PRK), laser assisted *in-situ* keratomileusis (LASIK) for correction of refractive errors and phototherapeutic keratectomy (PTK) for corneal diseases such as band-shaped keratopathy.

CRYOTHERAPY IN OPHTHALMOLOGY

Cryopexy means to produce tissue injury by application of intense cold (–40 °C to –100 °C). This is achieved by a cryoprobe from a cryo-unit (Fig. 18.1).

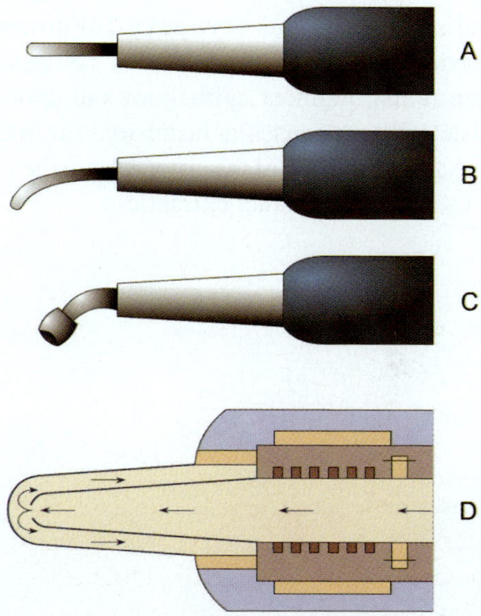

Fig. 18.1. Cryoprobes : A and B, for cataract extraction-straight and curved, respectively; C, for cyclocryopexy; and D, internal structure.

Principle

Working of cryoprobes is based on the Joule Thompson principle of cooling.

Cryounit

The cryounit uses freon, nitrous oxide or carbon dioxide gas as cooling agent. Cryoprobes are available in different sizes such as 1 mm for intravitreal use, 1.5 mm straight or curved probe for cataract extraction, 2.5 mm for retina and 4 mm for cyclocryopexy

(Fig. 18.2). Temperature produced depends upon the size of the cryoprobe tip, duration of freezing process and the gas used.

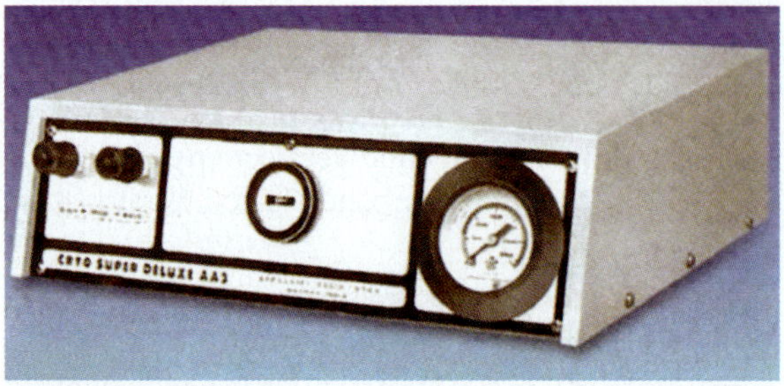

Fig. 18.2. Ophthalmic cryo unit.

Modes of action

Cryopexy produces the required therapeutic effect by different modes which include *tissue necrosis* (as in cyclocryopexy and cryopexy for tumours), production of adhesions between tissues (e.g. between retina, pigment epithelium and choroid in retinal detachment), vascular occlusions (as in Coats' disease) and adherence of the cryoprobe to the iceball in the tissue (as in cataract extraction).

Uses

1. *Lids.* Cryosurgery may be used for following lesions: (i) Cryolysis for trichiasis, (ii) Cryotherapy for warts and *Molluscum Contagiosum*, (iii) Cryotherapy for basal cell carcinoma and haemangioma.
2. *Conjunctiva.* Cryotherapy is used for hypertrophied papillae of vernal catarrh.
3. *Cornea.* Herpes simplex keratitis may be treated by cryotherapy.
4. *Lens.* Cryoextraction of the lens used to be the best intracapsular technique. However, now-a-days intracapsular cataract extraction (ICCE) is no more performed.
5. *Ciliary body.* Cyclocryopexy for absolute glaucoma and neovascular glaucoma.
6. *Retina.* (i) Cryopexy is widely used for sealing retinal holes in retinal detachment. (ii) Prophylactic cryopexy to prevent retinal detachment in certain prone cases. (iii) Anterior retinal cryopexy (ARC) in retinal ischaemic disease e.g., retinopathy of prematurity to prevent neovascularization. (iv) Cryo-treatment of retinoblastoma and angioma.

19 CHAPTER

Systemic Ophthalmology

OCULAR MANIFESTATIONS OF SYSTEMIC DISEASES

INTRODUCTION

Ocular involvement in systemic disorders is quite frequent. It is imperative for the ophthalmologists as well as physicians to be well conversant with these. Many a time, the ocular manifestations may be the presenting signs and the ophthalmologist will refer the patient to the concerned specialist for diagnosis and/or management of the systemic disease. While, in other cases the opinion for ocular involvement may be sought for by the physician who knows to look for it.

Ocular lesions of the common systemic disorders are enumerated and a few important ones are described here.

OCULAR MANIFESTATIONS OF NUTRITIONAL DEFICIENCES

1. *Deficiency of vitamin A.* Ocular manifestations of vitamin A deficiency are referred to as xerophthalmia.
2. *Deficiency of vitamin B_1 (thiamine).* It can cause corneal anaesthesia, conjunctival and corneal dystrophy and acute retrobulbar neuritis.
3. *Deficiency of vitamin B_2 (riboflavin).* It can produce photophobia and burning sensation in the eyes due to conjunctival irritation and vascularisation of the cornea.
4. *Deficiency of vitamin C.* It may be associated with haemorrhages in the conjunctiva, lids, anterior chamber, retina and orbit. It also delays wound healing.
5. *Deficiency of vitamin D.* It may be associated with zonular cataract, papilloedema and increased lacrimation.

XEROPHTHALMIA

The term xerophthalmia is now reserved (by a joint WHO and USAID Committee, 1976) to cover all the ocular manifestations of vitamin A deficiency, including not only the structural changes affecting the conjunctiva, cornea and occasionally retina, but also the biophysical disorders of retinal rods and cones functions.

Etiology

It occurs either due to *dietary deficiency* of vitamin A or its *defective absorption* from the gut. It has long been recognised that vitamin A deficiency does not occur as an isolated problem but is almost invariably accompanied by protein-energy malnutrition (PEM) and infections.

WHO classification (1982)

The new xerophthalmia classification (modification of original 1976 classification) is as follows:

XN	Night blindness
X1A	Conjunctival xerosis
X1B	Bitot's spots
X2	Corneal xerosis
X3A	Corneal ulceration/keratomalacia affecting less than one-third corneal surface
X3B	Corneal ulceration/keratomalacia affecting more than one-third corneal surface.
XS	Corneal scar due to xerophthalmia
XF	Xerophthalmic fundus.

Clinical features

1. *X N (night blindness).* It is the earliest symptom of xerophthalmia in children. It has to be elicited by taking detailed history from the guardian or relative.

2. *X1A (conjunctival xerosis).* It consists of one or more patches of dry, lustreless, nonwettable conjunctiva (Fig. 19.1), which has been well described as 'emerging like sand banks at receding tide' when the child ceases to cry. These patches almost always involve the inter-palpebral area of the temporal quadrants and often the nasal quadrants as well. In more advanced cases, the entire bulbar conjunctiva may be affected. Typical xerosis may be associated with conjunctival thickening, wrinkling and pigmentation.

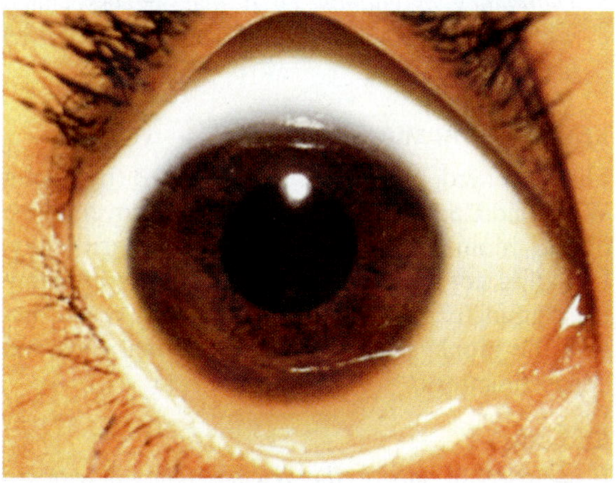

Fig. 19.1. Xerophthalmia, stage XIA: Conjunctival xerosis.

3. *X1B (Bitot's spots).* It is an extension of the xerotic process seen in stage X1A. The Bitot's spot is a raised, silvery white, foamy, triangular patch of keratinised epithelium, situated on the bulbar conjunctiva in the inter-palpebral area (Fig. 19.2). It is usually bilateral and temporal, and less frequently nasal.

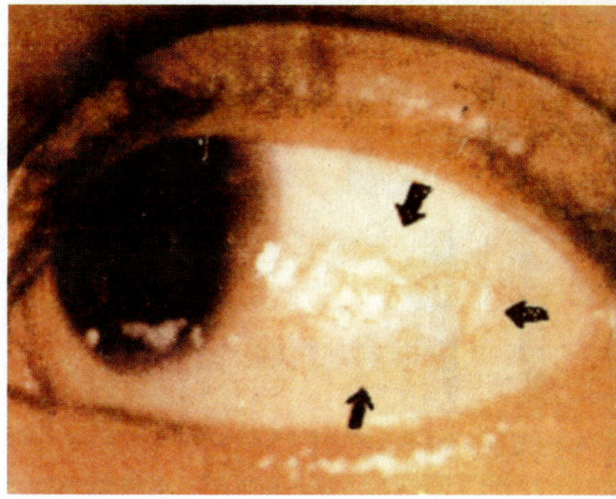

Fig. 19.2. Xerophthalmia, stage XIB: Bitot spots.

4. *X2 (corneal xerosis).* The earliest change in the cornea is punctate keratopathy which begins in the lower nasal quadrant, followed by haziness and/or granular pebbly dryness (Fig. 19.3). Involved cornea lacks lustre.

5. *X3A and X3B (corneal ulceration/keratomalacia),* Stromal defects occur in the late stage due to colliquative necrosis and take several forms. Small ulcers (1-3 mm) occur peripherally; they are characteristically circular, with steep margins and are sharply demarcated (Fig. 19.4). Large ulcers and areas of necrosis may extend centrally or involve the entire cornea. If appropriate therapy is instituted immediately, stromal defects involving less than one-third of corneal surface (X3A) usually heal, leaving some useful vision. However, larger stromal defects (X3B) (Fig. 19.5) commonly result in blindness.

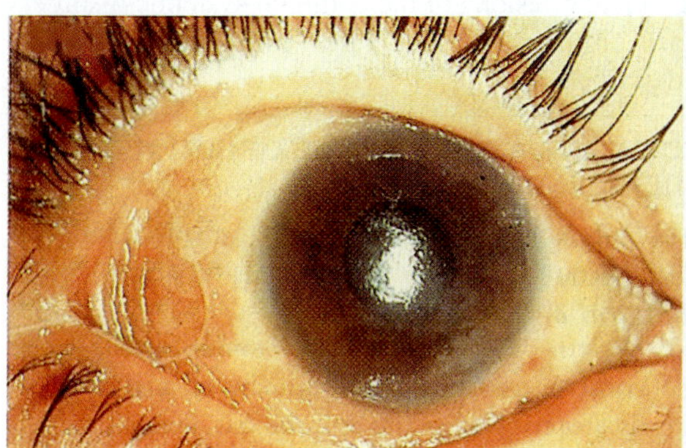

Fig. 19.3. Xerophthalmia, stage X2: Corneal xerosis.

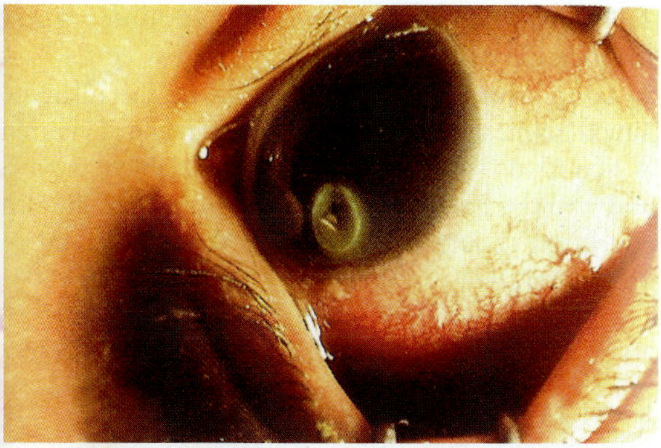

Fig. 19.4. Xerophthalmia, stage X3A: Keratomalacia involving less than one-third of corneal surface.

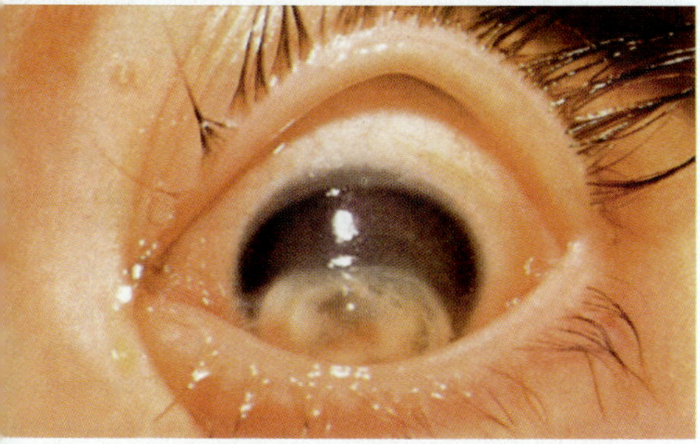

Fig. 19.5. Xerophthalmia, stage X3B: Keratomalacia involving more than one-third of corneal surface.

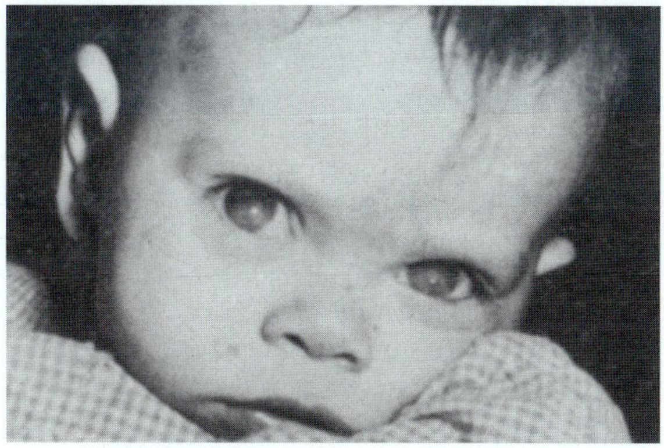

Fig. 19.6. Xerophthalmia, stage XS: Corneal scars.

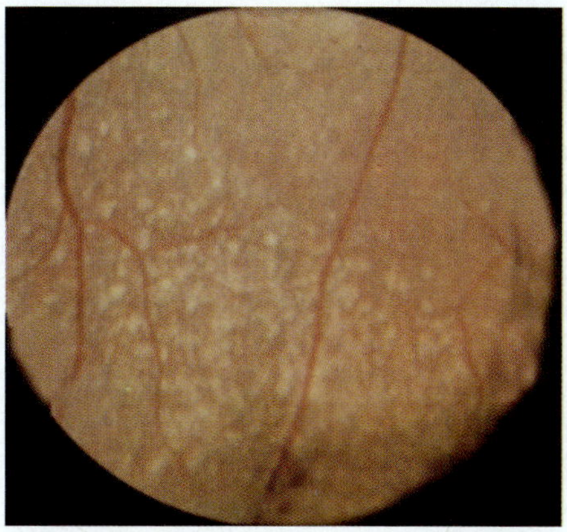

Fig. 19.7. Xerophthalmia, stage XF: Xerophthalmic fundus.

6. *XS (corneal scars).* Healing of stromal defects results in corneal scars of different densities and sizes which may or may not cover the pupillary area (Fig. 19.6). A detailed history is required to ascertain the cause of corneal opacity.

7. *XFC (Xerophthalmic fundus).* It is characterized by typical seed-like, raised, whitish lesions scattered uniformly over the part of the fundus at the level of optic disc (Fig. 19.7).

Treatment

It includes local ocular therapy, vitamin A therapy and treatment of underlying general disease.

1. *Local ocular therapy.* For conjunctival xerosis artificial tears (0.7 percent hydroxypropyl methyl cellulose or 0.3 percent hypromellose) should be instilled every 3-4 hours. In the stage of keratomalacia, full-fledged treatment of bacterial corneal ulcer should be instituted (see pages 98-100).

2. *Vitamin A therapy.* Treatment schedules apply to all stages of active xerophthalmia viz. XN, X1A, X1B, X2, X3A and X3B. Oral administration is the recommended method of treatment. However, in the presence of repeated vomiting and severe diarrhoea, intramuscular injections of water-miscible preparation should be preferred. The WHO recommended schedule is as given below:

i. *All patients above the age of 1 year* (except women of reproductive age): 200,000 IU of vitamin A orally or 100,000 IU by intramuscular injection should be given immediately on diagnosis and repeated the following day and 4 weeks later.

ii. *Children under the age of 1 year and children of any age who weigh less than 8 kg* should be treated with half the doses for patients of more than 1 year of age.

iii. *Women of reproductive age, pregnant or not:* (a) *Those having night blindness* (XN), conjunctival xerosis (X1A) and Bitot's spots (X1B) should be treated with a daily dose of 10,000 IU of vitamin A orally (1 sugar coated tablet) for 2 weeks.
(b) *For corneal xerophthalmia,* administration of full dosage schedule (described for patients above 1 year of age) is recommended.

3. *Treatment of underlying conditions* such as PEM and other nutritional disorders, diarrhoea, dehydration and electrolyte imbalance, infections and parasitic conditions should be considered simultaneously.

Prophylaxis against xerophthalmia

The three major known intervention strategies for the prevention and control of vitamin A deficiency are:

1. *Short-term approach.* It comprises periodic administration of vitamin A supplements. WHO recommended, universal distribution schedule of vitamin A for prevention is as follows:

i.	Infants 6-12 months old and any older children who weigh less than 8 kg.	100,000 IU orally every 3-6 months.
ii.	Children over 1 year and under 6 years of age	200,000 IU orally every 6 months.
iii.	Lactating mothers	20,000 IU orally once at delivery or during the next 2 months. This will raise the concentration of vitamin A in the breast milk and therefore, help to protect the breastfed infant.
iv.	Infants less than 6 months old, not being breastfed.	50,000 IU orally should be given before they attain the age of 6 months.

A revised schedule of vitamin A supplements being followed in India since August 1992, under the programme named as 'Child Survival and Safe Motherhood (CSSM)' is as follows:

- First dose (1 lakh I.U.)—at 9 months of age along with measles vaccine.
- Second dose (2 lakh I.U.)—at 18 months of age along with booster dose of DPT/OPV.
- Third dose (2 lakh I.U.)—at 2 years of age.

2. *Medium-term approach.* It includes food fortification with vitamin A.

3. *Long-term approach.* It should be the ultimate aim. It implies promotion of adequate intake of vitamin A rich foods such as green leafy vegetables, papaya and drum-sticks (Fig. 19.8). Nutritional health education should be included in the curriculum of school children.

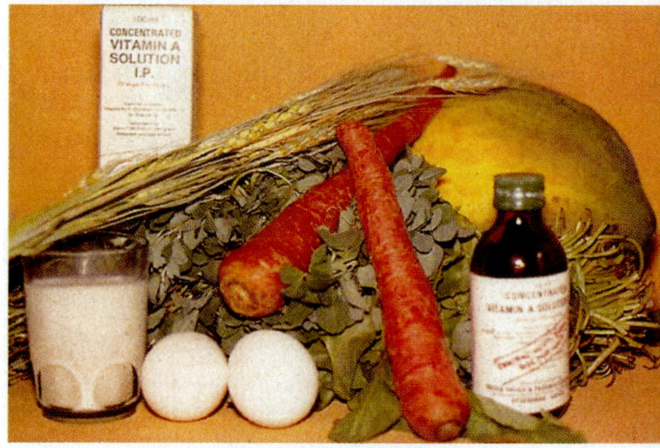

Fig. 19.8. Rich sources of vitamin A.

Note. The short-term approach has been mostly in vogue especially in Asia. The best option perhaps is a combination of all the three methods with a gradual weaning away of the short-term approach.

OCULAR MANIFESTATIONS OF SYSTEMIC INFECTIONS

A. VIRAL INFECTIONS

Measles. Ocular lesions are: catarrhal conjunctivitis, Koplik's spots on conjunctiva, corneal ulceration, optic neuritis and retinitis.

Mumps. Ocular involvement may occur as conjunctivitis, keratitis, acute dacryoadenitis and uveitis.

Rubella. Ocular lesions seen in rubella (German measles) are congenital microphthalmos, cataract, glaucoma, chorioretinitis and optic atrophy.

Whooping cough. There may occur subconjunctival haemorrhages and rarely orbital haemorrhage leading to proptosis.

Ocular involvement in AIDS

AIDS (Acquired Immune Deficiency Syndrome) is caused by Human immuno deficiency virus (HIV) which is an RNA retrovirus.

Modes of spread include:

- Sexual intercourse with an infected person,
- Use of infected hypodermic needles,
- Transfusion of infected blood and
- Transplacental spread to foetus from the infected mothers.

Pathogenesis of AIDS. The HIV infects T-cells, T-helper cells, macrophages and B-cells and thus interferes with the mechanism of production of immune bodies thereby causing immunodeficiency.

Immune deficiency renders the individuals prone to various infections and tumours, which involve multiple systems and finally cause death.

Ocular manifestations. These occur in about 75 percent of patients and sometimes may be the presenting features of AIDS in an otherwise healthy person or the patient may be a known case of AIDS when his eye problems occur. Ocular lesions of AIDS may be classified as follows:

1. *Retinal microvasculopathy.* It develops from vaso-occlusive process which may be either due to direct toxic effects of virus on the vascular endothelium or immune complex deposits in the precapillary arterioles.

It is characterised by non-specific lesions (Fig. 19.9):

- Multiple 'cotton-wool spots' occur in 50 percent cases,
- Superficial and deep retinal haemorrhages occur in 15-40 percent cases.
- Microaneurysms and telangiectasia may also be seen rarely.

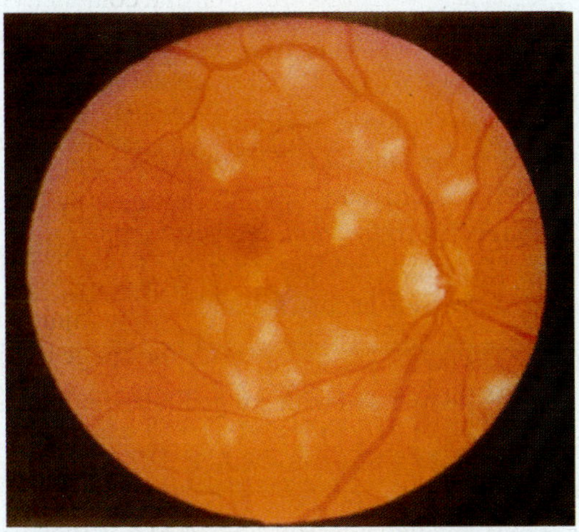

Fig. 19.9. Retinopathy in AIDS.

2. *Usual ocular infections.* These are also seen in healthy people, but occur with greater frequency and produce more severe infections in patients with AIDS. These include:

- Herpes zoster ophthalmicus,
- Herpes simplex infections,
- Toxoplasmosis (chorioretinitis),
- Ocular tuberculosis, syphilis and fungal corneal ulcers.

3. *Opportunistic infections of the eye.* These are caused by microorganisms which do not affect normal patients. They can infect someone whose cellular immunity is suppressed by HIV infection or by other causes such as leukaemia. These include: cytomegalovirus (CMV) retinitis (see page 253 Fig 11.5), candida endophthalmitis, cryptococcal infections and pneumocystis carini, choroiditis.

4. *Unusual neoplasms.* Kaposi's sarcoma is a malignant vascular tumour which may appear on the eyelid or conjunctiva as multiple nodules. It is seen in about 3 percent cases of AIDS. Burkitt's lymphoma of the orbit is also seen in a few patients.

5. *Neuro-ophthalmic lesions.* These are thought to be due to CMV or other infections of the brain. These include isolated or multiple cranial nerve palsies resulting in paralysis of eyelids, extraocular muscles, loss of sensory supply to the eye and optic nerve involvement causing loss of vision.

Management. It consists of the measures directed against the associated infection/lesions. For example:

- *CMV infections* can be treated by zidovudine, ganciclovir and foscarnet (see page 450).
- *Kaposi's sarcoma* responds to radiotherapy.
- *Horpes zoster ophthalmicus*, is treated by acyclovir.

B. BACTERIAL INFECTIONS

1. *Septicaemia.* Ocular involvement may occur in the form of metastatic retinitis, uveitis or endophthalmitis.
2. *Diphtheria.* There may occur: membranous conjunctivitis, corneal ulceration, paralysis of accommodation and paralysis of extraocular muscles.
3. *Brucellosis.* It may involve the eye in the form of iritis, choroiditis and optic neuritis.

4. *Gonococcal ocular lesions* are: ophthalmia neonatorum, acute purulent conjunctivitis in adults and corneal ulceration.
5. *Meningococcal infection* may be associated with: metastatic conjunctivitis, corneal ulceration, paresis of extraocular muscles, optic neuritis and metastatic endophthalmitis or panophthalmitis.
6. *Typhoid fever.* It may be complicated by optic neuritis and corneal ulceration due to lagophthalmos.
7. *Tuberculosis.* Ocular lesions seen are granulomatous conjunctivitis, phlyctenular keratoconjunctivitis, interstitial keratitis, nongranulomatous and granulomatous uveitis, Eales' disease, optic atrophy (following chiasmal arachnoiditis secondary to meningitis), and papilloedema (due to raised intracranial pressure following intracranial tuberculoma).
8. *Syphilitic lesions* (acquired) seen in *primary stage* are conjunctivitis and chancre of conjunctiva. In *secondary stage* there may occur iridocyclitis. *Tertiary stage* lesions include chorioretinitis and gummata in the orbit. *Neurosyphilis* is associated with optic atrophy and pupillary abnormalities. Ocular lesions of *congenital syphilis* are: interstitial keratitis, iridocyclitis and chorioretinitis.
9. *Leprosy.* Ocular lesions of leprosy include cutaneous nodules on the eyelids, madarosis, interstitial keratitis, exposure keratitis, granulomatous uveitis and dacryocystitis.

C. PARASITIC INFECTIONS

1. *Toxoplasmosis* is known to produce necrotising chorioretinitis (see page 163).
2. *Taenia echinococcus* infestation may manifest as hydatid cyst of the orbit, vitreous and retina.
3. *Taenia solium* infestation. Cysticercus cysts are known to involve conjunctiva, vitreous, retina, orbit and extra-ocular muscles.
4. *Toxocara* infestation may be associated with endophthalmitis (see page 164).
5. *Onchocerciasis* is a common cause of blindness in African countries. Its ocular features include sclerosing keratitis, uveitis, chorioretinitis and optic neuritis invariably ending in optic atrophy.

D. FUNGAL INFECTIONS

Systemic fungal infections may be associated with corneal ulceration and endophthalmitis.

OCULAR MANIFESTATIONS OF COMMON ENDOCRINAL AND METABOLIC DISORDERS

Gout

Ocular lesions of gout include:

- Episcleritis,
- Scleritis, and
- Uveitis.

Diabetes mellitus

Ocular involvement in diabetes is very common. Structure-wise ocular lesions are as follows:

1. *Lids.* Xanthelasma and recurrent stye or internal hordeolum.
2. *Conjunctiva.* Telangiectasia, sludging of the blood in conjunctival vessels and subconjunctival haemorrhage.
3. *Cornea.* Pigment dispersal at back of cornea, decreased corneal sensations (due to trigeminal neuropathy), punctate kerotapathy, Descemet's folds, higher incidence of infective corneal ulcers and delayed epithelial healing due to abnormality in epithelial basement membrane.
4. *Iris.* Rubeosis iridis (neovascularization).
5. *Lens.* Snow-flake cataract in patients with IDDM, posterior subcapsular cataract, early onset and early maturation of senile cataract.
6. *Vitreous.* Vitreous haemorrhage and fibre-vascular proliferation secondary to diabetic retinopathy
7. *Retina.* Diabetic retinopathy and lipaemia retinalis (see page 274).
8. *Intraocular pressure.* Increased incidence of POAG, neovascular glaucoma and hypotony in diabetic ketoacidosis (due to increased plasma bicarbonate levels).
9. *Optic nerve.* Optic neuritis.
10. *Extraocular muscles.* Ophthalmoplegia due to diabetic neuropathy.
11. *Changes in refraction.* Hypermetropic shift in hypoglycemia, myopic shift in hyperglycemia and decreased accommodation.

Galactosemia

It is usually associated with congenital cataract (page 181).

Homocystinuria

It is associated with bilateral subluxation of lens (page 214).

Mucopoly saccharidosis

Ocular lesions include:
- Corneal opacification,
- Pigmentary retinopathy,
- Glaucoma, and
- Optic atrophy

Hyperthyroidism

Ocular lesions include:
- Thyroid ophthalmopathy (see page 417)
- Superior limbic keratoconjunctivitis (page 113), and
- Optic disc oedema

Hypoparathyroidism

Ocular lesions include:
- Fasciculation
- Cataract and
- Optic disc oedema

Wilson disease

Ocular lesions include:
- Kayser - Fleisher ring
- Sunflower cataract

OCULAR MANIFESTATIONS OF COMMON DISORDERS OF SKIN AND MUCOUS MEMBRANES

1. *Atopic dermatitis.* It may be associated with conjunctivitis, keratoconus and cataract.
2. *Rosacea.* Its ocular lesions include blepharitis, conjunctivitis, keratitis and rosacea pannus.
3. *Dermatitis herpetiformis.* Its ocular complications include recurrent bullae, ulceration and cicatrization.
4. *Epidermolysis bullosa.* Ocular complications, when they occur, take the form of cicatrizing conjunctivitis and keratitis.
5. *Stevens-Johnson syndrome.* Stevens-Johson syndrome is an acute illness often caused by hypersensitivity to drugs, particularly sulphonamides. It is characterized by acute ulceration of the conjunctiva and other mucous membranes like that of mouth and vagina. Conjunctival ulceration is followed by cicatrizing conjunctivitis. The clinical picture at this stage is the same as in ocular pemphigoid.

OCULAR MANIFESTATIONS OF HAEMATOLOGICAL DISEASES

1. *Anaemias.* Anaemic retinopathy may occur in severe anaemia of any etiology (see page 279).

2. *Leukaemias.* Ocular involvement in leukaemias may occur in the form of:
- *Proptosis* due to leukaemic deposits in the orbital tissue.
- *Leukaemic retinopathy* is of common occurrence in lymphocytic as well as myeloid leukaemias (see page 279).

3. *Sickle cell disease.* Ocular involvement may occur as:
- Dilated conjunctival vessels and
- Sickle cell retinopathy (see page 279)

4. *Lymphomas* may cause following ocular lesions:
- Lid and/or orbital deposits, and
- Uveitis

OCULAR ABNORMALITIES IN TRISOMIES

Trisomy 13 (D Trisomy or Patau Syndrome)

- Microphthalmos
- Colobomas (almost 100%)
- Retinal dysplasia
- Cataract
- Corneal opacities
- Optic nerve hypoplasia
- Cyclopia
- Intra-ocular cartilage

Trisomy 18 (E trisomy or Edwards syndrome)

- Blepharophimosis
- Ptosis
- Epicanthal fold
- Hypertelorism
- Microphthalmos
- Uveal coloboma
- Congenital glaucoma
- Corneal opacities

Trisomy 21 (G Trisomy or Down's syndrome)

- Upward slanting palpebral fissure (Mongoloid slant)
- Almond-shaped palpebral fissure
- Epicanthus

- Telecanthus
- Narrowed interpupillary distance
- Esotropia (35% cases)
- High refractive errors
- Cataract
- Iris hypoplasia
- Keratoconus

Ocular abnormalities in chromosomal deletion syndromes

Cri-du-Chat syndrome (5p.)

- Hypertelorism
- Epicanthus
- Antimongoloid slant
- Strabisums

Cri-du-Chat syndrome (11 p.)

- Aniridia
- Glaucoma
- Foveal hypoplasia
- Nystagmus
- Ptosis

Cri-du-Chat syndrome (13 q.)

- Retinoblastoma
- Hypertelorism
- Microphthalmos
- Epicanthus
- Ptosis
- Coloboma
- Cataract

De Grouchy syndrome (18q.)

- Hypertelorism
- Epicanthus
- Ptosis
- Strabismus
- Myopia
- Glaucoma
- Microphthalmos (with or without cyst)
- Coloboma
- Optic atrophy
- Corneal opacity

Turner syndrome (XO)

- Antimongoloid slant
- Epicanthus
- Ptosis
- Strabismus
- Blue sclera
- Eccentric pupils
- Cataract
- Colour blindness
- Pigmentary disturbances of fundus

ADVERSE OCULAR EFFECTS OF COMMON SYSTEMIC DRUGS

C.V.S. drugs

- *Digitalis:* Disturbance of colour vision, scotomas
- *Quinidine:* Optic neuritis (rare)
- *Thiazides:* Xanthopsia (yellow vision), Myopia
- *Carbonic anhydrase inhibitors:* Ocular hypotony, Transient myopia
- *Amiodarone:* Corneal deposits
- *Oxprenolol:* Photophobia, Ocular irritation

G.I.T. drugs

- *Anticholinergic agents:* Risk of angle-closure glaucoma due to mydriasis, Blurring of vision due to cycloplegia (Occasional).

C.N.S. drugs

- *Barbiturates:* Extraocular muscle palsies with diplopia, Ptosis, Cortical blindness
- *Chloral hydrate:* Diplopia, Ptosis, Miosis
- *Phenothiazines:* Deposits of pigment in conjunctiva, cornea, lens and retina, Oculogyric crisis
- *Amphetamines:* Widening of palpebral fissure, Dilatation of pupil, Paralysis of ciliary muscle with loss of accommodation
- *Monoamine oxidase inhibitors:* Nystagmus, Extraocular muscle palsies, Optic atrophy
- *Tricyclic agents:* Pupillary dilatation (glaucoma risk), Cycloplegia
- *Phenytoin:* Nystagmus, Diplopia, Ptosis, Slight-blurring of vision (rare)
- Neostigmine: Nystagmus, Miosis
- Morphine: Miosis
- Haloperidol: Capsular cataract
- Lithium carbonate: Exophthalmos, Oculogyric crisis
- Diazepam: Nystagmus.

Hormones

Female sex hormones

- Retinal artery thrombosis
- Retinal vein thrombosis
- Papilloedema
- Ocular palsies with diplopia
- Nystagmus
- Optic neuritis and atrophy
- Retinal vasculitis
- Scotomas
- Migraine
- Mydriasis
- Cyloplegia
- Macular oedema

Corticosteroids

- Cataract (posterior subcapsular)
- Local immune suppression causing susceptibility to viral (herpes simplex), bacterial and fungal infections
- Steroid-induced glaucoma

Antibiotics

- *Chloramphenicol:* Optic neuritis and optic atrophy
- *Streptomycin:* Optic neuritis
- *Tetracycline:* Pseudotumour cerebri, Transient myopia

Antimalarial

Chloroquine

- Macular changes (Bull's eye maculopathy)
- Central scotomas
- Pigmentary degeneration of the retina
- Chloroquine keratopathy
- Ocular palsies
- Ptosis
- Electroretinographic depression

Amoebicides

- *Diiodohydroxy quinoline:* Subacute myelo optic neuropathy (SMON), optic atrophy

Chemotherapeutic agents

- *Sulfonamides:* Stevens-Johnson syndrome
- *Ethambutol:* Optic neuritis and atrophy
- *Isoniazid:* Optic neuritis and optic atrophy

Heavy metals

- *Gold salts:* Deposits in the cornea and conjunctiva
- *Lead:* Optic atrophy, Papilloedema, Ocular palsies

Chelating agents

- *Penicillamine:* Ocular pemphigoid, Ocular neuritis, Ocular myasthenia

Oral hypoglycemic agents

- *Chloropropamide:* Transient change in refractive error, Diplopia, Stevens-Johnson syndrome

Vitamins

Vitamin A

- Papilloedema
- Retinal haemorrhages
- Loss of eyebrows and eyelashes
- Nystagmus
- Diplopia and blurring of vision

Vitamin D

- Band-shaped keratopathy

Antirheumatic agents

- Salicylates: Nystagmus, Retinal haemorrhages, Cortical blindness (rare)
- Indomethacin: Corneal deposits
- Phenylbutazone: Retinal haemorrhages

20 CHAPTER

Community Ophthalmology

INTRODUCTION

Community ophthalmology, over the years, has leveloped as an important branch of community nedicine. Its activities emphasize the prevention of ocular diseases and visual impairment; reduction of ocular disability; and promotion of ocular health, quality of life and efficiency of a group of people at he community level. Thus, it can be defined as a system (rather than a branch of community medicine) which utilises the full scope of ophthalmic knowledge and skill, methodology of public health and services of other medical and non-medical agencies to promote ocular health and prevent blindness at the community evel with an active, recognised and crucial role of community participation.

The concept of community ophthalmology has become more relevant and essential to achieve the goal of 'Vision 2020: The Right to Sight' and to, accomplish the theme behind 'Vision for the Future (VFTF)'.

BLINDNESS AND ITS CAUSES

DEFINITION OF BLINDNESS

Different definitions and terms for blindness such as total blindness, economic blindness, legal blindness and social blindness are in vogue in different countries so much so that 65 definitions of blindness are listed in a WHO publication (1966)[1]. In ophthalmology, the term blindness strictly refers to the inability to perceive light (PL absent).

WHO definition of blindness. In order to have comparable national and international statistics, the WHO in 1972 proposed a uniform criterion and defined blindness as, "*Visual acuity of less than 3/60 (Snellen) or its equivalent*"[2]. In order to facilitate the screening of visual acuity by non-specialised persons, in the absence of appropriate vision charts, WHO in 1979 added the "*Inability to count fingers in day-light at a distance of 3 metres*" to indicate vision less than 3/60 or its equivalent[3].

Visual field less than 10º, irrespective of the level of visual acuity is also labelled as blindness (WHO, 1977)[4].

NPCB definition of blindness. Under national programme for control of blindness (NPCB) in India, blindness is defined as presenting distance visual acuity of < 6/60 or central visual fields < 20° in the better eye.

Other definitions of blindness in vogue are:

- *Economic blindness:* vision in better eye <6/60 to 3/60
- *Social blindness:* Vision in better eye <3/60 to 1/60.
- *Legal blindness:* Vision in better eye <1/60 to perception light
- *Total blindness:* No light perception (PL -ve).

Categories of visual impairment.

In the Ninth Revision (1977) of the International Classification of Diseases (ICD), the visual impairment (maximum vision less than 6/18 Snellen) has been divided into 5 categories. Categories 1 and 2 constitute "*low vision*" and categories 3, 4 and 5 constitute "*blindness*" (Table 20.1). Patients with the visual fields between 5° and 10° are placed in category 3 and those with less than 5° in category 4.

Table 20.1. Categories of visual impairment (WHO, 1977)[4]

Category of visual impairment		*Level of visual acuity (Snellen)*
Normal vision	0	6/6 to 6/18
Low vision	1	Less than 6/18 to 6/60
	2	Less than 6/60 to 3/60
Blindness	3	Less than 3/60 (FC at 3 m) to 1/60 (FC at 1m) or visual field between 5°and 10°
	4	Less than 1/60 (FC at 1 m) to light perception or visual field less than 5°
	5	No light perception

Avoidable blindness

The concept of avoidable blindness includes both preventable blindness and curable blindness.

- *Preventable blindness* is that which can be easily prevented by attacking the causative factor at an appropriate time. For example, corneal blindness due to vitamin A deficiency and trachoma can be prevented by timely measures.
- *Curable blindness* is that in which vision can be restored by timely intervention, e.g., cataract blindness can be cured by surgical treatment.

MAGNITUDE OF BLINDNESS

Magnitude of global blindness

The number of blinds across the globe is not within the exact realms of counts. However, from time to time, the World Health Organization (WHO) provides the estimates.

Statistics of blindness. According to WHO estimates is as below:

i. Blind due to eye diseases : 37 million
ii. Blind due to refractive errors : 08 million
iii. Blind due to all causes (*i* + *ii*) : 45 million
iv. Low vision due to eye diseases : 124 million
v. Low vision due to refractive errors : 145 million
vi. Low vision (all causes) (*iv* + *v*) : 269 million
vii. Total visual impairment (blindness + low vision due to all causes) (*iii* + *vi*) : 314 million

- 90% of the world's blind live in developing countries
- More than 50% of world's blind due to eye diseases live in: India (9 million), Africa (7 million) and China (6 million)
- Of the 37 million blinds due to eye diseases, the age wise distribution is: 0-14 yrs: 1.4 million 15-49 yrs: 5.2 million, 50 yrs. or above: 30.3 million
- Female to male blindness ratio varies from 1.5 to 2.2 : 1.
- About 85% of all visual impairment is avoidable globally.
- Every 5 seconds, one person in our world goes blind.
- Every minute one child goes blind.
- 75 millions will be blind due to eye diseases by 2020 (if trend continues)

Geographical distribution of global blindness.

About 90% of the world's blinds live in developing countries and around 60% of them reside in sub-Saharan Africa, China and India. There is a significant difference in the level of blindness in the developing countries as compared to the developed countries of the world, as there are:

- 3 blind people/1000 population in developed countries of Europe, America and Japan,
- 9 blind people/1000 population in Asia, and
- 12 blind people/1000 population in Africa.

Regional burden of blindness

For having an easy means of comparison among different regions of the world, a ratio referred to as the Regional Burden of Blindness (RBB) was evolved. This means the ratio of the proportion of the number of blind in a particular region to the global number of blind and the proportion of the regional population to the world population. The sub-Saharan Africa, India and other Asia and Islands have RBB ratio greater than unity[6]. This indicates that in these regions, the burden of blindness is to be taken into special consideration in terms of fixing priorities on a global scale.

Magnitude of blindness in India

While the problem of blindness is global, its magnitude is much higher in India. Of the estimated 45 million, India alone has 9 million blind people, which comes to one-fifth of the total in the world[5]. The prevalence of blindness in India, as determined by the three major surveys conducted in the last 3 decades and a Rapid Assessment of Avoidable Blindness (RAAB) in India 2007 is as below:

Prevalence	*Source*
1.38%	ICMR (1971 - 74)[7]
1.49%	WHO-NPCB (1986-89)[8]
1.1%	NPCB (2001-2002)[9]
1%	RAAB (2006-2007)[10]

Constraints in controlling blindness in India

The Working Group identified following major constraints in controlling blindness in India:

- Inequitable distribution of eye surgeons
- Sub-optimal utilization of human resources
- Inadequate number of paramedical eye care personnel
- Variation in quality
- Sub-optimal coverage
- Overemphasis on cataract
- Lack of public awareness
- Prevalence of infections.
- Man-made blindness due to quack practice and home remedies.

CAUSES OF BLINDNESS

Causes of global blindness

Major causes of blindness and the estimated number of blinds (%) due to them are as under[5]:

- Cataract 17.6 million (39%)
- Glaucoma 4.5 million (10%)
- Corneal scarring including trachoma 1.3 million (3%)
- Age related macular degeneration 3.2 million (7%)
- Diabetic retinopathy 1.8 million (4%)
- Childhood blindness including xerophthalmia >1.4 million (3%)
- Onchocerciasis 0.3 million (0.7%)
- Others 10 million

Causes of blindness in India

The problem of blindness in India is not only of its gigantic size, but also of its causes, which are largely preventable or curable with the present available knowledge and skill. Three major population based surveys and one rapid assessment of avoidable

Table 20.2. Major causes of blindness in India

RAAB Survey (2006-07)[10]		*NPCB Survey (2001-02)[9]*		*WHO-NPCB Survey (1986-89)[8]*		*ICMR Survey (1971-74)[7]*	
Disease condition	*Percent blindness*	*Disease condition*	*Percent blindness*	*Disease condition*	*Percent blindness*	*Disease condition*	*Percent blindness*
Cataract	72.2	Cataract	62.6	Cataract	80.1	Cataract	55
Refractive errors (0.7%) + aphakia (5.6%)	6.3	Refractive errors	19.7	Refractive errors	7.35	Malnutrition	2
Glaucoma	4.4	Glaucoma	5.8	Glaucoma	1.7	Glaucoma	0.5
Complications of cataract surgery	3.0	Posterior segment disorders	4.7	Trachoma	0.39	Trachoma and associated infections	20
Corneal opacity including trachoma	6.5	Surgical complications	1.2	Aphakic blindness	4.67	Injuries	1.2
Posterior segment disorders (DR, 0.1% + ARMD 0.7% + others 2.2%)	3.0	Corneal blindness	0.9	Corneal opacity	1.52	Small pox seaquele	3
		Others	5.0	Others	4.25	Others	18

blindess (RAAB) survey have been carried out in India to estimate the magnitude and causes of blindness. These surveys have shown that trends in blindness continue to change, though the major causes of blindness still continue to be the same (Table 20.2)[7,8,9,10].

Developed versus developing countries

The main causes of blindness in developed countries are different from those of developing countries.

- *In developed countries*, 50 percent of all blindness is because of age related macular degeneration (ARMD), while another 10-20 percent each is because of glaucoma, diabetic retinopathy and cataract.
- *In developing countries* the frequent causes are cataract, infectious diseases, xerophthalmia, injuries, glaucoma, and onchocerciasis.

GLOBAL INITIATIVES FOR PREVENTION OF BLINDNESS

The concept of avoidable blindness (i.e., preventable or curable) has gained increasing recognition during the last three decades. Inter-national Agency for the Prevention of Blindness (IAPB) formed in 1975, is an international non-governmental agency which has a close and complementary relationship with WHO (an international inter-governmental agency in the field of prevention of blindness).

The major global initiatives taken for prevention of blindness are:

- WHO: Prevention of Blindness Programme (PBP), (1978)
- Vision 2020: The Right to Sight (1999), and
- Vision For the Future (VFTF) (2001).

WHO PREVENTION OF BLINDNESS PROGRAMME

The WHO launched the 'Prevention of Blindness Programme (WHO : PBL)' in 1978. In accordance with which many countries have already come up with a 'National Blindness Control Programme'.

Control strategies suggested by WHO include:

1. Assessment of common blinding disorders at local, regional and national levels.
2. Establishment of national level programmes for control of blindness suited to the national and local needs.
3. Training of eye care providers.
4. Operational research to improve and apply appropriate technology.

VISION 2020: THE RIGHT TO SIGHT

'Vision 2020: The Right to Sight'[11], is a global initiative launched by WHO in Geneva on Feb. 18,1999 in a broad coalition with a 'Task Force of International Non-Governmental Organisations (NGOs)' to combat the gigantic problem of blindness in the world.

Partners of Vision 2020: Right to Sight include:

I. World Health Organisation (WHO),

II. Task Force of International NGOs, which has following members:

- International Agency for Prevention of Blindness (IAPB)
- Christopher Blindness Mission (CBM)
- Helen Keller International
- ORBIS International
- Sight Savers International
- Al Noor Foundation
- International Federation of Ophthalmological Societies
- Lions Clubs International Foundation
- Operation Eye Sight Universal
- The Carter Centre

Objective of vision 2020. Objective of this new global initiative is to eliminate avoidable blindness by the year 2020 and to reduce the global burden of blindness which currently affects an estimated 45 million people worldwide.

Implementation of vision 2020. Vision 2020 is being implemented through four phases of five year plans, the first one started in 2000, second in 2005 and third in 2010. The last phase of implementation will commence from 2015.

STRATEGIC APPROACHES: GLOBAL PERSPECTIVE

Strategic approaches of Vision 2020: Right to Sight (Global perspective) are:

- Disease prevention and control,
- Training of eye health personnel,
- Strengthening of existing eye care infrastructure,
- Use of appropriate and affordable technology,

and
- Mobilization of resources.

Disease prevention and control

Globally, WHO has identified five major blinding eye conditions, for immediate attention to achieve the goals of Vision 2020, which are:
- Cataract
- Childhood blindness,
- Trachoma,
- Refractive errors and low vision, and
- Onchocerciasis.

These conditions have been chosen on the basis of their contribution to the burden of blindness, feasibility and affordability of interventions to control them. Each country will decide on its priorities based on the magnitude of specific blinding conditions in that country.

Cataract

Cataract remains the single largest cause of blindness. There is an estimated figure of 17.6 million (39%) people worldwide who are blind because of curable cataract[5].

Aim under 'Vision 2020' is to eliminate avoidable blindness due to cataract by the year 2020 by performing cataract extraction with intraocular lens (IOL), implantation.

Strategy to achieve the aim to measure the increase in the cataract surgery rate (CSR), i.e., number of cataract surgeries per million population per year as below:

Year	*Global cataract surgical rate targets*	*Global number of cataract operation targets (million)*
2000	2000	12
2010	3000	20
2020	4000	32

Emphasis is to be placed on achieving:
- High success rates in terms of restored vision and quality-of-life outcome.
- Affordable and accessible services
- Measures to overcome barriers and increased use of services.

Childhood blindness

Childhood blindness is considered a priority area due to the number of years of blindness that ensues.

Prevalence is 0.5-1 per 1000 children, aged 0-15 years. There are 1.4 million blind children estimated in the world of whom 1 million live in Asia and 3 lakhs in Africa. There are 5 lakh children going blind each year (one per minute) also.

Causes of childhood blindness vary from place to place and change over time. The main causes include: Vitamin A deficiency, measles, conjunctivitis, ophthalmia neonatorum, congenital cataract and retinopathy of prematurity (ROP).

Aim is to eliminate avoidable causes of childhood blindness by the year 2020.

Strategies. Vision 2020 envisages following strategies:
- *Strengthening primary eye care programmes* within primary healthcare to eliminate preventable causes.
- *Developing therapeutic and surgical support services* to deal effectively with curable eye problem.
- *Establishing optical and low vision services*

Activities. Under the global initiative vision 2020 include:

I. *Elimination of preventable blindness* by:
   - Measles immunisation,
   - Vitamin A supplementation (see page 466),
   - Monitoring use of oxygen in the premature new born,
   - Avoidance of harmful traditional practices,
   - Promoting school screening programmes for diagnosis and management of common conditions like refractive errors and trachoma in endemic areas, and
   - Promoting eye health education in schools.

II. *Management of surgically avoidable causes* of childhood blindness such as cataract, glaucoma, and retinopathy of prematurity (ROP).

Trachoma blindness

Trachoma is a leading cause of preventable blindness worldwide with an estimated 5.9 million persons blind or at immediate risk because of trichiasis[11]. The disease accounts for nearly one-sixth of the global burden of blindness. In India, blindness due to trachoma (0.39%, WHO-NPCB 1986-89) is on the decline when compared with previous figures (20%,

ICMR 1975). The RAAB survey (2006-07) have reported trachoma blindness to be 0.6%.

Effective interventions have been demonstrated in developing nations using the **SAFE** strategy:

- **S**urgery to correct lid deformity and prevent blindness,
- **A**ntibiotics for acute infections and community control,
- **F**acial hygiene, and
- **E**nvironmental change including improved access to water and sanitation and health education.

Elimination of blindness due to trachoma is considered feasible, eradication of trachoma is not. Trachoma has disappeared from North America and Europe because of improved socio-economic conditions and hygiene. Research needs include validation of rapid community assessment techniques, identification of barriers to the acceptance of preventive surgical procedure, studying effectiveness of annual treatment cycles and cost-effective studies. W.H.O. has organized an Alliance for **G**lobal **E**limination of **T**rachoma by the year 2020 (GET 2020).

Refractive errors and low vision

Aim is to eliminate visual impairment (visual acuity less than 6/18) and blindness due to refractive errors or other causes of low vision. It is estimated that there are 35 million people in the world who require low vision care and 8 million (18%) are blind due to refractive errors[5].

Strategies recommended under 'Vision 2020' initiative include:

- *Create awareness* for refractive errors and demand for refractive services.
- *Screening* to identify individuals with poor vision which can be improved by spectacles or other optical devices.
- *Refraction services* to be made available to individuals identified with significant refractive errors.
- *Ensure optical services* to provide affordable spectacles for individuals with significant refractive errors.
- *Low vision services and low vision aids* to be provided for all those in need.

Onchocerciasis

Onchocerciasis (river blindness) is known to be endemic in 37 countries. An estimated 17 million people are infected with onchocerciasis. Approximately 0.3 million (0.7%) people are blind from the disease worldwide[5]. About 95% of infected persons reside in Africa, where the disease is most severe along the major rivers in 30 countries. Outside Africa, the disease occurs in Mexico, Guatemala, Ecuador, Columbia, Venezuela and Brazil in the America, and in Yemen in Asia.

Aim is to eliminate blindness due to onchocerciasis by the year 2020.

Target is to develop 'National Onchocerciasis Control Programme' with satisfactory coverage in all the 37 countries where disease is endemic.

Strategy is to introduce community directed treatment with annual doses of Mectizan (ivermectin). The disease in expected to be brought under control by the year 2010, if present efforts in endemic countries are successfully implemented.

STRATEGIC PLAN FOR 'VISION 2020': THE RIGHT TO SIGHT IN INDIA

It is described under National Programme for Control of Blindness in India (page 451).

VISION FOR THE FUTURE (VFTF)

Vision for the future (VFTF): International Ophthalmology Strategic Plan to Preserve and Restore Vision[12], launched in Feb 2001, is another global initiative (in addition to Vision 2020) for prevention of blindness.

Implementation of this program is being done by International Council of Ophthalmology (ICO) by working closely with other international, supranational and national organizations. It is parallel to and complementary of 'Vision 2020'. Care is being taken to avoid duplication.

Top priorities for action of this programme are:

- Enhancement of ophthalmology residency training around the world, particularly through definition of principles, guidelines and curricula.
- Development of model guidelines and recommendations for ophthalmic clinical care in critical disease areas.

- Dissemination of sample curricula for training of medical students and allied health personnel.
- Advocacy and support for 'Vision 2020: Right to Sight', particularly by encouraging national ophthalmologic societies to support the initiative and become involved.
- Helping national ophthalmologic societies develop more effective organizations.

NATIONAL PROGRAMME FOR CONTROL OF BLINDNESS (NPCB) IN INDIA

India was the first country in the world to launch the 'National Programme for Control of Blindness (NPCB)' in year 1976 as 100 percent centrally sponsored programme with the following ***goals***:

- To provide comprehensive eye care facilities for primary, secondary and tertiary levels of eye healthcare, and
- To reduce the prevalence of blindness in population from 1.38% (ICMR 971-74) to 0.31 by 2000 AD.

Major flips in NPCB include:

- *Inclusion in 'Prime Minister's-20 point programme'* in 1982, was the first major flip for NPCB.
- *Launching of 'Cataract Blindness Control Project'* assisted by World Bank from 1994-2001 was another major flip for NPCB. This project was launched to reduce the cataract back-log in 7 States which were identified to have the highest prevalence of cataract blindness by WHO-NPCB survey (1986-89). These, in descending order, are: Uttar Pradesh, Tamil Nadu, Madhya Pradesh, Maharashtra, Andhra Pradesh, Rajasthan and Orissa.
- *Adoption of vision 2020: Right to Sight* in 2001 is the most prestigious major flip for NPCB. It has been adopted with the objective to eliminate avoidable blindness by the year 2020.

OBJECTIVES

Present objectives of the NPCB include:

- *Reduction in the backlog of blindness* through identification and treatment of blinds.
- *Development of comprehensive eyecare facilities* in every district
- *Development of human resources* for providing eye care services.
- *Improvement in quality of service* delivery
- *Securing participation* of voluntary organizations and private practitioners in eye care.
- *Enhancement in community awareness* on eye care.
- *Setting up of mechanism* for referral, coordination and feedback between organizations dedicated to prevention, treatment and rehabilitation.

PROGRAMME ORGANIZATION

Various programme activities implemented at central, state and district levels are as follows[13]:

1. Central level

At the central level, programme organization is the responsibility of the 'National Programme Management Cell' located in the office of Director General Health Services (DGHS), Department of Health, Government of India (GOI). To oversee the implementation of the programme three national bodies have been constituted as below:

- National Blindness Control Board, chaired by Secretary Health to GOI.
- National Programme Co-ordination Committee, chaired by Additional Secretary to GOI.
- National Technical Advisor Committee, headed by Director General Health Services, GOI.

Central level activities include:

1. Procurement of goods (major equipments, bulk consumables, vehicles, etc.)
2. Non-recurring grant-in-aid to NGOs.
3. Organizing central level training courses.
4. Information, education and communication (IEC) activities (prototype development and mass media).
5. Development of MIS, monitoring and evaluation.
6. Procurement of services and consultancy.
7. Salaries of additional staff at the central level.

2. State level

The NPCB is implemented through the State Government. A 'State Programme Cell' is already in place for which five posts including that of a Joint Director (NPCB) have been created.

State-level activities include:

1. Execution of civil works for new units.
2. Repairs and renovation of existing units/ equipments.
3. State level training and IEC activities.
4. Management of State Project Cell.
5. Salaries for additional staff.

'State Blindness Control Society' (SBCS) is being established in each state for monitoring and implementing the programme at the state level. The SBCS will release grant-in-aid to District Blindness Control Societies (DBCS) for various activities.

3. District level

To organize the programme at district level, 'District Blindness Control Societies' have been established.

District blindness control society

The concept of 'District Blindness Control Society (DBCS)' has been introduced, with the primary purpose to plan, implement and monitor the blindness control activities comprehensively at the district level under overall control and guidance of the 'National Programme for Control of Blindness'. This concept has been implemented after pioneering work by DANIDA in five pilot districts in India.

Objective of DBCS establishment is to achieve the maximum reduction in avoidable blindness in the district through optimal utilisation of available resources in the district.

Need for establishment of DBCS was considered because of the following factors:

1. To make control of blindness a part of the Government's policy of designating the district as the unit for implementing various development programmes.
2. To simplify administrative and financial procedures.
3. To enhance participation of the community and the private sector.

Composition of DBCS. Each DBCS will have a maximum of 20 members, consisting of 10 ex-officio and 10 other members with following structure:

- *Chairman*: Deputy Commissioner/District Magistrate.
- *Vice-Chairman:* Civil Surgeon/District Health Officer.
- *Member Secretary*: District Programme Manager (DPM) or District Blindness Control Co-ordinator (DBCC), who is appointed by the Chairman. DPM will co-ordinate the activities of the programme between the government and non-government organizations (NGOs).
- *Members* will include District Eye Surgeon, District Education Officer, President local IMA branch, President Rotary Club, representatives of various NGOs and local voluntary action groups. The ex-officio members will be the members of the society as long as they hold the post. The term of other members is notified by the Chairman.
- *Advisor of the society* is the State Programme Manager.
- *Technical guidance* is provided by the Chief Ophthalmic Surgeon/Head of the Ophthalmology Department of Medical College.

Present status. Till date more than 600 DBCSs have been established.

Revised strategies adopted for implementation of programme at district level are:

1. Annual district action plan is to be submitted by DBCS. Funding will be in two instalments through GOI/SBCS.
2. NGO participation made accountable; allotted area of operation.
3. Revised guidelines for DBCS — capping of expenditure; phasing out contract managers.
4. Emphasis on utilization of existing government facilities.
5. Gradual shift from camp surgery to institutional surgery.
6. Development of infrastructure and manpower for IOL surgery.

PLAN OF ACTION AND ACTIVITIES

The basic plan of action and activities of NPCB, since its inception in 1976, includes the following[13]:

I. ***Extension of eye care services***

II. ***Establishment of permanent infrastructure*** for :

- *Primary Eye Care*, at peripheral level (PHCs and subcentres) is being strengthened by:
  – Providing necessary equipment,
  – Posting a paramedical ophthalmic assistant, and
  – Organising refresher courses for doctors and other staff of PHC on prevention of blindness.

Community ophthalmic practice at primary care level is summarized in Table 20.3. Currently, the programme implementation is sub-sumed under 'National Rural Health Mission' (NRHM).

Table 20.3. Community Ophthalmology Practice at Primary Level

Promotive	*Preventive*	*Curative*	*Rehabilitative*
• Nutrition Education • Improved maternal and child nutrition • Health education • Face washing • Good antenatal care • Safe water • Improved – environmental sanitation	• Ocular prophylaxis at birth • Vitamin A doses • Measles vaccine • Perinatal care • Avoid medication in pregnancy • Avoid hypoxia at birth • Examine neonate's eyes • Nutrition supplementation	• Vision screening • Treatment for vitamin A def. • Referral for surgery • Emergency management • Treatment for trachoma • Treatment for other common eye diseases	• Provision of low vision services • Community based rehabilitation • Counselling of the incurable blind • Certification of blind by eye surgeon • Sensitise about concessions

- *Secondary Eye Care*, at intermediate level,
- *Tertiary Eye Care*, at central level, and
- *Center of Excellence*, at apex level for high quality tertiary eye care, and to provide guidance and leadership for technical matters.

III. *Intensification of eye health education.*

Note: For the above activities Government of India has adopted 'Vision 2020: Right to Sight' under 'National Programme for Control of Blindness' at a meeting held in Goa on October 10-13, 2001 and constituted a working group to plan the action and activities.

STRATEGIC PLAN FOR VISION 2020: THE RIGHT TO SIGHT IN INDIA

The draft plan of action submitted by the 'Working Group' to the Ministry of Health and Family Welfare Govt. of India in August, 2002 includes following strategies[14]:

A. Strengthening advocacy
B. Reduction of disease burden
C. Human resource development, and
D. Eye care infrastructure development

A. Strengthening advocacy

To strengthen advocacy and generate public awareness various activities are proposed at national, state, and district level under Vision 2020 initiative in India.

National and State Level

- Public awareness and information about eye care and prevention of blindness by:
  - Frequent press releases and articles in leading newspapers of the country,
  - Increased frequency of broadcast and telecast of messages on eye care, and
  - Introduction of topics on eye care in school curricula.
- Involvement of professional organizations such as All India Ophthalmological Society (AIOS), Eye Bank Association of India (EBAI) and Indian Medical Association (IMA) in the National Programme for Control of Blindness.
- Publishing quarterly newsletters, articles in scientific journals and developments of prototype print materials.

District Level

- To strengthen the functioning of District Blindness Control Society (DBCS).
- To enhance involvement of NGOs, local community societies and community leaders.
- To strengthen hospital retrieval programmes for eye donation through effective grief counselling by involving volunteers, Forensic Deptt., Police etc.
- Public awareness activities based on local needs through effective media.
- Strong interpersonnel communication through village-based link workers, aphakic motivators and community leaders.
- Multisectoral approach particularly involving departments of education, social welfare, media etc.

B. Reduction of disease burden (disease-specific approach)

Target diseases identified for intervention under 'Vision 2020' initiative in India include:

- Cataract,
- Childhood blindness,
- Refractive errors and low vision,
- Corneal blindness,
- Diabetic retinopathy,
- Glaucoma, and
- Trachoma (focal)

Cataract

Cataract continues to be the single largest cause of blindness. According to latest National Survey in India (1999-2001), 62.6% of blindness in 50+ population of India was found to be cataract related. During 'Rapid Assessment of Avoidable Blindness (RAAB)' conducted in 2006-07, the cataract is reported to be responsible for 72.2% of blindness in 50+ population.

Objective. To improve the quantity and quality of cataract surgery.

Targets include:

- The targets fixed for the Cataract Surgery Rate (CSR) in the vision 2020 strategy were 4500 per match the year by 2005, 5000 by 2010, 5500 by 2015 and 6000 by 2020.
- To improve the visual outcome of surgery to match the standards set by WHO (i.e., 80% to have visual outcome 6/18 or >6/18 after surgery).
- IOL surgery for >80% by the year 2005 and for all by the year 2010.
- YAG capsulotomy services at all district hospitals by 2010.

Strategic activities to clear backlog of cataract include:

- *Primary screening* by community health worker to identify persons with visual impairment (finger counting <6 m in any eye).
- *Case selections* by eye surgeons at screening camps and at base level (district hospital).
- *Cataract extraction with IOL implantation* to be done free of cost for bilateral cases, underserved poor people, especially women.
- *Reduction in disparities* based on geographical, socio-economic and gender based.

Grant-in aid for cataract surgery may continue to be released through DBCS.

Childhood blindness

Childhood blindness is an important public health problem in developing countries due to its social and economic implications. Though prevalence of childhood blindness is low as compared to blindness in the aged, it assumes significance due to large number of disability years of every child remaining blind.

Extent and causes of problem. Prevalence of childhood blindness in India has been projected to be 0.8/1000 children by using the correlation between under five mortality rate and prevalence. Currently, there are about 270,000 blind children in India.

Common causes of childhood blindness are vitamin A deficiency, measles, conjunctivitis, ophthalmia neonatorum, injuries, congenital cataract, retinopathy of prematurity (ROP), and childhood glaucoma.

Refractive errors are the commonest cause of visual impairment in children.

Aim is to eliminate avoidable causes of childhood blindness by the year 2020.

Strategies and activities under Vision 2020: Right to Sight initiative in India include:

1. *Detection of eye disorders.* Following schedule of ophthalmic examination of children is recommended to identify early childhood disorders, refractive errors, squint, amblyopia and corneal diseases:
   - At the time of primary immunization,
   - At school entry, and
   - Periodic check up every 3 years for normal and every year for those with defects.
2. *Preventable childhood blindness* to be taken care of through cost effective measures:
   - *Prevention of xerophthalmia* is of utmost value in preventing childhood blindness (see page 466).
   - *Prevention and early treatment of trachoma by active intervention* (see page 65 and 478).
   - *Refractive errors* to be corrected at primary eye care centres.
   - *Childhood glaucomas* to be treated promptly.
   - *Harmful traditional practices* need to be avoided.
   - *Prevention of ROP* by proper screening and

monitoring use of oxygen in premature new borns.

3. *Curable childhood blindness* due to cataract, ROP, corneal opacity and other causes to be taken care of by the experts at secondary and tertiary level eye care services.

Targets include:

- *Establishment of Paediatric Ophthalmology units.* In India, 50 Pediatric Ophthalmology units are to be established by 2010 for effective management of childhood diseases.
- *Establishment of refraction services and low vision centers* (see below).

Refractive errors and low vision

According to 'Rapid Assessment of Avoidable Blindness (RAAB)' conducted in 2006-2007, refractive errors including uncorrected aphakia were responsible for 6.3% of blindness and 35.6 (32.9 + 2.7) % of low vision.

Aim and strategies are same as described for 'Vision 2020' Global initiative (see page 477)

Targets. To combat refractive error and low vision following targets have been set in India:

- *Refraction services* to be available in all primary health centres by 2010. Availability of low-cost, good quality spectacles for children to be insured.
- *Low vision service centres* are to be established at 150 tertiary level eye care institutions. 50 such centres are to be developed by 2010, another 50 by 2015 and the final 50 by 2020.

Glaucoma

As per the 'National Survey on Blindness' (1999-2001, Govt. of India Report 2002)[9] glaucoma is responsible for 5.8% cases of blindness in 50+ population and as per RAAB (2006-07) the corresponding figure is 4.4%[10]. Effective intervention for prevention of glaucoma resultant blindness is quite difficult. Failure of early detection of the disease poses a management problem towards controlling glaucomatous blindness. Population based screening of glaucoma is not recommended as a strategy in developing countries. Following measures are recommended for ***opportunistic glaucoma screening*** (case detection) by tonometry and fundus examination:

- *Opportunistic screening at eye care institutions* should be done in all persons above the age of 35 years, those with diabetes mellitus, and those with family history of glaucoma.
- *Community based referral* by multi-purpose workers of all persons with dimunition of vision, coloured haloes, rapid change of glasses, ocular pain and family history of glaucoma.
- *Opportunistic screening at eye camps* in all patients above the age of 35 years.

Diabetic retinopathy

Diabetic retinopathy (DR) is emerging as an important cause out of 4.7% cases of blindness due to posterior segment disorders in 50+ population (National Survey 1999-2001)[9]. To prevent visual loss occurring from diabetic retinopathy a periodic follow-up (see page 277) is very important for timely intervention. Following recommendations are made:

- Awareness generation by health workers.
- All known diabetics to be examined and referred to Eye Surgeon by the Ophthalmic Assistant.
- Confirmation by fundus fluorescein angiography (FFA) and laser treatment of diabetic retinopathy at tertiary level.
- The strategy must be to bring down the medical management of DR at the secondary level.

Corneal blindness

Background. A significant number of cases of visual impairment and gross degree of loss of vision occur due to diseases of the cornea. According to NPCB survey (2001-02)[9], corneal blindness accounts for 0.9% of total blindness while according to RAAB (2006-07) corneal opacities including trachoma account for 6.5% cases of blindness. It is reported that there is an addition of 25,000 to 30,000 corneal blindness cases every year in the country. Majority of these persons are affected in the first and second decade of life. The major causes of this blindness are corneal ulcers due to infections, trachoma, ocular injuries and keratomalacia caused by nutritional deficiencies. Thus, corneal blindness is one of the outstanding problems in the field of preventive and community ophthalmology and is a great challenge to the medical profession in general and ophthalmolgists in particular. This challenge can be faced boldly by the combined efforts of the public and the government; especially the education department, school teachers, general medical practitioners and ophthalmologists.

Objective regarding corneal blindness under 'Vision 2020' in India is:

- To reduce prevalence of preventable and curable corneal blindness.

Strategies for control of corneal blindness

I. *General strategies* include:

- *Identification of infants* at risk in co-operation with RCH programme to take appropriate measures.
- *Identification of pre-school children* at risk by door to door survey.
- *Identification of school children* through school health services.
- *Identification of senior citizens* with post cataract surgery bullous keratopathy.
- *To ensure supply of essential drugs* required for primary care such as: Tetracycline eye ointment, antibiotic eye drops, and vitamin A supplements.

II. *Disease-specific strategies* are as below:

1. *Eye infections* including *ophthalmia neonatorum.* Ocular prophylaxis at birth with broad-spectrum antibiotics is very important. Health education and improvement in personal hygiene will reduce the incidence of conjunctivitis, corneal ulcer and other eye infections. Early treatment of eye infections will prevent corneal blindness.
2. *Eye injuries.* Education of people regarding avoidance of ocular trauma like cracker blast, industrial accidents, road accidents and other trauma, thereby reducing irreversible corneal blindness. Ocular trauma cases should be immediately referred to specialists for effective management. Facilities for administrating general anaesthesia for ocular trauma patients at secondary eye care level.
3. *Trachoma Blindness.* In India, the corneal blindness due to trachoma (0.39% WHO-NPCB, 1986-88) is on the decline when compared with previous figures (20% ICMR 1975). RAAB (2006-07) reports 0.6% incidence of trachoma blindness. However, in isolated pockets (focal) blindness related to trachoma continues to be important. (For prevention of trachoma blindness see page 66 and 478).
4. *Prevention of Xerophthalmia* will make a strong dent in the number of corneal blinds. The three major known intervention strategies for the prevention and control of vitamin A deficiency are described on page 466.
5. *A total ban should be placed on the ophthalmic practice by quacks* and sale of harmful eye medicines especially various 'surmas'.
6. *Protective measures* for the eyes of industrial workers and agriculturists should include use of goggles and eye shades.

III. *Keratoplasty and Eye Banking.* There is a need of around 1 lakh corneas per year for transplantation to clear the backlog of corneal blindness. Currently we are collecting around 25000 eyes per year. As keratoplasty operation can restore vision in a significant number of corneal blinds, an intensive publicity and cooperation of government and non-government agencies is needed to enhance the voluntary eye donations. Under NPCB, eye donation fortnight is organized from 25th August to 8th Sept. every year to promote eye donation. More eye banks should be established and more ophthalmic surgeons should be trained for corneal grafting. *Under Vision 2020: Indian initiative* emphasis is on hospital retrieval system to get better donor material. Death certificates should bear one line on eye donations.

C. Human resource development

For 'Vision 2020' initiative in India, the human resource needs identified to combat blindness by 2020 are depicted in Table 20.4.

Mid-Level Ophthalmic Personnel (MLOP). The term MLOP has been introduced to include all categories of paramedics who work full time in eye care. Broadly two streams of such personnels are envisaged:

1. *Hospital-based MLOP.* These include ophthalmic nurses, ophthalmic technicians, optometrists, and orthoptists etc.
2. *Community-based MLOP* include those with out-reach/field functions such as primary eye care workers and ophthalmic assistants.

D. Eye care infrastructure development

Based on the recommendations of WHO, there is a need to develop the infrastructure pyramid which includes (Fig. 20.1):

1. *Primary level Vision Centres.* There is a need to develop 20,000 vision centres, each with one Ophthalmic Assistant or equivalent (Community based MLOP) covering a population of 50,000.
2. *Service Centres.* There is need to develop 2,000 service centres at secondary level—each with two ophthalmologists and 8 paramedics (Hospital based MLOP), covering a population of 5,00,000.

Table 20.4. Human resource needs for the country to combat blindness by 2020

Sr. No.	Category	2001 numbers	Required by the year 2005	2010	2015	2020
1.	Ophthalmic surgeons	12000	15000	18000	21000	25000
2.	Ophthalmic assistants (community)	6000	10000	15000	20000	25000
3.	Ophthalmic paramedics (Hospital)	18000	30000	36000	42000	48000
4.	Eye-care managers	200	500	1000	1500	2000
5.	Community eye health specialists	20	50	100	150	200

One eye care manager will be required at each service centre.

3. *Training Centres.* There is a need to develop 200 'Training Centres' for the training of Ophthalmologists. Each tertiary level training centre will cater to a population of 5 million.
4. *Centre of Excellence (COE).* There is need to develop 20 COE with well developed all sub specialities of Ophthalmology. Each advanced tertiary level center of excellence will cater to a population of 50 millions.

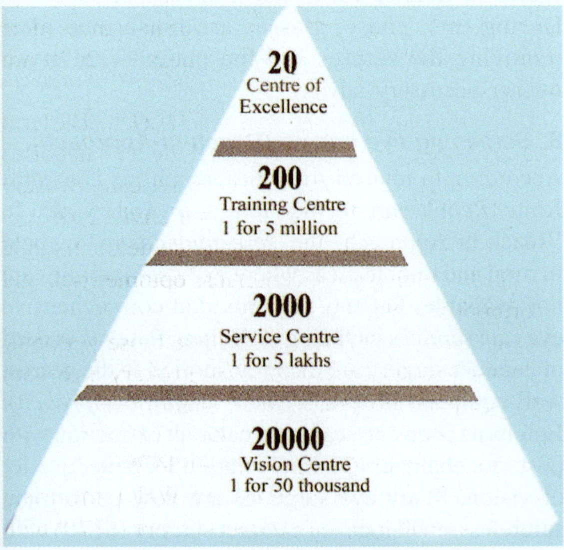

Fig. 20.1. The infrastructure pyramid, based on the recommendations of WHO.

ROLE OF EYE CAMPS IN PREVENTION OF BLINDNESS

Objectives

Eye camp approach for prevention of blindness still plays a vital role in the developing countries where infrastructure is not fully established. It is particularly more relevant keeping in view the fact that still 62.6% of blindness in India is due to cataract which can be very well cured in eye camps.

Organization of an eye camp

Presently two types of eye camps are held:

- Comprehensive eye care camps with 'Reach-out-Approach', and
- Screening eye camps (Reach-in-Approach with comprehensive eye care).

As mentioned earlier the recent emphasis is on the 'Reach-in-Approach'.

I. *Comprehensive eye care camps with 'Reach-Out-Approach'*

A. ***Preparatory phase*** is most important for the successful organization of an eye camp. Activities during this phase are:

1. *Finalization of organizers and medical team.* Presently, most of the eye camps are planned and co-ordinated by the DBCS. Usually, the organizers are voluntary organizations of repute. The medical team is either from district mobile ophthalmic units or charitable hospitals or state mobile ophthalmic units.
2. *Permission to hold eye camp.* Permission is sought by the organizers from the Chief Medical Officer/Civil Surgeon of the district.
3. *Selection of the camp site.* The eye camps should preferably be held at CHC/PHC/charitable hospitals/civil hospital, so that available operation theatre facilities can be used.
4. *Publicity and mobilisation of community resources.* These are most important aspects for

the success of an eye camp. Publicity should start at least a fortnight prior to the actual camp dates. Method of publicity should include public announcements, radio broadcast and display of banners and posters at prominent places like bus-stands, railway stations, schools etc.

5. *Other activities.* These include arrangement for medicines and food for the patients, stay arrangements for the medical team and mobilization of volunteers and social workers, for rendering assistance to the camp team.

B. *Intensive phase.* Eye camps should last 7 days out of which 2-3 days should be set apart for intensive phase, during which following activities need to be performed:

1. The medical team comprising at least one resident doctor, 2 nurses, 2 operation theatre assistants and 2 paramedical personnel should reach the camp site an evening before the scheduled commencement of the camp. They should set up the OPD, ward and operation theatre. The OT room should be fumigated with formalin vapours and kept closed overnight.
2. Patients are provided comprehensive eye care services including refraction. Those requiring surgical intervention for cataract or other diseases are admitted in the ward. For performing ophthalmic surgery, following *guidelines laid down by Govt. of India* should be adhered to:
   - At least one anaesthetist with arrangements to meet common emergencies should be available.
   - At least one, preferably two, operating surgeons should be there and each surgeon should not perform more than thirty operations in a day.
   - Presently extracapsular cataract extraction by any technique preferably manual small incision cataract surgery (SICS) or phacoemulsification with posterior chamber intraocular lens implantation is the recommended method.
   - Ideally the number of operations performed per day should not exceed 50 and in a camp should not exceed 200 to maintain quality and safety of sterilization, surgery and post-operative care.
   - Both the eyes should never be operated at one go.
   - Cases with poor surgical risk such as severe diabetics, severe hypertensives and those having cardiac problems should not be operated in camps. The cases associated with problems like these should be referred to the base hospitals.
3. Along with curative and preventive services, eye health education is also carried out simultaneously.

C. *Consolidation phase* of 4-5 days follows the intensive phase with following activities:

- Care of operated and other admitted patients.
- Out-patient's care including refraction.
- Community eye health and morbidity surveys with greater emphasis on school children.

D. *Culmination and retrieval phase.* On the morning of last day, each patient is very carefully examined and discharged after proper guidance. After this, the men and material resources are packed up and transported back to the base hospital.

E. *Follow-up phase.* One ophthalmic surgeon with the help of one ophthalmic assistant, one staff nurse and paramedical personnel conducts the follow-up examination after 4-6 weeks of closing of the camp. During this, phase, glasses are prescribed after removing the sutures and the patients are given further necessary advice.

II. *Screening eye camps (Reach-in-Approach)*

According to revised strategies, emphasis is to shift from '*Reach-out*' to the '*Reach-in-Approach*'. In 'Reach-in-Approach', the '*screening camps*' are held in rural and remote areas where eye-care facilities are not available. Patients are provided comprehensive eye care services including refraction. Patients in need of cataract surgery are then transported to the nearest well-equipped hospitals *(Base hospital approach)*. Emphasis is on extracapsular cataract extraction with posterior chamber IOL implantation for better quality of vision. Many eye surgeons are now performing sutureless small incision cataract surgery (SICS) with posterior chamber intraocular lens implantation. The trained surgeons are even performing the cataract surgery by latest technique i.e., phacoemulsification in eye camps.

Documentation, monitoring and evaluation

A complete and meticulous record of the patients treated in the eye camp alongwith the post-operative complications noted and managed should be kept.

Each eye camp should be monitored by the competent authorities and evaluated in terms of various activities assigned to such camps and the results obtained.

EYE BANKING

Eye bank is an organization which deals with the collection, storage and distribution of cornea for the purpose of corneal grafting, research and supply of the eye tissue for other ophthalmic purposes.

Functions of an eye bank include:

1. *Promotion of eye donation* by increasing awareness about eye donation to the general public.
2. *Registration* of the pledger for eye donation.
3. *Collection* of the donated eyes from the deceased.
4. *Receiving and processing* the donor eyes.
5. *Preservation* of the tissue for short, intermediate, long or very long term.
6. *Distribution* of the donor tissues to the corneal surgeons.
7. *Research activities* for improvement of the preservation methodology, corneal substitute and utilisation of the other components of eye.

Eye bank personnel include:

1. *Eye bank incharge.* He should be a qualified ophthalmologist to evaluate, process and distribute the donor tissue.
2. *Eye bank technician.* The duties of a trained eye bank technician are:
   - To keep the eye collection kits ready.
   - To assist in enucleation of donor eyes.
   - To record data pertaining to donor material and waiting list of patients.
   - To process and treat the donor eyes with antibiotics.
   - To assist in corneal preservation and storage.
   - To maintain asepsis in the eye bank.
3. *Clerk-cum-storekeeper.* The duties are:
   - To maintain meticulous records.
   - To coordinate with other eye banks.
   - To deal with other eye banks and exert with efficiency regarding donor's correspondence.
   - To distribute cornea to eye surgeons/eye banks.
4. *Medical social worker or public relation officer* is required:
   - To supply publicity material to common public
   - To promote voluntary eye donation.

   He may be a voluntary or paid worker.
5. *Driver-cum-projectionist* is required:
   - To maintain vehicle of the eye bank.
   - To screen films of eye donation promotion in the community.

Eye collection centres. These are the peripheral satellites of an eye bank for better functioning. One collection centre is viably located at an urban area with a population of more than 200,000. About 4-5 collection centres are attached with each eye bank.

Functions of eye collection centre are:

- Local publicity for eye donation.
- Registration of voluntary donors.
- Arrangement for collection of eyes after death.
- Initial processing, packing and transportation of collected eyes to the attached eye bank.

Personnel needed for eye collection centre are:

- Ophthalmic technician trained in eye bank.
- Local honorary workers/voluntary agencies like Lions club, Rotary club etc. to boost the eye donation campaign.
- Services of honorary ophthalmic surgeon or medical officer trained in enucleation available on call.

Legal aspect. The collection and use of donated eyes come under the preview of 'The Transplantation of Human Organs Act, 1994'.

Facts about eye donation

- Almost anyone at any age can pledge to donate eyes after death; all that is needed is a clear healthy cornea.
- The eyes have to be removed within six hours of death.
- Eye donation gives sight to two blind persons as one eye is transplanted to one blind person.
- The eyes can be pledged to an eye bank and can be actually donated to any nearest eye bank at the time of death.
- The donated eyes are never bought or sold.
- Eye donation is never refused.
- The eyes cannot be removed from a living human being inspite of his/her consent and wish.

REHABILITATION OF THE BLIND

Rehabilitation of the blind is as important as the prevention and control of blindness; spiritually speaking even more. A blind person needs the following types of rehabilitation:

1. *Medical rehabilitation.* By low vision aids (LVA) many visually handicapped can have a useful vision.
2. *Training and psychosocial rehabilitation.* It is the most important aspect. First of all the blinds should be assured and made to feel that they are equally useful and not inferior to the sighted persons. Their training should include:
   - Mobility training with the help of a stick.
   - Training in daily living skills such as bathing, washing, putting on clothes, shaving, cooking and other household work.
3. *Educational rehabilitation.* It includes education avenues in 'Blind Schools' with the facility of Braille system of education.
4. *Vocational rehabilitation.* It will help them to earn their livelihood and live as useful citizens. Blinds can be trained in making handicrafts, canning, book binding, candle and chalk making, cottage industries and as telephone operators.

To conclude, it should never be forgotten that, one of the basic human rights is the right to see. The strategicians MUST ensure that:

- No citizen goes blind needlessly due to preventable causes.
- All avenues are exhausted to restore the best possible vision to curable blinds.
- Blinds not amenable to curable measures receive comprehensive rehabilitation.

REFERENCES

1. WHO (1966). Epi and Vital Statis. Rep., 19: 437.
2. The Prevention of Blindness. Report of a WHO Study Group. Geneva, World Health Organization, 1973 (WHO Technical Report Series, No. 518).
3. WHO (1979). WHO Chronicle 33: 275.
4. WHO (1977). International Classification of Diseases. Vol. 1, p. 242.
5. Changing patterns in global blindness: 1988-2008. Community Eye Health; 21(67):37-39, Sept. 2008.
6. Thylefors B et al. Global Data on Blindness. Bull. WHO 1995; 73: (1) 115-121.
7. Indian Council of Medical Research : Collaborative study on Blindness (1971-74).
8. Report of National Workshop (1989). National Programme for Control of Blindness. Director General Health Services, Ministry of Health and Family Welfare, New Delhi.
9. Govt. of India, National Survey on Blindness: 1999-2001, Report 2002.
10. Rapid Assessment of Avoidable Blindness (RAAB) in India (2006-07); PLoS One 2008 Aug. 6; 3(8): e2867.
11. Strategic plan for Vision 2020: The Right to Sight WHO Report. SEA-Ophthal 177, 2000
12. Vision for the Future, International ophthalmology strategic plan to preserve and Restore Vision, 2001.
13. Govt. of India (1992), Present Status of National Programme for Control of Blindness, Ophthalmology Section, DGHS, New Delhi, 1992.
14. Strategic plan for Vision 2020: The Right to sight initiative in India, National Programme for control of blindness, Director General of Health Services, Ministry of Health and Family Welfare Govt. of India.

Section-II

Practical Ophthalmology

INTRODUCTION TO PRACTICAL OPHTHALMOLOGY

Medical graduates have to apply the knowledge gained during their five and a half years of exhaustive study course, for the management and care of a patient in one or the other way. Therefore, it is imperative for them to learn and practise the art of medicine. Consequently the practical examinations have been given equal importance to that of theory examinations during the entire study course. Practical training is thus supplementary and complementary to the lecture course.

Practical examinations in ophthalmology are conducted with the main aims to evaluate a student for his or her capability to identify and diagnose common eye diseases to provide primary eye care and to timely refer the patients needing secondary and tertiary level services to the eye hospitals as per the indications.

To assess the students for the above-mentioned capabilities, the practical examinations are conducted under the following heads:

1. CLINICAL CASE PRESENTATION

Under this section, students are assessed for their knowledge and art of a meticulous history taking, methods of examination, diagnostic skills and plan of management of an ophthalmic patient. For this purpose, the students are supposed to work up a long case and/or 2 to 3 short cases with common eye disorders. The approach to clinical work of an ophthalmic patient is given in Chapter 21 of the book. The clinical case presentation along with the related viva questions have been described in Chapter 22 of this book.

2. DARKROOM EXAMINATIONS

Students are evaluated for their knowledge of basic principles, clinical applications, procedures and the equipment required for the commonly performed darkroom procedures. These procedures along with relevant viva questions have been described in Chapter 23 of this book.

3. OPHTHALMIC INSTRUMENTS AND OPERATIVE OPHTHALMOLOGY

The aim of this part of practical examination is to assess the students for their exposure and acquaintance with functioning of the ophthalmic operation theatre. Students should be able to identify and tell the utility of common eye instruments. They should be able to describe the techniques of local ocular anaesthesia and to enumerate the main steps of a few common eye operations. Students are also supposed to be familiar with the commonly used ophthalmic equipment including use of cryo and lasers in ophthalmology. Subject matter relevant to this part of practical examinations is described in Chapter 24 of this book.

4. SPOTTING

In some centres, spotting also forms a part of practical examinations. This allows an overall objective evaluation of the candidate, so also called as, 'objectively structured clinical examination (OSCE)'. Commonly employed spots in ophthalmology practical examinations include : a typical photograph of any common eye disorder, an instrument, photograph of any ophthalmic equipment, a darkroom appliance, a fundus photograph or a visual field chart.

5. VIVA QUESTIONS

Viva questions form an integral and important part of each section of the practical examination, viz. clinical case presentation, darkroom examination and description of ophthalmic instruments. Therefore, relevant questions have been described in the concerned sections.

The main aim of the examiner during the session of viva questions is to assess the student's overall familiarity with common disorders of the eye, their management and important recent developments in the field of ophthalmic practice.

CHAPTER 21

Clinical Methods in Ophthalmology

HISTORY AND EXAMINATION

HISTORY

The importance of painstaking meticulous history cannot be overemphasized. The complete history-taking should be structured as:

- Demographic data
- Chief presenting complaints
- History of present illness
- History of past illness
- Family history

Demographic data

Demographic data should include patient's name, age, sex, occupation and religion.

Name and address. Name and address are primarily required for patient's identification. It also proves useful for demographic research.

Age and sex. In addition to the utility in patient's identification, knowledge of age and sex of the patient is also useful for noting down and ruling out the particular diseases pertaining to different age groups and a particular sex.

Occupation. An information about patient's occupation is helpful since ophthalmic manifestations due to occupational hazards are well known, e.g.:

- Ocular injuries and trauma due to foreign bodies have typical pattern in factory workers, lathe workers, farmers and sport persons.
- Computer vision syndrome is emerging as a significant ocular health problem in computer professionals.
- Heat cataract is known in glass factory workers.
- Photophthalmitis is known in welders not taking adequate protective measures.

In addition, information about the patient's occupation is useful in providing ocular health education and patient's visual rehabilitation.

Religion. Recording the religion of the patient may be helpful in ascertaining the diseases which are more common in a particular community. It also helps in knowing the aptitude and practices prevalent in different communities for various common eye problems.

Chief presenting complaints

Chief presenting complaints of the patients should always be recorded in a chronological order with their duration. Common presenting ocular complaints are:

- Defective vision
- Watering and/or discharge from the eyes
- Redness
- Asthenopic symptoms
- Photophobia
- Burning/itching/foreign body sensation
- Pain (eyeache and/or headache)
- Deviation of the eye
- Diplopia
- Black spots in front of eyes
- Coloured halos
- Distorted vision

History of present illness

The patients should be encouraged to narrate their complaints in detail and the examiner should be a patient listener. While history taking, the examiner should try to make a note of the following points about each complaint:

- Mode of onset with duration
- Severity
- Progression
- Accompaniment of each symptom

History of past illness

A probe into history of past illness should be made to know:

- History of similar ocular complaint in the past. It is specially important in recurrent conditions such as *herpes simplex keratitis, uveitis* and *recurrent corneal erosions.*
- History of similar complaints in other eye is important in bilateral conditions such as *uveitis, senile cataract* and *retinal detachment.*
- History of trauma to eye in the past may explain occurrence of lesions such as delayed rosette cataract and retinal detachment.
- It is important to know about history of any ocular surgery in the past.
- History of any systemic disease in the past such as tuberculosis, syphilis, leprosy may sometimes explain the occurrence of present ocular disease.
- History of drug intake and allergies is also important.

Family history

Efforts should be made to establish familial predisposition of inheritable ocular disorders like congenital cataract, ptosis, squint, corneal dystrophies, glaucoma and refractive error.

Common ocular symptoms and their causes

1. *Defective vision.* It is the commonest ocular symptom. Enquiry should reveal its onset (sudden or gradual), duration, whether it is painless or painful, whether it is more during the day, night or constant, and so on. Important causes of defective vision can be grouped as under:

Sudden painless loss of vision

- Central retinal artery occlusion
- Massive vitreous haemorrhage
- Retinal detachment involving macular area
- Ischaemic central retinal vein occlusion

Sudden painless onset of defective vision

- Central serous retinopathy
- Optic neuritis
- Methyl alcohol amblyopia
- Non-ischaemic central retinal vein occlusion

Sudden painful loss of vision

- Acute congestive glaucomas (primary or secondary)
- Acute iridocyclitis
- Chemical injuries to the eyeball
- Mechanical injuries to the eyeball

Gradual painless defective vision

- Progressive pterygium involving pupillary area
- Corneal degenerations
- Corneal dystrophies
- Developmental cataract
- Senile cataract
- Optic atrophy
- Chorioretinal degenerations
- Age-related macular degeneration
- Diabetic retinopathy
- Refractive errors

Gradual painful defective vision

- Chronic iridocyclitis
- Corneal ulceration
- Chronic simple glaucoma

Transient loss of vision (Amaurosis fugax)
- Carotid artery disease
- Papilloedema
- Giant cell arteritis
- Migraine
- Raynaud's disease
- Severe hypertension
- Prodromal symptom of CRAO

Night blindness (Nyctalopia)
- Vitamin A deficiency
- Retinitis pigmentosa and other tapetoretinal degenerations
- Congenital night blindness
- Pathological myopia
- Peripheral cortical cataract

Day blindness (Hamarlopia)
- Central nuclear or polar cataracts
- Central corneal opacity
- Central vitreous opacity
- Congenital deficiency of cones (rarely)

Diminution of vision for near only
- Presbyopia
- Cycloplegia
- Internal or total ophthalmoplegia
- Insufficiency of accommodation

2. *Other visual symptoms*. Visual symptoms other than the defective vision are as follows:

Black spots or floaters in front of the eyes may appear singly or in clusters. They move with the movement of the eyes and become more apparent when viewed against a clear surface e.g., the sky. Common causes of black floaters are:
- Vitreous haemorrhage
- Vitreous degeneration. e.g.,
  - senile vitreous degeneration
  - vitreous degeneration in pathological myopia
- Exudates in vitreous
- Lenticular opacity

Flashes of light in front of the eyes (photopsia). Occur due to traction on retina in following conditions:
- Posterior vitreous detachment
- Prodromal symptom of retinal detachment
- Vitreous traction bands
- Sudden appearance of flashes with floaters is a sign of a retinal tear
- Retinitis
- Migraine

Distortion of vision
- Central chorioretinitis
- Central serous chorioretinopathy
- ARMD
- CNVM
- Keratoconus
- Corneal irregularity

Glare
- Early cataract
- Corneal oedema
- Status postrefractive surgery

Photophobia
- Corneal abrasion
- Acute conjuctivitis
- Keratitis
- Anterior uveitis
- Dilated pupil

Coloured halos. Patient may perceive coloured halos around the light. It is a feature of:
- Acute congestive glaucoma
- Corneal edema e.g. bullous keratopathy
- Early stages of cataract
- Mucopurulent conjunctivitis

Diplopia, i.e., perceiving double images of an object is a very annoying symptom. It should be ascertained whether it occurs even when the normal eye is closed (uniocular diplopia) or only when both eyes are open (binocular diplopia). Common causes of diplopia are:

Uniocular diplopia
- Subluxated lens
- Double pupil
- Incipient cataract
- Keratoconus
- Eccentric IOL

Binocular diplopia
- Paralytic squint
- Myasthenia gravis
- Diabetes mellitus
- Thyroid disorders
- Blow-out fracture of floor of the orbit
- Anisometropic glasses (e.g., uniocular aphakic glasses)
- After squint correction in the presence of abnormal retinal correspondence (paradoxical diplopia).

3. *Watering from the eyes.* Watering from the eyes is another common ocular symptom. Its causes can be grouped as follows:
Excessive lacrimation, i.e., excessive formation of tears occurs in multiple conditions (see page 391).
Epiphora, i.e., watering from the eyes due to blockage in the flow of normally formed tears somewhere in the lacrimal drainage system (see page 392).

4. *Discharge from the eyes.* When a patient complains of a discharge from the eyes, it should be ascertained whether it is mucoid, mucopurulent, purulent, serosanguinous or ropy. Discharge from the eyes is a feature of conjunctivitis, corneal ulcer, stye, burst orbital abscess, and dacryocystitis.

5. *Itching, burning and foreign body sensation in the eyes.* These are very common ocular symptoms. Their causes are:
- Conjunctivitis (e.g., allergic, chronic simple, and GPC)
- Blepharitis
- Dry eye
- Trachoma and other conjunctival inflammations
- Trichiasis and entropion

6. *Redness of the eyes.* It is a common presenting symptom in many conditions such as conjunctivitis, keratitis, iridocyclitis, acute glaucomas, conjunctivital or corneal foreign body, trichiasis, episcleritis, scleritis, sub-conjunctivial haemorrhage, endophthalmitis.

7. *Ocular pain.* Pain in and around the eyes should be probed for its onset, severity, and associated symptoms. It is a feature of ocular inflammations and acute glaucoma. Ocular pain may also occur as referred pain from the inflammation of surrounding structures such as sinusitis, dental caries and abscess.

8. *Asthenopic symptoms.* Asthenopia refers to mild eyeache, headache and tiredness of the eyes which are aggravated by near work. Asthenopia is a feature of extraocular muscle imbalance and uncorrected mild refractive errors especially astigmatism.

9. *Other ocular symptoms* are as follows:
- Deviation of the eyeball (squint)
- Protrusion of the eyeball (proptosis)
- Drooping of the upper lid (ptosis)
- Retraction of the upper lid
- Sagging down of the lower lids (ectropion)
- Swelling on the lids (e.g., chalazion and tumours)

(These specific symptoms have been discussed in the concerned chapters).

GENERAL PHYSICAL AND SYSTEMIC EXAMINATION

General physical and systemic examination should be carried out in each case. Sometimes it may help in establishing the aetiological diagnosis, e.g., ankylosing spondylitis may be associated with uveitis. Further, it is essential to treat associated diseases like bronchial asthma, hypertension, diabetes and urinary tract problems before taking up the patient for cataract surgery.

OCULAR EXAMINATION

- Testing of visual acuity
- External ocular examination
- Fundus examination
- Visual field examination

I. *TESTING OF VISUAL ACUITY*

Visual acuity should be tested in all cases, as it may be affected in numerous ocular disorders. In real sense acuity of vision is a retinal function (to be more precise of the macular area) concerned with the appreciation of form sense.

Distant and near visual acuity should be tested separately.

The distant visual acuity

Snellen's test types. The distant central visual acuity is usually tested by Snellen's test types. The fact that two distant points can be visible as separate only when they subtend an angle of 1 minute at the nodal point of the eye, forms the basis of Snellen's test-types. It consists of a series of black capital letters on a white board, arranged in lines, each progressively diminishing in size. The lines comprising the letters have such a breadth that they will subtend an angle of 1 min at the nodal point. Each letter of the chart is so designed that it fits in a square, the sides of which are five times the breadth of the constituent lines. Thus, at the given distance, each letter subtends an angle of 5 min at the nodal point of the eye (Fig. 21.1). The letters of the top line of Snellen's chart (Fig. 21.2) should be read clearly at a distance of 60 m. Similarly, the letters in the subsequent lines should be read from a distance of 36, 24, 18, 12, 9, 6, 5 and 4 m, respectively.

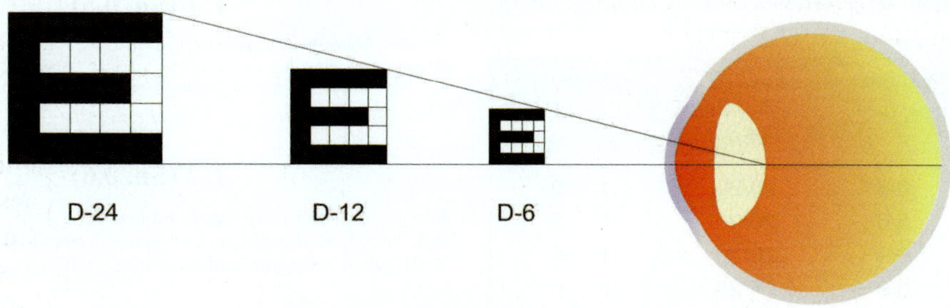

Fig. 21.1. Principle of Snellen's test types.

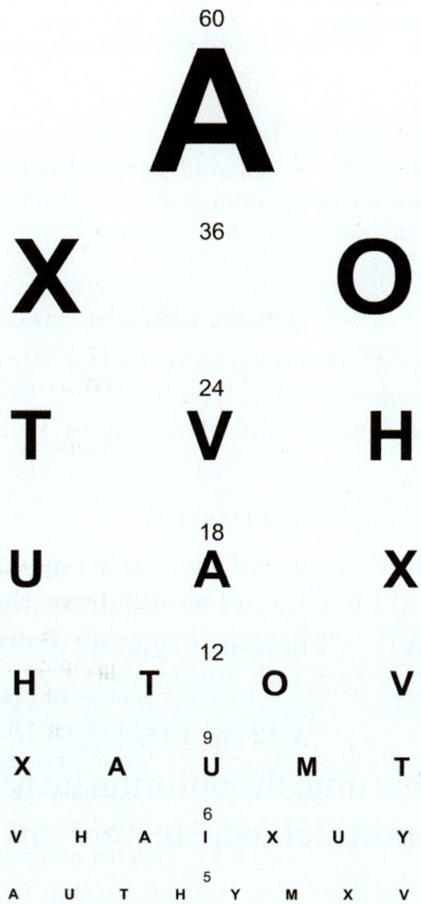

Fig. 21.2. Snellen's test types.

Procedure of testing. For testing distant visual acuity, the patient is seated at a distance of 6 m from the Snellen's chart, so that the rays of light are practically parallel and the patient exerts minimal accommodation. The chart should be properly illuminated (not less than 20 ft candles). The patient is asked to read the chart with each eye separately and the visual acuity is recorded as a fraction, the numerator being the distance of the patient from the letters, and the denominator being the smallest letters accurately read.

When the patient is able to read up to 6 m line, the visual acuity is recorded as 6/6, which is normal. Similarly, depending upon the smallest line which the patient can read from the distance of 6 m, his vision is recorded as 6/9, 6/12, 6/18, 6/24, 6/36 and 6/60, respectively. If he cannot see the top line from 6 m, he is asked to slowly walk towards the chart till he can read the top line. Depending upon the distance at which he can read the top line, his vision is recorded as 5/60, 4/60, 3/60, 2/60 and 1/60, respectively.

If the patient is unable to read the top line even from 1 m, he is asked to count fingers (CF) of the examiner. His vision is recorded as CF-3', CF-2', CF-1' or CF close to face, depending upon the distance at which the patient is able to count fingers. When the patient fails to count fingers, the examiner moves his hand close to the patient's face. If he can appreciate the hand movements (HM), visual acuity is recorded as HM +ve. When the patient cannot distinguish the hand movements, the examiner notes whether the patient can perceive light (PL) or not. If yes, vision is recorded as PL +ve and if not it is recorded as PL –ve.

Other tests which are based on the same principle as Snellen's test types are as follows:

(a) Simple picture chart: used for children > 2 years
(b) Landolt's C-chart: used for illiterate patients
(c) E-chart: used for illiterate patients

Visual acuity equivalents in some common notations are depicted in Table 21.1.

Table 21.1. Visual acuity equivalents in some common notations

Decimal resolution system	*Snellen 6-m table*	*Snellen 20-foot table*	*Angle table*
1.0	6/6	20/20	1 . 0
0.8	5/6	20/25	1 . 3
0.7	6/9	20/30	1 . 4
0.6	5/9	15/25	1 . 6
0.5	6/12	20/40	2 . 0
0.4	5/12	20/50	2 . 5
0.3	6/18	20/70	3 . 3
0.1	6/60	20/200	1 0 . 0

Visual acuity for near

Near vision is tested by asking the patient to read the near vision chart (Fig. 21.3), kept at a distance of 35 cm in good illumination, with each eye separately. In near vision charts, a series of different sizes of printer type are arranged in increasing order and marked accordingly. Commonly used near vision charts are as follows:

1. *Jaeger's chart.* In this chart, prints are marked from 1 to 7 and accordingly patient's acuity is labelled as J1 to J7 depending upon the print he can read.
2. *Roman test types.* According to this chart, the near vision is recorded as N5, N8, N10, N12 and N18 (Printer's point system) (Fig. 21.3).
3. *Snellen's near vision test types.*

II. *EXTERNAL OCULAR EXAMINATION*

External ocular examination should be carried out as follows:

A. *Inspection in diffuse light* should be performed first of all for a preliminary examination of the eyeballs and related structures viz. lids, eyebrows, face and head.

B. *Focal (oblique) illumination examination* should be carried out for a detailed examination under magnification. It can be accomplished using a magnifying loupe (uniocular or binocular) and a focussing torch light or preferably a slit-lamp.

C. *Special examination* is required for measuring intraocular pressure (tonometry) and for examining angle of the anterior chamber (gonioscopy).

J. 1 (Sn. 0.5) **N5.**

As she shoke Moses came slowly on foot, and aweating under the deal box which he had strapt round his shoulders like a pediar "Welcome, welcome, Moses! well, my boy, what have you brought us from the fair?—"I have brought

J. 2 (Sn. 0.6) **N6**

five shillings and twopence is no bad day's work. come, let us have it then."—"I have brought back no money," cried Moses again. "I have laid it all out in a bargain and here it is, "pulling out a bundle from his

J. 4 (Sn. 0.8) **N9**

mother," cried the boy, "why won't you listen to reason. I had them a dead bargain, or I should not have brought them. The silver rims alone will sell for double the money"—"A fig for

J. 6 (Sn. 1) **N12**

the rims, for they are not worth sixpence; for I perceive they are only copper varnished over."—"What! cried my wife," not silver! the rims not silver?"—"No,"

J. 8 (Sn. 1.25) **N18**

with copper rims and shagreen cases? A murrain take such trumpery! The blockhead has been imposed upon, and should have know his

J. 10 (Sn. 1.5) **N24**

the idiot!" returned she, "to bring me such stuff: if I had them I would throw them in the fire."—"There again you are wrong, my

J. 12 (Sn. 1.75) **N36**

By this time the unfortunate Moses was undeceived. He now saw that

J. 14 (Sn. 2.25) **N48**

asked the circumstances of his deception. He sold the

Fig. 21.3. Near vision chart.

Scheme of external ocular examination is described here. (For details of the examination techniques see page 509-523). Scheme of examination includes the structures to be examined and the signs to be looked for. Further, the important causes of the common signs are also listed to fulfill the prerequisite that '*the eyes see what the mind knows*'. Both eyes should be examined in each case.

The external ocular examination should proceed in the following order:

1. Examination for the head posture

Position of the head and chin should be noted first of all. Head posture may be abnormal in a patient with paralytic squint (head is turned in the direction of the action of paralysed muscle to avoid diplopia) and in complete ptosis (chin is elevated to uncover the pupillary area in a bid to see clearly).

2. Examination of forehead

- Forehead may show increased wrinkling (due to overaction of frontalis muscle) in patient with ptosis.
- Complete loss of wrinkling in one-half of the forehead is observed in patients with lower motor neuron facial palsy.
- Facial asymmetry may be noted in patient with Bell's palsy and facial hemiatrophy.

3. Examination of eyebrows

- Level of the two eyebrows may be changed in a patient with ptosis (due to overaction of frontalis).
- Cilia of lateral one-third of the eyebrows may be absent (madarosis) in patients with leprosy or myxoedema.

4. Examination of the eyelids

All the four eyelids should be examined for their position, movements, condition of skin and lid margins.

i. *Position*. Normally the lower lid just touches the limbus while the upper lid covers about 1/6th (2 mm) of cornea.

- In ptosis, upper lid covers more than 1/6th of cornea.
- Upper limbus is visible due to lid retraction as in thyrotoxicosis and sympathetic overactivity.

ii. *Movements of lids.* Normally the upper lid follows the eyeball in downward movement but it lags behind in cases of thyroid ophthalmopathy.

- *Blinking* is involuntary movement of eyelids. Normal rate is 12-16 blinks per minute. It is increased in local irritation. Blinks are decreased in trigeminal anaesthesia and absent in those with 7th nerve palsy.
- *Lagophthalmos* is a condition in which the patient is not able to close his eyelids. Causes of lagophthalmos are:
  - Facial nerve palsy
  - Extreme degree of proptosis
  - Symblepharon

iii. *Lid margin*. Note presence of any of the following:

- *Entropion* (inward turning of lid margin).
- *Ectropion* (outward turning of lid margin).
- *Eyelash abnormalities* such as:
  - *Trichiasis* i.e., misdirected cilia rubbing the eyeball. Common causes are trachoma, blepharitis, stye and lid trauma.
  - *Distichiasis* i.e., an abnormal extra row of cilia taking place of meibomian glands.
  - *Madarosis* i.e., absence of cilia may be seen in patients with chronic blepharitis, leprosy and myxoedema.
  - *Poliosis* i.e., greying of cilia is seen in old age and also in patients with Vogt-Koyanagi-Harada's disease.
- *Scales* at lid margins are seen in blepharitis.
- *Swelling* at lid margin may be stye, papilloma or marginal chalazion.

iv. *Abnormalities of skin.* Common lesions are herpetic blisters, molluscum contagiosum lesions, warts, epidermoid cysts, ulcers, traumatic scar etc.

v. *Palpebral aperture*. The exposed space between the two lid margins is called *palpebral fissure* which measures 28-30 mm horizontally and 8-10 mm vertically (in the centre). Following abnormalities may be observed:

- *Ankyloblepharon* is usually seen following adhesions of the two lids at angles, e.g., after ulcerative blepharitis and burns. It results in horizontally narrow palpebral fissure.
- *Blepharophimosis* (all around narrow palpebral fissure) is usually a congenital anomaly.
- *Vertically narrow palpebral fissure* is seen in:

- Inflammatory conditions of conjunctiva, cornea and uvea due to blepharospasm
- Ptosis (drooping) of upper eyelid
- Enophthalmos (sunken eyeball)
- Anophthalmos (absent eyeball)
- Microphthalmos (congenital small eyeball)
- Phthisis bulbi
- Atrophic bulbi

- *Vertically wide palpebral fissure* may be noted in patients with:
  - Proptosis
  - Large-sized eyeball (e.g. buphthalmos)
  - Retraction of upper lid
  - Facial nerve palsy

5. Examination of lacrimal apparatus

A thorough examination of lacrimal apparatus is indicated in patients with epiphora, corneal ulcer and in all patients before intraocular surgery. The examination should include:

- *Inspection of lacrimal sac area* for redness, swelling or fistula
- *Inspection of the lacrimal puncta,* for any defect such as eversion, stenosis, absence or discharge.
- *Regurgitation test.* It is performed by pressing over the lacrimal sac area just medial to the medial canthus and observing regurgitation of any discharge from the puncta. Normally it is negative. A *positive regurgitation test* indicates dacryocystitis. A *false negative regurgitation test* may be observed in internal fistula, wrong method of performing regurgitation test, patient might have emptied the sac just before coming to the examiner's chamber, encysted mucocele.
- *Lacrimal syringing.* It is done to locate the probable site of blockage in patients with epiphora (see page 392).
- Other tests such as *Jone's dye test I and II,* dacryocystography etc. can be performed when indicated (see page 393).

6. Examination of eyeball as a whole

Observe the following points:

i. *Position of eyeballs*. Normally, the two eyeballs are symmetrically placed in the orbits in such a way that a line joining the central points of superior and inferior orbital margins just touches the cornea. Abnormalities of the position of eyeball can be:

(a) *Proptosis/exophthalmos* i.e., bulging of eyeballs; note whether proptosis is:
- axial or eccentric
- reducible or non-reducible
- pulsatile or non-pulsatile

(b) *Enophthalmos* (sunken eyeball)

ii. *Visual axes of eyeballs*. Normally the visual axes of the two eyes are simultaneously directed at the same object which is maintained in all the directions of gaze. Deviation in the visual axis of one eye is called *squint* (complete evaluation of a case of squint is a specialised examination) (see pages 342, 347).

iii. *Size of eyeball*. Obvious abnormalities in the size of eyeball can be detected clinically. However, precise measurement of size can only be made by ultrasonography (A-scan). The size of eyeball is increased in conditions like buphthalmos and unilateral high myopia. *The causes of small-sized eyeball are*: congenital microphthalmos, phthisis bulbi, and atrophic bulbi.

iv. *Movements of eyeball* should be tested uniocularly (ductions) as well as binocularly (versions) in all the six cardinal directions of gaze (see pages 335-336).

7. Examination of conjunctiva

i. *Bulbar conjunctiva* can be examined by simply retracting the upper lid with index finger and lower lid with thumb of the left hand.

ii. *Lower palpebral conjunctiva and lower fornix* can be examined by just pulling down the lower lid and instructing the patient to look up (Fig. 21.4).

iii. *Upper palpebral conjunctiva* can be examined only after everting the upper eyelid. Eversion of upper lid can be carried out by one-hand or two-hand technique.

- *One-hand technique.* In it patient looks down and the examiner grasps the lid margin alongwith lashes with left index finger and thumb. Then swiftly everts the upper lid by making index finger a fulcrum. This, however, requires some practice.
- *Two-hand technique.* It is comparatively easier. Procedure is same as above, except that here the lid is rotated around a fixed probe which is held

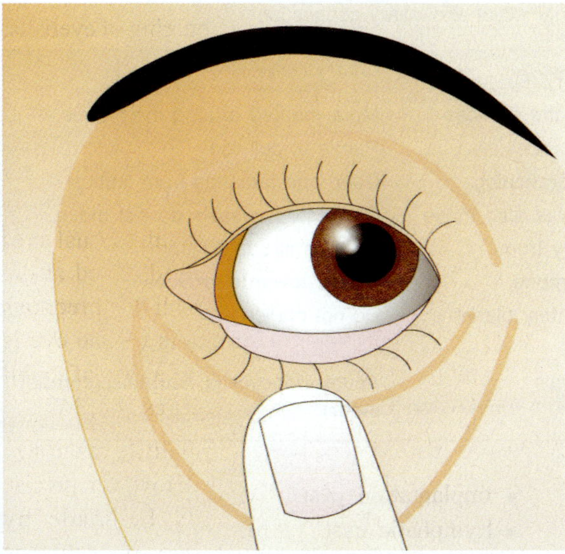

Fig. 21.4. Examination of the lower fornix and lower palpebral conjunctiva.

above the level of tarsal plate with right hand (Fig. 21.5). In slight modification of two-hand technique, index finger of right hand can be used instead of probe.

iv. *Examination of superior fornix* requires double eversion of upper lid using Desmarre's lid retractor.

Conjunctival signs

Normal conjunctiva is a thin semi-transparent structure. A fine network of vessels is distinctly seen in it. Following signs may be observed:

i. *Discoloration* of conjunctiva may be brownish in melanosis and argyrosis (silver nitrate deposits), greyish due to *surma* deposits, pale in anaemia, bluish in cyanosis and bright red due to subconjunctival haemorrhage.

ii. *Congestion of vessels.* Congestion may be superficial (in conjunctivitis) or ciliary/circumcorneal/deep (in iridocyclitis, and keratitis) or mixed (in acute congestive glaucoma). Differences between conjunctival and ciliary congestion are depicted in Table 21.2.

iii. *Conjunctival chemosis* (oedema) may be observed in allergic and infective inflammatory conditions.

iv. *Follicles.* These are seen as greyish white raised areas (mimicking boiled sago-grains) on fornices and palpebral conjunctiva. Follicles represent areas of aggregation of lymphocytes. Follicles may be seen in following conditions:
- Trachoma
- Acute follicular conjunctivitis
- Chronic follicular conjunctivitis
- Benign (School) folliculosis

v. *Papillae* are seen as reddish raised areas with flat tops and velvety appearance. These represent areas of vascular and epithelial hyperplasia. Papillae are seen in the following conditions:
- Trachoma
- Spring catarrh

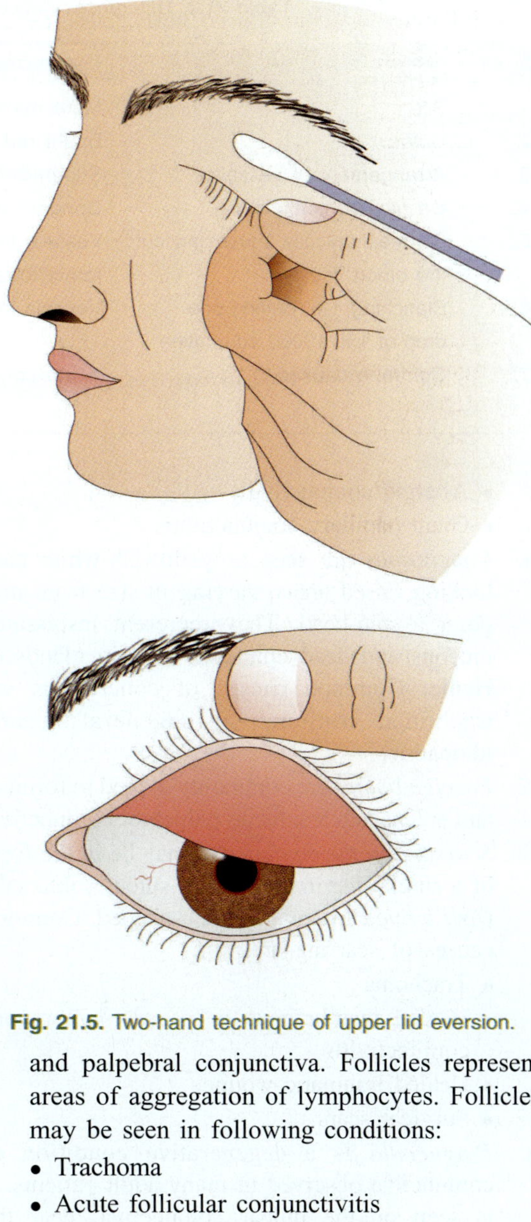

Fig. 21.5. Two-hand technique of upper lid eversion.

Table 21.2. Differences between conjunctival and ciliary congestion

S. no.	Feature	Conjunctival congestion	Ciliary congestion
1.	Site	More marked in the fornices	More marked around the limbus
2.	Colour	Bright red	Purple or dull red
3.	Arrangement of vessels	Superficial and branching	Deep and radiating from limbus
4.	On moving conjunctiva	Congested vessels also move	Congested vessels do not move
5.	On mechanically squeezing out the blood vessels	Vessels fill slowly from fornix towards limbus	Vessels fill rapidly from limbus towards fornices
6.	Blanching, i.e., putting one drop of 1 in 10000 adrenaline	Vessels immediately blanch	Do not blanch
7.	Common causes	Acute conjunctivitis	Acute iridocyclitis, keratitis (corneal ulcer)

- Allergic conjunctivitis
- Giant papillary conjunctivitis

vi. *Concretions* are seen as yellowish-white hard looking raised areas, varying in size from pin-point to pin-head. They represent inspissated mucous and dead epithelial cells in glands of Henle. Common causes of concretions are trachoma, conjunctival degeneration and idiopathic.

vii. *Foreign bodies* are commonly lodged in fornices and sulcus subtarsalis on palpebral conjunctiva.

viii. *Scarring on the conjunctiva* may be in the form of a single line in the area of sulcus subtarsalis (*Arlt's line*), irregular, or star-shaped. Common causes of scarring are:
- Trachoma
- Healed membranous or pseudomembranous conjunctivitis
- Healed traumatic wounds
- Surgical scars

ix. *Pinguecula* is a degenerative condition of conjunctiva observed in many adult patients. It is seen on the bulbar conjunctiva, near the limbus, in the form of a yellowish triangular nodule resembling a fat drop.

x. *Pterygium* is a degenerative conjunctival fold which encroaches on the cornea in the palpebral area. It must be differentiated from pseudopterygium (an inflammatory fold of conjunctiva encroaching the cornea).

xi. *Conjunctival cysts* which may be observed are:
- Retention cyst
- Implantation cyst
- Lymphatic cyst
- Cysticercosis.

xii. *Conjunctival tumours.* A few common tumours are dermoids, papillomas and squamous cell carcinoma.

8. Examination of sclera

Normally anterior part of sclera covered by bulbar conjunctiva can be examined under diffuse illumination. Following abnormalities may be seen:

i. *Discoloration*. Normally sclera is white in colour. It becomes yellow in jaundice. Bluish discoloration may be seen as an isolated anomaly or in association with osteitis deformans, Marfan's syndrome, pseudo-xanthoma elasticum. Pigmentation of sclera is also seen in naevus of Ota, and melanosis bulbi.

ii. *Inflammation*. A superficial localised pink or purple circumscribed flat nodule is seen in *episcleritis.* While a deep, dusky patch associated with marked inflammation and ciliary congestion is suggestive of *scleritis.*

iii. *Staphyloma* is a thinned out bulging area of sclera which is lined by the uveal tissue. Depending upon its location, scleral staphylomas may be intercalary, ciliary, equatorial and posterior.

iv. *Traumatic perforations* in blunt trauma are usually seen in the region of limbus or at the equator.

9. Examination of cornea

Loupe and lens examination or preferably slit-lamp biomicroscopy is a must to delineate corneal lesions.

While examining the cornea, a note of following points should be made:

i. *Size*. The anterior surface of normal cornea is elliptical with an average horizontal diameter of 11.7 mm and vertical diameter of 11 mm. Abnormalities of corneal size can be:

- *Microcornea,* when the anterior horizontal diameter is less than 10 mm. It may occur isolated or as a part of microphthalmos.
- Corneal size also decreases in patients with phthisis bulbi.
- *Megalocornea* is labelled when the horizontal diameter is more than 13 mm. Common causes are congenital megalocornea and buphthalmos.

ii. *Shape (curvature)*. Normal cornea is like a watch glass with a uniform posterior curve in its central area. In addition to biomicroscopy, keratometry and corneal topography is required to confirm changes in corneal curvature. Abnormalities of corneal shape (curvature) are:

- *Keratoglobus.* It is an ectatic condition in which cornea becomes thin and bulges out like a globe.
- *Keratoconus.* It is an ectatic condition in which cornea becomes cone shaped.
- *Cornea plana* i.e., flat curvature of cornea which may occur in patients with severe hypotony and phthisis bulbi and rarely as a congenital anomaly.

iii. *Surface.* Smoothness of corneal surface is disturbed due to abrasions, ulceration, ectatic scars and facets. Changes in smoothness of surface can be detected by slit-lamp biomicroscopy, window reflex test and Placido's disc examination.

Placido's keratoscopic disc. It is a disc painted with alternating black and white circles (Fig. 21.6). It may be used to assess the smoothness and curvature of corneal surface. Normally, on looking through the hole in the centre of disc a uniform sharp image of the circles is seen on the cornea (Fig. 21.7). Irregularities in the corneal surface cause distortion of the circles (Fig. 21.8).

iv. *Sheen.* Normal cornea is a bright shining structure. Sheen of corneal surface is lost in 'dry eye' conditions. A loss of the normal polish of the corneal surface causes loss in the sharpness of the outline of the image of circles on *Placido's disc test.*

v. *Transparency* of cornea is lost in corneal oedema, opacity, ulceration, dystrophies, degenerations,

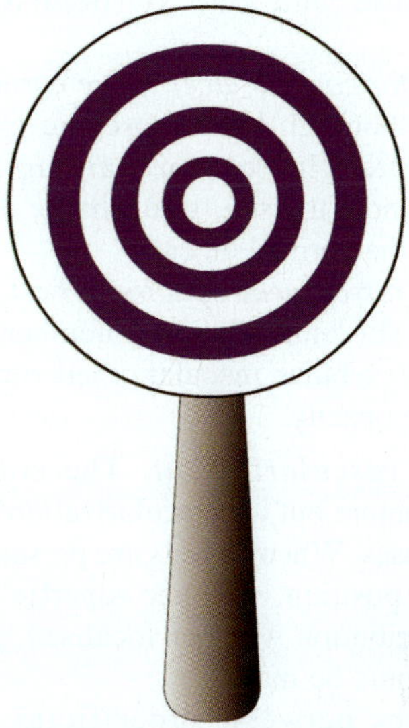

Fig. 21.6. Placido's disc.

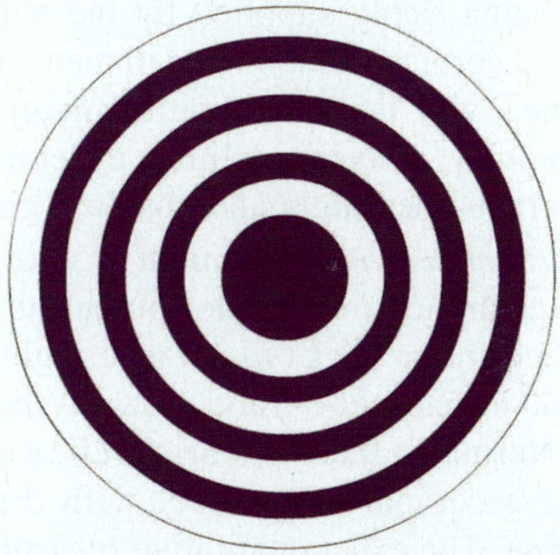

Fig. 21.7. Placido's disc reflex from normal cornea.

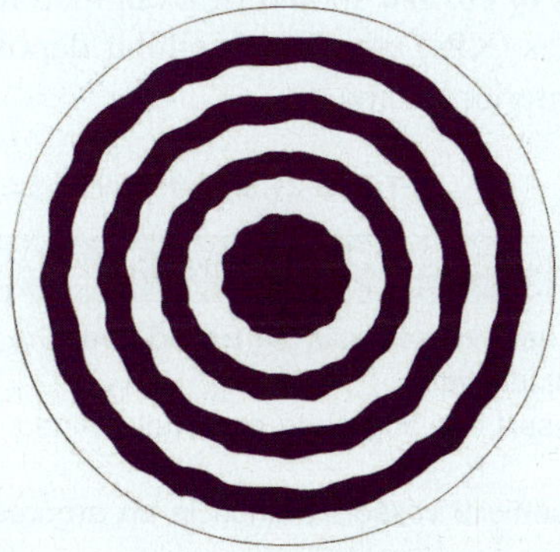

Fig. 21.8. Placido's disc reflex from irregular corneal surface.

vascularization and due to deposits in the cornea.

Examination for corneal ulcer. Once corneal ulcer is suspected, a thorough biomicroscopic examination before and after fluorescein staining should be performed to note the site, size, shape, depth, floor and edges of the corneal ulcer.

Examination for corneal opacity is best done with the help of a slit-lamp. Note the number, site, size, shape, density (nebular, macular or leucomatous) and surface of the opacity.

vi. *Corneal vascularization.* The cornea is an avascular structure but its vascularization may occur in many diseases. When vessels are present, an exact note of their position, whether superficial or deep and their distribution whether localised, general, or peripheral should be made.

Differences between superficial and deep vascularization of cornea are shown in Table 21.3.

vii. *Corneal sensations.* Cornea is a very sensitive structure, being richly supplied by the nerves. The sensitivity of cornea is diminished in many affections of the cornea, viz., herpetic keratitis, neuroparalytic keratitis, leprosy, diabetes mellitus, trigeminal block for post-herpetic neuralgia and absolute glaucoma.

Testing corneal sensations. Patient is asked to look ahead; the examiner touches the corneal surface with a fine twisted cotton wick (which is brought from the side to avoid menace reflex) and observes the blinking response. Normally, there is a brisk reflex closure of lids. Always compare the effect with that on the opposite side. The exact qualitative measurement of corneal sensations is made with the help of an aesthesiometer.

viii. *Back of cornea* should be examined for keratic precipitates (KPs) which are cellular deposits and a sign of anterior uveitis.

KPs can be of different types such as fine, pigmented, or mutton fat (see page 151).

ix. *Corneal endothelium.* It is examined with specular microscope which allows a clear morphological study of endothelial cells including photographic documentation. The cell density of endothelium is around 3000 cells/mm^2 in young adults, which decreases with advancing age.

Biomicroscopic examination after staining of cornea with vital stains

1. *Fluorescein staining* of cornea is carried out either using one drop of 2 percent freshly prepared aqueous solution of the dye or a disposable autoclaved filter paper strip impregnated with the dye. The area denuded of epithelium due to abrasions or corneal ulcer when stained with fluorescein appear brilliant green. When examined using cobalt blue light, the stained area appears opaque green.
2. *Bengal rose* (1%) stains the diseased and devitalized cells red, e.g., as in superficial punctate keratitis and filamentary keratitis. Bengal rose dye is very irritating. Therefore, a drop of 2% xylocaine should be instilled before using this dye.
3. *Alcian blue* dye stains the excess mucus selectively, e.g., as in keratoconjunctivitis sicca.

10. Examination of anterior chamber

It is best done with the help of a slit-lamp.

i. *Depth of anterior chamber.* Normal depth of anterior chamber is about 2.5 mm in the centre (slightly shallow in childhood and in old age). On slit-lamp biomicroscopy, an estimate of depth is made from the position of iris. Anterior chamber may be normal, shallow, deep or irregular in depth.

Table 21.3. Differences between superficial and deep corneal vascularization.

	Superficial corneal vascularization	*Deep corneal vascularization*
1.	Corneal vessels can be traced over the limbus into the conjunctiva.	Corneal vessels abruptly end at the limbus.
2.	Vessels are bright red and well-defined.	Vessels are ill-defined and cause only a diffuse reddish blush.
3.	Superficial vessels branch in an arborescent manner.	Deep vessels run parallel to each other in a radial fashion.
4.	Superficial vessels raise the epithelium and make the corneal surface irregular.	Deep vessels do not disturb the corneal surface.

Causes of shallow anterior chamber
- Primary narrow angle glaucoma
- Hypermetropia
- Postoperative shallow anterior chamber (after intraocular surgery due to wound leak or cilio-choroidal detachment).
- Malignant glaucoma
- Anterior perforations (perforating injuries or perforation of corneal ulcer).
- Anterior subluxation of lens
- Intumescent (swollen) lens

Causes of deep anterior chamber
- Aphakia/Pseudophakia
- Total posterior synechiae
- Myopia
- Keratoglobus
- Buphthalmos
- Keratoconus
- Anterior dislocation of lens into the anterior chamber.
- Posterior perforation of the globe.

Causes of irregular anterior chamber
- Adherent leucoma
- Iris bombe formation due to annular synechiae
- Tilting of lens in subluxation

ii. *Contents of anterior chamber.* Anterior chamber contains transparent watery fluid—the aqueous humour. Any of the following abnormal contents may be detected on examination:
- *Aqueous flare* in anterior chamber occurs due to collection of inflammatory cells and protein particles in patients with iridocyclitis. Aqueous flare is demonstrated in fine beam of slit-lamp light as fine moving (Brownian movements) suspended particles. It is based on the Tyndall phenomenon (see page 151).
- *Hypopyon* i.e. *Pus* in the anterior chamber may be seen in cases of infectious corneal ulcer, iridocyclitis, toxic anterior segment syndrome (TASS), endophthalmitis and panophthalmitis.
- *Pseudohypopyon* due to collection of tumour cells in anterior chamber and seen in patients with retinoblastoma.
- *Foreign bodies*—wooden, iron, glass particles, stone particles, cilia etc., may enter the anterior chamber after perforating trauma.
- *Crystalline lens* may be observed in anterior chamber after anterior dislocation of lens.
- *Lens particles* in anterior chamber after trauma, planned extracapsular cataract extraction (ECCE) is a frequent observation.
- *Blood* in the anterior chamber is called *hyphaema* and may be seen after ocular trauma, surgery, herpes zoster and gonococcal iridocyclitis, blood dyscrasias, clotting disorder and intraocular tumours. (e.g. retinoblastoma, angioma).
- *Parasitic cyst* e.g., cysticercus cellulosae has been demonstrated in anterior chamber.
- *Artificial lens.* Anterior chamber intraocular lens may be observed in patients with pseudophakia.

iii. *Examination of angle of anterior chamber* is performed with the help of a gonioscope and slit lamp. Gonioscopy is a specialized examination required in patients with glaucoma (see page 578).

11. Examination of the iris

It should be performed with reference to following points:

i. *Colour of the iris.* It varies in different races; it is light blue or green in caucasians and dark brown in orientals. Heterochromia iridum (different colour of two iris) and heterochromia iridis (different colour of sectors of the same iris) may be present in some individuals. Heterochromia may be either due to involved iris being lighter or darker than the normal.
- *Causes of iris lighter than normal* are: congenital heterochromia, congenital Horner's syndrome, Fuch's heterochromic iridocyclitis, atrophic patches in chronic uveitis, juvenile xantho-granuloma, metastatic carcinoma and Wardenburg syndrome.
- *Causes of darker iri*s include, iris naevi, ocular melanocytosis or oculodermal melanocytosis, haemosiderosis, siderosis bulbi, retained iris foreign body, malignant melanoma of iris and lymphoma.
- Darkly pigmented spots (naevi) are common freckles on the iris.

ii. *Pattern of normal iris* is peculiar due to presence of collarette, crypts and radial striations on its anterior surface. This pattern is disturbed due to 'muddy iris' in acute iridocyclitis and due to atrophy of iris in healed iridocyclitis.

iii. ***Persistent pupillary membrane*** (PPM) is seen sometimes as abnormal congenital tags of iris tissue adherent to the collarette area.

iv. ***Synechiae*** i.e., adhesions of iris to other intraocular structures may be seen. Synechiae may be anterior (in adherent leucoma) or posterior (in iridocyclitis). Posterior synechiae may be total, annular (ring), or segmental.

v. ***Iridodonesis*** (tremulousness of the iris). It is observed when its posterior support is lost as in aphakia and subluxation of lens.

vi. ***Nodules on the iris surface***. These are observed in granulomatous uveitis (Koeppe's and Busacca's nodules), melanoma, tuberculoma and gumma of the iris.

vii. ***Rubeosis iridis*** (new vessel formation on the iris). It may occur in patients with diabetic retinopathy, central retinal vein occlusion (CRVO) , branch retinal vein occlusion (BRVO), ocular ischaemic syndrome, chronic uveitis, chronic retinal detachment, intraocular tumours e.g. retinobalstoma.

viii. ***A gap or hole in the iris***. It may be congenital coloboma or due to iridectomy (surgical coloboma). Separation of iris from ciliary body is called *iridodialysis*.

ix. ***Aniridia or irideremia*** (complete absence of iris). It is a rare congenital condition.

x. ***Iris cyst***. It may be seen near the pupillary margin in patients using strong miotic drops.

12. Examination of pupil

Note the following points:

i. ***Number.*** Normally there is only one pupil. Rarely, there may be more than one pupil. This congenital anomaly is *called polycoria*.

ii. ***Location.*** Normally pupil is placed almost in the centre (slightly nasal) of the iris. Rarely, it may be congenitally eccentric (corectopia).

iii. ***Size.*** Normal pupil size varies from 3 to 4 mm depending upon the illumination. But it may be abnormally small (*miosis)* or large (*mydriasis).*

Causes of miosis

- Effect of local miotic drugs (parasympathomimetic drugs).
- Effect of systemic morphine.
- Iridocyclitis (narrow, irregular, non-reacting pupil).
- Horner's syndrome.
- Head injury (pontine haemorrhage).
- Senile rigid miotic pupil.
- Due to effect of strong light.
- During sleep pupil is pinpoint.

Causes of mydriasis

- Effect of topical sympathomimetic drugs (e.g., adrenaline and phenylephrine).
- Effect of topical parasympatholytic drugs (e.g., atropine, homatropine, tropicamide and cyclopentolate).
- Acute congestive glaucoma (vertically oval large immobile pupil).
- Absolute glaucoma.
- Optic atrophy.
- Retinal detachment.
- Internal ophthalmoplegia.
- 3rd nerve paralysis.
- Belladonna poisoning.

iv. ***Shape.*** Normal pupil is circular in shape.

- *Irregular narrow pupil* is seen in iridocyclitis.
- *Festooned pupil* is the name given to irregular pupil obtained after patchy dilatation (effect of mydriatics in the presence of segmental posterior synechiae).
- *Vertically oval pupil* (pear-shaped pupil or updrawn pupil) may occur post-operatively due to incarceration of iris or vitreous in the wound at 12 O'clock position.

v. ***Colour.*** Of course, pupil is a hole in the iris, but the pupillary area does exhibit colour depending upon the condition of the structures located behind it. Pupil looks:

- *Greyish black* normally,
- *Jet black* in aphakia;
- *Greyish white* in immature senile cortical cataract;
- *Pearly white* in mature cortical cataract;
- *Milky white* in hypermature cataract;
- *Brown* in cataracta brunescence, and
- *Brownish black* in cataracta nigra.
- *Leucocoria* (white reflex in pupil) in children is seen in congenital cataract, retinoblastoma, retrolental fibroplasia (retinopathy of prematurity), persistent primary hyperplastic vitreous and toxocara endophthalmitis. The yellowish white, semidilated, non-reacting pupil seen in retinoblastoma and pseudogliomas is also called as *amaurotic cat's eye reflex.*

- *Greenish hue* is observed in pupillary area in some patients with glaucoma.
- *Dirty white exudates* may occlude the pupil *(occlusio pupillae)* in patients with iridocyclitis.

vi. ***Pupillary reactions.*** Note as follows:

- *The direct light reflex.* To elicit this reflex the patient is seated in a dimlighted room. With the help of a palm one eye is closed and a narrow beam of light is shown to other pupil and its response is noted. The procedure is repeated for the second eye. A normal pupil reacts briskly and its constriction to light is well maintained.
- *The consensual light reflex.* To determine consensual reaction to light, patient is seated in a dimly-lighted room and the two eyes are separated from each other by an opaque curtain kept at the level of nose (either hand of examiner or a piece of cardboard). Then one eye is exposed to a beam of light and pupillary response is observed in the other eye. The same procedure is repeated for the second eye. Normally, the contralateral pupil should also constrict when light is thrown onto one pupil.
- *Swinging flash light test.* It is performed when relative afferent pathway defect is suspected in one eye (unilateral optic nerve lesion with good vision). To perform this test, a bright flash light is shone on to one pupil and constriction is noted. Then the flash light is quickly moved to the contralateral pupil and response is noted. This swinging to-and-fro of flash light is repeated several times while observing the pupillary response. Normally, both pupils constrict equally and the pupil to which light is transferred remains tightly constricted. In the presence of relative afferent pathway defect in one eye, the affected pupil will dilate when the flash light is moved from the normal eye to the abnormal eye. This response is called '*Marcus Gunn pupil*' or a relative afferent pupillary defect (RAPD). It is the earliest indication of optic nerve disease even in the presence of normal visual acuity.
- *The near reflex.* In it pupil constricts while looking at a near object. This reflex is largely determined by the reaction to convergence but accommodation also plays a part.

  To determine the near reflex, patient is asked to focus on a far object and then instructed suddenly to focus at an object (pencil or tip of index finger) held about 15 cm from patient's eye. While the patient's eye converges and focuses the near object, observe the constriction of pupil.

Abnormal pupillary reactions include (i) amaurotic pupil, (ii) efferent pathway defect, (iii) Wernicke's hemianopic pupil, (iv) Marcus Gunn pupil, (v) Argyll Robertson pupil, and (vi) the tonic pupil (for details see page 312).

13. Examination of the lens

A thorough examination of the lens can be accomplished with the help of oblique illumination, slit-lamp biomicroscopy and distant direct ophthalmoscopy with fully-dilated pupils. Following points should be noted:

i. ***Position.*** A normal lens is positioned in the patellar fossa (space between the vitreous and back of iris) by the zonules. Abnormalities of position may be:

- *Dislocation of lens* i.e., lens is not present in its normal position (i.e., patellar fossa) and all its supporting zonules are broken. In *anterior dislocation* the intact lens (clear or cataractous) is present in the anterior chamber. While in *posterior dislocation* the lens is present in vitreous cavity where it might be floating (*lensa nutans)* or fixed to the retina (*lensa fixata).*
- *Subluxation of lens* i.e., lens is partially displaced from its position. Here zonules are intact in some quadrant and lens is shifted on that side. With dilated pupil, edge of the subluxated lens is seen as shining golden crescent on focal illumination and as a dark line (due to total internal reflection) on distant direct ophthalmoscopy. In the presence of substantial degree of subluxation, half pupil may be phakic and half aphakic (and patient may experience unilateral diplopia). Common causes of subluxation of lens are trauma. Marfan's syndrome, homocystinuria, Weill-Marchesani syndrome.
- *Aphakia* (absence of lens) is diagnosed by jet black pupil, deep anterior chamber, empty patellar fossa on slit lamp biomicroscopy, hypermetropic eye on ophthalmoscopy, retinoscopy and absence of 3rd and 4th Purkinje images.
- *Pseudophakia.* When posterior chamber IOL is present it is diagnosed by a black pupil, deep anterior chamber, shining reflexes from the anterior surface of IOL and presence of all the four

Purkinje's images. Examination after dilatation of pupil confirms pseudophakia.

ii. *Shape of lens.* Normal lens is a biconvex structure, which is nicely demonstrated in an optical section of the lens on slit-lamp examination (Fig. 21.9). The optical section of the lens shows from within outward embryonic, foetal, infantile and adult nuclei, cortex and capsule. An anterior Y-shaped and posterior inverted Y-shaped sutures may also be seen.

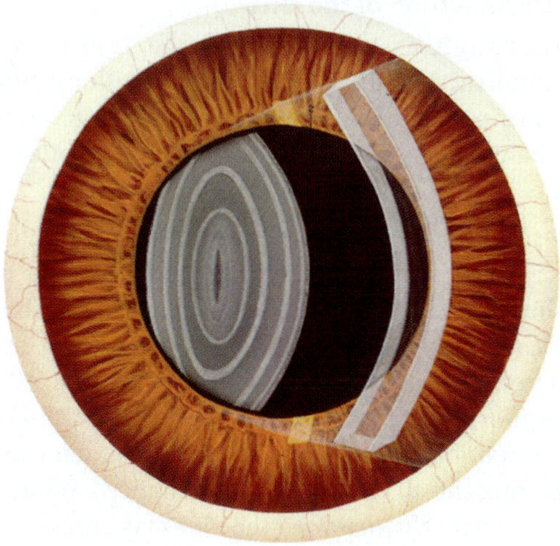

Fig. 21.9. Optical section of the cornea and adult lens as seen on slit-lamp examination.

Abnormalities of the lens shape include:

- Spherophakia i.e., spherical lens.
- Lenticonus anterior i.e., an anterior cone-shaped bulge in the lens as seen in Alport syndrome. (see page 216).
- Lenticonus posterior i.e., a cone-shaped bulge in the posterior aspect of lens (see page 216).
- Coloboma of lens i.e., a notch in the lens (see page 216).

iii. *Colour.* On focal illumination the normal lens in young age appears almost clear or gives a faint blue hue.

- *In old age* even the clear lens gives greyish white hue due to marked scattering of light as a result of increased refractive index of the lens with advancing age. It is usually mistaken for cataract.
- *In cortical cataract* lens may be greyish white, pearly white or milky white in colour in immature, mature and hypermature cataracts, respectively.
- In *nuclear cataract* lens may look amber, brown or black in colour.
- *A rusty (orange) discoloration* is seen in cataractous lens with siderosis bulbi (due to retained intraocular iron foreign body).

iv. *Transparency.* Normal lens is a transparent structure. Any opacity in the lens is called *cataract,* which looks greyish or yellowish white on focal illumination. On *distant direct ophthalmoscopy* the lenticular opacities appear black against a red fundal reflex. On slit-lamp biomicroscopy the morphology of cataract can be studied in detail:

- *Complicated cataract* in the early stages exhibits polychromatic lustre and gives bread crumb appearance.
- *True diabetic cataract* presents *'snow flake'* opacities.
- *Sunflower cataract* is typically seen in disorder of copper metabolism (Wilson's disease).
- *Rosette-shaped cataract,* early as well as late, is typical of concussion injury of lens.

v. *Deposits on the anterior surface of lens* may be:

- *Vossius ring.* It is a small ring-shaped pigment dispersal seen on the anterior surface of lens after blunt trauma. It corresponds in shape and size to the miosed pupil i.e. smaller than the pupil.
- *Pigmented clumps* may be deposited on the anterior surface of lens in patients with iridocyclitis.
- *Dirty white exudates* may be present on the anterior surface of lens in patients with uveitis and endophthalmitis.
- *Rusty deposits* i.e. deposition of ferrous ions just below the anterior capsule is seen in siderosis bulbi.
- *Greenish deposits* i.e. deposition of copper ions is seen in chalcosis.

vi. *Purkinje images test.* This test does not have much significance and thus is not frequently employed in clinical practice. However, it is described as a tribute to the original worker who used this test to diagnose mature cataract and aphakia. Normally, when a strong beam of light is shown to the eye, four images (Purkinje images) are formed from the four different reflecting surfaces, viz., anterior and posterior surfaces of cornea and anterior and posterior surfaces of lens (Fig. 21.10). In patients with mature cataract, fourth image (formed by posterior surface of the lens)

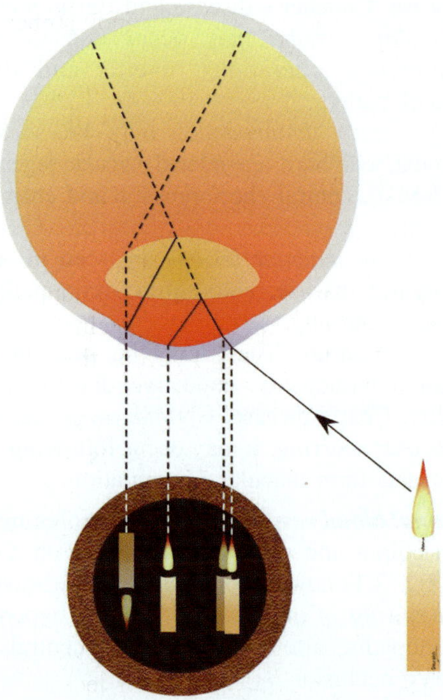

Fig. 21.10. Purkinje images.

is absent i.e., three Purkinje images are formed. In aphakia, third and fourth Purkinje images (formed by anterior and posterior surface of lens) are absent i.e., only two images are formed.

14. The intraocular pressure (IOP)

The measurement of IOP (ocular tension) should be made in all suspected cases of glaucoma and in routine after the age of 40 years. A rough estimate of IOP can be made by *digital tonometry.* For this procedure patient is asked to look down and the eyeball is palpated by index fingers of both the hands, through the upper lid, beyond the tarsal plate. One finger is kept stationary which feels the fluctuation produced by indentation of globe by the other finger (Fig. 21.11). It is a subjective method and needs experience. When IOP is raised, fluctuation produced is feeble or absent and the eyeball feels firm to hard. When IOP is very low eye feels soft like a partially filled water bag.

The exact measurement of IOP is done by an instrument called *tonometer.* Indentation (Schiotz tonometer) and applanation (e.g., Goldmann's tonometer) tonometers are frequently used (for detailed techniques see pages 510-512).

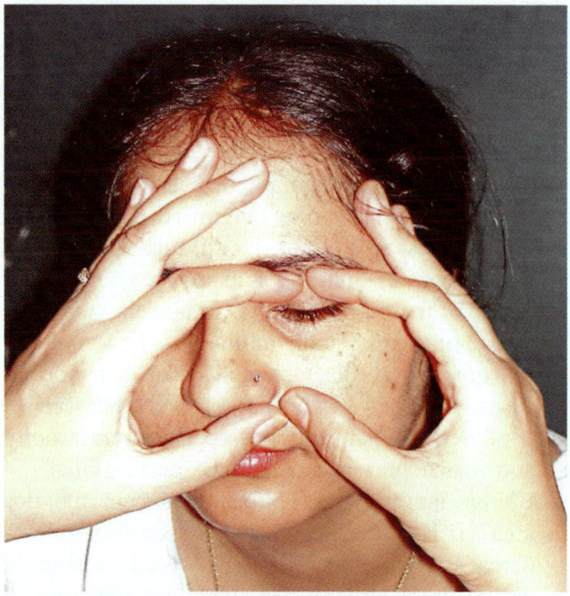

Fig. 21.11. Technique of digital tonometry.

- *Normal IOP range* is 10-21 mm of Hg with an average tension of 16 ± 5.0 mm of Hg.
- *Hypotony* is labelled when IOP is less than 10 mm Hg. Causes of hypotony include ruptured globe, phthisis bulbi, retinal/choroidal detachment, iridocyclitis, ocular ischaemia, post-operative wound leak and traumatic ciliary body shut down.
- Glaucoma should be suspected when IOP is more than 21 mm of Hg and such patients should be thoroughly investigated.

III. *FUNDUS EXAMINATION*

This is essential to diagnose the diseases of the vitreous, optic nerve head, retina and choroid. For thorough examination of the fundus pupils should be dilated with 5 per cent phenylephrine and/or 1 per cent tropicamide eye drops. The fundus examination can be accomplished by ophthalmoscopy (see page 596) and slit-lamp biomicroscopic examination (see page 600).

Observations during fundus examination

During fundus examination following observations should be made:

1. *Media*. Normally the ocular media is transparent. Opacities in the media are best diagnosed by distant direct ophthalmoscopy, where the opacities look black against the red glow.

Causes of opacities in media are: corneal opacity, lenticular opacity, vitreous opacities (may be exudates, haemorrhage, degeneration, foreign bodies and vitreous membranes).

2. *Optic disc*

- *Size (diameter)* of the optic disc is 1.5 mm which looks roughly 15 times magnified during direct ophthalmoscopy. Disc is slightly smaller in hypermetropes and larger in myopes.
- *Shape* of the normal disc is circular. In very high astigmatism, disc looks oblong.
- *Margins* of the disc are well defined in normal cases. Blurring of the margins may be seen in papilloedema, papillitis, postneuritic optic atrophy and in the presence of opaque nerve fibres.
- *Colour.* Normal disc is pinkish with central pallor area. (i) Hyperaemia of disc is seen in papilloedema and papillitis, (ii) Paler disc is a sign of partial optic atrophy, (iii) Chalky-white disc is seen in primary optic atrophy, (iv) Yellow-waxy disc is typical of consecutive optic atrophy.
- *Cup-disc ratio.* Normal cup disc ratio is 0.3. (i) Large cup may be physiological or glaucomatous. (ii) Cup becomes full in papilloedema and papillitis.
- *Splinter haemorrhages* on the disc may be seen in primary open angle glaucoma, normal tension glaucoma and papilloedema.
- *Neovascularization* of the disc may occur in diabetic retinopathy, CRVO and sickle-cell retinopathy.
- *Opticociliary shunt* is a sign of orbital meningioma.
- *Peripapillary* crescent is seen in myopia.
- *Kesten-Baum index* refers to ratio of large blood vessels versus small blood vessels on the disc. Normal ratio is 4:16. This ratio is decreased in patients with optic atrophy.

3. *Macula.* The macula is situated at the posterior pole with its centre (foveola) being about 2 disc diameters lateral to temporal margin of disc. Normal macula is slightly darker than the surrounding retina. Its centre imparts a bright reflex (foveal reflex). Following abnormalities may be seen on the macula:

- *Macular hole.* It looks red in colour with punched-out margins.
- *Macular haemorrhage* is red and round.
- *Cherry red spot* is seen in central retinal artery occlusion, Tay-Sach's disease, Niemann-Pick's disease, Gaucher's disease and Berlin's oedema.
- *Macular oedema* may occur due to trauma, intraocular operations, uveitis and diabetic maculopathy.
- *Pigmentary disturbances* may be seen after trauma, solar burn, age-related macular degeneration (ARMD), central chorioretinitis and chloroquine toxicity.
- *Bull's eye macular lesions* are seen in ARMD, Stargardt disease, chloroquine retinopathy, and cone dystrophy.
- *Hard exudates.* These may be seen in hypertensive retinopathy, exudative diabetic maculopathy, Coat's disease, CNVM.
- *Macular scarring.* It may occur following trauma and disciform macular degeneration.

4. *Retinal blood vessels.* Normal arterioles are bright red in colour and veins are purplish with a caliber ratio of 2 : 3. Following abnormalities may be detected:

- *Narrowing of arterioles* is seen in hypertensive retinopathy, arteriosclerosis, and central retinal artery occlusion.
- *Tortuosity of veins* occurs in diabetes mellitus, central retinal vein occlusion and blood dyscrasias.
- *Sheathing* of vessels may be seen in periphlebitis retinae, (Eale's disease, sarcoidosis, syphillis, tuberculosis, Behcet's disease, AIDS) and hypertensive retinopathy.
- *Vascular pulsations. Venous pulsations* may be seen at or near the optic disc in 10-20% of normal people and can be made manifest by increasing the intraocular pressure by slight pressure with the finger on the eyeball. Venous pulsations are conspicuously absent in papilloedema. *Arterial pulsations* are never seen normally and are always pathological. The true arterial pulsations may be noticed in patients with aortic regurgitation, aortic aneurysm and exophthalmic goitre. True arterial pulsations are not limited to disc. While a pressure arterial pulse which is seen in patients with very high IOP or very low blood pressure is limited to the optic disc.

5. *General background.* Normally the general background of fundus is pinkish red in colour. Physiological variations include dark red background in black races and tessellated or tigroid fundus due to excessive pigment in the choroid. Following abnormal findings may be seen in various pathological states:

- *Superficial retinal haemorrhage* may be found in hypertension, diabetes, trauma, venous occlusions, and blood dyscrasias.
- *Deep retinal haemorrhages* are typically seen in diabetic retinopathy.
- *Cotton wool spots (old name soft exudates)* appear as whitish fluffy spots with indistinct margins. These may occur in hypertensive retinopathy, toxaemic retinopathy of pregnancy, diabetic retinopathy, anaemias and collagen disorders like DLE, PAN and scleroderma.
- *Hard exudates* are small, discrete yellowish, waxy areas with crenated margins. Common causes are diabetic retinopathy, hypertensive retinopathy, Coats' disease and circinate retinopathy.
- *Colloid bodies* also called *drusens* occur as numerous minute, whitish, refractile spots, mainly involving the posterior pole. They are seen in senile macular degeneration and Doyne's honeycomb dystrophy.
- *Pigmentary disturbances* may be seen in tapetoretinal dystrophies e.g., retinitis pigmentosa and healed chorioretinitis.
- *Microaneurysms* are seen as multiple tiny dot-like dilatations along the venous end of capillaries. They are commonly found in diabetic retinopathy. Other causes include hypertensive retinopathy, retinal vein occlusions, Eales' disease and sickle cell disease.
- *Neovascularization of retina* occurs in hypoxic states like diabetic retinopathy, Eales' disease, sickle-cell retinopathy, and following central retinal vein occlusion.
- *Tumours of fundus* include retinoblastoma, astrocytoma and melanomas.
- *Peripheral retinal degenerations* include lattice degeneration, paving stone degeneration, white areas with and without pressure.
- *Retinal holes* are seen as punched out red areas with or without operculum. These may be round or horse-shoe in shape or giant tears.
- *Proliferative retinopathy* is seen as disorganized mass of fibrovascular tissue in patients with proliferative diabetic retinopathy, sickle cell retinopathy, following trauma, in Eales' disease and retinopathy of prematurity.
- *Retinal detachment.* Retina looks grey, raised and folded.

(IV) *VISUAL FIELD EXAMINATION*

Examination of visual fields is important in many eye diseases. Technique of visual field examination is described on Page 513. Common types of field defects and their causes are mentioned below :

- *Altitudnal field defects*: Ischaemic optic neuropathy, optic disc disease, high myopia and optic neuritis
- *Enlargement of blind spot*: glaucoma, papillodema, optic disc drusen, coloboma of optic disc, medullated nerve fibers, and myopic disc with a crescent .
- *Central scotoma*: Macular disease, optic neuritis, toxic amblyopia, tumours compressing the nerve.
- *Constriction of peripheral fields*: Glaucoma, retinitis pigmentosa, after panretinal photocoagulation, central retinal artery occlusion with cilioretinal artery sparing, and chronic papillodema .
- *Homonymous hemianopia*: lesion of the optic tract, lateral geniculate body, optic radiations in temporal, parietal or occipital lobe lesions of the brain such as stroke, tumours, aneurysm and trauma.
- *Bitemporal hemianopia*: Lesions involving optic chiasma, such as pituitary adenoma, meningioma, craniopharyngioma and glioma .
- *Binasal field defects*: tumours or aneurysm compressing both optic nerves, or chiasma, chiasmatic arachnoiditis, bilateral occipital disease, bitemporal retinal disease (e.g. retinitis pigmentosa) and glaucoma.
- *Arcuate scotoma*: glaucoma, optic disc drusen, high myopia , ischaemic optic neuropathy and optic neuritis.

RECORD OF OPHTHALMIC CASE

Both right and left eye should be examined and findings should be recorded in ophthalmic clinical case sheet (Appendix I, page 496).

TECHNIQUES OF OCULAR EXAMINATION AND DIAGNOSTIC TESTS

OBLIQUE ILLUMINATION

(See page 575).

TONOMETRY

The intraocular pressure (IOP) is measured with the help of an instrument called *tonometer*. Two basic types of tonometers available are: indentation and applanation.

Indentation tonometery

Indentation (impression) tonometry is based on the fundamental fact that a plunger will indent a soft eye more than a hard eye. The indentation tonometer in current use is that of Schiotz, who devised it in 1905 and continued to refine it through 1927. Because of its simplicity, reliability, low price and relative accuracy, it is the most widely used tonometer in the world.

Schiotz tonometer. It consists of (Fig. 21.12):

- *Handle* for holding the instrument in vertical position on the cornea;
- *Footplate* which rests on the cornea;
- *Plunger* which moves freely within a shaft in the footplate;
- *Bent lever* whose short arm rests on the upper end of the plunger and a long arm which acts as a pointer needle. The degree to which the plunger indents the cornea is indicated by the movement of this needle on a scale; and
- *Weights*: a 5.5 g weight is permanently fixed to the plunger, which can be increased to 7.5 and 10 gm.

Technique of Schiotz tonometry. Before tonometry, the footplate and lower end of plunger should be sterilized. For repeated use in multiple patients it can be sterilized by dipping the footplate in ether, absolute alcohol, acetone or by heating the footplate in the flame of spirit.

After anaesthetising the cornea with paracaine or 2-4 per cent topical xylocaine, patient is made to lie supine on a couch and instructed to fix at a target on

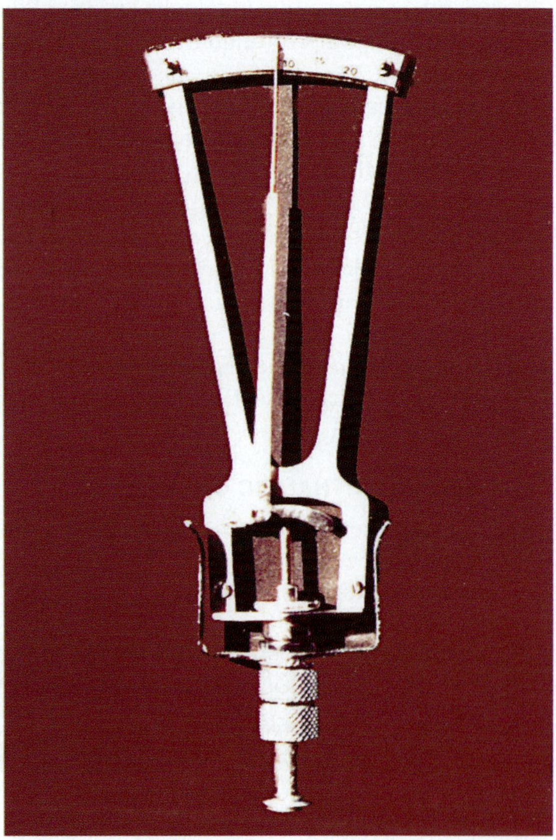

Fig. 21.12. Schiotz tonometer.

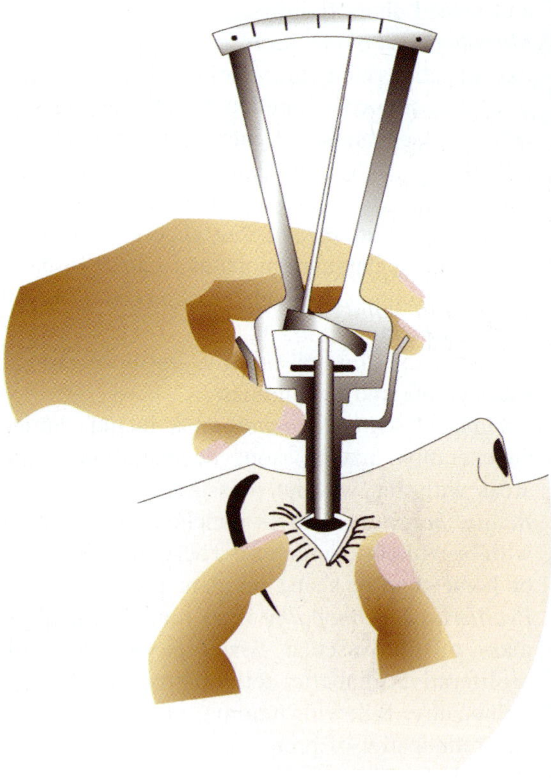

Fig. 21.13. Technique of Schiotz tonometry.

the ceiling. Then the examiner separates the lids with left hand and gently rests the footplate of the tonometer vertically on the centre of cornea. The reading on scale is recorded as soon as the needle becomes steady (Fig. 21.13).

It is customary to start with 5.5 gm weight. However, if the scale reading is less than 3, additional weight should be added to the plunger to make it 7.5 gm or 10 gm, as indicated; since with Schiotz tonometer the greatest accuracy is attained if the deflection of lever is between 3 and 4. In the end, tonometer is lifted and a drop of antibiotic is instilled. A conversion table is then used to derive the intraocular pressure in mm of mercury (mm Hg) from the scale reading and the plunger weight.

The main *advantages of Schiotz tonometer* are that it is cheap, handy and easy to use. Its *main disadvantage* is that it gives a false reading when used in eyes with abnormal scleral rigidity. False low levels of IOP are obtained in eyes with low scleral rigidity as seen in high myopes and following ocular surgery.

Applanation tonometry

The concept of applanation tonometry was introduced by Goldmann is 1954. It is based on *Imbert-Fick law* which states that the pressure inside a sphere (P) is equal to the force (W) required to flatten its surface divided by the area of flattening (A); i.e., P = W/A.

The commonly used applanation tonometers are:

1. *Goldmann tonometer*. Currently, it is the most popular and accurate tonometer. It consists of a double prism mounted on a standard slit-lamp. The prism *applanates* the cornea in an area of 3.06 mm diameter.

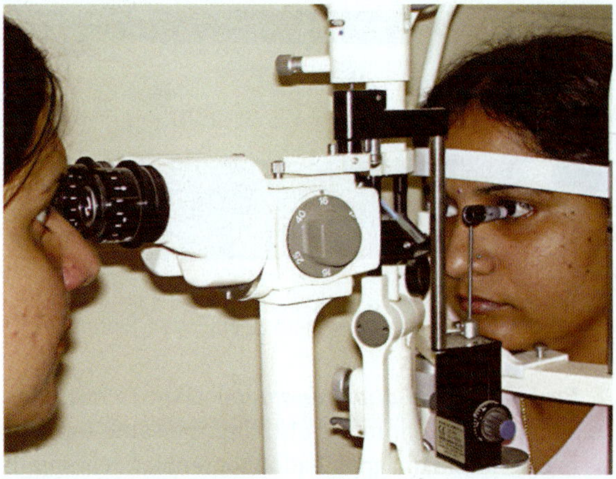

Fig. 21.14. Technique of applanation tonometry.

Technique (Fig. 21.14). After anaesthetising the cornea with a drop of 2 per cent xylocaine and staining the tear film with fluorescein patient is made to sit in front of slit-lamp. The cornea and biprisms are illuminated with cobalt blue light from the slit-lamp. Biprism is then advanced until it just touches the apex of cornea. At this point two fluorescent semicircles are viewed through the prism. Then, the applanation force against cornea is adjusted until the inner edges of the two semicircles just touch (Fig. 21.15). This is the end point. The intraocular pressure is determined by multiplying the dial reading with ten.

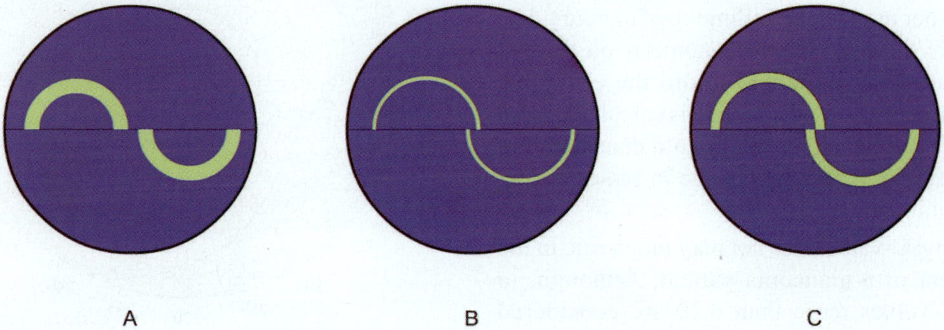

Fig. 21.15. End point of applanation tonometry. (A) too small; (B) too large; (C) end point.

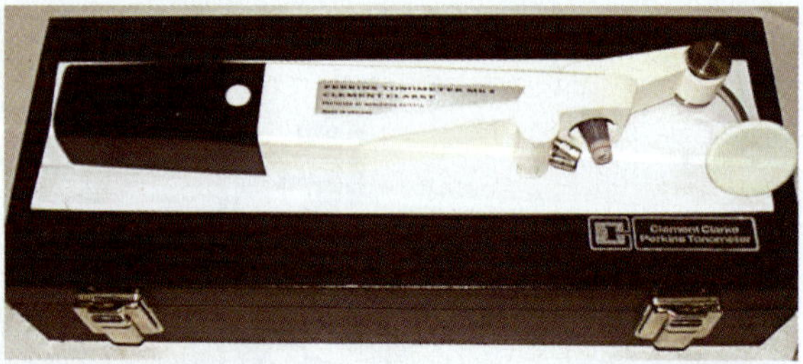

Fig. 21.16. Perkin's hand-held applanation tonometer.

2. ***Perkin's applanation tonometer*** (Fig. 21.16). This is a hand-held tonometer utilizing the same biprism as in the Goldmann applanation tonometer. It is small, easy to carry and does not require slit lamp. However, it requires considerable practice before, reliable readings can be obtained.

3. ***Pneumatic tonometer.*** In this, the cornea is applanated by touching its apex by a silastic diaphragm covering the sensing nozzle (which is connected to a central chamber containing pressurised air). In this tonometer, there is a pneumatic-to-electronic transducer, which converts the air pressure to a recording on a paper-strip, from where IOP is read.

4. ***Pulse air tonometer*** is a hand-held, non-contact tonometer that can be used with the patient in any position.

5. ***Tono-Pen*** is a computerised pocket tonometer. It employs a microscopic transducer which applanates the cornea and converts IOP into electric waves.

Tonography

Tonography is a non-invasive technique for determining the facility of aqueous outflow (C-value). The C-value is expressed as aqueous outflow in microlitres per minute per millimetre of mercury. It is estimated by placing Schiotz tonometer on the eye for 4 minutes. For a graphic record the electronic Schiotz tonometer is used. C-value is calculated from special tonographic tables taking into consideration the initial IOP (P_0) and the change in scale reading over the 4 minutes.

Clinically, C-value does not play much role in the management of a glaucoma patient. Although, in general, C-values more than 0.20 are considered normal, between 0.2 and 0.11 border line, and those below 0.11 abnormal.

TECHNIQUES OF FUNDUS EXAMINATION

A. Ophthalmoscopy, and

B. Slit-lamp biomicroscopic examination of the fundus by:
- Indirect slit-lamp biomiscroscopy,
- Hruby lens biomicroscopy,
- Contact lens biomicroscopy

(For details see page 596-600).

PERIMETRY

The visual field is a three-dimensional area of a subject's surroundings that can be seen at any one time around an object of fixation. Iraquir described it as an "island of vision surrounded by a sea of darkness". The extent of normal visual field with a 5 mm white colour object is superiorly 50°, nasally 60°, inferiorly 70° and temporally 90° (Fig. 21.17). The field for blue and yellow is roughly 10° less and that for red and green colour is about 20° less than that for white. Perimetry with a red colour object is particularly useful in the diagnosis of bitemporal hemianopia due to chiasmal compression and in the central scotoma of retrobulbar neuritis.

The visual field can be divided into central, and peripheral field (Fig. 21.17):

- *Central field* includes an area from the fixation point to a circle 30° away. The central zone contains physiologic blind spot on the temporal side.

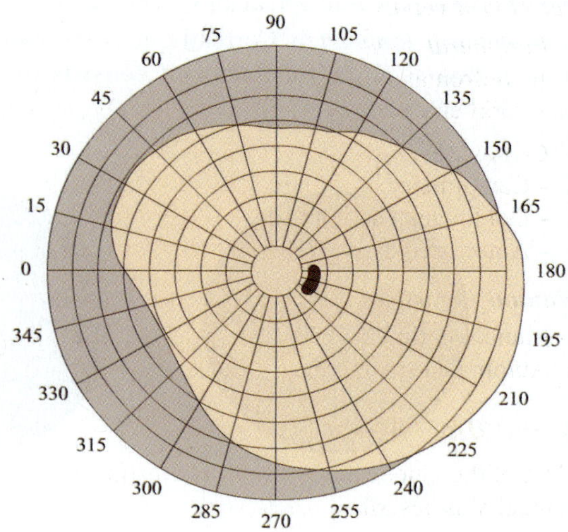

Fig. 21.17. Extent of normal visual field.

- *Peripheral field of vision* refers to the rest of the area beyond 30° to outer extent of the field of vision.
- *Isopter.* Visual field i.e., the three dimensional hill of vision can be divided into many isopters depending upon the perception sensitivity. Thus each isopter can be defined as a threshold line forming points of equal sensitivity on a visual field chart .
- *Scotoma refers* to an area of loss of vision totally (*absolute scotoma*) or partially (*relative scotoma*) in the visual field.

Methods of estimating the visual fields

Perimetry. It is the procedure for estimating extent of the visual fields. It can be classified as below:

Kinetic versus static perimetry

- *Kinetic perimetry.* In this the stimulus of known luminance is moved from a peripheral non-seeing point towards the centre till it is perceived to establish the isopters. Various methods of kinetic perimetry are: confrontation method, Lister's perimetery, tangent screen scotometry and Goldmann's perimetry.
- *Static perimetry.* This involves presenting a stimulus at a predetermined position for a preset duration with varying luminance in the field of vision. Various methods of static perimetry adopted are Goldmann perimetry, Friedmann perimetry, automated perimetry.

Peripheral versus central field charting

- *Peripheral field charting*
  - Confrontation method
  - Perimetry: Lister's, Goldmann's and automated.
- *Central field charting*
  - Campimetry or scotometry
  - Goldmann's perimetry
  - Automated field analysis

Manual versus automated perimetry

- Manual perimetry
- Automated perimetry

A. MANUAL PERIMETRY

Most of the kinetic methods of field testing are done manually as described below:

1. *Confrontation method.* This is a rough but rapid and extremely simple method of estimating the peripheral visual field. Assuming the examiner's fields to be within the normal range, they are compared with patient's visual fields.

The patient is seated facing the examiner at a distance of 1 metre. While testing the left eye, the patient covers his right eye and looks into the examiner's right eye. The examiner occludes his left eye and moves his hands in from the periphery keeping it midway between the patient and himself. The patient and the examiner ought to see the hand simultaneously, for the patient's field to be considered normal. The hand is moved similarly from above, below and from right and left.

2. *Lister's perimeter* (Fig. 21.18). It has a metallic semicircular arc, graded in degrees, with a white dot for fixation in the centre. The arc can be rotated in different meridians. Though not in much use now-a-days, the Lister's perimeter is useful for peripheral field charting.

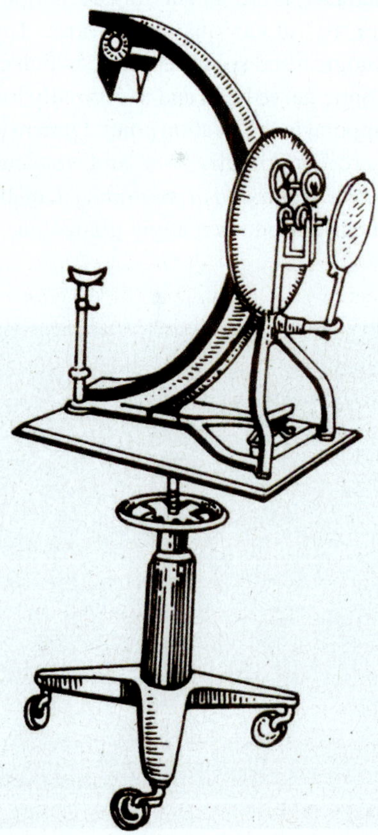

Fig. 21.18. Lister's perimeter.

The patient is seated facing the arc with his chin firmly in the chin-rest. With one eye occluded, he fixates the white dot in the centre. A test object (usually white and of size 3 to 5 mm) is moved along the arc from extreme periphery towards the centre, and the point at which the patient first sees the object is registered on a chart. The arc is moved through 30° each time and 12 such readings are taken. The details of the object regarding its colour and size are noted.

3. *Campimetry* (scotometry), though not used now-a-days, it is useful to evaluate the central and paracentral area (30°) of the visual field. For it, the Bjerrum's screen of either1 metre or 2 metres square is used (Fig. 21.19). Accordingly, the patient is seated at a distance of 1 metre or 2 metres, respectively. The screen has a white object for fixation in its centre, around which are marked concentric circles from 5° to 30°. The patient fixates at the central dot with one eye, the other being occluded. A white target (1-10 mm diameter) is brought in from the periphery towards the centre in various meridians. Initially the physiologic blind spot is charted, which corresponds to the optic nerve head and is normally located about 15° temporal to the fixation point. Dimensions of blind spots are horizontally 7-8° and vertically 10-11°.

Central/paracentral scotomas can be found in optic neuritis and open angle glaucoma.

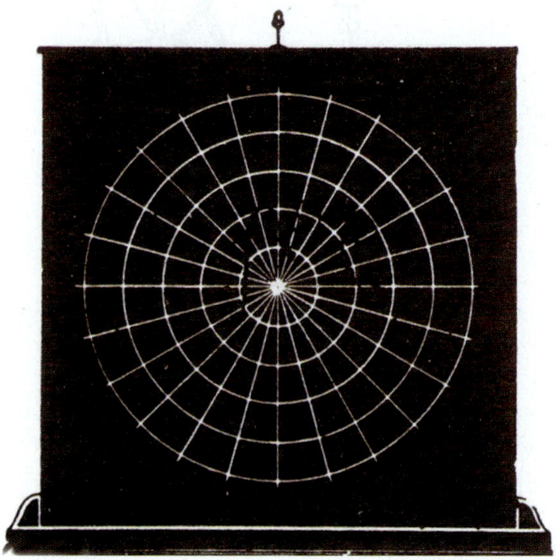

Fig. 21.19. Bjerrum's screen.

4. *Goldmann's perimeter* (Fig. 21.20). It consists of a hemispherical dome. Its main advantage over the tangent screen is that the test conditions and the intensity of the target are always the same. It permits greater reproducibility.

Note: Presently, the Goldman perimeter is not in much use.

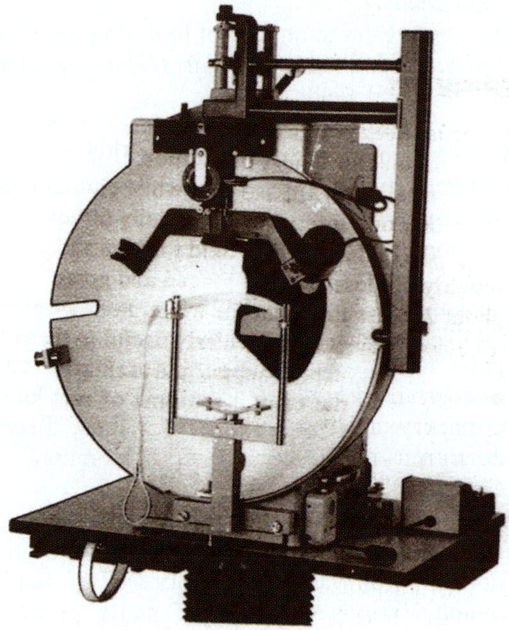

Fig. 21.20. Goldmann's perimeter.

B. AUTOMATED PERIMETRY

Automated perimeters are computer assisted and test visual fields by a static method. The automated perimeters automatically test suprathreshold and threshold stimuli and quantify depth of field defect. Commonly used automated perimeters are: Octopus, Field Master and Humphrey field analyser (Fig. 21.21).

Advantages of automated perimetry over manual perimetry

Presently, automated perimetry has almost completely replaced the manual perimetry because of the following advantages:

- Automated computerized perimetry offers an unprecedented flexibility, a level of precision and consistency of test method that are not generally possible with manual perimetry.

- Other important advantages of automated perimeters are data storage capability, ease of operation, well controlled fixation, menu driven software and on line assistance making them easy to learn and use.
- Automated perimetry also provides facility to compare results statistically with normal individuals of the same age group and with previous tests of the same individual.

Interpretation of automated perimetry print out field charts

Before embarking on the interpretation of automated perimetry printout field charts, it will be worthwhile to have a knowledge about:

- Automated perimeter variables and
- Testing strategies and programmes

The following description is mainly based on Humphrey's field Analyser (HFA).

Automated perimeter variables

1. *Background illumination*. HFA uses 31.5 apostilb (asb) background illumination. Apostilb (asb) is a unit of brightness per unit area (and is defined as 35^{-1} candela / m^2).

2. *Stimulus intensity.* HFA uses projected stimuli which can be varied in *intensity* over a range of more than 5% log units (51 decibels) between 0.08 and 10,000 asb. In decibel notation (db), the value refers to retinal sensitivity rather than to stimulus intensity. Therefore, 0 db corresponds to 10,000 asb and 51 db to 0.08 asb (Fig. 21.22). In contrast to kinetic perimetry, the higher numbers indicate a logarithmic reduction in test object brightness, and hence greater sensitivity of vision (Fig. 21.22).

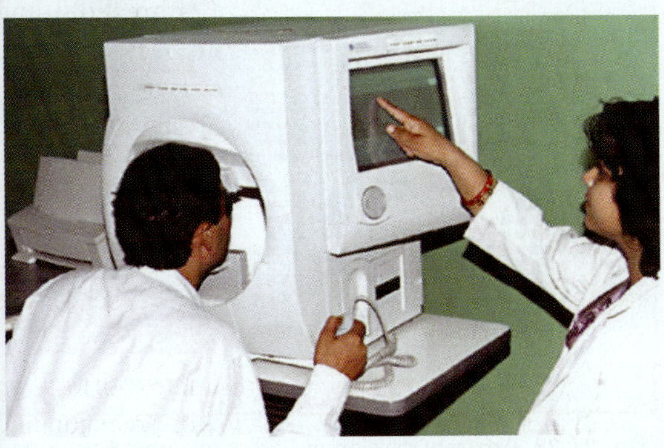

Fig. 21.21. Humphrey field analyser (automated perimeter).

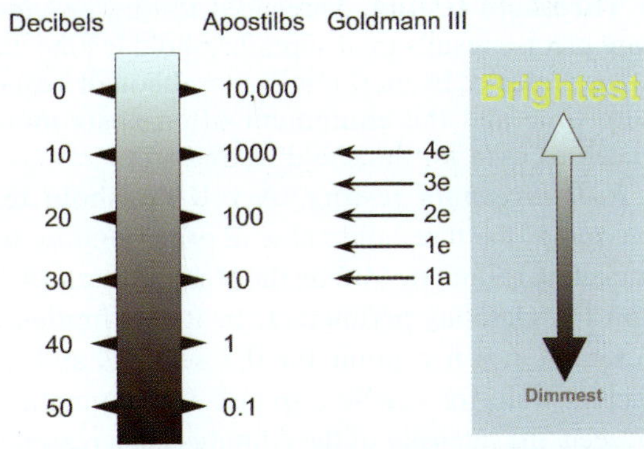

Fig. 21.22. Stimulus intensity scales compared.

3. *Stimulus size.* HFA usually offers five sizes of stimuli corresponding to the Goldmann perimeter stimuli I through V. Unless otherwise instructed, the standard target size for automated perimetry is equivalent to Goldmann size III (4 mm^2) white target.

4. *Stimulus duration.* Stimulus duration should be shorter than the latency time for voluntary eye movements (about 0.25 seconds). HFA uses a stimulus duration of 0.2 sec. while octopus has 0.1 sec.

Testing strategies and programmes

The visual threshold is the physiologic ability to detect a stimulus under defined testing conditions. The normal threshold is defined as the mean threshold in normal people in a given age group at a given location in the visual field. It is against these values that the machine compares the patient's sensitivity. Thresholds are reported in decibels in a range of 0-50. Fifty decibels (db) is the dimmest target the perimeter can project. 0 db is the brightest illumination the perimeter can project. The lower the decibel value the lower the sensitivity; the higher the decibel value, the higher is the sensitivity.

Two basic testing strategies are used in automated static perimetry:

A. Suprathreshold testing. It uses targets that are well above the brightness that the patient should be able to see (suprathreshold). It is simply a screening procedure to detect gross defects. It should not be used to monitor glaucoma. Strategies for supra-threshold testing include:

- Screening central > 6 points.
- Full field 120 points.

B. Threshold testing. Threshold testing provides more precise results than suprathreshold testing and is thus preferred by most clinicians, although it takes more time and the equipment often costs more. Strategies used for threshold testing are:

1. *Full threshold testing.* A full threshold test determines the threshold value at each point by the bracketing technique (4-2 on the Humphrey and 4-2-1 on the Octopus perimeter). In it, a stimulus is presented at a test point for 0.2 seconds and the machine waits for Yes/No response. If the stimulus is not seen, the intensity of the stimulus is increased in 4 db steps till it is seen. Once the threshold is crossed, the stimulus intensity is decreased in 2 db steps till the stimulus is not seen. A full threshold test is appropriate for a patient's first test, because it crosses the threshold twice (first with a 4 dB increment). Accurately determined threshold values make subsequent tests easier because it allows the perimeter to begin with the previous threshold values for determining future data points. Full threshold test is, however, a time consuming process.

2. *Fast Pac.* It is a more rapid testing strategy where the threshold is only crossed once (in 3 dB increments), but this strategy is often not appropriate.

3. *SITA* (Swedish Interactive Threshold Algorithm). It is a strategy of threshold testing which dramatically reduced test time. It is available as SITA - standard and SITA-fast.

Test programmes

The standard test programmes used with static threshold strategy on the *Humphrey's Field Analyser (HFA)* can be grouped as below:

A. *Central field tests*
- Central 30 - 2 test,
- Central 24 - 2 test,
- Central 10 - 2 test, and
- Macular test

B. *Peripheral field tests*
- Peripheral 30/60-1,
- Peripheral 30/60-2,
- Nasal step, and
- Temporal crescent

C. *Speciality tests*
- Neurological -20,
- Neurological -50,
- Central 10-12, and
- Macular test

D. *Custom tests*

Central field tests are more commonly required. These include:

1. *Central 30-2 test.* It offers the most comprehensive form of visual field assessment of the central 30 degrees. It consists of 76 points 6 degrees apart on either side of the vertical and horizontal axes, such that the inner most points are three degrees from the fixation point.

2. *Central 24-2 test.* In it, 54 points are examined. It is near similar to the 30-2 test except that the two peripheral nasal points at 30 degrees on either side of the horizontal axis are not included while testing the central 24 degrees.

3. *Central 10-2 test.* When most points in the *arcuate region* between 10 and 30 degrees show marked depression then this test helps to assess and follow-up 68 points 2 degrees apart in the central 10 degree are examined.

4. *Macular grid test* is used when the field is limited to central 5 degrees. This test examines 10 points

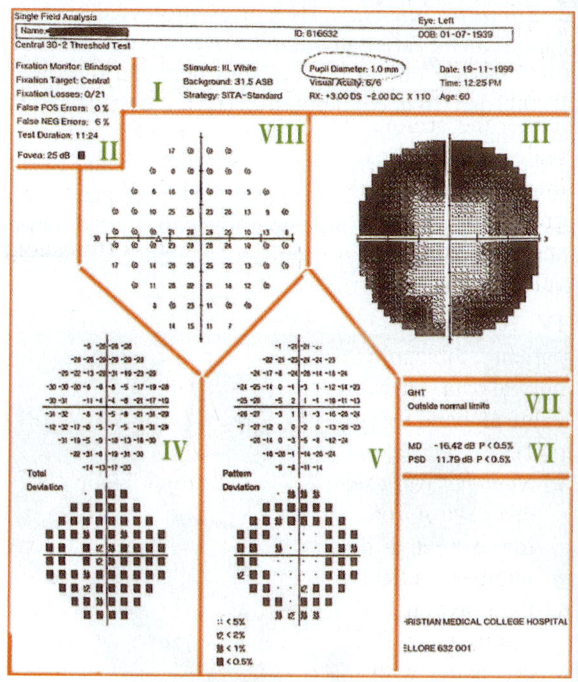

Fig. 21.23. Arbitraty division of humphry single field print out (statpac printout) with central 30-2 test in sparts (zones) for the purpose of discription and understanding.

spaced on a 29 degree square grid centred on the point of fixation.

Evaluation of Humphrey single-field print-out

The standard HFA single field printout is obtained using a software called *Statpac printout*. For the purpose of evaluation, the Humphrey single-field printout (Statpac printout) with central 30-2 test can be studied in eight parts or zones I to VIII as described below (Fig. 21.23):

I. *Patient data and test parameters.* At the top of printout page (part I or zone I) are printed:

- *Patients data* (name, date of birth, eye (right/left) pupil size visual acuity).
- *Test parameters* (test name, strategy, stimulus used, background).

II. *Reliability indices.* The part II or zone II of the printout shows the reliability indices and test duration (Fig. 21.23). The visual field examination is considered unreliable if three or more of the following reliability indices have below mentioned values:

- Fixation losses ≥ 20%,
- False positive error ≥ 33%,
- False negative error ≥ 33%,
- Short-term fluctuations ≥ 4.0 dB,
- Total questions ≥ 400.

III. *Gray scale* simulation of the test data is depicted in zone III or part III of the printout (Fig. 21.23). The darker the printout, the worse is the field. The gray scale provides the field defects at a glance. However, in general we do not make a diagnosis based on the grey scale. The main emphasis on statistical help shows in zone IV to VIII of the printout (threshold values).

IV. *Total deviation plots* provide the deviation of patient's threshold values from that of age corrected normal data. The two total deviation plots are numeric value plot and the probability plot (grey scale symbol plot).

- *Numeric value plot* represents the differences in decibels. A zero value means that the patient has the expected threshold for that age. Positive numbers reflect points that are more sensitive than average for that age; whereas negative numbers reflect points that are depressed compared with the average.
- *Probability plot* (grey scale symbol plot). In the lower part of zone IV of the printout, the total deviation plot is represented graphically. The darker the graphic representation the more significant it is.

  Note: In general, the total deviation plot is an indicator of the general depression and is not capable of revealing the hidden scotomas that may be present in the overall depressed field.

V. *Pattern deviation plots.* The two pattern deviation plots (*numeric pattern deviation plot and probability pattern deviation plot*) shown in zone V of the printout are similar to the total deviation plots except that here Statpac software has corrected the results for the changes caused by cataract, small pupil, etc.

VI. *Global indices* are depicted in the zone VI of the printout. Global indices refer to some calculations made by Statpac to provide overall guidelines to help the practitioner assess the field results as a whole rather than on point-to-point basis as shown in the total deviation and pattern deviation plots.

Below mentioned four global indices are provided with the full threshold program which summarize the status of the visual field at a glance. Principally, the global indices are used to monitor progression of glaucomatous damage rather than for initial diagnosis.

1. *Mean deviation (MD).* This is the mean difference (in decibel value) between the normative data for that age compared with that of collected data. It is more an indicator of the general depression of the field. Worse than normal value is indicated by a negative value.
2. *Pattern standard deviation (PSD).* It is a measure of variability within the field i.e. it measures the difference between a given point and adjacent points. It actually points out towards localized field loss and is most useful in identifying early defects. It loses its advantage in marked depression.
3. *Short-term fluctuation (SF).* It is a measure of the variability between two different evaluations of the same 10 points in the field. It is not available with SITA strategy. A high SF means either decreased reliability or an early finding indicative of glaucoma.
4. *Corrected pattern standard deviation (CPSD).* It is the PSD corrected for SF. It indicates the variability between adjacent points that may be due to disease rather than due to intra-test variability.

VII. ***Glaucoma hemifield test (GHT)*** compares the five clusters of points in the upper field (above the horizontal midline) with the five mirror images in the lower field. These clusters of points have been developed based on the anatomical distribution of the nerve fibres and are specific to the detection of glaucoma. Depending upon the differences between the upper and lower clusters of points the following five messages may be displayed:

- *Outside normal limits.* The GHT outside normal limits denotes that either the values between upper and lower clusters differ to an extent found in less than 1% of the population or any one pair of clusters is depressed to the extent that would be expected in less than 0.5% of the population.
- *Border line.* The GHT is considered border line when the difference between any one of the upper and lower mirror clusters is what might be expected in less than 3% of population.
- *General reduction in sensitivity.* The GHT is considered to have general reduction in sensitivity if the best part of visual field is depressed to an extent expected in less than 0.5% of the population.
- *Abnormally high sensitivity* is labelled when the best part of the visual field is such as would be found in less than 0.5% of the population.
- *Within normal limits.* GHT is considered within normal limits when none of the above criteria is met.

VIII. ***Actual threshold values*** shown in part VIII of the printout (Fig. 21.23) may be inspected for any pattern or scotoma when clinical features are suspeciant and even if all the seven other parts of the printout are normal. A scotoma by definition is the depressed part of the field as compared to the surrounding and not as compared to normals. When the actual test threshold values are below 15 dB, the sensitivity of the test is lost.

Diagnosis of glaucoma field defects on HFA single-field printout

(See page 233).

FUNDUS FLUORESCEIN ANGIOGRAPHY

Fundus flourescein angiography (FFA) is a valuable tool in the diagnosis and management of a large number of fundus disorders.

Basically, FFA gives information by allowing the examiner to study the changes, produced by various fundus disorders, in the flow of fluorescein dye along the vasculature of the retina and choroid.

Indications. It is indicated in many disorders of ocular fundus, viz., (1) Diabetic retinopathy (2) Vascular occlusions; (3) Eales' disease. (4) Central serous retinopathy, (5) Cystoid macular oedema.

Contraindications include renal impairment and known allergy to fluorescein.

Technique. The technique of FFA comprises rapidly injecting 5 ml of 10 per cent solution of sterile sodium fluorescein dye in the antecubital vein and taking serial photographs (with fundus camera) of the fundus of the patient who is seated with pupils fully dilated. The fundus camera has a mechanism to use blue light (420-490 nm wavelength) for exciting the fluorescein present in blood vessels and to use yellow-green filter for receiving the fluorescent light (510-530 nm wavelength) back for photography.

The first photograph is taken after 5 seconds, then every second for next 20 seconds and every 3-5 seconds for next one minute. The last pictures are taken after 10 minutes.

Complications. FFA is a comparatively safe procedure. Minor side effects include: discoloration of skin and urine, mild nausea and rarely vomiting. Anaphylaxis or cardiorespiratory problems are extremely rare. However, a syringe filled with dexamethasone and antihistaminic drug alongwith other measures should be kept ready to deal with such catastrophy.

Phase of angiogram. Normal angiogram consists of following overlapping phases:

1. *Pre-arterial phase.* Since the dye reaches the choroidal circulation 1 second earlier than the retinal arteries, therefore in this stage choroidal circulation is filling, without any dye in retinal arteries.
2. *Arterial phase.* It starts 1 second after prearterial phase and lasts until the retinal arterioles are completely filled.
3. *Arteriovenous phase.* This is a transit phase and involves the complete filling of retinal arterioles and capillaries with a laminar flow along the retinal veins (Fig. 21.24).

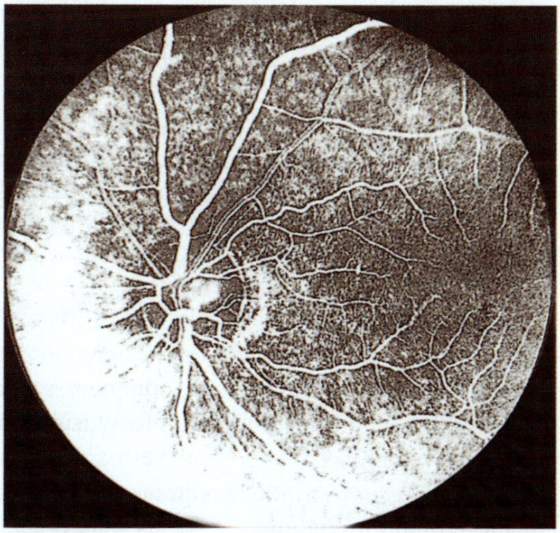

Fig. 21.24. Normal fluorescein angiogram (arteriovenous phase).

4. *Venous phase.* In this phase, veins are filling and arterioles are emptying. This phase can be subdivided into early, mid, and late venous phase.

Abnormalities detected by FFA. In the blood fluorescein is readily bound to the albumin. Normally the dye remains confined to the intravascular space due to the barriers formed by the tight junctions between the endothelial cells of retinal capillaries (inner blood-retinal barrier) and that between the pigment epithelial cells (outer blood-retinal barrier).

In diseased states abnormalities in the form of hyperfluorescence and hypofluorescence may be detected on FFA.

1. *Hyperfluorescence.* The causes are:

- *Window defect* in RPE due to atrophy shows background choroidal fluorescence.
- *Pooling of dye* under detached RPE e.g. ARMD.
- *Pooling of dye* under sensory retina after breakdown of the outer blood-retinal barrier as occur in central serous retinopathy (CSR).
- *Leakage of dye* into the neurosensory retina due to the breakdown in inner blood-retinal barrier e.g., as seen in cystoid macular edema (CME).
- *Leakage of dye* from the choroidal or retinal neovascularization e.g., as seen in cases of proliferative diabetic retinopathy, and subretinal neovascular membrane in age-related macular degeneration.
- *Staining* i.e., long retention of dye by some tissues e.g., as seen in the presence of drusen.
- *Leakage of dye* from optic nerve head as seen in papilloedema.

2. *Hypofluorescence.* The causes are:

- Blockage of background fluorescence due to abnormal deposits on retina e.g., as seen due to the presence of retinal haemorrhage, hard exudates and pigmented clumps.
- Occlusion of retinal or choroidal vasculature, e.g., as seen in central retinal artery occlusion and occlusion of capillaries in diabetic retinopathy.
- Loss of vasculature as occurs in patients with choroideremia and myopic degeneration.

ELECTRORETINOGRAPHY AND ELECTRO-OCULOGRAPHY

The electrophysiological tests allow objective evaluation of the retinal functions. These include: electroretinography (ERG), electro-oculography (EOG), and visually-evoked response (VER).

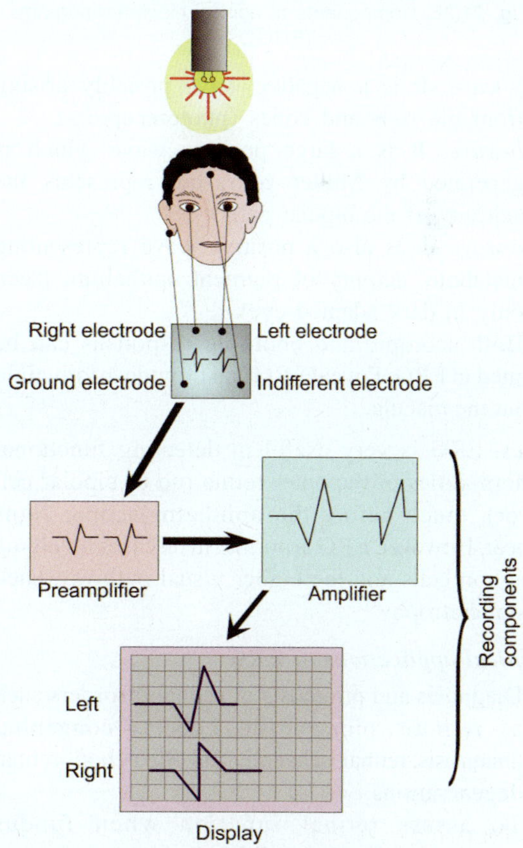

Fig. 21.25. Technique of electroretinogram (ERG) recording.

Electroretinography (ERG)

Electroretinography (ERG) is the record of changes in the resting potential of the eye induced by a flash of light. It is measured in dark adapted eye with the active electrode (fitted on contact lens) placed on the cornea and the reference electrode attached on the forehead (Fig. 21.25).

Normal record of ERG consists of the following waves (Fig. 21.26):

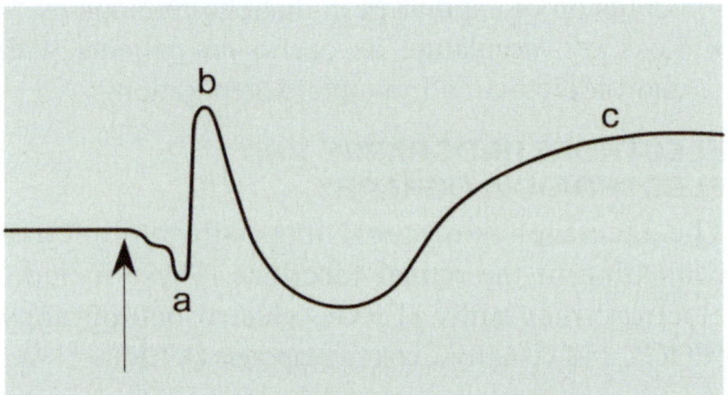

Fig. 21.26. Components of normal electroretinogram (ERG).

- *a-wave.* It is a negative wave possibly arising from the rods and cones (photoreceptors).
- *b-wave.* It is a large positive wave which is generated by Muller cells, but represents the acitivity of the bipolar cells.
- *c-wave.* It is also a positive wave representing metabolic activity of pigment epithelium (seen only in dark adapted eye).

Both scotopic and photopic responses can be elicited in ERG. Foveal ERG can provide information about the macula.

Uses. ERG is very useful in detecting functional abnormalities of the outer retina (up to bipolar cell layer), much before the ophthalmoscopic signs appear. However, ERG is normal in diseases involving ganglion cells and the higher visual pathway, such as optic atrophy.

Clinical applications of ERG

1. Diagnosis and prognosis of retinal disorders such as retinitis pigmentosa, Leber's congenital amaurosis, retinal ischaemia and other chorioretinal degenerations.
2. To assess retinal function when fundus examination is not possible, e.g., in the presence of dense cataract and corneal opacity.
3. To assess the retinal function of the babies where possibilities of impaired vision is considered.

Abnormal ERG response. It is graded as follows:

1. *Subnormal response.* b-wave response is subnormal in early cases of retinitis pigmentosa even before the appearance of ophthalmoscopic signs. A subnormal ERG indicates that a large area of retina is not functioning.
2. *Extinguished response* is seen when there is complete failure of rods and cones function e.g., advanced retinitis pigmentosa, complete retinal detachment, central retinal artery occlusion and advanced siderosis.
3. *A negative response* indicates gross disturbances of the retinal circulation.

Electro-oculography (EOG)

Electro-oculography is based on the measurement of resting potential of the eye which exists between the cornea (+ve) and back of the eye (–ve).

Technique (Fig. 21.27). Electrodes are placed over the orbital margin near the medial and lateral canthi. The patient is asked to move the eye sideways (medially and laterally) and keep there for few seconds, during which recording is done. In this procedure, the electrode near the cornea (e.g.,

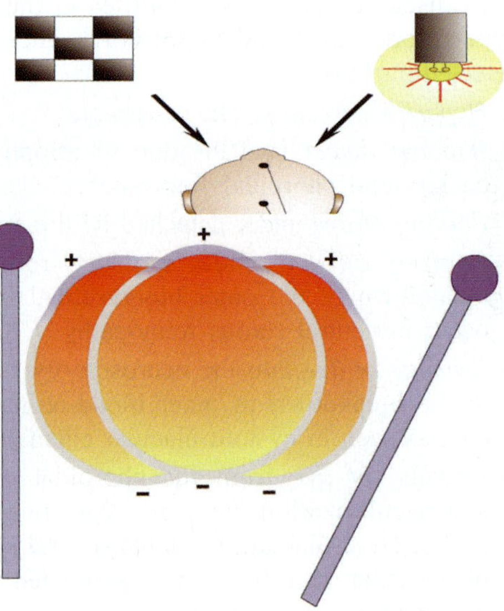

Fig. 21.27. Technique of electro-oculography (EOG) and record of normal electro-oculogram.

electrode placed near lateral canthus, when the eye is rotated laterally) becomes positive. The recording is done every minute for 12 minutes. This procedure is performed first in the dark adapted stage and then repeated for light adapted stage.

Normally, the resting potential of the eye decreases during dark adaptation and reaches its peak in light adaptation.

Interpretation of results. Results of EOG are interpreted by finding out the Arden ratio as follows:

$$\text{Arden ratio} = \frac{\text{Maximum height of light peak}}{\text{Minimum height of dark trough}} \times 100$$

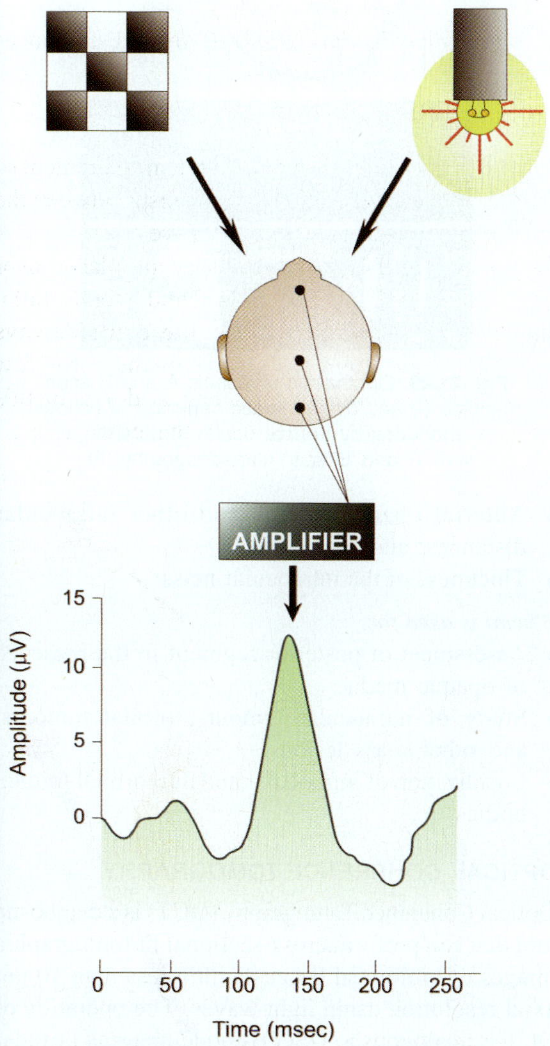

Fig. 21.28. Technique of recording visually evoked response (VER) and record of normal VER pattern.

- *Normal curve* values are 185 or above.
- *Subnormal curve* values are less than 150.
- *Flat curve* values are less than 125.

Uses. Since the EOG reflects the presynaptic function of the retina, any disease that interferes with the functional interplay between the retinal pigment epithelium (RPE) and the photoreceptors will produce an abnormal or absent light rise in the EOG. Thus, EOG is affected in diseases such as retinitis pigmentosa, vitamin A deficiency, retinal detachment and toxic retinopathies. Hence, EOG serves as a test that is supplementary and complementary to ERG and in certain states is more sensitive than the ERG e.g. in diagnosis of Best's disease.

VISUALLY EVOKED RESPONSE (VER)

As we know when light falls on the retina, a series of nerve impulses are generated and passed on to the visual cortex via the visual pathway. The changes produced in the visual cortex by these impulses can be recorded by electroencephalography (EEG) (Fig. 21.28). Thus, visually-evoked response (VER) is nothing but the EEG recorded at the occipital lobe. VER is the *only clinically objective technique available to assess the functional state of the visual system beyond the retinal ganglion cells.* Since there is disproportionately large projection of the macular area in the occipital cortex, the VER represents the macula-dominated response. VER is of two types depending upon the techniques used.

1. *Flash VER*. It is recorded by using an intense flash stimulation. It merely indicates that light has been perceived by the visual cortex. It is not affected by the opacities in the lens and cornea.

Clinical uses. (i) It can assess the integrity of macula and visual pathway in infants, mentally retarded and aphasic patients. (ii) It can distinguish between cases of organic and psychological blindness (e.g., malingering and hysterical blindness). (iii) It can detect visual potentials in eyes with opaque media.

2. *Pattern reversal VER*. It is recorded using some patterned stimulus, as in the checker board. In it the pattern of the stimulus is changed (e.g., black squares go white and white become black) but the overall illumination remains same. The pattern reversal VER depends on form sense and thus may give a rough estimate of the visual acuity.

Normal versus abnormal record of VER. In normal VER record, a positive wave occurs at a latency of about 100 ms (P_{100}). Negative deflections occur at 75 ms (N_{75}) and 135 ms (N_{135}). Amplitude of the positive deflection normally, is the order of 10-25 μV (Fig. 21.28). It is fully established by the age of 6 months.

In the lesions affecting the conduction of the nerve impulse by visual pathway (e.g., retrobulbar neuritis) the amplitude is reduced and there is delay in the transmission time. The timing of the response is more reliable than the amplitude. Increased latency is also common in macular dysfunction; therefore, a delayed VEP should not be considered pathognomic of optic nerve disease.

OCULAR ULTRASONOGRAPHY

Ultrasonography has become a very useful diagnostic tool in ophthalmology. The diagnostic ophthalmic ultrasound is based upon 'pulse-echo' technique. Ultrasonic frequencies in the range of 10 MHz are used for ophthalmic diagnosis. Rapidly repeating short bursts of ultrasonic energy are beamed into the ocular and orbital structures. A portion of this signal is returned back to the examining probe (transducer) from areas of reflectivity. The echoes detected by the transducer are amplified and converted into display form. The processed signal is displayed on cathode ray tubes in one of the two modes: A-scan or B-scan (Fig. 21.29).

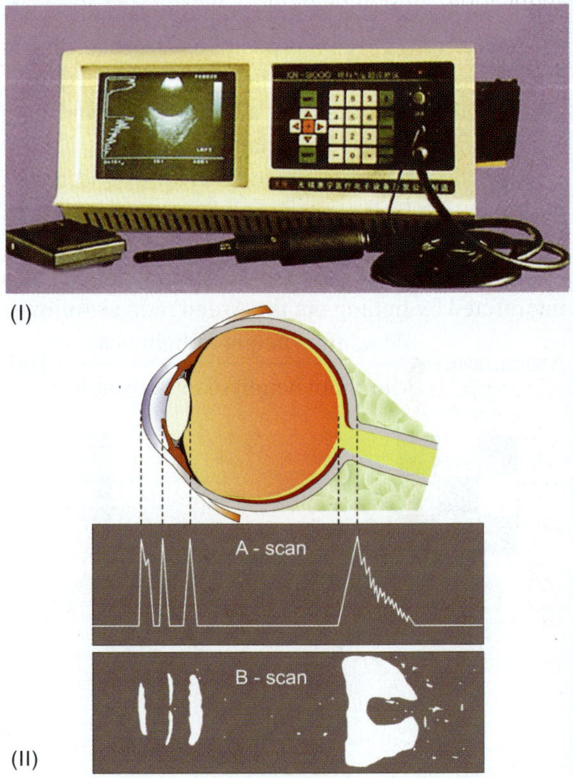

(I)
(II)

Fig. 21.29. Ophthalmic ultrasonic A and B scan machine (I) and diagrammatic depiction of echoes produced by normal ocular structures with 'A' and 'B' scan ultrasonography (II).

A-scan (Time amplitude). The A-scan produces a unidimensional image and echoes are plotted as spikes.

Interpretation of A-scan. (i) The distance between the two echo spikes provides an indirect measurement of tissue such as eyeball length or anterior chamber depth and lens thickness.

(ii) *The height of the spike* indicates the strength of the tissue sending back the echo. The cornea, lens and sclera produce very high amplitude spikes, while the vitreous membrane and vitreous haemorrhage produce lower spikes.

B-scan (intensity modulation). B-scan produces two-dimensional dotted section of the eyeball. The location, size and configuration of the structures is easy to interpret.

Clinical uses of ocular ultrasound

A scan is used for measurement of:

- Axial length, mainly for IOL power calculation (biometry),
- Anterior chamber depth and other intraocular distances, and
- Thickness of the intraocular mass

B scan is used for:

- Assessment of posterior segment in the presence of opaque media.
- Study of intraocular tumours, orbital tumours, and other mass lesions.
- Localization of intraocular and intraorbital foreign bodies.

OPTICAL COHERENCE TOMOGRAPHY

Optical Coherence Tomography (OCT) is a diagnostic tool that can perform cross-sectional or tomographic images of biological tissues within less than 10 μm axial resolution using light waves. The operation of OCT is analogous to USG B-mode imaging or radar except that light is used rather than acoustic or radiowaves. OCT is specially suited for diagnostic applications in ophthalmology because of the ease of optical access to the anterior and posterior segment of the eye. The information provided by OCT is akin to *in-vivo* histopathology of the structure.

Principle. OCT utilizes the interferometry and low-coherence light in near infra red range.

OCT machine (Fig 21.30) comprises: Fundus viewing unit, Interferometric unit, computer display, control panel and colour inkjet printer.

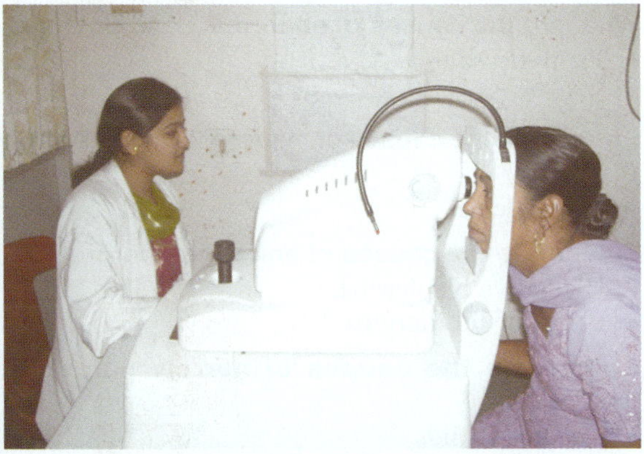

Fig. 21.30. Examination on OCT machine

OCT machine is available as:

- Anterior segment OCT machine,
- Posterior segment OCT machine, and
- Combined anterior segment and posterior segment OCT machine.

Types of OCT machines are:

- Time domain OCT (TD-OCT).
- Frequency domain OCT (FD-OCT).
- Specially encoded frequency domain OCT(SEFD-OCT).
- Time encoded frequency domain OCT (TEFD-OCT).

Normal OCT scan of retina shows cross-sectional study of macula (Fig 21.31A), and optic nerve head (ONH) region including retinal nerve fiber layer (RNFL) of the peripapillary region (Fig 21.31B).

Clinical applications of OCT :

I. ***Applications of anterior segment OCT***

- Imaging of the anterior chamber angle,
- Pachymetry,
- Imaging of trabeculotomy blebs,
- Assessment of tumours and cysts of iris and ciliary body.

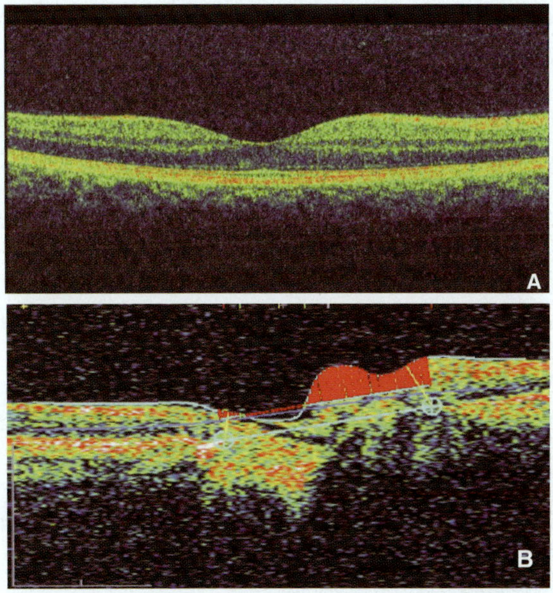

Fig. 21.31. Normal OCT scan of retina: A. Macular region; B. Optic disc region

II. ***Applications of posterior segment OCT***

1. *Macular disorders.* OCT is very useful in confirming macular pathologies such as macular hole, (Fig. 11.27), cystoid macular edema (Fig. 11.25B), age related macular degeneration(ARMD) (Fig. 11.26D), central serous retinopathy (CSR) (Fig. 11.23C) and epiretinal membrane (ERM) etc.
2. *Glaucoma diagnosis.* Optic disc scan (Fig. 9.10c) is very useful in diagnosing and monitoring the glaucomatous changes. It is also useful in evaluating the RNFL for early (pre-perimetric) glaucoma detection.

RELATED QUESTIONS

Enumerate the causes of sudden painless loss of vision.

(See page 492)

Enumerate the causes of sudden painful loss of vision.

(See page 492)

Enumerate causes of gradual painless loss of vision.

(See page 492)

Enumerate the causes of gradual painful loss of vision.

(See page 492)

What are the causes of transient loss of vision (amaurosis fugax) ?

(See page 493)

Enumerate the causes of night blindness (nyctalopia).

(See page 493)

Enumerate the causes of day blindness (hamarlopia).

(See page 493)

What are the causes of defective vision for near only?

(See page 493)

Name the common causes of black spots in front of the eyes.

(See page 493)

What are the causes of flashes of light in front of the eyes (photopsia)?

(See page 493)

What is the most common cause of micropsia (small size of objects), macropsia (large size of objects) and metamorphopsia (distorted shape of objects)?

- Central chorioretinitis

Enumerate the causes of coloured halos.

(See page 493)

Enumerate the causes of diplopia.

(See page 493)

What are the causes of watering from the eyes?

(See page 391)

Enumerate the common causes of redness of eyes.

- Conjunctivitis
- Keratitis
- Iridocyclitis
- Acute glaucomas
- Subconjunctival haemorrhage
- Endophthalmitis
- Panophthalmitis
- Ocular injuries

What are the common causes of pain in eyes?

- Inflammatory conditions of lids, conjunctiva, cornea, uvea, sclera, endophthalmitis, panophthalmitis
- Acute glaucomas
- Refractive errors
- Ocular injuries
- Asthenopia

Enumerate the causes of the foreign body sensation.

- Conjunctival or corneal foreign bodies
- Trichiasis
- Corneal abrasion

Itching in the eyes is a feature of which disease?

- Allergic conjunctivitis (marked itching is pathognomonic of spring catarrh).

COMMON OCULAR SIGNS

What are the causes of abnormal head posture?

- Paralytic squint
- Severe ptosis

Enumerate the causes of madarosis of eyebrows.

- Leprosy
- Myxoedema

Enumerate the causes of ankyloblepharon.

- Ulcerative blepharitis
- Burns of lid margins

Enumerate the causes of narrow palpebral fissure.

- Oedema of lids
- Ptosis
- Enophthalmos
- Anophthalmos
- Microphthalmos
- Phthisis bulbi
- Atrophic bulbi

Enumerate the causes of wide palpebral aperture.

- Proptosis
- Buphthalmos
- Congenital cystic eyeball
- Upper, lid retraction
- Facial nerve palsy

Enumerate the causes of lagophthalmos.

- Facial nerve palsy
- Leprosy
- Myxoedema

Enumerate the causes of poliosis (greying of eye lashes).

- Vogt-Koyanagi-Harada's disease
- Old age
- Vitiligo
- Albinism

Enumerate the causes of circumcorneal congestion.

- Acute glaucomas
- Keratitis and corneal ulcer
- Acute iridocyclitis

Enumerate the causes of conjunctival follicles.

- Trachoma
- Acute follicular conjunctivitis
- Chronic follicular conjunctivitis
- Benign folliculosis

Enumerate the causes of conjunctival papillae.

- Trachoma
- Spring catarrh
- Allergic conjunctivitis
- Giant papillary conjunctivitis

Enumerate the causes of concretions.

- Trachoma
- Degenerative conditions
- Idiopathic

Enumerate the causes of decreased corneal sensations.

- Herpes simplex keratitis
- Neuroparalytic keratitis
- Leprosy
- Herpes zoster ophthalmicus
- Absolute glaucoma
- Acoustic neuroma

Enumerate the causes of superficial corneal vascularization.

- Trachoma
- Phlyctenular keratoconjunctivitis
- Rosacea keratitis
- Superficial corneal ulcer

Enumerate the causes of deep corneal vascularization.

- Interstitial keratitis
- Deep corneal ulcers
- Chemical burns
- Sclerosing keratitis
- After keratoplasty

Enumerate the causes of increased corneal thickness.

- Corneal oedema

Enumerate the causes of abnormal corneal surface.

- Corneal abrasion
- Corneal ulcer
- Keratoconus

Enumerate the causes of shallow anterior chamber.

- Primary angle-closure glaucoma
- Hypermetropia
- Malignant glaucoma
- Postoperative shallow anterior chamber due to
  - Leaking wound
  - Ciliochoroidal detachment
- Corneal perforation
- Intumescent (swollen cataractous) lens
- Iris bombe formation
- Adherent leucoma

Enumerate the causes of deep anterior chamber.

- Aphakia
- Total posterior synechiae
- Myopia
- Keratoglobus
- Keratoconus
- Anterior dislocation of lens in the anterior chamber
- Posterior perforation of the globe
- Buphthalmos

Enumerate the causes of nodules on the iris surface.

- Granulomatous uveitis (Koeppe's and Busacca's nodules)
- Melanoma of the iris
- Tuberculoma
- Gumma

Enumerate the causes of rubeosis iridis (neovascularization of iris).

- Diabetes mellitus
- Central retinal vein occlusion
- Chronic iridocyclitis
- Sickle-cell retinopathy
- Retinoblastoma

Enumerate the causes of iridodonesis.

- Dislocation of lens
- Aphakia
- Hypermature shrunken cataract
- Buphthalmos

Enumerate the causes of hyphaema.

- Ocular injuries
- Postoperative
- Herpes zoster iritis

- Gonococcal iritis
- Intraocular tumour
- Spontaneous (from rubeosis iridis).

Enumerate the causes of hypopyon.

- Corneal ulcer
- Iridocyclitis
- Retinoblastoma (pseudohypopyon)
- Endophthalmitis
- Panophthalmitis

What is diameter of normal pupil?

- Diameter 3 to 4 mm
- In infancy pupil is smaller than at birth
- Myopes have larger pupil than hypermetropes

Enumerate the causes of miosis.

- Effect of miotic drugs (parasympathomimetic drugs, e.g., pilocarpine)
- Effect of systemic morphine
- Iridocyclitis (narrow, irregular non-reacting pupil)
- Horner's syndrome
- Head injury (pontine haemorrhage)
- Senile rigid miotic pupil
- During sleep
- Argyll Robertson pupil
- Poisonings
  - Alcohol
  - Barbiturates
  - Organophosphorus compounds
  - Morphine
  - Carbolic acid
- Hyperpyrexia

Enumerate the causes of mydriasis.

- Topical sympathomimetic drugs such as adrenaline and phenylephrine
- Topical parasympatholytic drugs such as atropine, homatropine, cyclopentolate, tropicamide
- Acute congestive glaucoma (vertically oval, large, immobile pupil)
- Absolute glaucoma
- Optic atrophy
- Retinal detachment
- Internal ophthalmoplegia
- Third nerve paralysis
- Belladonna poisoning
- Coma
- Sympathetic stimulation
  - Aortic aneurysm
  - Cervical rib
  - Mediastinal sarcoma, lymphosarcoma, Hodgkin's disease and pulmonary carcinoma
  - Emotional excitement
- Severe anaemia
- Adie's tonic pupil is larger than its fellow

Enumerate the causes of leukocoria (white reflex in pupillary area).

- Congenital cataract
- Retinoblastoma
- Persistent hyperplastic primary vitreous
- Retrolental fibroplasia
- Toxocara endophthalmitis
- Coat's disease

Enumerate the causes of Marcus Gunn pupil.

(In swinging flashlight test, the pupil on the diseased side dilates on transferring light to it)

- Optic neuritis
- Optic atrophy
- Retinal detachment
- Central retinal artery occlusion
- Central retinal vein occlusion

Enumerate the causes of subluxation of lens.

- Trauma
- Marfan's syndrome
- Homocystinuria
- Weill-Marchesani syndrome

Enumerate the causes of deposits on anterior surface of lens.

- Vossius ring — pigmented ring seen after blunt trauma
- Pigment clumps in iridocyclitis
- Rusty (orange) deposits in siderosis bulbi

Enumerate the causes of cherryred spot.

- Central retinal artery occlusion
- Commotio retinae (Berlin's oedema)
- Tay-Sachs' disease
- Niemann-Pick's disease
- Gaucher's disease

Enumerate the causes of macular oedema.

- Trauma
- Intraocular operations

- Uveitis
- Diabetic maculopathy

Enumerate the causes of superficial retinal haemorrhages.

- Hypertensive retinopathy
- Diabetic retinopathy
- Central retinal vein occlusion
- Anaemic retinopathy
- Leukaemic retinopathy
- Retinopathy of AIDS

Enumerate the causes of soft exudates on the retina.

- Hypertensive retinopathy
- Retinopathy of toxaemia of pregnancy
- Diabetic retinopathy
- Anaemic retinopathy
- LE, PAN and scleroderma
- Leukaemic retinopathy
- Retinopathy of AIDS

Enumerate the causes of hard exudates on the retina.

- Diabetic retinopathy
- Hypertensive retinopathy
- Coats' disease
- Circinate retinopathy

Enumerate the causes of neovascularization of retina.

- Diabetic retinopathy
- Eales' disease
- Sickle-cell retinopathy
- Central retinal vein occlusion

Enumerate the causes of proliferative retinopathy.

- Proliferative diabetic retinopathy
- Sickle cell retinopathy
- Eales' disease
- Ocular trauma

Differential diagnosis of salt and pepper appearance of fundus.

- Prenatal rubella
- Prenatal influenza
- Varicella
- Mumps
- Congenital syphilis

Enumerate the causes of arterial pulsations at the disc.

- Visible arterial pulsations are always pathological
- True pulse waves are seen in:
  - Aortic regurgitation
  - Aneurysm
  - Exophthalmic goitre
- Pressure pulse is seen in:
  - Glaucoma
  - Orbital tumours

What is the significance of venous pulsations at the disc?

- Are visible in 10 to 20% of normal people
- Are absent in papilloedema

In which condition capillary pulsations of the optic disc are seen?

- Are seen in aortic regurgitation as a systolic reddening and diastolic paling of the disc.

Enumerate the causes of enlargement of blind spot.

- Primary open-angle glaucoma
- Papilloedema
- Medullated nerve fibres
- Drusen of the optic nerve
- Juxtapapillary choroiditis

Enumerate the causes of tubular vision.

- Terminal stage of advanced glaucomatous field defect
- Advanced stage of retinitis pigmentosa

Enumerate the causes of ring scotoma.

- Glaucoma
- Retinitis pigmentosa

Enumerate the causes of central scotoma.

- Optic neuritis
- Tobacco amblyopia
- Macular hole, cyst, degeneration

Enumerate the causes of bitemporal hemianopia

Central lesions of chiasma:

- Pituitary tumours (common)
- Suprasellar aneurysms
- Craniopharyngioma
- Glioma of third ventricle
- Meningiomas at tuberculum sellae

Enumerate the causes of homonymous hemianopia.

- Optic tract lesions

Appendix-I

Ophthalmic Clinical Case Sheet

NAME AND ADDRESS

AGE AND SEX

OCCUPATION

RELIGION

CHIEF PRESENTING COMPLAINTS

HISTORY OF PRESENT ILLNESS

PAST HISTORY

PERSONAL HISTORY

FAMILY HISTORY

GENERAL PHYSICAL AND SYSTEMIC EXAMINATION

FACIAL SYMMETRY

HEAD POSTURE

FOREHEAD

OCULAR EXAMINATION

	RIGHT EYE	LEFT EYE
VISUAL ACUITY		
• DISTANCE (WITH AND WITHOUT GLASSES)		
• NEAR		
EYEBROWS		
• LEVEL		
• CILIA		
ORBIT		
• INSPECTION		
• PALPATION		
EYEBALLS		
• POSITION		
• SIZE		
• ALIGNMENT		
• MOVEMENTS		
– UNIOCULAR		
– BIOCULAR		
EYELIDS		
• POSITION		
• MOVEMENTS		
• LID MARGIN		
• EYELASHES		
• SKIN OF LIDS		

	RIGHT EYE	LEFT EYE
PALPEBRAL APERTURE • WIDTH • HEIGHT • SHAPE		
LACRIMAL APPARATUS • PUNCTA • LACRIMAL SAC AREA • REGURGITATION TEST • LACRIMAL SYRINGING		
CONJUNCTIVA • BULBAR CONJUNCTIVA • PALPEBRAL CONJUNCTIVA • FORNICES		
LIMBUS **SCLERA** • DISCOLORATION • NODULE • ECTASIA • ANY OTHER ABNORMALITY		
CORNEA • SIZE • SHAPE • SURFACE • TRANSPARENCY • ULCER • OPACITY • SENSATIONS • VASCULARIZATION • BACK OF THE CORNEA – KPs – PIGMENTATION – ENDOTHELIUM		
ANTERIOR CHAMBER • DEPTH • CONTENTS		
IRIS • COLOUR • PATTERN • SYNECHIAE • IRIDODONESIS • NODULES • NEOVASCULARIZATION • GAP OR HOLE • ANIRIDIA • IRIS CYST • ANY OTHER ABNORMALITY		

	RIGHT EYE	LEFT EYE
PUPIL		
• NUMBER		
• SIZE		
• SHAPE		
• POSITION		
• COLOUR		
• PUPILLARY MARGIN		
• PUPILLARY REACTIONS		
– DIRECT LIGHT REFLEX		
– CONSENSUAL LIGHT REFLEX		
– SWINGING FLASHLIGHT TEST		
– NEAR REFLEX		
LENS		
• POSITION		
– APHAKIA		
– PSEUDOPHAKIA		
– SUBLUXATION		
– DISLOCATION		
• SHAPE		
• TRANSPARENCY		
• COLOUR		
• DEPOSITS ON THE ANTERIOR SURFACE		
• PURKINJE-SAMSON IMAGES		
INTRAOCULAR PRESSURE		
• DIGITAL		
• SCHIOTZ TONOMETER		
• APPLANATION TONOMETER		
FUNDUS EXAMINATION		
• MEDIA		
• DISC		
• BLOOD VESSELS		
• MACULAR AREA		
• GENERAL BACKGROUND		

PROVISIONAL DIAGNOSIS:
OCULAR DIAGNOSTIC TESTS AND INVESTIGATIONS:
FINAL DIAGNOSIS:
TREATMENT:

22 CHAPTER Clinical Ophthalmic Cases

INTRODUCTION

Clinical case discussion is the most important method of assessing the students' clinical acumen. In ophthalmology practical examinations, the students are supposed to work-up a long case and/or 2 to 3 short cases with common eye disorders.

Presentation of a long case

Students are supposed to evaluate a long case under following headings:

1. Name, age, sex, occupation and address of the patient
2. Chief complaints
3. History
   i. History of present illness
   ii. History of past illness
   iii. Personal and professional history
   iv. Family history
4. General physical examination and relevant systemic examination
5. Ocular examination
6. Provisional diagnosis
7. Differential diagnosis, if any
8. List of diagnostic tests required
9. Line of management

List of long cases. During the eight weeks clinical posting in ophthalmology department, students should evaluate and write in their clinical case registers, the common long cases. These include a case of—cataract, aphakia, pseudophakia, glaucoma, iridocyclitis, corneal ulcer (bacterial, viral or fungal), corneal opacity, leukocoria, red eye, chronic dacryocystitis or epiphora and anterior staphyloma.

Presentation of a short case

Students are required to evaluate a short case under following headings:

1. Name, age, sex, occupation and address of the patient.
2. Chief complaints with only one or two relevant questions of history.
3. Ocular examination
4. Diagnosis and differential diagnosis if any
5. List of important diagnostic tests
6. Line of management

List of short cases. During clinical posting in the outdoor (OPD), students should see and evaluate the common short cases. These include a case of—chalazion, stye, trichiasis, entropion, ectropion, ptosis, blepharitis, symblepharon, pterygium, pinguecula, phlyctenular conjunctivitis, spring catarrh, trachoma, Bitot's spots, xerosis, red eye, corneal ulcer, corneal opacity, arcus senilis, band-shaped keratopathy, anterior staphyloma, proptosis, phthisis bulbi, senile cataract (immature, mature, hypermature, nuclear), congenital cataract, traumatic cataract, aphakia, pseudophakia, iridocyclitis, absolute glaucoma, fixed dilated pupil, miosed pupil, amaurotic cat's eye reflex, etc.

Description of clinical cases and viva questions

Description of common clinical cases and related viva questions and other miscellaneous viva questions are described chapterwise.

DISEASES OF THE CONJUNCTIVA

A CASE OF PTERYGIUM

CASE DISCRIPTION

Age and sex. More common in males than females (2:1) and usually occurs past-middle age.

Presenting symptoms. Patients usually present with:

- A cosmetically unacceptable dirty white growth on the cornea. Usually there are no other symptoms in early stages.
- Patient may experience slight irritation or foreign body sensation.
- Diminution of vision may occur due to astigmatism produced by traction on the cornea. Gross diminution of vision occurs when it encroaches upon the pupillary area.
- Occasionally diplopia may occur due to limitation of ocular movements.
- Usually there is history of prolonged exposure to sunny, hot, dusty atmosphere.

Signs on examination. A wing-shaped fold of conjunctiva encroaching upon the cornea in the area of palpebral aperture is seen (Fig.4.28), more commonly on the nasal than the temporal side.

- A fully-developed pterygium consists of three parts: head (optical part present on the cornea), neck (limbal part) and body (scleral part extending between limbus and the canthus).
- Pterygium may be progressive or regressive.
  - *Progressive pterygium* is thick, fleshy and vascular with a few infiltrates in the cornea in front of the head (called *cap of pterygium*).
  - *Regressive pterygium* is thin, atrophic, attenuated with very little vascularity. There is no cap. Ultimately it becomes membranous (pterygium siccus) but never disappears.

Differential diagnosis Pterygium must be differentiated from pseudopterygium.

RELATED QUESTIONS

What is a pterygium?

Pterygium is degenerative condition of the subconjunctival tissue which proliferates as vascularized granulation tissue and is characterized by formation of a triangular fold of conjunctiva encroaching on the cornea.

What is a pseudopterygium; how does it differ from the pterygium?

Pseudopterygium is a fold of bulbar conjunctiva attached to the cornea. It is formed due to adhesions of chemosed bulbar conjunctiva to the marginal corneal ulcer. It usually occurs following chemical burns of the eye.

Differences between the pterygium and pseudopterygium are depicted in Table 22.1.

What complications can occur in an untreated case of pterygium?

- Cystic degeneration
- Neoplastic change (rarely) to: epithelioma, fibrosarcoma or malignant melanoma.

Table 22.1. Differences between pterygium and pseudopterygium

	Pterygium	*Pseudopterygium*
1. Aetiology	A degenerative process	Inflammatory process
2. Age	Usually occurs in elderly persons	Can occur at any age
3. Site	Always situated in the palpebral aperture	Can occur at any site
4. Stages	Either progressive, regressive or stationary	Always stationary
5. Probe test	Probe cannot be passed underneath	A probe can be easily passed under its neck

How can we prevent the recurrence after surgical excision of the pterygium?

Recurrence of the pterygium after surgical excision is the main problem (30-50%). It can be reduced by any of the following measures:

- Preoperative use of mitomycin-C
- Postoperative use of antimitotic drops such as mitomycin-C or thiotepa
- Surgical excision with bare sclera
- Surgical excision with mucous membrane grafts.
- Best method is surgical excision followed by limbal cell transplantation.

What is a pinguecula?

Pinguecula is a degenerative condition of the conjunctiva characterized by formation of a yellowish white triangular patch near the limbus.

What are the causes of conjunctival xerosis?

Depending upon the aetiology, conjunctival xerosis can be divided into two groups:

I. *Parenchymatous xerosis:* It occurs due to cicatricial disorganization of the conjunctiva as seen in following conditions:
   - Trachoma
   - Membranous conjunctivitis
   - Stevens-Johnson syndrome
   - Pemphigus
   - Pemphigoid
   - Conjunctival burns (thermal, chemical or radiational)
   - Prolonged exposure of conjunctiva as in lagophthalmos.

II. *Epithelial xerosis:* It occurs due to hypovitaminosis A.

What is pannus?

Pannus is infiltration of the cornea associated with vascularization. In progressive pannus, the infiltration is seen ahead of the parallel blood vessels, while in regressive pannus it stops short and the blood vessels extend beyond the corneal haze.

DISEASES OF THE CORNEA AND SCLERA

A CASE OF CORNEAL ULCER

CASE DESCRIPTION

Age and sex. May occur at any age in both the sexes. Comparatively males are more commonly affected due to higher chances of injury to the eyes and exposure to infection because of outdoor activity.

Presenting symptoms. A case of corneal ulcer presents with pain, photophobia, lacrimation, discharge, redness, swelling of eyelids and defective vision.

Predisposing factors. A meticulous history taking may reveal presence of any of the following predisposing factors:

- Injury to the eye by vegetative matter, nail, foreign body, etc.
- Chronic dacryocystitis.
- Acute or chronic conjunctivitis
- Chronic foreign body sensation in the eye as in trichiasis and concretions.
- Contact lens wear
- Use of topical steroids
- Diabetes mellitus.

General physical and systemic examination should be performed with specific aim to rule out presence of vitamin A deficiency, malnutrition, diabetes mellitus, source of infection in the body including nasal cavity, paranasal sinuses and teeth and gums.

Signs on ocular examination (Fig. 5.5 and 5.6):

- *Visual acuity* is diminished
- *Lids* show oedema, blepharospasm, lashes may be matted and trichiasis may be present sometimes.

- *Lacrimal sac.* Regurgitation test is positive when there is associated chronic dacryocystitis.
- *Conjunctiva* reveals conjunctival as well as circumcorneal congestion and chemosis. Concretions may be seen on tarsal conjunctiva due to old trachoma.
- *Cornea* on meticulous examination may reveal:
  - Loss of normal corneal transparency
  - Corneal ulcer (better seen after staining with 2% fluorescein dye) should be described with reference to its site, size, shape, depth, margins and floor. Typical features of the bacterial, fungal or viral ulcer may be seen.
  - Window reflex and Placido's disc reflex are distorted.
  - Corneal sensations may be diminished or absent.
  - Superficial peripheral corneal vascularization may be seen.
  - A descematocele may sometimes be seen in a deep ulcer.
- *Anterior chamber* may or may not show pus (hypopyon). It is a feature of bacterial as well as fungal corneal ulcers.
- *Iris* may be slightly muddy in colour.
- *Pupil* may be small due to associated toxin-induced iritis.
- *Intraocular pressure* is usually normal. IOP may be raised if hypopyon or associated uveitis is present.

(*Note:* To record IOP, Schiotz tonometer is never used in corneal ulcer. Always non-contact tonometer is used)

Differential diagnosis. Efforts should be made to describe the type of corneal ulcer whether bacterial, fungal, viral, degenerative or nutritional.

RELATED QUESTIONS

Define keratitis.

Keratitis refers to inflammation of the cornea. It is characterized by corneal oedema, cellular infiltration and conjunctival reaction. Keratitis may be either ulcerative or non-ulcerative.

Define corneal ulcer.

Corneal ulcer may be defined as discontinuation in the normal epithelial surface of the cornea associated with necrosis of the surrounding corneal tissue. Pathologically, it is characterized by oedema and cellular infiltration.

Classify keratitis

Keratitis can be classified in two ways: topographically and aetiologically.

Topograhical (morphological) classification

(A) *Ulcerative keratitis (corneal ulcer):* It can be further classified variously as follows:

1. Depending on location:
   (a) Central corneal ulcer
   (b) Peripheral corneal ulcer
2. Depending on purulence:
   (a) Purulent corneal ulcer or suppurative corneal ulcer (mostly bacterial and fungal corneal ulcers are purulent).
   (b) Non-purulent corneal ulcer (most of the viral, chlamydial, allergic and other non-infective corneal ulcers are non-suppurative).
3. Depending upon association of hypopyon:
   (a) Simple corneal ulcer (without hypopyon)
   (b) Hypopyon corneal ulcer
4. Depending upon depth:
   (a) Superficial corneal ulcer
   (b) Deep corneal ulcer
   (c) Corneal ulcer with impending perforation
   (d) Perforated corneal ulcer
5. Depending upon slough formation:
   (a) Non-sloughing corneal ulcer
   (b) Sloughing corneal ulcer

(B) *Non-ulcerative keratitis*

1. Superficial keratitis
   (a) Superficial punctate keratitis
   (b) Diffuse superficial keratitis
2. Deep keratitis
   (a) Non-suppurative
   - Interstitial keratitis
   - Disciform keratitis
   - Keratitis profunda
   - Sclerosing keratitis

   (b) Suppurative deep keratitis
   - Central corneal abscess
   - Posterior corneal abscess

Aetiological classification

1. Infective keratitis
   (a) Bacterial
   (b) Viral
   (c) Fungal
   (d) Chlamydial
   (e) Protozoal
   (f) Spirochaetal
2. Allergic keratitis
   (a) Phlyctenular keratitis
   (b) Vernal keratitis
   (c) Atopic keratitis
3. Trophic keratitis
   (a) Exposure keratitis
   (b) Neuroparalytic keratitis
4. Keratitis associated with diseases of the skin and mucous membranes.
5. Keratitis associated with systemic collagen vascular disorders.
6. Traumatic keratitis which may be due to mechanical trauma, chemical burns, radiational burns or thermal burns.
7. Idiopathic keratitis, e.g.,
   (a) Mooren's ulcer
   (b) Superior limbic keratoconjunctivitis
   (c) Superficial punctate keratitis of Thygeson.

Name the common bacteria responsible for corneal ulceration.

Common bacteria associated with corneal ulceration are: *Staphylococcus aureus, Pseudomonas pyocyanea, Streptococcus pneumoniae, E.coli, Proteus, Klebsiella, Neisseria gonorrhoeae, Neisseria meningitidis* and *Corynebacterium diphtheriae*.

What is the prerequisite for most of the infecting agents to produce corneal ulceration?

Damage to the corneal epithelium is a prerequisite for most of the infecting organisms to produce corneal ulceration. Damage to corneal epithelium may occur in following forms:

- *Corneal abrasion* due to small foreign body, misdirected cilia, trivial trauma, etc.
- *Necrosis of epithelium* as in keratomalacia.
- *Epithelial damage* due to trophic changes as in neuroparalytic keratitis.
- *Desquamation of epithelial cells* as a result of corneal oedema, corneal xerosis and exposure keratitis.

Name the bacteria which can invade the intact corneal epithelium and produce ulceration.

- *Neisseria gonorrhoeae*
- *Neisseria meningitidis*
- *Corynebacterium diphtheriae*

Name the layers of cornea.

1. Epithelium
2. Bowman's membrane
3. Corneal stroma
4. Descemet's membrane
5. Endothelium

What are the pathological stages of corneal ulceration?

1. Stage of progressive infiltration
2. Stage of active ulceration
3. Stage of regression
4. Stage of cicatrization

What are the characteristic features of bacterial corneal ulcer?

A clinical diagnosis of bacterial corneal ulcer is made in patients with a greyish white central or marginal ulcer associated with marked pain, photophobia, blepharospasm, lacrimation, circumcorneal congestion, purulent/mucopurulent discharge, presence or absence of hypopyon with or without vascularization.

What do you mean by hypopyon corneal ulcer?

A purulent corneal ulcer associated with collection of pus in the anterior chamber caused by *Pneumococcus* is called *hypopyon corneal ulcer.*

Name the common organisms responsible for hypopyon corneal ulceration.

1. Most fungal ulcers are associated with hypopyon.
2. Common bacteria producing hypopyon ulcer are *Pneumococcus, Pseudomonas, Gonococcus* and *Staphylococcus*.

What is ulcus serpens?

The characteristic hypopyon ulcer caused by pneumococcus is called *ulcus serpens.*

Name the complications of corneal ulcer.

1. Toxic iridocyclitis
2. Secondary glaucoma

3. Descemetocele
4. Corneal perforation, which may be complicated by:
   - Iris prolapse
   - Subluxation or dislocation of the lens
   - Anterior capsular cataract
   - Purulent iridocyclitis often leading to endophthalmitis or even panophthalmitis
   - Intraocular haemorrhage in the form of a vitreous haemorrhage or expulsive choroidal haemorrhage.
5. After healing of corneal ulcer following complications may be left as sequelae:
   - Keractasia
   - Corneal opacity which may be nebular, macular, leucomatous or adherent leucoma
   - Anterior staphyloma which usually follows a sloughing corneal ulceration.

What is a descemetocele?

When a corneal ulcer extends up to Descemet's membrane, it herniates (bulges out) as a transparent vesicle called the descemetocele or keratocele.

What are the signs of an impending corneal perforation?

Descemetocele formation associated with excessive corneal oedema are the signs of an impending corneal perforation.

What are the clinical features of perforation of corneal ulcer?

Following perforation of a corneal ulcer, immediately pain decreases and patient feels some hot fluid (aqueous) coming out of the eyes. Anterior chamber becomes shallow and iris prolapse may occur.

How will you manage a case of corneal ulcer?

Management of a case of corneal ulcer is as follows:

Clinical evaluation

1. *Meticulous history* should be taken and a thorough ocular examination including slit-lamp biomicroscopy should be carried out to reach the clinical diagnosis for the type of corneal ulcer.
2. *Regurgitation test* and syringing of lacrimal sac should be carried out to rule out associated dacryocystitis.
3. *General physical and systemic examination* should be carried out to elucidate the associated malnutrition, diabetes mellitus and any other chronic debilitating disease.

Laboratory investigations

1. *Routine laboratory investigations* such as haemoglobin, TLC, DLC, ESR, blood sugar and complete urine examination should be carried out in each case.
2. *Microbiological investigations:* Material is obtained by scraping the base and margins of the corneal ulcer (under topical anaesthesia) and is used for following investigations:
   - Gram and Giemsa-stained smears for possible identification of infecting organisms.
   - 10 per cent KOH wet preparation is made for identification of fungal hyphae
   - Culture on blood agar medium for aerobic organisms
   - Culture on Sabouraud's dextrose agar medium for fungi.

Treatment of uncomplicated corneal ulcer

I. *Specific treatment for the cause:* Bacterial corneal ulcer is treated by topical and systemic antibiotics.
   1. It is preferable to start concentrated amikacin (40-100 mg/ml) eyedrops along with fortified cephazolin (33 mg/ml) eyedrops every one hourly for first five days and then reduced to 2 hourly, 3 hourly, 4 hourly and 6 hourly.
   2. Antibiotic eye ointment should be applied at night.
   3. Subconjunctival injection of gentamicin 40 mg and cephazolin 125 mg once a day for 5 days should be given in sloughing corneal ulcer.

II. *Non-specific treatment* includes:
   1. Cycloplegic drugs, e.g., 1 per cent atropine, 0.5 per cent homatropine or cyclopentolate.
   2. Systemic analgesics and anti-inflammatory drugs to relieve the pain and oedema.
   3. Vitamins (A, B-complex and C) help in early healing of the ulcer.

III. *Physical and general measures:*
   1. Hot fomentation gives comfort, reduces pain and causes vasodilatation.
   2. Rest and good diet are useful for smooth convalescence.

What do you mean by a non-healing corneal ulcer? Enumerate its common causes.

When a corneal ulcer does not start healing despite the best therapy for about 7 to 10 days it is labelled as a non-healing corneal ulcer. Common causes of non-healing corneal ulcers are as follows:

Local causes

- Associated raised intraocular pressure
- Multiple large concretions
- Misdirected cilia
- An impacted foreign body
- Dacryocystitis
- Wrong diagnosis, e.g., fungal ulcer being treated as a bacterial ulcer
- Lagophthalmos
- Excessive vascularization of the ulcer area

Systemic causes

- Diabetes mellitus
- Severe anaemia
- Malnutrition
- Chronic debilitating diseases
- Immunocompromised patients
- Patients on systemic steroids.

How will you treat a case of non-healing corneal ulcer?

1. Removal of any known cause of non-healing: A thorough search should be made to find out any already missed cause of non-healing and when found it should be removed.
2. Mechanical debridement of the ulcer to remove necrosed material may hasten the healing.
3. Chemical cauterization with pure carbolic acid or 10 to 20 per cent trichloroacetic acid may be considered in indolent cases.
4. Peritomy, i.e., severing of perilimbal conjunctival vessels may be useful in the presence of excessive corneal vascularization.
5. Conjunctival flap may be used to cover and support the weak tissue.
6. Bandage soft contact lenses are also useful.
7. Therapeutic keratoplasty, when available, is considered the best mode of treatment.

What extra measures will you take for the treatment of impending perforation?

1. Patient should be advised to avoid strain during sneezing, coughing, passing stool, etc.
2. Pressure bandage should be applied to give some external support.
3. Lowering of intraocular pressure by simultaneous use of acetazolamide 250 mg qId orally, 0.5 per cent timolol eyedrops twice a day and intravenous mannitol (20%) drip stat. Even paracentesis with slow evacuation of the aqueous from the anterior chamber may be done, if required.
4. Tissue adhesive glue such as cyanoacrylate is helpful in preventing perforation.

How will you treat a case of perforated corneal ulcer?

The best treatment is an immediate therapeutic keratoplasty. However, short of it, depending upon the size and location of the perforation measures like use of a tissue glue (cyanoacrylate), bandage soft contact lens or conjunctival flap may be used over and above the conservative management with pressure bandage.

What is a marginal catarrhal ulcer?

Marginal catarrhal ulcer is a superficial ulcer situated near the limbus, usually seen in association with chronic staphylococcal blepharo-conjunctivitis. It is thought to be caused by hypersensitivity reaction to staphylococcal toxins.

Name the common fungi associated with mycotic corneal ulceration.

The fungi most commonly responsible for mycotic corneal ulceration are: *Aspergillus*, *Candida* and *Fusarium*.

What are the predisposing factors for a mycotic corneal ulcer?

1. Injury by vegetative material.
2. Immunosuppressed patients are prone to secondary fungal ulcers.
3. Excessive use of topical antibiotics and steroids predispose the cornea for fungal infections.

What are the characteristic features of a fungal corneal ulcer?

1. A typical fungal corneal ulcer is dry looking, greyish white with elevated rolled-out margins and delicate feathery finger-like extensions into the surrounding stroma under the intact epithelium.
2. A sterile immune ring (yellow line of demarcation) may be present where fungal antigen and host antibodies meet.
3. Multiple, small satellite lesions may be present around the ulcer.

4. Usually a massive and thick hypopyon is present even if the ulcer is very small.
5. A history of trauma (especially by vegetative material) and clinical signs out of proportion to the symptoms, i.e., less marked photophobia and lacrimation with intense ciliary and conjunctival congestion support a fungal origin.

How will you confirm the diagnosis of a fungal corneal ulcer?

Confirmation is made by laboratory investigations, which include examination of a wet KOH, Gram's and Giemsa-stained films for fungal hyphae and culture on Sabouraud's dextrose agar medium.

Name the ocular antifungal drugs.

I. Polyene antifungals, e.g.,
   1. Nystatin 3.5 per cent eye ointment
   2. Amphotericin-B (0.75 to 3% eyedrops)
   3. Natamycin 5 per cent suspension
II. Imidazole antifungal drugs, e.g., ketoconazole, fluconazole miconazole, clotrimazole and econazole
III. Pyrimidine, e.g., flucytosine
IV. Silver compounds, e.g., silver sulphadiazine eyedrops.

Enumerate the ocular lesions of herpes simplex.

Ocular involvement by herpes simplex virus (HSV) occurs in two forms:

I. *Primary herpes* – It is characterized by:
   1. Vesicular lesions involving the skin of lids
   2. Acute follicular conjunctivitis
   3. Fine or coarse epithelial punctate keratitis
II. *Recurrent herpes* – Its lesions are as follows:
   1. Punctate epithelial keratitis
   2. Dendritic ulcer
   3. Geographical or amoeboid ulcer
   4. Disciform keratitis.

Describe the characteristic features of recurrent herpetic keratitis.

Dendritic ulcer is a typical epithelial lesion of the recurrent herpetic keratitis. The ulcer is of an irregular zigzag linear branching shape (Fig. 5.9). The branches are generally knobbed at the ends. Floor of the ulcer stains with fluorescein and the virus laden cells at the margin take up rose bengal stain. There is an associated marked diminution of the corneal sensations.

Sometimes, the branches of the dendritic ulcer enlarge and coalesce to form a large epithelial ulcer typically known as *geographical* or *amoeboid ulcer*.

What are the features of herpes simplex virus (HSV)?

Herpes simplex virus is an epitheliotropic, DNA virus. It is of two types: HSV type-1 which typically causes infection above the waist (herpes labialis) and HSV type-II which causes infection below the waist (herpes genitalis).

Name the predisposing/precipitating stress stimuli which trigger an attack of herpetic keratitis.

- Fever, especially malaria
- General ill health
- Exposure to ultraviolet rays
- Mild trauma
- Use of topical and systemic steroids
- Immunosuppression.

What is disciform keratitis?

Disciform keratitis is stromal keratitis which occurs due to delayed hypersensitivity reaction to the HSV antigen. It is characterized by a focal disc-shaped patch of stromal oedema without necrosis. Associated diminished corneal sensations and fine keratic precipitates differentiate it from other causes of stromal oedema.

Name the antiviral drugs.

Idoxuridine (IDU), trifluorothymidine (TFT), adenine arabinoside (vidarabine) and acyclovir.

Which antiviral drug is effective for stromal viral keratitis?

- Acyclovir

Enumerate the causes of decreased corneal sensations.

Viral keratitis, neuroparalytic keratitis, diabetic neuropathy and leprosy.

What is herpes zoster ophthalmicus?

Herpes zoster ophthalmicus is an acute infection of the gasserian ganglion of the fifth cranial nerve by varicella zoster virus. In it, frontal nerve is more frequently affected than the lacrimal and nasociliary nerve. About 50 per cent cases of herpes zoster ophthalmicus develop ocular complications.

Ocular involvement in herpes zoster ophthalmicus is associated with involvement of which nerve?

- Nasociliary nerve.

What are the characteristic features of herpes zoster?

1. Fever and malaise occur at the onset
2. The vesicular eruptions are preceded by severe neuralgic pain along the course of the involved nerves
3. The lesions are strictly limited to one side of the midline of head (pathognomic feature).

Enumerate the ocular lesions of herpes zoster ophthalmicus.

Conjunctivitis, keratitis, episcleritis, scleritis, iridocyclitis and secondary glaucoma.

What is Mooren's ulcer?

Mooren's ulcer (chronic serpiginous or rodent ulcer) is a peripheral degenerative ulcerative keratitis of unknown aetiology. It is characterized by a shallow furrow-shaped ulcer having whitish overhanging margin at the advancing edge (Fig. 5.13).

What are the features of neuroparalytic keratitis?

1. No pain, no lacrimation and complete loss of corneal sensations
2. Marked ciliary congestion
3. Corneal sheen is dull
4. Corneal ulcer is usually superficial and involves the interpalpebral area.

What are the causes of exposure keratitis?

1. Extreme proptosis
2. Bell's palsy
3. Symblepharon
4. Patients in deep coma.

What is superficial punctate keratitis; name a few of its causes?

Superficial punctate keratitis (SPK) refers to occurrence of multiple, spotty lesions in superficial layer of cornea. Its common causes are:

1. Viral infections, e.g., adenovirus infection, epidemic keratoconjunctivitis, herpes zoster keratitis, herpes simplex keratitis, and pharyngo-conjunctival fever
2. Chlamydial infections, e.g., trachoma
3. Toxic, e.g., in association with blepharo-conjunctivitis
4. Trophic lesions, e.g., exposure keratitis and neuroparalytic keratitis
5. Allergic lesions, e.g., vernal keratitis
6. Keratoconjunctivitis sicca
7. Specific type of idiopathic SPK, e.g., Thygeson's SPK and superior limbic keratoconjunctivitis
8. Photophthalmitis.

What is photophthalmia?

Photophthalmia refers to occurrence of multiple epithelial erosions due to exposure to ultraviolet rays having a wavelength of 290-311 mμ. It occurs in the following conditions:

1. Exposure to naked arc light as in industrial welding
2. Exposure to bright light of a short circuit
3. Snow blindness due to reflected ultraviolet rays from the snow surface.

What is filamentary keratitis/keratopathy? Name its few important causes.

Filamentary keratitis is a type of superficial punctate keratitis associated with formation of corneal epithelial filaments. Its common causes are:

1. Keratoconjunctivitis sicca (KCS)
2. Recurrent corneal erosion syndrome
3. Herpes simplex keratitis
4. Thygeson's superficial punctate keratitis
5. Prolonged patching of the eye particularly following ocular surgery like cataract
6. Trachoma.

What is interstitial keratitis? What are its common causes?

Interstitial keratitis is inflammation of the corneal stroma without primary involvement of the epithelium or endothelium. Its common causes are: congenital syphilis, tuberculosis, acquired syphilis, Cogan's syndrome (interstitial keratitis with acute tinnitus, vertigo and deafness).

What are corneal dystrophies?

Corneal dystrophies are inherited disorders characterized by development of corneal haze in otherwise normal eyes that are free of inflammation or vascularization. These are classified as follows:

1. *Anterior dystrophies* which primarily affect epithelium and Bowman's membrane, e.g., recurrent corneal erosion syndrome.
2. *Stromal dystrophies:* These include: granular dystrophy, macular dystrophy and lattice dystrophy
3. *Posterior dystrophies* which primarily affect the corneal endothelium and Descemet's membrane, e.g., cornea guttata, Fuchs' dystrophy
4. *Ectatic dystrophies* e.g., keratoconus, keratoglobus.

What is Fuchs' dystrophy?

Also called as *epithelial endothelial dystrophy,* affects females more than the males between 5th and 7th decade of life. It is a slowly progressive bilateral condition. Its clinical features can be divided into following four stages:

- Stage of cornea guttata
- Oedematous stage or stage of endothelial decompensation
- Stage of bullous keratopathy
- Stage of scarring

Define keratoconus and describe its treatment.

Keratoconus is a non-inflammatory ectatic condition of the cornea. It is usually bilateral and manifests at puberty with gradual loss of vision.

The high myopic irregular astigmatic refractive error seen in keratoconus may be treated by hard contact lens in early stages. Ultimately penetrating keratoplasty is required.

A CASE OF CORNEAL OPACITY

CASE SUMMARY

Presenting symptoms. A patient with corneal opacity usually presents with a whitish scar, causing defective vision as well as cosmetic blemish.

History may reveal a history of trauma to the eye or symptoms suggestive of healed corneal ulceration.

Examination reveals an opacity on the cornea (Fig. 5.20) which may be nebular, macular or leucomatous. The location, size, shape and density of the opacity must be described.

RELATED QUESTIONS

What is a corneal opacity?

The term corneal opacity is used for the loss of corneal transparency due to scarring.

What are common causes of corneal opacity?

1. Congenital opacities
2. Healed corneal wounds
3. Healed corneal ulcers

What are the types of corneal opacity?

1. *Nebular corneal opacity.* It is a faint opacity which results due to scars involving up to a few superficial lamellae of corneal stroma.
2. *Macular opacity.* It is a dense opacity produced by scars involving up to about half the thickness of the stroma.
3. *Leucomatous corneal opacity* (leucoma- simplex). It is a very dense, white opacity, which results due to scarring of more than half thickness of corneal stroma.
4. *Adherent leucoma.* It results when healing occurs after perforation of cornea with incarceration of the iris.

Name the secondary changes which can occur in a long standing case of corneal opacity.

1. Hyaline degeneration
2. Calcareous degeneration
3. Pigmentation
4. Atheromatous ulceration

How will you treat a case with corneal opacity?

1. *Optical iridectomy.* It may be performed in cases with central macular or leucomatous corneal opacities; provided vision improves with pupillary dilatation.
2. *Keratoplasty.* It provides good visual results in uncomplicated cases with corneal opacities; where optical iridectomy is not of much use.
3. *Tattooing of scar.* It used to be performed for cosmetic purposes. It is suitable only for firm scars in a quite eye without useful vision. Presently it is sparingly done.

How do you perform tattooing?

First of all, the epithelium covering the opacity is removed under topical anaesthesia. Then a piece of blotting paper of the same size and shape soaked in 4 per cent gold chloride (for brown eyes) or 2 per cent platinum chloride (for dark colour) is applied over it. After 2 to 3 minutes the piece of blotting paper is removed and a few drops of freshly-prepared hydrazine hydrate (2%) solution are poured over it. Lastly, eye is irrigated with normal saline and patched after instilling antibotic and atropine eye ointment. Epithelium grows over the pigmented area.

What are the causes of corneal vascularization?

Normal cornea is avascular. In pathological states, superficial or deep corneal vascularization may occur (Fig. 5.22).

1. *Superficial corneal vascularization.* In it, vessels are arranged in an arborizing pattern, present below the epithelium and their continuity can be traced with the conjunctival vessels. Its common causes are:
   - Trachoma
   - Phlyctenular keratoconjunctivitis
   - Superficial corneal ulcers
   - Rosacea keratitis
2. *Deep corneal vascularization.* In it, the vessels are generally derived from the anterior ciliary arteries and lie in the corneal stroma. These vessels are usually straight, not anastomosing and their continuity cannot be traced beyond the limbus. Its common causes are:
   - Interstitial keratitis
   - Disciform keratitis
   - Deep corneal ulcers
   - Chemical burns
   - Sclerosing keratitis
   - Corneal graft vascularization

What is keratoplasty?

Keratoplasty is an operation in which the patient's diseased cornea is replaced by the donor's healthy clear cornea. It is of two types:

1. *Lamellar keratoplasty* (partial thickness).
   - Anterior lamellar keratoplasty (ALK), and
   - Deep lamellar keratoplasty (DLK)
2. *Penetrating keratoplasty* (full thickness).

Name the indications for keratoplasty.

Anterior Lamellar keratoplasty

Indolent corneal ulcer, superficial corneal opacity and lattice dystrophy.

Penetrating keratoplasty

1. *Optical*, i.e., to improve vision in patient with corneal opacity, bullous keratopathy, corneal dystrophies and advanced keratoconus
2. *Therapeutic*, i.e., to replace inflamed cornea not responding to treatment (indolent deep ulcer)
3. *Tectonic grafts*, i.e., to restore the integrity of eyeball in corneal perforation and marked corneal thinning
4. *Cosmetic*, i.e., to improve appearance of the eye in deep leucomas with no vision in the eye.

What is the optimum time for the removal of donor eyes from the body of a deceased?

The donor eyes should be removed as early as possible (within 6 hours of death) and should be stored under sterile conditions.

What are the methods of corneal preservation?

1. *Short-term storage* (up to 48 hours): The whole globe is preserved at 4°C in a moist chamber.
2. *Intermediate storage* (up to 2 weeks): The donor corneal button is prepared and stored in McCarey-Kaufman (MK) medium and various chondroitin sulphate-enriched media such as optisol.
3. *Long-term storage* (up to 35 days): It is done by organ culture method or cryopreservation.

Enumerate the complications of keratoplasty operation.

I. *Early complications* are: flat anterior chamber, iris prolapse, infection, secondary glaucoma, epithelial defects, primary graft failure

II. *Late complications* are: graft rejection, recurrence of disease, marked astigmatism and cystoid macular oedema.

From which sources cornea derives its nutrition?

- Perilimbal capillaries
- Aqueous humour
- Oxygen from atmosphere

What is the nerve supply of cornea?

Cornea is supplied by the nasociliary branch of ophthalmic division of the trigeminal nerve.

What is a corneal facet?

A corneal facet is a transparent depressed scar. On slit-lamp examination light beam appears to dip in the area of a facet.

What is kerotomalacia?

Keratomalacia refers to corneal necrosis due to vitamin A deficiency. In this condition, there is no inflammatory reaction.

What is arcus senilis?

Arcus senilis is a degenerative condition of cornea characterized by an annular lipid infiltration concentric to the limbus. The ring of opacity is about 1 mm wide and is separated from the limbus by a clear zone (lucid interval of Vogt).

A CASE OF ANTERIOR STAPHYLOMA

CASE SUMMARY

Presenting symptoms. Patient presents with loss of vision, bluish discoloration and bulging of anterior part of the eyeball.

History is suggestive of symptoms of corneal ulceration (pain, redness, photophobia, watering, loss of vision and whitish discoloration) followed by bluish discoloration and bulging of anterior part of the eye.

Examination reveals that cornea is replaced by a lobulated ectatic scar tissue which is blackened due to the iris plastered behind it (Fig. 5.21).

RELATED QUESTIONS

What is a staphyloma?

Staphyloma refers to the localized bulging of weak and thin outer tunic of the eyeball (cornea or sclera) lined by uveal tissue which shines through the thinned-out fibrous coat.

What are the types of staphyloma?

1. Anterior staphyloma
2. Ciliary staphyloma
3. Intercalary staphyloma
4. Equatorial staphyloma
5. Posterior staphyloma.

How is an anterior staphyloma formed?

In a patient with sloughing corneal ulcer when the whole cornea sloughs out, the inflamed iris is covered with exudates. Ultimately these exudates organize and form a fibrous layer over which the conjunctival or corneal epithelium rapidly grows and thus a pseudocornea is formed. Since the pseudocornea is thin and cannot withstand the intraocular pressure, it usually bulges forward along with the plastered iris tissue. This ectatic cicatrix is called anterior staphyloma.

What is the treatment of anterior staphyloma?

1. Most of the times there is no chance of getting useful vision in such eyes. Therefore, treatment is carried out to improve the cosmetic appearance. *Localized staphylectomy* under heavy doses of steroids may be carried out. After healing, cosmetic artificial shell may be advised.
2. In patients where there is a chance of getting useful vision, *keratoplasty* (wherever possible) or *keratoprosthesis* may be performed.

What are the causes of posterior staphyloma?

- Pathological myopia
- Posterior scleritis
- Perforating injuries.

What is episcleritis? Describe features of a nodule of episcleritis.

Episcleritis is a benign recurrent inflammation of episclera, involving the overlying Tenon's capsule but not the underlying sclera.

A typical nodule of episcleritis is flat, pink or purple, surrounded by injection and is usually situated 2 to 3 mm away from the limbus.

What is the differential diagnosis of nodular episcleritis?

- Inflamed pinguecula
- Foreign body embedded in the bulbar conjunctiva
- Scleritis.

DISEASES OF THE UVEAL TRACT

A CASE OF ACUTE IRIDOCYCLITIS

CASE DESCRIPTION

Presenting symptoms. A patient with acute iridocyclitis (anterior uveitis) presents with moderate to severe pain which radiates all over the distribution of trigeminal nerve, photophobia, watering, redness and some diminution of vision of sudden onset.

History of present illness. In addition to the details about the presenting symptoms, the history of present illness should also explore the following associations:

- History of allergic conditions like bronchial asthma, hay fever, allergic rhinitis, allergic skin conditions
- History of joint pains to rule out rheumatoid disease
- History suggestive of urethritis
- History of any dental problem
- History of chronic rhinitis and/or sinusitis
- History of trauma to eye

Past history should include enquiries about:
- History of *similar attacks* in the past
- History of chronic *systemic infections* such as tuberculosis, syphilis, leprosy, measles, mumps and any other infection
- History of *non-infectious systemic disorders* such as diabetes, gout, rheumatoid arthritis and collagen disorder
- History of allergic and autoimmune disorders.

General physical and systemic examination should be conducted to rule out systemic diseases enumerated in the history. Special care should be given to dental, ENT, lymph nodes and joint examinations.

Ocular examination may reveal following signs (Fig. 7.8):
- *Visual acuity* is diminished.
- *Lids* may show slight oedema.
- *Circumcorneal congestion* is marked.
- *Cornea* may be slightly hazy due to oedema and KPs at the back of cornea which are seen on slit-lamp examination.
- *Anterior chamber* shows aqueous cells and aqueous flare, hypopyon may also be present
- *Iris* may show loss of normal pattern, muddy colour, posterior synechiae, iris nodules and patches of atrophy
- *Pupil* is narrow, irregular and sluggishly reacting. Exudates may be present in pupillary area, occlusio pupillae and seclusio pupillae may be seen in some cases.
- *Lens*. Pigment dispersal, exudates and iris adhesion may be seen on anterior capsule. Complicated cataract may also occur.
- *IOP* may be normal, low or raised. It is raised firstly in hypertensive uveitis and secondly in pupillary block secondary glaucoma.

A CASE OF CHRONIC IRIDOCYCLITIS

CASE DESCRIPTION

Presenting symptoms are mild to moderate dull ache in the eye, mild photophobia and diminution of vision.

History of present illness and past history should explore the diseases mentioned in a case of acute iridocyclitis.

Ocular examination may reveal mild circumcorneal flush, keratic precipitates, aqueous flare, aqueous cells, iris atrophic patches, iris nodules, posterior synechial neovascularization and irregular pupil.

RELATED QUESTIONS

Define uveitis.

Uveitis refers to inflammation of any part or whole of the uveal tract. Uveal tract includes iris, ciliary body and choroid.

How do you classify uveitis?

I. *Anatomical classification*
   1. Anterior uveitis (iridocyclitis)
   2. Intermediate uveitis (pars planitis)
   3. Posterior uveitis (choroiditis)
   4. Panuveitis

II. *Clinical classification*
   1. Acute uveitis
   2. Chronic uveitis

III. *Pathological classification*
   1. Suppurative or purulent uveitis
   2. Non-suppurative uveitis, which may be:
      (i) Non-granulomatous uveitis
      (ii) Granulomatous uveitis

IV. *Aetiological classssification (Duke-Elder's)*
   1. Infective uveitis
   2. Allergic uveitis
   3. Toxic uveitis
   4. Traumatic uveitis
   5. Uveitis associated with non-infective systemic diseases
   6. Idiopathic uveitis

What is the differential diagnosis of acute iridocyclitis?

Acute iridocyclitis must be differentiated from other causes of acute red eye; especially acute congestive glaucoma and acute conjunctivitis. The differentiating features are shown in Table 7.1.

What are the differences between granulomatous and non-granulomatous uveitis?

These are shown in Table 7.2.

What are the common causes of acute anterior uveitis?

1. Microbial allergy, e.g., allergy to tubercular proteins, streptococcal proteins, spirochaetal proteins, etc.

2. Atopic uveitis
3. HLA associated uveitis, e.g., HLA-B_{27}: Anterior uveitis is associated with ankylosing spondylitis and Reiter's syndrome.
4. Idiopathic.

What are the causes of granulomatous uveitis?

- Tuberculosis
- Syphilis
- Sarcoidosis
- Leprosy
- Vogt-Koyanagi-Harada's disease
- Sympathetic ophthalmia.

What are the common causes of unilateral iridocyclitis?

- Traumatic uveitis
- Herpes zoster uveitis
- Fuchs' heterochromic cyclitis
- Retinal detachment
- Haemophthalmitis
- Iridocyclitis secondary to intraocular tumours.

What are the keratic precipitates; what are their types and significance?

Keratic precipitates are proteinaceous-cellular deposits occurring at the back of cornea (Fig. 7.9). These are of the following types:

1. *Fine KPs* are characteristic of Fuchs' cyclitis and herpes zoster uveitis.
2. *Small and medium size* KPs are seen in acute and chronic non-granulomatous uveitis. These are composed of lymphocytes and may number in hundreds (usually 40-60).
3. *Mutton fat KPs.* These typically occur in granulomatous iridocyclitis and are composed of epithelioid cells and macrophages. They are large, thick, fluffy, lardaceous KPs, having a greasy or waxy appearance. They are usually few (10-15) in number.

What are iris nodules?

Iris nodules typically occur in granulomatous uveitis. Nodules situated at pupillary border are known as Koeppe's nodules, while those seen near the collarette are called Busacca's nodules (Fig. 7.12).

What are synechiae? Describe their types.

Synechiae are adhesions of the iris with other intraocular structures. These can be divided into following types:

1. *Anterior synechiae:* These include anterior peripheral synechiae seen in the angle of anterior chamber and anterior central synechiae seen in adherent leucoma.
2. *Posterior synechiae:* These refer to adhesions of posterior surface of iris to the anterior surface of crystalline lens or intraocular lens implant or posterior capsule or anterior phase of the vitreous. These are of the following types:
   - Posterior segmental synechiae (Fig. 7.8)
   - Annular synechiae (Fig. 7.13), and
   - Total posterior synechiae (Fig. 7.14).

What is seclusio pupillae and iris bombe?

Annular or ring synechiae are 360° adhesions of pupillary margin to anterior capsule of the lens. These prevent the circulation of aqueous humour from posterior to anterior chamber (seclusio pupillae). Thus, the aqueous collects behind the iris and pushes it anteriorly (leading to iris bombe formation).

What is occlusio pupillae?

Occlusio pupillae refers to occlusion of pupil by the exudates.

What is festooned pupil?

When atropine is instilled in the presence of segmental posterior synechiae, the pupil does not dilate in the areas of synechiae, but dilates in the areas without synechiae. This results in an irregular and dilated pupil known as festooned pupil.

Name the various types of HLA associated uveitis.

HLA-B_{27}:	Anterior uveitis seen with ankylosing spondylitis and Reiter's syndrome
HLA-B_5:	Behcet's disease
HLA-BW_{54}:	Glaucomatocyclitic crisis
HLA-BW_{22}:	Vogt-Koyanagi-Harada's syndrome

What are the causes of diminution of vision in a patient with iridocyclitis?

One or more of the following factors cause diminution of vision:

- Corneal oedema
- Aqueous haze
- Exudates in the pupillary area
- Complicated cataract

- Cyclitic membrane
- Vitreous haze
- Papillitis
- Macular oedema.

What are the complications of iridocyclitis?

- Complicated cataract (Fig. 7.15)
- Secondary glaucoma
- Cyclitic membrane
- Cystoid macular oedema
- Secondary periphlebitis retinae
- Band-shaped keratopathy
- Phthisis bulbi.

What is the treatment of iridocyclitis?

I. *Non-specific treatment*

a) Local therapy

1. Mydriatic-cycloplegic drugs, e.g., 1 percent atropine, eyedrops or ointment; or percent homatropine eyedrops .
2. Corticosteroid eyedrops such as dexamethasone eyedrops 4 times a day.

b) Systemic therapy

1. Corticosteroids are quite useful in severe cases.
2. Non-steroidal anti-inflammatory drugs (NSAIDs) such as aspirin and phenylbutazone are used when steroids are contraindicated.
3. Immunosuppressive drugs are used in desperate and extremely serious cases.
4. Adrenocorticotropic hormone (ACTH) may be required in recalcitrant cases.

c) Physical measures

1. Hot fomentation. It is very soothing, diminishes pain and increases circulation.
2. Dark goggles give feeling of comfort by reducing photophobia.

II. *Specific treatment*

It consists of treatment of the cause when discovered, e.g., antitubercular drugs for the underlying Koch's disease, adequate treatment of associated syphilis, toxoplasmosis, etc.

What are the features of Fuchs' uveitis?

Fuchs' uveitis is a chronic non-granulomatous type of low-grade anterior uveitis. It is unilateral and affects middle-aged persons. The disease is characterized by:

- Heterochromia of iris
- Fine KPs at the back of cornea
- Faint aqueous flare
- Absence of posterior synechiae
- A fairly common rubeosis iridis
- Comparatively early development of complicated cataract and secondary glaucoma.

What are the features of glaucomatocyclitic crisis (Posner-Schlossman syndrome)?

It typically affects young adults and is characterized by:

- Recurrent attacks of acute rise of IOP (40-50 mm of Hg) without shallowing of anterior chamber
- Fine KPs at the back of cornea without any posterior synechiae
- Epithelial corneal oedema
- A dilated pupil
- A white eye (no congestion).

What is sympathetic ophthalmitis?

Sympathetic ophthalmitis is rare bilateral granulomatous panuveitis which occurs following penetrating ocular trauma usually associated with incarceration of uveal tissue in the wound. The injured eye is called *exciting eye* and the fellow eye which also develops uveitis is called *sympathizing eye*.

What are Dalen-Fuchs' nodules?

Dalen-Fuchs' nodules are proliferation of the pigment epithelium of iris and ciliary body to form nodular aggregations in sympathetic ophthalmitis.

What is Behcet's disease?

Behcet's disease is an idiopathic multisystem disease associated with HLA-B_5. It is characterized by:

- Recurrent acute iridocyclitis associated with hypopyon
- Aphthous ulceration
- Genital ulceration
- Erythema multiforme

What are ocular lesions of sarcoidosis?

1. Sarcoid plaque on the skin of the eyelids
2. Granulomatous infiltration of the lacrimal gland with xerosis
3. Conjunctival sarcoid nodules
4. Episcleritis
5. Iridocyclitis may occur as:
   - Acute iridocyclitis

- Chronic granulomatous iridocyclitis (more common) with Koeppe's and Busacca's nodules on the iris and mutton fat KPs
- Uveoparotid fever (Heerfordt's syndrome)

6. Vitritis with snowball opacities
7. Choroidal and retinal granulomas
8. Secondary periphlebitis retinae with candle wax droppings.

What is VKH Syndrome?

Vogt-Koyanagi-Harada's (VKH) syndrome is an idiopathic multisystem disorder associated with HLA-BW22. It is characterized by:

- *Cutaneous lesions* such as: alopecia, poliosis and vitiligo
- *Neurological lesions* include meningism, encephalopathy, tinnitus, vertigo and deafness
- *Ocular features* are: chronic granulomatous anterior uveitis, posterior uveitis and exudative retinal detachment.

What is endophthalmitis? Enumerate common causes of purulent endophthalmitis.

Endophthalmitis is inflammation of the inner structures of the eyeball which include uveal tissue, retina and vitreous. Purulent endophthalmitis is a dreaded complication. Its common causes are:

1. *Exogenous infections* following:
   - Perforating injuries
   - Perforation of corneal ulcer
   - Intraocular operations such as cataract surgery and glaucoma surgery
2. *Endogenous or metastatic endophthalmitis* may occur rarely through blood stream from some septic focus in the body such as caries teeth, puerperal sepsis and generalized speticaemia.

What is panophthalmitis? Describe its treatment.

Panophthalmitis is an intense purulent inflammation of the whole eyeball including the Tenon's capsule.

Since there is little hope of saving such an eye, evisceration operation should be performed to remove the pus and infected intraocular contents leaving behind the sclera.

Which is the most common presenting symptom in a patient with choroiditis?

Floaters, i.e., moving small black spots in front of the eyes is the most common presenting symptom in a patient with choroiditis. Floaters occur due to pouring of exudates in the vitreous.

What are the symptoms of central choroiditis?

- Defective vision
- Floaters
- Micropsia (patient complains of seeing the objects smaller than normal) due to separation of cones of macula due to oedema)
- Metamorphopsia (patient perceives distorted images of the objects) results due to alteration in the retinal contour caused by a raised patch of choroiditis
- *Macropsia,* i.e., perception of the objects larger than they are, may occur due to crowding together of cones
- *Photopsia,* i.e., a subjective sensation of flashes of light may result due to irritation of cones by inflammatory oedema.

What is the most common cause of central choroiditis?

- Toxoplasmosis.

What is pathognomic feature of fungal endophthalmitis?

Flufy ball opacities in the vitreous are pathognomic of fungal endophthalmitis.

At what stage vitrectomy operation should be performed in a patient with endophthalmitis?

Vitrectomy is the treatment of choice for fungal endophthalmitis. In bacterial endophthalmitis it should be performed when the condition does not improve with intensive conservative therapy for 48 hours.

What is Reiter's syndrome?

Reiter's syndrome is characterized by a triad of urethritis, arthritis and conjunctivitis. In 20 to 30 per cent cases, acute non-granulomatous uveitis is also associated.

What are the causes of a patch of iris atrophy?

- Senile
- Post-inflammatory
- Glaucomatous
- Neurogenic, in lesions of ciliary ganglion
- Essential iris atrophy

DISEASES OF THE LENS

A CASE OF SENILE CATARACT

CASE DESCRIPTION

Age and sex. It is seen equally in persons of either sex, usually above the age of 45 years (average 50-60 years).

Presenting symptoms. Patient usually presents with a gradual, painless and progressive loss of vision. In the early stages there may or may not be associated history of coloured haloes, uniocular polyopia, glare and misty vision.

History of present illness. In addition to the details about the presenting symptoms, the history of present illness should be taken:

- *To rule out other cause of acquired cataract* e.g., history of exposure to radiations (radiation cataract) excessive heat in industrial workers especially in glass workers and iron workers (heat cataract), history of injury to the affected eye (traumatic cataract), history of diabetes mellitus (diabetic cataract), history of atopic diseases (atopic cataract), history of steroid intake (steroid cataract), history suggestive of anterior uveitis (complicated cataract) etc.
- *To rule out diseases affecting surgical treatment* such as history of hypertension, diabetes mellitus, bronchial asthma.

Ocular signs observed in different types of senile cataract are shown in Table 8.1, page 179

General physical and systemic examination (see page 194).

Ocular examination. In addition to ocular examination to note signs of different types of cataract, the following useful information is essential before the patient is considered for surgery (see page 194):

- Retinal function tests,
- Search for local source of infection,
- Slit-lamp examination for anterior segment status, and
- IOP measurement.

RELATED QUESTIONS

What is your diagnosis?

Senile cataract (immature, mature, hypermature or nuclear, depending upon the type of cataract).

Define cataract.

Normal crystalline lens is a transparent structure. Any opacity in the lens or its capsule is called a cataract.

How do you classify cataracts?

I. *Aetiological classification*
   1. Congenital and developmental cataract
   2. Acquired cataract
      1. Senile cataract
      2. Traumatic cataract
      3. Complicated cataract
      4. Metabolic cataract
      5. Electric cataract
      6. Radiational cataract
      7. Toxic cataract, e.g.,
         a) Corticosteroid-induced cataract
         b) Miotics-induced cataract
         c) Copper-and iron-induced cataracts (in chalcosis and siderosis respectively)
      8. Cataract associated with skin diseases (dermatogenic cataract)
      9. Cataract associated with osseous diseases
      10. Cataract associated with miscellaneous syndromes e.g.,
          - Dystrophia myotonica
          - Down's syndrome

II. *Morphological classification* (Fig. 8.4)
   1. Capsular cataract: It involves the capsule and may be:
      a) Anterior capsular cataract
      b) Posterior capsular cataract
   2. Cortical cataract: It involves the cortex of the lens
   3. Nuclear cataract: It involves the nucleus of the crystalline lens
   4. Polar cataract: It involves the capsule and superficial part of the cortex in the polar region and may be:
      a) Anterior polar cataract
      b) Posterior polar cataract

What are the types of senile cataract?

- Cortical cataract
- Nuclear cataract

Name the stages of maturation of senile cortical cataract.

- Stage of lamellar separation
- Stage of incipient cataract

- Stage of immature senile cataract (cuneiform or cupuliform)
- Stage of mature senile cataract
- Stage of hypermature senile cataract (Morgagnian or sclerotic type).

What do you mean by nuclear sclerosis?

Nuclear sclerosis is an aging process in which lens nucleus becomes inelastic and hard. Refractive index of the lens is increased resulting in myopia. These changes begin centrally and spread peripherally. On oblique illumination pupillary area looks greyish.

How will you differentiate immature senile cataract (ISC) from nuclear sclerosis without cataract changes?

(See Table 8.3, Page 191).

Name the complications which can occur during maturation of cortical cataract.

(a) Lens-induced glaucoma, which may be:

1. *Phacomorphic glaucoma* (secondary narrow-angle glaucoma). It occurs due to intumescent (swollen) lens causing blockage of the angle of anterior chamber and pupil
2. *Phacolytic glaucoma* (secondary open-angle glaucoma). It occurs due to blockage of trabecular meshwork by macrophages laden with lens proteins leaked from the Morgagnian hypermature cataract

(b) Phacoanaphylaxis
(c) Subluxation or dislocation of the lens.

What are the characteristics of diabetic cataract?

A true diabetic cataract is characterized by appearance of bilateral snowflake-like opacities hence the name 'snowflake cataract' or 'snow-storm cataract'.

What are the characteristics of a complicated cataract?

A typical complicated cataract is characterized by 'bread-crumb' appearance of the opacities situated in the posterior subcapsular area, which exhibit 'polychromatic lustre' on slit-lamp examination.

Enumerate the indications for extraction of a cataractous lens.

1. Grossly diminished vision hampering easy living
2. Medical indications, e.g.,
   - Lens-induced glaucoma
   - Phacoanaphylaxis
   - Patient having diabetic retinopathy or retinal detachment, treatment of which is hampered by the presence of lens opacities
3. Cosmetic indication. Some patients may insist for cataract extraction (even with no hope of getting useful vision) in order to obtain a black pupil.

What preoperative evaluation would you like to carry out before cataract surgery?

1. General physical and systemic examination to rule out: diabetes mellitus, hypertension, obstructive lung disorders and any potential source of infection in the body such as septic gums, urinary tract infection, etc.
2. Ocular examination with special reference to:
   1. Retinal function tests
   2. Search for local source of infection, i.e., conjunctivitis, dacryocystitis, blepharitis, etc.
   3. Intraocular pressure measurement.

Name the retinal function tests that you would like to carry out before planning cataract surgery?

1. Light perception (PL)
2. Projection of light rays (PR)
3. A test for Marcus Gunn pupillary response
4. Two-light discrimination test.

What is the most accurate method of predicting the macular potential for visual acuity in the presence of advanced cataract?

- Laser interferometry.

Name the objective tests for evaluating posterior segment of eye in a cataract patient.

1. Ultrasonography (A and B scan)
2. Electroretinography
3. Electro-oculography
4. Visually-evoked response.

Surgical management of adulthood cataracts

For questions related to surgical management of cataract, see page 619.

A CASE OF CONGENITAL/ DEVELOPMENTAL CATARACT

CASE DESCRIPTION

Age and sex. Congenital cataract is present since birth. Developmental cataract may occur any time from infancy to adolescence. It is equally common in both sexes.

Presenting symptoms. Parents may bring the child with one or more of the following complaints:

- White reflex in the pupillary area (leukocoria)
- Inability of the child to see well which may be noticed by the parents
- Wandering movements of the eyes
- Deviation (squint) in one eye
- Nystagmus

History of present illness should include:

- Details about the time of appearance and progress of the above symptoms
- *Obstetrical history* to explore occurrence of rubella, malnutrition, diabetes mellitus, exposure to radiations and drug intake during pregnancy.
- *Birth history* should include information about: home or hospital delivery; full-term or premature birth; normal or low birth weight (LBW) for age; history of birth trauma; and history of ocular infections after birth
- *Family history* should include history of similar complaints in the family, history of any other ocular or systemic defects in the family, history of diabetes mellitus and history of consanguinous marriage.

General physical and systemic examination should be carried out thoroughly with special attention for any associated mental retardation, cerebral palsies, features of rubella, features of galactosaemia, hepatosplenomegaly and cardiovascular anomalies such as patent ductus arteriosus (PDA), ventricular septal defect (VSD) and pulmonary stenosis (PS).

Ocular examination. Conspicuous sign is leukocoria (white reflex in pupillary area). Make special note of visual acuity (if possible), any associated squint, nystagmus and other congenital anomalies such as microphthalmos, microcornea, aniridia, iris coloboma, and persistent pupillary membrane. Lens should be examined in detail after dilation of the pupil. If possible fundus should be examined to know the status of the posterior segment.

RELATED QUESTIONS

Name the types of congenital cataract.

- Cataracta centralis pulverulenta (embryonic nuclear cataract)
- Lamellar (zonular) cataract
- Sutural cataract
- Anterior polar cataract
- Posterior polar cataract
- Coronary cataract
- Blue dot punctate cataract
- Total congenital cataract.

Enumerate the aetiological factors associated with congenital cataract.

1. Heredity (about 3 per cent cases)
2. Maternal factors, e.g.,
    - Malnutrition during pregnancy
    - Rubella infection
    - Toxoplasmosis
    - Cytomegalo inclusion disease
    - Drug ingestion during pregnancy, e.g., thalidomide, corticosteroids
3. Fetal or infantile factors, e.g.,
    - Anoxia due to placental haemorrhage
    - Metabolic disorders, e.g., galactosaemia, neonatal hypoglycaemia
    - Lowe's syndrome
    - Myotonia dystrophica
    - Birth trauma
    - Malnutrition in early infancy
4. Idiopathic (about 50 per cent cases).

What are the features of zonular (lamellar) cataract?

Zonular cataract typically occurs in a zone of fetal nucleus surrounding the embryonic nucleus (Fig. 8.5). The area of the lens internal and external to the zone of cataract is clear, except for small linear opacities like spokes of a wheel (riders) which run outwards towards the equator. It is usually bilateral and frequently causes severe visual defect.

What is the differential diagnosis of a white pupillary reflex?

1. Congenital cataract
2. Retinoblastoma
3. Retinopathy of prematurity (retrolental fibroplasia)
4. Persistent hyperplastic primary vitreous
5. Parasitic endophthalmitis
6. Exudative retinopathy of Coats.

How will you manage a case of congenital cataract?

1. Small stationary lens opacities which do not interfere with vision can safely be ignored
2. Incomplete central stationary cataracts may be treated by optical iridectomy or use of mydriatics to improve the vision considerably
3. Complete cataracts should be removed surgically as early as possible

Name the surgical procedures in vogue for management of childhood cataracts

1. Discission (needling) operation (almost obsolete)
2. Anterior capsulotomy and irrigation aspiration of the lens matter
3. Lensectomy

How should paediatric aphakia be corrected?

1. Children above the age of 5 years can be corrected by implantation of posterior chamber intraocular lens during surgery
2. Those below the age of 5 years should preferably be treated by extended wear contact lens. Spectacles can be prescribed in bilateral cases. At a later stage secondary IOL implantation may be considered
3. Epikeratophakia and keratophakia are still under trial

A CASE OF APHAKIA

CASE DESCRIPTION

Presenting symptoms. Patient usually gives history of cataract extraction operation (postoperative aphakia). Sometimes patient may present with such a situation following trauma to the eye (aphakia due to traumatic posterior dislocation of lens) and rarely without any cause (aphakia due to spontaneous posterior dislocation of lens).

- Patient usually has marked loss of vision both for distance and near due to high hypermetropia and absence of accommodation, respectively.
- Patient may complain of seeing red (erythropsia) and blue (cyanopsia) images. This occurs due to excessive entering of ultraviolet and infrared rays in the absence of crystalline lens.

Signs of aphakia seen on ocular examination:

- *Limbal scar* may be seen in surgical aphakia
- *Anterior chamber* is deeper than normal
- *Iridodonesis,* i.e., tremulousness of the iris can be demonstrated
- *Pupil* is jet black in colour
- *Purkinge image test* shows only two images (normally four images are seen)
- *Fundus examination* shows hypermetropic small disc
- *Retinoscopy* reveals high hypermetropia

A CASE OF PSEUDOPHAKIA

CASE DESCRIPTION

Presenting symptoms

- Patient usually gives a history of cataract operation and may also be aware of the intraocular lens (IOL) implantation.
- Patient may give history of normal far vision (emmetropia produced by IOL) but defective near vision due to loss of accommodation.
- Some patients may give history of normal near vision but defective far vision (due to 2-3 D myopia produced by a high power IOL).
- Some patients are uncomfortable due to defective vision both for distance and near. This occurs due to hypermetropia produced by a low power IOL and loss of accommodation.

Signs of pseudophakia

- *Surgical limbal scar* may be seen
- *Anterior chamber* is slightly deeper than normal
- When implanted, the angle supported anterior chamber IOL (Fig. 8.23) and iris claw IOL (Fig. 8.25) are seen in the anterior chamber.
- *Mild iridodonesis* (tremulousness of iris) may be demonstrated
- *Purkinje image test* shows four images
- *Pupil* is blackish in colour. When light is thrown in pupillary area, shining reflexes are observed. When examined under magnification after dilating the pupil, the presence of posterior chamber IOL when implanted is confirmed (Fig. 8.26)
- *Visual status* and refraction of the patient will vary depending upon the power of IOL implanted as described above.

RELATED QUESTIONS

Define aphakia.

Aphakia literally means absence of the crystalline lens from the eye. However, from the optical point of view, it may be considered as a condition in which the lens is absent from the pupillary area and does not take part in refraction. Optically aphakia may be:

- *Complete aphakia* i.e, whole of the lens is absent from its normal position.
- *Partial aphakia,* i.e. part of the lens is present in the pupillary area. In this situation aphakic and phakic portions are seen simultaneously in pupillary area.

Enumerate the refractive changes which occur in an aphakic eye.

1. Eye becomes highly hypermetropic.
2. Total power of the eye is reduced to +44 DS from +60 DS.
3. Anterior focal distance becomes 23 mm (from 15 mm in normal phakic eye).
4. Posterior focal distance becomes 31 mm (from 24 mm in normal phakic eye).
5. There is anterior shift of nodal point and principal focus.
6. There is complete loss of accommodation due to absence of lens.
7. Astigmatism is induced due to corneal/limbal scar.

Name the various modalities for correction of aphakia and enumerate advantages and disadvantages of each.

1. *Spectacles*

Advantages: It is cheap, easy and safe method of correcting aphakia.

Disadvantages: (i) Image is magnified by 30 per cent, so not useful in unilateral aphakia (produces diplopia), (ii) problems of spherical and chromatic aberrations may be troublesome, (iii) field of vision is limited, (iv) prismatic effect of thick glasses causes, 'roving ring scotoma' (v) cosmetic blemish, especially in young aphakics.

2. *Contact lenses*

Advantages: (i) Less magnification (5%) of the image, (ii) elimination of aberrations and prismatic effect of thick glasses, (iii) wider and better field of vision, (iv) cosmetically better accepted by young persons.

Disadvantages: (i) more cost, (ii) cumbersome to wear, especially in old age and in childhood, (iii) corneal complications may occur.

3. *Intraocular lens implantation*

It is the best available method of treatment.

Advantage: It offers all the advantages which the contact lenses offer over the spectacles. In addition, the disadvantages of contact lenses are also taken care of.

Disadvantages: It requires more skilled surgeons and costly equipment.

4. *Refractive corneal surgery*

It is still under trial and includes keratophakia and epikeratophakia.

What are fundus findings in a patient with high hypermetropia?

Fundus examination in a patient with high hypermetropia may show:

- Pseudopapillitis
- Shot silk appearance of the retina

Enumerate the signs of aphakia.

- Deep anterior chamber
- Iridodonesis
- Jet black pupil
- Purkinje's image test shows only two images (normally four)
- Fundus examination shows small optic disc.
- Retinoscopy, reveals high hypermetropia.

What is the average standard power of the lenses required for spectacle correction of aphakia?

In preoperative emmetropic patient, the standard power of the lenses required for spectacle correction of aphakia for distance vision is +10 DS with an additional cylindrical lens for acquired astigmatism. For near vision correction an additional +3 DS is required as the accommodation is absent in an aphakic eye.

What is pseudophakia?

Pseudophakia refers to presence of an intraocular lens in the pupillary area.

What is the refractive position of the pseudophakic eye?

A pseudophakic eye may be emmetropic, myopic or hypermetropic depending upon the power of the IOL implanted.

What is the average standard power of the posterior chamber IOL?

Exact power of an IOL to be implanted varies from individual to individual and is calculated by biometry using keratometer and A-scan ultrasound.

What is the average weight of an IOL?

Average weight of an IOL in air is 15 mg and in aqueous humour is about 5 mg.

What is the power of the IOL in air vis-a-vis in the aqueous humour?

Power of an IOL in air is much more (about +60D) than that in the aqueous humour (about + 20D).

What is the difference in the power of an anterior chamber IOL versus posterior chamber IOL?

Equivalent power of an anterior chamber IOL is less (say about +18D) than that of posterior chamber IOL (+20D).

Surgical management of cataract

For questions related to surgical management of a cataract patient, see page 619.

GLAUCOMA

A CASE OF PRIMARY ANGLE CLOSURE GLAUCOMA

CASE DESCRIPTION

Age and sex. Primary narrow-angle glaucoma usually presents between 50 and 60 years of age. It occurs more commonly in females than males in a ratio of 4:1.

Presenting symptoms depend upon the stage of the disease as follows:

1. *Primary angle-closure suspect* (PACS). Patient does not present in this stage as there are no symptoms. It is diagnosed:

- On routine slit-lamp examination in patients presenting with some other eye disease, and
- In fellow eye of the patients presenting with subacute or acute angle-closure glaucoma.
- On glaucoma screening.

2. *Primary angle-closure* (PAC). Patient presents with transient blurring of vision, coloured haloes around the light due to corneal oedema and mild headache. These symptoms are due to transient rise in intra- ocular pressure (IOP) and occur in intermittent attacks at irregular intervals. The attacks are usually precipitated by overwork in the evening, anxiety and fatigue.

Acute primary-angle closure (*Acute PAC*). Patient presents with an attack of sudden onset of very severe pain in the eye which radiates along the branches of fifth nerve. Frequently there is history of associated nausea, vomiting and prostrations. There is history of rapidly progressive loss of vision, redness, photophobia and watering. About 5 per cent patients give history of typical previous intermittent attacks.

3. *Primary angle-closure glaucoma* (PACG). Patients may have dull pain and discomfort in the eye along with marked diminution of vision. Patients may or may not give history of preceding attack of acute PAC.

4. *Absolute glaucoma.* Such patients present with:

- Pain in the eye which is severe and irritating
- Constant headache
- Watering and redness of the eye
- Complete loss of vision (no perception of light)

  This stage results if PACG is left untreated.

Ocular examination. The signs observed on ocular examination depend upon the stage of glaucoma (See page 228-234):

1. *Primary angle-closure suspect* (PACS). The eye is white and quiet. Anterior chamber is shallow. Gonioscopy reveals narrow angle. IOP is usually normal.

2. *Primary angle-closure* (PAC). Usually the eye looks normal except for a shallow anterior chamber and narrow angle (on gonioscopy)

Acute primary angle-closure. Signs are as follows:

- *Lids* may be oedematous
- *Conjunctiva* is chemosed, and congested, (both conjunctival and ciliary vessels are congested).
- *Cornea* becomes oedematous and insensitive.
- *Anterior chamber* is very shallow. Aqueous flare or cells may be seen in anterior chamber.
- *Angle of anterior chamber* is completely closed as seen on gonioscopy.
- *Iris* may be discolored.
- *Pupil* is semidilated, vertically oval and fixed. It is non-reactive to both light and accommodation.
- *IOP* is markedly elevated, usually between 40 and 70 mm of Hg.
- *Optic disc* is oedematous and hyperaemic.
- *Fellow eye* shows shallow anterior chamber and a narrow angle.

3. *Primary angle-closure glaucoma* (PACG). Signs are as follows:

- *The IOP* remains constantly raised.
- Eye is painless and white like primary open-angle glaucoma.
- *Visual field defects* appear which are similar to those in POAG.
- *Optic disc* may show glaucomatous cupping.
- *Visual acuity* is decreased.
- *Gonioscopy* reveals angle closed by peripheral anterior synechiae.

4. *Absolute glaucoma.* Signs are as follows:

- *Lids* show mild oedema.
- *Palpebral aperture* is slightly narrow.
- The anterior *ciliary veins* are dilated with a slight ciliary flush around the cornea (*perilimbal reddish blue zone*).
- In long-standing cases, few prominent and enlarged vessels are seen in the form of '*caput medusae*'.
- Cornea in early cases is clear but insensitive. Slowly it becomes hazy and may develop epithelial bullae (*bullous keratopathy*) or filaments (*filamentary keratitis).*
- *Anterior chamber* is very shallow.
- *Iris* becomes atrophic.
- *Pupil* becomes fixed and dilated and gives a greenish hue.
- *Optic disc* shows glaucomatous optic atrophy.
- *Intraocular pressure* is high; eyeball becomes stony hard.

A CASE OF PRIMARY OPEN-ANGLE GLAUCOMA

CASE DESCRIPTION

An early case of primary open-angle glaucoma (POAG) is usually not given in undergraduate examinations. However, an advanced or a case of POAG which has been operated for trabeculectomy may be kept as short or long case.

Age and sex. POAG usually affects about 1 in 100 of the general population (of either sex) above the age of 40 years. The disease is essentially bilateral.

Presenting symptoms. The disease is insidious and usually asymptomatic. Mild symptoms experienced by the patients include:

- Mild headache and eyeache.
- Difficulty in reading (patients usually give history of frequent change in near vision glasses).
- Occasionally an observant patient may notice a defect in the visual field (scotoma).
- In late stages patient may complain of delayed dark adaptation.

Ocular examination. Anterior segment is usually normal. In advanced cases the pupils are sluggishly reacting. Fixed and dilated pupils are seen in absolute glaucoma. Diagnosis is usually made from triad of raised intraocular pressure (IOP), glaucomatous optic disc changes and visual field changes (see pages 228-234). In a case of POAG operated for trabeculectomy, a filteration conjunctival bleb is seen at the site of operation near the limbus.

A CASE OF PHACOMORPHIC GLAUCOMA

Presenting symptoms. Patient presents with a sudden onset of severe pain, redness, watering from the eyes and marked loss of vision. Usually there is associated nausea, vomiting, headache and prostration. Patient always gives history of preceding gradual painless loss of vision.

Ocular examination reveals following signs (Fig. 9.20):

- *Lids* may be oedematous.
- *Conjunctiva* is chemosed and congested (both conjunctival and ciliary vessels are congested).
- *Cornea* becomes oedematous and insensitive.
- *Anterior chamber* is very shallow (opposite eye normal). Aqueous flare and cells may be seen in the anterior chamber
- *Pupil* is semidilated, vertically oval and fixed.
- *Lens* is cataractous, swollen and bulging forward (intumescent cataract).
- *IOP* is markedly elevated.

A CASE OF PHACOLYTIC GLAUCOMA

CASE DESCRIPTION

The presenting symptoms and signs are similar to phacomorphic glaucoma except for following differences:

- *Anterior chamber* is not shallow. It is normal or slightly deep. Aqueous is turbid.
- *Lens* shows hypermature Morgagnian senile cataract.

RELATED QUESTIONS

What are normal values of intraocular pressure?

- Range: 10 to 21 mm of Hg
- Mean: 16 ± 2.5 mm of Hg

What is the normal amount of aqueous humour present in the eye?

Normal amount of aqueous humour present in the anterior chamber is about 0.25 ml and in posterior chamber is 0.06 ml.

What is the normal rate of aqueous production?

- 2.3 μl/minute.

What is the site of aqueous production?

- Ciliary processes.

Name the mechanisms concerned with aqueous production.

- Diffusion
- Ultrafiltration
- Active secretion

Define glaucoma.

Glaucoma is not a single disease but a group of disorders in which intraocular pressure is sufficiently raised (above the tolerance limit of the affected eye) to impair normal functioning of the optic nerve.

How do you classify glaucoma?

I. *Congenital/developmental glaucomas*
   1. Primary congenital glaucoma (without associated anomalies)
   2. Developmental glaucoma with other associated anomalies

II. *Primary glaucoma*
   1. Primary open-angle glaucoma (POAG)
   2. Primary angle-closure glaucoma (PACG)
   3. Primary mixed mechanism glaucoma

III. *Secondary glaucomas*

What is the incidence of primary angle-closure glaucoma?

- 1 in 1000 people over 40 years
- Male to female ratio is 1:4

Name the predisposing factors for PACG.

- Hypermetropic eyes
- Small corneal diameter
- Relative large size of the crystalline lens
- Short axial length of eyeball
- Shallow anterior chamber
- Plateau iris configuration

Name the precipitating factors for an attack of acute congestive glaucoma.

- Dim illumination
- Emotional stress, anxiety and excitement
- Use of mydriatics

Describe the mechanism of rise in IOP in acute narrow-angle glaucoma.

Mid-dilated pupil — increased contact between the lens and relative iris pupil block – physiological iris bombe formation — appositional angle closure (causing transient rise in IOP) — synechial angle closure — prolonged rise in IOP.

Name the clinical stages of primary angle-closure glaucoma.

1. Primary angle-closure suspect (PACS)
2. Primary angle closure (PAC)
   - Acute primary angle-closure
3. Primary angle-closure glaucoma (PACG)
4. Absolute glaucoma.

Name the provocative tests used in primary angle-closure suspect (PACS) and primary angle closure (PAC) stage to confirm the diagnosis.

1. Darkroom test
2. Prone test
3. Prone darkroom test
4. Mydriatic test (10% phenylephrine test)
5. Mydriatic-miotic test (10% phenylephrine and 2% pilocarpine test).

Enumerate the sequelae of an attack of acute primary angle closure (Acute PAC).

- Sectoral iris atrophy
- Spiralling of iris fibres
- Iris hole (pseudopolycoria)
- Large irregular pupil
- Glaucomflecken
- Peripheral anterior synechiae
- Chronic corneal oedema

How will you treat a case of acute primary angle closure?

I. *Immediate medical treatment* to control pain and lower the intraocular pressure
   1. Injectable analgesic to relieve the severe pain
   2. Acetazolamide 500 mg stat and then 250 mg qId orally.
   3. Hyperosmotic agents, e.g., glycerol 1 to 2 g per kg body weight orally in lemon juice and/ or mannitol 1 to 2 g per kg body weight (20% solution) IV over 30 minutes
   4. Pilocarpine eyedrops 2 to 4 per cent every 15 minutes for one hour and then qId
   5. 0.5 per cent timolol maleate eyedrops bd
   6. Topical steroid 3 to 4 times a day to control the inflammation

II. *Surgical treatment*
   1. Peripheral iridectomy/laser iridotomy is sufficient when peripheral anterior synechiae (PAS) are formed in less than 50 percent of the angle.
   2. Filtration surgery (e.g., trabeculectomy) is performed when PAS are formed in more than 50 percent of the angle
   3. Peripheral iridectomy/laser iridotomy should also be considered as prophylaxis for the fellow eye.

Name the structures forming angle of the anterior chamber.

1. Root of the iris
2. Anterior most part of the ciliary body
3. Scleral spur
4. Trabecular meshwork
5. Schwalbe's line (prominent end of Descemet's membrane of cornea).

How will you grade the angle width gonioscopically?

Shaffer's grading system is as follows:

Grade 4 (Wide open angle)
- Angle width is 35°-45°
- Structures seen are from Schwalbe's line to ciliary body
- Closure impossible

Grade 3 (Open angle)
- Angle width is 20°-35°
- Structures seen are from Schwalbe's line to scleral spur
- Closure impossible

Grade 2 (Moderately narrow angle)
- Angle width is about 20°
- Structures seen are from Schwalbe's line to trabecular meshwork
- Angle closure is possible but unlikely

Grade 1 (Very narrow angle)
- Angle width is about 10°
- Structure seen is Schwalbe's line only
- High-angle closure risk

Grade 0 (Closed angle)
- Angle width is 0°
- None of the angle structures are seen (iridocorneal contact)
- Completely closed angle

Name the structures forming aqueous outflow system.

1. Trabecular meshwork
2. Schlemm's canal
3. Collector channels.

What is the incidence of primary congenital/ developmental glaucoma?

- Affects 1 in 10,000 live births
- Male to female ratio is 3:1.

What is the pathogenesis of developmental glaucoma?

Failure in the absorption of mesodermal tissue resulting in failure of development of the angle structures.

What are gonioscopic findings of developmental glaucoma?

- Barkan's membrane may be present
- Thickening of trabecular meshwork
- Insertion of iris above the scleral spur
- Peripheral iris stroma hypoplasia

What is buphthalmous?

This term is used when eyeball enlarges (corneal diameter becomes more than 13 mm) in children developing congenital glaucoma at an early age (before the age of 3 years).

What is the treatment of primary congenital glaucoma?

1. Goniotomy
2. Trabeculotomy
3. Trabeculectomy (with antifibrosis treatment)

What are the causes of secondary congenital glaucoma?

I. Glaucoma associated with mesodermal dysgenesis of the anterior ocular segment, e.g.:
   1. Posterior embryotoxon
   2. Axenfeld's anomaly
   3. Rieger's syndrome
   4. Peter's anomaly

II. Glaucoma associated with aniridia (50%)

III. Glaucoma associated with ectopia lentis syndrome
   1. Marfan's syndrome
   2. Weill-Marchesani's syndrome
   3. Homocystinuria

IV. Glaucoma associated with phacomatoses:
   1. Sturge-Weber syndrome (50% cases)
   2. Von Recklinghausen's neurofibromatosis (25% cases)

V. Miscellaneous conditions
   1. Lowe's syndrome (50% cases)
   2. Naevus of Ota
   3. Nanophthalmos
   4. Congenital microcornea (60%)
   5. Congenital rubella syndrome (10% cases).

What is the incidence of primary open-angle glaucoma?

- It affects 1 in 100 population (of either sex) above the age of 40 years.
- It forms about one-third cases of all glaucomas.

What are the features of glaucomatous cupping of the disc?

These include (Fig. 9.9 and 9.10) the following:

1. Cup/disc ratio is increased (normal 0.3 to 0.4), asymmetry of more than 0.2 is suspicious
2. Notching of the rim
3. Nasal shift of the vessels at disc
4. Pallor area on the disc
5. Presence of splinter haemorrhages on or near the disc margin

Name the predisposing factors for POAG.

1. Heredity (positive family history)
2. Age (between 5th and 7th decade)
3. High myopia
4. Diabetes mellitus

What is the characteristic triad of POAG?

1. Intraocular pressure more than 21 mm of Hg
2. Glaucomatous cupping of the disc
3. Glaucomatous field defects

What is ocular hypertension?

Ocular hypertension or glaucoma suspect is the term used when a patient has an IOP constantly more than 23 mm of Hg but no optic disc or visual field changes.

What is low-tension glaucoma (LTG)?

This term is used when typical glaucomatous disc cupping with or without visual field changes is associated with an IOP constantly below 21 mm of Hg.

What are the other ocular associations of POAG?

1. High myopia
2. Fuchs' dystrophy
3. Retinitis pigmentosa
4. Central retinal vein occlusion (CRVO)
5. Primary retinal detachment

What are glaucomatous field defects?

1. Baring of the blind spot
2. Paracentral scotoma in Bjerrum's area (an arcuate area extending above and below the blind spot upto between 10° and 20° of fixation point)
3. Seidel scotoma
4. Arcuate or Bjerrum's scotoma
5. Double arcuate scotoma
6. Roenne's central nasal step
7. Advanced field defects with tubular vision

What is the treatment for primary open-angle glaucoma?

1. *Medical treatment:* It is still the initial therapy. Topical timolol maleate 0.25 per cent BD which may be increased to 0.5 per cent BD Pilocarpine TDS 2 per cent which may be increased to 4 per cent BD was previously used as drug of second choice. Recently latanoprost (0.005%, OD) is being considered the drug of first choice (provided

patients can afford to buy it. Dorzolamide (2%, 2-3 times/day) has replaced pilocarpine as the second drug of choice and even as adjunct drug. If the patient does not respond to a single drug the two drugs can be combined. If still the IOP is not controlled, tablet acetazolamide 250 mg TDS may be added.

2. *Argon laser trabeculoplasty:* It may be considered as an alternative to medical therapy or as an additional measure in patients not responding to medical therapy alone.
3. *Surgical therapy:* It is usually undertaken when patient does not respond to maximal medical therapy alone or in combination with laser trabeculoplasty. Recently it is also being considered as the primary line of treatment. Surgical treatment mainly consists of filtration surgery trabeculectomy.

What are secondary glaucomas?

In secondary glaucomas, intraocular pressure is raised due to some other primary ocular or systemic disease.

Depending upon the causative primary disease, secondary glaucomas are classified as follows:

1. Lens-induced glaucomas
2. Glaucomas associated with uveitis
3. Pigmentary glaucoma
4. Neovascular glaucoma
5. Pseudoexfoliative glaucoma (glaucoma capsulare)
6. Glaucomas associated with intraocular haemorrhages
7. Steroid-induced glaucoma
8. Traumatic glaucoma
9. Glaucoma in aphakia
10. Glaucoma associated with intraocular tumours
11. Glaucomas associated with iridocorneal endothelial (ICE) syndromes
12. Ciliary block glaucoma (malignant glaucoma)

What are lens-induced glaucomas?

1. *Phacomorphic glaucoma:* Herein IOP is raised due to secondary angle closure and/or pupil block by:
   - Intumescent (swollen) cataractous lens (Fig. 9.20)
   - Anterior subluxated lens
   - Spherophakia
2. *Phacolytic glaucoma:* Here in IOP is raised due to clogging of trabecular meshwork by the macrophages laden with the leaked lens proteins, usually in hypermature cataract.
3. *Lens particle glaucoma:* It occurs due to blockage of trabeculae by the lens particles following rupture of the lens or after ECCE.
4. *Phacoanaphylactic glaucoma:* Sensitization of eye or its fellow to lens proteins. Inflammatory material clogs trabecular meshwork.
5. *Phacotoxic glaucoma:* Herein IOP is raised due to lens matter induced uveitis.

What is malignant glaucoma?

Malignant or ciliary block glaucoma occurs rarely as a complication of any intraocular operation. Classically, it occurs following peripheral iridectomy or filtration operation for primary narrow angle glaucoma. Its pathogenesis includes cilio-lenticular or ciliovitreal block.

It is characterized by a markedly raised intraocular pressure, persistent flat anterior chamber and a negative Seidel's test.

What is differential diagnosis of acute congestive glaucoma?

- Acute conjunctivitis
- Acute iridocyclitis
- Secondary acute congestive glaucomas
  - Phacomorphic glaucoma
  - Phacolytic glaucoma
  - Glaucomatocyclitic crisis

What is post-inflammatory glaucoma?

Postinflammatory glaucoma refers to rise in intraocular pressure due to following complications of anterior uveitis:

- Annular synechiae
- Occlusio pupillae
- Angle closure following iris bombe formation
- Angle closure due to organization of the inflammatory debris

What is pigmentary glaucoma?

Pigmentary glaucoma refers to raised IOP in patients with pigment dispersion syndrome. It typically affects young myopic males. Its features are similar to POAG with associated pigment deposition on corneal endothelium (Krukenberg's spindle) trabecular meshwork, iris, lens and zonules.

What is neovascular glaucoma?

Neovascular glaucoma refers to raised IOP occurring due to formation of a neovascular membrane involving angle of the anterior chamber. Usually, stimulus to new vessel formation is retinal ischaemia as seen in diabetic retinopathy, CRVO, Eales' disease. Other rare causes are chronic uveitis, intraocular tumours, old retinal detachment, CRAO and retinopathy of prematurity.

What is pseudoexfoliation glaucoma?

Pseudoexfoliation glaucoma is a type of secondary open-angle glaucoma associated with pseudo-exfoliation (PEX) syndrome. PES refers to amyloid like deposits on pupillary border, anterior lens surface, posterior surface of iris, zonules and ciliary processes.

What is steroid-induced glaucoma?

Steroid-induced glaucoma is secondary open-angle glaucoma having features similar to POAG. It probably occurs due to deposition of mucopolysaccharides in the trabecular meshwork in patients using topical steroid eyedrops. Roughly 5 per cent of general population is high steroid responder (develop marked rise of IOP after about 6 weeks of steroid therapy), 35 per cent are moderate and 60 per cent are non-responders.

Enumerate the causes of glaucoma in aphakia.

- Raised IOP due to postoperative hyphaema, inflammation, vitreous filling the anterior chamber.
- Angle closure due to flat anterior chamber
- Pupil block with or without angle closure
- Undiagnosed pre-existing POAG
- Steroid-induced glaucoma
- Epithelial in growth
- Aphakic malignant glaucoma

DISEASES OF THE EYELIDS

A CASE OF BLEPHARITIS

CASE DESCRIPTION

Age and sex. Though more common in children, blepharitis may occur at any age equally in both sexes.

Presenting symptoms. Patients usually complain of deposits at the lid margin, associated with irritation, discomfort, occasional watering and history of falling of cilia or gluing of cilia.

Ocular examination may reveal signs of either seborrhoeic or ulcerative (Fig. 14.8) or mixed blepharitis.

- *Signs of seborrhoeic blepharitis are:* accummulation of white dandruff-like scales on the lid margin. On removing these scales underlying surface is found to be hyperaemic (no ulcers). Lashes fall out easily. In long standing cases lid margin is thickened and the sharp posterior lid border tends to be rounded leading to epiphora.
- *Signs of ulcerative blepharitis.* Yellow crusts are seen at the root of cilia which glue them together. Small ulcers, which bleed easily, are seen on removing the crusts. In between the crusts, the anterior lid margin may show dilated blood vessels (rosettes).

RELATED QUESTIONS

What is blepharitis and how do you classify it?

Blepharitis is a chronic inflammation of the lid margins. It can be divided into four classical types:

1. Seborrhoeic or squamous blepharitis
2. Ulcerative blepharitis
3. Mixed ulcerative with seborrhoeic blepharitis
4. Posterior blepharitis or meibomitis.

How will you differentiate squamous blepharitis from ulcerative blepharitis?

1. In squamous blepharitis white dandruff-like scales are seen at the lid margin while in ulcerative blepharitis yellow crusts are seen.
2. On removing the white scales underlying surface is found to be hyperaemic in squamous blepharitis. While in ulcerative blepharitis, small ulcers which bleed easily are seen on removing the crusts.
3. Cilia may be glued together in ulcerative blepharitis, but not so in squamous belpharitis.

What are the complications of ulcerative blepharitis?

When not treated for a long time, the following complications may occur:

1. Chronic conjunctivitis
2. Trichiasis

3. Madarosis (sparseness or absence of lashes)
4. Poliosis (greying of cilia)
5. Tylosis (thickening of lid margin)
6. Eversion of punctum leading to epiphora
7. Recurrent styes

How will you treat a case of squamous blepharitis?

1. Scales should be removed from the lid margin with the help of lukewarm solution of 3 per cent soda-bicarb or some baby shampoo.
2. Combined steroid and broad spectrum eye ointment should be rubbed at the lid margin twice daily.
3. Associated seborrhoea should be treated adequately.

How will you treat a case of ulcerative blepharitis?

1. Hot compresses.
2. Crusts should be removed after softening with 3 percent soda bicarb.
3. Antibiotic ointment should be applied at lid margin immediately after removal of crusts.
4. Antibiotic eye drops should be instilled 3 to 4 times a day.
5. Oral antibiotics such as amoxycillin, cloxacillin, erythromycin or tetracycline may be useful.

A CASE OF CHALAZION (MEIBOMIAN CYST)

CASE DESCRIPTION

Presenting symptoms. Patient usually presents with a painless swelling near the lid margin. Patient may be concerned about the cosmetic disfigurement caused and may also feel mild heaviness in the lids. Sometimes, mild defective vision may occur due to astigmatism caused by pressure of chalazion on the cornea.

Ocular examinations reveal a small, firm to hard, non-tender swelling present slightly away from the lid margin (Fig. 14.12). Overlying skin is normal and mobile. The swelling usually points on the conjunctival side as red, purple or grey area seen on everting the lid. Sometimes, the main bulk of swelling may project on the skin side and occasionaly on the lid margin.

Differential diagnosis. Chalazion needs to be differentiated from meibomian gland carcinoma, tuberculomata and tarsitis.

A CASE OF STYE

Presenting symptoms include acute pain and swelling in the lid. Patient also experiences heaviness in the eyelid, mild photophobia and watering.

Ocular examination during stage of cellulitis reveals tender swelling, redness and oedema of the affected lid margins (Fig. 14.11). During *stage of abscess formation* a visible plus point on the lid margin in relation to the roof of affected cilia is formed.

Differential diagnosis. Stye (hordeolum externum) should be differentiated from hordeolum internum.

RELATED QUESTIONS

What is a chalazion?

Chalazion is also known as *tarsal* or *meibomian cyst.* It is a chronic non-infective granulomatous inflammation of the meibomian gland.

What is hordeolum externum (stye)?

Hordeolum externum is an acute suppurative inflammation of one of the Zeis' glands.

It is characterized by a localized, hard, red, tender swelling at the lid margin (PI.IV.I). In advanced stage, a pus point is visible at the lid margin.

What is hordeolum internum? How will you differentiate it from hordeolum externum?

Hordeolum internum is a suppurative inflammation of the meibomian gland associated with blockage of the duct. It may occur as primary staphylococcal infection of the meibomian gland or due to secondary infection in a chalazion (infected chalazion).

Its symptoms are similar to hordeolum externum except that pain is more intense due to the swelling being deeply embedded in the dense fibrous tissue. On examination it can be differentiated from hordeolum externum by the facts that in it, the point of maximum tenderness and swelling is away from the lid margin and that pus usually points on the tarsal conjunctiva (seen as a yellowish area on everting the lid) and not on the root of cilia.

When not treated, what complications can occur in a case of chalazion?

1. A large chalazion of the upper lid may press on the cornea and may cause blurred vision due to induced astigmatism.

2. A large chalazion of the lower lid may rarely cause eversion of the punctum or even ectropion and epiphora.
3. Occasionally, a chalazion may burst on the conjunctival side forming a fungating mass of granulation tissue.
4. Due to secondary infection the chalazion may be converted into hordeolum internum.
5. Calcification may occur, though very rarely.
6. Malignant change into meibomian gland carcinoma may be seen occasionally in elderly people.

How do you treat a case of chalazion?

1. *Conservative treatment* in the form of hot fomentation, topical antibiotic eyedrops and oral anti-inflammatory drugs may lead to self-resolution in a small, soft and recent chalazion.
2. *Intralesional injection* of long acting steroid (triamcinolone) is reported to cause resolution in about 50 per cent cases.
3. *Incision and curettage* is the conventional and effective treatment for chalazion.

Describe the steps of incision and curettage of a chalazion.

1. Local anaesthesia is obtained by topical instillation of 4 percent Xylocaine drops in the conjunctival sac and infiltration of the lid in the region of chalazion with 2 per cent Xylocaine.
2. A chalazion clamp is applied with its fenestrated side on the conjunctival side and the lid is everted.
3. A vertical incision is made to avoid injury to the other meibomian glands.
4. The contents are curetted out with the help of a chalazion scoop.
5. To avoid recurrence its cavity should be cauterized with carbolic acid.
6. An antibiotic eye ointment is instilled and eye is padded.

What is the treatment of a marginal chalazion?

Destruction by diathermy is the treatment of choice for a marginal chalazion.

A CASE OF TRICHIASIS AND ENTROPION

DESCRIPTION OF A CASE OF TRICHIASIS

Presenting symptoms. Patients may present with a foreign body sensation, photophobia, irritation and lacrimation. Sometimes patient may experience troublesome pain.

Past history of the disease causative of trichiasis such as cicatrizing trachoma, ulcerative blepharitis, membranous conjunctivitis, mechanical injuries, burns and operation of the lid margin may be explored.

Ocular examination reveals one or more misdirected cilia touching the eyeball (Fig. 14.16). There may or may not be signs of the causative disease.

DESCRIPTION OF A CASE OF ENTROPION

Presenting symptoms and past history exploration are similar to a case of trichiasis.

Ocular examination reveals inturned lid margin (Fig. 14.17). Depending upon the degree of inturning the entropion can be divided into three grades. In grade I entropion, only the posterior lid border is inrolled. Grade II entropion includes inturning up to the intermarginal strip, while in grade III, the whole lid margin including the anterior lid border is inturned.

Examination may also reveal signs of the causative disease.

RELATED QUESTIONS

Define trichiasis.

Trichiasis refers to inward misdirection of cilia which rub against the eyeball.

What are the common causes of trichiasis?

1. Cicatrizing trachoma
2. Ulcerative blepharitis
3. Healed membranous conjunctivitis
4. Healed hordeolum externum
5. Mechanical injuries
6. Burns and operative scars on the lid margin

When not treated in time, what complications can occur in a case of trichiasis?

1. Corneal abrasions
2. Superficial corneal opacities
3. Corneal vascularization
4. Non-healing corneal ulceration

What is distichiasis?

Distichiasis is condition of an extra posterior row of cilia which occupy the position of meibomian glands.

How will you treat a case of trichiasis?

1. *Epilation:* It is a temporary measure.

2. *Electrolysis:* After local infiltration of anaesthesia, a current of 2 milliampere is passed for about 10 seconds through a fine needle inserted into the lash root. The loosened cilia with destroyed follicles are then removed with the help of an epilation forceps.
3. *Cryoepilation:* After infiltration anaesthesia, the cryoprobe (–20°C) is applied for 20 to 25 seconds to the external lid margin. The loosened lash is pulled with an epilation forceps.
4. *Surgical correction:* It is similar to cicatricial entropion and should be employed when many cilia are misdirected.

Define entropion.

Entropion refers to turning in of the lid margin.

What are the types of entropion?

Depending upon the cause, entropion may be of the following types:

1. Congenital entropion
2. Cicatricial entropion
3. Spastic entropion
4. Mechanical entropion

What are the causes of cicatricial entropion?

1. Trachoma
2. Membranous conjunctivitis
3. Chemical burns
4. Pemphigus
5. Stevens-Johnson syndrome

Name the surgical techniques employed for correcting cicatricial entropion.

1. Resection of skin and muscle
2. Resection of skin, muscle and tarsus
3. Modified Burow's operation
4. Jaesche-Arlt's operation
5. Modified Ketssey's operation

Name the surgical techniques used to correct a senile (involutional) entropion.

1. Modified Wheeler's operation
2. Bick's procedure with Reeh's modification
3. Weiss operation
4. Tucking of inferior lid retractors (Jones, Reeh and Webing operation).

A CASE OF ECTROPION

CASE DESCRIPTION

Presenting symptoms include watering (epiphora) and cosmetic disfigurement. Patients may also have symptoms of associated chronic conjunctivitis which include irritation, discomfort and mild photophobia.

Ocular examination. The lid margin is outrolled (Fig. 14.24). Depending upon the degree of outrolling, ectropion can be divided into three grades. In grade I ectropion, only the punctum is everted. In grade II ectropion lid margin is everted and palpebral conjunctiva is visible while in grade III the fornix is also visible.

Examination may also reveal signs of aetiological condition such as scar in cicatricial ectropion (Fig. 14.25) and seventh nerve palsy in paralytic ectropion.

RELATED QUESTIONS

What is ectropion?

Outrolling or outward turning of the lid margin is called ectropion.

What are the types of ectropion?

1. Senile ectropion
2. Paralytic ectropion
3. Cicatricial ectropion
4. Spastic ectropion

What is the treatment of senile ectropion?

Depending upon the severity of the ectropion, following three operations are commonly performed:

1. Medial conjunctivoplasty
2. Horizontal shortening
3. Byron-Smith's modified Kuhnt-Szymanowski operation.

What is a symblepharon?

Symblepharon is a condition in which lids become adherent with the eyeball. It results from healing of the kissing raw surfaces of the palpebral and bulbar conjunctiva.

What are the common causes of symblepharon?

1. Chemical burns
2. Thermal burns
3. Membranous conjunctivitis
4. Conjunctival injuries
5. Ocular pemphigus
6. Stevens-Johnson syndrome

What do you mean by ankyloblepharon?

Ankyloblepharon refers to the adhesions between margins of the upper and lower lids. It may be congenital or may result after healing of chemical or thermal burns.

What is blepharophimosis?

In blepharophimosis vertical as well as horizontal extent of the palpebral fissure is decreased.

What is lagophthalmos? Enumerate its common causes.

Lagophthalmos refers to the inability to voluntarily close the eyelids. Its common causes are:

1. Paralysis of seventh nerve
2. Marked proptosis
3. Cicatricial contraction of the lids
4. Following over-resection of the levator palpebrae superioris
5. Symblepharon
6. Comatosed patient

What is belpharospasm?

Belpharospasm refers to the involuntary, sustained and forceful closure of the eyelids. It is of two types: essential belpharospasm and reflex blepharospasm.

A CASE OF PTOSIS

CASE DESCRIPTION

Age and sex. Ptosis may be congenital or acquired. Acquired ptosis may occur at any age in either sex.

History. It should include age of onset, family history, history of trauma, eye surgery, and variability in degree of ptosis.

Examination should include:

1. *Inspection* to note:
   - True ptosis or pseudoptosis
   - Unilateral or bilateral ptosis
   - Eyelid crease and function of orbicularis
   - Presence of Jaw winking phenomenon
   - Associated weakness of extraocular muscles
   - Bell's phenomenon
2. Measurement of degree of ptosis
3. Assessment of levator function
4. Special investigations for acquired ptosis (For details see page 380).

RELATED QUESTIONS

What is ptosis?

Abnormal drooping of the upper eyelids is called ptosis. Normally upper lid covers about upper one-sixth (2 mm) of the cornea. Therefore, in ptosis it covers more than 2 mm.

What are the types of ptosis?

I. Congenital ptosis which may be:
   1. Simple congenital ptosis (not associated with any other anomaly) (Fig. 14.32A).
   2. Congenital ptosis with associated weakness of the superior rectus muscle.
   3. As a part of blepharophimosis syndrome (Fig. 14.32B).
   4. Congenital synkinetic ptosis (Marcus Gunn jaw winking ptosis).

II. Acquired ptosis includes:
   1. Neurogenic ptosis
   2. Myogenic ptosis
   3. Aponeurotic ptosis
   4. Mechanical ptosis

How do you grade ptosis?

Depending upon the amount of ptosis in mm, it is graded as follows:

1. Mild ptosis (2 mm)
2. Moderate ptosis (3 mm)
3. Severe ptosis (4 mm).

How do you grade levator function?

Depending upon the amount of lid excursion caused by levator muscle (Burke's method), its function is graded as follows:

Normal	:	15 mm
Good	:	8 mm or more
Fair	:	5-7 mm
Poor	:	4 mm or less

Which test is carried out to confirm the diagnosis in a patient with ptosis suspected of myasthenia gravis?

- Tensilon or edrophonium test.

Which test is carried out in a patient suspected of Horner's syndrome?

- Phenylephrine test.

Name the three basic surgical procedures for ptosis correction.

1. Fasanella - Servat operation
2. Levator resection operation
3. Frontalis sling operation

Name the common lid tumours.

I. Benigu tumours
   1. Simple papilloma
   2. Naevus
   3. Haemangioma
   4. Neurofibroma

II. Precancerous conditions
   1. Solar keratosis
   2. Carcinoma *in-situ*
   3. Xeroderma pigmentosa

III. Malignant tumours
   1. Squamous-cell carcinoma
   2. Basal-cell carcinoma
   3. Malignant melanoma
   4. Sebaceous gland carcinoma.

Which is the most common malignant tumour of the lids?

- Basal-cell carcinoma.

Which is the most common site for occurrence of basal cell carcinoma?

- Medial canthus.

What is the structure of an eyelid?

Each eyelid from anterior to posterior consists of the following layers:

1. Skin
2. Subcutaneous areolar tissue
3. Layer of striated muscle (orbicularis oculi and levator palpebrae superioris in upper lid only)
4. Submuscular areolar tissue
5. Fibrous layer (tarsal) plate and septum orbitale
6. Layer of non-striated muscle fibres (Muller's muscle)
7. Conjunctiva

Name the glands of the eyelids.

1. Meibomian glands
2. Glands of Zeis
3. Glands of Moll
4. Accessory lacrimal glands of Wolfring

What are the causes of pseudoproptosis?

- Anophthalmos
- Enophthalmos
- Phthisis bulbi
- Atrophic bulbi
- Trachoma (stage of sequelae)
- Any tumour or nodule of upper lid

DISEASES OF THE LACRIMAL APPARATUS

A CASE OF CHRONIC DACRYOCYSTITIS

CASE DESCRIPTION

Age and sex. The disease may occur at any age and in any sex. However, in general, females are much more commonly affected than males and the disease is more common between 40 and 60 years of age.

Presenting symptoms. A patient presents with a long standing history of watering from the eyes which may or may not be associated with a swelling at the inner canthus.

Ocular examination may reveal any of the following signs:

- No swelling is seen at the medial canthus but regurgitation test is positive, i.e., a reflux of mucopurulent discharge from the puncta when pressure is applied over the lacrimal sac area.
- A swelling may be seen at the medial canthus (Fig. 15.8). Milky or gelatinous mucoid fluid regurgitates from the lower punctum on pressing the swelling (lacrimal mucocele).
- Sometimes on pressing the swelling, a frank purulent discharge flows from the lower punctum (lacrimal pyocele).
- Sometimes a swelling is seen at the inner canthus with a negative regurgitation test (encysted mucocele).

RELATED QUESTIONS

What are the causes of a watering eye?

Watering from the eyes may occur either due to excessive lacrimation or may result from obstruction to the outflow of normally secreted tears (epiphora). The common causes of watering eye are listed at page 367.

Name the tests which you would like to carry out to evaluate a case of watering eye.

1. Examination with diffuse illumination under magnification to rule out causes of hyper-lacrimation and punctal causes of epiphora
2. Regurgitation test for chronic dacryocystits
3. Fluorescein dye disappearance test (FDDT)
4. Lacrimal syringing test
5. Jone's dye test I and II
6. Dacryocystography
7. Lacrimal scintillography

What is regurgitation test?

In regurgitation test a steady pressure with index finger is applied over the lacrimal sac area above the medial palpebral ligament. Reflux of mucopurulent discharge (a positive regurgitation test) indicates chronic dacryocystitis with obstruction at the lower end of sac or nasolacrimal duct.

What are the causes of a negative regurgitation test?

Causes of a negative regurgitation test are:

- Normal sac (no dacryocystitis)
- Wrong site of pressure
- Patient might have emptied the sac just before coming to the examiner's chamber
- Encysted mucocele
- Internal fistula

Name the indications of lacrimal syringing.

1. Diagnostic indications:
   - Epiphora
   - For dacryocystography
2. Therapeutic indications:
   - Congenital dacryocystitis
   - Early cases of chronic catarrhal dacryocystitis
3. Prognostic:
   After DCR operation

Describe the procedure and interpretations of the results of lacrimal syringing.

1. Topical anaesthesia is obtained by instilling 4 per cent Xylocaine in the conjunctival sac
2. Lower punctum is dilated with a punctum dilator
3. Normal saline is pushed into the lacrimal sac through the lower punctum with the help of a syringe and lacrimal cannula (Fig. 3.7-2) and results are interpreted as follows:
   - A free passage of saline through lacrimal passages into the nose indicates either no obstruction or partial obstruction.
   - In the presence of obstruction no fluid passes into the nose. When obstruction is in the nasolacrimal duct, the sac fills with the normal saline which refluxes from the upper punctum.
   - In case of lower canalicular obstruction, there will be immediate reflux of the saline through the lower punctum. Under these circumstances the procedure should be repeated through the upper punctum. A free passage of saline into the nose will confirm the blockage in the lower canaliculus while regurgitation back through the same punctum will indicate block at the level of common canaliculus.

What is dacryocystitis, how will you classify it?

Dacryocystits is inflammation of the lacrimal sac. It can be classified as follows:

1. Congenital dacryocystitis
2. Adult dacryocystitis which may occur as:
   - Chronic dacryocystitis, and
   - Acute dacryocystitis

What is the aetiology of congenital dacryocystitis? How will you treat it?

Congenital dacryocystitis follows stasis of secretions in the lacrimal sac due to congenital blockage in the nasolacrimal duct (usually a membranous occlusion at the lower end of NLD).

Its treatment, depends upon the age at which child is brought (see page 394).

What is the treatment of choice in adulthood chronic dacryocystitis?

Dacryocystorhinostomy (DCR) operation is the operation of choice since it re-establishes the lacrimal drainage. When DCR is contraindictated, dacryocystectomy may be performed.

What is dacryocystectomy? Enumerate its indications.

Dacryocystectomy is the excision of the lacrimal sac. It should be performed only when DCR is contraindicated as in following conditions:

1. Too young (less than 4 years) or too old (more than 60 years) a patient
2. Markedly shrunken and fibrosed sac

3. Tuberculosis, syphilis, leprosy or mycotic infection of the sac
4. Tumours of the sac
5. Gross nasal diseases like atrophic rhinitis
6. An unskilled surgeon, because it is said that a good 'DCT' is always better than a badly done 'DCR'.

What are tears?

Tears form the aqueous layer of tear film and are secreted by the accessory and main lacrimal glands. Tears mainly comprise water and small quantities of salts such as sodium chloride, sugar, urea and proteins. Therefore, it is alkaline and saltish in taste. It also contains antibacterial substances like lysozyme, betalysin and lactoferrin.

What are the layers of tear film?

Wolf described the following three layers of tear film:

1. *Mucous layer:* It is the innermost and thinnest layer of tear film. It consists of mucin secreted by the conjunctival goblet cells. It converts the hydrophobic corneal surface into a hydrophilic one.
2. *Aqueous layer:* It consists of tears secreted by the main and accessory lacrimal glands and forms the main bulk of the tear film.
3. *Lipid or oily layer:* It consists of secretions of the meibomian, Zeis and Moll's glands. It prevents the overflow of tears and retards their evaporation.

What are the functions of tear film?

1. It keeps the cornea and conjunctiva moist
2. Provides oxygen to the corneal epithelium
3. It washes away debris and noxious irritants
4. It prevents infection due to presence of antibacterial substances
5. It facilitates movement of the lids over the globe.

What is dry eye?

Dry eye per se is not a disease entity but a symptom complex occurring as a sequela to deficiency or abnormalities of the tear film.

What are the causes of dry eye?

1. *Aqueous deficiency dry eye (*keratoconjunctivitis sicca — KCS)
   - Congenital alacrimia
   - Sjogren's syndrome
   - Riley-Day syndrome
   - Idiopathic hyposecretion
2. *Mucin deficiency dry eye*
   - Hypovitaminosis A (xerophthalmia)
   - Stevens-Johnson syndrome
   - Trachoma
   - Chemical burns
3. *Lipid abnormalities*
   - Chronic blepharitis
   - Chronic meibomitis
4. *Impaired eyelid function*
   - Bell's palsy
   - Exposure keratitis
   - Ectropion
5. *Epitheliopathies* of corneal surface

Name the important tear film tests performed to diagnose the dry eye.

- Tear film break-up-time (BUT)
- Schirmer 1 test
- Rose bengal staining

What is tear film break-up time?

Tear film break-up time is the interval between a complete blink and appearance of the first randomly distributed dry spot on the corneal surface. Its normal values range between 15 and 35 seconds. Values less than 10 seconds employ an unstable tear film.

What is Schirmer 1 Test?

Schirmer test measures the total tear secretions with the help of 5 × 35 mm strip of Whatman No. 42 filter paper. Its normal values are more than 15 mm of wetting of the filter paper strip in 5 minutes. Values between 5 and 10 mm are suggestive of mild to moderate keratoconjunctivitis sicca (KCS) and less than 5 mm of severe KCS.

What is Sjogren's syndrome?

Sjogren's syndrome is an autoimmune disease usually occurring in women between 40 and 50 years of age. Its main feature is an aqueous deficiency dry eye (KCS). It occurs in two forms:

1. *Primary Sjogren's syndrome:* In it, KCS is combined with xerostomia (dry mouth)
2. *Secondary Sjogren's syndrome:* In it dry eye and /or dry mouth is associatcd with an autoimmunc disease, commonly rheumatoid arthritis.

What is the treatment of dry eye?

1. *Supplementation by artificial tear* solution such as: 0.7 percent methylcellulose, 0.3 percent hypromellose or 1.4 percent polyvinyl alcohol.
2. *Preservation of existing tears* by punctal occlusions with collagen implants or electrocauterization
3. *Mucolytics* such as 5 percent acetylcysteine help by dispersing the mucous threads.

DISEASES OF THE ORBIT

A CASE OF PROPTOSIS

CASE DESCRIPTION

Presenting symptoms. A patient presents with a history of the bulging of the eyeball which may be gradually or rapidly progressive. It may or may not be associated with visual loss, diplopia, pain or other symptoms.

Ocular examination reveals outward protusion of the eyeball which may be:

- Unilateral (Fig. 16.7) or bilateral (Fig. 16.11),
- Axial or eccentric
- Pulsatile or non-pulsatile
- Reducible or non-reducible
- May or may not be associated with lagophthalmos

RELATED QUESTIONS

What is proptosis and exophthalmos?

Proptosis refers to forward displacement of the eyeball beyond the orbital margin. Though the word exophthalmos (out eye) is synonymous with proptosis; somehow it has become customary to use the term exophthalmos for the displacement associated with thyroid eye disease.

What are the causes of unilateral proptosis?

1. Congenital conditions
   - Dermoid cyst
   - Congenital cystic eyeball
   - Teratoma
2. Traumatic lesions
   - Orbital haemorrhage
   - Retained intraorbital foreign body
   - Traumatic aneurysm
3. Inflammatory lesions
   - Orbital cellulitis or abscess
   - Panophthalmitis
   - Cavernous sinus thrombosis
   - Pseudotumour
4. Circulatory disturbances and vascular lesions
   - Orbital varix
   - Aneurysm
5. Cysts of the orbit
   - Implantation cyst
   - Hydatid cyst
   - Cysticercus cellulosae
6. Tumours of the orbit, which may be
   - Primary tumours (arising from the various intraorbital structures)
   - Secondary tumours (invading from the surrounding structures)
   - Metastatic tumours from the distant primary tumours.

Enumerate the causes of bilateral proptosis.

1. Developmental anomalies of the skull
   - Oxycephaly
2. Inflammatory conditions
   - Mikulicz's syndrome
   - Late stage of cavernous sinus thrombosis
3. Endocrine exophthalmos (most common cause) (Fig. 16.11)
4. Orbital tumours, e.g.:
   - Lymphoma or lymphosarcoma
   - Secondaries from:
     - Neuroblastoma
     - Nephroblastoma
     - Ewing's sarcoma
     - Leukaemic infiltration
5. Systemic diseases, e.g.:
   - Histiocytosis-X
   - Systemic amyloidosis
   - Xanthomatosis
   - Wegener's granulomatosis

What are the causes of acute proptosis?

1. Orbital emphysema following fracture of medial orbital wall
2. Orbital haemorrhage
3. Rupture of ethmoidal mucocele

What are the causes of intermittent proptosis?

1. Orbital varix (most common cause)
2. Periodic orbital oedema
3. Highly vascular tumour

What are the causes of pulsatile proptosis?

1. Caroticocavernous fistula (most common cause)
2. Saccular aneurysm of ophthalmic artery
3. Congenital orbital meningocele or meningo-encephalocele
4. Hiatus in the orbital roof due to trauma, operation or that associated with neurofibromatosis

How will you investigate a case of proptosis?

Evaluation of a case of proptosis includes the following:

I. *Clinical evaluation*
   a) History
   b) Local examination
      (1) Inspection; (2) palpation; (3) auscultation; (4) transillumination; (5) visual acuity; (6) pupillary reactions; (7) fundoscopy; (8) ocular motility; (9) exophthalmometry
   c) Systemic examination

II. *Laboratory investigations*
   - Thyroid function tests
   - Haematological tests
   - Stool examination for cysts and ova
   - Urine analysis

III. *Roentgen examination*
   1. Plain radiograph of orbit
   2. CT Scanning
   3. Ultrasonography
   4. Magnetic resonance imaging (MRI)
   5. Carotid angiography

IV. *Histopathological studies*
   1. Fine-needle aspiration biopsy (FNAB)
   2. Incisional biopsy
   3. Excisional biopsy

What is enophthalmos? Enumerate its causes.

Enophthalmos is the inward displacement of the eyeball. Its common causes are:

1. Congenital microphthalmos
2. Congenital maxillary hypoplasia
3. Traumatic blow-out fractures of the orbital floor
4. Post-inflammatory cicatrization of the extraocular muscles as in pseudotumour syndromes
5. Paralytic enophthalmos as seen in Horner's syndrome
6. Atrophy of the orbital contents, e.g., senile atrophy of orbital fat, atrophy following irradiation of malignant tumours.

What is Graves' ophthalmopathy?

This is a term coined to denote typical ocular changes which include: lid retraction, lid lag and proptosis (Fig. 16.11). These changes are also known as endocrine exophthalmos, dysthyroid ophthalmopathy, thyroid ophthalmopathy and ocular Graves' disease (OGD).

Name the extraocular muscle most frequently affected in Graves' ophthalmopathy.

- Inferior rectus.

What is American Thyroid Association classification of Graves' ophthalmopathy?

American Thyroid Association (ATA) has classified Graves' ophthalmopathy irrespective of the hormonal status into the following classes; characterized by the acronym 'NOSPECS':

Class 0 : No signs and symptoms.

Class 1 : Only signs, no symptoms. Signs are limited to lid retraction with or without lid lag and mild proptosis.

Class 2 : Soft tissue involvement with signs of class 1 and symptoms including lacrimation, photophobia, lid or conjunctival swelling.

Class 3 : Proptosis is well established.

Class 4 : Extraocular muscle involvement (limitation of movements and diplopia).

Class 5 : Corneal involvement (exposure keratitis)

Class 6 : Sight loss due to optic nerve involvement with disc pallor or papilloedema.

What are the two clinical types of Graves' ophthalmopathy?

1. *Thyrotoxic exophthalmos* (exophthalmic goitre): In this form, a mild exophthalmos is associated with lid signs and all signs of thyrotoxicosis which include: tachycardia, muscle tremors and raised basal metabolism
2. *Thyrotropic exophthalmos* (exophthalmic ophthalmoplegia): In this marked exophthalmos and an infiltrative ophthalmoplegia is associated with euthyroidism or hypothyroidism.

What are the causes of pseudoproptosis?

1. Buphthalmos
2. Lid retraction
3. High-axial myopia
4. Staphyloma
5. Enophthalmos of the opposite eye

What are the causes of reducible proptosis?

- Early stages of ocular Graves' disease
- Haemangioma
- Orbital varix
- Caroticocavernous fistula

Which is the most common primary tumour of the orbit presenting as proptosis?

- Cavernous haemangioma

Name the most common primary orbital tumour of childhood.

- Rhabdomyosarcoma

DISORDERS OF OCULAR MOTILITY

A CASE OF SQUINT

CASE DESCRIPTION

Presenting symptoms. Patient presents with deviation of one eye which may be on medial side (convergent squint) or lateral side (divergent squint).

History of present illness must include following important points:

- Age of onset
- Mode of onset, sudden or gradual
- Precipitating factors such as, systemic illness ocular cause, emotional breakdown, trauma
- History of diplopia
- Birth history is important in early childhood onset deviation.
- History of use of glasses

Family history is also important in a case of strabismus.

Ocular examination should reveal:

- Whether the manifest squint is convergent (Fig. 13.14) or divergent (Fig. 13.15).
- Abnormal head posture associated or not.
- Whether the squint is unilateral or alternating
- Ocular movements are normal (concomitant squint) or limited (paralytic or non-concomitant squint).
- Angle of squint on corneal reflex test (Hirschberg's test).

Note: Detailed orthoptic examination is not expected from an undergraduate student.

RELATED QUESTIONS

Name the various extraocular muscles.

- Superior rectus
- Inferior rectus
- Medial rectus
- Lateral rectus
- Superior oblique
- Inferior oblique

What is the origin of rectus muscles?

The rectus muscles originate from a common tendinous ring (annulus of Zinn), which is attached at the apex of the orbit.

Where are the rectus muscles inserted?

The rectus muscles are inserted into the sclera by flat tendons at different distances from the limbus as under:

- Medial rectus – 5.5 mm
- Inferior rectus – 6.5 mm
- Lateral rectus – 6.9 mm
- Superior rectus – 7.7 mm

What is the nerve supply of extraocular muscles?

The extraocular muscles are supplied by third, fourth and sixth cranial nerves. The third cranial nerve (oculomotor) supplies the superior, medial and inferior recti and inferior oblique muscles. The fourth cranial nerve (trochlear) supplies the superior oblique muscle, and sixth cranial nerve supplies the lateral rectus muscle.

What are the actions of extraocular muscles?

Action of each extraocular muscle is as below:

Muscle	*Primary action*	*Secondary action*	*Tertiary action*
Medial rectus	Adduction	–	–
Lateral rectus	Abduction	–	–
Superior rectus	Elevation	Intorsion	Adduction
Inferior rectus	Depression	Extorsion	Adduction
Superior oblique	Intorsion	Depression	Abduction
Inferior oblique	Extorsion	Elevation	Abduction

Describe uniocular movements of the eyeball.

Uniocular movements of the eyeball are called *ductions.* These are as follows:

1. *Adduction.* It is medial rotation along the vertical axis
2. *Abduction.* It is lateral rotation along the vertical axis
3. *Infraduction.* It is downward movement (depression) along the horizontal axis
4. *Supraduction.* It is upward movement (elevation) along the horizontal axis
5. *Incycloduction (Intorsion).* It is rotatory movement along the anteroposterior axis in which superior pole of cornea (12 O'clock point) moves medially
6. *Excycloduction (Extorsion).* It is rotatory movement along the anteroposterior axis in which superior pole of cornea (12 O'clock point) moves laterally

What are version movements of the eyeball?

Versions also known as *conjugate movements,* are synchronous (simultaneous) symmetric movements of both the eyes in the same direction. For example:

- Dextroversion is the movement of both eyes to the right.
- Levoversion is the movement of both eyes to the left.

What are vergence movements of the eyeball?

Vergences, also called as *disjugate movements,* are synchronous and symmetric movements of both eyes in opposite directions, e.g.:

- Convergence is simultaneous inward movement of both the eyes.
- Divergence is simultaneous outward movement of both the eyes.

Define synergists, antagonists and yoke muscles.

1. *Synergists* are the muscles which have a similar primary action in the same eye, e.g., superior rectus and inferior oblique of the same eye act as synergistic elevators.
2. *Antagonists* are the muscles which have opposite actions in the same eye, e.g., superior and inferior recti are the antagonists to each other in the same eye.
3. *Yoke muscles* (contralateral synergists) are a pair of muscles (one from each eye) which contract simultaneously during version movements. Different pairs of yoke muscles are as follows:
   - Right medial rectus and left lateral rectus
   - Right lateral rectus and left medial rectus
   - Right superior rectus and left inferior oblique
   - Right inferior rectus and left superior oblique
   - Right superior oblique and left inferior rectus
   - Right inferior oblique and left superior rectus

What is Hering's law of equal innervation?

According to it, an equal and simultaneous innervation flows from the brain to a pair of muscles which contract simultaneously (yoke muscles) in different binocular movements, e.g., during dextroversion, right lateral rectus muscles and left medial rectus muscle, receiving an equal and simultaneous flow of innervation.

What is Sherrington's law of reciprocal innervation?

According to it, during ocular movements an increased flow of innervation to the contracting muscles is accompanied by a simultaneous decreased flow of innervation to the relaxing antagonists. For example, during dextroversion an increased innervational flow to the right lateral rectus and left medial rectus is accompanied by a decreased flow to the right medial rectus and left lateral rectus muscles.

What is the primary position of gaze?

It is the position assumed by the eyes when fixing a distant object (straight ahead) with the erect position of head.

What are the secondary positions of gaze?

These are the positions assumed by the eyes while looking straight up, and down to the right and to the left.

What are the cardinal positions of gaze?

These are the positions which allow examination of each of the 12 extraocular muscles in their main field of action. There are six cardinal positions of gaze, viz. dextroversion, levoversion, dextroelevation, levoelevation, dextrodepression and levodepression.

What are the three grades of binocular single vision?

Grade 1. Simultaneous macular perception (SMP): It is the power to see two dissimilar objects which can be superimposed to form a joint picture. For example, when the picture of a lion is projected onto the right eye and that of a cage to the left eye, an individual with presence of SMP will see the lion in the cage.

Grade II. Fusion: It consists of the power to superimpose two incomplete but similar images to form one complete image.

Grade III. Stereopsis: It consists of the ability to perceive the third dimension (depth perception).

What is squint; how do you classify it?

Normally visual axes of the two eyes are parallel to each other in the primary position of gaze and this alignment is maintained in all positions.

A misalignment of the visual axes of the two eyes is called squint or strabismus. Broadly it can be classified as:

1. Apparent squint or pseudostrabismus
2. Latent squint (heterophoria)
3. Manifest squint (heterotropia), which includes:
   i. Concomitant squint
   ii. Incomitant squint.

What is heterophoria; what are its types?

Also known as *latent squint,* it is a condition in which the tendency of the eyes to deviate is kept latent by fusion. Therefore, when the influence of fusion is removed the visual axis of one eye deviates.

Common types of heterophoria are:

1. *Esophoria:* It is a tendency to converge when binocularity is broken by any means
2. *Exophoria:* It is a tendency to diverge
3. *Hyperphoria:* It is a tendency to deviate upwards, while hypophoria is a tendency to deviate downwards. However, in practice it is customary to use the term right or left hyperphoria, depending on the eye which remains up as compared to the other.

Name a few tests by which heterophoria can be diagnosed.

1. Cover-uncover test
2. Maddox rod test
3. Maddox wing test

What is suppression?

Suppression is a temporary active cortical inhibition of the image of an object formed on the retina of the squinting eye. This phenomenon occurs only during binocular vision (with both eyes open). It can be tested by Worth's four-dot test.

What is abnormal retinal correspondence?

Normally, fovea of the two eyes act as corresponding points and have the same visual direction (normal retinal correspondence). Sometimes in a patient with squint, fovea of the normal eye and an extra foveal point on the retina of the squinting eye acquire a common visual direction, i.e., become the corresponding points. This adjustment is called abnormal retinal correspondence (ARC).

Name a few methods by which angle of squint can be measured.

1. Hirschberg's corneal reflex test
2. Prism bar cover test (PBCT)
3. By synoptophore (major amblyoscope)
4. Krimsky's corneal reflex test
5. Perimeter method

Describe Hirschberg's corneal reflex test.

Hirschberg's corneal reflex test is a rough but handy method to estimate the angle of manifest squint. In this, the patient is asked to fixate at a light point held at a distance of 33 cm and the deviation of the corneal light reflex from the centre of pupil is noted in the squinting eye. Roughly, the angle of squint is 15° and 45° when the corneal light reflex falls on the border of pupil and limbus, respectively.

What is a concomitant squint?

Concomitant squint is a type of manifest squint in which the angle of deviation remains constant in all the directions of gaze; and there is no associated limitation of ocular movements.

How do you classify concomitant esotropia?

1. Infantile esotropia
2. Accommodative esotropia
3. Non-accommodative esotropia

What is accommodative esotropia?

Accommodative esotropia occurs due to overaction of convergence associated with accommodation reflex. Refractive type of accommodative esotropia is associated with high hypermetropia (+4 to +7D).

How do you classify concomitant exotropia (divergent squint)?

1. Congenital exotropia
2. Primary exotropia
   a. Intermittent

b. Constant
   - Unilateral
   - Alternating
3. Secondary (sensory deprivation) exotropia
4. Consecutive exotropia

What is paralytic squint?

Paralytic squint is a type of incomitant squint in which ocular deviation results from complete or incomplete paralysis of one or more extraocular muscles.

What are the features of paralytic squint?

1. History of diplopia and confusion.
2. Secondary deviation is greater than primary deviation.
3. Ocular movements are restricted towards the action of paralyzed muscle.
4. Head is turned towards the action of paralyzed muscle.

What are the features of complete third cranial nerve palsy?

These include the following (Fig. 13.25):
1. Ptosis due to paralysis of levator muscle
2. Eyeball is deviated out and slightly down
3. Ocular movements are restricted in all the directions except outward
4. Pupil is fixed and dilated
5. Accommodation is completely lost
6. Crossed diplopia is elicited on raising the eyelid

What are the differences between paralytic and non-paralytic squint?

Feature	*Paralytic squint*	*Non-paralytic squint*
1. Onset	Usually sudden	Usually slow
2. Diplopia	Usually present	Usually absent
3. Ocular movements	Limited in the direction of action of paralysed muscle	Full
4. False projection	It is positive, i.e., patient cannot correctly locate the object in space when asked to see in the direction of paralyzed muscle in early stages.	False projection in negative
5. Head posture	A particular head posture depending upon the muscle paralyzed may be present	Normal
6. Nausea and vertigo	Present	Absent
7. Secondary deviation	More than the primary deviation	Equal to primary deviation
8. In old cases pathological sequelae in the muscles	Present	Absent

What is nystagmus?

Nystagmus is defined as to-and-fro oscillatory movements of the eyes.

What are pendular and jerk nystagmus?

In pendular nystagmus, movements are of equal velocity in each direction. In jerk nystagmus, the movements have a slow component in one direction and a fast component in the other direction. The direction of jerk nystagmus is defined by direction of the fast component.

What are clinical types of nystagmus?

1. Physiological nystagmus, e.g., optokinetic nystagmus
2. Congenital nystagmus, e.g.,
   - Congenital jerk nystagmus
   - Latent nystagmus
   - Spasmus nutans
3. Acquired nystagmus, e.g.,
   - Acquired ocular nystagmus
   - Peripheral vestibular nystagmus
   - Central vestibular nystagmus
   - See-saw nystagmus

OCULAR INJURIES

A CASE OF BLUNT OCULAR TRAUMA

CASE DESCRIPTION

Age and sex. Trauma to the eyeball may occur at any age in either sex. However, in general, ocular trauma is more common in children than adults and in males than females.

Presenting symptoms and history. Patient usually presents with a direct blow to the eyeball by a large blunt object (tennis ball, cricket ball, fist etc) or injuries in a road side accident. There may be associated:

- Visual loss
- Pain and swelling of varying degree

Ocular examination may reveal varying signs depending upon the extent of trauma. In general the traumatic lesions produced by blunt trauma can be grouped as below:

- Closed globe injury
- Globe rupture
- Extraocular lesions

(For details see page 431).

RELATED QUESTIONS

What are the common sites for retention of an extraocular foreign body?

- Sulcus subtarsalis
- Fornices
- Bulbar conjunctiva
- Cornea

How do you remove a corneal foreign body?

- Eye is anaesthetized with topical instillation of 2 to 4 percent Xylocaine.
- Lids are separated with universal eye speculum.
- An attempt should be made to remove the foreign body with the help of a cotton swab stick. If it fails then foreign body spud or hypodermic needle should be used.
- After removal of the foreign body, pad and bandage with antibiotic eye ointment is applied for 24 to 48 hours.

How do you classify mechanical ocular injuries?

(see page 429)

Enumerate the lesions which can result from a blunt trauma to the eye (contusional injury).

1. *Lids*: Ecchymosis, Black eye, Avulsion of the lid, Traumatic ptosis
2. *Orbit*: Fracture of the orbital walls, Orbital haemorrhage, Orbital emphysemas
3. *Lacrimal apparatus:* Laceration of canaliculi, Dislocation of lacrimal gland
4. *Conjunctiva:* Subconjunctival haemorrhage, Chemosis, Lacerating tears of the conjunctiva
5. *Cornea:* Abrasion, Partial or complete corneal tear, Deep corneal opacity
6. *Sclera:* Scleral tear
7. *Anterior chamber:* Traumatic hyphaema, Collapse of the anterior chamber following perforation
8. *Iris, pupil and ciliary body:* Traumatic miosis, Traumatic mydriasis, Radiating tears in iris stroma, Iridodialysis, Traumatic aniridia, Traumatic cyclodialysis, Traumatic uveitis
9. *Lens:* Vossius ring, Concussion cataract, Early rosette cataract, Late rosette cataract, Total cataract, Subluxation of the lens, Dislocation of the lens
10. *Vitreous:* Traumatic vitreous degeneration, Traumatic vitreous detachment, Vitreous haemorrhage
11. *Choroid:* Rupture of the choroid, Choroidal haemorrhage, Choroidal detachment, Traumatic choroiditis
12. *Retina:* Commotio retinae (Berlin's oedema), Retinal haemorrhages, Retinal tears, Retinal detachment, Traumatic macular oedema, Traumatic macular degeneration
13. *Optic nerve*
    - Laceration of the optic nerve
    - Optic nerve sheath haemorrhage
    - Avulsion of the optic nerve

What are the effects of a perforating ocular injury?

1. *Mechanical effects* in the form of wounds of different parts of the eyeball
2. *Introduction of infection* may result in:
    - Purulent iridocyclitis
    - Endophthalmitis
    - Panophthalmitis
3. Post-traumatic iridocyclitis
4. Sympathetic ophthalmitis

What is siderosis bulbi?

Siderosis bulbi refers to the degenerative changes produced by an iron foreign body retained inside the eyeball.

The iron particles undergo electrolytic dissociation. The iron ions combine with the intracellular proteins and produce degenerative changes. Epithelial structures of the eye are most affected.

What are the features of siderosis bulbi?

1. Orangish or rusty deposits arranged radially in a ring in the anterior capsule and anterior epithelium of the lens

2. Greenish or reddish brown staining of the iris
3. Pigmentary degeneration of the retina
4. Secondary open-angle glaucoma due to degenerative changes in the trabecular meshwork

What is chalcosis?

Chalcosis refers to the specific changes produced by the alloy of copper in the eye.

Copper ions from the alloy are dissociated electrolytically and deposited under the membraneous structures of the eye. Unlike iron ions, these do not enter into chemical combination with intracellular proteins and thus produce no degenerative changes.

What are clinical manifestations of chalcosis?

1. Kayser-Fleischer ring in cornea
2. Sunflower cataract
3. Deposition of golden plaques in retina

What are the methods of localizing an intraocular foreign body (IOFB):

1. Radiographic localization
   1. Limbal ring method
   2. Specialized radiographic techniques, e.g., Sweet and Dixon's method
2. Ultrasonographic localization
3. CT Scan

What are the predisposing factors favouring development of sympathetic ophthalmitis?

1. A perforating wound
2. Wounds in the ciliary region (the so-called dangerous zone) are more prone to it.
3. Wounds with incarceration of the uveal tissue are more vulnerable
4. It is more common in children than in adults
5. It is more common in the absence of suppuration. In fact, it does not occur when actual suppuration develops in the injured eye

What are the early features of sympathetic ophthalmitis?

- Photophobia
- Lacrimation
- Transient blurring of near vision
- Mild ciliary tenderness
- A few fine keratic precipitates

Name the measures to prevent occurrence of sympathetic ophthalmitis?

1. Early excision of the injured eye with no vision
2. Meticulous repair of the wound under microscope followed by systemic and topical steroids should be undertaken in an eye with hope of saving useful vision.

Why alkali burns are more serious than the acid burns?

Alkalies penetrate deep into the tissues unlike acids (which cause instant coagulation of all the proteins which then acts as a barrier and prevents deep penetration) and thus produce more damage.

What are the effects of ultraviolet radiations on the eye?

1. May produce photophthalmia
2. May be responsible for senile cataract

What are the effects of infra-red radiations on the eye?

- Photoretinitis (solar macular burn or eclipse burn)

23

CHAPTER

Darkroom Procedures

OBLIQUE ILLUMINATION, GONIOSCOPY AND TRANSILLUMINATION

Oblique illumination
- Loupe and lens examination
- Slit-lamp examination

Gonioscopy

Transillumination

RETINOSCOPY

Objective refraction
- Retinoscopy
- Refractometry
- Keratometry

Subjective refraction
- Subjective adjustment of refraction
- Subjective refinement of refraction
- Subjective binocular balancing
- Correction for near vision

TECHNIQUES OF FUNDUS EXAMINATION

Ophthalmoscopy
- Distant direct ophthalmoscopy
- Direct ophthalmoscopy
- Indirect ophthalmoscopy

Slit-lamp biomicroscopic examination of the fundus

Darkroom procedures (DRPs) form an essential part of examination of the eyes in modern ophthalmic practice. Consequently, this section has been given a special slot in the undergraduate as well as postgraduate examinations. Most of the darkroom procedures have been described vividly with the support of self-explanatory illustrations. Common darkroom procedures are:

- Oblique illumination examination
  - Loupe and lens examination
  - Slit-lamp biomicroscopy
- Gonioscopy
- Transillumination
- Retinoscopy
- Ophthalmoscopy

OBLIQUE ILLUMINATION, GONIOSCOPY AND TRANSILLUMINATION

OBLIQUE ILLUMINATION

Oblique illumination also known as focal illumination, is a method for examination of the structures of the anterior segment of the eye. Karl Himly (1806) was the first to employ the technique of oblique illumination examination. In it, a zone of light is made to fall upon the structure to be examined so that it is brilliantly illuminated and stands out with special clarity as compared to the surroundings which remain in shadow.

There are two main methods of focal illumination:
- Loupe and lens examination; and
- Slit-lamp examination.

Loupe and lens examination

Optical principle. It is based on the principle that when an object is placed between a convex lens and its focal point, its image formed is virtual, erect, magnified and on the same side as the object.

Prerequisites. (1) Darkroom, (2) source of light, (3) condensing lens of +13 D, (4) corneal loupe of +41 D, made with two planoconvex lenses each of 20.5 D (×10 magnification) (Fig. 23.1).

Procedure. (1) Light source is placed about 2 feet away, laterally and slightly in front of the patient's eye (2) Light is focused on the structure to be examined with the help of +13 D condensing lens, held in one hand (3) The examination is carried out with the help of corneal loupe. The loupe is held between thumb and forefinger of the second hand, the fourth and fifth fingers are supported on the patient's forehead, while the middle finger is used for elevating the upper lid (Fig. 23.2). The loupe is brought close to the patient's eye till the illuminated area is focused. The observer should also move his or her eyes as close to the loupe as possible to have a better view (4). By changing the position of the condensing lens and loupe, various structures of the anterior segment can be examined one by one.

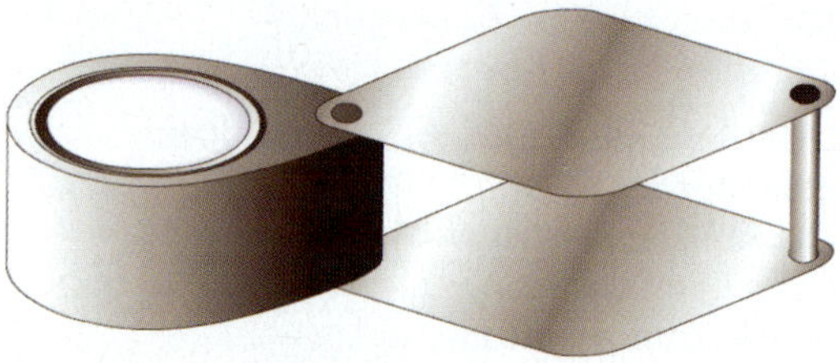

Fig. 23.1. Corneal loupe.

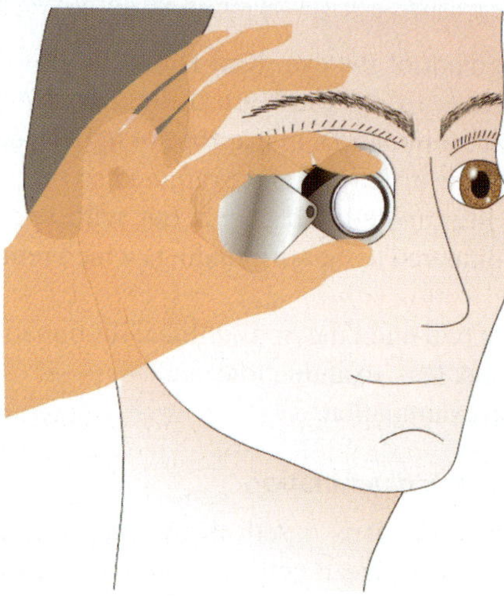

Fig. 23.2. Technique of loupe and lens examination.

Use of binocular loupe. The corneal loupe may be replaced by a binocular loupe (Fig. 23.3), which gives the added advantage of stereoscopic view and easy manoeuvring, as normally it is fixed to the examiner's head by a band. However, the magnification achieved with binocular loupe is much less than that of uniocular corneal loupe.

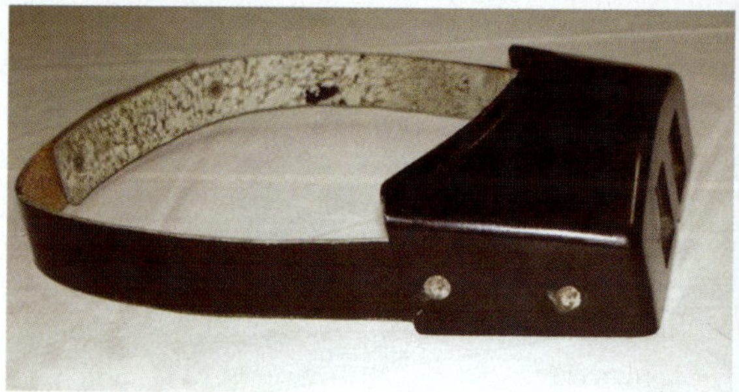

Fig. 23.3. Binocular loupe.

Slit-lamp examination

Slit-lamp biomicroscope was invented in 1911 by Gullstrand. Today, biomicroscopy forms an invaluable and indispensable part of ophthalmological examination.

Parts. Slit-lamp consists of following three parts (Fig. 23.4):

1. Observation system (Microscope)
2. Illumination system (Slit-lamp)
3. Mechanical system (Engineering support)

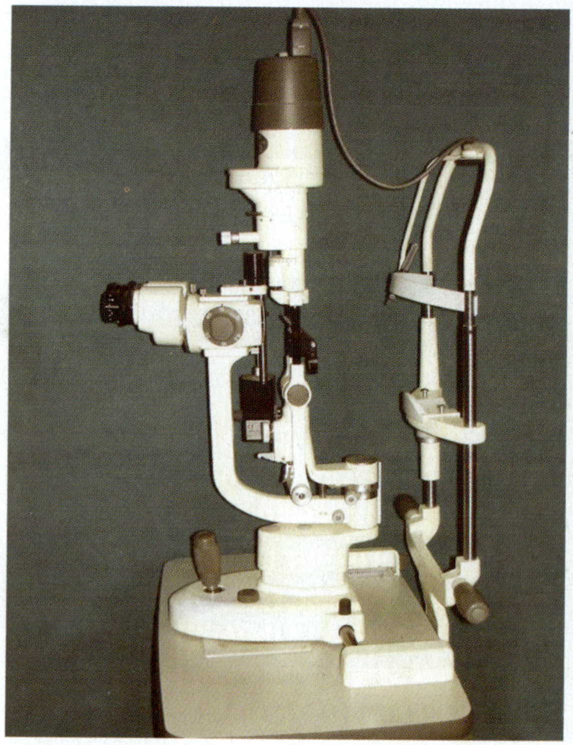

Fig. 23.4. The slit-lamp.

Optics
- It works on the same principle as a compound microscope.
- The objective lens (+22 D) is towards the patient, whose eye forms the object. The objective lens consists of two planoconvex lenses with their convexities facing towards each other.
- The eyepiece is +10 to +14 D and is towards the examiner.
- The illuminating system can be adjusted to vary the width, height and angle of incidence of the light beam.

Slit-lamp biomicroscopy routine. While performing slit-lamp biomicroscopy, following routine may be adopted (Fig. 23.5):

1. *Patient adjustment*. Patient should be positioned comfortably in front of the slit-lamp with his/her chin resting on the chin rest and forehead opposed to head rest.
2. *Instrument adjustment*. The height of the table housing the slit-lamp should be adjusted according to patient's height. The microscope and illumination system should be aligned with the patient's eye to be examined. Fixation target should be placed at the required position.
3. *Beginning slit-lamp examination*. Some points to be kept in mind are:

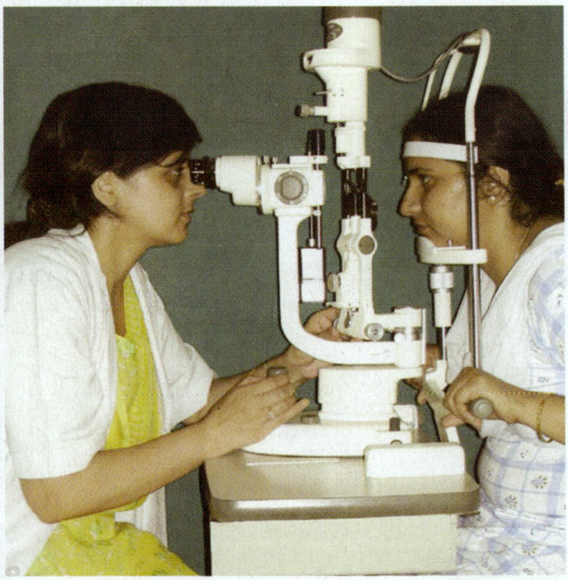

Fig. 23.5. Technique of slit-lamp examination.

   i. Examination should be carried out in semidark room so that the examiner's eyes are partially dark adapted to ensure sensitivity to low intensities of light.
   ii. Diffuse illumination should be used for a short time as necessary.
   iii. There should be a minimum exposure of retina to light.
   iv. Medications like ointments and anaesthetic eyedrops produce corneal surface disturbances which can be mistaken for pathology.
   v. Low magnification should be first used to locate the pathology and higher magnification should then be used to examine it.

   Start with diffuse illumination and examine the lid margins, bulbar conjunctiva, limbus, cornea, tear film, aqueous, iris and the lens one by one.

Methods of illumination. There are 7 basic methods of illumination using the slit-lamp as described by Berliner:

1. *Diffuse illumination*. A diffuse broad beam of light is used, and a general view of the anterior segment of eye is observed.
2. *Direct illumination*. The slit beam and microscope are focused on the same area, and examination is performed. Changes in the corneal stroma and epithelium are better noted by this technique.
3. *Indirect illumination*. The slit beam is focused on a position just beside the area to be examined. Corneal microcysts and vacuoles can be best observed by this method.
4. *Retroillumination*. Light is reflected off the iris or fundus, while the microscope is focused on the cornea. This technique is especially helpful in detecting corneal oedema, neovascularization, microcysts and infiltrates.
5. *Specular reflection*. Here the angle between the slit-lamp and microscope is increased to 60°, i.e., angle of incidence = angle of reflection. Changes in the endothelium like polymegathism, guttate, etc. can be viewed by this method.
6. *Sclerotic scatter*. It utilizes the phenomenon of total internal reflection. The slit beam is focused at the temporal limbus, and as it passes through the cornea, it outlines any subtle stromal or epithelial opacities which may lie in its path.

7. *Oscillatory illumination of Koeppe*. In this, the beam is given an oscillatory movement by which it is often possible to see minute objects or filaments, especially in the aqueous which would otherwise escape detection.

GONIOSCOPY

Owing to lack of transparency of corneoscleral junction and total internal reflection of light (emitted from angle structures) at anterior surface of cornea it is not possible to visualize the angle of anterior chamber directly. Therefore, a device (goniolens) is used to divert the beam of light and this technique of biomicroscopic examination of the angle of anterior chamber is called *gonioscopy*.

***Types of goniolens*.**: (i) *Indirect* goniolens provides a mirror image of the opposite angle, e.g., Goldmann (Fig. 23.6) and the Zeiss goniolens; (ii) *direct* goniolens provides a direct view of the angle. *Koeppe goniolens* is the most popular type.

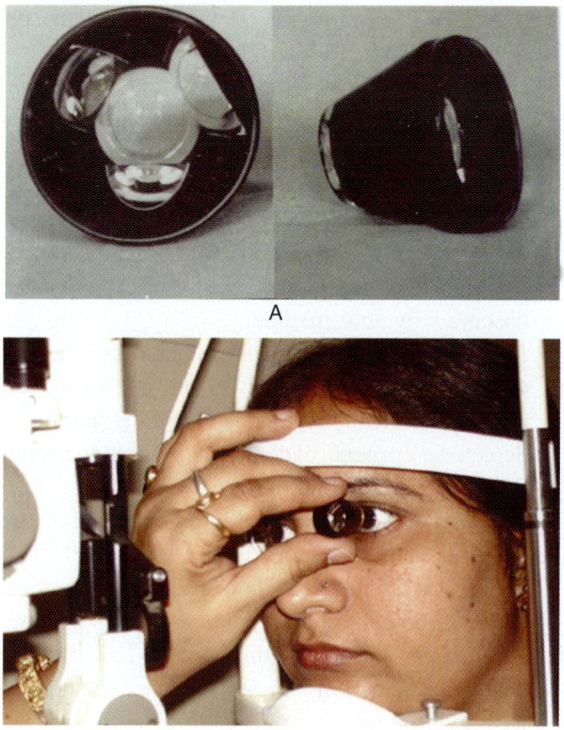

A

B

Fig. 23.6. Goldmann's goniolens (A) and technique of gonioscopy (B)

***Procedure*.** The patient is seated upright on the slit-lamp. A drop of 1 percent methylcellulose is placed in the concavity of the goniolens and with the patient looking up, one edge of the lens is positioned in the lower fornix. The upper lid is elevated and the patient is instructed to look straight ahead. The lens is rotated into position against the eye. When checking the lateral and medial angles, the slit beam should be horizontal and when checking the superior and inferior angles, the slit beam should be vertical.

The angle structures (Fig. 23.7) seen from behind forwards are:

1. Root of the iris,
2. Anteromedial surface of the ciliary body (ciliary band),
3. Scleral spur,
4. Trabecular meshwork and Schlemm's canal and
5. Schwalbe's line

Applications of gonioscopy

1. Classification of glaucoma into open angle and closed angle based on configuration of the angle.
2. Localization of foreign bodies, abnormal blood vessels or tumours in the angle.
3. Demonstration of extent of peripheral anterior synechiae (PAS) and hence planning of glaucoma surgery.
4. Direct goniolens is used during goniotomy.

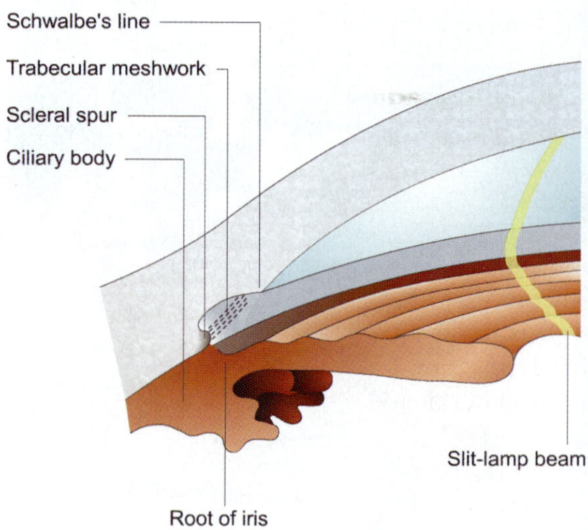

Fig. 23.7. Structures forming angle of the anterior chamber.

Gonioscopic grading of angle width

(See page 217-218).

TRANSILLUMINATION

Herein an intense beam of light is thrown through the conjunctiva and sclera or pupil and illumination is observed in the pupillary area.

1. *Trans-scleral techniques.* The beam of light is thrown through the sclera. Normally, the pupil emits a red glow but in the presence of a solid mass (e.g., intraocular tumour) in the path of light, the pupil remains black as the beam is obstructed by the mass.
2. *Transpupillary technique.* The beam of light is allowed to pass obliquely through the dilated pupil. Normally the pupil is well illuminated but in detached retina, a grayish reflex is seen.

RELATED QUESTIONS

Who invented the technique of oblique illumination examination?

Karl Himly (1806) was the first to employ the technique of oblique illumination examination.

Who invented the slit-lamp?

Gullstrand

What is the power of the condensing lens used in loupe and lens examination technique?

+13Ds

What is the power of a corneal loupe?

+41Ds

What is the magnification of a corneal loupe?

10x

What are the advantages and disadvantages of a binocular loupe over the monocular corneal loupe?

Advantages

- Binocular loupe provides stereoscopic vision.
- It is easier to use.

Disadvantages

- Magnification is less.

What is the optical principle of oblique illumination?

It is based on the principle that when an object is placed between a convex lens and its focal point, the image formed is virtual, erect, magnified and on the same side.

What are the prerequisites for loupe and lens examination technique?

- A darkroom
- Source of light
- A condensing lens of +13 Ds
- A corneal loupe of +41 Ds

Where is the source of light placed in oblique illumination examination?

The source of light is placed slightly laterally and 2 feet in front of the patient's eye.

Enumerate the structures which can be examined with a slit-lamp without any additional aid?

- Lid margin
- Conjunctiva
- Cornea
- Sclera
- Anterior chamber
- Iris and pupil
- Lens
- Anterior part of vitreous

What are the advantages and disadvantages of slit-lamp examination over loupe and lens examination?

Advantages

1. Magnification can be increased and decreased.
2. Stereoscopic vision improves depth perception.
3. Aqueous flare can be better demonstrated.
4. Applanation tonometry and gonioscopy can be performed with the slit-lamp.

Disadvantages

1. Slit-lamp is very costly.
2. It is not handy.

Enumerate a few ocular conditions where transillumination test helps in the diagnosis.

1. Intraocular tumour
2. Retinal detachment
3. Vitreous haemorrhage

RETINOSCOPY

The procedure of determining and correcting refractive errors is termed as *refraction*. It is an art that can only be mastered by practice. The refraction comprises two complementary methods, objective and subjective.

OBJECTIVE REFRACTION

The objective methods of refraction include retinoscopy, refractometry and keratometry.

RETINOSCOPY

Definition

Retinoscopy also called *skiascopy* or *shadow test* is an *objective method* of finding out the error of refraction by the method of neutralization.

Principle

Retinoscopy is based on the fact that when light is reflected from a mirror into the eye, the direction in which the light will travel across the pupil will depend upon the refractive state of the eye.

Prerequisites for retinoscopy

1. *Darkroom,* preferably 6 m long, or which can be converted into 6 m by use of a plane mirror.
2. *Trial box* containing spherical and cylindrical lenses of variable plus and minus powers, a pinhole, an occluder and prisms.
3. *Trial frame* (Fig. 23.8) preferably of adjustable type which can be used in children as well as adults.
4. *Vision box.* A Snellen's self-illuminated vision box (Fig. 23.9).
5. *Retinoscope.* It is a simple device to perform the retinoscopy. Broadly, retinoscopes available are of two types:

(a) *Mirror retinoscopes* are cheap and the most commonly employed. A source of light is required when using mirror retinoscope, which is kept above and behind the head of the patient. A mirror retinoscope may consist of a single plane mirror (Fig. 23.10A) or a combination of plane and concave mirrors (*Pristley-Smith mirror*–Fig. 23.10B).

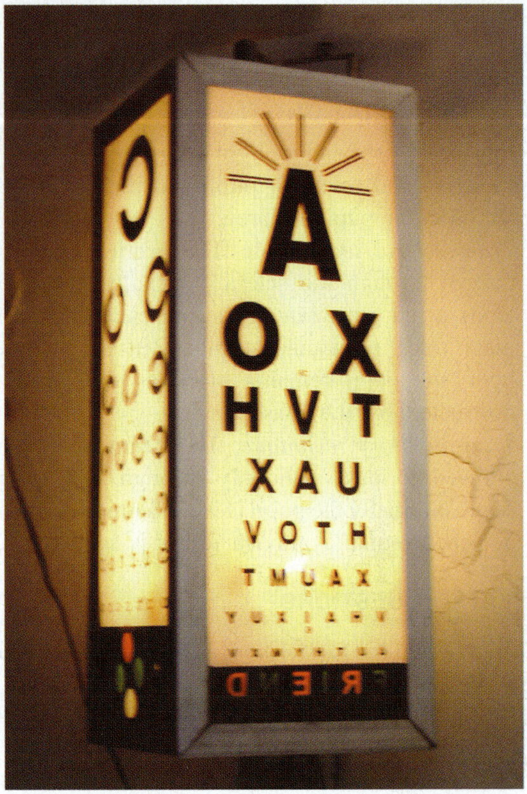

Fig. 23.9. Snellen's vision box.

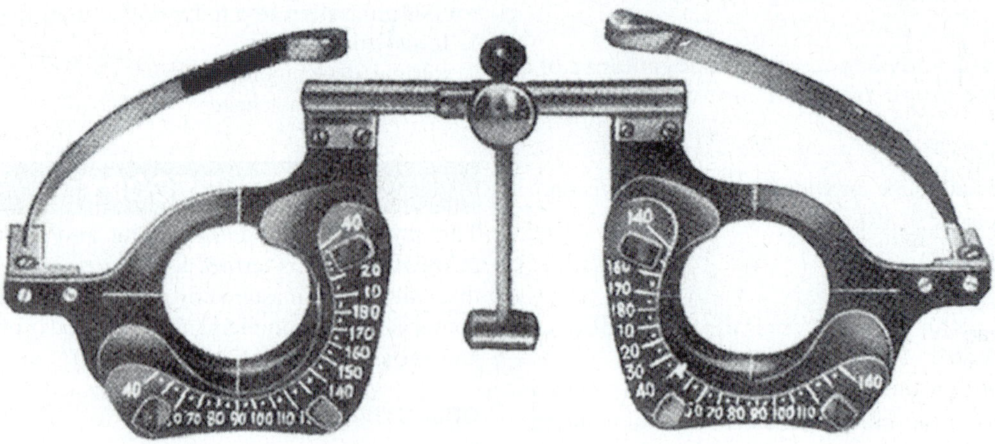

Fig. 23.8. Trial frame.

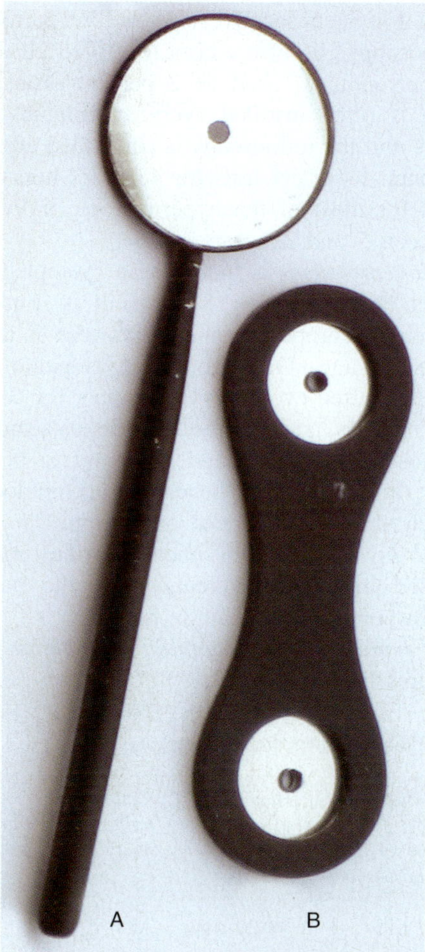

Fig. 23.10. Mirror retinoscopes: A, plane mirror; B, Pristley-Smith, mirror.

(b) *Self-illuminated retinoscopes* are costly but handy. Two types of self-illuminated retinoscopes available are: a spot retinoscope and a streak retinoscope (Fig. 23.11). The streak retinoscope is more popular. In it the usual circular beam of light is modified to produce a linear streak of light by using a planocylindrical retinoscopy mirror. The streak retinoscopy is more sensitive than spot retinoscopy in detecting astigmatism.

Plane versus concave mirror retinoscope

In practice, plane mirror is used for retinoscopy. In patients with hazy media and high degree of ametropia concave mirror is more useful.

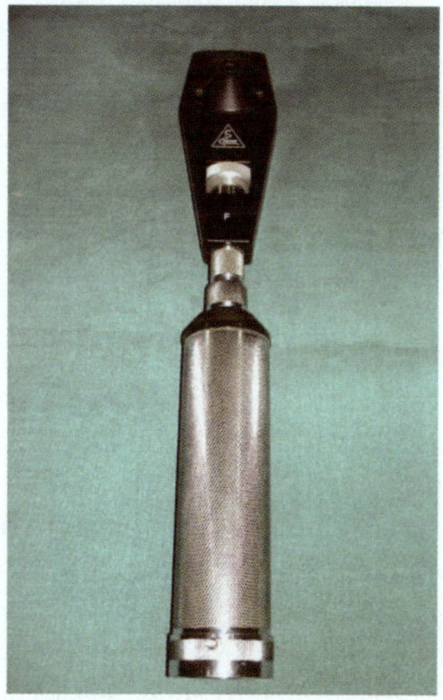

Fig. 23.11. Streak retinoscope.

Procedure

The patient is made to sit at a distance of 1 m from the examiner (Fig. 23.12). With the help of a retinoscope, light is thrown onto the patient's eye, who is instructed to look at a far point (to relax the accommodation). However, when a cycloplegic has been used, the patient can look directly into the light and have the refraction assessed along the actual visual axis. Through a hole in the retinoscope's mirror, the examiner observes a red reflex in the pupillary area of the patient. Then the retinoscope is moved in horizontal and vertical meridia keeping a watch on the red reflex (which also moves when the retinoscope is moved).

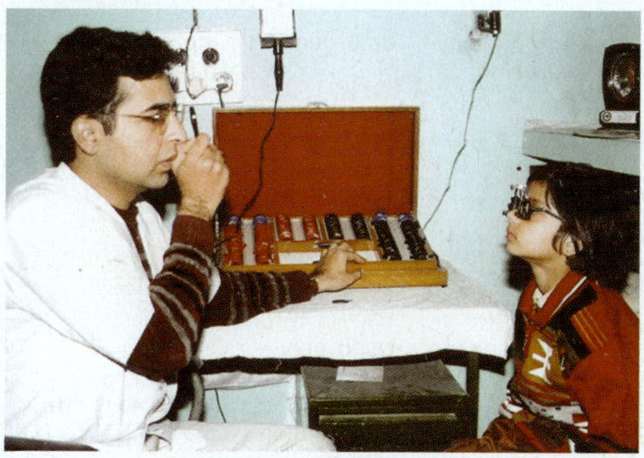

Fig. 23.12. Procedure of retinoscopy.

In low degrees of refractive errors the shadow (red reflex) seen in the pupillary area is faint and moves rapidly with the movement of the mirror; while in high degrees of ametropia it is very dark and moves slowly. In the presence of astigmatism, when the axis does not correspond with the movement of the mirror, the shadow appears to swirl around.

Use of cycloplegics in retinoscopy

Cycloplegics are the drugs which cause paralysis of accommodation and dilate the pupil (cycloplegia). These are used for retinoscopy, when the examiner suspects that accommodation is abnormally active and will hinder the exact retinoscopy. Such a situation is encountered in young children and hypermetropes. When retinoscopy is performed after instilling cycloplegic drugs it is termed as *wet retinoscopy* in converse to *dry retinoscopy* (without cycloplegics). The commonly employed cyclopegics are as follows:

1. *Atropine is* indicated in children below the age of 5 years. It is used as 1 percent ointment thrice daily for 3 consecutive days before performing retinoscopy. Its effect lasts for 10 to 20 days.
2. *Homatropine* is used as 2 percent drops. One drop is often instilled every 10 minutes for 6 times and the retinoscopy is performed after 1 to 2 hours. Its effect lasts for 48 to 72 hours. It is used for most of the hypermetropic individuals between 5 and 25 years of age.
3. *Cyclopentolate* is a short acting cycloplegic. Its effect lasts for 6 to 18 hours. It is used as 1 percent eyedrops in patients between 8 and 20 years of age. One drop of cyclopentolate is instilled after every 10-15 minutes for 3 times (Havener's recommended dose) and the retinoscopy is performed about 60 to 90 min. later, (after estimating the residual accommodation which should not exceed one dioptre).
4. Only *mydriatic* (10% phenylephrine) may be needed in elderly patients when the pupil is narrow or media is slightly hazy.

Salient features of the common cycloplegic drugs are summarized in Table 23.1.

Table 23.1. Salient features of common cycloplegic and mydriatic drugs

Sl. no.	*Name of the drug*	*Age of the patient when indicated*	*Dosage of instillation*	*Peak effect*	*Time of performing retinoscopy*	*Duration of action*	*Period of postcyclo-plegic test*	*Tonus allowance*
1.	Atropine sulphate (1% ointment)	< 5 year	TDS × 3 day	2-3 days	4th day	10-20 days	After 3 weeks of retinoscopy	1D
2.	Homatropine hydrobromide (2% drops)	5-8 years	One drop every 10 min. for 6 times	60-90 min.	After 90 min. of instillation of first drop	48-72 hours	After 3 days of retinoscopy	0.5D
3.	Cyclopentolate hydrochloride (1% drops)	8-20 years	One drop every 15 min. for 3 times	80-90 min.	After 90 min. of instillation of first drop	6-18 hours	After 3 days of retinoscopy	0.75D
4.	Tropicamide (0.5%, 1% drops)	Not used as cycloplegic for retino-scopy; used only as mydriatic	One drop every 15 min. for 3 to 4 times	20-40 min.	—	4-6 hours	—	—
5.	Phenylephrine (5%, 10% drops)	Used only as mydriatic alone or in combination with tropica-mide	One drop every 15 min. for 3 to 4 times	30-40 min.	—	4-6 hours	—	—

Note: The mydriatics should be used with care in adults with shallow anterior chamber, owing to the danger of an attack of narrow-angle glaucoma. In older people, mydriasis should be counteracted by the use of miotic drug (2% pilocarpine).

Observations and inferences

Depending upon the movement of the red reflex (Fig. 23.13) when a plane mirror retinoscope is used at a distance of 1 metre) the results are interpreted as:

1. *No movement* of red reflex indicates myopia of 1D.
2. *With movement of red reflex* along the movement of the retinoscope, indicates either emmetropia or hypermetropia or myopia of less than 1 D.
3. *Against movement* of red reflex to the movement of the retinoscope implies myopia of more than 1 D.

Above assertions can be easily remembered from the Fig. 23.14.

Neutralization

When the red reflex moves with or against the movement of retinoscope we do not exactly know the amount of refractive error. However, when the red glow in the pupil does not move then we know for certain that patient has myopia of 1D. Therefore, to estimate the degree of refractive error, the movement of red reflex is neutralized by addition of increasingly convex (+) spherical lenses (when the red reflex was moving with the movement of plane mirror) or concave (–) spherical lenses (when the red reflex was moving against the movement of plane mirror). When a simple spherical error alone is present, the movements of red reflex will be neutralized in both vertical as well as the horizontal meridia. However, in the presence of an astigmatic refractive error, one meridian is neutralized by adding appropriate cylindrical lens with its axis at right angle to the meridian to be neutralized. It is important to note that sometimes, especially, when pupil is dilated, two light reflexes—one central and other peripheral—may be seen. Under such circumstances one should neutralize the central glow because the central parts of cornea and lens are more important in forming the image on the retina.

The end point of retinoscopy

- *With simple plane mirror retinoscope* the end point of retinoscopy is neutralization of red reflex in all the meridia, i.e., either no movement or just reversal of the movement.
- *With a streak retinoscope* at the end point streak disappears and the pupil appears completely illuminated or completly dark (Fig. 23.13).

Problems in retinoscopy

Certain difficulties encountered during the procedure of retinoscopy are summarized below:

1. *Red reflex may not be visible or may be poor.* This may happen with small pupil, hazy media and high degree of refractive error. In most cases, this difficulty is overcome by causing mydriasis and/or use of converging light with concave mirror retinoscope.

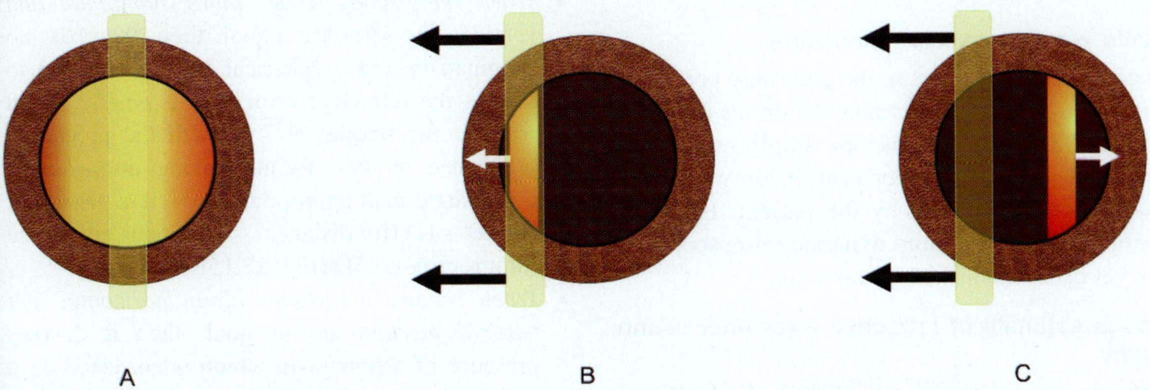

Fig. 23.13. Red reflex during streak retinoscopy: A, Neutralization point; B, With movement; C, Against movement.

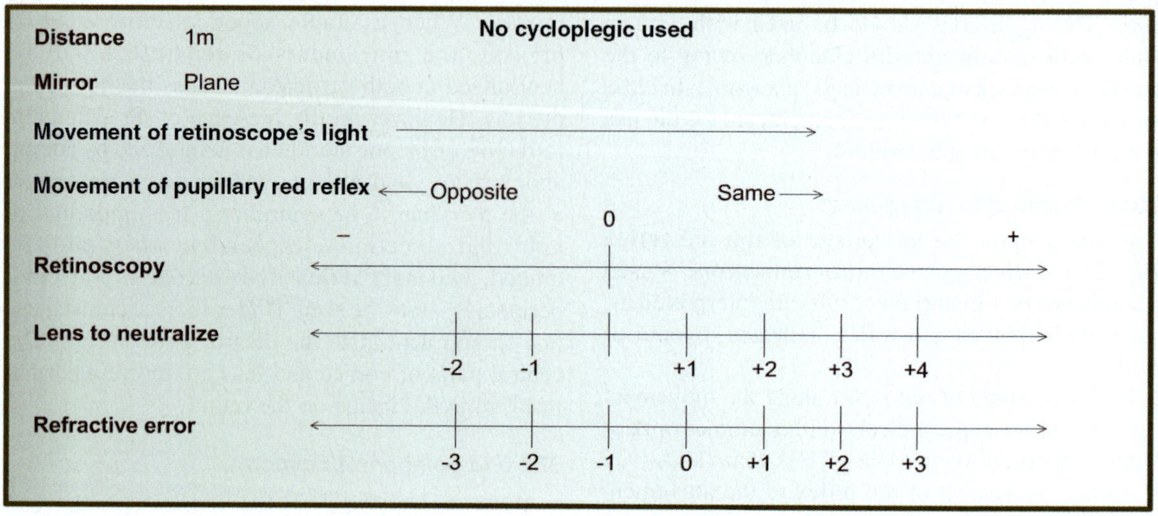

Fig. 23.14. Diagrammatic depiction of the relation of movement of pupillary red reflex with the error of refraction.

2. ***Changing retinoscopy findings*** are observed due to abnormally active accommodation and is corrected by use of cycloplegia.

3. ***Scissors shadows*** may sometimes be seen in patients with regular astigmatism with dilated pupils. Mostly this difficulty is diminished with the undilated pupil.

4. ***Conflicting shadows*** moving in various directions in different parts of the pupillary area are seen in patients with irregular astigmatism.

5. ***Triangular shadow*** may be observed in patients with conical cornea (keratoconus), with its apex at the apex of cone. On moving the mirror the triangular reflex appears to swirl around its apex (*yawning reflex*).

Static versus dynamic retinoscopy

Static retinoscopy refers to the procedure performed without active use of accommodation (as described above). Dynamic retinoscopy implies when the procedure is performed for near vision with active use of accommodation by the patient. However, usefulness of performing dynamic retinoscopy has not yet been established in refraction.

Rough estimate of refractive error after retinoscopy

Objectively a rough estimate of error of refraction is made by taking into account the retinoscopic findings, deductions for distance (e.g., 1D for 1 m and 1.5 D when retinoscopy is performed at 2/3rd m distance) and deduction for the cycloplegic when used (e.g., 1 D for atropine, 0.5 D for homatropine and 0.75 D for cyclopentolate).

Amount of refractive error is equal to the retinoscopic findings minus deduction for the distance and deduction for tonus allowance for the cycloplegic drug used.

It is customary to do retinoscopy both vertically and horizontally and note the values separately (Fig. 23.15). In Fig. 23.15 A, X denotes retinoscopy value along horizontal meridian and Y denotes the value along the vertical meridian.

- *When retinoscopy values along horizontal and vertical meridia* are equal then there is no astigmatism and a spherical lens is required to correct the refractive error. *For example:* When retinoscopic finding is 7 D with the procedure preformed at 1 m distance using atroprine as cycloplegic than appropriate refractive error will be: 7D – 1D (for distance) – 1D (tonus allowance for atroprine) = 5D (Fig. 23.15B).
- *When retinoscopy values along horizontal and vertical meridia* are unequal, then it denotes presence of astigmatism which is corrected by a cylindrical lens alone or in combination with a spherical lens (Figs. 23.15C and D).

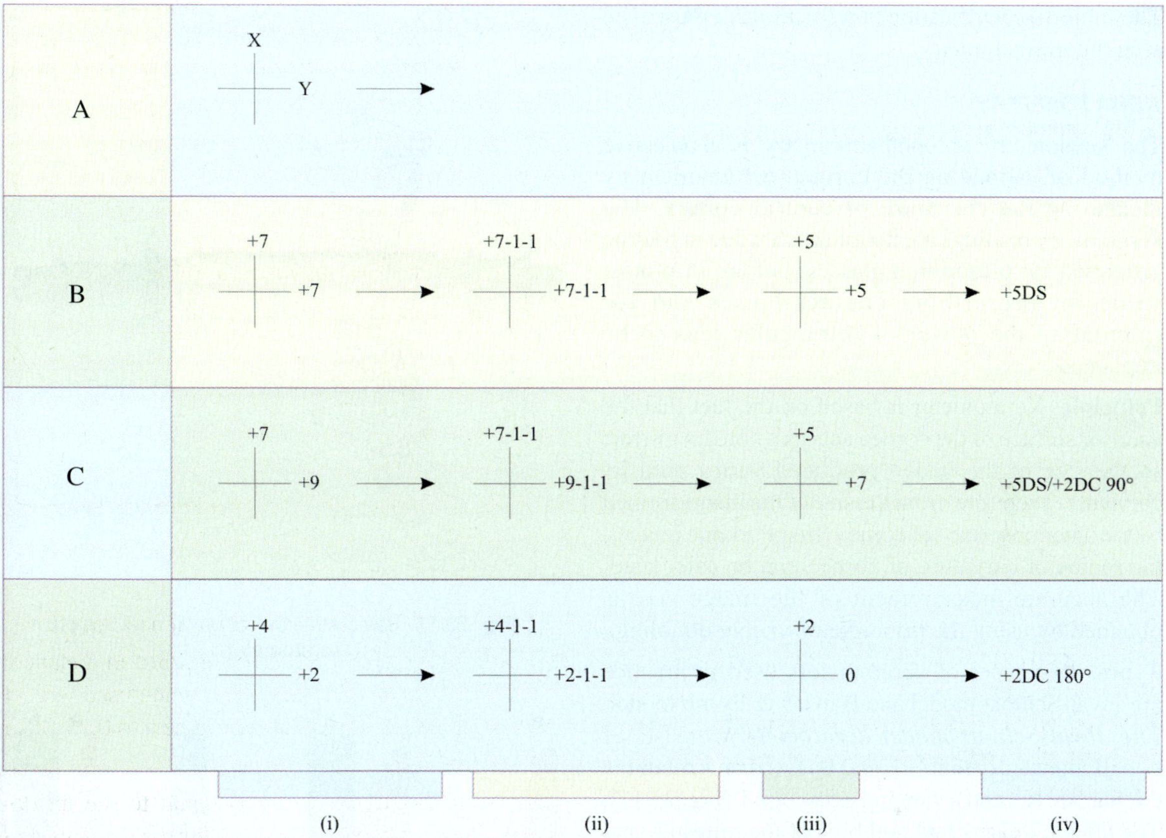

Fig. 23.15. A: Customary way of writing retinoscopic findings, B, C and D: Calculation for rough estimate of refractive error: (i) Retinoscopic findings, when performed at 1 m distance under atropine cycloplegia; (ii) Deduction of –1D for distance and –1D for the atropine from the retinoscopic findings. (iii) Rough estimate of refractive error along horizontal and vertical meridian; and (iv) Prescription required.

REFRACTOMETRY

The refractometry (optometry) is an objective method of finding out the error of refraction by use of an equipment called *refractometer* (optometer). Refractometry utilizes the principles of indirect ophthalmoscopy. The conventional refractometers include dioptron, ophthalmometron, Henker's parallax refractometer and coincidence-refractometer. Presently, the *computerized autorefractometers* (Fig. 23.16) are being used increasingly. The computerized, autorefractometer quickly gives information about the refractive error of the patient in terms of sphere, cylinder with axis and interpupillary distance. This method is a good alternative to retinoscopy in busy practice. It is also advantageous for mass screening, research programmes and epidemiological studies.

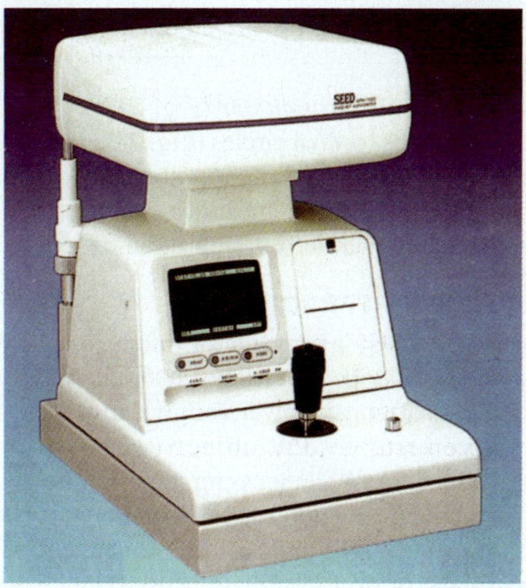

Fig. 23.16. Computerized autorefractometer.

The subjective verification of refraction is a must even after autorefractometry.

KERATOMETRY

The 'keratometry' or 'ophthalmometry' is an objective method of estimating the corneal astigmatism by measuring the curvature of central cornea. The keratometry readings are not of much value in routine refraction for prescribing glasses; but are of utmost value for prescribing contact lenses and for calculating the power of intraocular lens to be implanted.

Principle. Keratometer is based on the fact that the anterior surface of the cornea acts as a convex mirror; so the size of the image produced varies with its curvature. Therefore, from the size of the image formed by the anterior surface of cornea (first Purkinje image), the radius of curvature of cornea can be calculated. The accurate measurement of the image size is obtained by using the principle of visible doubling.

Types. Two types of keratometers used in practice are Javal-Schiotz model and Bausch & Lomb model. ***The Javal-Schiotz model keratometer*** consists of two illuminated 'mires' (A and B) fixed on a rotatable circular arc (C) and a viewing telescope T (Fig. 23.17). The double images (aa^1 and bb^1) of the mires (A and B) are formed on the cornea. Keratometry readings are obtained by coinciding the images a^1 and b as shown in Fig. 23.18. The readings are noted first in the horizontal meridian and then the arc is rotated by 90° and the readings are noted in the vertical meridian.

Bausch & Lomb keratometer (Fig. 23.19). In it, the 'mires' are in the form of circles (Fig. 23.20). With this keratometer the radius of curvature of cornea in horizontal and vertical meridia can be measured simultaneously without rotating the mires.

SUBJECTIVE REFRACTION

Subjective refraction is meant for finding out the most suitable lenses to be prescribed. It should always be carried out after getting a rough estimate of the refractive error by the objective refraction as described above. When a cycloplegic has been used the subjective refraction (postmydriatic test) should be carried out preferably after 3 to 4 days (when homatropine or cyclopentolate is used) and 3 weeks (when atropine is used).

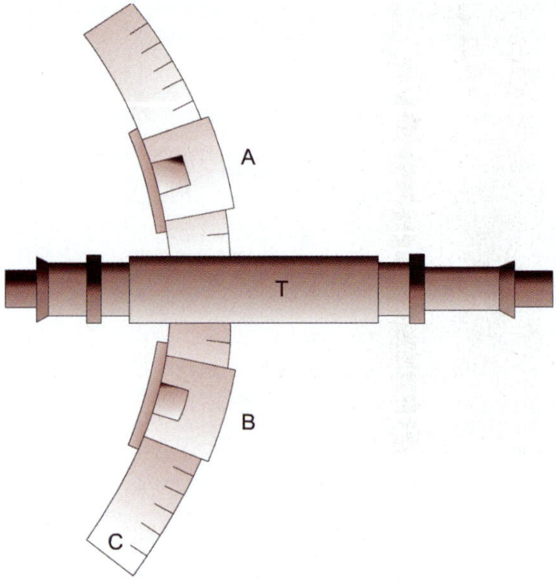

Fig. 23.17. Basic structure of Javal and Schiotz keratometer.

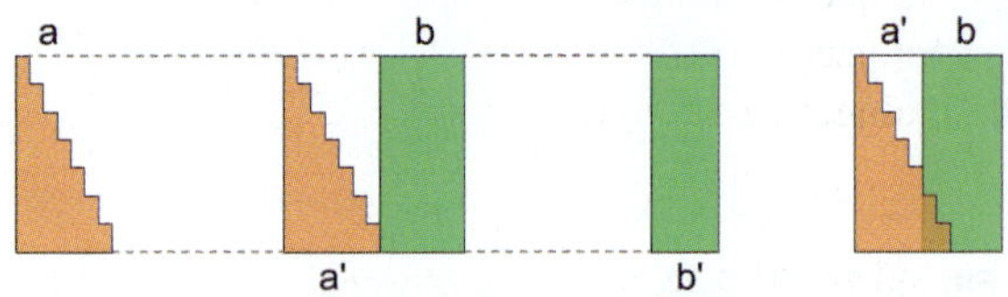

Fig. 23.18. Mires during keratometry with Javal-Schiotz Keratometer.

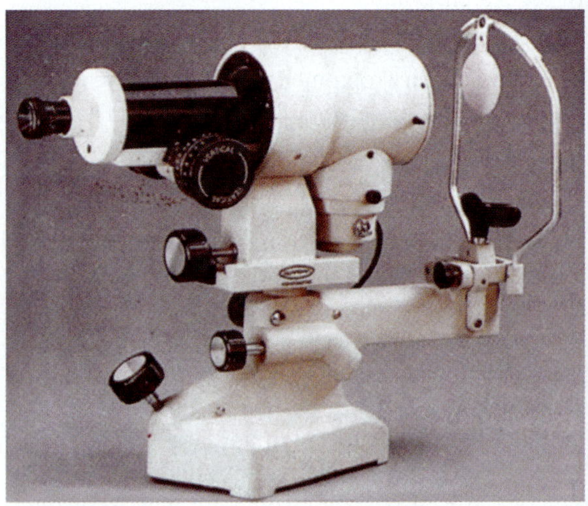

Fig. 23.19. Bausch and Lomb Keratometer.

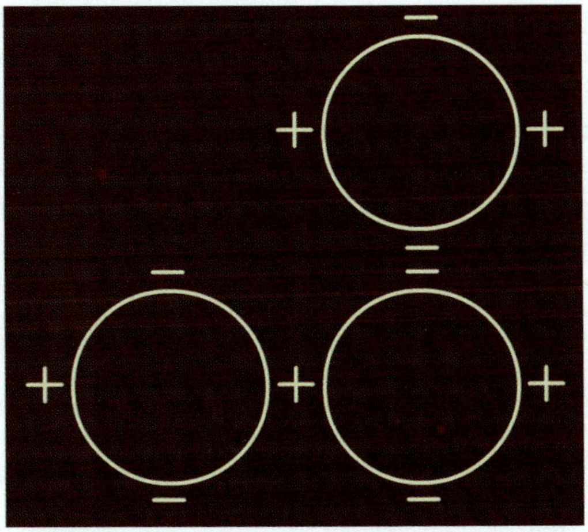

Fig. 23.20. Mires during keratometry with Bausch & Lomb keratometer.

The technique of subjective refraction requires the patient's cooperation in arriving at the proper estimation of the refractive error. The proper subjective refraction includes three steps:

I. Subjective adjustment of refraction.
II. Subjective refinement of refraction, and
III. Subjective binocular balancing.

I. The subjective adjustment of refraction

The subjective adjustment of refraction can be performed by: the *'trial-and-error' method*. For this, the patient is seated at a distance of 6 metres from the Snellen's vision chart. A trial frame is put on the face of the patient and the visual acuity is noted for both the eyes, separately. Then an occluder is put in front of one eye and the appropriate lens combination (as indicated by retinoscopy or automated refractometry) is placed in front of the other eye. By increasing or decreasing the power of lens the most suitable spherical lens is chosen (the strongest convex lens and the weakest concave lens providing best vision should be chosen in patients with hypermetropia and myopia, respectively). Then the axis of the cylinder and finally its strength should by finalized using the same 'trial-and-error' method. The similar procedure is repeated for the second eye.

II. Subjective refinement of refraction

The most suitable combination of lenses chosen after the subjective adjustment of refraction is refined before the final prescription is made. It is always better to first refine the cylinder and then sphere.

1. Refining the cylinder. Cylinder can be refined by either use of Jackson's crosscylinder (more commonly) or by astigmatic fan test.

i. Jackson's crosscylinder test. It is used to verify the strength and axis of the cylinder prescribed. The crosscylinder is a combination of two cylinders of equal strength but with opposite sign placed with their axes at right angles to each other and mounted in a handle (Fig. 23.21). The commonly used crosscylinders are of ±0.25 D and ±0.5 D.

- *Verification of strength of the cylinder.* To check the power of the cylinder, the crosscylinder of ± 0.25 D is placed with its axis parallel to the axis of the cylinder in the trial frame first with the same sign and then with opposite sign. In the first position, the cylindrical correction is enhanced by 0.25 D and in the second it is diminished by the same amount. When the visual

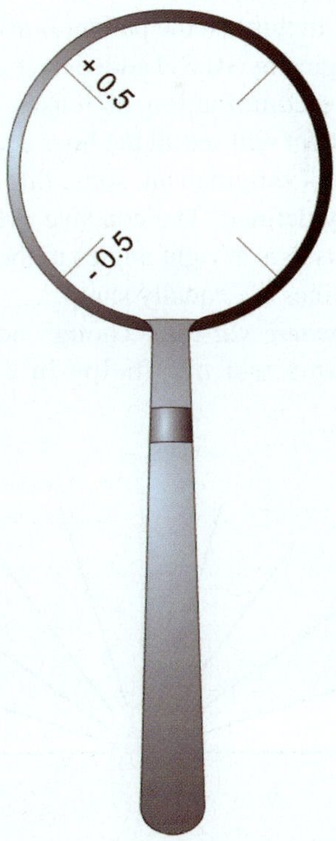

Fig. 23.21. Jackson's crosscylinder.

acuity does not improve, in either of the positions the power of cylinder in trial frame is correct. However, if the visual acuity improves in any of the positions a corresponding correction should be made and reverified till final correction is attained.

- *Verification of axis of the cylinder.* Crosscylinder (±0.5 D) is placed before the eye with its axis at 45° to the axis of cylinder in trial frame (first with –0.5 D cylinder and then +0.5 D cylinder or vice-versa) and the patient is asked to tell about any change in the visual acuity. If the patient notices no difference between the two positions, the axis of the correcting cylinder in the trial frame is correct. However, if the visual improvement is attained in one of the positions, a 'plus' correcting cylinder should be rotated in the direction of the plus cylindrical components of the crosscylinder (and vice-versa). The test is then repeated several times until the neutral point is reached.

ii. The *astigmatic fan test*. It is used to confirm the cylindrical correction. The astigmatic fan consists of a dial of lines radiating at 10° interval to one another (Fig. 23.22). In this test the patient is asked to see the fan after fogging by +0.5 D added over and above the best suitable combination of lenses chosen. The stigmatic patient will see all the lines equally clear. In the presence of astigmatism, some lines will be seen more sharply defined. The concave cylinder is then added with its axis at right angles to the clearest line until all the lines are equally sharp.

iii. *A stenopaeic slit-test*. Though not practically used now, this test also helps in checking the correction of astigmatism. The 1 mm wide stenopaeic slit (Fig. 23.23) when placed in front of the eye allows clearest vision when it is rotated into the axis of astigmatism and the refraction will then be indicated by the strongest convex lens which allows full vision in this axis and again in the axis perpendicular to it.

2. Refining the sphere. The spherical correction is refined after refining the cylinder power and axis. Refining of the sphere is done by using following tests:

i. *The fogging technique*. After the cylinder power and axis have been refined, the eye to be tested is fogged by insertion of about +2D spherical lens in myopic patients and about +4D in hypermetropic patients over the previously verified sphere. The patient is instructed to see the distant test types through this, and gradually the additional convex lens is reduced (by about 1/2 D at a time) until full vision is restored. This method is more useful in hypermetropia.

ii. *Duochrome test*. It is based on the principle of chromatic aberration. In this, the patient is asked to read the *red* and *green* letters. In an emmetropic eye the green rays are focused slightly anterior and red rays slightly posterior to the retina. Therefore, to an emmetropic patient letters of both colours look equally sharp. When the patient tells that he or she sees *red* letters more clearly than the *green*, it indicates that he or she is slightly myopic. His or her spherical lenses should be adjusted such that he or she sees letters of both colours with equal clarity.

iii. *Pin-hole test*. It helps in confirming whether the optical correction in the trial frame is correct or not.

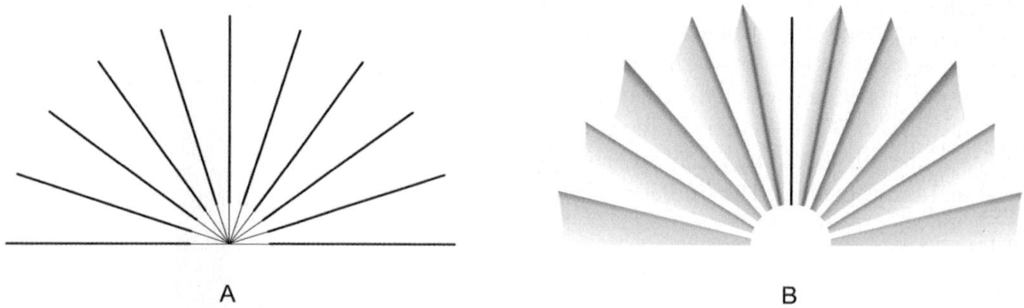

Fig. 23.22. Astigmatic fan: A, As seen by an emmetropic person; B, As seen by a patient with astigmatism at horizontal axis.

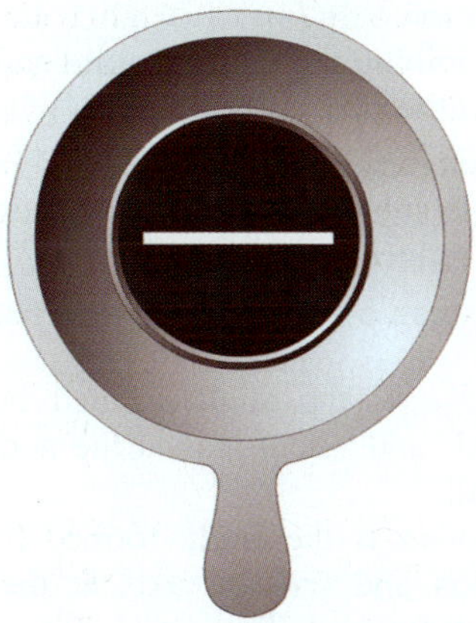

Fig. 23.23. Stenopaeic slit.

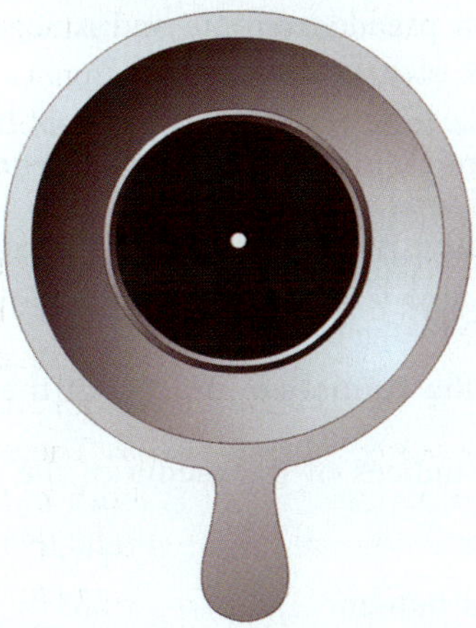

Fig. 23.24. Pin-hole.

An improvement in visual acuity while looking through a pin hole (Fig. 23.24) indicates that optical correction in the trial frame is incorrect.

III. Subjective binocular balancing

The final step in the subjective refraction is binocular balancing—a process sometimes known as 'equalizing the accommodative effort' or 'equalization of vision'. This allows both eyes to have the retinal image simultaneously in focus. The details of the techniques of binocular balancing are beyond the scope of this book.

Correction for near vision

Correction for near vision is indicated usually after the age of 40 years. When the distance vision has been satisfactorily corrected, the visual acuity at working distance of the patient should be estimated using any of the near vision charts (Jaeger's chart or Snellen's reading test types or number points types standardized by the faculty of ophthalmologists, N5 to N48). In case near vision is defective, a suitable convex lens addition (tested separately for each eye) should be made over the distant correction. The near correction added should be such that about one-third of the amplitude of accommodation should remain as reserve. *In general, it is better to undercorrect than to overcorrect the presbyopia (also see page 42).*

RELATED QUESTIONS

LIGHT AND GEOMETRICAL OPTICS

What is the wavelength of visible spectrum of the light?

Between 390 and 700 nm.

Which light rays are absorbed by the cornea and crystalline lens of the eye?

Cornea absorbs rays having wavelength shorter than 295 nm and the crystalline lens of the eye absorbs rays having wavelength shorter than 350 nm.

White light consists of how many colours?

Seven, viz. violet, indigo, blue, green, yellow, orange and red (VIBGYOR).

What do you mean by reflection of light?

Reflection of light is a phenomenon of change in the path of light rays without any change in the medium.

What are the features of an image formed by a plane mirror?

It is: (i) virtual, (ii) erect and laterally inverted, (iii) of the same size as object, and (iv) at the same distance behind the mirror as the object is in front.

What do you mean by refraction of light?

Refraction of light is a phenomenon of change in the path of light when it goes from one medium to another.

Describe the features of the images formed by a concave mirror for different positions of the object.

(See Table 3.1)

What is total internal reflection?

When a ray of light travelling from an optically denser medium to an optically rarer medium is incident at an angle greater than the critical angle of the pair of media in contact, the ray is totally reflected back into the denser medium. This phenomenon is called total internal reflection.

What is the critical angle?

Critical angle refers to the angle of incidence in the denser medium corresponding to which angle of refraction in the rarer medium is 90°.

What do you mean by Sturm conoid focal interval of Sturm and circle of least diffusion?

Sturm conoid refers to the configuration of the light rays refracted through an astigmatic (toric) surface. The parallel rays of light when refracted through a toric surface are not focused at one point but form two focal lines. Distance between the two lines is called *focal interval of Sturm. Circle of least diffusion* is formed between these two lines.

Why a patient with mixed astigmatism has comparatively better vision?

Because in such patients the circle of least diffusion is formed on the retina.

OPTICS OF THE EYE

What is a 'reduced eye'?

The focusing system of the eye is composed of cornea, aqueous humour, crystalline lens and vitreous humour, the optics of which, otherwise is very complex. However, listing has chosen a simple data to understand the optics of eye. This is called Listing's reduced eye. Its cardinal points are:

- Single nodal point situated (in the posterior part of crystalline lens) is 7.2 mm behind the anterior surface of cornea.
- Anterior focal point is 15.7 mm in front of the anterior surface of cornea.
- Posterior focal point (on the retina) is 24.4 mm behind the anterior surface of cornea.
- Total dioptric power is about +60D.

What is the nodal point of the eyeball?

It is the optical centre of the entire focusing system of the eye consisting of cornea, aqueous and lens when considered as one lens.

What is optical axis of the eyeball?

It is a line passing through the centre of cornea and centre of the lens which meets the retina on the nasal side of fovea.

What is visual axis?

It is a line joining the fixation object, nodal point and the fovea.

What is fixation axis?

It is the line joining the fixation point and the centre of rotation of the eye.

What is visual angle?

It is the angle subtended by an object on the nodal point of the reduced eye.

What are angles alpha, gamma and kappa of the eye- ball?

1. *Angle alpha* is the angle formed between the optical axis and visual axis at the nodal point of the eyeball.
2. *Angle gamma* is the angle formed between the optical axis and fixation axis at the centre of rotation of the eyeball.
3. *Angle kappa* is formed between the visual axis and control pupillary line. A positive angle kappa results in pseudoexotropia and a negative angle kappa is seen in esotropia.

What is the total refractive power of the eyeball and how much is contributed by cornea and the crystalline lens.

Total refractive power of the eyeball is about +60D; out of this +44 D is contributed by the cornea and about +16D by the crystalline lens.

What are the refractive indices of the media of the eye?

Refractive indices of the media of the eye are as follows:

Cornea	:	1.37
Aqueous humour	:	1.33
Crystalline lens	:	1.42
Vitreous humour	:	1.33

REFRACTIVE ERRORS

What is emmetropia?

Emmetropia (optically normal eye) is a state of refraction when the parallel rays of light coming from infinity are focused at the sensitive layer of retina with accommodation at rest.

Define ametropia.

Ametropia (a condition of refractive error) is defined as a state of refraction when the parallel rays of light coming from infinity are focused either in front or behind the retina. It includes myopia, hypermetropia and astigmatism.

Define hypermetropia (long-sightedness).

Hypermetropia is the refractive state of the eye wherein parallel rays of light coming from infinity are focused posterior to the retina, with accommodation at rest.

What is the refractive status of the eye at birth?

At birth the eyeball is relatively short and thus most infants are born with +2 to +3 D hypermetropia. This is gradually reduced and by the age of 5 to 7 years usually the eye becomes emmetropic.

What are aetiological types of ametropic refractive errors?

1. *Axial ametropia:* There is abnormal axial length of the eyeball, too long in myopia and too short in hypermetropia.
2. *Curvatural ametropia:* There is abnormal curvature of the cornea or lens or both; too strong in myopia and too weak in hypermetropia.
3. *Index ametropia:* There is abnormal refractive index of the media; too high in myopia and too low in hypermetropia.
4. *Positional ametropia:* Forward displacement of the lens causes myopia and backward displacement results in hypermetropia.

What are the components of the hypermetropia?

Total hypermetropia = latent + manifest (facultative + absolute)

1. *Total hypermetropia:* It is the total amount of refractive error estimated after complete cycloplegia with atropine.
2. *Latent hypermetropia* is that which is corrected by inherent tone of the ciliary muscle.
3. *Manifest hypermetropia:* It is the remaining portion of total hypermetropia, which is not corrected by the ciliary tone.

Name the most common factor responsible for myopia and hypermetropia.

Too long axial length and too short axial length are responsible for myopia and hypermetropia, respectively.

Name the complications which may occur in non-treated cases of hypermetropia.

1. Recurrent styes and blepharitis,
2. Accommodative convergent squint,
3. Amblyopia.

Define aphakia.

Aphakia literally means absence of the crystalline lens from the eye. However, from the optical point of view, it may be considered as a condition in which the lens is absent from the pupillary area and does not take part in refraction.

Enumerate the refractive changes which occur in an aphakic eye.

1. Eye becomes highly hypermetropic.
2. Total power of the eye is reduced to +44Ds from +60 Ds
3. Anterior focal distance becomes 23 mm (from 15 mm in normal phakic eye)
4. Posterior focal distance becomes 31 mm (from 24 mm in normal phakic eye).

Name the various modalities for correction of aphakia and enumerate advantages and disadvantages of each.

1. *Spectacles*

Advantages: It is cheap, easy and safe method of correcting aphakia.

Disadvantages: (i) Image is magnified by 30 percent, so not useful in unilateral aphakia (produce diplopia), (ii) problems of spherical and chromatic aberrations may be troublesome, (iii) field of vision is limited, (iv) prismatic effect of thick glasses causes, 'roving ring scotoma' (v) cosmetic blemish, especially in young aphakics.

2. *Contact lenses*

Advantages: (i) Less magnification (5%) of the image, (ii) Elimination of aberrations and prismatic effect of thick glasses, (iii) Wider and better field of vision, (iv) Cosmetically better accepted by young persons.

Disadvantages: (i) More cost, (ii) Cumbersome to wear, especially in old age and in childhood, (iii) Corneal complications may occur.

3. *Intraocular lens implantation*

It is the best available method of treatment.

Advantage: It offers all the advantages which the contact lenses offer over the spectacles. In addition, the disadvantages of contact lenses are also taken care of.

Disadvantages: It requires more skilled surgeons and costly equipments.

4. *Refractive corneal surgery*

It is still under trial and includes keratophakia and epikeratophakia.

What are fundus findings in a patient with high hypermetropia?

Fundus examination in a patient with high hypermetropia may show:

- Pseudopapillitis
- Shot silk appearance of the retina.

Enumerate the signs of aphakia.

- Deep anterior chamber
- Iridodonesis
- Jet black pupil
- Purkinje's image test shows only two images (normally four)
- Fundus examination shows small optic disc
- Retinoscopy reveals high hypermetropia

What is pseudophakia?

Pseudophakia refers to presence of an intraocular lens in the pupillary area.

What is the refractive position of the pseudophakic eye?

A pseudophakic eye may be emmetropic, myopic or hypermetropic depending upon the power of the IOL implanted.

What is the average standard power of the posterior chamber IOL?

Exact power of an IOL to be implanted varies from individual to individual and is calculated by biometry using keratometer and A-scan ultrasound.

What is the average weight of an IOL?

Average weight of an IOL in air is 15 mg and in aqueous humour is about 5 mg.

What is the power of the IOL in air vis-a-vis in the aqueous humour?

Power of an IOL in air is much more (about +60D) than that in the aqueous humour (about + 20D).

What is the difference in the power of an anterior chamber IOL versus posterior chamber IOL?

Equivalent power of an anterior chamber IOL is less (say about +18D) than that of posterior chamber IOL (+20D).

What is myopia (short-sightedness)?

Myopia is a refractive error in which parallel rays of light coming from infinity are focused in front of the retina when accommodation is at rest.

Name the clinical varieties of myopia.

1. Congenital myopia
2. Simple myopia
3. Pathological or degenerative myopia
4. Acquired myopia which may be: (i) post-traumatic, (ii) post-keratitis, (iii) space myopia, and (iv) consecutive myopia (following overcorrection of aphakia by intraocular lens).

Enumerate the fundus changes in pathological myopia.

1. Optic disc appears large, pale and at its temporal edge characteristic myopic crescent is present.
2. Chorioretinal degeneration.
3. Foster-Fuchs' spot at the macula.
4. Vitreous shows synchysis and syneresis.
5. Posterior staphyloma may be seen.

Name the surgical treatment of myopia.

1. Radial keratotomy
2. Photorefractive keratectomy (PRK) using excimer laser.
3. Automated microlamellar keratectomy (ALK)
4. Removal of clear crystalline lens by extracapsular cataract extraction (ECCE) is recommended in unilateral very high myopia.

Name the complications of pathological myopia.

1. Complicated cataract
2. Choroidal haemorrhage
3. Tears and haemorrhage in the retina
4. Vitreous haemorrhage
5. Retinal detachment

Name the diseases which can be associated with myopia.

1. Microphthalmos
2. Congenital glaucoma
3. Microcornea
4. Retrolental fibroplasia
5. Marfan's syndrome
6. Turner's syndrome
7. Ehlers-Danlos syndrome

What is the basic principle of radial keratotomy operation for myopia?

In radial keratotomy operation, multiple radial incisions are given in the periphery of cornea (leaving central 4 mm optical zone) in order to flatten the curvature of cornea.

What is the principle of photorefractive keratectomy (PRK) operation for myopia?

In it, superficial keratectomy (reshaping) is performed in the central part of cornea with the help of excimer laser.

What is ALK operation for myopia?

It is automated lamellar keratectomy. In it a small disc of corneal stroma is removed with the help of an automated machine.

What is LASIK operation for myopia?

It is laser-assisted *in-situ* keratomileusis. It is performed using ALK machine and the excimer laser. This procedure is good for myopia of more than – 8D.

Define astigmatism.

Astigmatism is a type of refractive error, wherein the refraction varies in the different meridia. Consequently, the rays of light entering in the eye cannot converge to a point focus but form focal lines.

What are the clinical types of astigmatism?

1. *Regular astigmatism*, which may be:
   (i) With-the-rule (WTR) astigmatism, wherein the vertical meridian is more curved than the horizontal.
   (ii) Against-the-rule (ATR) astigmatism, wherein the horizontal meridian is more curved than the vertical meridian.
   (iii) Oblique astigmatism, wherein the two principal meridia are not the horizontal and vertical though these are at right angles to one another (e.g., 45° and 135°).
   (iv) Bioblique astigmatism, wherein the two principal meridia are not at right angle to each other, e.g., one may be at 30° and the other at 100°.
2. *Irregular astigmatism:* In it refraction varies in multiple meridia which admits no geometrical analysis. It commonly follows corneal scarring.

What is the treatment of irregular astigmatism?

Contact lens prescription, which replaces the anterior surface of the cornea for refraction.

What is simple, compound and mixed astigmatism?

1. *Simple astigmatism.* Herein the rays of light entering the eye are focused on the retina in one meridian and either in front (*simple myopic astigmatism*, or behind (*simple hypermetropic astigmatism)* the retina in other meridian.
2. *Compound astigmatism.* In this type of astigmatism, light rays are focused in both the principal meridia either in front (*compound myopic astigmatism)* or behind (*compound hypermetropic astigmatism)* the retina.
3. *Mixed astigmatism.* In this condition, light rays are focused in front of the retina in one meridian and behind the retina in the other meridian.

What is the most common cause of irregular astigmatism?

Irregular corneal scars.

What is anisometropia?

In it, total refraction of the two eyes is unequal. Practically a difference of more than 2.5 D (which causes more than 5% difference in the retinal images of the two eyes) poses problem of anisometropia.

What is aniseikonia?

Aniseikonia is defined as a condition, wherein the images projected to the visual cortex from the two retinae are abnormally unequal in size and shape.

How much image magnification is caused by one dioptre anisometropia?

One dioptre anisometropia produces image magnification by 2 percent. An image difference up to 5 percent to 7 percent is well tolerated.

What are the common causes of aniseikonia?

Aniseikonia may be *optical* (due to high anisometropia), *retinal* (due to stretching or crowding of retina in macular area) or *cortical* (due to abnormal cortical perception of the images).

ACCOMMODATION AND ITS ANOMALIES

Define accommodation.

Accommodation is a mechanism by which the eyes can focus the diverging rays coming from a near object on the retina. In it, there occurs increase in the power of crystalline lens.

What is presbyopia?

Presbyopia is not an error of refraction but a condition of physiological insufficiency of accommodation resulting from the decreased elasticity and plasticity of the lens due to advancing age (usually after the age of 40 years) leading to failing vision for near.

What is near point of the eye?

The nearest point at which small objects can be seen clearly is called near point or *punctum proximum*. Its value varies with age; being about 7 cm at 10 years of age and about 25 cm at about 40 years of age.

What is far point of the eye?

The farthest point from where objects can be seen by the eye is called far point or *punctum remotum.* In an emmetropic eye, far point is at infinity.

Enumerate the causes of premature presbyopia.

1. Uncorrected hypermetropia
2. Premature hardening of the lens
3. General debility causing premature senile weakness of the ciliary muscle
4. Chronic simple glaucoma

What is range of accommodation?

Range of accommodation is the distance between the near point and far point of the eye.

What is amplitude of accommodation?

Amplitude of accommodation is the difference between the dioptric power needed to focus at near and far point.

What do you mean by insufficiency of accommodation? Enumerate its causes.

Insufficiency of accommodation refers to a significant decrease in accommodation power than the normal physiological limit for the patient's age. Common *causes* of insufficiency of accommodation are:

- Premature sclerosis of the lens.
- Weakness of ciliary muscle associated with chronic debilitating disease, anaemia, malnutrition, pregnancy, stress and so on.
- Primary open-angle glaucoma.

DETERMINATION AND CORRECTION OF REFRACTIVE ERRORS

Enumerate objective methods of refraction.

- Retinoscopy
- Autorefractometry
- Keratometry

Name some subjective methods of refraction.

- Trial and error method
- Fogging method
- Tests for confirming refraction subjectively
  - Duochrome test
  - Astigmatic fan test
  - Jackson's crosscylinder test
  - Pin-hole test

Define retinoscopy (skiascopy or shadow test).

Retinoscopy is an objective method of finding out the error of refraction by the method of neutralization.

What is the principle of retinoscopy?

Retinoscopy is based on the fact that when light is reflected from a mirror into the eye, the direction in which light will travel across the pupil will depend upon the refractive state of the eye.

What are the prerequisites for retinoscopy?

1. A darkroom preferably 6-m long or which can be converted into 6 metres by the use of a plane mirror.
2. A trial box containing spherical and cylindrical lenses of variable plus and minus powers, a pinhole, an occluder and prisms.
3. A trial frame
4. A Snellen's self-illuminated vision box
5. A retinoscope

What are the common types of retinoscopes?

1. Mirror retinoscopes, which may consist of a simple plane mirror or a combination of a plane mirror (on one end) and a concave mirror (on the other end) e.g., Pristley-Smith's mirror.
2. Self-illuminated streak retinoscope.

What are the advantages of a streak retinoscope over a simple plane mirror retinoscope?

The streak retinoscope is more sensitive than the spot retinoscope in detecting astigmatism.

Name the conditions where concave mirror retinoscopy is more useful.

1. Patient with hazy media.
2. Patient with very high degree of refractive error.

What are the indications of using cycloplegic drugs for retinoscopy?

Cycloplegics are used before retinoscopy in patients where the examiner suspects that accommodation is abnormally active and will hinder the exact retinoscopy. Such a situation is encountered in young children especially hypermetropes.

What do you mean by wet retinoscopy and dry retinoscopy?

When retinoscopy is performed after instilling a cycloplegic, it is termed 'wet-retinoscopy' in converse to dry retinoscopy (without cycloplegic).

Name the commonly used cycloplegics.

1. Atropine
2. Homatropine
3. Cyclopentolate

At what distance retinoscopy is performed?

One meter or two-third metre.

When retinoscopy is performed with a plane mirror at a distance of 1 m; what inferences are drawn?

Depending upon the movement of the red reflex vis-a-vis movement of the plane mirror, following inferences are drawn:

1. *No movement* of the red reflex indicates myopia of 1 D.
2. *With movement* of the red reflex indicates either emmetropia or hypermetropia or myopia of less than 1 D.
3. *Against movement* indicates myopia of more than 1D.

What inferences are drawn from the movement of the red reflex when concave mirror retinoscope is used?

The inferences drawn while using a concave mirror are reverse to that of plane mirror.

What is the point of neutralization while using a simple plane mirror retinoscope?

The end point of neutralization is either no movement or just reversal of the movement of the pupillary shadow.

What is the end point of neutralization while using a streak retinoscope?

At the end point, the streak disappears and the pupil appears completely illuminated or completely dark.

While performing retinoscopy, if the shadow appears to swirl around, what does it indicate?

Astigmatism.

While performing retinoscopy with dilated pupil, one central and another peripheral shadow may be seen. It is important to neutralize which shadow?

Central shadow.

When a cycloplegic retinoscopy has been performed, how many dioptres should be deducted to compensate for the ciliary tone?

- 1 D for atropine
- 0.75 D for cyclopentolate
- 0.5 D for homatropine

What is an autorefractometer?

It is a computerized refractometer which quickly estimates the refractive error of the patient objectively in terms of sphere, cylinder with its axis and interpupillary distance. The subjective verification is a must even after autorefractometry.

What is a duochrome test?

Duochrome test is based on the principle of chromatic aberrations. It helps in verifying the spherical correction subjectively. In it, the patient is asked to tell the clarity of the letters with red background vis-a-vis green background. To an emmetropic patient, letters of both the colours look equally sharp; while to a slightly myopic patient the red letters appear sharper and to a slightly hypermetropic patient the green letters look sharper.

Name common problems which can arise while performing retinoscopy.

Red reflex may not be visible. It occurs in:

1. small pupil,
2. hazy media, and
3. high degree of refractive errors.

DARKROOM APPLIANCES

What is a prism and what are its uses in ophthalmology?

Prism is a refracting medium, having two plane surfaces inclined at an angle. Its uses are:

1. Objective measurement of angle of squint (prism bar cover test, Krimsky's test).
2. Measurement of fusional reserve.
3. Diagnosis of microtropia.
4. Used in ophthalmic equipment such as gonioscope, keratometer, applanation tonometer, etc.

What are the uses of a convex spherical lens?

Its uses are:

1. For correction of hypermetropia, aphakia and presbyopia
2. In oblique illumination examination
3. In indirect ophthalmoscopy
4. As a magnifying lens

How will you identify a convex lens?

A convex lens can be identified from following features:

1. It is thicker at the centre.
2. An object held close to it appears magnified.
3. When it is moved, the objects seen through it move in the opposite direction.

How will you identify a concave lens?

A concave lens can be identified from following features:

1. It is thin at the centre and thick at the periphery.
2. An object seen through it appears minified.
3. When it is moved, the objects seen through it move in the same direction of the lens.

What are the uses of concave lens?

1. For correction of myopia
2. As Hruby lens for fundus examination.

How will you identify a cylindrical lens?

1. When it is rotated around its optical axis, objects seen through it become distorted.
2. It acts only in one axis, i.e., when it is moved up and down or sideways the object seen through it moves only in one direction (with the lens in a convex cylinder and against the lens in a concave cylinder).

What are the uses of cylindrical lenses?

Cylindrical lens is prescribed to: (i) correct astigmatic refractive error, (ii) it is used as a crosscylinder to check the power and axis of the cylindrical lens prescribed, subjectively.

What is a crosscylinder and what are its uses?

The Jackson's crosscylinder is a combination of two cylindrical lenses of equal strength but with opposite sign placed with their axis at right angles to each other and mounted in a handle. The crosscylinder effect is obtained by combining a spherical lens with a cylindrical lens (double the power of spherical lens) with opposite sign –0.25 D spherical and +0.5 D cylindrical. Commonly used crosscylinders are a combination of 0.25 D and 0.5 D.

A crosscylinder is used to verify the strength and axis of the cylinder subjectively.

What are the uses of red and green glasses or filters?

These are used for:

1. Diplopia charting
2. Worth's four-dot test
3. Malingering test

While testing, the red glass is kept in front of the right eye and the green glass is kept in front of the left eye.

Which glass is used most commonly for making spectacles?

Crown glass with refractive index 1.5223 is most commonly used for making spectacles.

What are the types of contact lenses you know of?

1. Hard contact lenses
2. Soft contact lenses
3. Rigid gas-permeable (RGP) contact lenses

What are the advantages and disadvantages of hard contact lenses?

Hard contact lenses are made up of PMMA (polymethylmethacrylate) which is a light weight, non-toxic but of hydrophobic material.

Advantages
Cheap, durable and have high optical quality.

Disadvantages
Can cause corneal hypoxia and corneal abrasions.

What are the advantages and disadvantages of soft contact lenses?

Soft contact lenses are made up of HEMA (hydroxy-ethylmethacrylate) which is hydrophilic.

Advantages
Being soft and oxygen permeable, they are most comfortable and so well tolerated.

Disadvantages
Problems of proteinaceous deposits, getting cracked, limited life, inferior optical quality, more chances of corneal infections, and inability to correct astigmatism of more than one dioptre.

TECHNIQUES OF FUNDUS EXAMINATION

Techniques of fundus examination include:

A. Ophthalmoscopy, and
B. Slit-lamp biomicroscopic examination of the fundus by:
   - Indirect slit-lamp biomiscroscopy
   - Hruby lens biomicroscopy
   - Contact lens biomicroscopy

A. OPHTHALMOSCOPY

Ophthalmoscopy is a clinical examination of the interior of the eye by means of an ophthalmoscope. It is primarily done to assess the state of fundus and detect the opacities of ocular media. The ophthalmoscope was invented by Babbage in 1848, however its importance was not recognized, and it was re-invented by von Helmholtz in 1850. Three methods of examination in vogue are: (1) distant direct ophthalmoscopy, (2) direct ophthalmoscopy, and (3) indirect ophthalmoscopy.

1. *DISTANT DIRECT OPHTHALMOSCOPY*

It should be performed routinely before the direct ophthalmoscopy, as it gives a lot of useful information (vide infra). It can be performed with the help of a self-illuminated ophthalmoscope or a simple plain mirror with a hole at the centre.

Procedure. The light is thrown into patient's eye sitting in a semi-darkroom, from a distance of 20-25 cm and the features of the red glow in the pupillary area are noted.

Applications of distant direct ophthalmoscopy

i. To *diagnose opacities in the refractive media.* Any opacity in the refractive media is seen as a black shadow in the red glow. The exact location of the opacity can be determined by observing the parallactic displacement. For this, the patient is asked to move the eye up and down while the examiner is observing the pupillary glow. The opacities in the pupillary plane remain stationary, those in front of the pupillary plane move in the direction of the movement of the eye and those behind it will move in opposite direction (Fig. 23.25).
ii. *To differentiate between a mole and a hole of the iris.* A small hole and a mole on the iris appear as a black spot on oblique illumination. On distant direct ophthalmoscopy, the mole looks black (as earlier) but a red reflex is seen through the hole in the iris.
iii. *To recognize detached retina or a tumour arising from the fundus.* A grayish reflex seen on distant direct ophthalmoscopy indicates either a detached retina or a tumour arising from the fundus.

2. DIRECT OPHTHALMOSCOPY

It is the most commonly practised method for routine fundus examination.

Optics. The modern direct ophthalmoscope (Fig. 23.26) works on the basic optical principle of glass plate ophthalmoscope introduced by von Helmholtz. Optics of direct ophthalmoscopy is depicted in Fig. 23.27.

A convergent beam of light is reflected into the patient's pupil (Fig. 23.27, dotted lines). The emergent rays from any point on the patient's fundus reach the observer's retina through the viewing hole in the ophthalmoscope (Fig. 23.27, continuous lines). The emergent rays from the patient's eye are parallel and brought to focus on the retina of the emmetropic observer when accommodation is relaxed. However, if the patient or/and the observer is/are ametropic, a correcting lens (equivalent to the sum of the patient's and observer's refractive error) must be interposed (from the system of plus and minus lenses, inbuilt in the modern ophthalmoscopes).

Characteristics of image formed. In direct ophthalmoscopy, the image is erect, virtual and about 15 times magnified in emmetropes (more in myopes and less in hypermetropes).

Technique. Direct ophthalmoscopy should be performed in a semi-darkroom with the patient seated and looking straight ahead, while the observer standing or seated slightly over to the side of the eye to be examined (Fig. 23.28). Patients right eye should be examined by the observer with his or her right eye and left with the left eye.

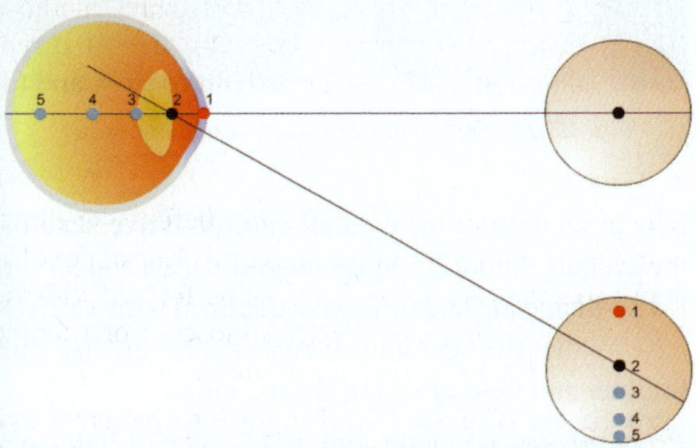

Fig. 23.25. Parallactic displacement on distant direct ophthalmoscopy.

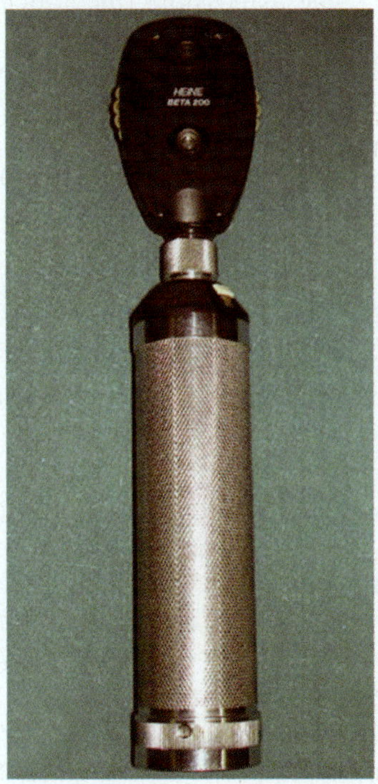

Fig. 23.26. Direct ophthalmoscope.

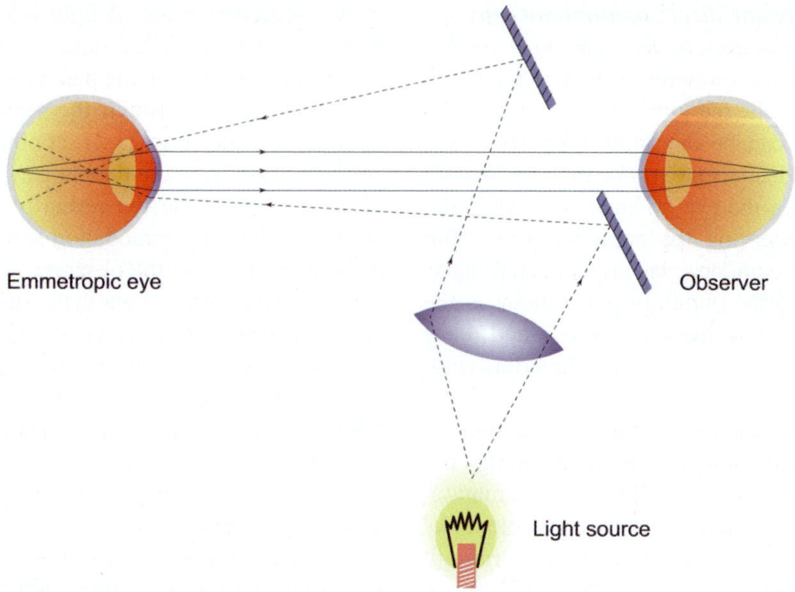

Fig. 23.27. Optics of direct ophthalmoscopy.

The observer should reflect beam of light from the ophthalmoscope into patient's pupil. Once the red reflex is seen the observer should move as close to the patient's eye as possible (theoretically at the anterior focal plane of the patient's eye, i.e., 15.4 mm from the cornea). Once the retina is focused the details should be examined systematically starting from disc, blood vessels, the four quadrants of the general background and the macula. (see page 507-509 for systematic observations to be made on ophthalmoscopy)

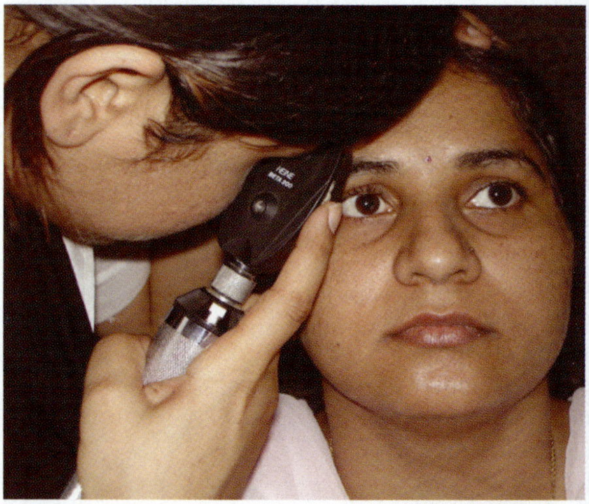

Fig. 23.28. Technique of direct ophthalmoscopy.

3. INDIRECT OPHTHALMOSCOPY

Indirect ophthalmoscopy introduced by Nagel in 1864, is now a very popular method for examination of the posterior segment.

Optical principle. The principle of indirect ophthalmoscopy is to make the eye highly myopic by placing a strong convex lens in front of patient's eye so that the emergent rays from an area of the fundus are brought to focus as a real, inverted image between the lens and the observer's eye, which is then studied (Fig. 23.29).

Characteristics of image. The image formed in indirect ophthalmoscopy is real, inverted and magnified. Magnification of image depends upon the dioptric power of the convex lens, position of the lens in relation to the eyeball and refractive state of the eyeball. About 2.5 times magnification and 35° or 8 disc-diameter field of view is obtained with a +20 D lens. With a stronger lens, image will be smaller, but brighter and field of vision will be more.

Prerequisites. (i) Darkroom, (ii) Source of light and concave mirror or self-illuminated indirect ophthalmoscope, (iii) Convex lens (now-a-days commonly

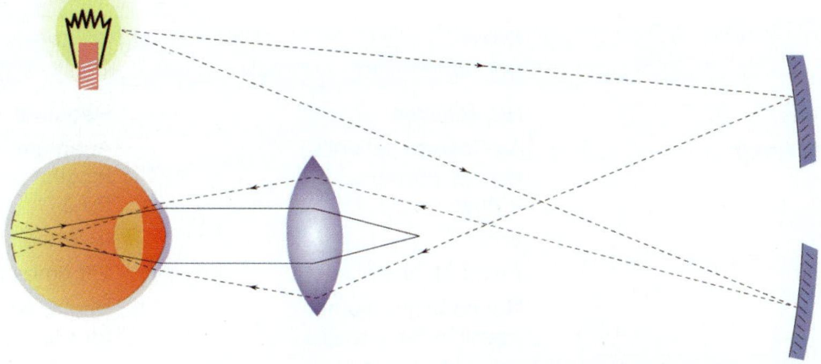

Fig. 23.29. Optics of indirect ophthalmoscopy.

employed lens is of +20 D), (iv) Pupils of the patient should be dilated.

Technique. Patient is made to lie in the supine position, with one pillow on a bed or couch and instructed to keep both eyes open. The examiner throws the light into patient's eye from an arm's distance (with the self-illuminated ophthalmoscope). In practice, binocular ophthalmoscope with head band or that mounted on the spectacle frame is employed most frequently (Fig. 23.30). Keeping his or her eyes on the reflex, the examiner then interposes the condensing lens (+20 D, routinely) in the path of beam of light, close to patient's eye, and then slowly moves the lens away from the eye (towards himself) until the image of the retina is clearly seen. The examiner moves around the head of the patient to examine different quadrants of the fundus. He or she has to stand opposite the clock hour position to be examined, e.g., to examine inferior quadrant (around 6 O'clock meridian) the examiner stands towards patient's head (12 O'clock meridian) and so on. By asking the patient to look in extreme gaze, and using scleral indenter, the whole peripheral retina up to ora serrata can be examined.

Applications. Indirect ophthalmoscopy is essential for the assessment and management of retinal detachment and other peripheral retinal lesions.

Difficulties

1. The technique is difficult and can be mastered by hours of practice.
2. Reflexes from the corneal surface can be decreased by holding the condensing lens at a distance equal to its focal length from the anterior focus of the eye.
3. Formation of reflexes by the two surfaces of convex lens can be eliminated by slightly tilting the lens and use of aspheric lens.

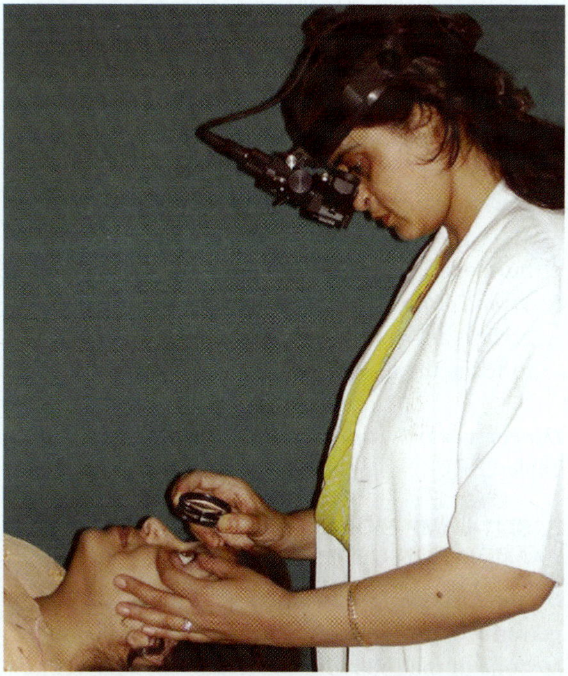

Fig. 23.30. Technique of indirect ophthalmoscopy.

Advantages of the binocular indirect ophthalmoscope

1. *Visualization through hazy media* is possible due to strong in built illumination system.
2. *Field of view is much larger* than direct ophthalmoscopy.

Table 23.2. Direct versus indirect ophthalmoscopy

Sr. no.	*Feature*	*Direct ophthalmoscopy*	*Indirect ophthalmoscopy*
1.	Condensing lens	Not required	Required
2.	Examination distance	As close to patient's eye as possible	At an arm's length
3.	Image	Virtual, Erect	Real, Inverted
4.	Magnification	About 15 times	2.5 times (with +20D lens)
5.	Illumination	Not so bright; so not useful in hazy media	Bright; so, useful for hazy media
6.	Area of field in focus	About 2 disc diameter	About 8 disc diameter
7.	Stereopsis	Absent	Present
8.	Accessible fundus view	Slightly beyond equator	Up to ora serrata
9.	Examination through hazy media	Not possible	Possible

3. *Examination of peripheral retina* up to Ora-serrata is possible
4. *Depth perception of the lesion is possible* due to stereopsis with binocular indirect ophthalmoscope.
5. *Visualization of fundus in very high refractive error* is also possible, where it may not be possible to focus the lesion with direct ophthalmoscope.

Direct versus indirect ophthalmoscopy. (See Table 23.2).

B. SLIT-LAMP BIOMICROSCOPIC EXAMINATION OF THE FUNDUS

Biomicroscopic examination of the fundus can be performed after full mydriasis using a slit-lamp and any one of the following lenses:

1. *Indirect slit-lamp biomicroscopy.* *Using +78 D or +90 D small diameter lens* (Fig. 23.31A) is presently the most commonly employed technique for biomicroscopic examination of the posterior pole of fundus. Similar to binocular indirect ophthalmoscopy, the image formed is inverted, real and magnified. This technique is being considered a better alternative to all the below discussed techniques for slip lamp biomicroscopy of the fundus.

2. *Hruby lens biomicroscopy.* Hruby lens is a planoconcave lens with dioptric power 58.6D (Fig. 23.31B). This lens provides a small field with low magnification and cannot visualize the fundus beyond equator.

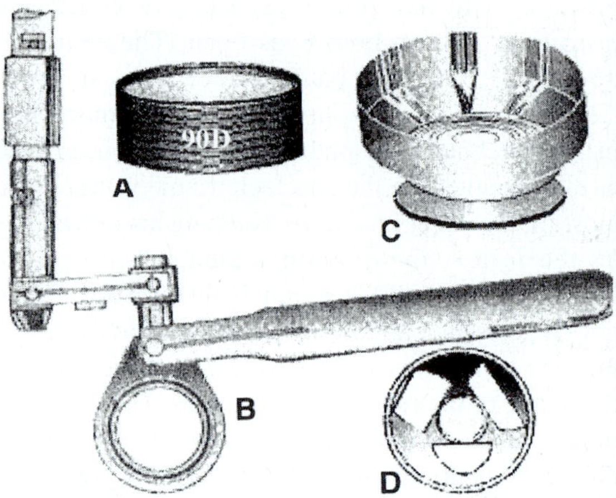

Fig. 23.31. Lenses used for slit-lamp biomicroscopic examination of fundus: A, +78D or +90D, small diameter lens. B, Hruby lens; C, Posterior fundus contact lens (modified Koeppe's lens); D, Goldmann's three-mirror contact lens.

3. *Contant lens biomicroscopy* can be performed by following lenses:

- *Posterior fundus contact lens* is a modified Koeppe's lens (Fig. 23.31C). The image produced by it is virtual and erect.
- *Goldmann's three-mirror contact lens* consists of a central contact lens and three mirrors placed in the cone, each with different angles of

inclination (Fig. 23.31D). With this the central as well as peripheral parts of the fundus can be visualized.

RELATED QUESTIONS

Define ophthalmoscopy.

It is a darkroom procedure carried out to examine the fundus oculi.

What are the types of ophthalmoscopy?

Ophthalmoscopy is of three types:

1. Distant direct ophthalmoscopy.
2. Direct ophthalmoscopy
3. Indirect ophthalmoscopy

What are the other methods of fundus examination?

In addition to ophthalmoscopy fundus can also be examined by focal illumination using a slit-lamp biomicroscope and any of the following lenses:

- Hruby lens
- Posterior fundus contact lens
- Goldmann's three-mirror contact lens
- +78 D and +90 D small diameter lenses.

When and who invented the direct ophthalmoscope?

Babbage in 1848.

Who reinvented and popularised the ophthalmoscope?

von Helmholtz in 1850.

At what distance distant direct ophthalmoscopy is performed?

20-25 cm.

What are the uses (applications) of distant direct ophthalmoscopy?

1. To diagnose opacities in the ocular media
2. To differentiate between a mole and a hole of the iris.
3. To recognize a detached retina
4. To recognize a subluxated lens.

At what distance 'direct ophthalmoscopy' should be performed?

As near to the patient's eye as possible.

What are the features of the image formed in direct ophthalmoscopy?

The image formed is erect, virtual and about 15 times magnified in an emmetrope.

When and who invented the indirect ophthalmoscopy?

Nagel in 1864.

What is the principle of indirect ophthalmoscopy?

The principle of indirect ophthalmoscopy is to make the eye highly myopic by placing a strong convex lens in front of the patient's eye so that emergent rays from an area of the fundus are brought to focus as a real, inverted image between the lens and the observer's eye.

What is the power of the convex lens most commonly used in indirect ophthalmoscopy?

+20 D.

What are the characteristics of the image formed in indirect ophthalmoscopy?

It is real, inverted, magnified about 2.5 times when +20 D lens is used and is formed between the convex lens and the observer.

What are the advantages of indirect ophthalmoscopy over direct ophthalmoscopy?

1. It allows a stereoscopic view of the fundus.
2. It allows examination in hazy media.
3. Periphery of the retina up to ora serrata can be examined.

What are the advantages of direct ophthalmoscopy over indirect ophthalmoscopy?

1. It is a handy procedure
2. Easy to perform
3. Allows examination of the minute details of the approachable lesion, since image formed is 15 times magnified.
4. Orientation and understanding of the lesion is easy as the image formed is erect.

Name the common diseases of the optic disc which can be diagnosed on direct ophthalmoscopy.

- Papillitis
- Papilloedema
- Optic atrophy
- Glaucomatous cupping

Name few common retinal disorders diagnosed on direct/ indirect ophthalmoscopy.

- Diabetic retinopathy
- Hypertensive retinopathy
- Retinal detachment
- Retinitis pigmentosa

24

CHAPTER

Ophthalmic Instruments and Operative Ophthalmology

INTRODUCTION

To perform well in this section of practical examinations, students are supposed to be well versed with the following topics:

- Anaesthesia for ocular surgery
- Ophthalmic equipment
- Ophthalmic instruments
- Sterilization techniques
- Surgical steps of common eye operations
  - Cataract surgery (see page 199-208)
  - Glaucoma surgery (see page 252)
  - Enucleation operation (see page 304)
  - Evisceration operation (see page 171)
- Lasers and cryotherapy in ophthalmology (see page 460-462).

ANAESTHESIA FOR OCULAR SURGERY

Ocular surgery may be performed under topical, local or general anaesthesia. Local anaesthesia is more frequently employed as it entails little risk and is less dependent upon patient's general health. It is easy to perform, has got rapid onset of action and provides a low intraocular pressure with dilated pupil. Above all, in developing countries like India, with a large number of cataract cases, it is much more economical.

REGIONAL (LOCAL) ANAESTHESIA

Indications. Almost all ocular operations, namely, cataract extraction, glaucoma surgery, keratoplasty and other corneal surgeries, iridectomy, squint and retinal detachment surgery in adults can be performed under local anaesthesia.

Goals. The main goals of regional anaesthesia for successful ocular surgery are: globe and conjunctival anaesthesia, orbicularis akinesia, ocular akinesia and low intraocular and intraorbital pressure.

These goals can be achieved by a local anaesthesia comprising either surface anaesthesia, facial block and retrobulbar block or a combination of surface anaesthesia and peribulbar block.

Surface (Topical) anaesthesia

Surface anaesthesia is achieved by topical instillations of 2 to 4 percent xylocaine or 1 percent amethocaine. Usually a drop of anaesthetic solution instilled 4 times after every 4 minutes, is sufficient to produce conjunctival and corneal anaesthesia. Cataract surgery by phacoemulsification can be performed even under topical anaesthesia only.

Facial block

For intraocular surgery it is necessary to block the facial nerve which supplies the orbicularis oculi muscle, so that patient cannot squeeze the eyelids.

Orbicularis akinesia can be achieved by blocking the facial nerve at its terminal branches (van Lint block), superior branches (Atkinson block) or proximal trunk (O'Brien or Nadbath block).

1. *Blocking the peripheral branches of facial nerve (van Lint's block):* This technique blocks the terminal branches of the facial nerve, producing localized akinesia of the orbicularis oculi muscle without associated facial paralysis.

In this technique, 2.5 ml of anaesthetic solution is injected in deeper tissues just above the eyebrow and just below the inferior orbital margin, through a point about 2 cm behind the lateral orbital margin, level with outer canthus (Fig. 24.1).

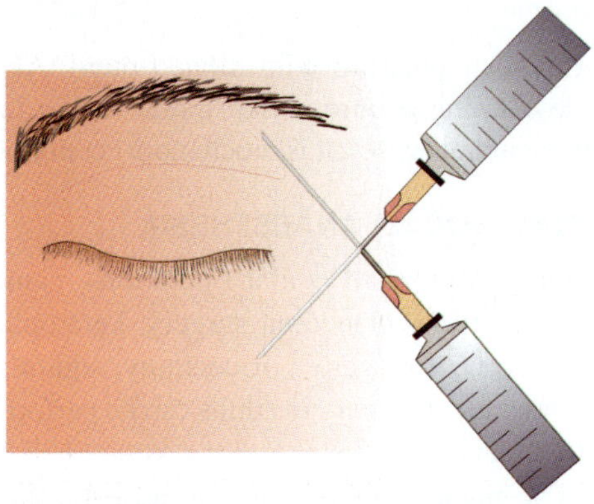

Fig. 24.1. Technique of van Lint's block.

2. *Facial nerve trunk block:* At *the neck of mandible (O'Brien's block)*. In it, facial nerve is blocked near the condyloid process. The condyle is located 1 cm anterior to the tragus. It is easily palpated if the patient is asked to open and close the mouth with the operator's index finger located across the neck of the mandible. At this point the needle is inserted until contact is made with the periosteum and then 4 to 6 ml of local anaesthetic is injected while the needle is withdrawn (Fig. 24.2).

This technique is associated with pain at the injection site and unwanted facial paralysis.

3. *Nadbath block:* In this technique, the facial nerve is blocked as it leaves the skull through the stylomastoid foramen. This block is also painful.

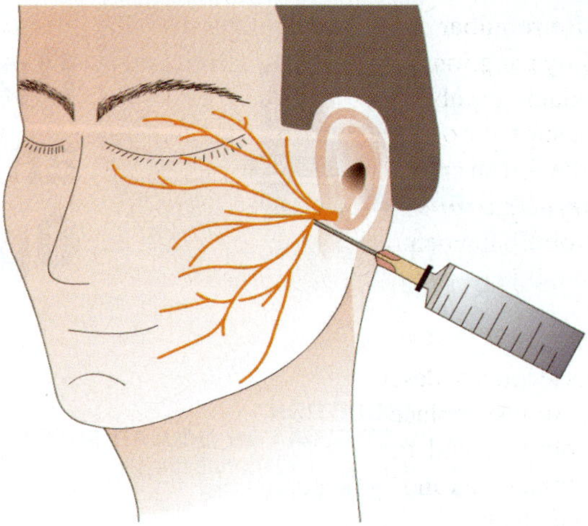

Fig. 24.2. Diagrammatic distribution of the facial nerve and technique of O'Brien's block.

4. *Atkinson's block:* In it superior branches of the facial nerve are blocked by injecting anaesthetic solution at the inferior margin of the zygomatic bone.

Retrobulbar block

Retrobulbar block was introduced by Herman Knapp in 1884. It is administered by injecting 2 ml of anaesthetic solution (2% xylocaine with added hyaluronidase 5 IU/ ml and with or without adrenaline one in one lac) into the muscle cone behind the eyeball (Fig. 24.3 'A'). It is usual to give the injection through the inferior fornix or the skin of outer part of lower lid with the eye in primary gaze (Fig. 24.4 'A'). The needle is first directed straight backwards then slightly upwards and inwards towards the apex of the orbit, up to a depth of 2.5 to 3 cm.

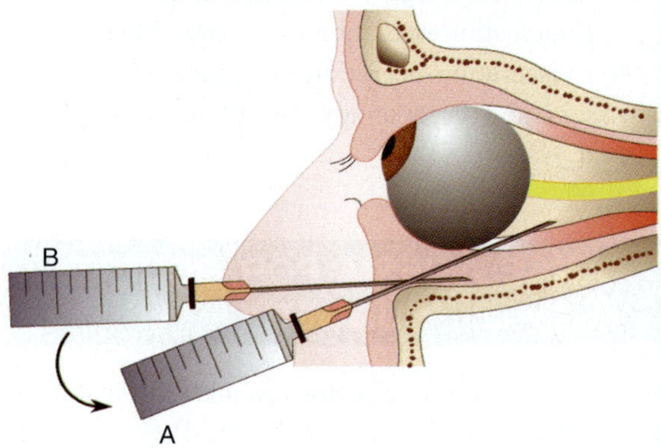

Fig. 24.3. (A) Position of needle for retrobulbar block in the muscle cone, (B) for peribulbar block in the peripheral orbital space.

Retrobulbar block anaesthetizes the ciliary nerves, ciliary ganglion and third and sixth cranial nerves thus producing globe akinesia, anaesthesia and analgesia. The superior oblique muscle is not usually paralyzed as the fourth cranial nerve is outside the muscle cone. ***Complications*** encountered with it include retrobulbar haemorrhage, globe perforation, optic nerve injury, and extraocular muscle palsies.

Peribulbar block

This technique described in 1986 by Davis and Mandel has almost replaced the time-tested combination of retrobulbar and facial blocks, because of its fewer complications and by obviating the need for a separate facial block.

Primarily the technique involves the injection of 6 to 7 ml of local anaesthetic solution in the peripheral space of the orbit (Fig. 24.3 position 'B'), from where it diffuses into the muscle cone and lids; leading to globe and orbicularis akinesia and anaesthesia. Classically, the peribulbar block is administered by two injections; first through the upper lid (at the junction of medial one-third and lateral two-third) and second through the lower lid (at the junction of lateral one-third and medial two third) (Fig. 24.4 'B'). After injection orbital compression for 10 to 15 minutes is applied with superpinky or any other method.

The *anaesthetic solution* used for peribulbar anaesthesia consists of a mixture of 2 per cent lignocaine, and 0.5 to 0.75 per cent bupivacaine (in a ratio of 2:1) with hyaluronidase 5 IU/ml and adrenaline one in one lac.

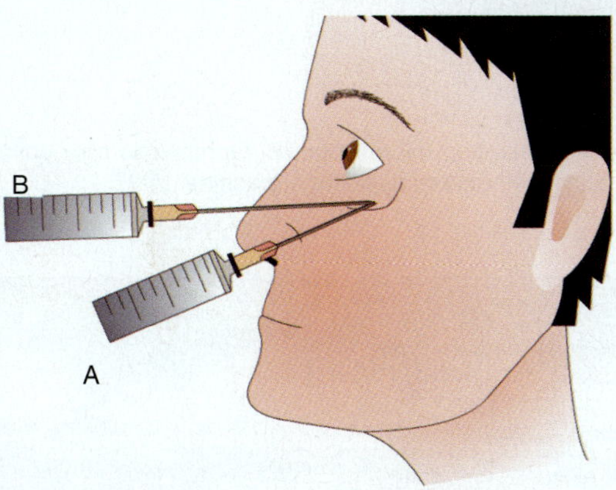

Fig. 24.4. (A) Position of the needle on the skin for retrobulbar block, (B) for peribulbar block.

GENERAL ANAESTHESIA

Indications include infants and children, anxious, non co-operative and mentally retarded adults, perforating ocular injuries, major operations like exenteration and the patients willing for operation under general anaesthesia.

Important points. During general anaesthesia for ocular surgery, use of relaxants, endotracheal intubation and controlled respiration is preferred. Under general anaesthesia, it must be ensured that patient does not develop carbon dioxide retention. When this occurs, choroid swells to many times its normal value and ocular contents prolapse as soon as the eye is opened.

In perforating injuries and other ocular emergency cases, use of suxamethonium should always be preferred over non-depolarizing relaxants as the risk of vomiting and regurgitation of stomach contents is less with it.

OPHTHALMIC EQUIPMENT AND INSTRUMENTS

ESSENTIAL EQUIPMENT FOR OPHTHALMIC OPERATION THEATRE

In addition to the basic requirements of general operation theatre with equipment for general anaesthesia and facilities to deal with the cardiorespiratory emergency situations, a modern ophthalmic operation theatre should also have the following equipment:

- An operating microscope (Fig. 24.5A),
- An ophthalmic cryo unit (Fig. 24.5B),
- A wet-field bipolar cautery (Fig. 24.5C),
- An electrolysis machine,
- An electromagnetic unit for removal of intraocular foreign bodies,
- A vitrectomy unit (Fig. 24.5D), and
- Phacoemulsification machine (Fig. 24.5E) for modern cataract surgery.

OPHTHALMIC INSTRUMENTS

Commonly used ophthalmic instruments can be grouped as under:

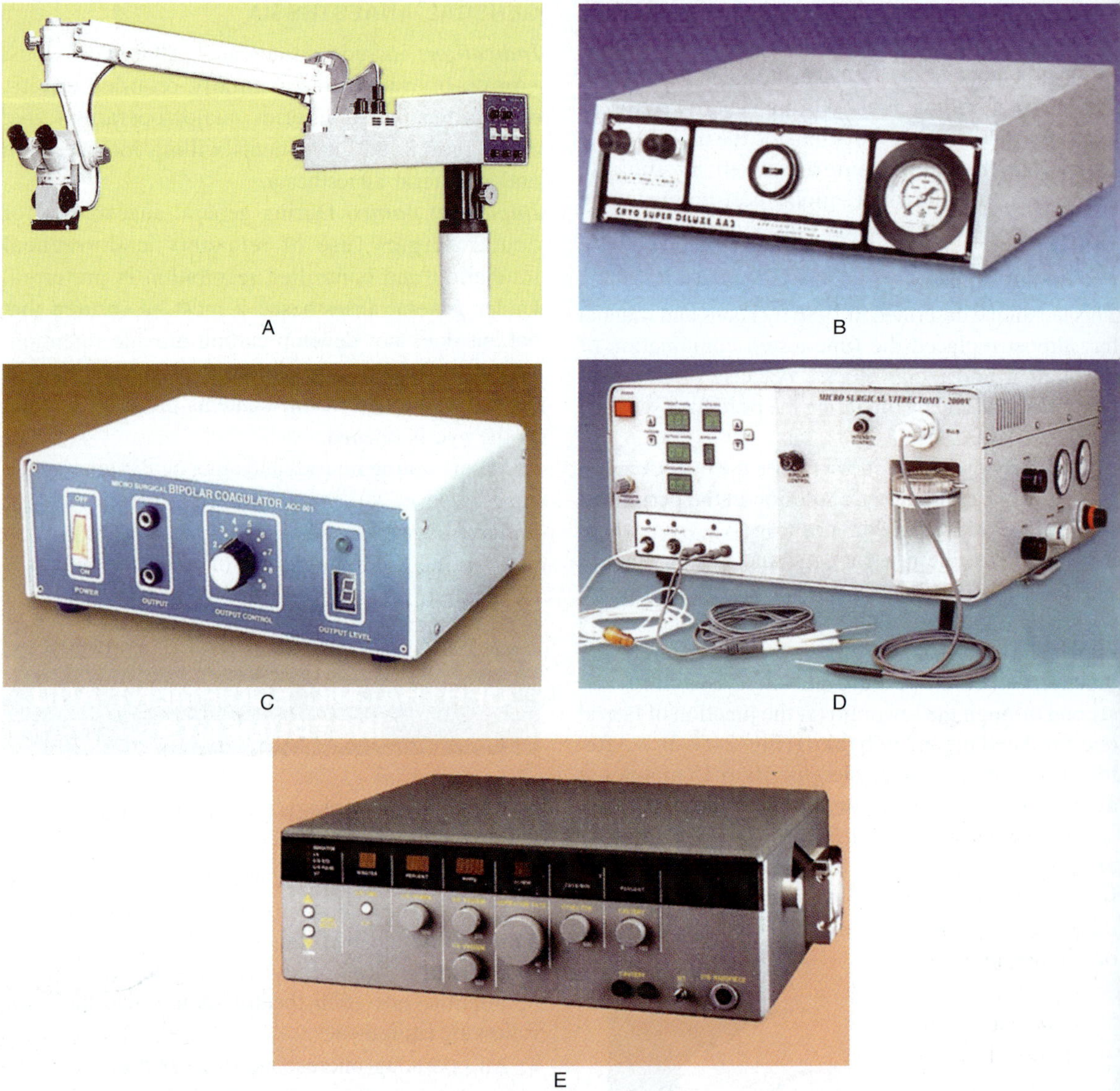

Fig. 24.5. Essential equipment for ophthalmic operation theatre: A, Operating microscope; B, Ophthalmic cryo unit; C, Wet field bipolar cautery; D, Vitrectomy unit; and E, Phacoemulsification machine.

I. Lid speculums

Three types of speculums are in use:

1. *Universal metallic eye speculum* (Fig. 24.6). It is called universal eye speculum because it can be used for both eyes i.e., right as well as left. It has two limbs and a spring mechanism with a screw to adjust the limbs. Its blades are open.

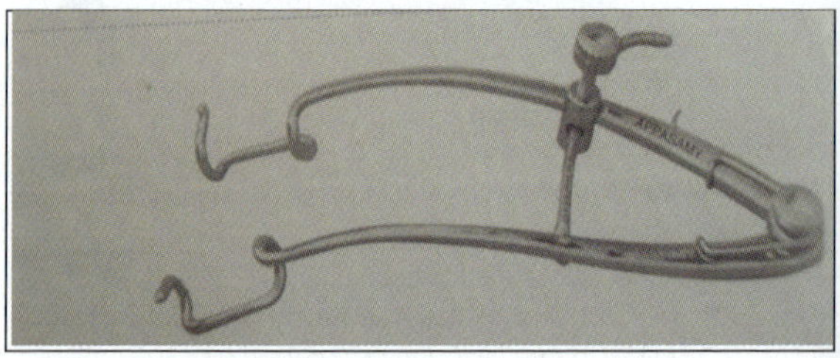

Fig. 24.6.

2. *Eye speculum with guard or with solid blades* (Fig. 24.7). It retracts the lids and its solid blades keep the lashes away from the field of operation.

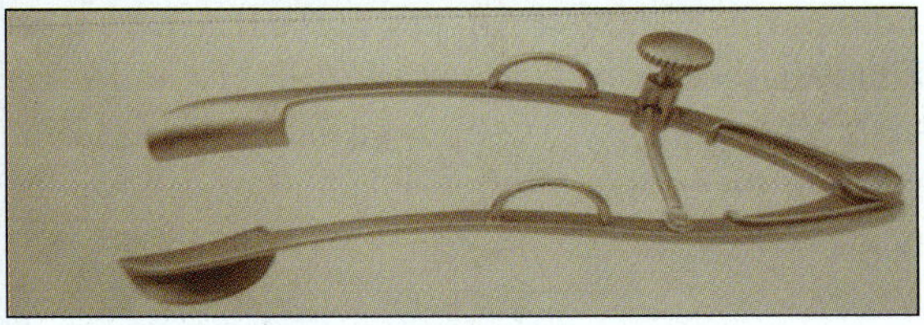

Fig. 24.7.

3. *Wire speculum* (Fig. 24.8). It is very light and causes minimal pressure on the eyeball. It is also universal.

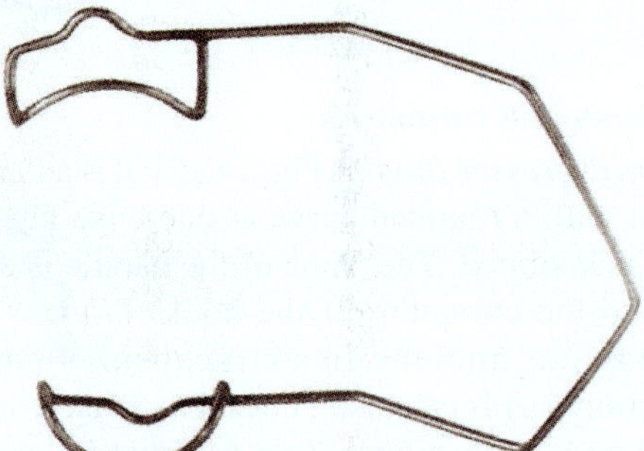

Fig. 24.8.

Uses. Eye speculums are used to keep the lids apart during:

- Intraocular operations such as cataract surgery, glaucoma surgery and keratoplasty.
- Extraocular surgery e.g., squint surgery, pterygium surgery.
- Enucleation and evisceration operation.
- Removal of conjunctival and corneal foreign bodies.
- Cauterization of corneal ulcer.
- Examination of the eye in a patient with blepharospasm.

II. Forceps

Many kinds of forceps are available for different purposes. A few common ones are mentioned here.

1. *Plain forceps* (Fig. 24.9). It is simple forcep without any teeth. Serrations (either horizontal or vertical) are present near the tip. ***Uses:*** (i) To hold the conjunctiva during any surgical procedure. (ii) To tie sutures. (iii) To hold scleral flap in trabeculectomy. (iv) To hold skin during eyelid surgery. (v) To hold nasal mucosal flaps and lacrimal sac flaps in DCR operation.

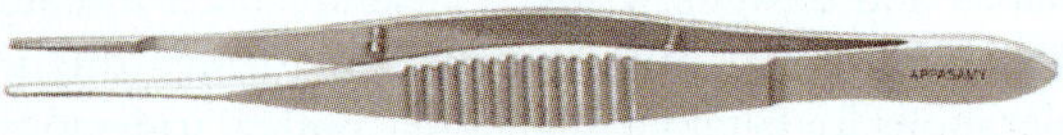

Fig. 24.9.

2. *Globe fixation forceps* (Fig. 24.10). It has 2 × 3 or 3 × 4 teeth at the tip. It is applied near the limbus to hold the conjunctiva and episcleral tissue together. ***Uses:*** (i) To fix the eyeball during operations on the eyeball. (ii) To hold the eyeball during forced-duction test.

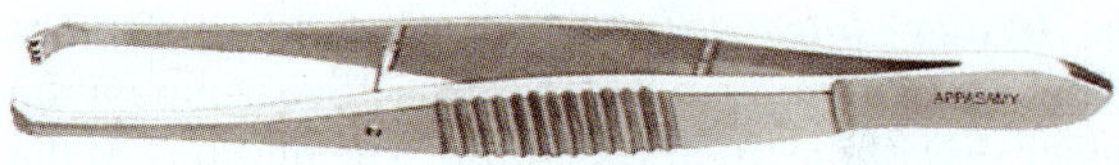

Fig. 24.10.

3. *Superior rectus holding forceps* (Fig. 24.11). It is a toothed forceps (1 × 2 teeth) with S-shaped double curve near the tip. ***Uses:*** It is used to hold the superior rectus muscle while passing a bridle suture under it; to stabilize the eyeball during any operation such as cataract surgery, glaucoma surgery, corneal surgery, etc.

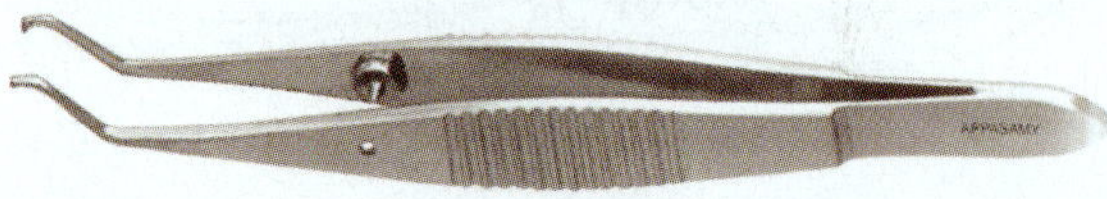

Fig. 24.11.

4. *Corneo-scleral forceps*. These are available in many shapes and designs. Commonly used are *Colibri forceps* (Fig. 24.12 A) and *Lim's forceps* (Fig. 24.12 B). These are the forceps with very fine teeth (1 × 2) at the tip. ***Uses:*** These are used to hold the cornea or scleral edge (of incision) for suturing during cataract, glaucoma, repair of corneal and/or scleral tears and keratoplasty operations.

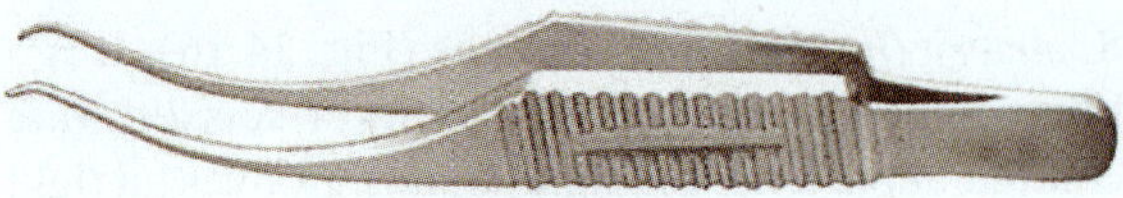

Fig. 24.12 A

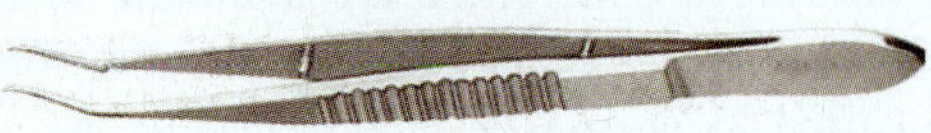

Fig. 24.12 B

5. ***Iris forceps*** (Fig. 24.13). These are small and delicate forceps having fine 1 × 2 teeth on the inner side of the limbs. These are also available in various shapes and designs. ***Uses:*** These are used to catch the iris for the purpose of iridectomy during operations for cataract, glaucoma, optical iridectomy and excision for iris prolapse, tumours and entangled foreign bodies.

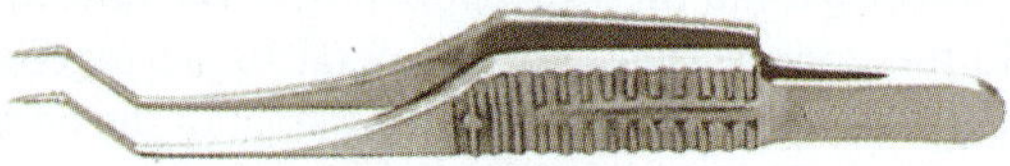

Fig. 24.13

6. ***Arruga's intracapsular (capsule holding) forceps*** (Fig. 24.14). Intracapsular forceps have a cup on the inner side of the tip of each limb. The margins of the cup are very smooth which do not damage the lens capsule when applied. ***Uses***: Not used now-a-days. In the era of intracapsular cataract extraction (ICCE) it was used to hold the lens capsule (usually at 6 O'clock position) during capsule forceps method of lens delivery in intracapsular cataract extraction and to grasp and remove the capsular remnants after accidental extracapsular lens extraction.

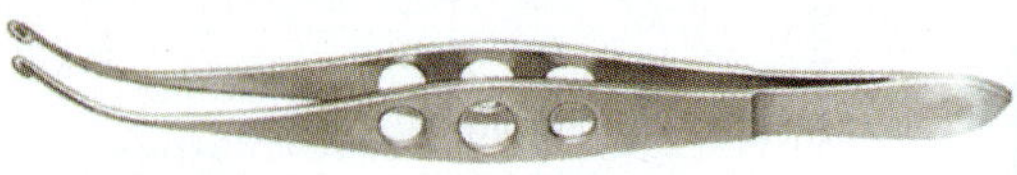

Fig. 24.14

7. ***Epilation forceps*** (Fig. 24.15). These are small stout forceps with blunt and flat ends. ***Uses***: These are used to epilate the cilia in trichiasis and stye, to remove cilia after electrolysis and cryolysis and to remove cilia lodged in the punctum.

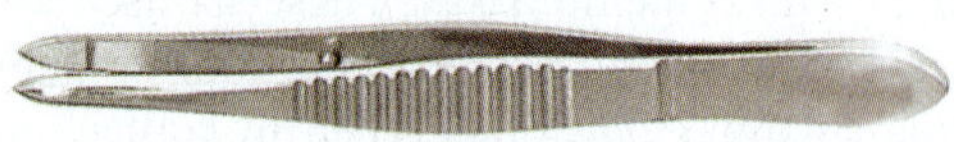

Fig. 24.15

8. ***Artery (haemostatic) forceps*** (Fig. 24.16). It is a blunt-tipped stout forceps having a scissors-like configuration. It has multiple straight grooves (at right angle to the limbs) near the tip and a locking mechanism near the ringed end. These are available in large, medium and small size. The small-sized artery forceps, also called as *mosquito artery forceps* are more commonly used in ophthalmology. These can be straight or with curved ends. ***Uses***: (i) To catch the bleeding vessels during operations of the lids and lacrimal sac. (ii) To hold the skin and muscle stay sutures. (iii) To hold small 'pea-nut' gauze pellets for blunt dissection in lacrimal sac surgery and other extraocular surgery. (iv) To hold gauze pieces while packing the socket after enucleation or exentration operation.

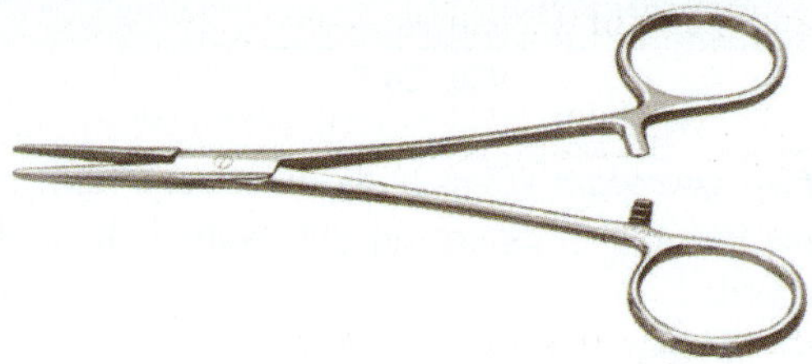

Fig. 24.16

III. Hooks and retractors

1. ***Lens expressor (hook)*** (Fig. 24.17). It is a flat metal handle with a rounded curve at one end. Tip of the curve is knobbed. The plane of the handle is at right angle to the curvature of the hook. ***Uses:*** (i) To express the nucleus in extracapsular cataract extraction. (ii) It can also be used as muscle hook if the latter is not available. (iii) Also used along with wire vectis to extract out the dislocated lens. (iv) In the era of ICCE it was used to apply pressure on the limbus at the 6 O'clock position during the delivery of lens in intracapsular cataract extraction with Smith's (tumbling) and capsule forceps techniques.

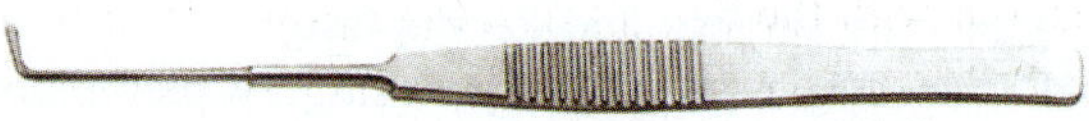

Fig. 24.17

2. ***Muscle (strabismus) hook*** (Fig. 24.18). It is similar to the lens expressor in appearance but has a blunt gaurding knob at the end to prevent muscle slippage. The plane of the handle is the same as that of the curvature of the hook. ***Uses***: (i) It is used to engage the extraocular muscles during surgery for squint, enucleation, and retinal detachment. (ii) In the absence of lens expressor, it may be used in its place.

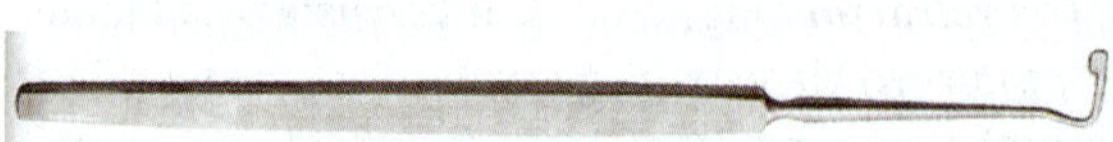

Fig. 24.18

3. ***Desmarre's retractor*** (Fig. 24.19). It is a saddle-shaped instrument folded on itself at one end. It is

available in two sizes: small (paediatric) and large (adult). ***Uses:*** It is used to retract the lids during examination of the eyeball in cases of blepharospasm in children, in cases with marked swelling and ecchymosis, removal of corneoscleral sutures, removal of corneal foreign body and for double eversion of upper lid to examine the superior fornix. *Advantages.* Allows continuous adjustment of the lids and width of the palpebral aperture.

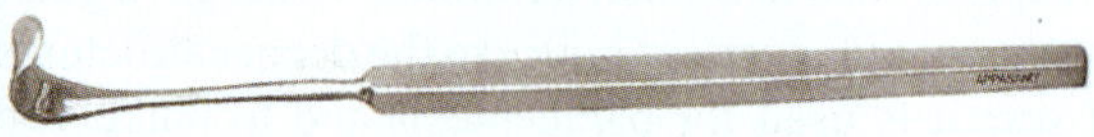

Fig. 24.19

Disadvantages. It is not self-retaining, so an assistant is needed to hold it.

4. *Cat's paw lacrimal wound retractor* (Fig. 24.20). It is a fork-like instrument with the terminals bent inward. ***Uses:*** It is used to retract the skin during lacrimal sac and lid surgery.

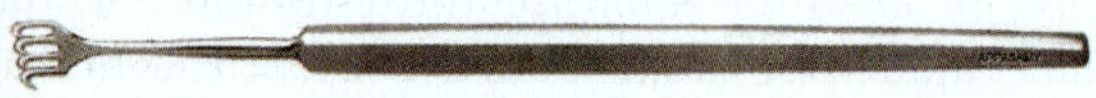

Fig. 24.20

5. *Self-retaining lacrimal wound (Muller's) retractor* (Fig. 24.21). It is made up of two limbs with three curved pins on each for engaging the edges of the skin incision. The limbs are kept in a retracted position with the help of a fixing screw. ***Uses:*** It is used to retract the skin during surgery on the lacrimal sac (e.g., DCT or DCR).

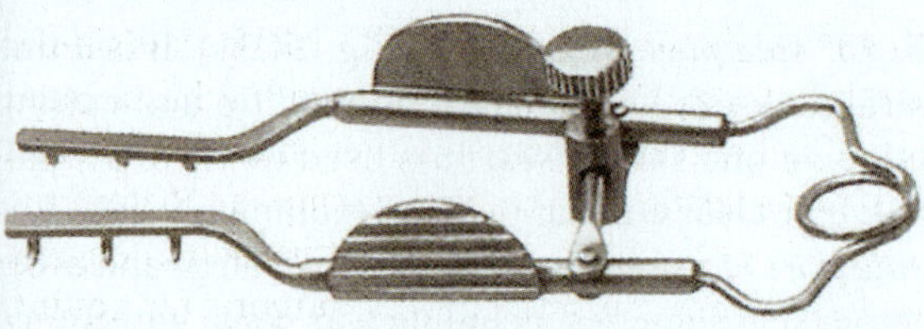

Fig. 24.21

6. *Iris retractor* (Fig. 24.22). It consists of a handle with a curved blade (which conforms to the pupillary margin) at one end. Its edges and corners are rounded so as not to damage either the iris or the lens capsule. ***Uses*:** To retract the upper edge of pupil in cryoextraction technique of ICCE and also to aspirate the lens matter from behind the iris at 12 O'clock position in ECCE.

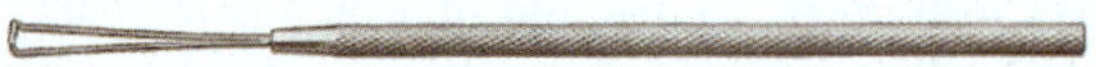

Fig. 24.22

IV. Needle holders

1. *Spring action (Barraquer's type) needle holder* (Fig. 24.23). These are available in various sizes with straight or curved tips, in different shapes and may be with or without locking system. The jaws of the needle holder are finely serrated to hold the fine needles firmly. ***Uses*:** Spring type needle holders are used for passing sutures in the conjunctiva, cornea, sclera and extraocular muscles.

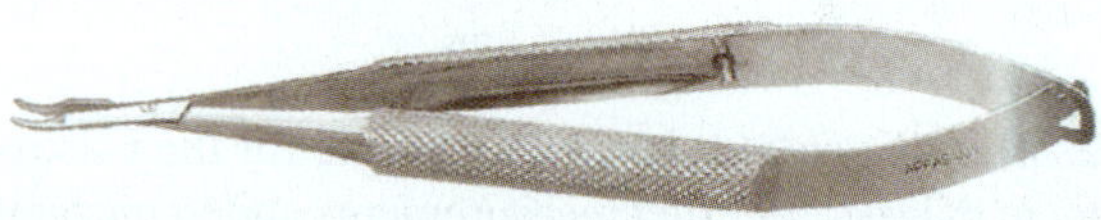

Fig. 24.23

2. *Castroviejo's needle holder* (Fig. 24.24). It is a medium-sized spring action needle holder with a S-shaped locking system. ***Uses.*** It is generally used in extraocular surgery e.g., conjunctival suturing, squint surgery etc. It can also be used for intraocular surgery.

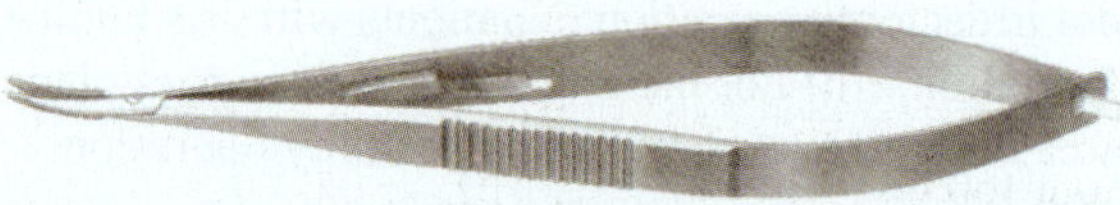

Fig. 24.24

3. *Arruga's, Stevens', Silcock's and Kelt needle holder* (Fig. 24.25). These are large needle holders and all are of similar type with slight model differences. The upper shank of these needle holders has a flat and broad plate to accommodate the surgeon's thumb. These are available with and without locking device. ***Uses*:** These are very commonly used in lid surgery and also for passing superior rectus suture.

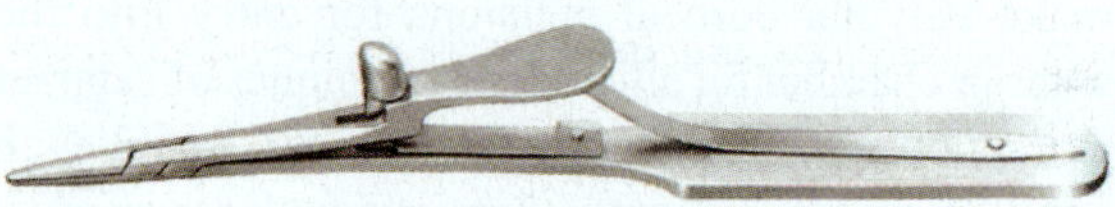

Fig. 24.25

V. Callipers and rules

1. ***Castroviejo calliper*** (Fig. 24.26). It is a divider-like instrument, to one arm of which is attached a graduated scale (in mm). Its other arm can be moved by a screw over the scale. ***Uses:*** It is used to take measurements during squint, ptosis, retinal detachment and pars plana vitrectomy surgery. It is also used to measure corneal diameter and visible horizontal iris diameter.

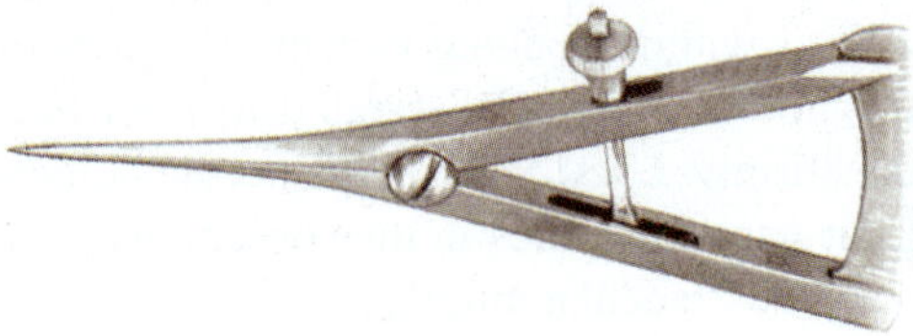

Fig. 24.26

2. ***Metallic rule***: It is used as a scale for the Castroviejo calliper for exact measurements and to measure the palpebral aperture width.

V. Knives and knife-needles

1. ***Von Graefe's knife*** (Fig. 24.27). It is a long, narrow, thin and straight blade with a sharp tip and cutting edge on one side. It is not used presently. ***Uses:*** (i) Previously it was used for making an abinterno corneoscleral incision during cataract surgery and for iridectomy operation. (ii) It is also used for four-dot iridectomy operation in patients with iris bombe formation. (iii) For making a puncture in pars plana area during lensectomy and vitrectomy operation.

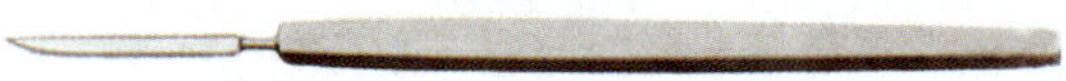

Fig. 24.27

2. ***Keratomes*** (Fig. 24.28). A keratome has a thin diamond-shaped blade with a sharp apex and two cutting edges. Straight as well as curved keratomes are available in various sizes (2.8 mm, 3 mm, 3.5 mm, 5.5 mm). Presently disposable curved keratomes are more commonly used. ***Uses.*** Keratomes are used to make valvular corneal incisions for entry into the anterior chamber for all modern techniques of cataract extraction viz. phacoemulsification, SICS and even conventional ECCE and other intraocular surgeries, e.g., iridectomies and paracentesis.

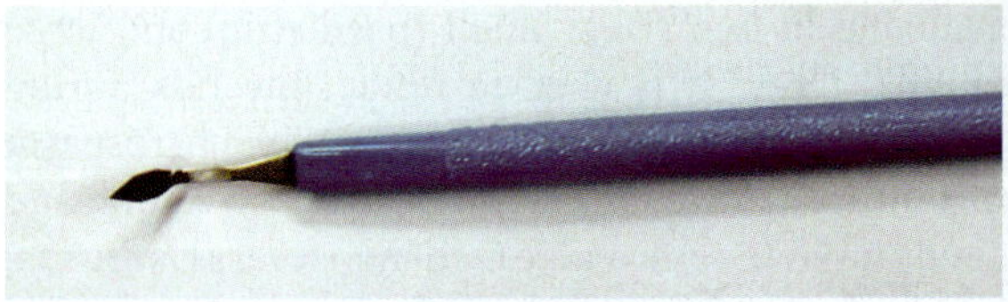

Fig. 24.28

3. ***Paracentesis needle*** (Fig. 24.29). It is a small lancet-shaped needle with sharp cutting edges resembling in appearance to a small keratome. It has got a guard to prevent inadvertent injury to the deeper structures. ***Uses:*** It is used for paracentesis and to make very small corneoscleral incisions.

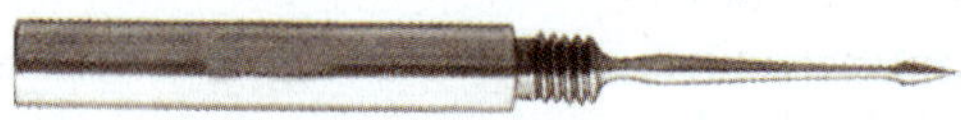

Fig. 24.29

4. ***Tooke's knife*** (Fig. 24.30). It has a short flat blade with a semicircular blunt dissecting edge, which is bevelled on both the surfaces like a chisel. ***Uses:*** (i) It can be used to separate the conjunctiva and subconjunctival tissue from the sclera and limbus when limbal based flap is made for trabeculectomy surgery. (ii) It can also be used to separate partial thickness lamellae of sclera during trabeculectomy. (iii) To separate pterygium head or limbal dermoid from the underlying corneal lamellae. (iv) To separate corneal lamellae in lamellar keratoplasty.

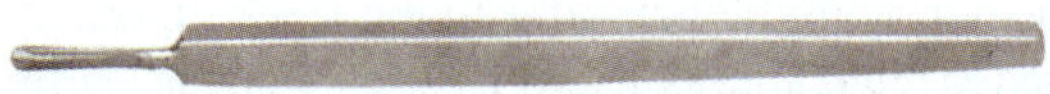

Fig. 24.30

5. ***15° side port entry blade*** (Fig. 24.31). It is a fine straight knife with a sharp pointed tip and cutting edge on one side. ***Uses.*** It is used to make a small valvular clear corneal incision (commonly called as *side port incision*) in phacoemulsification and other intraocular surgeries including pars plana vitrectomy.

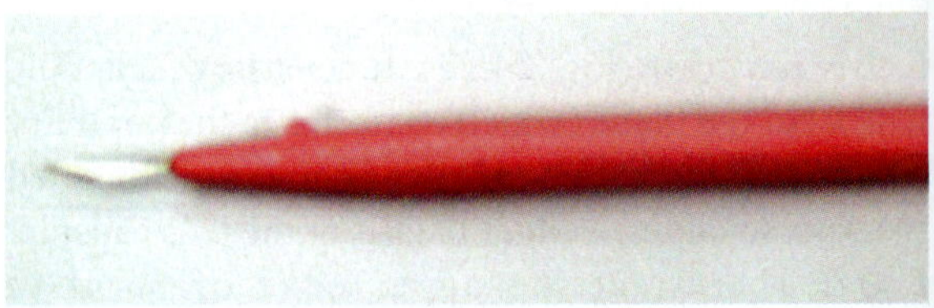

Fig. 24.31

6. *MVR or V lance blade* (Fig. 24.32). It is a fine straight but triangular knife similar to 15° side port entry blade but with cutting edges on both sides. ***Uses.*** Its uses are similar to 15° side port entry blade.

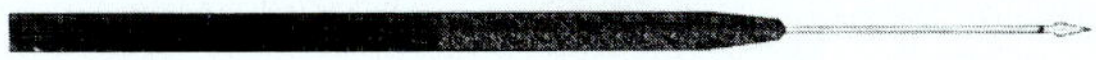

Fig. 24.32

7. *Cystitome or capsulotome* (Fig. 24.33). It is a small needle knife with a bent tip which is sharp on both the edges. Presently disposable cystitome is prepared by bending the disposable 26 gauge or 30 gauge hypodermic needle. ***Uses:*** It is used for doing anterior capsulotomy or capsulorhexis during extracapsular cataract extraction.

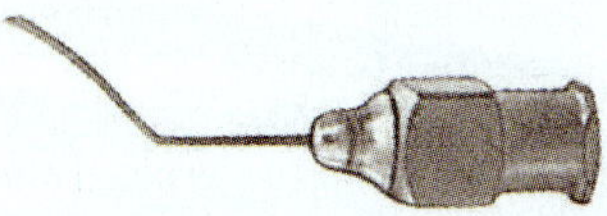

Fig. 24.33

8. *Foreign body spud* (Fig. 24.34). It has a small, stout and flat blade with blunt tip and edges on both sides. ***Uses:*** It is used to remove corneal foreign body.

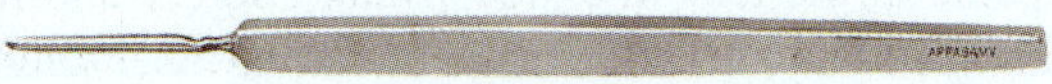

Fig. 24.34

9. *Razor blade fragment with blade holder*. Razor blade fragment holder (Fig. 24.35) is designed to hold the razor blade fragment firmly in its jaws and has a locking device. The razor blade fragments broken to a uniform size and shape have the sharpest possible metal edge with an absolute point. Presently pre-sterilized razor blade fragments mounted on a disposable plastic handle (Fig. 24.36) are also being preferred. ***Uses:*** It is the most commonly used cutting device for making incisions in cataract, glaucoma, keratoplasty, sclerotomy, pterygium and many other operations.

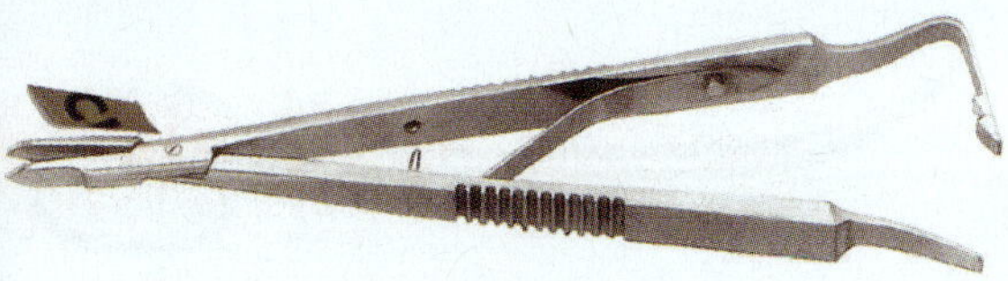

Fig. 24.35

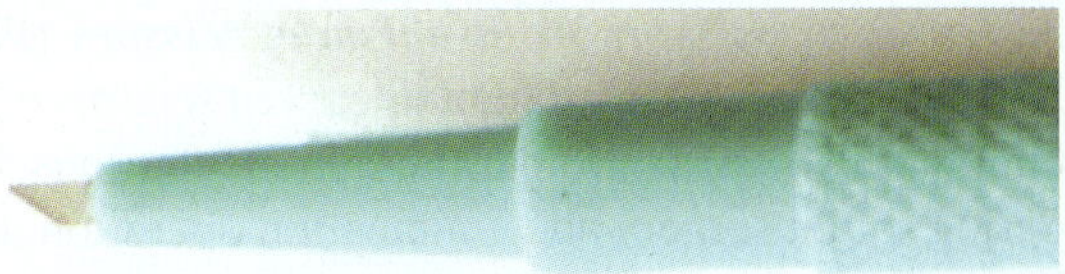

Fig. 24.36

10. *Crescent knife* (Fig. 24.37). It is blunt-tipped, bevel up knife having cut-splitting action at the tip and at both sides. Its blade is curved and either mounted on a plastic handle (disposable) or can be fixed with metallic handle. ***Uses:*** It is used to make tunnel incision in the sclera and cornea for phacoemulsification, manual small incision cataract surgery (SICS), and sutureless trabeculectomy.

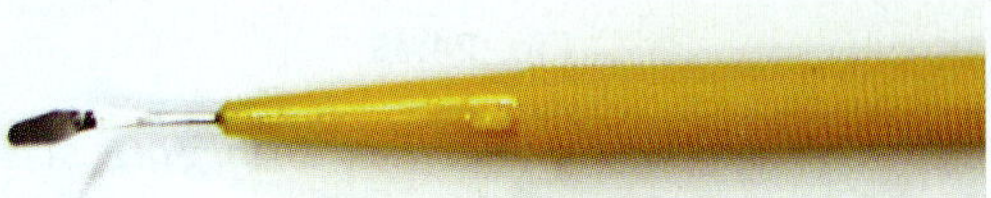

Fig. 24.37

VI. Scissors

1. *Plain straight scissors (ringed)* (Fig. 24.38): It is a fine pointed scissors with straight sharp cutting blades. ***Uses:*** It is used to cut conjunctival sutures, eyelashes, and muscles.

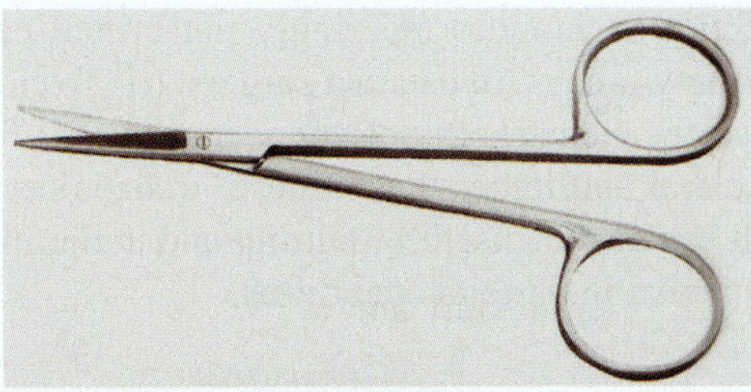

Fig. 24.38

2. *Plain curved scissors (ringed)* (Fig. 24.39). It is a fine pointed scissors with curved, sharp cutting blades. ***Uses:*** It is used to cut and undermine conjunctiva in various operations and to undermine skin during operations on lids and lacrimal sac.

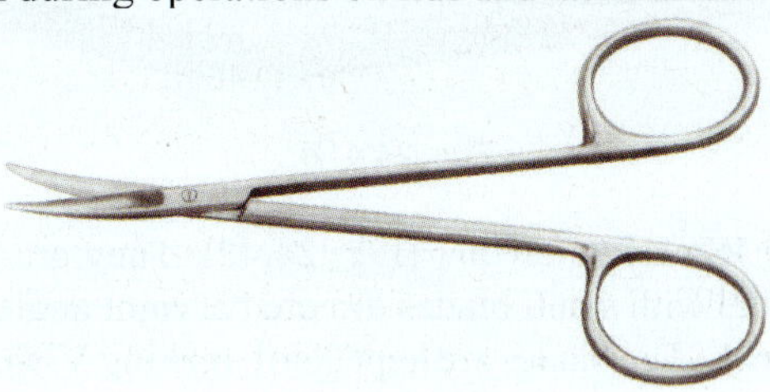

Fig. 24.39

3. ***Tenotomy scissors or strabismus scissors*** (Fig. 24.40). They are plain straight or curved scissors with blunt ends. ***Uses:*** (i) To cut the extraocular muscles during squint surgery and enucleation operation. (ii) To separate the delicate tissues without damaging the surrounding area in oculoplastic operations and squint surgery.

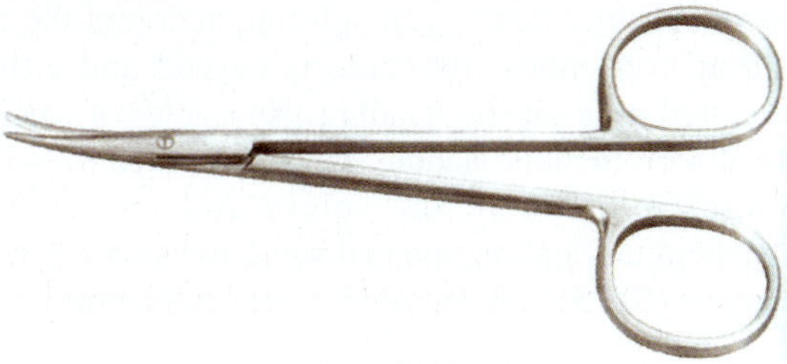

Fig. 24.40

4. ***Corneal scissors or section enlarging scissors*** (Fig. 24.41 A and B). They are fine curved scissors. Their cutting blades are kept apart by spring action. They are available in various shapes and sizes. The universal corneal scissors can be used for both sides while right and left curved corneal scissors are separated for the two sides. ***Uses:*** (i) These are used to enlarge corneal or corneoscleral incision for conventional intracapsular and extracapsular cataract extraction techniques (sparingly performed procedures now-a-days) of cataract surgery. (ii) To enlarge corneal incision in keratoplasty operation. (iii) To cut the scleral and trabecular tissue in trabeculectomy. (iv) It can also be used for cutting and undermining conjunctiva in various operations.

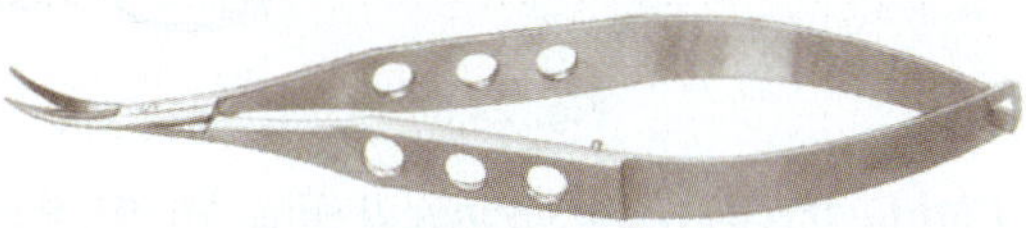

Fig. 24.41A

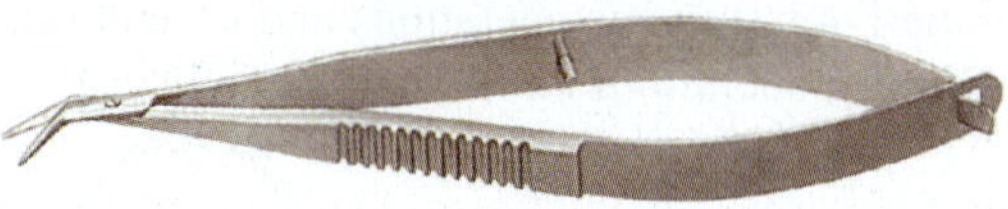

Fig. 24.41B

5. ***de Wecker's scissors*** (Fig. 24.42). They are fine scissors with small blades directed at right angles to the arms. The blades are kept apart, making V-shape, by spring action. ***Uses:*** It is used to perform iridectomy, iridotomy and to cut the prolapsed form vitreous and pupillary membrane.

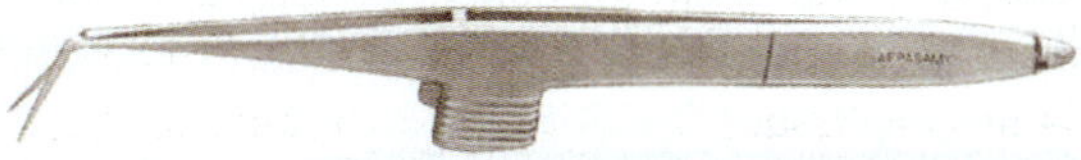

Fig. 24.42

6. ***Spring scissors (Westcott's)*** (Fig. 24.43). They are stout scissors available with straight or curved blades with sharp or blunt tips. The blades are kept apart by spring action. ***Uses:*** They are used as a handy alternative to plain straight and plain curved ringed scissors for cutting and undermining conjunctiva in various operations and to cut sutures.

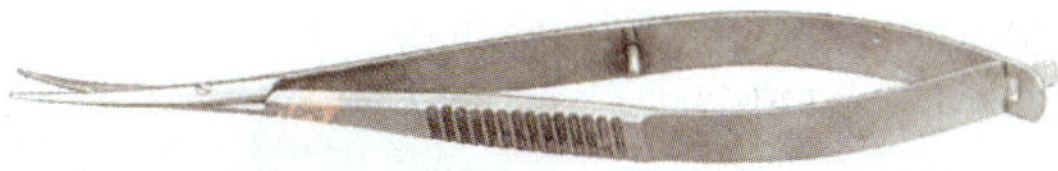

Fig. 24.43

7. ***Vannas scissors*** (Fig. 24.44). These are very fine delicate scissors with small cutting blades kept apart by spring action. The blades may be straight or curved. ***Uses:*** (i) These are used for cutting anterior capsule of the lens in extracapsular surgery and for cutting 10-0 nylon sutures. (ii) For cutting inner scleral flap in trabeculectomy. (iii) For doing pupillary sphincterotomy. (iv) For performing iridectomy. (v) For cutting pupillary membrane.

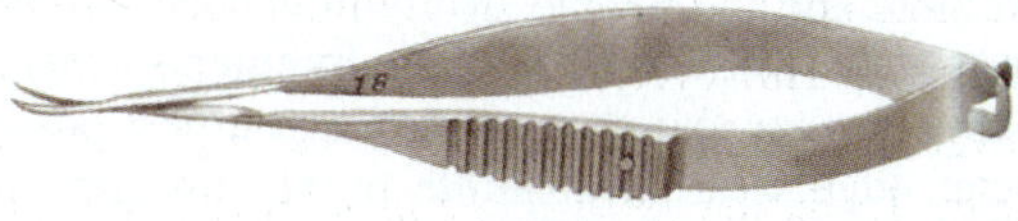

Fig. 24.44

8. ***Enucleation scissors*** (Fig. 24.45). They are large, stout and strong scissors having curved sharp blades with blunt ends. ***Uses:*** They are used to cut the optic nerve during enucleation operation.

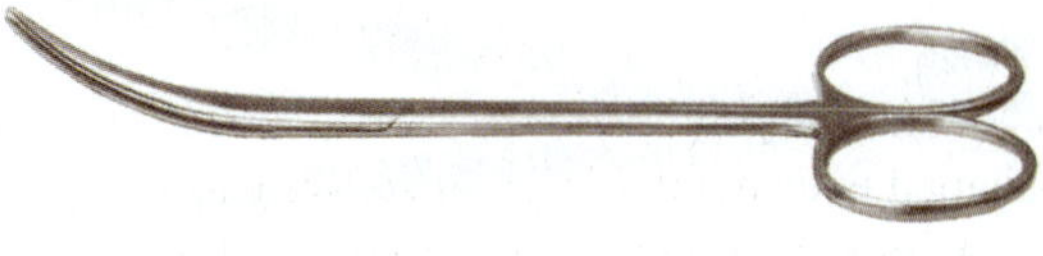

Fig. 24.45

VII. Clamps

1. ***Lid clamp or entropion clamp*** (Fig. 24.46). It consists of a D-shaped plate opposed by a U-shaped rim, which when tightened with the help of a screw, clamps the tissues. Two clamps are required; one can be used for right upper and left lower lid and the second for right lower and left upper lid. While applying the lid clamp, the plate is kept towards the conjunctival side, the rim on the skin side, and the handle is always situated on the temporal side. ***Advantage over lid spatula:*** It is a self-retaining instrument and does not need an assistant to hold. ***Disadvantages:*** (i) Operative field is less. (ii) Pressure necrosis can occur if fitted tightly. ***Uses:*** It is used in lid surgery e.g., entropion, and ectropion corrections. It protects the eyeball, supports the lid tissue and provides haemostasis during surgery.

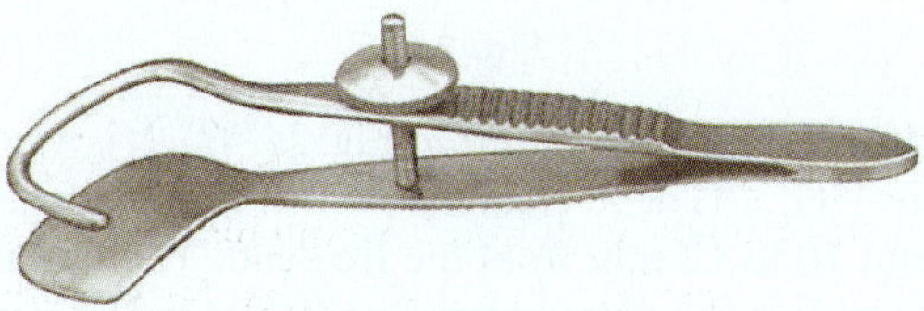

Fig. 24.46

2. ***Chalazion clamp*** (Fig. 24.47). It consists of two limbs like a forceps, which can be clamped with the help of a screw. The tip of one limb is flattened in the form of round disc while the tip of the other arm has a small circular ring. Usually the flat disc is applied on the skin side and ring on the conjunctival side of the chalazion. However, rarely when the chalazion points towards the skin, the ring side is applied to the skin. ***Uses:*** To fix the chalazion and achieve haemostasis during the incision and curettage operation.

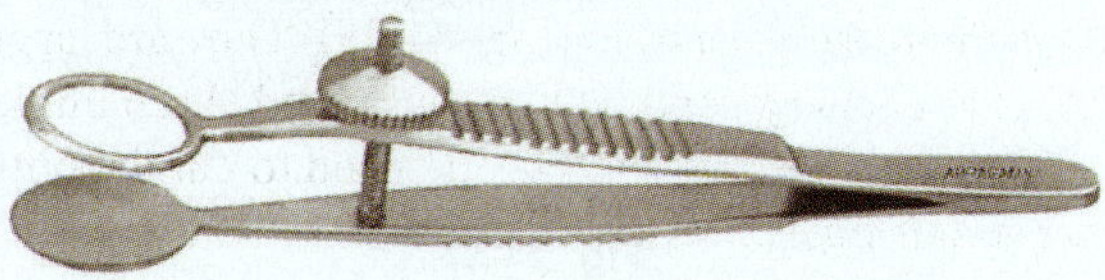

Fig. 24.47

3. ***Ptosis clamp*** (Fig. 24.48). It is like a forceps with J-shaped ends having internal serrations. The clamp has a locking mechanism. ***Use:*** To hold levator palpebrae superioris muscle during ptosis surgery.

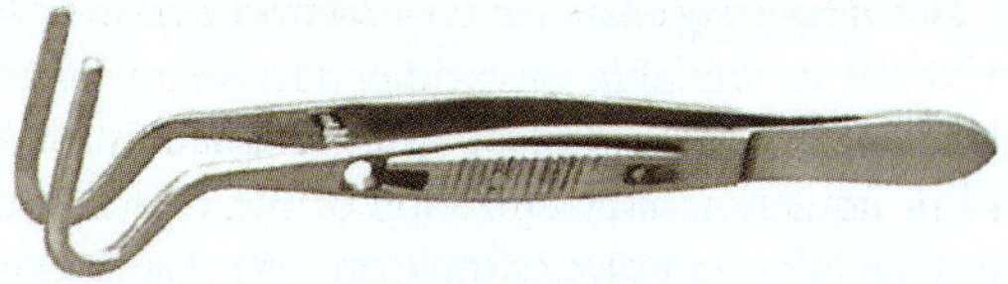

Fig. 24.48

VIII. Additional instruments for cataract surgery

1. ***Lens spatula*** (Fig. 24.49). It is a flat metallic handle with tiny spoon-shaped ends. It is used to apply counter-pressure at 12 O'clock position during expression of nucleus in extracapsular cataract extraction. In the era of ICCE, it was used in a similar way to extract cataractous lens in Smith's technique.

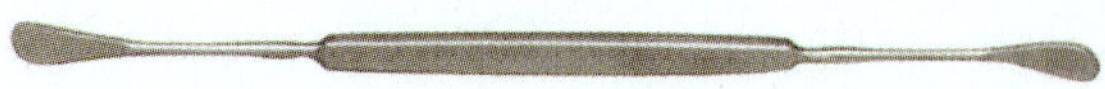

Fig. 24.49

2. ***Wire vectis*** (Fig. 24.50). It is a wire loop attached to a metallic handle. ***Uses:*** It is used to remove subluxated lens and anteriorly dislocated lens in ICCE technique and the nucleus in ECCE technique.

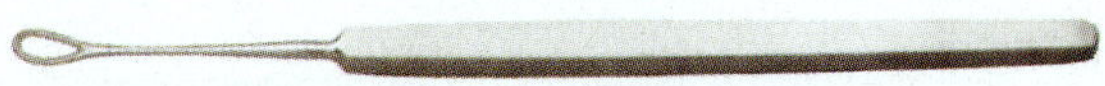

Fig. 24.50

3. ***Irrigating wire vectis*** (Fig. 24.51). It is a modified vectis in which the loop is made of a thick hollow wire. The anterior end of the loop has three 0.3 mm openings. The posterior end of the loop is continuous with a hollow handle. The posterior end of the hollow handle has a hub similar to that of a hypodermic needle to which is attached a syringe or infusion set. The size of the loop of the vectis is variable. In commonly used wire vectis the loop is 4 mm in width and about 8-9 mm in length. The superior surface of the loop has a slight concavity to accommodate the lens nucleus. ***Uses.*** Irrigating wire vectis is most commonly used to deliver nucleus in the manual small incision cataract surgery (SICS) and in conventional ECCE by hydroexpression or viscoexpression technique.

Fig. 24.51

4. *Two-way irrigation and aspiration cannula* (Fig. 24.52). It is available in various designs, commonly used are Simcoe's classical or reverse cannula. ***Uses:*** (i) For irrigation and aspiration of the lens matter in extracapsular cataract extraction. (ii) Aspiration of hyphaema.

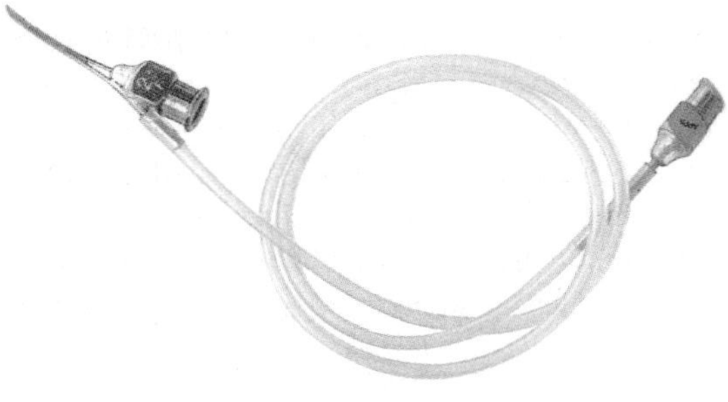

Fig. 24.52

5. *Iris repositor* (Fig. 24.53). It consists of a delicate, flat, malleable, straight or bent blade with blunt edges and tip attached to a handle. ***Uses:*** (i) To reposit the iris in the anterior chamber in any intraocular surgery. (ii) To break synechiae at the pupillary margin.

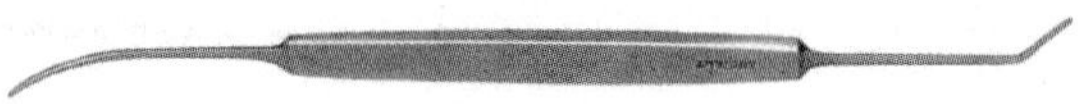

Fig. 24.53

IX. Additional instruments for intraocular lens implantation

For IOL implantation, the cataract surgery set should contain the following basic additional instruments:

1. *IOL holding forceps* (Fig. 24.54). It is a spring-action forceps with short, blunt and curved blades having smooth edges and tips with platform (no teeth or serrations). ***Use:*** To hold optic of non-foldable PMMA IOL during implantation.

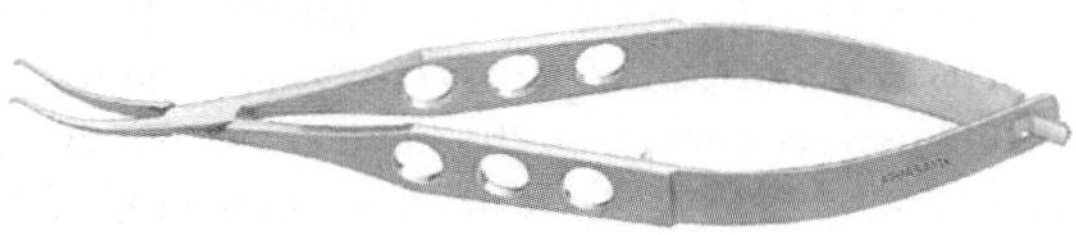

Fig. 24.54

2. *Kelman-McPherson forceps* (Fig. 24.55). These are fine forceps with bent limbs. ***Uses:*** (i)To hold the superior haptic of IOL during its placement. (ii) To tear off the anterior capsular flap in ECCE. (iii) Can be used for suture tying.

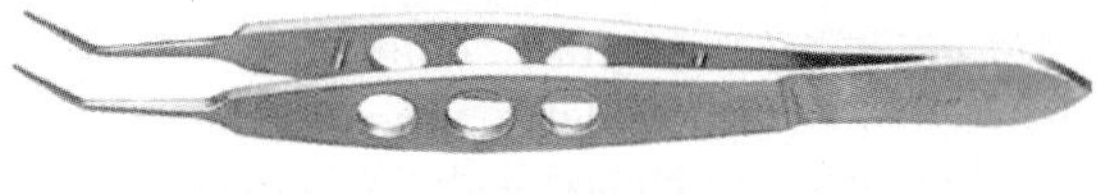

Fig. 24. 55

3. *Sinskey hook or IOL dialer* (Fig. 24.56). It is a fine but stout instrument with a bent tip. The tip engages the dialing holes of the IOL. ***Uses:*** (i) It is used to dial the PMMA non-foldable IOL for proper positioning in the capsular bag or ciliary sulcus. (ii) It can also be used to manipulate the nucleus in phacoemulsification surgery. Nucleus manipulation may be in the form of nucleus rotation in the capsular bag, cracking of the nucleus and feeding of the nuclear fragments into the phaco tip.

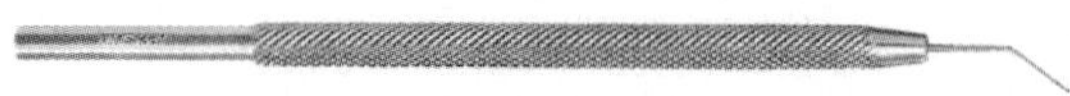

Fig. 24.56

4. *Hydrodissection cannula* (Fig. 24.57). It is a single bore 25G, 27G or 30 G cannula with a 45° angulation at about 10 to 12 mm from the free end. The tip at the free end can be flattened or bevelled. ***Uses.*** It is used to perform hydrodissection (separation of cortex from the posterior capsule) and hydrodelineation (separation of cortex from the nucleus) in phaco-emulsification and manual SICS. This cannula is attached to the syringe carrying irrigating fluid. For hydrodissection its tip is introduced beneath the anterior capsular margin after capsulorhexsis and fluid is injected to obtain subcapsular dissection.

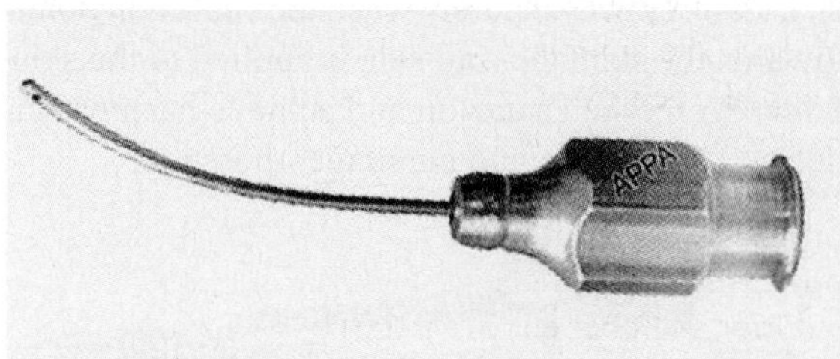

Fig. 24.57

5. *Chopper* (Fig. 24.58). The chopper is a fine instrument resembling sinskey hook in shape. The inner edge of the bent tip is cutting and may have different angles. ***Uses.*** It is used to split or chop the nucleus into smaller pieces and also for nuclear manipulation in phacoemulsification surgery.

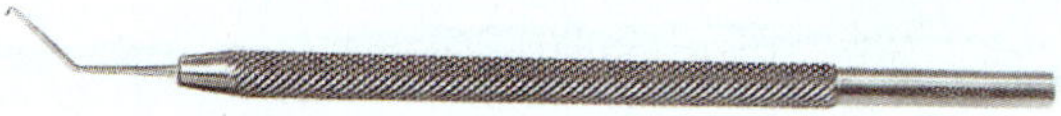

Fig. 24.58

6. ***Ring capsule polisher or posterior capsule polishing curette*** (Fig. 24.59). It consists of a long handle and a bent slender neck. The tip of the instrument has a tiny circular ring. ***Uses.*** It is used to clear and polish the posterior lens capsule to make it more clear in the extracapsular cataract surgery. It is specially used when a plaque or sticky cortex is adhered to the posterior capsule.

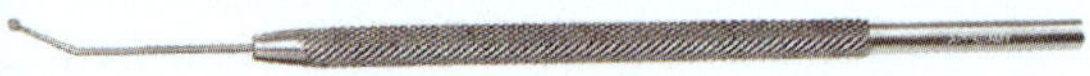

Fig. 24.59

X. Additional instruments for glaucoma surgery

1. ***Scleral punch*** (Fig. 24.60). It is similar in shape to corneal scissors with spring action mechanism. Its one blade is sharp and thick which presses into the second blade which is a hollow rectangular frame. ***Use:*** To perform punch sclerectomy during glaucoma surgery.

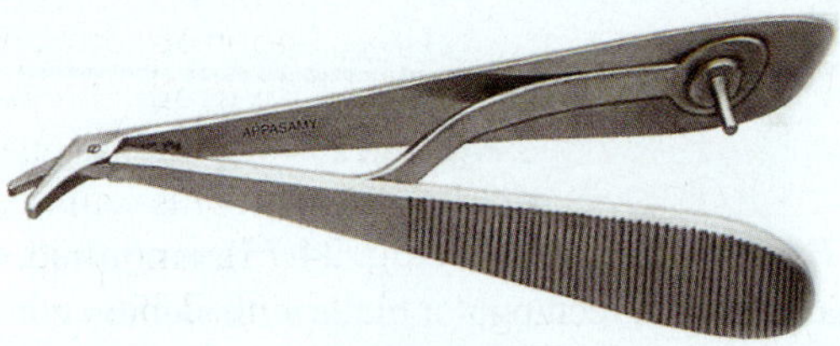

Fig. 24.60

2. ***Kelley's punch*** (Fig. 24.61). It consists of two blades. The inner larger blade is a stout thin rod with a cup like depression having sharp margins and facing backward. The outer smaller blade is a hollow tube which slides with a spring mechanism around the inner blade. While in use during trabeculectomy operation, its punch cuts the posterior lip of the anterior chamber entry site (see page 254).
Uses. It is used to punch out trabecular tissue in conventional as well as sutureless trabeculectomy operation.

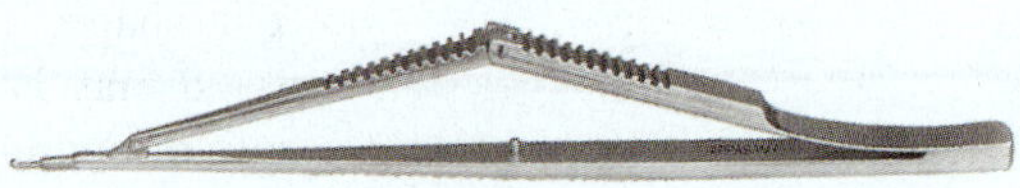

Fig. 24.61

XI. Additional instruments for lid surgery

1. ***Chalazion scoop*** (Fig. 24.62). It has a small cup with sharp margins attached to a narrow handle. ***Use:*** To scoop out contents of the chalazion during incision and curettage.

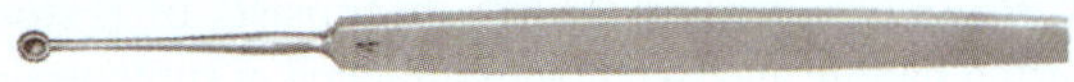

Fig. 24.62

2. ***Lid spatula*** (Fig. 24.63). It is a simple metal plate having slightly convex surfaces at either end. ***Uses:*** To protect the globe and support the lid during entropion, ectropion, ptosis and other lid surgeries.

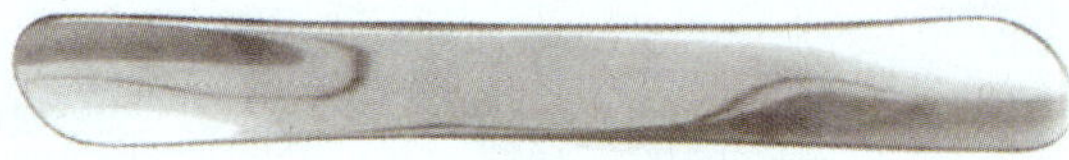

Fig. 24.63

XII. Additional instruments for lacrimal sac surgery (DCT and DCR)

1. ***Punctum dilator (Nettleship's)*** (Fig. 24.64). It has a cylindrical corrugated metal handle with a conical pointed tip. ***Uses***: To dilate the punctum and canaliculus during syringing, probing, dacryocystography, DCT and DCR procedures.

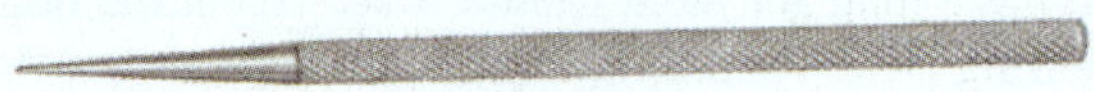

Fig. 24.64

2. ***Lacrimal probes (Bowman's)*** (Fig. 24.65). These are a set of straight metal wires of varying thickness (size 0-8) with blunt rounded ends and flattened central platform. ***Uses:*** (i) To probe nasolacrimal duct in congenital blockage. (ii) To identify the lacrimal sac during DCT and DCR operations.

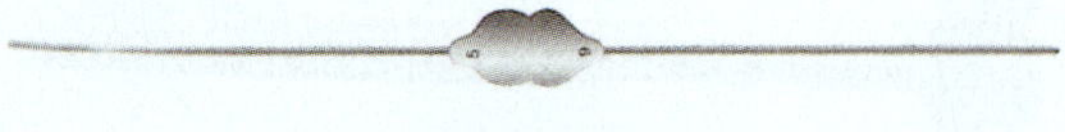

Fig. 24.65

3. ***Lacrimal cannula*** (Fig. 24.66). It is a long curved hypodermic needle with blunt tip. ***Uses:*** (i) For syringing the lacrimal passages. (ii) As AC cannula for putting air, tryphan blue dye, pilocarpine and balanced salt solution in the anterior chamber during intraocular surgery.

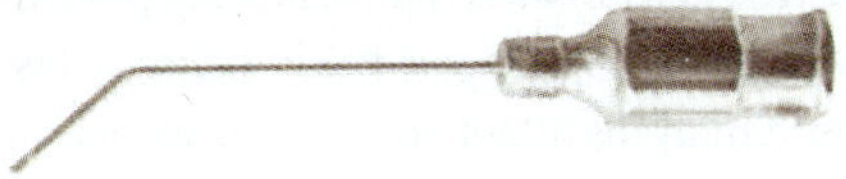

Fig. 24.66

4. ***Bone punch*** (Fig. 24.67). It consists of a stout spring handle and two blades attached at right angle. The upper blade has a small hole with a sharp cutting edge. The lower blade has a cup-like depression. ***Uses:*** It is used to enlarge the bony opening during DCR operation by punching the bone from margins of the opening. Carelessness during this step can cause accidental damage to the nasal mucosa and the nasal septum.

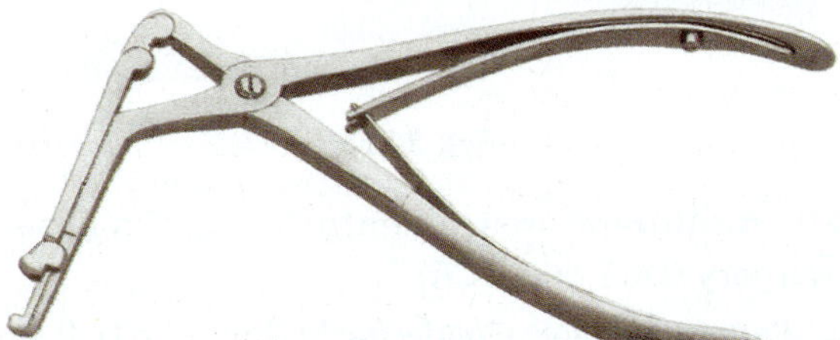

Fig. 24.67

5. ***Chisel*** (Fig. 24.68). It consists of a blade having a sharp-cutting straight edge with one surface bevelled. It has a long and stout handle. ***Use:*** To cut the bone during DCR and orbitotomy operations.

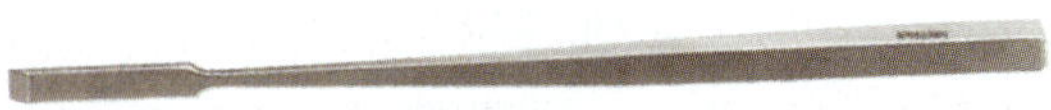

Fig. 24.68

6. ***Hammer*** (Fig. 24.69). It is a small steel hammer attached to a corrugated handle. ***Use:*** To hammer the chisel during DCR and orbitotomy operations.

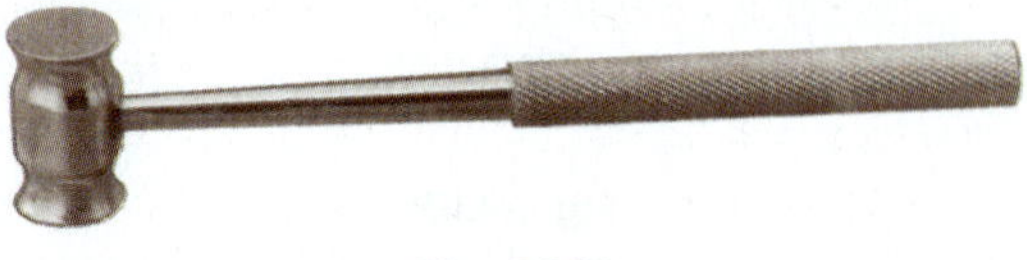

Fig. 24.69

7. ***Lacrimal sac dissector and curette*** (Fig. 24.70). It is a cylindrical instrument, one end of which is a blunt-tipped dissector and the other end is curetted. ***Use:*** In lacrimal sac surgery.

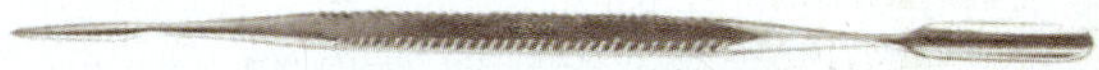

Fig. 24.70

8. ***Bone gouge*** (Fig. 24.71). It consists of a stout metallic handle, one end of which is longitudinally scooped. The edges of the scoop are sharp. ***Use:*** To smoothen the irregularly cut margins of the bone by nibbling small projecting bone and in DCR operation and in orbitotomy operation.

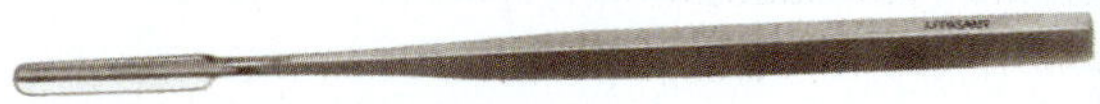

Fig. 24.71

XIII. Additional instruments for enucleation and evisceration

1. ***Optic nerve guide (enucleation spoon)*** (Fig. 24.72). It is a spoon-shaped instrument with a central cleavage. ***Use:*** To engage the optic nerve during enucleation.

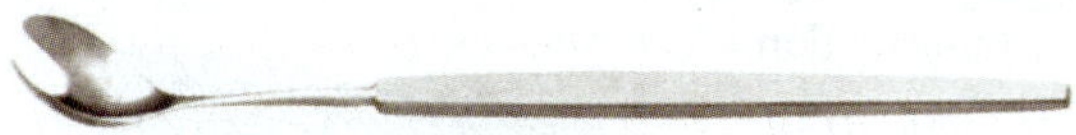

Fig. 24.72

2. ***Evisceration spatula*** (Fig. 24.73). It consists of a small but stout rectangular blade with slightly convex surface and blunt edges attached to a handle. ***Use:*** To separate out the uveal tissue from the sclera during evisceration operation.

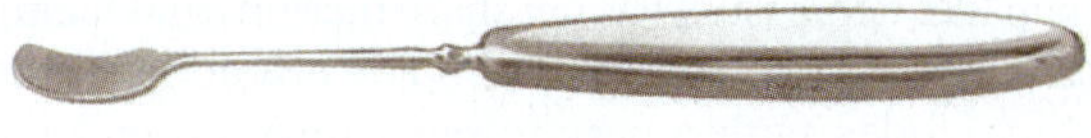

Fig. 24.73

3. ***Evisceration curette*** (Fig. 24.74). It consists of an oval or rounded shallow cup with blunt margins attached to a stout handle. ***Use:*** To curette out the intraocular contents during evisceration operation.

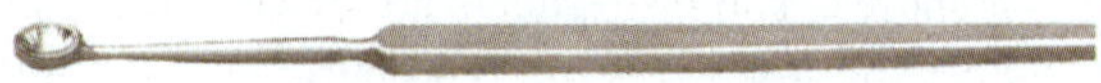

Fig. 24.74

STERILIZATION, DISINFECTION AND FUMIGATION

STERILIZATION AND DISINFECTION

It is a process which kills or removes all micro-organisms including bacterial spores from an article, surface or medium. It must be differentiated from disinfection which destroys pathogenic micro-organisms but does not kill or remove spores.

Sterilization can be accomplished by *physical agents* (viz. sunlight, heat, filtration and radiation) and *chemical agents* (such as alcohols, aldehydes, halogens, phenol, surface acting agents and gases).

Methods

(A) *Heat sterilization*

Both dry and moist heat can be used.

Dry heat sterilization methods

1. *Flaming.* It can be used to sterilize points of forceps, hypodermic needles, tips of AC cannula and scraping spatulas. The instrument is held in a bunsen flame till it becomes red hot.
2. *Incineration.* It is used to destroy soiled dressings, beddings and pathological materials.
3. *Hot air oven.* It is the most commonly used method of sterilization by dry heat. It kills bacteria, spores and viruses. This method is employed to sterilize instruments like forceps, scissors, scalpels, glass syringes, glassware etc. The item must be double wrapped and kept at 150° C for 2 hours.

Moist heat sterilization methods

1. *Boiling.* It kills bacteria and viruses. Heavier metallic ophthalmic instruments, e.g., Bard-Parker handles, lid guards etc. can be sterilized by boiling in water for 30 minutes. This method, however, blunts the cutting instruments.
2. *Steaming.* It kills most bacteria and viruses, but not spores. The instruments are placed on a shelf above the level of water and steamed for about 30 minutes. Most of the metallic instruments e.g., scissors and knives can be sterilized by this method.
3. *Autoclaving (steam under pressure).*It is the most widely used method for sterilization. It is based on the principle that at boiling point of water, the vapour pressure equates the atmospheric pressure. So, if the pressure is increased, boiling point tends to rise, which increases the penetrating power of the steam.

Autoclaving at 121° C under 15 1b/in^2 pressure for 20 min. or at 116° C under 10 1b/in^2 pressure for 40 min. kills bacteria, spores and viruses. This method is suitable for sterilizing various instruments, linen, glasswares, rubber goods, gowns, towels, gloves dressings and eyedrops.

(B) *Chemical sterilization*

1. *Savlon.* It comprises of cetavlon or cetrimide and chlorhexidine. Cetavlon is a surface active agent and chlorhexidine is a phenol. It is active against most Gram-positive organisms. It is used for cleaning/preparation of skin. Scissors, catheters, knives etc. may also be sterilized with it.
2. *Spirit (95% alcohol).* It kills bacteria and spores, but not viruses. It is mostly used with savlon.
3. *Methylated spirit.* It is 70 percent isopropyl alcohol. Schiotz tonometer can be sterilized by it.
4. *Formaldehyde*
   i. *Formalin.* 10 percent solution of formalin has a marked bactericidal, sporicidal and some viricidal activity. It is suitable for cryoextractor probes and heat sensitive instruments.
   ii. *Formaldehyde gas.* It may be used for fumigating wards, sick rooms and laboratories. But this gas is irritant and toxic when inhaled.
5. *Glutaraldehyde (2%).* It is available as 'Cidex' solution. It has a special activity against tubercle bacilli, fungi and viruses. It is mostly used for sterilising endoscopes because it has no damaging effect on the lenses. It can be safely used for catheters, face-masks, anaesthetic tubes and metal instruments. However, it is not suitable for silicone tubing. It is specially used to sterilize sharp instruments, as it does not affect the sharpness. In three hours, the instruments are free of pathogens and spores. Instruments should be thoroughly washed with sterile distilled water before use.

6. *Hydrogen peroxide.* 3 percent solution of H_2O_2 is used for sterilisation of applanation tonometers, prisms and ophthalmoscopy lenses. It is specially active against AIDS and herpes viruses.
7. *Ethylene oxide gas:* It is a highly inflammable gas and is usually mixed with an inert gas like nitrogen or carbon dioxide. It denatures the protein molecules. It is effective against almost all bacteria, spores and viruses. Goniotomy lenses, indirect ophthalmoscopy lenses, DCR tubings and cryoprobes can be sterilized with it.
8. *Acetone.* Use of acetone is a quick and cheap method of sterilising instruments. Instruments should be kept in acetone for 5 minutes and then thoroughly washed with sterile water before use.

(C) Radiation sterilization

1. ***Ionising radiations**:* These include X-rays, gamma-rays, cosmic rays. They are highly lethal to DNA and thus kill all types of micro-organisms. They can penetrate solids and liquids without raising the temperature appreciably (cold sterilisation). They are used for sterilizing plastic syringes, swabs, catheters, tubings etc.

2. ***Non-ionising radiations**:* They act as a form of hot air sterilization since they are absorbed as heat. They include the infrared rays which is used for rapid mass sterilization of disposable syringes.

FUMIGATION OF OPERATION THEATRE

Fumigation refers to disinfection of the operating room by exposure to the fumes of a vaporised disinfectant. *Formaldehyde* is an effective agent commonly used to sterilize the operating room. For optimum disinfection, formaldehyde fumigation is recommended fortnightly as a routine and at the end of an operating session of a grossly infected case.

Method of fumigation involves following steps:

- *Cleaning and scrubing* of the operating room is done thoroughly.
- *Carbolisation* of the floor is carried out after the cleaning.
- *Sealing* of all the apertures in the room is done prior to fumigation leaving only one door open.
- *Generation of formaldehyde* is done by addition of 150 gm of potassium permanganate ($KMnO_4$) to 280 ml of formalin in a steel bucket for every 1000 cubic feet of room volume. Alternatively, 500 ml of 40% formaldehyde in one litre of water is put into an electric boiler or in a large bowl placed on a electric hot plate with safety cut-out when dry on boiling.
- *Closure and sealing of the door* is done quickly. After formaldehyde vapour is generated the room should be left closed for 24 to 48 hours.
- *Neutralization of formaldehyde* is then carried out with ammonium solution left in the operating room for a few hours. One litre of ammonium solution plus one litre of water is required to neutralize every litre of 40% formaldehyde used.
- *Replacement of left out formalin with air.* Subsequently the room doors may be opened for a short period or the air-conditioning be switched on to replace the formalin with air.

RELATED QUESTIONS

ANAESTHESIA FOR OCULAR SURGERY

How topical ocular anaesthesia is achieved? What are its indications?

Topical ocular anaesthesia is achieved by instillation of 2 to 4% xylocaine or 1% amethocaine, 4 times every 4 minute.

Indications

- For minor procedures like removal of corneal foreign body, removal of stitches etc.
- Along with retrobulbar block.
- Recently, phacoemulsification operation is being done under topical anaesthesia.

What are various techniques of facial block anaesthesia?

- *Van Lint's block:* Terminal branches of facial nerve are blocked by injecting 2.5 ml of anaesthetic solution in deeper tissues just above the eyebrows and just below the inferior orbital margin.
- *O'Brien's block:* Facial nerve is blocked at the neck of mandible
- *Nadbath block:* Facial nerve is blocked near the stylomastoid foramen.
- *Atkinson's block:* Only superior branches of facial nerve are blocked by an injection at the inferior margin of zygomatic bone.

Where injection is made for retrobulbar block?

For a retrobulbar block, 2 ml of 2% xylocaine is injected into the muscle cone.

What are the effects of retrobulbar block ?

- Ciliary nerve and ciliary ganglion block
- Ocular akinesia
- Ocular anaesthesia and analgesia
- Dilatation of the pupil
- Ocular hypotony

Enumerate complications of retrobulbar block.

- Retrobulbar haemorrhage
- Globe perforation
- Optic nerve injury
- Extraocular muscle palsies

What is the technique of peribulbar block?

An anaesthetic solution, 6 to 9 ml (a mixture of 2% xylocaine and 0.5-0.75% bupivacaine) in a ratio of 2:1 with hyaluronidase 5 I.U./ml with or without adrenaline 1:1 lac is injected into the peripheral orbital space.

What are the advantages of peribulbar block?

- No separate facial block is required.
- Complications associated with retrobulbar block are almost eliminated.

OPHTHALMIC INSTRUMENTS AND EYE OPERATIONS

Usually a student is asked to describe a particular ophthalmic instrument in reference to following aspects:

- Identification of the instrument
- Methods of its sterilization
- Uses of the instrument
- Advantages or disadvantages of the use of any particular instrument.

OPERATIONS FOR CATARACT EXTRACTION

Name the instruments required for the basic intraocular surgery set.

The instruments required include superior rectus holding forceps, Stevens' needle holder, artery forceps, plane forceps, curved ringed scissors, heat cautery or wet-field cautery, razor–blade fragment holder, corneo scleral suturing forceps, corneoscleral section enlarging scissors, iris forceps, deWecker's iridectomy scissors, lens spatula, lens hook, anterior chamber cannula, iris repositor, spring action fine needle holder.

These instruments form the basic intraocular surgery set.

Name the additional instruments required for extracapsular cataract extraction.

Cystitome, Vannas' scissors, McPherson's forceps, two-way irrigation-aspiration cannula; posterior capsule polisher.

Name (pick up) the additional instruments required for an intraocular lens implantation.

Anterior chamber cannula for injecting viscoelastic substance, intraocular lens (implant) holding forceps, foldable IOL injector and intraocular lens dialer.

What are the advantages of ECCE over ICCE?

1. Extracapsular cataract extraction is a universal operation and can be performed at all ages, except when zonules are not intact. While ICCE cannot be performed below 40 years of age.
2. Posterior chamber IOL can be implanted after ECCE, while it cannot be implanted after ICCE.
3. Postoperative vitreous-related problems (such as herniation in anterior chamber, pupillary block and vitreous touch syndrome) associated with ICCE are not seen after ECCE.
4. Incidence of postoperative complications such as endophthalmitis, cystoid macular oedema and retinal detachment is much less after ECCE as compared to that after ICCE.

What are the advantages of ICCE over ECCE?

1. The technique of ICCE as compared to ECCE is simple, cheap, easy and does not need sophisticated microinstruments.
2. Postoperative opacification of posterior capsule is seen in a significant number of cases after ECCE. No such problem is there after ICCE.
3. ICCE is less time consuming and hence more useful than ECCE for mass scale operations in eyecamps.

Name the different techniques of extracapsular cataract extraction.

1. Discission or needling (obsolete)
2. Linear extraction or curette evacuation (obsolete)
3. Modern extracapsular cataract extraction (ECCE)
4. Small incision cataract surgery (SICS)
5. Lensectomy
6. Phacoemulsification

What are the main steps of lens removal in ECCE operation ?

1. Anterior capsulotomy
2. Removal of nucleus
3. Aspiration of the cortical lens matter

Name the techniques of anterior capsulotomy

1. Can-opener technique
2. Linear capsulotomy (envelope technique)
3. Continuous circular capsulorhexis (CCC)

What is phacoemulsification ?

Phacoemulsification is a technique of extracapsular cataract extraction in which after the removal of anterior capsule (by capsulorhexis), the lens nucleus is emulsified and aspirated with the probe of a phacoemulsification machine.

What are the advantages of phacoemulsification over the conventional ECCE operation?

1. Corneoscleral incision required is very small (3 mm). Therefore, sutureless surgery is possible with a self-sealing scleral tunnel incision
2. Early visual rehabilitation of the patient
3. Very less astigmatism

What are the main types of intraocular lenses (IOL)?

The major classes of IOL based on the method of fixation in the eye are as follows:

1. Anterior chamber IOL, e.g., 'Kelman multiflex IOL'
2. Iris supported lenses, e.g., Singh-Worst's iris claw lens
3. Posterior chamber IOL

When and who preformed the first successful intraocular implant operation?

Harold Ridley, a British ophthalmologist, performed the first IOL implantation on November 29, 1949.

Name a few per operative complications of cataract operation.

1. Injury to cornea (Descemet's detachment)
2. Accidental rupture of the lens capsule
3. Vitreous loss
4. Expulsive choroidal haemorrhage

Name some early postoperative complications of cataract extraction.

1. Hyphaema
2. Iris prolapse
3. Striate keratopathy
4. Flat (shallow) anterior chamber
5. Bacterial endophthalmitis

What are delayed complications of cataract extraction?

1. Cystoid macular oedema (CME)
2. Retinal detachment (RD)
3. Epithelial ingrowth
4. After-cataract

What are the types of after-cataract?

1. Thin membranous after-cataract (thickened posterior capsule).
2. Dense membranous after-cataract
3. Soemmerring's ring after-cataract
4. Elschnig's pearls

Name the IOL-related complications.

1. Malpositions of the IOL, e.g., inferior subluxation (Sunset syndrome), superior subluxation (Sunrise syndrome), dislocation of IOL in the vitreous cavity (lost lens syndrome)
2. Toxic lens syndrome (IOL-induced iritis).

What are the advantages of an IOL implantation over spectacle correction of aphakia?

1. No magnification of the object.
2. No problem of anisometropia in uniocular aphakia.
3. Elimination of aberrations and prismatic effect of thick glasses.
4. Wider and better field of vision.
5. Cosmetically more acceptable.

What is postoperative management of cataract operation ?

1. The patient is asked to lie quietly upon his/her back for about one hour and advised to take nil orally.
2. For mild to moderate postoperative pain, injection diclofenac sodium (Voveran) may be given intramuscularly.
3. In the morning after about 24 hours of operation, bandage is removed and the eye is inspected thoroughly for any postoperative complication. Under normal circumstances, eye is opened with the use of one drop of 1 percent cyclopentolate, one drop of antibiotic and steroid drops and tinted glasses are advised.
4. Antibiotic steroid eyedrops are continued for four times, three times, two times and then once a day for 2 weeks each.
5. Final spectacles are prescribed after about 8 weeks of operation

What do you understand by primary and secondary IOL implantation?

Primary IOL implantation refers to the use of IOL during surgery for cataract, while secondary IOL is implanted to correct aphakia in a previously operated eye.

How will you calculate the power of posterior chamber IOL to be implanted?

The power of the IOL to be implanted can be calculated using keratometry and A-scan ultrasound. SRK formula commonly employed to calculate IOL power is as follows:

$P = A - 2.5L - 0.9K$; where P = IOL power in dioptres, A = specific constant of the IOL, L= axial length of the eyeball in mm and K= average keratometric reading.

IRIDECTOMY OPERATION

What is iridectomy and what are its types?

Iridectomy is an abscission of a part of the iris. It is of the following types:

- Peripheral iridectomy
- Key-hole iridectomy
- Broad or sector iridectomy

What are the indications of iridectomy operation?

1. Abscission of the prolapsed iris
2. For optical purposes (optical iridectomy)
3. As a part of glaucoma operation
4. For removal of foreign body, cyst or tumour of the iris

What is iridotomy and how is it performed?

Iridotomy means just incising a part of the iris. It can be performed by two methods:

- Surgical iridotomy
- Laser iridotomy

What are indications of iridotomy operation?

1. Laser iridotomy for primary narrow-angle glaucoma
2. Four-dot iridotomy for iris bombe

SURGICAL PROCEDURES FOR GLAUCOMA

Name the various surgical procedures for glaucoma.

1. Peripheral iridectomy
2. Goniotomy
3. Trabeculotomy
4. Filtration operations
5. Seton operation (glaucoma valve operation)
6. Cycloablative procedures

Peripheral iridectomy operation is performed for which type of glaucoma?

- Primary angle closure suspect (PACS) with positive provocative test.
- PAC suspect in fellow eye of patient with PAC glaucoma in other eye.
- Primary angle closure (manifest).
- Primary angle closure glaucoma.

What are filtration operations for glaucoma?

In filtration operations, passage is made for the drainage of aqueous humour into the subconjunctival space. Trabeculectomy is presently the most frequently performed filtration surgery. Other filtration operations which are not performed now included: Elliot's sclerocorneal trephining, punch sclerectomy, iridencleisis, Scheie's thermal sclerostomy and cyclodialysis.

What are the indications of trabeculectomy operation?

1. Primary angle-closure glaucoma with peripheral anterior synechiae involving more than half of the angle.
2. Primary open-angle glaucoma.
3. Congenital and development glaucoma where trabeculotomy and goniotomy fail.
4. Selective cases of secondary open angle glaucoma and secondary narrow-angle glaucoma.

What are the advantages of trabeculectomy over other filtration operations?

1. Incidence of postoperative shallow or flat anterior chamber is very less.
2. Incidence of postoperative hypotony is very low.
3. Chances of postoperative infection through the filtration bleb are low.
4. Quality of filtration bleb formed is good.

What is Seton operation?

In this operation, a valvular synthetic tube is implanted which drains the aqueous humour from the anterior chamber into the subconjunctival space.

It is performed for neovascular glaucoma and intractable cases of primary and other secondary glaucomas where medical treatment and conventional filtration surgery fail.

What are cycloablative procedures ?

In these procedures, ciliary epithelium is destroyed to control the intraocular pressure. These procedures are used for absolute glaucoma. Commonly employed cycloablative procedures include: cyclocryopexy, cyclophotocoagulation and cyclodiathermy.

Cyclodialysis operation is useful in which type of glaucoma?

- Glaucoma in aphakes

ENUCLEATION AND EVISCERATION OPERATIONS

What is enucleation operation?

It is complete excision of the eyeball.

Enumerate indications of enucleation.

Absolute indications are:

- Retinoblastoma
- Malignant melanoma

Relative indications are:

- Painful blind eye
- Mutilating ocular injury
- Phthisis bulbi
- Anterior staphyloma

Indication for eye donation. Removal of eyes from the cadaver is presently the most common indication for enucleation.

What precautions should be taken while performing enucleation in a patient with retinoblastoma?

During enucleation the longest possible piece of optic nerve should be excised.

What is evisceration operation?

It is removal of the contents of the eyeball leaving behind the sclera. Frill evisceration is preferred over simple evisceration. In this, only about 3 mm frill of the sclera is left around the optic nerve.

What are the indications of evisceration?

- Panophthalmitis
- Expulsive choroidal haemorrhage
- Bleeding anterior staphyloma

How can the cosmetic appearance be improved after enucleation or evisceration operation?

For best results, an orbital implant should be implanted at the time of surgery and an artificial eye of plastic should be worn after about 2 weeks of surgery. A delay in the use of artificial eye may lead to a contracted socket.

OPERATIONS ON EYELIDS

For important questions related to eyelid operations see page 558-563.

LACRIMAL APPARATUS OPERATIONS

Questions related to operations on the lacrimal apparatus are described on page 563-566.

LASERS AND CRYOTHERAPY IN OPHTHALMOLOGY

What are the properties of laser light?

- Monochromaticity
- Coherence
- Collimation

Name the different types of lasers and their mechanism of action.

Type of laser	*Mechanism of action*
Argon	Photocoagulation
Krypton	Photocoagulation
Diode	Photocoagulation
Frequency doubled Nd-YAG	Photocoagulation
Nd-YAG	Photodisruption
Excimer	Photoablation

Enumerate uses of argon/diode laser.

In glaucoma

1. Laser trabeculoplasty for primary open-angle glaucoma.
2. Laser goniopuncture for developmental glaucoma.
3. Laser iridotomy for narrow-angle glaucoma.
4. Cyclophotocoagulation for absolute glaucoma.

In lesions of retina

1. Diabetic retinopathy
2. Eales' disease
3. Coats' disease
4. Sickle-cell retinopathy
5. Exudative age-related macular degeneration

What are the therapeutic uses of Nd-YAG laser?

1. Capsulotomy for thickened posterior capsule
2. Membranectomy for pupillary membranes

What are therapeutic applications of excimer laser?

1. LASIK for correction of refractive errors.
2. Photorefractive keratectomy (PRK) for correction of myopia and hypermetropia.
3. Phototherapeutic keratectomy (PTK) for corneal diseases such as band-shaped keratopathy.

Describe the laser treatment for diabetic retinopathy.

Photocoagulation by frequency doubled Nd-YAG laser (532 nm) is employed as follows:

1. *Panretinal photocoagulation* (PRP) is indicated in severe cases of preproliferative and proliferative diabetic retinopathy.
2. *Focal laser burns* are applied in the centre of the hard exudate's ring in focal exudative maculopathy.
3. *Grid pattern laser burns* are applied in diffuse exudative maculopathy.

What do you mean by cryopexy ?

Cryopexy means to produce tissue injury by application of extremely low temperature (–100°C to – 40°C). This is achieved by a cryoprobe from a cryo-unit.

On what principle is the working of a cryoprobe based?

Working of a cryoprobe is based on the Joule-Thompson principle of cooling.

Which gas is used in a cryo-machine?

The cryounit uses freon, nitrous oxide or carbon-dioxide gas as a cooling agent.

Enumerate the applications of cryo in ophthalmology?

1. *Lids:* (i) cryolysis for trichiasis, (ii) cryotherapy for warts and molluscum contagiosum, (iii) cryotherapy for basal cell carcinoma and haemangioma
2. *Conjunctiva:* Cryotherapy for hypertrophied papillae of vernal catarrh
3. *Lens:* Cryoextraction of the cataractous lens by ICCE technique was done in olden days (not done now-a-day)
4. *Ciliary body:* Cyclocryopexy for absolute glaucoma and neovascular glaucoma
5. *Retina:* (i) Cryopexy is widely used for sealing retinal breaks in retinal detachment, (ii) Prophylactic cryopexy to prevent retinal detachment in certain prone cases, (iii) Anterior retinal cryopexy (ARC) for neovascularization and, (iv) Cryotreatment of retinoblastoma.

Index

B

C

D

E

F

G

H

I

J

K

L

M

P

Q

R

S

W

X

Y

Z